RHEUMATOLOGY

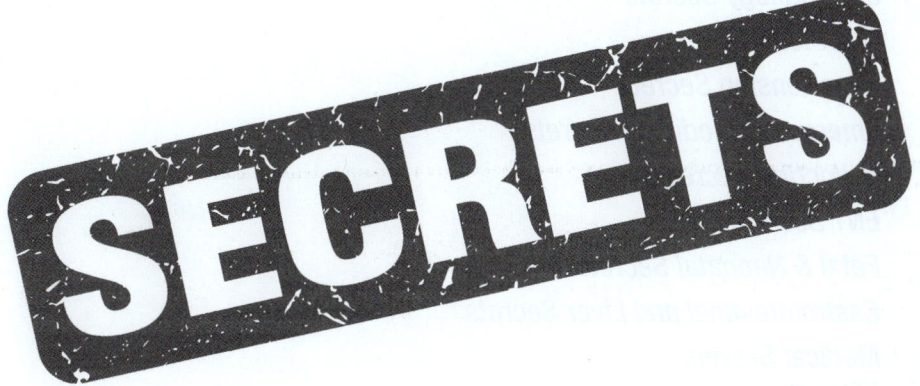

Volumes in the Secrets Series

RHEUMATOLOGY

JASON R. KOLFENBACH, MD, FACR
Professor of Medicine
Department of Medicine
Division of Rheumatology
University of Colorado School of Medicine
Aurora, Colorado

STERLING G. WEST, MD, MACP, MACR
Professor of Medicine
Department of Medicine
Division of Rheumatology
University of Colorado School of Medicine
Aurora, Colorado

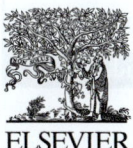

ELSEVIER

Elsevier
1600 John F. Kennedy Blvd.
Ste 1800
Philadelphia, PA 19103-2899

RHEUMATOLOGY SECRETS, FIFTH EDITION

ISBN: 978-0-443-12794-6

Previous editions copyrighted 2020, 2015, 2002, 1996.

Senior Content Strategist: Marybeth Thiel
Senior Content Development Specialist: Jinia Dasgupta
Publishing Services Manager: Deepthi Unni
Project Manager: Manchu Mohan
Design Direction: Renee Duenow

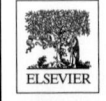 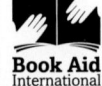

Working together to grow libraries in developing countries

www.elsevier.com • www.bookaid.org

Printed in India

Last digit is the print number: 9 8 7 6 5 4 3 2 1

To my wife, Brenda, my best friend.
To my children, Dace and Matthew, the joys of my life.
To my amazing grandchildren, Aidan, Eva, Owen, and Stella.

Sterling G. West, MD

To my three kids, Bella, Hayden, and Dylan:
you have lived with this book for most of your lives,
and I'm thankful for your patience with the many months required
to bring it into publication.

To my wife, Lauren: I dedicate this book to you.
In the past year you have taught me about the courage to take risks in life
and pushing beyond our comfort levels when important work is at hand.
Thank you for your encouragement and support in all things,
and for walking together with me through this life.

Jason R. Kolfenbach, MD

Contributors

Venu Akuthota, MD
Professor
Physical Medicine and Rehabilitation
University of Colorado
Denver, Colorado

Meghan J. Anderson, DO
Assistant Professor
Department of Rheumatology
University of Pennsylvania
Philadelphia, Pennsylvania

Brendan Antiochos, MD
Assistant Professor
Rheumatology
Johns Hopkins
Baltimore, Maryland

Ramon A. Arroyo, MD
Rheumatology Staff
Department of Rheumatology
San Antonio Military Medical Center
Ft. Sam Houston, Texas
Associate Professor
Department of Medicine
Uniform University of Health Science
Bethesda, Maryland

Kristina Barber, MD
Resident Physicain
Physical Medicine & Rehabilitation
University of Colorado
Aurora, Colorado

Amrita Bath, MBBS, RhMSUS, FACR
Assistant Professor
Divison of Allergy Immunologyand
  Rheumatology, Department of Internal
  Medicine
University of Kansas Medical Center
Kansas City, Kansas

David B. Beck, MD, PhD
Assistant Professor
Center for Human Genetics and Genomics
New York University School of Medicine
New York, New York

Jessica L. Bloom, MD, MSCS
Assistant Professor
Department of Pediatrics
University of Colorado School of Medicine
Aurora, Colorado

Jonathan T. Bravman, MD
Orthopaedic Surgeon
Department of Orthopaedic Surgery
University of Colorado
Aurora, Colorado

Mary Elizabeth Buchanan, MD
Assistant Professor
Musculoskeletal Radiology
CU Anschutz
Aurora, Colorado

Lindsay Burke, MD
Psychiatric Nurse Practitioner
Physical Medicine & Rehabilitation
Hospital for Special Surgery
New York, New York

Amy C. Cannella, MD, MS, RhMSUS, FACR
Professor
Internal Medicine and Rheumatology
University of Nebraska Medical Center
Omaha, Nebraska

Liron Caplan, MD, PhD
Section Head, Rheumatology
Rocky Mtn Regional Veterans Affairs Medical
  Center
Associate Professor
Division of Rheumatology
University of Colorado School of Medicine
Aurora, Colorado

Laura C. Cappelli, MD, MHS
Associate Professor of Medicine
Infectious Disease, Department of Medicine
Johns Hopkins School of Medicine
Baltimore, Maryland

Guiset Carvajal Bedoya, MD, FACR
Rheumatology
Billings Clinic
Billings, Montana

Bradley G. Changstrom, MD, CAQSM
Associate Professor
Department of Medicine, Division of General
  Internal Medicine
University of Colorado School of Medicine
Aurora, Colorado

Walter Winn Chatham, MD
Professor
Internal Medicine, Rheumatology
University of Nevada, Las Vegas
Las Vegas, Nevada
Professor (retired)
Medicine, Clnical Immunology and Rheumatology
University of Alabama at Birmingham
Birmingham, Alabama

Lisa Christopher-Stine, MD, MPH
Professor of Medicine (Rheumatology)
  and Neurology
Director, Johns Hopkins Myositis Center
Johns Hopkins University School of Medicine
Baltimore, Maryland

Sharon A. Chung, MD, MAS
Professor of Clinical Medicine
Department of Medicine, Division of
  Rheumatology
University of California, San Francisco
San Francisco, California

Lyndsey Dyan Cole, MD, FACR
Assistant Professor
Department of Pediatrics, Sections of
  Rheumatology and Infectious Diseases
University of Colorado Anschutz Medical
  Campus
Aurora, Colorado

Kathleen Jo E. Corbin, MD, MHS
Associate Professor
Pediatrics
Yale University School of Medicine
New Haven, Connecticut

Lisa Criscione-Schreiber, MD, MEd
Professor
Department of Medicine, Division of
  Rheumatology and Immunology
Vice Chair for Education
Department of Medicine
Duke University School of Medicine
Durham, North Carolina

Randy Q. Cron, MD, PhD
Professor of Pediatrics
Pediatrics
University of Alabama at Birmingham Heersink
  School of Medicine
Director of Pediatric Rheumatology
Pediatrics
Children's of Alabama
Birmingham, Alabama

Megan L. Curran, MD
Associate Professor
Pediatrics
University of Colorado
Aurora, Colorado

Laura Damioli, MD
Associate Professor
Infectious Disease,
Department of Medicine
University of Colorado
Aurora, Colorado

Lisa Anne Davis, MD, MsCS, FACR
Associate Professor of Medicine
Rheumatology
Denver Health
Denver, Colorado
Associate Program Director, Rheumatology
University of Colorado
Aurora, Colorado

Kevin D. Deane, MD, PhD
Professor of Medicine
Division of Rheumatology
University of Colorado School of Medicine
  Anschutz Medical Campus
Aurora, Colorado

M. Kristen Demoruelle, MD, PhD, FACR
Associate Professor
Division of Rheumatology
University of Colorado School of Medicine
Aurora, Colorado

Sarah L. Dill, MD
Rheumatology
St. Luke's Clinic-Boise & Meridian
Boise, Idaho

Stacy Dixon, MD, PhD
Assistant Professor
Neurology
University of Colorado School of Medicine
Aurora, Colorado

Anisha B. Dua, MD, MPH
Professor
Medicine
Northwestern University
Chicago, Illinois

Jared J. Eddy, MD, MSc
Assistant Professor of Medicine
Medicine
National Jewish Health
Denver, Colorado

Alan R. Erickson, MD
Associate Professor
Rheumatology
University of Nebraska
Omaha, Nebraska

Doruk Erkan, MD, MPH
Rheumatology
Hospital for Special Surgery
Professor of Medicine
Weill Cornell Medicine
New York, New York

Michael G. Feely, MD
Associate Professor
Internal Medicine,
Division of Rheumatology
University of Nebraska Medical Center
Omaha, Nebraska

Elizabeth D. Ferucci, MD, MPH
Rheumatologist
Research Services
Alaska Native Tribal Health Consortium
Anchorage, Alaska
Affiliate Professor, Medicine/Rheumatology
University of Washington School of Medicine
Seattle, Washington

Jason Friedrich, MD
Associate Professor
PM&R
University of Colorado School of Medicine
Aurora, Colorado

Robert C. Fuhlbrigge, MD, PhD
Professor
Department of Pediatrics
Section Head for Rheumatology
University of Colorado School of Medicine
Chair, Rheumatology
Children's Hospital Colorado
Aurora, Colorado

Alison M. Gizinski, MD, MS, FACR
Assistant Professor
Internal Medicine, Division of Rheumatology
Emory University School of Medicine
Atlanta, Georgia

Sarah Goglin, MD
Associate Professor
Department of Medicine
University of California San Francisco
San Francisco, California

Melissa Griffith, MD, RhMSUS, FACR
Associate Professor
Rheumatology
University of Colorado
Aurora, Colorado

Michael Haden, MD
Assistant Professor
Department of Medicine, Division of Infectious
  Diseases
University of Colorado, Anschutz Medical
  Campus
Aurora, Colorado

Nathaniel J. Harris, MD, PhD
Assistant Professor
Department of Medicine, Division of
  Rheumatology
Duke University
Durham, North Carolina

Lindsay N. Helget, MD
Assistant Professor
Rheumatology
University of Nebraska Medical Center
Omaha, Nebraska

Craig Hogan, MD, FAAOS
Associate Professor, Orthopedics
Department of Orthopedics
University of Colorado
Aurora, Colorado

Laura K. Hummers, MD, ScM
Associate Professor of Medicine
Division of Rheumatology
Co-Director
Johns Hopkins Scleroderma Center
Johns Hopkins University
Baltimore, Maryland

Timothy Kaniecki, MD
Assistant Professor
Medicine, Division of Rheumatology
Johns Hopkins University School of Medicine
Baltimore, Maryland

Liudmila Kastsianok, MD, RhMSUS, FACR
Associate Professor
Department of Medicine
University of Colorado Anschutz Medical
  Campus Division of Rheumatology
Aurora, Colorado

Jason R. Kolfenbach, MD, FACR
Professor
Rheumatology & Ophthalmology
University of Colorado
Aurora, Colorado

Kristine A. Kuhn, MD, PhD
Professor
Department of Medicine, Division of
  Rheumatology
University of Colorado Anschutz Medical
  Campus
Aurora, Colorado

Bharat Kumar, MD, MMEd, FACR
Clinical Assistant Professor of Internal Medicine,
  Immunology
University of Iowa Hospitals and Clinics
Iowa City, Iowa

Audrey Leung, MD
Deputy Assistant Chief of Staff
Department of Spinal Cord Injury
John Cochran Veterans Administration
St. Louis, Washington

David L. Leverenz, MD, MEd
Associate Professor of Medicine
Department of Medicine, Division of
  Rheumatology and Immunology
Duke University School of Medicine
Durham, North Carolina

Tiffany Lin, MD
Associate Professor
Medicine
University of Wisconsin School of Medicine and
  Public Health
Madison, Wisconsin

Mary K. Lowry, MD
Associate Professor
Radiology
University of Colorado
Denver, Colorado

Kyle D. Maier, MD
Service Chief, Associate Program Director,
  Department of Medicine
Brooke Army Medical Center
Ft. Sam Houston, Texas

Daniele Marcy, MD
Fellow
Rheumatology
University of Colorado
Aurora, Colorado

Sara S. McCoy, MD, PhD, RhMSUS, FACR
Assistant Professor of Rheumatology
Department of Medicine, Division of
  Rheumatology
University of Wisconsin School of Medicine and
  Public Health
Madison, Wisconsin

Michael T. McDermott, MD
Professor of Medicine and Clinical Pharmacy
Department of Medicine, Division of
  Endocrinology
Lucas Family Endowed Chair in Endocrinology
  and Diabetes
University of Colorado Denver School of
  Medicine
Denver, Colorado

Trevor McKown, MD
Assistant Professor (CHS)
Division of Rheumatology, Department of
  Medicine
University of Wisconsin–Madison
Madison, Wisconsin

Ted R. Mikuls, MD, MSPH
Stokes Shackleford Professor of Rheumatology
Department of Internal Medicine
University of Nebraska Medical Center
Rheumatologist
VA Nebraska-Western Iowa Health Care System
Omaha, Nebraska

Katharine F. Moore, MD
Associate Professor of Pediatrics
Department of Pediatrics
University of Colorado School of Medicine
Department of Pediatric Rheumatology
Children's Hospital Colorado
Aurora, Colorado

Meredith Morcos, MD
Assistant Professor
Department of Rheumatology
University of Colorado
Aurora, Colorado

Larry W. Moreland, MD, MACR
Professor of Medicine
Department of Medicine
University of Colorado
Denver, Colorado

Vivek K. Murthy, MD, MSc, FACR
Associate Professor
Department of Medicine
University of California San Francisco School of
  Medicine
San Francisco, California

Katherine D. Nowicki, MD
Assistant Professor
Department of Pediatrics - Section of
  Rheumatology
University of Colorado
Aurora, Colorado

Alan G. Palestine, MD
Professor
Department of Ophthalmology
University of Colorado Anschutz Campus
Aurora, Colorado

Dianna Quan, MD
Professor
Department of Neurology
University of Colorado Denver
Director, Electromyography Laboratory
Department of Neurology
University of Colorado Hospital
Aurora, Colorado

Itziar Quinzaños Alonso, MD
Assistant Professor
Department of Medicine Division of
  Rheumatology
University of Colorado School of Medicine
Aurora, Colorado
Department of Medicine Division of
  Rheumatology
Denver Health and Hospital
Denver, Colorado

Amit K. Reddy, MD
Assistant Professor
Department of Ophthalmology
University of Colorado Anschutz School of
  Medicine
Aurora, Colorado

Bradley Reeves, MD
Resident
Department of Orthopaedic Surgery
University of Colorado
Denver, Colorado

Manuel L. Ribeiro Neto, MD
Department of Pulmonary Medicine
Cleveland Clinic
Cleveland, Ohio

Eileen C. Rife, MD MPH
Pediatric and Adult Rheumatologist
Department of Pediatric Rheumatology
University of Alabama–Birmingham
Birmingham, Alabama

Rouhin Sen, MD, MS
Assistant Professor
Division of Clinical Immunology and
  Rheumatology
University of Alabama–Birmingham
Birmingham, Alabama

Philip Seo, MD, MHS
Associate Professor of Medicine
Division of Rheumatology
Johns Hopkins University School of Medicine
Baltimore, Maryland

Ami A. Shah, MD, MHS, FACR
Professor of Medicine
Division of Rheumatology
Johns Hopkins University School of Medicine
Baltimore, Maryland

Emily Shelkowitz, MD
Assistant Professor
Department of Pediatrics
University of Washington
Seattle, Washington

Jeffrey Shen, MD
Medical Instructor
Department of Rheumatology
Duke University
Durham, North Carolina

Joel Brian Shirley, DO
Associate Professor of Clinical Practice
Department of Pediatrics, Division of
  Rheumatology
University of Colorado School of Medicine
Aurora, Colorado

Namrata Singh, MD, MSCI
Adjunct Assistant Professor
Department of Epidemiology
Assistant Professor
Division of Rheumatology
University of Washington
Seattle, Washington

Tara Skorupa, MD
Instructor
Department of Medicine; Division of
  Rheumatology, Division of General Medicine,
  Beth Israel Deaconess Medical Center, Harvard
  Medical School
Boston, Massachusetts

Marcus H. Snow, MD
Associate Professor
Department of Internal Medicine
University of Nebraska Medical Center
Omaha, Nebraska

Jennifer B. Soep, MD
Professor
Department of Pediatric Rheumatology
University of Colorado
Denver, Colorado

Jack Spittler, MD
Associate Professor
Department of Family Medicine and Orthopedics
University of Colorado
Aurora, Colorado

Jennifer Stichman, MD
Associate Professor
Department of Medicine, Divisions of General
  Internal Medicine and Rheumatology
Denver Health Medical Center
Denver, Colorado

John H. Stone, MD, MPH
Professor of Medicine
Department of Medicine, Division of Rheumatology
Harvard Medical School
The Edward A. Fox Chair in Medicine
Massachusetts General Hospital
Boston, Massachusetts

Colin Strickland, MD
Associate Professor
Department of Radiology
University of Colorado
Aurora, Colorado

Christopher C. Striebich, MD, PhD
Associate Professor
Department of Medicine
University of Colorado School of Medicine
Aurora, Colorado

Christine M. Swanson, MD, MCR, CCD
Associate Professor
Department of Medicine, Division of
  Endocrinology, Metabolism and Diabetes
University of Colorado
Aurora, Colorado

Tho Quy Truong, MD, FACR
Associate Professor
Department of Allergy and Immunology
University of Colorado
Aurora, Colorado

Kim Nguyen Tyler, MD
Assistant Clinical Professor
Division of Rheumatology
University of Colorado School of Medicine
Aurora, Colorado

Patompong Ungprasert, MD, MS, FACR
Department of Rheumatology
Cleveland Clinic
Cleveland, Ohio

Seth J. VanDerVeer, DO, RhMSUS, FACR
Staff Rheumatologist
Department of Rheumatology
Mike O'Callaghan Military Medical Center
Nellis Air Force Base, Nevada

Zachary S. Wallace, MD, MSc
Physician-Investigator
Department of Rheumatology
Massachusetts General Hospital
Boston, Massachusetts

Carly A. Wanglin, MD
Fellow Physician
Department of Rheumatology
University of California San Francisco
San Francisco, California

Elena Weinstein, MD
Associate Professor
Department of Medicine, Division of
  Rheumatology
University of Colorado
Aurora, Colorado

Matthew S. West, MD
Assistant Professor
Department of Molecular, Cellular, and
  Developmental Biology
University of Colorado
Aurora, Colorado

Sterling G. West, MD, MACP, MACR
Professor of Medicine
Division of Rheumatology
University of Colorado School of Medicine
Aurora, Colorado

Matthew Wicklund, MD, FAAN
Professor
Department of Neurology
UT Health San Antonio
San Antonio, Texas

Timothy M. Wilson, MD
Assistant Professor
Division of Rheumatology
Thomas Jefferson University
Philadelphia, Pennsylvania

Yusuf Yazici, MD
Clinical Associate Professor of Medicine,
  Department of Rheumatology
NYU Grossman School of Medicine
New York, New York

JoAnn Zell, MD
Associate Professor
Department of Rheumatology
University of Colorado
Aurora, Colorado

Lisa Zickuhr, MD, MHPE
Associate Professor of Medicine
Department of Medicine
Washington University in St. Louis School of
  Medicine
St. Louis, Missouri

Preface

Newton's words are often cited in the context of mentor-mentee relationships, and indeed, they have rung true in my own career. Influential mentors, perhaps most importantly my co-editor Dr. Sterling West, have enriched my career and opened countless doors of opportunity.

In a similar fashion, this fifth edition of *Rheumatology Secrets* was also built on the shoulders of prior contributors, researchers, and clinicians. Updates on the evaluation and management of rheumatic disease have been included, as well as "evergreen" educational concepts (such as laboratory interpretation and physical examination) that are considered foundational to the practice of rheumatology. Through four previous editions, *Rheumatology Secrets* has provided medical trainees and practicing rheumatologists with tools to improve their understanding of autoimmune diseases and enhance the care of patients with rheumatic disease.

Many important advances in rheumatology have occurred since the last edition of this book, and we have extensively reviewed and March 2025. New authors were invited for 35 chapters in this edition, including a new chapter on IgG4-related disease by Dr. John Stone, broadening the clinical insight found in the subsequent pages of this book. As in the previous editions, *Rheumatology Secrets, 5th Edition*, is presented in the Socratic question-and-answer format that is the hallmark of *The Secrets Series*. Common and uncommon rheumatic disease conditions encountered in clinical practice, discussed during teaching rounds, and found on board examinations are covered. Each chapter reviews basic immunology and pathophysiology, important disease manifestations, and practical management issues. The book also contains a wealth of mnemonics, lists, tables, figures, and illustrations to emphasize important clinical pearls.

As with the fourth edition, this book includes access to over 150 online board-review questions. These questions are intended to solidify concepts covered in each chapter rather than serve as a comprehensive repository of board-style questions. In my own training (which continues to this day!), the previous editions of *Rheumatology Secrets* were enjoyable to read and provided quick insights during a busy clinic. I hope readers find the fifth edition similarly impactful to their own training and in daily clinical practice.

Jason R. Kolfenbach, MD

Acknowledgments

The editors would like to thank:

All the contributors for their valuable time and effort in writing the chapters in this edition.

The staff at Elsevier for their patience and help, and for providing us with the opportunity to edit *Rheumatology Secrets*.

To our patients, teachers, and students for continuing to teach us about the amazing field of rheumatology.

Contents

SECTION IV   The Vasculitides and Related Disorders

SECTION V   Seronegative Spondyloarthropathies

SECTION XIII   Miscellaneous Rheumatic Disorders

SECTION XIV   Management of the Rheumatic Diseases

SECTION XV   Final Secrets

SECTION XVI   eAppendix Board-Style Questions

CHAPTER 1

Top 100+ Rheumatology Secrets

Sterling G. West, MD and Jason R. Kolfenbach, MD

A physician is judged by the three A's—ability, availability, and affability.

—Paul Reznikoff, MD (1896–1984)

Rheumatology can be confusing to many physicians during their housestaff training (and beyond!). Often the patient's presentation is not according to the "textbook." That is what makes rheumatology fun—diagnosing unusual presentations of the disease! In addition to having interesting diseases, we now have many more effective therapies. Although nothing in medicine is 100%, we have found the following useful and cost-effective when evaluating a patient with a rheumatic/musculoskeletal problem:

1. **A good history and physical examination, coupled with musculoskeletal anatomy knowledge, is the most important part of the evaluation of a patient with rheumatic symptoms.**
   You have to examine the patient! The answer is typically sitting on the examination table rather than in the electronic medical record. That means taking off their shoes and socks, examining their feet, and watching them walk if they have lower extremity (hip, knee, ankle, and foot) complaints.
   * Joint effusion and limited range of motion are the most specific signs for arthritis.
   * True hip joint pain is in the groin. In a young patient who cannot flex their hip greater than 90 degrees, rule out femoroacetabular impingement syndrome.
   * Feel both the knees with the back of your hand for temperature differences and compare them with the temperature of the lower extremity. The knee should be cooler than the skin over the tibia. If the knee is warmer, then there is ongoing knee inflammation.

2. **Soft tissue rheumatism.**
   * Most shoulder pain is periarticular (i.e., bursitis or tendinitis). Rule out impingement in patients with recurrent shoulder tendinitis.
   * Causes of olecranon or prepatellar bursitis: trauma, infection, gout, rheumatoid arthritis (RA).
   * Olecranon bursitis presents as swelling and warmth at the extensor tip of the elbow, overlying the olecranon process (Popeye elbow); full extension and supination/pronation are typically not painful in contrast to true elbow effusions.
   * Eccentric stretching (flex bar) is an effective treatment for lateral epicondylitis; avoid corticosteroid injection, given the limited benefit and risk of post-injection flare.
   * Recalcitrant trochanteric bursitis: rule out leg length discrepancy, hallux rigidus with an abnormal gait, gluteus medius/minimus tear, and lumbar radiculopathy. Corticosteroid injections of the trochanteric bursa are best done with a spinal needle due to the distance the bursa is from the skin.
   * Greater trochanteric pain syndrome (GTPS): often referred to as trochanteric bursitis (20% of cases); pain in this region more commonly stems from gluteal muscle tendinopathy and iliotibial band thickening.
   * Similar to rotator cuff tendinopathy, GTPS that is treated with corticosteroid injection alone without stretching/strengthening exercises is doomed to recur.
   * Recalcitrant medial knee pain: rule out anserine bursitis.
   * Recalcitrant patellofemoral syndrome: rule out pes planus/hypermobility causing patellar maltracking.
   * Due to risk of rupture, do not inject corticosteroids for therapy of Achilles tendinitis/enthesitis. Use iontophoresis.

3. Back pain.

- Patients with significant low back pain cannot do a sit-up.
- Most back pain is nonsurgical; never advise surgery for mechanical low back pain without objective evidence for radiculopathy or spinal stenosis unresponsive to conservative therapy.
- Epidural steroids may provide short-term benefits (2–4 weeks) for radicular symptoms, but not necessarily spinal pain.
- Magnetic resonance imaging (MRI)/computed tomography (CT) scans of lumbar spine are abnormal in 30% of young patients with no symptoms, and 60–70% of older patients. Do not automatically attribute a patient's symptoms to an abnormal radiograph.
- Spinal Phalen's test is useful to diagnose spinal stenosis. Patients with spinal stenosis have more pain walking downhill due to spinal extension making the spinal canal smaller. Straight leg raise test and electromyography (EMG)/nerve conduction velocities (NCVs) are often normal or nonspecific.

4. Nerves.

- Cervical radiculopathy

Nerve (Frequency)	Motor Weakness	Sensory Loss	Reflex
C5 (5%)	Deltoid, **(deal five cards)** biceps	Lateral upper arm	Biceps
C6 (35%)	Wrist extensors, biceps	Lateral forearm, thumb, index finger **(six-shooter)**	Brachioradialis (supinator jerk)
C7 (35%)	Wrist flexor, finger extensors **(forms a 7)**, triceps	Middle finger	Triceps
C8 (25%)	Finger flexors **(forms an 8)**, thumb extensor, hand intrinsics	Medial forearm, ring and little finger	None

- Lumbar radiculopathy

Nerve (Frequency)	Motor Weakness	Sensory Loss	Reflex
L4 (5%)	Tibialis anterior (ankle dorsiflexion)	Anterior leg, medial foot	Patellar **(quads = 4)**
L5 (67%)	Extensor hallucis longus (great toe extension)	Lateral leg, web of great toe, **(5 toes)**	Medial hamstring
S1 (28%)	Peroneus muscles (foot eversion)	Posterior leg, lateral foot	Achilles **(ends in S)**

Mononeuritis multiplex is seen in patients with vasculitis and presents with painful asymmetric weakness (e.g., wrist drop, foot drop) and sensory changes involving individual nerves.

5. Do not order a laboratory test unless you know why you are ordering it and what you will do if it comes back abnormal.

6. Laboratory tests.

- Laboratory tests should be used to confirm your clinical diagnosis, not make it.
- All patients with a positive rheumatoid factor (RF) do not have RA, and all patients with a positive antinuclear antibody (ANA) do not have systemic lupus erythematosus (SLE).
- Low complement (C3, C4) levels in a patient with systemic symptoms suggest an immune complex-mediated disease and narrow your diagnosis: SLE, cryoglobulinemia (types II and III), urticarial vasculitis (HepB and C1q autoantibodies), subacute bacterial endocarditis, poststreptococcal or membranoproliferative glomerulonephritis, IgG4 disease (tubulointerstitial nephritis), hydralazine-associated vasculitis. Caveat: patients with end-stage liver disease and poor synthetic function.
- An undetectable (not just low) CH50 activity may indicate a disease associated with a specific hereditary complement component deficiency: autoimmune disorder (C1, C4, C2), infection (C3), *Neisseria* infection (C5 to C8).

- Separating iron deficiency from anemia of chronic disease is best done by measuring the ferritin level. Ferritin is an acute-phase reactant; so in a patient with inflammation (i.e., elevated C-reactive protein), a ferritin level of >100 ng/mL rules out iron deficiency.

7. Failure to aspirate, prepare to litigate!

Patients with acute inflammatory monoarticular arthritis need a joint aspiration to rule out septic arthritis and crystalline arthropathy.

- Atraumatic monoarticular arthritis is secondary to crystalline disease (75–80% of cases) or infection (10–15%) until proven otherwise.
- A red, hot joint is not typical of inflammatory arthritis in RA and other autoimmune conditions. Its presence, even in a patient with established disease, demands aspiration.
- To reduce the pain associated with an aspiration or injection, have the patient do the Valsalva maneuver when inserting the needle.
- Joint aspiration is generally safe up to an international normalized ratio (INR) of 4.5. However, if septic arthritis is possible, the joint should be aspirated regardless of the INR.

8. The synovial fluid analysis is a liquid biopsy of the joint.

Send any aspirated synovial fluid for cell count, crystal examination, Gram stain, and culture. Never send it for uric acid or lactate dehydrogenase (LDH).

- One can estimate the synovial fluid white blood cell (WBC) count by using the equation that one WBC per high-power field (HPF; 40 ×) equals 500 cells/μL. Thus, 6 WBCs/HPF estimates a synovial fluid WBC count of 3000 cells/μL, which is inflammatory.
- **Crystal mnemonic: ABC** = **A**lignment **B**lue **C**alcium. If the long axis of the crystal is aligned with the first-order red compensator and is blue, then it is a calcium pyrophosphate crystal. Uric acid crystals are yellow when aligned.
- If you cannot find uric acid crystals initially, let the slide dry for 3 hours and reexamine it. Hydrated crystals may not be visible initially.

9. Most patients with chronic inflammatory monoarticular arthritis of >8 weeks' duration, whose evaluation has failed to define an etiology for the arthritis, need a synovial biopsy to rule out an unusual cause (indolent infection, etc.).

10. In response to the Choosing Wisely initiative of the American Board of Internal Medicine (ABIM), the American College of Rheumatology (ACR) recommended the following five tests/treatments not be done in adult rheumatology patients.

- Do not test ANA subserologies (anti-dsDNA, anti-Sm, anti-RNP, anti-SS-B, anti-Scl-70) without a positive ANA and clinical suspicion of immune-mediated disease. Anti-SS-A may be an exception to this recommendation.
- Do not test for Lyme disease as a cause of musculoskeletal symptoms without an exposure history and appropriate examination findings.
- Do not perform an MRI of the peripheral joints to routinely monitor inflammatory arthritis.
- Do not prescribe biologics for RA before a trial of methotrexate (or other conventional synthetic disease-modifying antirheumatic drugs [csDMARDs]).
- Do not routinely repeat dual-energy X-ray absorptiometry (DXA) scans more often than once every 2 years.

11. In response to the Choosing Wisely initiative of the ABIM, the ACR recommended the following five tests/treatments not be done in pediatric rheumatology patients.

- Do not order autoantibody panels without a positive ANA and evidence of a rheumatic disease.
- Do not test for Lyme disease as a cause of musculoskeletal symptoms without an exposure history and appropriate examination findings.
- Do not routinely perform surveillance joint radiographs to monitor juvenile idiopathic arthritis (JIA) disease activity.
- Do not perform methotrexate toxicity laboratory tests more than every 12 weeks on stable doses.
- Do not repeat a confirmed positive ANA in patients with established JIA or SLE.

12. **In response to the Choosing Wisely initiative of the ABIM, the American Association of Orthopedic Surgeons recommended the following treatments not be done in patients (only those that apply to rheumatology patients are listed).**
    - Do not use needle lavage for long-term relief in symptomatic osteoarthritis (OA) treatment.
    - Do not use lateral wedge or neutral insoles to treat patients with medial knee OA.
    - Do not use glucosamine and chondroitin sulfate to treat patients with symptomatic knee OA.

13. **In response to the Choosing Wisely initiative of the ABIM, the North American Spine Society recommended the following tests/treatments not be done in patients with back pain.**
    - Do not order MRI of the spine within the first 6 weeks in patients with nonspecific low back pain in the absence of red flags (trauma, use of corticosteroids, unexplained weight loss, progressive neurologic signs, age >50 years or <17 years, fever, intravenous drug use, pain unrelieved by bed rest, history of cancer).
    - Do not perform elective spinal injections without imaging guidance.
    - Do not order EMG/NCVs to determine the cause of neck and back pain without radicular symptoms.
    - Do not recommend bed rest for >48 hours when treating low back pain.

14. **A few other "do nots" in rheumatology.**
    - Except for anti-dsDNA, do not repeat ANA subserologies in patients with an established connective tissue disease (CTD) diagnosis.
    - Do not perform serial measurements of RF and anti-cyclic citrullinated peptide in patients with documented seropositive RA, or serial ANAs in patients with a documented positive ANA and a CTD diagnosis (e.g., SLE).
    - Do not order a human leukocyte antigen (HLA)-B27 unless you suspect an undifferentiated spondyloarthritis based on history and examination and have nondiagnostic radiographs.
    - Do not check CH50 to follow lupus disease activity.
    - Do not order an MRI before ordering plain films in a patient presenting with joint or back pain.
    - Do not use intraarticular hyaluronic acid injections for advanced knee OA (i.e., bone on bone).
    - Do not treat low bone mass in patients at low risk for fracture (T score >−2.5, no history of fragility fracture, no steroids, low FRAX).
    - Do not order serial yearly plain radiographs in a patient with good clinical control of their arthritis (symptoms, examination, laboratory tests) unless you are willing to change therapy for minor radiographic disease progression.

15. **The innate immune system is critical to the activation of the adaptive immune system.**

16. **Osteoarthritis**
    - Cracking knuckles does not cause OA.
    - Obesity is the major modifiable risk factor for OA; the association is strongest with knee and hand OA (non-weight-bearing joint, suggesting a greater role than simply increased biomechanical stress).
    - The joints typically involved in primary OA are distal interphalangeal joints (DIPs) (Heberden's nodes), proximal interphalangeal joints (PIPs) (Bouchard's nodes), first carpometacarpal (CMC), hips, knees, first metatarsophalangeal joint (MTP), the cervical, and lumbosacral spine.
    - Patients with OA affecting multiple joints not normally affected by primary OA (i.e., metacarpophalangeals, wrists, elbows, shoulder, ankles) need to be evaluated for secondary causes of OA (i.e., calcium pyrophosphate disease [CPPD], metabolic diseases [e.g. hemochromatosis], others).
    - Erosive OA is an inflammatory subset of OA (10% of patients) primarily affecting the hands (DIPs, PIPs, first CMC) and causing the "seagull" sign on radiographs. It is more disabling than primary OA.

17. Knee and hip OA.
- Over 50% of patients aged >65 years have radiographic knee OA, but only 25% have symptoms. Do not rely on the radiograph to make the diagnosis of the cause of knee pain.
- Recurrent, large, noninflammatory knee effusions are frequently due to an internal derangement (e.g., meniscal tear).
- Nonsteroidal antiinflammatory drugs (NSAIDs) work better than acetaminophen if a patient has an effusion, which suggests more inflammation (wet OA).
- Intra-articular corticosteroids can be effective for OA in patients with a knee effusion and are cheaper than viscosupplementation (hyaluronic acid).
- Drain any knee effusion before giving corticosteroids. The injection works better when there is less fluid.
- Incidental and asymptomatic meniscal tears are common (>20%) in patients with knee OA. Meniscal repair and/or arthroscopic debridement and washout are not helpful unless there are signs of locking.
- Femoroacetabular impingement is a common cause of hip pain in young patients who develop early OA (congenital abnormalities such as Legg–Calvé–Perthes disease and slipped capital femoral epiphysis often present earlier for clinical evaluation but are also associated with early OA).

18. Extraarticular manifestations are often the most important findings to make a diagnosis in a patient with polyarthritis.

19. Myopathies tend to cause proximal and symmetric weakness, whereas neuropathies cause distal and asymmetric weakness and atrophy of muscles.

20. Cardiac disease occurs 10 years earlier in patients with inflammatory rheumatic disease than in normal individuals with the same cardiac risk factors.
This must be considered during the preoperative evaluation. Multiply the risk factor calculator (e.g. Framingham) value by 1.5 (RA, PsA) and by 2.0 (SLE) to assess cardiac risk.

21. Fever in a patient with known systemic rheumatic disease is an infection or nonrheumatic etiology (drug reaction, other illness [e.g., thrombotic thrombocytopenic purpura, lymphoma]) until proven otherwise.
Infection may cause death in patients with rheumatic disease more often than the underlying rheumatic disease does, especially later in the disease course.

22. RA is the most common inflammatory arthritis presenting with symmetric involvement of the small joints of the hands (MCPs, PIPs), wrists, and feet (MTPs).
If a patient carries a diagnosis of RA and is seronegative or only has large joint involvement, always reassess to ensure that the patient does not have another diagnosis (e.g. CPPD).

23. If a patient has seronegative RA, the "extraarticular manifestation" is probably not due to RA.

24. Seronegative RA is a difficult diagnosis in patients without erosions on radiographs.
Always consider CPPD in these patients.

25. Treat to target.
Early therapy with the goal of low disease activity is essential to RA therapy (and many other rheumatic diseases).
- It does not matter which disease activity measure you use (e.g., Clinical Disease Activity Index, Routine Assessment of Patient Index Data 3 [RAPID3], etc.), just pick one and use it to document if your therapy is achieving low disease activity or remission.

26. The development of drug-induced autoantibodies (usually anti-histone) is much more common than the development of lupus-like disease due to a drug.

27. **NSAIDs and SLE do not always mix well together.**
    - With new onset photosensitivity, rule out NSAIDs and/or thiazide diuretic as the cause.
    - In a patient with SLE with worsening renal function, rule out over-the-counter NSAIDs.
    - NSAIDs (especially ibuprofen) are associated with aseptic meningitis, which may be confused with central nervous system (CNS) lupus.

28. **Systemic sclerosis (SSc).**
    New onset hypertension, falling platelet count, and schistocytes on blood smear in a patient with diffuse SSc heralds the onset of scleroderma renal crisis (SRC). New-onset disease (< 2 years), diffuse scleroderma (dcSSc) subset, anti-RNA polymerase III antibody, rapid skin and/or pulmonary progression, tendon friction rubs, and exposure to corticosteroids (>15mg daily) or calcineurin inhibitors are risk factors for SRC. Angiotensin-converting enzyme (ACE) inhibitors work better than angiotensin-receptor blockers.
    - RNA polymerase III antibody is associated with elevated malignancy risk.
    - Pulmonary arterial hypertension (PAH) and interstitial lung disease (ILD) are the chief causes of scleroderma-related death; vigilant screening assessments are indicated in all patients with SSc.
    - Pulmonary function tests can be useful for identifying high risk of PAH: a declining diffusing capacity for carbon monoxide (DLCO) over time and a % forced vital capacity (FVC)/%DLCO ratio of >1.6 is associated with a high risk of PAH.
    - An FVC <70% and/or a high-resolution CT scan of the lung showing >20% fibrosis signifies "extensive" ILD. This subset is associated with: (1) 5-year survival of only 60% to 65%, (2) elevated risk of progressive ILD, (3) identifies a group with a greater response to immunosuppressive (cyclophosphamide) therapy than in patients with milder ILD.

29. **One should suspect a disease mimicking scleroderma (e.g. scleromyxedema, eosinophilic fasciitis, others) in any patient with skin induration who lacks Raynaud phenomenon, nailfold capillary abnormalities, sclerodactyly, and autoantibodies**
    - Scleredema and scleromyxedema cause mucinous deposition in the skin and may be associated with monoclonal gammopathies
    - When ordering a skin biopsy, request specific stains for mucin and consider full thickness biopsy to include deeper tissue structures (especially for eosinophilic fasciitis)
    - Morphea (localized scleroderma) does not evolve into SSc (occurrence of transition is not higher than background incidence rate of SSc)

30. **Patients with Raynaud phenomenon are unlikely (<5%) to develop SSc if they have normal nailfold capillaroscopy and negative scleroderma-associated antibodies.**

31. **Inflammatory myositis should be highly considered in all patients with proximal muscle weakness, an elevated creatine phosphokinase (CPK), an elevated CK-MB fraction of total CPK (>2% of total), and an elevated aspartate aminotransferase.**
    - Always measure CPK in a patient with an unexplained elevation of "liver-associated enzymes".
    - Look for mechanic's hand on radial aspect of index finger and get a CPK in any patient presenting with ILD. Rule out antisynthetase antibody syndrome (e.g. anti-Jo-1).
    - Patients with antisynthetase antibody syndrome who also have anti-SS-A/Ro antibodies have a worse prognosis (the SS-A antibody is also associated with worse prognosis in other ILD subsets, including MDA-5-associated ILD)

32. **Skin ulcerations, anti-TIF1γ or anti-NXP2 antibodies, older age, and disease persistence despite adequate immunosuppression, are all associated with underlying malignancy risk in a patient with dermatomyositis. Patients with immune-mediated necrotizing myositis and anti-HMGCoA reductase antibodies that are not due to a statin also have an increased risk of an underlying cancer.**

33. **Steroid myopathy does not cause an elevated CPK.**

34. **Statins can cause myalgias without an elevated CPK, myalgias with an elevated CPK, and necrotizing myopathy with anti-HMGCoA reductase antibodies.**
    - Myalgia can be improved with coenzyme Q.
    - Hydrophilic statins (pravachol, rosuvastatin) cause less myopathy than lipophilic statins (simvastatin).

35. **All patients with MCTD should have Raynaud phenomenon and high-titer antibodies against U1-RNP.**

36. **Up to 25% of all patients presenting with a CTD will be undifferentiated, and a similar percentage of those will evolve into a defined CTD within 3 years.**
    Patience and follow-up are important.

37. **Sjögren disease (SjD) is the most common autoimmune disease in middle-aged women and should be considered in any patient with unexplained symptoms and a positive ANA.**

38. **One in five rule: 20% of deep venous thromboses, 20% of young adult (<50 years old) strokes, and 20% of recurrent miscarriages are due to the antiphospholipid antibody (aPL ab) syndrome.**

39. **"Triple positive" (positive lupus anticoagulant, anticardiolipin antibodies, and anti-β2 glycoprotein I antibodies) aPL patients are the most likely to have clots.**

40. **aPL abs plus a surgical insult or obstetrical delivery deserves short-term anticoagulation.**
    - All patients with significantly positive (and persistent) aPL abs should have prophylactic anticoagulation if they undergo a surgical procedure and/or following pregnancy delivery, even if they have never had a clot.
    - Surgical release of tissue factor is the second hit in the "two-hit" hypothesis for clots in aPL ab-positive patients.
    - Always have the placenta assessed (clinically and/or pathologically) for evidence of damage in patients with aPL ab regardless of pregnancy outcome. If placental damage is present, the patient needs anticoagulation during any future pregnancy.
    - All lupus patients should be screened for aPL abs, regardless of clot history, so counseling can occur regarding: prophylactic anticoagulation in high-risk scenarios (above), pregnancy risks/prognosis, choice of contraception (avoidance of estrogen-containing agents), and safety of hormone replacement therapy in the setting of aPL abs

41. **Still's disease should be considered in any patient with a quotidian fever (decreases to normal or below once a day), rash, and joint pain.**
    A ferritin level >1000 ng/mL supports the diagnosis.

42. **Patients with polymyalgia rheumatica (PMR) should respond completely to 20 mg daily of prednisone and normalize their erythrocyte sedimentation rate (ESR) within a month.**
    The presence of fever or failure to respond to prednisone clinically and serologically suggests giant cell arteritis (GCA) or another diagnosis such as lymphoma.

43. **After ruling out infection and malignancy, consider vasculitis in any patient with multisystem disease who has an ESR >100 mm/hour and a C-reactive protein >10 times the upper limit of normal.**
    The **primary** vasculitides (i.e., vasculitis not due to another disease such as SLE or cryoglobulinemia) are not associated with positive serologies (ANA, RF, low complements), neutropenia, or thrombocytopenia. If one of these is present, consider another diagnosis.

44. **GCA is the most common vasculitis in the elderly, and jaw claudication is the most specific symptom.**
    - Clinical presentations may include: (1) cranial symptoms (headache, scalp tenderness), (2) common ocular presentations (amaurosis fugax, double vision), and (3) claudication symptoms (tongue and jaw).
    - Other presentations include fever of unknown origin (without an elevated WBC count), large vessel involvement, stroke (frequently basilar/vertebral), and persistent unexplained cough.
    - GCA, GPA, and Behcet's are the only vasculitides thought to cause ulcers on the lateral aspect of the mid-tongue.

45. **Listen for subclavian bruits in all patients suspected of having GCA as it may be their only clinical finding.**
    - Asymmetric blood pressure should be tested for in all patients being evaluated for GCA.
    - Large vessel involvement puts them at increased (17 ×) risk for aortic dissections and aneurysms.

46. **Do not delay starting prednisone in a patient suspected to have GCA.**
    It will not affect the temporal artery biopsy results for at least a week. Evidence of inflammation on ultrasound ('halo sign') may resolve in less than a week following corticosteroid therapy.

47. **When the suspected diagnosis is primary vasculitis of the CNS, it is probably incorrect.**
    Rule out other diseases with a brain biopsy.

48. **Granulomatosis with polyangiitis (GPA) should be considered in any adult who develops otitis media.**
    - GPA predominantly affects the upper and lower respiratory tracts and kidneys and is associated with proteinase 3-antineutrophil cytoplasmic antibody (ANCA).
    - Strawberry gums are characteristic.
    - Necrotic ears, positive ANCA (especially discordant ANCA-IFA & specific ELISA PR3 and/or MPO testing results), and low neutrophil count suggest levamisole-laced cocaine as the etiology.

49. **Microscopic polyangiitis should be considered in all patients presenting with pulmonary–renal syndrome and is associated with myeloperoxidase-ANCA.**

50. **Skin biopsy in IgA vasculitis (IgA-V) shows leukocytoclastic vasculitis with predominantly IgA deposition in vessel walls on direct immunofluorescence.**
    - IgA-V is the most common small vessel vasculitis in childhood.
    - Scrotal swelling is common in males.

51. **Urticarial lesions lasting longer than 24 hours is not typical of idiopathic urticaria/ hives.**
    - Cutaneous lesions resolving with hyperpigmentation are likely to be vasculitic: rule out urticarial vasculitis and hypocomplementemic urticarial vasculitis (HUVS).
    - Other causes of recurrent and prolonged urticarial lesions not due to vasculitis: cryopyrin-associated periodic syndromes, Schnitzler's syndrome, and autoimmune thyroid disease.

52. **Most patients with mixed cryoglobulinemia will present with palpable purpura, arthralgia, and weakness/myalgias (Meltzer's triad).**
    A positive RF and low C4 level support the diagnosis before the cryoglobulin screen has returned.

53. **"Refractory" vasculitis is an infection until proven otherwise.**

54. **Behçet disease is the only vasculitis that causes pulmonary aneurysms and affects the venous system (venulitis) more than the arterial system.**
    Venous thrombosis can be seen in 15–30%; immunosuppression reduces subsequent clot risk.

55. **Relapsing polychondritis can be associated with an underlying disorder in one-third of cases, especially vasculitis and myelodysplastic syndromes.**
    In males with relapsing polychondritis, macrocytosis, and thrombocytopenia, *UBA1* genetic testing has a 100% sensitivity and 96% specificity for VEXAS syndrome.

56. **Enthesitis is the hallmark of seronegative spondyloarthritis.**

57. **HLA-B27 risk should be put into perspective.**
    - Even though HLA-B27 increases a person's risk of developing spondyloarthritis 50 times, only 1 out of every 50 (2%) HLA-B27-positive individuals without a family history will develop ankylosing spondylitis during their lifetime.
    - If the person has a family history, the risk increases to one in five (20%).
    - Approximately 50% of HLA-B27-positive patients with recurrent unilateral acute anterior uveitis have or will develop an underlying spondyloarthritis.

58. **A patient aged <40 years old with chronic low back pain (> 12 weeks), with three of the following has a high likelihood of inflammatory back pain: (1) morning stiffness of at least 30 minutes, (2) improvement of back pain with exercise but not rest, (3) awakening because of back pain and stiffness during second half of the night only, and (4) alternating buttock pain.**

59. **Inflammatory arthritis is most likely to occur in Crohn's disease patients with extensive colonic involvement.**
    These patients may present with prominent arthritis but few gastrointestinal symptoms. Unexplained iron deficiency anemia may be a hint.

60. **Pancreatic cancer can release enzymes, which cause fat necrosis, resulting in a triad of lower extremity arthritis, tender nodules, and eosinophilia (Schmidt's triad).**

61. **Reactive arthritis is a sterile, inflammatory arthritis that is typically preceded by a gastrointestinal or genitourinary infection occurring 1 to 4 weeks previously.**
    The arthritis can improve with prolonged antibiotics only if it is due to *Chlamydia*.

62. **Inflammation of the DIP joints and finger dactylitis are highly characteristic of psoriatic arthritis.**
    Differential diagnosis of DIP arthritis: psoriatic, OA, multicentric reticulohistiocytosis, and primary biliary cirrhosis. In a patient with OA who gets an inflamed DIP–rule out gout.

63. **Any patient with fever, arthralgias, and tenosynovitis should be evaluated for a disseminated gonococcal infection (DGI).**
    The majority of females develop DGI within 1 week of menses and genitourinary symptoms may be absent.

64. **Suspect coinfection with babesia or anaplasma in any Lyme disease patient with hemolysis, neutropenia, and/or thrombocytopenia.**
    - A minority (10%) of patients with confirmed Lyme disease arthritis may have continued synovitis despite adequate antibiotic treatment (including two courses). These patients should be treated with NSAIDs, intraarticular steroids, or csDMARDs such as hydroxychloroquine.
    - A minority of patients (<10%) with Lyme disease will develop post-treatment Lyme disease syndrome, a fibromyalgia-like and chronic fatigue-like illness, despite initial treatment with antibiotics for Lyme. Additional antibiotics are not helpful in this setting.

65. **The chest radiograph is normal in 50% of patients who have tuberculous septic arthritis, which most commonly presents as chronic inflammatory monoarticular arthritis involving the knee.**
    The diagnosis of tuberculous arthritis is best confirmed by synovial biopsy and culture because synovial fluid acid-fast bacilli stain is positive in only 20%.

66. Parvovirus is the most common viral arthritis and should be considered in any patient presenting with fever, rash, and arthritis, particularly if they have exposure to children.

67. Hepatitis C is the most common cause of cryoglobulinemia.

Overall, 50% of hepatitis C patients have cryoglobulins, but only 5% develop cryoglobulinemic vasculitis. With the availability of more effective therapies for the treatment of hepatitis C, its contribution to the development of cryoglobulinemia is expected to diminish.

68. Gout is the most common cause of inflammatory arthritis in men aged >40 years.

- It should not occur in premenopausal females in the absence of chronic kidney disease.
- Gout occurring in the context of renal insufficiency, encephalopathy/cognitive impairment, and microcytic anemia should raise suspicion for lead intoxication (saturnine gout)
- Consumption of alcohol (particularly beer), red meats, fructose (including energy drinks) and seafood increase serum urate levels and are associated with increased gout risk; in contrast, coffee, vitamin C, and low-fat dairy products appear to promote uricosuria and decrease gout risk.
- Major risk factors for allopurinol hypersensitivity syndrome include inheritance of HLA-B*5801, renal insufficiency, and higher starting dose of allopurinol.

69. Uric acid is less soluble in the cold.

- Consequently, gout occurs in the cooler distal joints (e.g. foot) and is rare in the spine or joints near the spine.
- The foot is always the first location involved in the patient's initial gout attack.
- If you do not get any fluid when you tap the first MTP joint, blow out the end of the needle onto a slide and examine the blood speck for uric acid crystals. If joint aspiration is not successful but tophi are present, consider using a 22-gauge needle for a "core biopsy" to blow out onto a slide.
- Dual-energy CT scan can be used to detect urate deposits in scenarios where joint aspiration is not successful and/or feasible.

70. In a patient with gout, the goal for uric acid lowering medications is to decrease the uric acid to <6.0 mg/dL.

Start allopurinol at a low dose (50-100mg/d) and increase monthly (50–100mg/d) to a maximum of 600mg/d. Larger patients may need a higher dose (4mg/kg/d dosing is associated with achieving goal uric acid concentration). Patients unable to lower their uric acid may have barriers to medication adherence (check a serum oxypurinol level and if low, address barriers to adherence).

71. CPPD disease is a disease of the elderly with onset and increasing frequency after the age of 55 years.

- Only patients with familial mutations or metabolic abnormalities (e.g., hemochromatosis, hypophosphatasia) get CPPD before the age of 55 years.
- Pseudogout occurs most commonly in the wrist and knee. It does not commonly occur in the foot.

72. CPPD should be considered in any elderly patient with a seronegative inflammatory or degenerative arthritis involving the MCPs, wrists, and shoulders.

CPPD can mimic seronegative RA, PMR, and OA (involving atypical joints), even in the absence of prior acute CPP crystal arthritis (pseudogout) attacks. CPPD can cause acute and severe neck pain (crowned dens syndrome).

73. The diabetic stiff hand syndrome is related to disease duration and therapy, and predicts microvascular complications of diabetes.

74. Hypothyroidism (thyroid-stimulating hormone [TSH] always >20 mIU/L with low free T4) should be ruled out in patients with muscle symptoms and an elevated creatine kinase.

75. **If a fracture is suspected as a cause of hemarthrosis, evaluate the synovial fluid for fat droplets, which indicates release of bone marrow elements through bony disruption.**

76. **When palmar fasciitis presents in a female, think ovarian carcinoma.**

77. **Leukocytoclastic vasculitis is the most common paraneoplastic vasculitis presentation, especially in patients with myelodysplastic syndromes (rule out VEXAS).**

78. **Osteoporosis.**
    - The major risk factors for fragility fractures are low bone mass, advancing age, previous fragility fractures, corticosteroid use, and the propensity to fall. The best predictor of a future fall is a fall within the previous 6 months. Screen the patient with the "get up and go" test.
    - Each decrease of -1.0 T-score on DXA correlates with a 12% loss of bone. At a T-score of -2.5, the patient has lost 30% of their bone mass, which is when osteopenia can reliably be detected on plain radiographs.
    - Rule out vitamin D insufficiency in all patients with a low bone mass. Consider celiac disease in any patient with an extremely low vitamin D level (< 10 ng/ml) even if they do not have diarrhea.
    - Pharmacologic therapy should be initiated in patients who have had a fragility fracture (regardless of T-score), a bone mineral density T-score ≤ -2.5 at any site, or a FRAX-derived 10-year risk of $\geq 3\%$ for hip fractures and $\geq 20\%$ for other major osteoporosis fractures (an adjustment should be made to the FRAX estimate for patients taking ≥ 7.5 mg daily of prednisone, and lower fracture risk thresholds may be considered in this setting as well).
    - Vertebroplasty and kyphoplasty are most effective when done within 6 months of onset of a severely symptomatic vertebral compression fracture and in patients with vertebral edema pattern on MRI.
    - A patient who meets criteria for osteoporosis treatment is 30 times more likely to get a fracture if untreated than they are to get osteonecrosis of the jaw or an atypical femoral fracture if they are treated with an antiresorptive (bisphosphonate or denosumab).

79. **Paget's disease of bone (PDB).**
    - The number of skeletal sites involved in PDB is stable over time.
    - Plain radiographs are the best modality to diagnose PDB, whereas nuclear medicine bone scan is the best study to evaluate the extent of disease.

80. **Musculoskeletal manifestations can be the presenting manifestation in up to 33% of patients with hemochromatosis.**
    Consider in any Caucasian male aged <40 years with "seronegative RA," degenerative changes of the second and third MCP joints, and/or hypogonadotrophic hypogonadism with low bone mass.

81. **Primary fibromyalgia does not typically occur for the first time in patients after the age of 55 years, nor is it likely to be the correct primary diagnosis in patients with musculoskeletal pain who also have abnormal laboratory values.**

82. **Fibromyalgia is a chronic noninflammatory, nonautoimmune central afferent processing disorder leading to a diffuse pain syndrome as well as other symptoms.**
    Narcotics and corticosteroids should not be used for treatment. Non-pharmacologic intervention has equivalent, if not more consistent, success than medication therapy.

83. **Obstructive sleep apnea (ask if they snore even if they are not obese), hypothyroidism (TSH >20 mIU/L), and vitamin D deficiency (25 OH vitamin D <5 ng/mL) should be ruled out in all fibromyalgia patients.**
    In patients with severe and refractory symptoms, ask about physical and/or sexual abuse. In fibromyalgia patients with concurrent sleep apnea, effective CPAP has been shown to decrease pain

symptoms and improve quality of life. Treatment of concurrent depression or sleep disturbance is critical for improvement in pain and functionality.

84. Growing pains do not occur during the daytime.

A limp in a child is pathologic until proven otherwise.

85. Malignancy is more likely than systemic JIA in any child who has fever, painful arthritis, an elevated LDH, and/or a low platelet count.

In patients with established systemic JIA, macrophage activation syndrome should be considered in any patient who develops a precipitous decrease in ESR (from hepatic dysfunction, decreased fibrinogen), decreased WBC and platelet counts, elevated liver-associated enzymes, elevated triglycerides, and extreme elevations of ferritin (especially if >10,000 ng/mL). An elevated sCD25 (interleukin-2 receptor) can help confirm the diagnosis.

86. Neck or back pain in a young child is never normal and demands an extensive workup.

87. ANA positivity, female sex, and age <6 years increase the risk of chronic uveitis regardless of the JIA subgroup.

88. Inflammatory myositis in childhood is almost always dermatomyositis and not polymyositis, whereas scleroderma in childhood is most commonly linear scleroderma.

89. Consider Kawasaki disease in any child aged <5 years presenting with prolonged high fevers and conjunctivitis.

Intravenous immunoglobulin within 10 days of disease onset is the treatment of choice.

90. Muscle cramps, pain, or myoglobinuria brought on by exercise suggests a metabolic myopathy.

- Muscle symptoms with short bursts of high-intensity exercise and the second wind phenomenon are characteristic of a glycogen storage disease. McArdle disease and acid maltase deficiency are most common.
- Muscle symptoms with prolonged low-intensity exercise and/or prolonged fasting suggest a defect in fatty acid oxidation. Carnitine palmitoyltransferase II (CPT II) deficiency is most common.
- The most common metabolic myopathies associated with myoglobinuria are CPT II deficiency and McArdle disease.
- The most common myopathies that are confused with polymyositis are acid maltase deficiency and limb-girdle muscular dystrophy.
- Children presenting with a muscle disease without rash almost always have a metabolic or genetic myopathy and not primary polymyositis.

91. Abdominal fat pad aspiration is the easiest and most sensitive method of obtaining tissue to examine for amyloid deposition (polarized microscopy of Congo red-stained tissue).

92. Uveitis is frequently a symptom of an underlying disease.

- Anatomic location (anterior, intermediate, posterior, panuveitis), laterality, and course (acute, chronic, recurrent) of uveitis attacks help develop a differential diagnosis.
- Most patients should be screened with the fluorescent treponemal antibody absorption test (syphilis), chest x-ray (CXR; tuberculosis [TB] and sarcoidosis) and consideration of TB screening (confirms exposure but not active ocular involvement). Additional targeted evaluation is based on the uveitis presentation and presence of extra-ocular symptoms.
- CT is more sensitive than CXR in the identification of suspected pulmonary sarcoidosis associated with uveitis.

- Nodular and necrotizing scleritis, and peripheral ulcerative keratitis (PUK), are non-uveitis inflammatory ocular conditions with high (50–75%) association with systemic rheumatic conditions. RA and ANCA-associated vasculitis are the most common rheumatic associations.

93. **A patient with acute, inflammatory arthritis involving bilateral ankles should always be evaluated for sarcoidosis.**
    - Erythema nodosum typically affects the anterior aspect of lower legs and never ulcerates. Subcutaneous nodules on the posterior aspect of calf or any that ulcerate should raise concern for vasculitis or infection.
    - Swelling and scaling of cosmetic tattoos can be caused by sarcoidosis.

94. **Patients with SLE and Sjögren disease who have anti-Ro (SS-A) and/or anti-La (SS-B) antibodies (and any mother with SS-A and/or SS-B, regardless of diagnosis) are at increased risk for having infants who develop the neonatal lupus syndrome and complete heart block (5–20%).**

95. **Autoinflammatory syndromes are characterized by episodes of fever, rash, arthritis, peritonitis, eye inflammation, lack of autoantibodies, and elevated acute-phase reactants in various combinations that normalize between flares.**
    The duration of flares differs between diseases: tumor necrosis factor-associated periodic fever syndrome > hyperimmunoglobulinemia D with periodic fever syndrome > familial Mediterranean fever > Muckle–Wells syndrome/familial cold autoinflammatory syndrome. Inhibition of interleukin-1 is the treatment of choice for most syndromes.

96. **Medications.**
    - Always rule out medication as the cause of musculoskeletal symptoms.
      - Perinuclear ANCA vasculitis: hydralazine, propylthiouracil, minocycline, cocaine (levamisole).
      - Fluoroquinolones: Achilles tendinitis and rupture.
      - Drug-induced lupus: hydralazine, minocycline, antitumor necrosis factor (TNF) agents, rifabutin, procainamide, and others.
    - All NSAIDs should be used with caution (if at all) in patients with underlying renal or cardiovascular disease.
    - All NSAIDs can cause photosensitivity.
    - NSAIDs can interfere with conception.
    - Hydrocortisone 20 mg = prednisone 5 mg = prednisolone 5 mg = methylprednisolone 4 mg = dexamethasone 0.75 mg.
    - Avascular necrosis (AVN) from corticosteroids is the most common reason a rheumatologist is sued for a medication adverse effect. Record in the chart that you counseled the patient on the following risk: for each 20 mg of prednisone taken for over a month, the risk of AVN is 5% (e.g., a 60-mg dose for a month confers a risk of 15% for AVN). Patients with SLE, those that have aPL abs, and those who rapidly become cushingoid are most at risk.
    - Choice of DMARD therapy is based on disease severity, comorbidities, and fertility plans.
    - Due to immunosuppression caused by many DMARDs it is necessary to make sure patients receive immunizations (influenza, pneumococcal, COVID, zoster, RSV, HPV) and are screened for viral (e.g., HPV) malignancies (cervical screening, etc).
    - Methotrexate is the most effective anchor drug for all combination therapies. An increase of the mean corpuscular volume by 5 fL correlates with a good methotrexate effect.
      - Patients on >15 mg/week of MTX should split their dose on the day they take it or switch to subcutaneous administration for better absorption.
      - Patients with MTX neurotoxicity may have less symptoms if taken with dextromethorphan (two tabs of Mucinex-DM) or a 10oz cup of caffeinated coffee on the day they take MTX.
    - Hydroxychloroquine (HCQ) is less effective in smokers, can cause dizziness and headache, and requires the patient to have eye examinations (recommended dose ≤5 mg/kg actual body weight; max 400 mg/day).

- Renal and hepatic insufficiency can cause elevated blood levels leading to eye disease. Whole blood levels should be monitored.
  - Split dose and coat pills with butter if generic HCQ tablets cause GI symptoms.
- Sulfasalazine can cause reversible azoospermia.
- Leflunomide has an extremely long half-life. In cases of toxicity or pregnancy, an elimination protocol with cholestyramine should be started.
  - Leflunomide can cause hypertension and neuropathy.
- Proton pump inhibitors can interfere with the absorption of mycophenolate mofetil.
- Patients on oral cyclophosphamide should take their dose in the morning (not at night) and drink several glasses of fluid to lessen chance of bladder toxicity.
  - Test for BK virus if develop hemorrhagic cystitis.
- Azathioprine is better used for maintenance of remission than for induction of remission. It should not be used in patients on allopurinol, febuxostat, or ampicillin (rash). It can cause resistance to coumadin effectiveness.
  - Switch to 6-mercaptopurine if patient has GI intolerance (not pancreatitis, hepatitis) with azathioprine.
- Dapsone can be associated with hemolytic anemia (avoid if glucose-6-phosphate dehydrogenase [G6PD]-deficient) and methemoglobinemia. Low-grade hemolysis can be seen on dapsone even with normal G6PD levels; folic acid 1 mg/day is recommended.
- Live vaccines should not be given to patients on biologic agents. Check for TB (purified protein derivative test, interferon-gamma release assay) and immunize patients before biologic therapy.
- Obesity and smoking lessen the effectiveness of anti-TNF agents.
- Stop anti-TNF agents if a patient has an open wound until it heals.
- Infliximab is most commonly associated with mycobacterial and fungal infections. Abatacept and rituximab are least associated.
- Tocilizumab may interfere with the effectiveness of birth control pills. Do not use in patients at risk for bowel perforations (history of diverticulitis).
- Rituximab works best in seropositive RA patients who have germinal centers in their synovium. Always send the synovial tissue at the time of any joint surgery to see if germinal centers are present.
- Most biologic therapies used during pregnancy do not cross the placenta to the fetus until the second trimester, due to lack of the neonatal Fc receptor during the first trimester.
- Patients on glucocorticoids (prednisone ≥ 20 mg/d for ≥ 3 weeks) or rituximab should be considered for pneumocystis jirovecii pneumonia (PJP) prophylaxis. The elderly and patients with lung disease are also at increased risk for PJP.
- All patients starting JAK inhibitors need the shingles vaccine.
  - JAK inhibitors can reversibly increase creatinine and CPK levels.
- Allopurinol hypersensitivity syndrome is more common in patients with the HLA-B*5801 gene, renal insufficiency, and higher starting doses of allopurinol.
- Avoid colchicine use in patients who are on cyclosporine/tacrolimus (myopathy risk), antifungals (e.g., ketoconazole), or HIV protease inhibitors. Do not use in patients on clarithromycin who have renal insufficiency.
- Pegloticase should not be used in patients with G6PD deficiency.
- Stop ACE inhibitors in patients with chronic regional pain syndrome; stop calcium channel blockers in patients with erythromelalgia.
- Direct oral anticoagulants (DOACs) can cause a false positive lupus anticoagulant test.
- Do not inject a joint or soft tissue area (tendon) with corticosteroids more than three to four times within a year and never within 2 months of a previous injection. If an injection does not last 4 months, find a different therapeutic approach instead of repeatedly injecting the joint, tendon area, or bursa.
- Voriconazole can cause nodular hypertrophic osteoarthropathy.

97. "ADEPTTS" (Ambulation, Dressing, Eating, Personal hygiene, Transfers, Toileting, Sleeping/sexual activities) is a useful mnemonic to screen for a patient's functional limitations.

98. Rehabilitative techniques.
- A properly fitted cane used in the contralateral hand can unweight a diseased hip by 25–40%.
- Fatigue for >1 hour or soreness for >2 hours after exercise indicates too much exercise for the arthritic patient.
- Up to heaven, down to hell. When a patient has a painful lower extremity joint, tell him/her to use the good leg to step up a stair (up to heaven) and use the painful leg to step down a stair (down to hell).

99. Surgery.
- There are two indications for joint replacement surgery: (1) pain unresponsive to medical therapy and (2) loss of joint function. Therefore, inability to walk more than one block, stand longer than 20 to 30 minutes due to pain, walk up stairs, or put on shoes/socks are indications for total hip and total knee replacement.
- Lumbar spine surgery is most successful in patients with radicular symptoms confirmed by clinical examination, EMG, and MRI findings who have failed conservative therapy. Success of surgery decreases by 33% for each one that does not confirm the other.
- Stop biologic agents for at least one administration cycle before major surgery and restart when staples/stitches are out.
- Take vitamin C 500 mg daily starting just before and for 50 days after carpal tunnel surgery to reduce the chance of developing chronic regional pain syndrome.
- *Cutibacterium acnes* is a common cause of delayed and late prosthetic joint infection and often takes 7 days to grow; therefore, alert the microbiology laboratory to hold the plates.

100. Most rheumatic disease patients are considering trying or are presently using complementary and alternative medicine (CAM) therapies.

Physicians should ask patients about CAM therapies and record them in the medical record because some interact with other medications or can cause bleeding during surgery.
- Cannabinoids can decrease the metabolism of warfarin and lessen the effectiveness of anesthesia. Ask your patients if they are using cannabinoids for pain control.

We are sure the readers of this book have other TOP SECRETS. Please send them to jason.kolfenbach@cuanschutz.edu for inclusion in the next edition.

CHAPTER 2

Classification and Health Impact of the Rheumatic Diseases

Sterling G. West, MD

When you are frustrated with me because of things I cannot do, just think how frustrated I must be because I am not able.

—One or more of the 107 million people in the United States with a musculoskeletal disorder

---

>> **KEY POINTS**

1. Approximately 33% of the US population has arthritis and/or back pain.
2. One out of every five office visits to a primary care provider and 10% of all surgeries are for a musculoskeletal problem.
3. Arthritis/back pain is the leading cause of chronic disability, the second leading cause of acute disability, and the most common reason for social security disability payments.

---

1. What is rheumatology?

A medical science devoted to the study of rheumatic and musculoskeletal disorders (RMDs). RMDs are diverse and include systemic autoimmune rheumatic disorders (SARDs, e.g., lupus), systemic autoinflammatory disorders (SAIDs, e.g., Familial Mediterranean fever), noninflammatory arthritides, diffuse and local soft tissue disorders, injuries, and osteoporosis.

2. What are the roots of rheumatology?

First century AD—The term *rheuma* first appears in the literature. Rheuma refers to "a substance that flows" and probably was derived from phlegm, an ancient primary humor, which was believed to originate from the brain and flow to various parts of the body causing ailments.

1642—The word "rheumatism" is introduced into the literature by the French physician Dr. G. Baillou who emphasized that arthritis could be a systemic disorder.

1928—The American Committee for the Control of Rheumatism is established in the United States of America by Dr. R. Pemberton. It was renamed the American Association for the Study and Control of Rheumatic Disease (1934), then American Rheumatism Association (ARA; 1937), and finally American College of Rheumatology (ACR; 1988).

1940s—The terms *rheumatology* and *rheumatologist* are first coined by Drs. Hollander and Comroe, respectively.

3. How many rheumatic/musculoskeletal disorders are there?

There are over 150–200 rheumatic/musculoskeletal disorders (https://www.uems.eu/areas-of-expertise/postgraduate-training).

4. How have these rheumatic/musculoskeletal disorders been classified over the years?

1904—Dr. Goldthwaite, an orthopedic surgeon, makes the first attempt to classify the arthritides into five categories: gout, infectious arthritis, hypertrophic arthritis (probably osteoarthritis), atrophic arthritis (probably rheumatoid arthritis), and chronic villous arthritis (probably traumatic arthritis).

1964—ARA classification.

1983—The ARA classification is revised based on the ninth edition of the International Classification of Disease (ICD 9).

2015—ICD 10 Diagnosis Codes are published. Chapter 13 (M00-M99) contains 6929 diagnosis codes related to diseases of the musculoskeletal system and connective tissue. Notably, there are other ICD 10 chapters that include diagnostic codes for other arthritides (e.g., psoriatic arthritis [L40.5], others]. ICD 11 is being developed.

5. The ICD 10 diagnostic codes and classification systems are overwhelming. Is there a simpler outline to remember?

Most of the rheumatic diseases can be grouped into 10 major categories:
1. Systemic connective tissue diseases
2. Vasculitides and related disorders
3. Seronegative spondyloarthropathies
4. Arthritis associated with infectious agents
5. Rheumatic disorders associated with metabolic, endocrine, and hematologic diseases
6. Bone and cartilage disorders
7. Hereditary, congenital, and inborn errors of metabolism associated with rheumatic syndromes
8. Nonarticular and regional musculoskeletal disorders
9. Neoplasms and tumor-like lesions
10. Miscellaneous rheumatic disorders

6. What is the origin and difference between a collagen vascular disease and a connective tissue disease?

1942—Dr. Klemperer introduces the term diffuse collagen disease based on his pathologic studies of systemic lupus erythematosus (SLE) and scleroderma/systemic sclerosis.

1946—Dr. Rich coins the term *collagen vascular disease* based on his pathologic studies in vasculitis, indicating that the primary lesion involved the vascular endothelium.

1952—Dr. Ehrich suggests the term *connective tissue diseases*, which has gradually replaced the term "collagen vascular diseases."

In summary, the two terms are used synonymously, although the purist would say that heritable collagen disorders (see Chapter 54: Heritable Connective Tissue Disease) are the only true "diffuse collagen diseases."

7. How common are rheumatic/musculoskeletal disorders in the general US population?

The number depends on which RMDs are included. A previous study estimated that 34% of the adult population (107.5 million) had a chronic musculoskeletal condition. Less than two-thirds of these patients have symptoms severe enough to cause them to seek medical care, so an estimated 21.2% of the adults (53.2 million) have doctor-diagnosed arthritis. The prevalence of musculoskeletal disorders increases with the age of the patient population (50.4% > age 65 years). Although noninflammatory RMDs are most common, a woman has a 1 in 12 risk and a man has a 1 in 20 risk of developing an inflammatory or autoimmune RMD during their lifetime.

8. What is the estimated prevalence of the various rheumatic/musculoskeletal disorders in the general population?

The estimated prevalence of rheumatic/musculoskeletal disorders in the US population is shown in Table 2.1.

9. What is the prevalence of autoimmune diseases in the general population?

Any organ system can be affected by autoimmunity. Presently there are over 100 autoimmune diseases with at least half of them considered rare. It is estimated that 4.5% to 7.0% of the population (14.7–23.5 million) have one or more autoimmune diseases. Approximately 40% of these patients (2–3% of the population) have an autoimmune rheumatic disease. Of all patients with an autoimmune rheumatic disease, about half will have rheumatoid arthritis and half will have one of the other autoimmune rheumatic diseases (e.g., SLE, polymyositis).

10. Which autoimmune diseases primarily affect women?

The most common autoimmune diseases target women 75% of the time, frequently during their reproductive years. Diseases suspected to be autoantibody mediated (Th2 diseases) have the highest female predominance (Table 2.2).

TABLE 2.1 Estimated Prevalence of Rheumatic/Musculoskeletal Disorders in the US Adult Population

NUMBER OF PATIENTS	PREVALENCE (ADULTS)	
All musculoskeletal disorders	34%	107.5 million[a]
Arthropathies		
Osteoarthritis	15%	32.5 million
Rheumatoid arthritis	0.6–1.0%	1.4–2.5 million
Crystalline arthritis (gout)	4%	9 million
Spondyloarthropathies	0.5–1.0%	1.3–2.5 million
Connective Tissue Disease		
Polymyalgia rheumatica	<0.2%	500,000–700,000
Poly/dermatomyositis	<0.03%	70,000–150,000
Antiphospholipid antibody syndrome	<0.04%	120,000-160,000
Systemic lupus erythematosus	<0.1%	200,000–260,000
Sjogren's syndrome	<0.2%	0.5–1.4 million
Scleroderma/systemic sclerosis	<0.025%	50,000–96,000
Other MSK Problems		
Back/neck pain: frequent	15%	33 million
Osteoporosis (age >50 years)	11%	12 million
Soft tissue rheumatism	3–5%	5–10 million
Fibromyalgia	2%[b]	3–5 million

[a]Overall 53.2 million (21.2%) adults have doctor-diagnosed arthritis, and 220,000 children have arthritis with juvenile idiopathic arthritis being the most common.
[b]Depending on the criteria used for diagnosis, the prevalence could be higher (i.e., 6%)

TABLE 2.2 The Female/Male Ratio of Autoimmune Diseases

DISEASE	FEMALE/MALE RATIO
Hashimoto's disease	9:1
Systemic lupus erythematosus	9:1
Sjögren's syndrome	9:1
Antiphospholipid syndrome	9:1
Mixed connective tissue disease	8:1
Graves' disease	7:1
Rheumatoid arthritis	3:1
Scleroderma/systemic sclerosis	3:1
Multiple sclerosis	2:1
Polymyositis	2:1

11. How often is one of the rheumatic/musculoskeletal disorders likely to be seen in an average primary care practice?

About 1 out of every 5 to 10 office visits to a primary care provider is for a musculoskeletal disorder. Interestingly, 66% of these patients are aged <65 years. The most common problems are osteoarthritis, back pain, gout, fibromyalgia, and tendinitis/bursitis.

BOX 2.1 Morbidity and Mortality of Rheumatic/Musculoskeletal Diseases

Percent of Population
- Symptoms of arthritis—30–40%
- Symptoms requiring medical therapy—20–25%
- Disability due to arthritis—5–10%
- Totally disabled from arthritis—0.5%
- Mortality from rheumatic disease—0.02%

12. How many rheumatologists are there in the United States?

In 2015, there were approximately 5595 adult rheumatologists (4997 FTEs) and 300 pediatric rheumatologists (287 FTEs), although not all are actively seeing patients. These numbers were projected to decrease (by 30% or more) by 2030. Consequently, the ACR has made efforts to support training more rheumatologists. In 2021, the AAMC survey reported 5416 rheumatologists (adult and pediatric) providing primarily patient care and another 1004 involved primarily in other activities (teaching, research, administration, and pharma) (www.aamc.org/data-reports/data/2021).

13. Discuss the impact of the rheumatic/musculoskeletal diseases on the general population in terms of morbidity and mortality.

Arthritis/back pain is the leading cause of chronic disability and the second leading cause of acute disability (behind respiratory illness) in the general population (Box 2.1). In 2018, of the estimated 54 million US adults with doctor-diagnosed arthritis, 23 million (42%) have arthritis-attributable activity limitations, which equates to 9% of all US adults having at least one limitation. Of working-age adults (aged 18–64 years) with doctor-diagnosed arthritis, 31% have arthritis-attributable work limitations. Due to lifestyle factors, the frequency of work limitations is more common in rural than in urban areas. Because these are prime working years, musculoskeletal conditions cause a significant loss of work productivity. Overall, one-quarter of social security disability payments are related to rheumatologic disorders, thus making it the leading cause of social security disability payments. Furthermore, 10% of all surgical procedures are for disabilities related to arthritis.

14. What is the economic impact of rheumatic/musculoskeletal diseases?

In 2014, the US Medical Expenditures Panel Survey reported that 107 million persons reported one or more musculoskeletal conditions. Three out of every four of these individuals also have another chronic medical condition. The total aggregate direct medical costs ($882.6 billion) and indirect costs due to lost earnings ($97.5 billion) were estimated to be $980.1 billion, which was equivalent to 5.76% of the gross domestic product. The total aggregate arthritis-attributable direct medical costs ($140 billion) and indirect costs ($164 billion) were estimated to be $304 billion.

BIBLIOGRAPHY

Battafarano DF, Ditmyer M, Bolster MB, et al. 2015 American College of Rheumatology Workforce Study: supply and demand projections of adult rheumatology workforce (2015–2030). *Arthritis Care Res (Hoboken)*. 2018;70:617–626.

Benedek TG. A century of American rheumatology. *Ann Intern Med*. 1987;106:304–312.

Fallon EA, Boring MA, Foster AL, et al. Prevalence of diagnosed arthritis-United States, 2019–2021. *MMWR*. 2023;72:1101–1107.

Jafarzadeh SR, Felson DT. Updated estimates suggest a much higher prevalence of arthritis in United States adults than previous ones. *Arthritis Rheumatol*. 2018;70:185–192.

Lites TD, Foster AL, Boring MA, et al. Arthritis among children and adolescents aged < 18 years-United States, 2017–2021. *MMWR*. 2023;72:788–792.

Murphy LB. Economic Impact of Arthritis and Rheumatic Conditions. In: Firestein GS, dd RS, Gabriel SE, Koretzky GA, McInnes IB, O'Dell JR, eds. *Firestein & Kelley's Textbook of Rheumatology*. 11th ed. Philadelphia: Elsevier; 2021:510–521.

Reynolds MD. Origins of the concept of collagen–vascular diseases. *Semin Arthritis Rheum*. 1985;15:127–131.

Roberts MH, Erdei E. Comparative United States autoimmune disease rates for 2010-2016 by sex, geographic region, and race. *Autoimmunity Rev*. 2020;19:102423.

Theis KA, Murphy LB, Guglielmo D, et al. Prevalence of arthritis and arthritis-attributable limitation – Unites States, 2016–2018. *MMWR*. 2021;70:1401–1407.

Van der Heide D, Daikh DI, Betteridge N, et al. Common language description of the term rheumatic and musculoskeletal diseases (RMDs) for use in communication with the lay public, healthcare providers, and other stakeholders endorsed by EULAR and the ACR. *Ann Rheum Dis*. 2018;77:829–832.

FURTHER READING

www.aarda.org.
www.usbji.org.
www.rheumatology.org.
www.arthritis.org.
www.boneandjointburden.org.
www.autoimmuneregistry.org.
www.allofus.nih.gov

Anatomy and Physiology of the Musculoskeletal System

Sterling G. West, MD

 KEY POINTS

1. Collagen is the most abundant protein in the body. Mutations of collagen types I and II can lead to musculoskeletal disorders.
2. Hyaline cartilage is the major cartilage of diarthrodial joints. It is avascular and aneural and composed mainly of type II collagen, hyaluronic acid, aggrecan, and water.
3. Synovial fluid is a selective transudate of plasma. It is made viscous by the secretion of hyaluronic acid by synoviocytes into the synovial fluid.
4. The Wnt/β-catenin signaling pathway is a critical pathway for osteoblast activation and bone mass regulation.
5. The receptor activator of the nuclear factory-κB ligand (RANKL)/RANK/osteoprotegerin (OPG) signaling pathway is critical for osteoclast differentiation/activation and bone remodeling.
6. Defects in cytoskeletal proteins that link myofibrils/actin cytoskeleton to laminin/collagen in the extracellular matrix cause various forms of muscular dystrophy.

1. Name two major functions of the musculoskeletal system.

Structural support and purposeful motion. The activities of the human body depend on effective interaction between joints and the neuromuscular units that move them.

2. Name the five components of the musculoskeletal system.

Muscles, tendons, ligaments, cartilages, and bones are the five components of the musculoskeletal system. All of these structures contribute to the formation of a functional and mobile joint.

3. The different connective tissues differ in their composition of macromolecules. List the major macromolecular "building blocks" of connective tissue.

Collagen, elastin, adhesins, and proteoglycans.

COLLAGEN

4. How many types of collagen are there? In which tissues is each type most commonly found?

Collagen is the most abundant body protein accounting for 25% to 30% of the total body protein. There are at least 29 different types of collagen; however, 90% of collagen in the human body is type I. The most common ones are listed in Table 3.1 and can be divided into seven subclasses. The unique properties and organization of each collagen type enable that specific collagen to contribute to the function of the tissue of which it is the principal structural component. Abnormalities of collagen types can cause several diseases.

5. Discuss the structural features common to all collagen molecules.

The definitive structural feature of all collagen molecules is the **triple helix.** This unique conformation is due to three polypeptide chains (α-chains) twisted around each other into a right-handed major helix. Extending from the amino and carboxyl terminal ends of both helical domains of the α-chains are nonhelical components, called telopeptides. In the major interstitial collagens, the helical domains are continuous, whereas in the other collagen classes, the helical domains may be interrupted by 1 to 12 nonhelical segments.

The primary structure of the helical domain of the α-chain is characterized by the repeating triplet Gly–*X*–*Y*. *X* and *Y* can be any amino acid though the most frequent are proline and hydroxyproline, respectively. Overall, approximately 25% of the residues in the triple helical domains consist of proline and hydroxyproline. Hydroxylysine is also commonly found. In the most abundant interstitial collagens (type I and II), the triple helical region contains about 1000 amino acid residues $(Gly–X–Y)_{333}$ (Fig. 3.1).

TABLE 3.1 Collagen Types, Tissue Distribution, and Diseases Caused by Mutations

CLASSES	TISSUE DISTRIBUTION	DISEASE
Fibril-forming (interstitial) collagens		
Type I	Bone, tendon, skin, joint capsule, synovium, arterial walls, cornea	OI, ED, Caffey's disease
Type II	Hyaline cartilage, disk, vitreous humor	CD, Stickler's
Type III	Blood vessels, skin, lung, granulation tissue	ED (vascular), Dupuytren's
Type V	Same as type I, placenta	ED (classical)
Type XI	Same as type II	SED, Stickler's
Network-forming and short-chain collagens		
Type IV[a]	Basement membrane	Alport syndrome
Type VIII	Endothelium, Descemet's membrane	Corneal dystrophy
Type X	Growth plate cartilage	MD
FACIT (fibril-associated collagens with interrupted triple helices)		
Type IX	Same as type II and type XI, cornea	MED
Type XII	Same as type I	–
Type XIV	Same as type I	–
Type XVI (FACIT-like)	Several tissues with types I/II	–
Type XIX	Rhabdomyosarcoma cells	–
Type XXI	Blood vessels	–
Beaded filament-forming collagen		
Type VI	Most connective tissues with type I	Rare muscle diseases
Collagen of anchoring fibrils		
Type VII	Dermoepidermal, cornea, oral mucosa	Epidermolysis bullosa dystrophica
MACIT (membrane-associated collagens with interrupted triple helices)		
Type XIII	Endomysium, placenta, meninges	–
Type XVII[a]	Skin, hemidesmosomes, cornea	–
Multiplexin (Multiple triple helix domains with interruptions)		
Type XV	Many tissues, especially muscle	–
Type XVIII	Many tissues Source of endostatin	Knobloch syndrome

CD, Chondrodysplasia; *ED,* Ehlers–Danlos syndrome; *MD,* metaphyseal dysplasia; *MED,* multiple epiphyseal dysplasia; *OI,* osteogenesis imperfecta; *SED,* spondyloepiphyseal dysplasia.
[a]Goodpasture syndrome results from an autoimmune response against collagen type IV; bullous pemphigoid results from an autoimmune response against collagen type XVII (BP180).

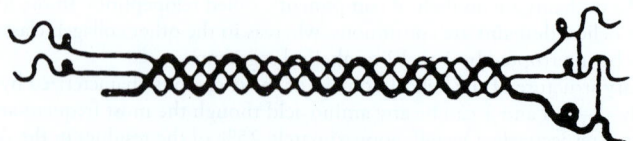

Fig. 3.1 Diagram of interstitial (fibrillar) collagen molecule demonstrating triple helix configuration with terminal telopeptides.

6. **Identify the major collagen classes and the types of collagen included in each class (Table 3.1).**
   - Fibril-forming (interstitial)—types I, II, III, V, and XI. Being the most abundant collagen class, these collagens form the extracellular fabric of the major connective tissues. They have the same tensile strength as steel wire.
   - Fibril-associated collagens with interrupted triple helices (FACIT)—types IX, XII, XIV, XVI, XIX, and XXI. These collagens are associated with the fibril-forming (interstitial) collagens and occur in the same tissues.
   - Nonfibrillar collagens with specialized structures or functions:
     Basement membrane collagen—type IV.
     Short-chain collagens—types VIII, X.
     Multiple triple helix domains with interruptions (Multiplexin)—types XV, XVIII.
     Membrane-associated collagens with interrupted triple helices (MACIT)—types XIII, XVII, XXIII.
     Microfibril forming collagens—type VI.
     Anchoring fibrils—type VII.

7. **How are the fibril-forming (interstitial) collagens synthesized?**
   1. There are at least 44 distinct genes that encode various collagen chains. In adults, collagen gene expression is subject to positive regulation (transforming growth factor [TGF]-β) and negative regulation (interferon-γ and tumor necrosis factor [TNF]-α). The collagen genes studied thus far contain coding sequences (exons) interrupted by large, noncoding sequences (introns). The DNA is transcribed to form a precursor mRNA, which is processed into functional mRNA by excising and splicing, which removes mRNA coded by introns. The processed mRNAs leave the nucleus and are transported to the polyribosomal apparatus in the rough endoplasmic reticulum for translation into polypeptide α-chains.
   2. The polypeptide α-chains (known as **preprocollagen**) are hydroxylated by prolyl hydroxylase and lysine hydroxylase to aid in the crosslinking of the α-chains. These enzymes require O_2, Fe^{2+}, α-ketoglutarate, and ascorbic acid (vitamin C) as cofactors. Hydroxyproline is critical to the stable formation of the triple helix. A decrease in the hydroxyproline content as seen in scurvy (ascorbic acid deficiency) results in unstable molecules that lose their structures and are broken down by proteases.
   3. Glycosylation of hydroxylysine residues by adding glucose or galactose monomers. Three of these hydroxylated and glycosylated polypeptide α-chains (preprocollagen) twist into a triple helix forming procollagen. Procollagen is packaged in vesicles that go to the Golgi apparatus. In the Golgi apparatus, oligosaccharides are added to the procollagen which is then secreted into the extracellular space.
   4. Outside the cell, procollagen peptidases on the cell membrane remove the amino and carboxyl-terminal telopeptides converting procollagen into tropocollagen. This step is absent in the vascular type of Ehlers–Danlos syndrome that fails to synthesize type III collagen.
   5. There is an assembly of these tropocollagen molecules by a quarter-stagger shift. In cartilage, cartilage oligomeric matrix protein (COMP) is important in this quarter-stagger arrangement. Lysyl oxidase, an extracellular, copper-dependent enzyme, acts on lysine and hydroxylysine producing aldehyde groups that form covalent bonds between the tropocollagen molecules. This polymer of tropocollagen molecules is called a collagen fibril. Mutations of COMP can cause achondroplasia and multiple epiphyseal dysplasia.

8. **Discuss end-to-end and lateral aggregation of collagen fibrils to form a collagen fiber.**
   Each collagen molecule measures 300 nm in length and 1.5 nm in width and has five charged regions 68 nm apart. The charged regions align in a straight line when the fibrils are formed, even though the individual molecules themselves are staggered a quarter of their lengths in relation to each other. One can easily see that there are multiple steps where defects in collagen biosynthesis could result in abnormalities leading to disease (Fig. 3.2; see also Chapter 54: Heritable Connective Tissue Disease).

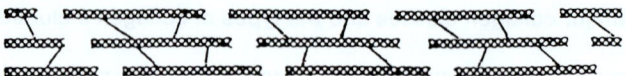

Fig. 3.2 Self-assembly of collagen molecules into fibrils with crosslinking.

9. Which enzymes are important in collagen degradation? How are they regulated?

The most important collagenolytic enzymes responsible for the cleavage of type I collagen belong to the matrix metalloproteinase (MMP) group. The collagenases are secreted in latent form and, when activated, cleave the collagen molecule at a single specific site following a glycine residue located about three quarters of the distance from the amino terminal end (between residues 775 and 776 of the α1[I] chain). Gelatinases and stromelysins then degrade the unfolded fragments.

Both α-macroglobulin and tissue inhibitors of metalloproteases (1–4) are capable of inhibiting collagenase activity. It is likely that other collagen types have type-specific collagenases capable of degrading them. Serum procollagen peptides, urinary hydroxyproline, urinary pyridinoline/deoxypyridinoline crosslinks, and serum *C*-telopeptides and urinary *N*-telopeptides are used as measures of collagen turnover.

ELASTIN AND ADHESINS

10. What is elastin, and where is it located?

Elastic fibers are connective tissue that can stretch when hydrated and return to their original length after being stretched. Elastic fiber is a mixture of elastin and fibrous fibrillin. Elastin is encoded by the ELN gene on chromosome 7. Elastin is synthesized by smooth muscle cells and less so by fibroblasts. Elastin comprises a significant portion of the dry weight of ligaments (up to 70–80%), lungs, larger blood vessels such as aorta (30–60%), and skin (2–5%). Elastin is a polymer of tropoelastin monomers, which contain 850 amino acids, predominantly valine, proline, glycine, and alanine. When tropoelastin molecules associate to form a fiber, lysine residues are crosslinked by the enzyme lysyl oxidase forming desmosine and isodesmosine, which are unique to elastin. Mutations in the elastin gene (ELN) can cause **cutis laxa** and **supravalvular aortic stenosis** among others. Elastases, which are serine proteases, are capable of degrading elastase. Elastases are located in tissues, macrophages, leukocytes, and platelets. Such elastases may contribute to blood vessel wall damage and aneurysm formation in the vasculitides. Urinary desmosine levels are used as a measure of elastin degradation.

11. What are fibrillin-1 and fibrillin-2?

These fibrillins are large glycoproteins coded for by a gene located on chromosome 15 (fibrillin-1) and chromosome 5 (fibrillin-2). They are secreted by fibroblasts into the extracellular matrix and become microfibrils. The microfibrils gather to form a hollow cylinder and tropoelastin is deposited in the space surrounded by the microfibrils. The tropoelastin which forms chemical bonds to fibrillin-1 is converted into elastin by lysyl oxidase. Fibrillin can also be found as isolated bundles of microfibrils in the skin, blood vessels, and several other tissues. Abnormalities in fibrillin-1 are thought to cause **Marfan's syndrome** (see also Chapter 54: Heritable Connective Tissue Disease), whereas abnormalities in fibrillin-2 cause **congenital contractural arachnodactyly.**

12. List the important adhesins (cell-binding glycoproteins) that can be present in intracellular matrices and basement membranes.

- Fibronectin—connective and many other tissues.
- Laminin—basement membrane.
- Entactin—basement membrane. It binds to type IV collagen
- Chondronectin—cartilage.
- Osteonectin—bone.
- Tenascin—embryonic connective tissue. It assists in cell migration.

These glycoproteins have specific adhesives and other important properties. They bind cells by attaching to integrins on cells. Some have the classical arginine–glycine–aspartic acid cell-binding sequence. In addition, there are **cadherins** that are transmembrane polypeptides that mediate cell–cell adhesion and recognition.

PROTEOGLYCANS

13. How do proteoglycans and glycosaminoglycan differ?

Proteoglycans are glycoproteins that contain one or more sulfated glycosaminoglycan (GAG) chains. They are classified according to their core protein, which is coded for by distinct genes.

GAGs make up part of the proteoglycans. GAGs are polysaccharides composed of sulfated and acetylated sugars with negative charges that can bind ions and large amounts of water. They are classified into four types: chondroitin sulfate/dermatan sulfate, heparan sulfate/heparin, keratan sulfate, and hyaluronic acid (hyaluronan). All GAGs except hyaluronic acid bind to proteins forming proteoglycans. **Hyaluronic acid** is the only GAG that is not sulfated. It is a giant polysaccharide composed of N-acetylglucosamine and glucuronic acid disaccharides. It is unique in that it forms in the plasma membrane (not Golgi) before release into the extracellular matrix and is widely distributed throughout the connective, epithelial, and neural tissues. It is important for cellular proliferation and migration in tissues.

14. How are proteoglycans distributed?

Proteoglycans are synthesized by all connective tissue cells. They can remain associated with these cells on their cell surface (syndecan, betaglycan), intracellularly (serglycin), or in the basement membrane (perlecan). These cell-associated proteoglycans commonly contain heparin/heparan sulfate or chondroitin sulfate as their major GAGs. Alternatively, proteoglycans can be secreted into the extracellular matrix (aggrecan, decorin, biglycan, fibromodulin, lumican). These matrix proteoglycans usually contain chondroitin sulfate, dermatan sulfate, or keratan sulfate as their major GAGs. **Aggrecan** binds noncovalently to a central hyaluronic acid filament in cartilage. Link protein stabilizes this linkage. Up to 100 aggrecan monomers can bind to a hyaluronic acid filament forming a large proteoglycan. Decorin helps bind type II collagen fibers together in cartilage, whereas fibromodulin and lumican bind type II collagen to type IX. Biglycan plays a role in osteoblast differentiation and bone mineralization.

15. How are proteoglycans metabolized in the body?

Proteoglycans are degraded by proteinases, which release the GAGs. The GAGs are taken up by cells by endocytosis, where they are degraded in lysosomes by a series of glycosidases and sulfatases. Defects in these degradative enzymes can lead to diseases called **mucopolysaccharidoses.**

MUSCULOSKELETAL SYSTEM

16. Discuss the classification of joints.

- **Synarthrosis:** suture lines of the skull where adjoining cranial plates are separated by thin fibrous tissue.
- **Amphiarthroses:** adjacent bones are bound by flexible fibrocartilage that permits limited motion. Examples include the pubic symphysis, part of the sacroiliac joint, and intervertebral discs.
- **Diarthroses** (synovial joints): These are the most common and most mobile joints. All have a synovial lining. They are subclassified into ball and socket (hip), hinge (interphalangeal), saddle (first carpometacarpal), and plane (patellofemoral) joints.

17. What major tissues comprise a diarthrodial (synovial) joint?

A diarthrodial joint consists of **hyaline cartilage** covering the surfaces of two or more opposing bones. These articular tissues are surrounded by a **capsule** that is lined by **synovium.** Some joints contain **menisci,** which are made of fibrocartilage. Note that the joint cavity is a potential space. The pressure within normal joints is negative (–5.7 cm H_2O) compared with ambient atmospheric pressure.

18. Describe the microanatomy of normal areolar synovium in diarthrodial joints.

Normal areolar synovium contains synovial lining (intimal) cells that are two to three cells deep. This synovium lines all intracapsular structures except the contact areas of articular cartilage. The synovial lining cells reside in a matrix rich in type I collagen and proteoglycans.

There are two main types of synovial lining (intimal) cells that can only be differentiated by electron microscopy. **Type A** cells are macrophage-like and have primarily a phagocytic function.

They are derived primarily from bone marrow via circulating monocytes. **Type B** cells are more abundant than type A cells. They are fibroblast-like and derived from the division of tissue-resident fibroblasts within the synovium. They produce hyaluronic acid (hyaluronan), which causes the increased viscosity of synovial fluid, as well as lubricin, which is the major boundary lubricant in joints.

Other cells found in the synovium include antigen-presenting cells (dendritic cells) and mast cells. The synovium does not have a limiting basement membrane but does have fenestrated capillaries below the synovial lining cells. The deeper synovial tissue matrix contains minor collagens, hyaluronic acid, small arterioles/venules, lymphatic vessels, and nerve fibers derived from the capsule and periarticular tissues.

19. Why is synovial fluid viscous?

Hyaluronic acid, synthesized by synovial lining cells (type B), is secreted into the synovial fluid, making the fluid viscous. Synovia means "like egg white," which describes the normal viscosity of synovial fluid.

20. What are the physical characteristics of normal synovial fluid from the knee joint?

- Color—colorless and transparent.
- Amount—thin film covering surfaces of synovium and cartilage within joint space.
- Cell count—<200/mm^3 with <25% neutrophils.
- Protein—1.3 to 1.7 g/dL (33% of normal plasma protein).
- Glucose—within 20 mg/dL of the serum glucose level after 6 hours of fasting.
- Temperature—32°C (peripheral joints are cooler than core body temperature).
- String sign (a measure of viscosity)—1 to 2 inches (2.5–5 cm).
- pH—7.4.

21. What are the function, structure, and composition of articular cartilage?

Articular cartilage is **avascular**, **aneural**, and **alymphatic.** It serves as a load-bearing connective tissue that can absorb impact and withstand shearing forces. This ability relates to the unique composition and structure of its extracellular matrix.

Normal cartilage is composed of a sparse population of specialized cells called **chondrocytes** that are responsible for the synthesis and replenishment of extracellular matrix. This matrix consists mainly of collagen and proteoglycans. Most of the collagen is type II (>90%), which makes up 50% to 60% of the dry weight of cartilage. Collagen forms a fiber network that provides shape, form, and tensile strength to the cartilage tissue.

Proteoglycans comprise the second largest portion of articular cartilage. The proteoglycan monomers (aggrecan) are large (molecular weight = 2–3 million) and contain mostly keratan sulfate and chondroitin sulfate GAGs. The proteoglycans are arranged into supramolecular aggregates consisting of a central hyaluronic acid filament to which multiple proteoglycan monomers (aggrecan) are noncovalently attached and stabilized by a link protein.

The entire structure looks like a large "bottle brush" and has a molecular weight of 200 million (Fig. 3.3). These proteoglycans are stuffed into the collagen framework. The negative charge of the proteoglycans causes them to spread out until the elastic forces are balanced by the tensile forces of the collagen. Note that other collagens (types V, VI, IX, X, XI), proteins (chondronectin, COMP, cartilage intermediate layer protein [CILP], proline/arginine-rich end leucine-rich repeat protein [PRELP], others), and lipids are also present in cartilage.

Water is the most abundant component of articular cartilage and accounts for 80% of the tissue wet weight. Water is held in cartilage by its interaction with the large matrix proteoglycan aggregates. This retained water is essential for cartilage to resist compression and distribute load.

22. What are the four zones of cartilage in diarthrodial joints?

The different molecular components of cartilage are highly organized into a structure that varies with the depth of cartilage. From top to bottom, these four zones include:

1. **Superficial (tangential/gliding) zone** (10%)—smallest zone (also called **lamina splendens**). Collagen fibers are thin and oriented horizontally to subchondral bone. This zone has a low GAG content but is enriched with lubricin (proteoglycan 4) that is important for lubrication.

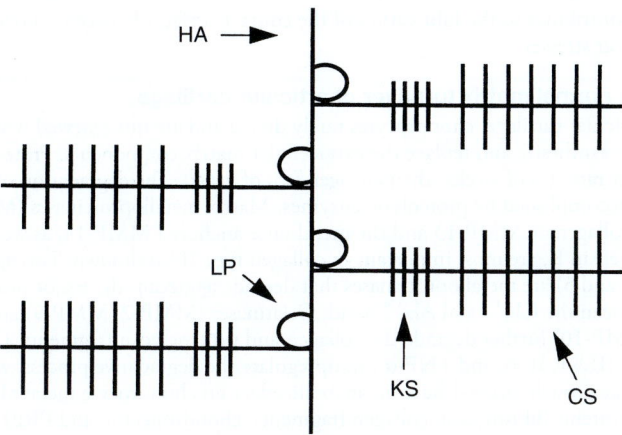

Fig. 3.3 Diagram of a proteoglycan aggregate in articular cartilage. Hyaluronate (HA) is the backbone of the aggregate. Proteoglycan monomers (aggrecan) arise at intervals from either side of the hyaluronate core. *CS,* Chondroitin sulfate; *KS,* keratin sulfate; *LP,* link protein.

2. **Middle (transitional, intermediate) zone** (50%)—largest zone. Collagen fibers are thicker and start to be arranged into radial bundles. This zone has high proteoglycan and water content.
3. **Deep (radial) zone** (20%)—largest collagen fibers arranged radially (perpendicular) to subchondral bone. This zone contains many chondrocytes.
4. **Calcified zone**—separates cartilage from subchondral bone. Collagen fibers penetrate into this zone and anchor the cartilage to the bone.

23. Since cartilage does not have a blood supply, how do chondrocytes obtain nutrition?

Adult cartilage is avascular, and chondrocytes obtain nutrients through diffusion. The nutrients are derived from synovial fluid. Diffusion is facilitated during joint loading. With joint loading, some of the water in the cartilage is squeezed out into the synovial space. When the joint is unloaded, the hydrophilic properties of the cartilage proteoglycans cause the water to be sucked back into the cartilage. As the water returns to the cartilage, diffusion of nutrients from the synovial fluid is facilitated enabling chondrocytes to obtain nutrition. Nutrients also enter articular cartilage through diffusion from subchondral blood vessels.

24. If cartilage is not innervated, why do patients with osteoarthritis have pain?

Patients experience pain due to irritation of the subchondral bone, which is exposed as the cartilage degenerates. Additionally, accumulation of synovial fluid can cause pain through distention of the innervated joint capsule and synovium. Mild synovial inflammation also causes pain.

25. Describe the lubrication of diarthrodial joints.

Diarthrodial (synovial) joints serve as mechanical bearings with coefficients of friction lower than the friction an ice skate generates as it glides over ice. The two major sources of lubrication are:
- **Fluid-film (hydrodynamic) lubrication:** Cartilage surfaces are separated by a noncompressible fluid film. Hyaluronic acid (hyaluronan) (HA) complexed to lubricin and phospholipids primarily provides this function. Water compressed from superficial and middle zones of cartilage during loading also contributes to this fluid film. During loading (i.e., knee joint during walking) the noncompressible fluid film is trapped between cartilage surfaces and prevents the surfaces from contacting each other. This stable film is 0.1 μm thick in normal joints.
- **Boundary layer lubrication:** a small glycoprotein called **lubricin** (proteoglycan 4), which is produced by synovial lining cells and chondrocytes, binds to the superficial zone of articular cartilage where it acts with HA and synovial fluid lipids to decrease the coefficient of friction between cartilage surfaces. This is important for reducing friction with non-weight-bearing loading (i.e., moving the knee to a different position while sitting).

HA also contributes to the lubrication of the contact surfaces between synovium and cartilage decreasing shear stresses.

26. Discuss the normal matrix turnover of articular cartilage.

In normal articular cartilage, chondrocytes rarely divide and are not renewed when they die. Chondrocytes synthesize and replace the extracellular matrix components. Proteoglycans have a faster turnover rate ($t_{1/2}$ of weeks) than collagen ($t_{1/2}$ of years). The degradation of these macromolecules is accomplished by proteolytic enzymes. Matrix metalloproteinases (MMPs), such as the secreted collagenase MMP-13 and the membrane-anchored MMP-14, as well as the lysosomal protease, cathepsin K, are most important in collagen type II breakdown. Two aggrecanases (ADAMTS 4 and 5) are metalloproteinases that degrade aggrecan, the major proteoglycan in cartilage, between the Glu^{373} and Ala^{374} bond. Gelatinases (MMP-2, MMP-9) and stromelysins (MMP-3, MMP-10) further degrade the collagen and proteoglycan fragments. Cytokines such as interleukin (IL)-1, IL-6, and TNF-α can upregulate the degradative process, whereas TGF-β and insulin-like growth factor-1 have an anabolic effect on chondrocyte metabolism. Extracellular matrix proteins (fibronectin, collagen fragments, chondronectin, and PRELP) interact with integrins or other cell surface receptors (syndecan), whereas hyaluronic acid interacts with CD44 to signal and regulate the chondrocyte's synthesis of extracellular cartilage matrix. Assays using monoclonal antibodies to measure type II collagen and proteoglycans (aggrecan, keratan sulfate, COMP) epitopes in bodily fluids have been used to detect cartilage breakdown.

27. What is the difference between a ligament and a tendon?

A **ligament** is a specialized form of connective tissue, which attaches one bone to another. It frequently reinforces the joint capsule and provides stability to the joint. A **tendon** attaches a muscle to a bone. Both are comprised mostly of type I collagen.

28. What is a bursa?

A **bursa** is a closed sac lined with mesenchymal cells. Bursae facilitate gliding of one tissue over another. There are approximately 160 in the body that form during embryogenesis. Trauma, overuse, and inflammation may lead to formation of new bursae or enlargement of existing ones.

29. How many bones are there in the skeleton? Discuss the types and composition of a bone.

- The human skeleton (from the Greek word, *skeletos*, "dried up") consists of 206 bones (126 appendicular bones, 74 axial bones, and 6 ossicles).
- Bone is a mineralized connective tissue, with two subtypes: **cortical** (or compact) bone and **cancellous** (or trabecular) bone. Cortical bone forms 80% of the skeleton weight and is increased in long bone shafts. Cancellous bone is in contact with bone marrow cells and is enriched in the vertebral bodies, pelvis, and proximal ends of femora, all of which are subject to osteoporosis and fractures. Bone remodeling normally replaces 25% of the trabecular bone and 3% of the cortical bone each year.
- Bone is comprised mainly of type I collagen and contains three cell types: **osteoclasts,** which resorb mineralized bone; **osteoblasts,** which synthesize the proteins of the bone matrix; and **osteocytes,** which are probably osteoblasts that have secreted bone matrix and become buried within it. Osteocytes communicate with each other through a canalicular system and play a role in response to mechanical loading. The skeleton contains 99% of the total calcium, 80–85% of the total phosphorus, and 66% of the total magnesium in the body.

30. Which pathway regulates bone metabolism though osteoblast signaling?

The **Wnt/β-catenin** signaling pathway (Fig. 3.4) is a critical component of bone mass regulation and is required for bones to respond to mechanical loading. The Wnt signaling cascade is triggered upon binding of members of the Wnt family of lipid-modified proteins (more than 12) to a coreceptor complex comprising low-density lipoprotein receptor-related proteins 5 or 6 (LRP 5 or 6) and frizzled protein (Frz). Activation of this receptor complex leads to activation of Dishevelled (Dsh), which then inactivates glycogen synthase kinase (GSK)-3β. This prevents GSK-3β from phosphorylating β-catenin which, when phosphorylated, is targeted for ubiquitination and proteasomal degradation. Thus, β-catenin is able to accumulate in the cytoplasm. Upon reaching

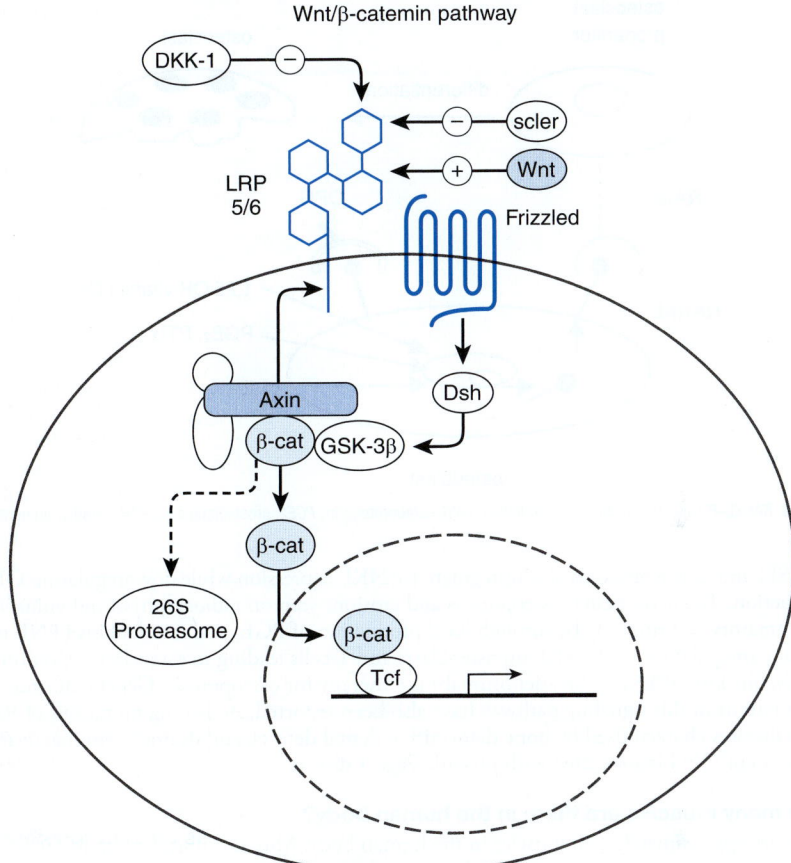

Fig. 3.4 Wnt/β-catenin pathway.

a certain concentration, the β-catenin translocates to the nucleus where it combines with the Tcf/ Lef family of transcription factors, which regulate the expression of specific osteoblastic genes necessary for bone formation. There are three extracellular proteins that regulate Wnt binding. One is secreted Frz protein which binds and neutralizes Wnt protein. The other two are sclerostin (Scler) and dickkopf (Dkk-1) proteins which are produced by osteocytes and bind to LRP5/6 and prevent Wnt signaling through these receptors. Notably, LRP5 mutations have been associated with both low and high bone mass. Sclerostin mutations have been linked to **osteosclerosis** (van Buchem syndrome) because of their inability to block Wnt signaling. Monoclonal antibodies against sclerostin (i.e., romosozumab) are used as a therapy for osteoporosis.

31. Which pathway regulates bone metabolism through osteoclast signaling?

The RANKL/RANK/OPG signaling pathway involves members of the TNF superfamily and is a critical pathway for the regulation of osteoclast activation and bone remodeling (Fig. 3.5). **RANKL** is a cell membrane-bound ligand (can also be secreted) on preosteoblasts, osteocytes, activated T cells, and other cells. It binds **RANK** on osteoclast precursors, which causes the osteoclast to differentiate and become activated. In most cases, RANKL is also assisted by macrophage colony-stimulated factor (M-CSF) as a cofactor for osteoclast differentiation. **OPG** is a soluble, regulatory cytokine secreted by osteoblasts that competitively binds RANKL and prevents its binding to RANK, thus inhibiting osteoclastogenesis. Expression of RANKL on osteoblasts is stimulated through vitamin D receptor (1,25 OH vitamin D_3), protein kinase A (prostaglandin E_2 [PGE_2], parathyroid hormone), and gp130 (IL-11). Cytokines (IL-1, IL-7, IL-17, TNF-α,

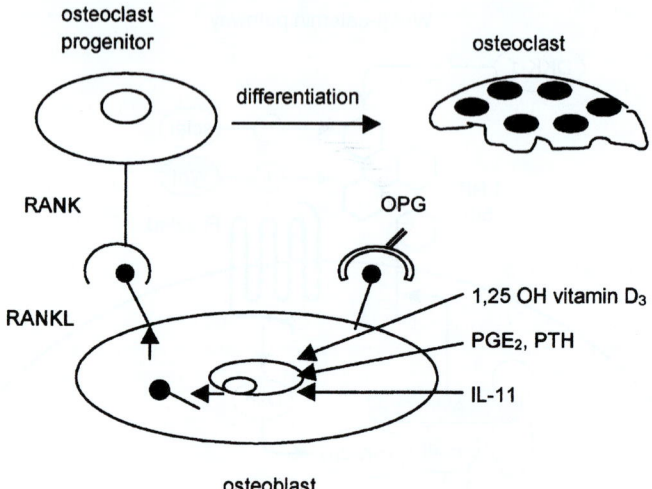

Fig. 3.5 RANKL–RANK–OPG system. *IL,* interleukin; *OPG,* osteoprotegerin; *PGE2,* prostaglandin E₂; *PTH,* parathyroid hormone.

M-CSF) and glucocorticoids also upregulate RANKL expression while downregulating OPG production. The periarticular osteoporosis and erosions seen on radiographs of individuals with inflammatory arthritis may be through local production of PGE_2 and interleukins (TNF-α, IL-1), causing upregulation of RANKL on osteoblasts and T cells leading to osteoclast activation. Conversely, blocking RANKL (i.e., denosumab) is a therapy for osteoporosis. Genetic disorders due to mutations in this signaling pathway have also been reported. Activating mutations of RANK cause diseases characterized by bone deformities, dental defects, and deafness. An inactivating mutation of OPG is associated with juvenile Paget's disease.

32. How many muscles are there in the human body?
There are approximately 660 muscles in the human body. Muscles constitute up to 40% of the adult body mass.

33. Discuss the morphology of human skeletal muscle.
- Each skeletal muscle is surrounded by an **epimysium**. Inside each skeletal muscle are cells called **fibers** which are organized into bundles called **fascicles**. Fascicles are surrounded by **perimysium** which contains blood vessels and nerves. Muscle fibers inside a fascicle are encased in connective tissue called **endomysium**.
- Muscle fibers are part of **motor units** that consist of a lower motor neuron originating from a spinal cord anterior horn cell and all the muscle fibers it innervates. All muscle fibers within a motor unit are of the same type. Different fibers within a single fascicle are innervated by different motor neurons.
- Muscle fibers are divided into three types based on their myosin heavy chain metabolism and response to stimuli: types 1, 2a, and 2x. Fiber type can be altered by reinnervation with a different motor neuron type, physical training (controversial), or disease processes. However, heredity is the most important determinant of fiber type distribution. On average, muscle contains 40% type 1 and 60% type 2 fibers. Each fascicle in a skeletal muscle contains all three types of fibers.
- Each muscle fiber is lined by a plasma membrane called a **sarcolemma** which is separate from the endomysium. Fibers contain numerous tubular **myofibrils**. Myofibrils are composed of repeating sections of **sarcomeres**. Sarcomeres are composed of **myofilaments** (myosin, actin, and others) which are contractile proteins. The myofilaments are bathed in sarcoplasm and organized into the myofibrils, which are enveloped by the sarcoplasmic reticulum. Communication between the sarcolemma and sarcoplasmic reticulum occurs through a channel network called the **T-tubule system.**

- Muscle force is transmitted to the exterior via protein cell adhesion complexes (integrins, dystroglycans) in the sarcolemma which connect muscle fibers to the extracellular matrix (ECM). Actin is linked through transmembrane integrins and via dystrophin to transmembrane dystroglycans which bind to laminins in the ECM. Defects in these cytoskeletal proteins lead to various types of muscular dystrophy.

34. Describe the characteristics of the three types of muscle fibers.
- **Type 1** (slow twitch, oxidative, red fibers): respond to electrical stimuli slowly; fatigue-resistant with repeated stimulation. These fibers have many mitochondria and higher lipid content. Endurance training (long-distance running, cycling) enhances the metabolism of these fibers.
- **Type 2a** (fast twitch, oxidative-glycolytic fibers): properties are intermediate between type 1 and type 2x. Important for longer sprints (400 m) and repeated weightlifting.
- **Type 2x** (very fast twitch, glycolytic, white fibers): respond rapidly and with greater force of contraction but fatigue rapidly. These fibers contain more glycogen and have higher myophosphorylase and myoadenylate deaminase activity. Strength training (maximal weightlifting, sprinters, and jumpers) leads to hypertrophy of these fibers.

35. How do muscle contraction and relaxation occur?
Muscle contraction occurs by shortening of myofilaments within muscle fibers. Stimulation causes an **action potential** to be transmitted along the sarcolemma, then through the T-tubule system to the sarcoplasmic reticulum. This causes the release of calcium into the sarcoplasm. As the calcium concentration increases, **actin** is released from a state of inhibition, allowing actin-myosin cross-linkage and shortening of the myofilaments. The muscle fiber shortens until calcium is actively pumped back into the sarcoplasmic reticulum by SERCA, which breaks the crosslinks causing the fiber to relax. ATP, electrolytes (Na, K, Ca, Mg), and three ATPase proteins contribute to normal fiber contraction and relaxation (see Chapter 71: Metabolic and Other Genetic Myopathies).

BIBLIOGRAPHY
Bozee A, Gruneboom A, Schett G. Biology, physiology, and morphology of bone. In: Firestein GS, Budd RC, Gabriel SE, Koretzky GA, McInnes IB, O'Dell JR, eds. *Firestein and Kelley's Textbook of Rheumatology*. 11th ed. Philadelphia: Elsevier; 2021:60–66.
Itoh Y. Proteinases and matrix degradation. In: Firestein GS, Budd RC, Gabriel SE, Koretzky GA, McInnes IB, O'Dell JR, eds. *Firestein and Kelley's Textbook of Rheumatology*. 11th ed. Philadelphia: Elsevier; 2021:109–131.
Liu J, Xiao Q, Xiao J, et al. Wnt/β-catenin signaling: function, biological mechanisms, and therapeutic opportunities. *Sig Transduct Target Ther*. 2022;7:3–26.
Miller MS, Debold EP, Toth MJ. Muscle: anatomy, physiology, and biochemistry. In: Firestein GS, Budd RC, Gabriel SE, Koretzky GA, McInnes IB, O'Dell JR, eds. *Firestein and Kelley's Textbook of Rheumatology*. 11th ed. Philadelphia: Elsevier; 2021:67–69.
Mobasheri A, Goldring MB, Loeser RF. Cartilage and chondrocytes. In: Firestein GS, Budd RC, Gabriel SE, Koretzky GA, McInnes IB, O'Dell JR, eds. *Firestein and Kelley's Textbook of Rheumatology*. 11th ed. Philadelphia: Elsevier; 2021:34–59.
Scanzello CR, Goldring SR. Biology of the normal joint. In: Firestein GS, Budd RC, Gabriel SE, Koretzky GA, McInnes IB, O'Dell JR, eds. *Firestein and Kelley's Textbook of Rheumatology*. 11th ed. Philadelphia: Elsevier; 2021:1–19.
Veale DJ, Firestein GS. Synovium. In: Firestein GS, Budd RC, Gabriel SE, Koretzky GA, McInnes IB, O'Dell JR, eds. *Firestein and Kelley's Textbook of Rheumatology*. 11th ed. Philadelphia: Elsevier; 2021:20–33.

CHAPTER 4

An Overview of the Immune Response, Inflammation, and Autoimmunity

Kristine A. Kuhn, MD, PhD

The origin of all science is in the desire to know causes.
—William Hazlitt, 1829

Science has been seriously retarded by the study of what is not worth knowing, and what is not knowable.
—Johann Wolfgang von Goethe, 1825

 KEY POINTS

1. The innate immune system is the first line of defense against invading organisms by recognizing specific molecular components found only in microbial pathogens.
2. The innate immune system is necessary to activate and instruct the adaptive immune system.
3. T-cell activation requires two signals: (1) contact of T-cell receptor (TCR) with major histocompatibility complex (MHC)-peptide and (2) engagement of costimulatory molecules.
4. T cells are critical for both humoral and cellular adaptive immunity.
5. Autoimmunity results when there is loss of tolerance to self-antigens.

1. What are the two broad categories of immunity involved in host defense?

The categories of immunity are given in Table 4.1.

2. What is the difference in function between the innate and adaptive immune systems?

Innate immunity is an inborn, phylogenetically conserved system that allows the host to rapidly respond to a pathogen within 20 to 30 minutes of exposure. This system is inflexible in that only specific pathogen features will result in a response. In contrast, adaptive immunity develops over 3 to 5 days following pathogen exposure. Yet, this system is flexible, allowing refinement of the lymphocytes' abilities to target the pathogen.

INNATE IMMUNITY

3. How is the innate immune system activated?

Innate immunity is activated by host signals called **alarmins** or pathogen signals called **pathogen-associated molecular patterns (PAMPs).** Alarmins are endogenous molecules that are constitutively available and passively released from necrotic cells upon infection or tissue injury. They are also secreted by stimulated leukocytes and epithelia. PAMPs are molecules produced only by microbes. Both alarmins and PAMPs activate innate immunity through **pattern recognition receptors (PRRs)** such as Toll-like receptors (TLRs). Alarmins and PAMPs activate and recruit cells of the innate immune system including dendritic cells (DCs).

4. Provide some examples of alarmins.

- **High-mobility group protein B1:** can be released from any cell type. They are proinflammatory when bound to other alarmins and PAMPs.
- **S100A8/A9/A12:** released by epithelial cells and phagocytes causing inflammation with increased neutrophil adhesion, migration, and release from bone marrow. Have some antibacterial activity. S100A8 and S100A9 form a heterodimer called calprotectin, often measured in feces as an indication of intestinal inflammation.
- **Heat-shock proteins** (HSP; HSP60 and HSP70): autoantigens stimulating pathways to suppress inflammation.

TABLE 4.1 Comparison Between Innate and Adaptive Immune Systems

	INNATE IMMUNITY	ADAPTIVE IMMUNITY
Physical barriers	Skin, mucous membranes, epithelia	
Cells	Monocytes/macrophages, neutrophils, dendritic cells, natural killer cells, innate lymphoid cells, eosinophils, basophils, mast cells	Lymphocytes (T cells, B cells, natural killer T cells)
Circulating factors	Complement, C-reactive protein, cytokines, chemokines, anti-microbial peptides	Antibodies, cytokines

- **Interleukin (IL)-33:** a member of the IL-1 family with proinflammatory properties through binding IL-1 receptor-like 1 (ST2) that is released by various cells including epithelia, fibroblasts, endothelial cells, osteoblasts, and immune cells.
- **Antimicrobial peptides (AMPs):** the main AMPs are **defensins,** bactericidal/permeability-increasing protein permeability-increasing protein, and cathelicidins. They are secreted by epithelial cells to form a microbial shield when the physical barriers (skin and mucous membranes) become injured. The AMPs integrate into outer cell membranes of invading microbes to form pores that disrupt the microbes' integrity. AMPs serve as chemoattractants for innate (neutrophils, DCs) and adaptive (lymphocytes) immune cells. AMPs can govern the composition of commensal microbes that colonize body surfaces. Abnormal AMP production may contribute to diseases such as psoriasis and Crohn's disease.

5. What are examples of PAMPs?

Examples of PAMPs include bacterial lipopolysaccharides (LPS), peptidoglycan, mannans, flagellin, and bacterial and viral DNA/RNA. These molecules are highly conserved structural motifs specific to microbes.

6. Name the PRRs that recognize PAMPs

There are two broad categories of PRRs.
- **Secreted PRRs and circulating PRRs:** these include lectins, pentraxins, LPS-binding proteins, collectins, and ficolins. Notable members of this group include:
  - **Mannan-binding lectin (MBL):** synthesized in the liver as an acute phase protein, MBL binds microbial carbohydrates and initiates the lectin pathway of complement (see Question #8). MBL-associated serine proteases (MASP-2) function like C1r and C1s to activate the classical complement pathway. MBL deficiency is associated with frequent infections.
  - **C-reactive protein (CRP):** as one of the pentraxin family members, CRP is also secreted as part of the acute phase response due to pro-inflammatory cytokines such as IL-6. CRP can fix C1q and activate complement to opsonize a pathogen for phagocytic clearance.
- **Cell-associated PRRs.**
  - **TLRs:** there are at least 10 human TLRs. TLRs 1, 2, 4, 5, and 6 are on cell surfaces, whereas TLRs 3, 7, 8, 9, and 10 localize to endosomes. They individually recognize different PAMPs. For example, TLR4 recognizes LPS and TLR5 recognizes flagellin, whereas TLR3 binds viral double-stranded RNA, TLR7/8 binds single-stranded RNA, and TLR9 binds CpG-DNA. Signaling through TLRs activates transcription factors (activator protein-1, nuclear factor-κB, interferon [IFN]-regulatory factors), resulting in the induction of inflammatory and immune response genes with subsequent production of IFNs, proinflammatory cytokines (IL-1, IL-6, tumor necrosis factor [TNF]), chemokines (IL-8), and other effector cytokines that attract innate immune cells and direct the adaptive immune response.
- **Intracellular PRRs:** in addition to the endosomal localized TLRs, there are nucleotide oligomerization domain **(NOD)-like receptors (NLRs)** and retinoic acid-inducible gene (RIG)-I-like family receptors that reside in the cytoplasm.
  - The NLRs include proteins NOD1 and NOD2 (also known as CARD15) and NOD leucine-rich repeat and pyrin domain containing (NLRPs). Upon PAMP binding to NLRs, an intracellular complex called the inflammasome forms, which contributes to the

processing and secretion of IL-1 and IL-18. Urate crystals and peptidoglycans are examples of PAMPs that activate NLRs. Polymorphisms of NOD2 gene are associated with Crohn's disease, and mutations in NLRPs have been associated with periodic fever syndromes.

- The **RIG-I-like receptor** family includes RIG 1, MDA5, and LGP2. These receptors react with virus-derived double-stranded RNA and mediate the production of type-1 IFN.

- **Receptors stimulating phagocytosis:** macrophages and DCs have **C-type lectin receptors** that bind microbial carbohydrates. This includes the **mannose receptor** that binds bacterial carbohydrates and facilitates phagocytic clearance, cytokine release, and activation of immune cells. **Dectin-1** is another C-type lectin receptor that binds fungal wall glucans. Mutations can lead to recurrent mucocutaneous fungal infections. **Formyl peptide receptor** is a G-coupled protein receptor on cells that binds N-formylmethionine from bacteria leading to release of chemoattractants, which facilitates phagocytosis. Finally, there are **scavenger receptors** on macrophages that facilitate removal of foreign substances by binding bacterial cell wall components, oxidized lipoproteins, and apoptotic cells.

7. What is the role of complement in the immune response?

Complement is a cascade of proteins that generate immune signals as well as come together to form a **membrane attack complex (MAC).** Complement proteins C5b with C6-9 create the MAC, which forms a pore in its target, resulting in lysis. Fig. 4.1 summarizes the complement cascade. Split products generated during this cascade function in several ways:

- C3b and C4b act as opsonins to target phagocytosis of bacterial particles by neutrophils and macrophages. C3b also binds receptors CR1 and CR2 to activate B-cell responses.

- C3a and C5a behave as chemoattractants that recruit neutrophils as well as anaphylatoxins that simulate mast cell and basophil degranulation of histamine, resulting in increased vascular permeability and augmentation of inflammation.

Deficiency in early complement components is associated with increased pyogenic infections (C3 deficiency) and increased risk of autoimmune disease (C1, C2, and C4 deficiencies), possibly due to an impaired ability to clear immune complexes. Deficiencies in components of the MAC (or targeted inhibition of C5 with therapeutics such as eculizumab) result in recurrent *Neisseria* infections, suggesting that this complex is important for defense against these organisms.

8. How is the complement system activated?

There are three pathways leading to complement activation with the generation of split products and the C5 convertase that results in MAC formation:

- **Classical pathway:** this pathway links adaptive immune responses with innate immunity. When the antibody isotypes of immunoglobulin (Ig) IgG and IgM are in complex with

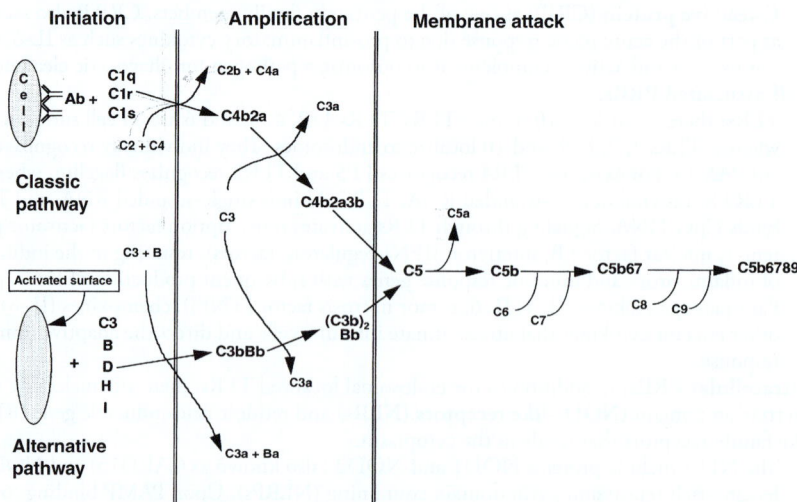

Fig. 4.1 Overview of the classical and alternative complement cascades.

antigen, C1q binds the Fc portion of Ig and activates C1r and C1s. The C1 complex then binds and activates C2, followed by C4. The C2C4 complex can cleave C3 into C3a and C3b and form the C5 convertase. Other proteins such as CRP, serum amyloid P, and C4 nephritic factor can also activate the classical pathway in the absence of an adaptive immune response.

- **Alternate pathway:** this pathway is activated in the absence of antibodies by LPS on bacterial cell membranes. C3b is generated by a natural "tickover" of C3 and binds LPS. Factor D cleaves factor B to generate factor Bb, which binds C3b, generates more C3b, and forms the C5 convertase.
- **Lectin pathway:** The liver synthesizes MBL, which can bind microbial carbohydrates. MBL resembles C1q and activates MASPs that are like C1r and C1s and can cleave C2 and C4. Like the alternate pathway, the lectin pathway is activated in the absence of an adaptive immune response.

9. **Which cells are important in the innate immune system?**
- **Phagocytes** contain PRRs and are critical effector cells of innate immunity by their ability to ingest microbes or cellular debris.
- **Neutrophils** are the first cells recruited to inflammation sites by various chemotactic signals (e.g., AMPs, N-formyl bacterial oligopeptide, C5a, leukotriene [LT] B4, IL-8). Neutrophils use at least two mechanisms to neutralize an invading microbe:
  - Neutrophils phagocytose invading microbes opsonized by the innate immune system. The microbe is ingested into the phagosome, which merges with intracellular granules containing microbicidal peptides, proteases, and highly reactive oxidizing agents generated by NADPH oxidase. The result is microbial death. Note that even in the absence of infection, billions of neutrophils normally leave the bone marrow, circulate, enter tissues, and die each day. When they die, they undergo apoptosis and are processed by macrophages, so they do not release their toxic constituents into normal tissues (efferocytosis). Macrophages that phagocytize the apoptotic neutrophils release anti-inflammatory cytokines to maintain homeostasis.
  - **Neutrophil extracellular traps (NETs)** are released from granules upon neutrophil activation. NETs contain complexes of proteins, histones, and DNA that bind and kill microbes extracellularly, independent of phagocytic uptake.
- **Monocytes and macrophages:** monocytes are the circulating precursors of macrophages; they differentiate into macrophages upon entry into specific tissues (e.g., Kupffer cells in the liver). Macrophages can be activated by PRRs and Fc receptors (that bind the constant region of antibody). Macrophage activation results in the phagocytosis of microbes, processing of microbial antigen for presentation to lymphocytes to initiate the adaptive immune response, and secretion of over 100 proteins including cytokines (both pro-inflammatory and anti-inflammatory) that mediate inflammation.
- **Natural killer cells (NK):** NK cells look like large granular lymphocytes and comprise 5% to 10% of the circulating lymphocyte population. They function as potent cytotoxic cells toward virally infected or malignant cells. They identify the target cells through the expression of killer cell immunoglobulin-like receptors (KIRs) that recognize MHC class I on healthy cells causing an inhibitory effect. Cells that are infected with viruses or are malignant upregulate stress ligands and downregulate their MHC class I receptors, which then cannot send an inhibitory signal via KIRs. Activating receptors on the NK cell include the characteristic cell surface markers CD16 (one type of Fc receptor) and CD56 as well as several PRRs. NK cells have granules with perforins and granzymes, which are released upon NK cell activation to kill the target cell. Activated NK cells also secrete IFN-γ in addition to other cytokines. DCs recruit and activate NK cells by secreting type I IFNs, IL-12, and IL-18.
- **Other cells exhibiting PRRs:** epithelial cells express PRRs and can react to infection and secrete AMPs and IL-8 (CXCL8), which are neutrophil chemoattractants. Mast cells have PRRs and release TNFα and IL-8. They also produce inflammatory mediators (histamine, LTs, platelet-activating factor), proteases (tryptase, chymase), and defensins. Platelets express PRRs and can produce cytokines recruiting leukocytes to sites of tissue damage. They also release microparticles that may modulate the immune response. Eosinophils are specialized leukocytes whose granules contain numerous toxic products, including major basic protein, eosinophil peroxidase, and eosinophil cationic protein. These products are especially toxic to helminths.

Activated eosinophils also produce large quantities of LTC$_4$ and transforming growth factor (TGF)-β that promote increased venular permeability and fibroblast-dependent fibrosis, respectively.

- **DCs:** these are "professional" antigen-presenting cells (APCs). They serve as a link between the innate and adaptive immune system. They are located in tissues in contact with the external environment including skin and mucous membranes of the respiratory, gastrointestinal, and genitourinary tracts. They are also present in lymphoid tissues and most solid organs. There are two major types of DCs: myeloid (mDCs) and plasmacytoid (pDCs). Most mDCs are derived from monocytes and a few from lymphoid cells. They display TLR2 and TLR4. The major cytokine that mDCs produce is IL-12, and it is the most important cell needed to activate naïve T cells. pDCs resemble plasma cells and comprise <1% of peripheral blood mononuclear cells. They display TLR7 and TLR9. They rapidly secrete large amounts of type I IFN (IFNα and IFNβ) following viral stimulation. Importantly, DCs can influence T-cell differentiation into Th1, Th2, Th17, and regulatory subtypes.
- **Innate lymphoid cells (ILCs):** these are innate immune cells derived from common lymphoid precursors. They respond to stress signals (alarmins), microbes (PAMPs), and cytokines in the environment by producing effector cytokines in patterns similar to T cells. There are three types: ILC1 cells produce IFNγ and play a role in cancer immunosurveillance; ILC2 cells produce Th2 cytokines (IL-4, IL-5, IL-13) and are important for helminth immunity, immune regulation, and wound healing; ILC3 cells produce IL-17 and IL-22, which are important for mucosal immunity. ILC3 cells are found in the lesional skin of patients with psoriasis.

10. What are the important endothelial adhesion molecules involved in the influx of neutrophils and mononuclear cells into damaged or infected tissue?

The important endothelial adhesion molecules involved in the influx of neutrophils and mononuclear cells into damaged or infected tissue are given in Table 4.2.

The time to adhesion molecule activation explains why neutrophils and monocytes/macrophages enter the inflammatory site first (acute inflammation), whereas lymphocytes enter later (chronic inflammation).

Targeting of adhesion molecules using monoclonal antibody therapeutics has been successful in the treatment of some inflammatory conditions. For example, vedolizumab targets MADCAM-1 (integrin α4β7) and prevents leukocyte recruitment to the intestines for the treatment of Crohn's disease.

11. Name the four cardinal signs of inflammation. What are the underlying mechanisms responsible for the signs of inflammation?

- Erythema (rubor).
- Warmth (calor).
- Swelling (tumor).
- Pain (dolor).

Local arteriolar dilation produces erythema and warmth. Permeability increases in the postcapillary venules, allowing vascular fluid to leak into the surrounding tissue to produce swelling

TABLE 4.2 Important Endothelial Adhesion Molecules Involved in the Influx of Neutrophils and Monocytes into Damaged or Infected Tissue

TIME TO ACTIVATION	LEUKOCYTE	ACTIVATED ENDOTHELIUM
<2 hours	L-selectin PSGL-1 (inactivated neutrophils/monos)	CD34, GlyCAM-1, MADCAM-1 (integrin α4β7), P-selectin
<4 hours	ESL-1	E-selectin (ELAM-1)
<12 hours	LFA-1 (CD11a/CD18) (activated neutrophils/monos)	ICAM-1 (CD54)
<24 hours	Mac-1 (CD11b/CD18) (activated neutrophils/monos) PECAM1	ICAM-1 Endothelial PECAM1
<48 hours	VLA-4 (CD49d/CD29) (lymphs, monos)	VCAM-1 (CD106)

TABLE 4.3 Classes of Inflammatory Mediators that Facilitate Inflammation During the Innate Immune Response

VASOACTIVE MEDIATORS	CHEMOTACTIC FACTORS	ENZYMES	PROINFLAMMATORY CYTOKINES
Histamine	Complement products (C3a, C5a)	Tryptase	IL-1, IL-6, IL-12, IL-17, IL-18, IL-23
Arachidonic acid products (prostaglandins, leukotrienes)	Leukotriene B$_4$	Chymase	TNFα
Platelet-activating factor	Platelet-activating factor		Type I interferons (e.g., IFNα), IFNγ
Kinins	Chemokines (IL-8, other CXCLs)		

IFN, Interferon; *IL,* interleukin; *TNF,* tumor necrosis factor.

(edema). Pain is a result of the action of numerous inflammatory mediators and inflammatory cell-derived products on local nerves. **Note that these symptoms and signs are the result of innate immune system activation.**

12. What are the major classes of inflammatory mediators that facilitate inflammation during the innate immune response?

See Table 4.3.

13. How are prostaglandins (PGs) and LTs formed?

Unlike histamine, which is a preformed and stored mediator, PGs and LTs require active synthesis. They are formed from arachidonic acid, an omega-6 polyunsaturated free fatty acid (PUFFA), which is liberated from phospholipids in the cell membrane by cytoplasmic phospholipase A$_2$. Arachidonic acid can then be metabolized by either of two enzyme pathways (Fig. 4.2):

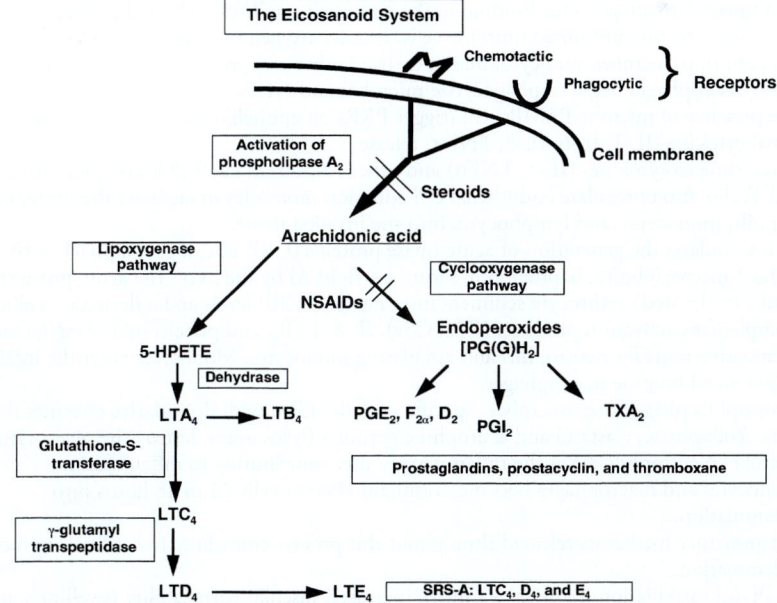

Fig. 4.2 Eicosanoid pathways. *HPETE,* Hydroperoxyeicosatetraenoic acid; *LT,* leukotriene; *NSAIDs,* nonsteroidal antiinflammatory drugs; *PG,* prostaglandin; *SRS-A,* slow-reacting substance of anaphylaxis; *TX,* thromboxane.

- The **cyclooxygenase (COX) pathway** results in PGs. The amount and type of PG made are determined by the expression levels of COX-1, COX-2, and cell-specific terminal synthase enzymes. As an example, platelets only make thromboxane A2 because platelets contain only COX-1 and thromboxane synthase.
- The **lipoxygenase (LOX) pathway** results in LTs and hydroxyeicosatetraenoic acids.

The synthesized PGs are exported from cells by the multidrug resistance-associated protein family of efflux transporters. Secreted PGs act on targets by binding to G-protein-coupled receptors. There are at least nine receptors mediating the various effects of PGs.

14. How do PGs and LTs promote inflammation?

PGs (especially PGD_2) induce local vasodilation and increased vascular permeability. PGE_2 is the most abundant PG at inflammation sites and can have both proinflammatory and anti-inflammatory effects depending on the receptor it activates. LTs fall into two classes: (1) LTC_4, LTD_4, and LTE_4 induce smooth muscle contraction, bronchoconstriction, and mucous secretion. They were once collectively called slow-reacting substances of anaphylaxis or SRS-A; (2) LTB_4 has none of the above properties but is a potent chemotactic factor for neutrophils.

Note that as the inflammatory process progresses, the same COX and LOX enzymes that initially produced PGs and LTs will shift to producing specialized pro-resolving mediators (SPMs) that dampen the inflammatory response. These SPMs include lipoxins enzymatically derived from arachidonic acid and resolvins and protectins from omega-3 PUFFA. Notably, omega-3 PUFFA from exogenous dietary sources can serve as substrates for COX and LOX resulting in the production of resolvins and protectins, which are anti-inflammatory.

15. Describe the initial events in chronological order resulting in an inflammatory response against a microbial pathogen.

- Microbes breach the physical epithelial barrier. The innate immune system response begins with the epithelial secretion of alarmins (S100A and antimicrobial defensins).
- The complement pathway is activated by C3 and factor B binding to the microbial membrane (alternate pathway) and/or mannan-binding protein interacting with the microbe (lectin pathway). This results in the generation of the MAC and chemoattractants C3a and C5a that will recruit cells of the innate immune system.
- N-Formylmethionyl peptides from microbes activate neutrophils and macrophages, which in turn upregulate integrins for binding to the endothelium. These cells will produce chemoattractants to recruit additional immune cells, reactive oxygen intermediates to kill microbes, NETs to trap microbes, and cytokines to activate other components of the immune response.
- Local macrophages begin to phagocytize microbes and NETs.
- The presence of microbe PAMPs will trigger PRRs on epithelial and innate immune cells to signal cytokine (IL-1, IL-6, IL-8, TNFα) release.
- In response to cytokines (IL-1, TNFα) and other stimuli, LTs and PGs are synthesized. IL-1 and TNFα also upregulate endothelial cell adhesion molecules to facilitate the influx of neutrophils, monocytes, and lymphocytes into the invaded tissue.
- IL-6 stimulates the generation of acute phase proteins (CRP, fibrinogen, alpha-1-antitrypsin, alpha-2 macroglobulin, haptoglobin, serum amyloid A) by the liver. The acute phase response results in elevated erythrocyte sedimentation rate and CRP levels and a decrease in albumin.
- Complement activation products (C3a, C5a), IL-8, LTB_4, and platelet-activating factor are chemoattractants for neutrophils and circulating monocytes. Monocytes enter the inflammatory site and become macrophages.
- Neutrophils phagocytize microbes. Specific granules filled with degradative enzymes (lysozyme, collagenase, elastase) and azurophilic granules (lysosomes) destroy the phagocytized microbe. Neutrophils die at the inflammatory site, contributing to inflammation.
- Monocytes and macrophages become dominant effector cells 24 to 48 hours into inflammation.
- Inflammatory mediators released throughout this process contribute to cardinal signs of inflammation.
  - PGE_2: vasodilation (redness, warmth), increased vascular permeability (swelling), and increased pain sensitivity to bradykinin.
  - Prostacyclin: vasodilation.

- Thromboxane A$_2$: platelet activation.
- Platelet-activating factor: vasodilation, increased vascular permeability, platelet activation.
- Bradykinin: activates nerve fibers (pain).
- APCs (DCs) present antigens bound to MHC molecules to activate acquired (adaptive) immune system (T and B lymphocytes), occurring 3 to 5 days after microbial invasion.

ADAPTIVE IMMUNITY

16. How does the innate immune system interact with the acquired immune system?

If innate immunity cannot handle the invading foreign antigen or microbe, then adaptive immunity responds. APCs in the tissue (e.g., skin, lung, and mucus membranes) endocytose antigen, becoming activated and upregulating the trafficking chemokine receptor CCR7 that causes migration toward the ligand CCL21 produced in the lymphoid tissues (e.g., spleen, lymph nodes, mucosal-associated lymphoid tissue [MALT]). In those lymphoid tissues, the adaptive immune response develops.

Antigen that has been endocytosed by APCs is processed in the endoplasmic reticulum where it is loaded onto MHC class I or II molecules depending upon the type of antigen. (See Question #18 below for more about MHC.) The MHC-antigen complex is then presented on the APC surface. Simultaneously, signals through TLRs and/or PRRs cause the APCs to upregulate costimulatory molecules such as CD80 (B7-1)/CD86 (B7-2) or CD40 on the cell surface. T cells within the lymphoid tissue recognize the MHC-presented antigen using the TCR as well as the costimulatory molecules using CD28 or CD40L, respectively. Both signals, the TCR (signal 1) and costimulation (signal 2) are required for T-cell activation. Note that self-antigens are not recognized by TLR/PRRs of the innate immune system and, therefore, do not induce the mandatory costimulatory molecules (signal 2) on APCs needed to activate T cells, ensuring that only pathogen-specific T cells are activated. Activated T cells then regulate B cells, other T cells, and other cells participating in the immune response.

17. Which cells are APCs? Where are they found?

Antigen-presenting cells are given in Table 4.4.

18. What is MHC and what does it do?

The MHC encodes the human leukocyte antigens (HLAs). MHC and HLA are often used interchangeably. There are three different classes—types I, II, and III. All are encoded on the short arm of chromosome 6 over a region of approximately 4 million base pairs. Class I and II molecules function to present antigens to T cells. There are over 1100 common polymorphisms of class I

TABLE 4.4 Antigen-Presenting Cells	
CELL TYPE	**LOCATION**
Macrophage	Connective tissue
Histiocyte	Connective tissue
Monocyte	Blood
Alveolar macrophage	Lung
Kupffer cell	Liver
Microglia	Central nervous system
Mesangial cell	Kidney
Osteoclast	Bone
Dendritic cell	Lymphoid tissue, mucous membranes, solid organs
Langerhans cell	Skin (dendritic cell)
B cell	Lymph nodes

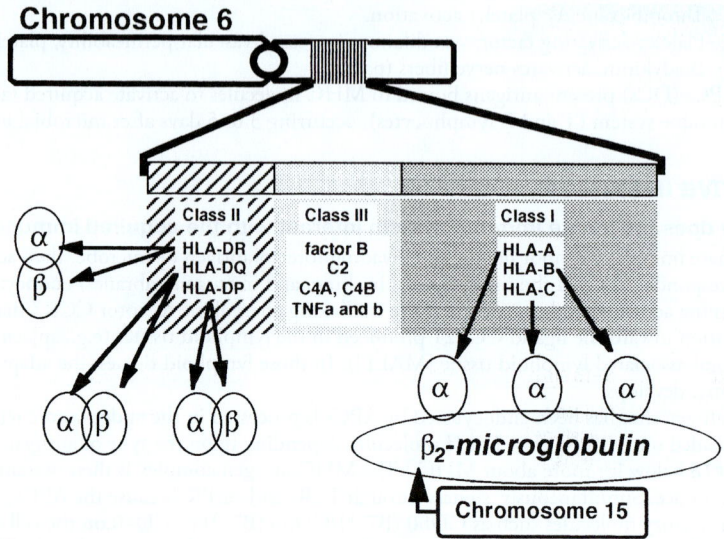

Fig. 4.3 The major histocompatibility complex. *HLA,* Human leukocyte antigen; *TNF,* tumor necrosis factor.

and II molecules in the general population. For the MHC class I region, over 200, 300, and 100 alleles have been identified for HLA-A, HLA-B, and HLA-C loci, respectively. Other class I genes (HLA-E, HLA-F, HLA-G) have limited function and polymorphisms. For the MHC class II region, over 250, 50, and 60 alleles have been identified for HLA-DRβ, HLA-DQ, and HLA-DP loci, respectively. Other genes in the class II region are involved in peptide processing, which includes peptide sizing (proteasome subunits LMP1 and 2), peptide transport (TAP1 and 2), and peptide loading onto class II molecules (DMA, DMB, DO/DN). The remainder of the MHC complex stretches between the class I and II regions and encodes various proteins that are not capable of presenting antigen. However, many of these MHC class III proteins are involved in the regulation of the immune response, and some have rheumatic disease associations. These include C2, C4A and C4B, and factor B of the complement system; TNFα and lymphotoxin; and some of the HSPs. Both MHC class I and II molecules are dimers. While the MHC encodes both α- and β-chains of class II molecules, it encodes only MHC class I α-chain. **β$_2$-microglobulin,** the β-chain shared by all MHC class I molecules, is encoded by a relatively invariant allele on chromosome 15. Note that in spite of the large number of HLA polymorphisms, each individual only codominantly inherits one allele at each locus from each parent, that is, two HLA-A alleles (one from father and one from mother), two HLA-B alleles, and so on. Fig. 4.3 summarizes the structure of Chromosomes 6 and 15 with the MHC genes.

19. How do the MHC class I and II molecules differ in function?

They are differ in their cellular distribution, the antigenic peptide fragments they present, and the type of T cell that recognizes and responds to the complex they present (Table 4.5).

20. How does the HLA protein bind its peptide antigen?

HLA proteins comprise two α-helical walls with a β-pleated sheet forming the floor of the binding site. In MHC class II molecules, the α- and β-chains together form this structure, whereas in MHC class I molecules, only the α-chain contributes to the peptide antigen-binding site.

The antigen binds at points on both the α-helical walls and the β-pleated floor. The three areas of greatest genetic diversity (**hypervariable regions**) are expressed in segments of each of the α-helices and β-pleated sheets. This genetic variation very specifically affects or "selects" which antigens can bind to specific molecules. In addition, it specifically "selects" which TCRs can interact with specific combinations of MHC-antigen complex.

TABLE 4.5 Function of Major Histocompatibility Complex (MHC) Class I and II Molecules

	MHC CLASS I	MHC CLASS II
Cellular distribution	All nucleated cells and platelets	Antigen-presenting cells: • B cells • Monocytes/macrophages • Dendritic cells • Thymic epithelial cells Some activated T cells Some cells in which MHC Class II is induced, particularly during chronic inflammation: • Endothelial cells • Synovial cells • Intestinal epithelia
Antigen size	8–13 amino acids in length	13–25 amino acids in length
Antigen type	Antigen peptides found inside the cell (self-peptides, intracellular pathogens, or tumor antigens)	Phagocytosed or receptor-mediated endocytosed antigen taken into the lysosome (extracellular pathogens)
T-cell recognition	CD8+ T cells	CD4+ T cells
T-cell response	Cell-mediated cytotoxicity of the cell presenting the antigen on MHC class I	T cell coordinated phagocytic and/or antibody response to eradicate the presented antigen

21. How do the MHC molecules control what the T cells see?

They do this in two ways. First, the sequence of amino acids in an HLA molecule, which is determined by an individual's genetic polymorphisms, determines which antigenic peptide fragments can bind to that molecule. Only those "selected" antigenic peptides that can bind to one of an individual's HLA molecules have the potential to be specifically recognized. Second, not all T cells can see all the HLA molecules. The peptides presented in the context of MHC class I molecules can only be seen by T cells that have CD8 molecules associated with their TCR, whereas the peptides presented in the context of MHC HLA class II molecules can only be seen by T cells that have CD4 molecules associated with their TCR.

22. What are the two main types of lymphocytes? How are they differentiated? What are their subtypes?

- **T lymphocytes,** or T cells, are **t**hymus-derived and express the TCR-CD3 complex on their surface. They can be separated from other lymphocytes by the use of monoclonal antibodies that recognize CD3, a component of the TCR that transduces the TCR signal across the lymphocyte membrane. T-cell subtypes include:
  - **CD4+ T cells:** Th1, Th2, Th17, regulatory T cells (Tregs), follicular T helper cells (Tfh).
  - **CD8+ T cells:** cytotoxic T lymphocytes (CTLs).
  - **Natural killer T cells (NKT):** T cells that express NK cell markers and have restricted TCRs that recognize lipids bound to the MHC-like molecule CD1d.
  - **Gamma-delta T cells:** use γ- and δ-chains to form the TCR. Most are double negative (lack CD4 and CD8). They make up 2% to 3% of circulating T cells and are primarily found in the skin and gut epithelium. These TCRs do not recognize antigen in context with MHC but rather recognize antigen directly or in association with MHC class I-like molecules such as CD1 (binds glycolipid antigens) and MICA/MICB in the gut. HSPs can directly activate these cells. They interact with alkyl phosphates found in mycobacteria and are expanded during certain infections. Notably, they are expanded in the small intestinal epithelium of individuals with celiac disease.
- **B lymphocytes,** or B cells, are **b**one marrow-derived antibody-secreting cells that express surface Ig (e.g., B-cell receptor [BCR]) on their surfaces. There are several subpopulations of B cells:
  - **B1 cells** develop earliest during ontogeny and are characterized as innate-like B cells. Most express CD5. They are activated by microbes through PRR, do not require T-cell help, do

not develop into memory B cells, and are the source of "natural" antibodies. These antibodies are low affinity, IgM, and polyreactive, recognizing both common pathogens and autoantigens. They are located predominantly in peritoneal and pleural cavities.

- **B2 cells** develop later in ontogeny and lack CD5 surface markers. Before encountering antigen, mature B2 cells coexpress IgM and IgD antibodies on their surfaces. With antigen stimulation and T-cell help, they secrete highly specific antibodies (IgM, IgG, IgA, or IgE) within the secondary lymphoid tissue. Follicular B cells can freely circulate and are organized into the primary follicles of B-cell zones focused around follicular dendritic cells (FDCs) in the white pulp of the spleen and the cortical areas of peripheral lymph nodes. They comprise 95% of B cells in lymph nodes and spleen. Marginal zone B cells are noncirculating B cells that are located in the marginal zone of the spleen. Memory B cells are CD27+, constitute 1% of the total B-cell population, and can be long-lived (years) with continued antigen stimulation. Plasma cells are terminally differentiated B cells that function to secrete antibodies.
- **Regulatory B cells** (Bregs, B10) subsets are found within the B1 and B2 populations. They secrete IL-10 to modulate the immune response.

23. Specific adaptive immune responses can be differentiated into two major categories based on whether B or T cells are primarily involved. What are these two categories?

1. **Humoral immunity** refers to immune responses involving antibodies that are produced by mature B cells and plasma cells. Important for defense against bacteria, especially those with a polysaccharide capsule (e.g., *Pneumococcus*, *Haemophilus influenzae*).
2. **Cellular immunity** is mediated by T cells that secrete cytokines and signal effector cells to direct an overall cell-mediated immune response. Important for defense against viruses, parasites, fungi, and mycobacteria.

24. How do T cells develop?

T-cell precursors from the bone marrow enter the thymus where they begin the process of becoming a naïve T cell. Nearly 99% of cells die in this process.

First, cells undergo **positive selection** in which the T cell must generate a TCR that, along with either CD4 or CD8, is capable of seeing antigens presented by MHC. The majority of circulating lymphocytes in the bloodstream are T cells with a TCR comprising an α-chain and a β-chain. To generate diversity, the TCR β-chain genes on chromosome 7 contain four segments (V, D, J, C), whereas the α-chain genes on chromosome 14 contain three segments (V, D, C). Each segment has several members to choose from (50-100V, 15D, 6-60 J, 1-2 C) in a process called gene recombination in which the T cell selects to use only one of each of these segments. This process of TCR gene rearrangement and the combination of the two TCR chains yield >10^8 possible combinations. After generating a TCR successfully, the T cell undergoes **negative selection**. In this case, T cells that bind too strongly to self-antigen or MHC and those that do not bind at all are eliminated.

T cells that survive the processes in the thymus are then released as naïve T cells into circulation where they will traffic to secondary lymphoid tissues to mature and differentiate.

25. Describe how CD4+ T cells are activated.

- DCs capture and process antigens from peripheral sites. They migrate to lymph nodes displaying the processed antigenic peptide in context with MHC.
- Naïve T cells continually recirculate through blood, spleen, lymph nodes, and MALT in search of DCs displaying a complementary MHC-peptide complex that can engage its TCR.
- If the naïve T cell TCR binds the MHC class II-peptide complex on the APC without engaging any costimulatory molecules, it becomes anergic (unresponsive) or undergoes apoptosis. However, if a naïve T cell TCR binds the MHC class II-peptide complex on the APC and the T cell is activated, then the T cell expresses CD40L, which binds to CD40 on the APC. This induces expression of CD80/CD86 on the APC, which binds to CD28 on the T cell, triggering the production of IL-2, which binds to the IL-2R on the T cell, causing a positive feedback loop and resulting in T-cell proliferation.

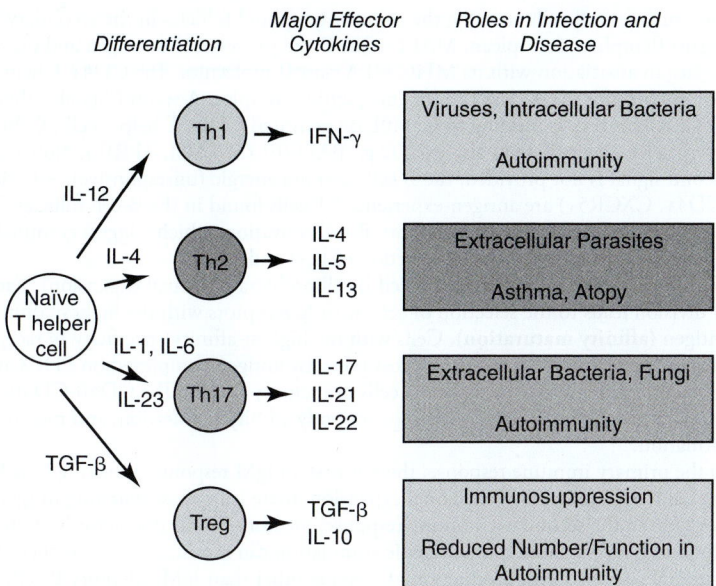

Fig. 4.4 Human CD4+ T helper differentiation pathways and roles in normal immunity and disease.

- Naïve T cells are activated to become one of the four distinct subpopulations of CD4+ T cells based on the cytokines produced by APCs in response to the antigen they are processing. The type of CD4+ T cell can be identified based on the cytokines it secretes (Fig. 4.4).
  - **Th1** responses promote the production of opsonizing antibodies (IgG1) and induction of cellular cytotoxicity and macrophage activation. Important against pathogens that replicate intracellularly (virus, intracellular bacteria).
  - **Th2** responses promote IgE and IgG4 production and stimulate eosinophil development. Important for helminth infections.
  - **Th17** responses are important for defense against chronic infections with extracellular bacteria and fungi.
  - **Tregs** are important for the establishment and maintenance of tolerance and suppression of immune response.
- The activated T cell proliferates and its progeny travel throughout the body until they reach where the antigen has invaded. They are restimulated by local APCs and release their cytokines (Fig. 4.4) that contribute to augmenting the immune response by activating monocytes/macrophages.
- Some activated T cells undergo further interactions with B cells in the lymphoid tissue, inducing a humoral immune response.
- Some activated T cells become long-lived memory T cells. Memory T cells are activated more easily and rapidly in a secondary immune response.

26. Describe how B cells can be stimulated to produce a humoral antibody response.

- **T cell-independent antigens:** mitogens and bacterial polysaccharides have repeating structures that enable them to crosslink surface Ig (BCR) causing B-cell activation that results in a predominantly IgM response.
- **T cell-dependent antigens:** the majority of protein and glycoprotein antigens require T-cell help to mount a humoral response against them. The steps for this to occur are:
  - Naïve T cells recognize antigens associated with MHC HLA class II molecules on APCs. The CD4+ T helper cell is activated and can provide help to a B cell for antibody production.
  - The BCR of a B cell binds and internalizes the antigenic peptide for which it is specific. This antigen is often provided by FDCs that present antigen–antibody complexes on

their surface to B cells entering the primary lymphoid follicles in the secondary lymphoid organs (lymph nodes, spleen, MALT). The B cell processes the antigen and puts it on its surface in association with its MHC HLA class II molecules. The CD4+ T helper cell TCR will bind to this HLA class II-antigenic peptide complex. A second signal is then provided by CD40 on B cells binding to CD40L on activated CD4+ T helper cells. Other costimu-latory activating pathways also exist (e.g., BAFF/BLYS, TACI, APRIL). Note that if a second signal is not provided, the B cell becomes anergic (unresponsive). Additionally, Tfh (CD4+, CXCR5+) are antigen-experienced T cells found in the B-cell follicles. They medi-ate antigen-specific naïve and memory B-cell activation, which triggers germinal center formation through the Tfh cell secretion of IL-4 and IL-21.

- Within germinal centers, the activated B cell proliferates (clonal expansion). Each cycle of division leads to the selection of cells with Ig receptors with the highest affinity for the antigen **(affinity maturation).** Cells with the highest-affinity/specificity Ig receptors on their surfaces have their receptors crosslinked by antigen complexed on FDCs and are selected to differentiate into plasma cells or memory B cells. The CD40-CD40L costimu-lation is critical for Ig class-switching, antibody affinity maturation, and memory B-cell formation.

- In the primary immune response, there is first an IgM response occurring 4 to 10 days after antigen exposure. With clonal expansion, there is Ig class-switching to IgG and other isotypes. In the secondary immune response, memory B cells that actively circulate from blood to lymph in search of antigenic stimulation can mount a much quicker (1–3 days) humoral response with production of isotypes other than IgM. Memory B cells require less antigens and less T-cell help than naïve B cells due to the high-affinity surface Ig receptors for their specific antigen.

- One activated B cell can generate up to 4000 plasma cells, which can produce up to 10^{12} antibody molecules per day.

27. Describe the structure of an Ig. How is antibody diversity generated?

Unlike TCRs that can only respond to linear antigenic peptides bound to an HLA molecule, Igs (antibodies) can bind to antigens in any formation (bound, soluble, linear, complex structures). The number of antigenic determinants (epitopes) that antibodies need to be able to bind is in bil-lions. This diversity is created by both the antibody's structure and genetic recombination.

An Ig is composed of four polypeptide chains, two identical heavy (H) and two identical light (L) chains. Each chain has a constant (C) and variable (V) domain. There are five different H-chain C regions (isotypes): IgM (μ), IgG (γ), IgA (α), IgE (ϵ), and IgD (δ) coded on chromo-some 14. The H-chain C region determines the Ig's ability to fix complement and to bind to Fc receptors. Th L-chains are designated kappa (κ) and lambda (λ) and coded for by chromosome 2 and 22, respectively. κ chains are used more often (65%) than λ chains.

Like the generation of TCR diversity, Ig genes undergo recombination. The H-chain V region genes contain three segments (V_H, D_H, J_H), whereas each of the L-chain genes contains two ($V\kappa$, $J\kappa$ or $V\lambda$, $J\lambda$). Each segment has several members to choose from ($38\text{-}46V_H$, $23D_H$, $9J_H$), ($31\text{-}35V\kappa$, $5J\kappa$), or ($29\text{-}32V\lambda$, $4\text{-}5J\lambda$). A single V(D)J is chosen from each segment and recom-bined by the enzymes RAG-1/RAG-2. The antigen-binding regions are formed by pairing the V domains of the L-chain to the V region of the H-chain. Within the V region of the Ig molecule are discrete regions, called **complementary determining regions (CDRs),** which contact the antigen specifically. Both the H- and L-chains contain three of these regions. The structure of the CDRs of an Ig is called the **idiotype.** The minimal antigenic determinant recognized by the CDRs is called the antigenic **epitope.** This process of generating Ig diversity occurs during B-cell maturation and is antigen-independent. After the B cell responds to the antigen, the BCR and Igs produced can undergo **somatic mutation** to increase the specificity of the antibody-binding site for the antigen.

28. Name the five major classes of antibodies. What specific role does each play in humoral immunity?

The mnemonic is GAMED:

- **G—IgG:** highest concentration in serum (70% of total Igs) and excellent penetration into tis-sues. Can cross the placenta by week 16 of pregnancy. Fixes complement. Four subtypes: IgG1 and IgG3 respond to protein antigens; polysaccharide antigens elicit IgG2 responses; IgG4 arises against nematodes and can dampen chronic inflammation.

- **A—IgA:** despite its low concentration in serum, more IgA is produced than any other Ig isotypes. Most IgA exists as secretory IgA in mucosal cavities and milk. There are two subclasses: IgA1 is a monomer in serum and IgA2 is a dimer/polymer and is the most important antibody for host defense at mucosal surfaces (sites of antigen entry). Dimer/polymeric IgA2 contains a J-chain. This complex is produced locally by plasma cells, captured by a receptor on the basolateral surface of epithelial cells, transported to the apical side, and cleaved from the receptor. IgA is released into secretions associated with a secretory component. This form (secretory IgA) is more resistant to enzymatic degradation.
- **M—IgM:** IgM is the first class of antibody made in the primary response to antigen. Pentameric form vigorously fixes complement and is very important in host defense against bloodborne antigens. IgM also associates with a J-chain, which allows its active transport to mucosal surfaces. A monomeric form of IgM complexed with Igα and Igβ on the surface of naïve B cells and serves as the BCR.
- **E—IgE:** binds to the surface of mast cells and basophils by high-affinity IgE Fc receptor, FcεR1. Crosslinking of IgE by antigen binding results in the release of the cells' granular contents (primarily histamine). Important in allergic diseases and host defense against parasites.
- **D—IgD:** found primarily as a membrane Ig on the surface of naïve B cells. B cells with IgD on their surface are more resistant to being tolerized.

29. How does antibody participate in immune and inflammatory responses?

There are three main ways in which antibody is immunologically active:

1. Antibodies can coat and neutralize invading organisms, not allowing the organism access to the host.
2. Two classes of antibodies (IgM and IgG) activate ("fix") complement by the classical pathway, resulting in cell chemotaxis, increased vascular permeability, and target cell lysis.
3. Antibody coats foreign particles, increasing the efficiency of phagocytosis by cells that contain surface Ig (Fc) receptors (neutrophils and macrophages). This process is called opsonization. Complement activation can also opsonize foreign particles facilitating removal through complement receptors.

30. How are CTLs activated?

Most CTLs are CD8+ T cells. A naïve CD8+ CTL first develops into a memory CD8+ CTL after engagement with an APC, usually a DC, which has been stimulated by an activated CD4+ helper T cell in lymphoid tissues. The CD4-activated DC presents intracellular antigen (e.g., viruses) on its surface in association with MHC-encoded HLA class I molecules. These engage with the CTL TCR (signal 1) as well as costimulatory molecules (signal 2), resulting in an activated CTL. On activation, CTLs divide and circulate to find infected/abnormal cells to kill. The CTL (CD8+) TCR specific for the antigen binds the HLA class I molecule containing the foreign peptide. Several other adhesion molecules also contribute to this interaction (e.g., CD2 [LFA-2]-CD58 [LFA-3]). Cytotoxicity occurs by:

- **Granule exocytosis:** granules containing granzymes from the CTL enter the target cell through pores in its membrane created by perforin. These proteases can cause apoptosis of the target cells.
- **Fas ligand (FasL)-induced apoptosis:** FasL on the CTL binds to Fas (CD95) on the target cell causing apoptosis.

CTLs can secrete cytokines (IFN-γ) and recruit macrophages into the area to augment the immune response. One CTL can lyse multiple cells.

31. What are NKT cells?

NKT cells are T cells that share properties of T cells (express αβ TCR) and NK cells (express CD16, 56, 161, and granzyme production) but are different from CTL and NK cells. They constitute 0.1% of all peripheral blood T cells. Most NKT cells are restricted to recognizing self and foreign lipids and glycolipids presented by CD1d molecules on target cells. Upon activation, NKT cells make IFN-γ, IL-4, granulocyte-macrophage colony-stimulating factor, and other cytokines (IL-2, TNFα). They are important in defense against mycobacterial infections.

ODDS AND ENDS

32. What pathways lead to cellular apoptosis?

Multiple triggers can lead to a cell undergoing apoptosis by one of two major pathways:

* **Death receptors** (Fas [CD95], TNF receptor 1 [TNFR1], DR4/5): all these receptors have a homologous intracellular region "death domain." These death domains bind to adaptor proteins (Fas and DR4/5 binds to FADD, TNFR1 to TRADD). These adaptor proteins can activate the cysteine protease, procaspase 8. This can be inhibited by FLIP. The activated caspase 8 activates the executioner caspases (3, 6, and 7), which in turn activates an endonuclease called caspase-activated DNAse as well as others. These endonucleases cleave DNA causing fragmentation and cell death. Caspases also activate proteases that act on actin microfilaments leading to blebbing of the membrane.
* **Mitochondria:** cellular stress causes Bax, Bak, and/or Bid to bind to mitochondria. This displaces Bcl-2 and Bcl-x, which are normally on the outer mitochondrial membrane and inhibit apoptosis. When this happens, cytochrome c is released from the mitochondria. Cytochrome c activates the adaptor protein, Apaf-1, which is in the cytosol. Apaf-1 activates procaspase-9, which activates caspases 3 and 7 causing apoptosis (as mentioned earlier). Akt inhibits this pathway. Many tumors have chronically activated Akt, so the tumor cell does not undergo apoptosis.
* **Others:** (1) cytotoxic cells (T and NK cells) inject granzyme B, which activates caspases 3 and 7. (2) DNA damage is detected by p53, resulting in activation of apoptosis.

33. Describe the differences between apoptosis, necrosis, and autophagy.

* **Apoptosis:** each day, 10 million cells undergo programmed cell death (apoptosis) in a healthy individual. The mechanism is necessary to control tissue size and homeostasis without inciting inflammation. The two pathways leading to apoptosis are listed in the previous question. During apoptosis, the chromatin condenses, cells shrink, and cell membranes form blebs that become apoptotic bodies containing organelles. The cell membrane is inverted and the phosphatidylserine in the membrane signals macrophages to phagocytose the apoptotic bodies causing them to release anti-inflammatory cytokines. Binding of C1q, collectins and MBL to apoptotic cells can facilitate their clearance.
* **Necrosis:** the cell swells and the plasma membrane ruptures releasing intracellular contents. This contributes to the inflammatory response.
* **Autophagy:** This is a degradation pathway for cellular components without killing the cell. Autophagosomes take in impaired organelles and unwanted cellular components and deliver them to lysosomes for degradation and recycling without causing apoptosis.

34. How is the immune response turned off after it is activated?

Once the immune response has been activated, it is important to restore immune homeostasis. This is done through various mechanisms:

* Negative regulation of the innate immune response.
  * **Efferocytosis:** activation of macrophages induces the secretion of not only proinflammatory molecules but also anti-inflammatory mediators (IL-10, TGF-β, and PGE$_2$) that downregulate macrophage and DC function. Macrophage ingestion of apoptotic cells (efferocytosis) that they identify by phosphatidylserine on the apoptotic cell's outer surface results in the release of anti-inflammatory mediators.
* Negative regulation of the adaptive cellular immune response.
  * **CTL-associated protein (CTLA-4):** after activation, T cells increase the expression of CTLA-4, which has higher affinity for CD80/CD86 than for CD28 leading to loss of costimulation. This results in cessation of T-cell proliferation and cytokine production.
  * **Activation-induced cell death:** the signals that activate T cells also result in upregulation of Fas and TNFR on their surface. When Fas binds to FasL on another cell, soluble TNFα binds to TNFR1, or transmembrane TNFα binds to TNFR2, the activated T cell undergoes apoptosis.
  * **Treg suppression:** Tregs release IL-10 and TGF-β, which suppress the immune response. Other suppressor T cells also exist (Tr1, Th3, CD8+, CD28+).

- **Breg suppression:** Bregs (B10) release IL-10, which suppresses T cells and DCs. Other subsets of Bregs exist.
- Negative regulation of the adaptive humoral immune response:
  - IgG binds antigens and eliminates them, so it no longer serves as an inducer of the immune response.
  - IgG binds antigen-forming immune complexes. These immune complexes can bind to FcγRII on B cells, which suppresses them.
  - Anti-idiotype antibodies may neutralize antibodies that are being made by binding to their idiotypic determinants.
- **Regulation of complement cascade:** C1 inhibitor, C1INH, binds C1r/C1s preventing C1 activation. C3 convertase (C4b2a and C3bBb) and C5 convertase (C4b2a3b and C3bBbC3b) are regulated by serum inhibitors (C4-binding protein and factor H) and membrane-bound factors (decay accelerating factor [DAF] and membrane cofactor protein [MCP]). C4b-binding protein inactivates C4b and the classical pathway, and factor H inactivates C3b and the alternative pathway by serving as cofactors for factor I-mediated cleavage of C4b and C3b, respectively. DAF causes release of C2a or Bb from cell surfaces leaving C4b and C3b to bind to MCP, which serves as a cofactor for factor I-mediated cleavage of C4b/C3b, halting the classical and alternative complement cascades. Complete deficiency and loss of function polymorphisms of factors H and I result in dysregulated complement activation and the atypical hemolytic uremic syndrome. Other complement regulatory proteins (vitronectin, CD59) block fluid phase and membrane-bound MAC. Note that all these regulatory proteins bind to glycosaminoglycans specific to host cells and not on microbes, therefore protecting host cells while allowing complement-mediated destruction of pathogens.

35. Using the classification developed by Gel and Coombs, immune responses causing immunopathology can be segregated into four main types. Name them.

Type I: IgE-mediated immediate hypersensitivity (e.g., allergic rhinitis or hay fever)
Type II: antibody-mediated tissue injury (e.g., autoimmune hemolytic anemia)
Type III: immune complex (antigen–antibody) formation (e.g., serum sickness, Arthus skin reaction)
Type IV: delayed-type hypersensitivity (e.g., immune response to mycobacterial antigens, positive purified protein derivative skin test).
A fifth type has been added where antibodies bind to receptors causing overstimulation (e.g., thyroid-stimulating Ig binds to thyrotropin receptor mimicking thyroid-stimulating hormone in Graves' disease).

AUTOIMMUNITY

36. What is tolerance?

Tolerance is the term used to describe the phenomenon of **antigen-specific unresponsiveness.** In other words, the immune system encounters certain antigens to which it is programmed specifically to not respond and, therefore, not eradicate.

37. Is tolerance innate or acquired?

The phenomenon of tolerance is present in both innate and adaptive immune systems. We are protected from the innate immune system by specific mechanisms that block its activities, such as membrane complement regulatory proteins that protect self-tissues from the alternative complement pathway. The adaptive immune system "learns" to be tolerant of some specific antigens, such as self-tissues, just as it learns to be "intolerant" of many foreign antigens. When discussing autoimmune disorders, we often narrow our perspective to the tolerance of **autoantigens,** such as an individual's own nucleoproteins or cell-surface molecules, by the adaptive immune system. However, the phenomenon of tolerance is not limited to autoantigens. In fact, tolerance to **exogenous antigens,** such as dietary proteins, is just as crucial for the survival of an individual as "self-tolerance."

38. What are the main pathogenetic mechanisms used to develop and maintain tolerance to self-antigens?

Most autoimmune diseases require the presence of self-reactive CD4+ T lymphocytes that have lost their tolerance to self-antigens. Mechanisms to maintain tolerance are:

- **Central tolerance.**
    - **Thymic selection of T cells:** during this process, the autoimmune regulator, the AIRE gene, is responsible for orchestrating intrathymic presentation of self-antigens bound to MHC HLA class I and II molecules. Those T cells that react too strongly with the MHC-self-antigen complexes are deleted (clonal deletion) during negative selection. This is particularly important for such antigens as major blood groups and MHC. T cells capable of reacting to other self-antigens may not be deleted and can gain access to the periphery.
    - **Receptor-editing of BCRs:** this process occurs during B-cell maturation in the bone marrow. B cells that interact too strongly with self-antigens undergo death by apoptosis. To avoid apoptosis, receptor editing modifies the sequence of L-chain (more than H-chain) V and J genes so that the BCR has a different specificity and will not recognize the self-antigen. Some estimate that 20% to 50% of B cells that come from the bone marrow have had receptor editing of their BCR. There is some evidence that TCRs may also undergo receptor editing.
- **Peripheral tolerance.**
    - **Clonal anergy:** self-reactive T cells that encounter self-antigen presented by HLA molecules in the periphery may not receive necessary second costimulatory signals. These T cells may be tolerized to the antigen and remain unresponsive. This anergic state may be terminated if costimulatory signals are upregulated during a nonspecific infection, tissue injury, or inflammatory state involving the innate immune system.
    - **Immunologic ignorance:** self-reactive T cells may not have a TCR that reacts well enough with the MHC/peptide complex to become activated. This anergic state may be breached if the antigen is changed in some manner such as during an infection.
    - **Tregs and Bregs:** some Tregs suppress self-reactive T cells by cell-to-cell contact with membrane-bound molecules like CTLA-4. Other Tregs are induced and exert suppressive effects by secreting cytokines, IL-10, and TGF-β. Some Bregs (e.g., B10 cells) secrete IL-10.
    - **Idiotype network theory:** a network of antibodies exists naturally or an anti-idiotypic antibody directed against the self-reactive antibody idiotype can be generated, which is capable of neutralizing self-reactive antibodies.

39. What is autoimmunity?

The term *autoimmunity* is commonly employed to describe conditions in which self-tolerance is broken and an individual becomes the victim of his or her own immune response. Just like immunity to foreign antigens, autoimmune disorders are antigen-driven processes that are characterized by specificity, high affinity, and memory. However, an autoimmune process involves the immune system's recognition of an antigen, either foreign or self, that is then followed by an assault on its own self-antigens (i.e., autoantigens). Typically, these processes develop in an individual who previously displayed tolerance to the same antigens that are now targeted by the immune response. Therefore, most autoimmune processes are better described not simply as an absence of tolerance but as a **loss of previously established tolerance.** Clinically, autoimmunity can be divided into two categories:

- **Organ-specific autoimmunity:** defined as an immune response against a single autoantigen or a restricted group of autoantigens within a given organ (e.g., myasthenia gravis [antibodies to acetylcholine receptor]).
- **Systemic autoimmunity:** defined as an immune response against multiple autoantigens resulting in clinical manifestations in multiple organs (e.g., systemic lupus erythematosus [SLE]).

40. What are the stages of an autoimmune disease?

Autoimmune diseases generally follow three stages:

1. Genetic risk: some genes contribute significant risk (e.g., HLA), whereas most genes (e.g., PTPN22, STAT4) confer a modest risk (usually two- to threefold), but in the aggregate, the risk is quite high in the setting of a combination of disease-promoting polymorphisms, which are usually (90%) in regulatory proteins and the "right" environmental exposure. **Epigenetics** (DNA methylation, histone modifications, microRNAs) also contribute to the genetic predisposition.

2. Autoimmunity: the development of autoimmune phenomena such as autoantibodies produced by B cells that have lost self-tolerance (and presumably driven by autoimmune T cells) but in a state wherein the individual still does not exhibit symptoms because the target organs have not yet become damaged to a sufficient level.

3. Disease: the third stage is the development of clinical symptoms that impair quality of life and require treatment. Although most autoimmune diseases are detected and treated only in the third phase, ongoing work in several diseases is expected to allow the detection of a "preclinical" disease state in which specific preventive therapies could be used.

41. Describe the mechanisms that may be involved in the pathogenesis of autoimmune disease.

Several mechanisms have been hypothesized. All center upon a genetically predisposed host who has had one or more environmental exposures that, over time, trigger the autoimmune process. The environmental trigger or triggers are usually not identifiable since they may have occurred years before the first clinical symptom develops (see previous question). More than one of the following possible mechanisms may contribute to the development of autoimmunity:

- **Superantigens:** these are foreign antigens, particularly of bacterial or viral origin, that are capable of binding to the TCR (typically V region of β chain) and MHC class II molecule outside the antigen-binding groove and, in turn, bind the two together. In the case of T cells, superantigens do not need to be processed and subsequently presented in the antigen-binding cleft of MHC molecules in order to stimulate T-cell activation. B-cell superantigens also exist that bind to regions of surface Ig that are common to various subtypes and cause polyclonal B-cell activation without the need for T-cell help.

- **T-B cell discordance with abnormal receptor-mediated feedback and suppression:** T cells responding normally to a foreign antigen release cytokines to augment the immune response. Self-reactive B cells in proximity are stimulated by the cytokine milieu. If these autoreactive B cells have defective receptors that do not respond to inhibitory signals needed to maintain self-tolerance, then they will survive, contribute to the inflammation, and become self-perpetuating. Additionally, abnormal Treg and Breg suppressive function can contribute to this autoimmune process.

- **Molecular mimicry:** an exogenous antigen may share structural similarities with a host antigen. Antibodies produced against this antigen can bind the host antigen causing amplification of the immune response.

- **Cytokine dysregulation:** innate immune system activation releases cytokines that activate the adaptive immune system. Excessive or defective cytokine production could result in an aberrant immune response and/or activation of anergic self-reactive T cells.

- **Defective apoptosis:** accelerated apoptosis of cells with increased release of self-antigens and/or defective presentation of apoptotic cell antigens to lymphocytes could lead to abnormal lymphocyte activation including self-reactive T and B cells.

- **Epitope spreading:** occurs when the immune reaction changes from targeting the primary epitope to also targeting other epitopes.

- **Cryptic epitope exposure:** the innate immune response is activated by an invading pathogen. The inflammatory response causes tissue damage with the release of self-antigens whose epitopes the immune system has not previously developed tolerance to. The adaptive immune system is recruited and continually stimulated by exposure to the new self-antigen released by the host tissue.

42. How might the microbiome influence the development of or ongoing immune responses during autoimmune and autoinflammatory diseases?

Recent data connect numerous diseases (rheumatologic and others) with changes in skin, oral, intestinal, and/or genitourinary microbiomes. The microbiome is comprised of trillions of microorganisms such as bacteria, viruses, and mycobiota that live in symbiosis with us. Alteration in this ecosystem is termed dysbiosis. Dysbiosis can affect the immune system by influencing specific innate and adaptive cellular development as well as influencing the secretion of AMPs and IgA at mucosal surfaces. Factors such as microbial metabolism of the diet (tryptophan, short-chain fatty acids) can generate metabolic products that directly regulate or activate immune functions as well as mucosal barrier permeability. These mechanisms may underlie the pathophysiology of both autoimmune and autoinflammatory diseases. Microbial translocation into mucosal tissues, circulation, and even the joint may stimulate the generation of T and B cell responses that initially target the organism, but through molecular mimicry or through epitope spreading, eventually target self-antigen, causing autoimmunity.

43. What is the difference between an autoinflammatory disease and an autoimmune disease?

Autoinflammatory diseases (e.g., familial Mediterranean fever, see Chapter 79: Familial Autoinflammatory Syndromes A) are diseases that have a chronic inflammatory response due to a defect in a component or regulation of the innate immune system. **Autoimmune diseases** (e.g., SLE) typically involve self-reactive CD4+ T lymphocytes and abnormalities in regulation of the adaptive immune system.

BIBLIOGRAPHY

Amulic B, Cazalet C, Hayes G, et al. Neutrophil function: from mechanisms to disease. *Ann Rev Immunol.* 2012;30:459–489.

Devitt A, Marshall LJ. The innate immune system and the clearance of apoptotic cells. *J Leukocyte Biology.* 2011;90:447–457.

DuPage M, Bluestone JA. Harnessing the plasticity of CD4+ T cells to treat immune-mediated disease. *Nat Rev Immunol.* 2016;16:3.

Galindo-Izquierdo M, Pablos Alvarez JL. Complement as a therapeutic target in systemic autoimmune diseases. *Cells.* 2021;10:148.

Iwasaki A, Medzhitov R. Control of adaptive immunity by the innate immune system. *Nat Immunol.* 2015;16:4.

Kaplan MJ, Radic M. Neutrophil extracellular traps: double-edged swords of innate immunity. *J Immunol.* 2012;189:2689.

Klein L, Kyewski B, Allen PM, Hogquist KA. Positive and negative selection of the T cell repertoire: what thymocytes see (and don't see). *Nat Rev Immunol.* 2014;14:6.

Kuballa P, Notte WM, Castoreno A, Xavier R. Autophagy and the immune system. *Ann Rev Immunol.* 2012;30:611–646.

Medzhitov R. The spectrum of inflammatory responses. *Science.* 2021;374:1070–1075.

Monach PA. Complement. *Arthritis Rheumatol.* 2024;76:1–8.

Nefla M, Holzinger D, Berenbaum F, Jacques C. The danger from within: alarmins in arthritis. *Nat Rev Rheumatol.* 2016;12:11.

Parish IA, Heath WR. Too dangerous to ignore: self-tolerance and the control of ignorant autoreactive T cells. *Immunol Cell Biol.* 2008;86:146.

Rich RR, Fleisher TA, Shroeder HW Jr, et al., eds. *Clinical Immunology.* 6th ed. Philadelphia: Elsevier; 2022.

Robinson MW, Hutchinson AT, Donnelly S. Antimicrobial peptides: utility players in innate immunity. *Front Immunol.* 2012;3:325.

Seymour BJ, Allen BE, Kuhn KA. Microbial mechanisms of rheumatoid arthritis pathogenesis. *Curr Rheumatol Rep.* 2024;26:124–132.

Sharpe AH. Mechanisms of costimulation. *Immunol Rev.* 2009;229:5.

CHAPTER 5

History and Physical Examination

Jason R. Kolfenbach, MD

Realize that the most important biomarkers in rheumatology are the history and physical examination.

Stephen A. Paget, MD

 KEY POINTS

1. A good history and physical examination evaluating for both articular and extraarticular features are the most important components in establishing a correct diagnosis of a rheumatic disorder.
2. If musculoskeletal pain is reproduced with direct palpation of a localized area and worsened by resistive maneuvers, then the source of pain is most likely periarticular (bursa or tendon).
3. The cardinal signs of musculoskeletal inflammation are pain, swelling, erythema, warmth, and limitation of motion. Of these, a joint effusion and limitation of motion are the most indicative of a true arthritis.

1. What should your history include when interviewing a patient with suspected rheumatic disease?

A chronologic history of symptom progression should include the joints that have been involved (including documentation of pain and/or swelling) as well as identifying precipitating factors, such as new drugs, recent infections, environmental exposures, diet, activity, travel history, or trauma. Determine responsiveness to prior therapeutic modalities. Has the joint involvement been episodic, additive, or migratory in nature? Is the pattern of joint involvement mono, oligo, or polyarticular and/or in a symmetrical distribution? Is axial spinal involvement present? Identify any constitutional symptoms that suggest systemic illness, vasculitis, or paraneoplastic disease such as fever, weight loss, or fatigue. A complete review of systems is necessary to determine the organ systems that may be involved (Table 5.1). Ask about functional losses including how their symptoms interfere with activities of daily living and ability to perform their job.

TABLE 5.1 The Rheumatologic Review of Systems

ORGAN SYSTEM	POTENTIAL CLINICAL MANIFESTATION
Skin	Malar rash, photosensitivity, alopecia, sclerodactyly, periungual erythema, Raynaud's phenomenon, digital ulcers, psoriasis, purpura, nodules, genital lesions
HEENT: head, ears, eyes, nose, and throat	Mucosal ulcers or perforation, sicca, ocular discomfort or decreased visual acuity, sinus drainage/nasal discharge, change in hearing, stridor
Cardiorespiratory	Dyspnea, cough, hemoptysis, pleurisy or pericardial pain, edema, pulmonary emboli
Gastrointestinal	Reflux, dysphagia, abdominal pain, diarrhea, hematochezia, jaundice
Renal	Renal insufficiency, proteinuria, hematuria, nephrolithiasis
Hematologic	Leukopenia, thrombocytopenia, anemia, fetal loss, deep vein thrombosis or pulmonary embolism, abnormal serologies
Neurologic	Neuropathies, weakness, transient ischemic attack, strokes, seizures, psychosis, cognitive deficits, temporal headaches

Family history: Ask about family history including various arthritides and other autoimmune diseases that tend to cluster in families.
Social History: Identify a history of drug use or unprotected sexual contact, as well as risk factors for HIV, Hep B, Hep C, gonococcal, or chlamydial infection.

TABLE 5.2 Inflammatory and Mechanical Rheumatic Disorder

FEATURE/SYMPTOMS	INFLAMMATORY	MECHANICAL
Morning stiffness	>1 hour	≤30 minutes
Fatigue	Significant	Minimal
Activity	May improve stiffness	May worsen symptoms
Rest	May cause gelling	May improve symptoms
Systemic involvement	Yes	No
Corticosteroid responsiveness	Yes	No

2. **What historical symptoms enable you to categorize a rheumatic disorder as inflammatory or mechanical (degenerative)?**
   See Table 5.2.

3. **List the five cardinal signs of inflammation.**
   - Swelling (*tumor*)
   - Warmth (*calor*)
   - Erythema (*rubor*)
   - Tenderness (*dolor*)
   - Loss of function (*functio laesa*)

4. **In a patient with inflammatory arthritis, what history is useful in assessing disease activity?**
   Duration of morning stiffness as well as the presence of night pain, joint swelling, or new joint involvement is more helpful than the severity of pain, which can be too subjective. The presence of the gelling phenomenon (joint stiffness after periods of inactivity) is also important to elicit. Inflammatory arthritis is characterized by joint pain and stiffness, whereas in noninflammatory arthritis the predominant feature is pain.

5. **Which signs of inflammation are suggestive of acute synovitis in a joint?**
   Joints affected by inflammatory arthritis commonly exhibit synovial distention, warmth, and limitation of range. The best indicator of synovitis is a distended joint capsule, especially if accompanied by warmth. Swelling due to joint effusions may also occur in the noninflammatory arthritides (e.g., osteoarthritis of knee). Inflamed joints are not typically erythematous, with the exception of acute septic and crystalline arthritis. If you encounter red, hot joints, particularly in a monoarticular distribution, your first thought should be "where is the needle?" (joint aspiration).

6. **How much pressure should you apply when palpating a joint for synovitis?**
   A good "rule of thumb" is to palpate with enough pressure to blanche your distal thumbnail (4 kg/cm^2). This standardizes the joint exam and ensures that adequate pressure is being applied to detect synovitis. Obviously, with overtly inflamed joints, this degree of pressure may be excessive.

7. **Describe the technique for performing a joint exam for the detection of synovitis.**
   Begin with a visual inspection. Look for findings suggestive of acute swelling such as loss of the "valley" between metacarpal heads when the patient makes a fist, loss of definition of the digital extensor tendons as they course over the metacarpophalangeal (MCP) and metatarsophalangeal (MTP) joint spaces, obliteration of the sulcus between the lateral epicondyle and olecranon process (elbow effusion), or the sulcus medial to the patella (knee effusion). Palpation of individual joints occurs at the joint line, so that the examiner can assess for the presence of a thickened overlying joint capsule as well as synovial effusion. Synovitis of the finger and wrist joints can be readily identified given their superficial nature (in contrast to deeper joints such as the shoulder), and these joints are a common site of involvement in rheumatoid arthritis (95%). As such, the evaluation for tender joint count and swollen joint count often starts here.

Technique for palpation at the proximal interphalangeal joint involves the examiner surrounding the joint on all four sides in order to maximize the potential to detect capsular inflammation and/or thickening (four-finger technique). A similar technique can be applied to the MCP joints (Fig. 5.1). An alternative approach to detection of synovitis at the MCP joint involves extension

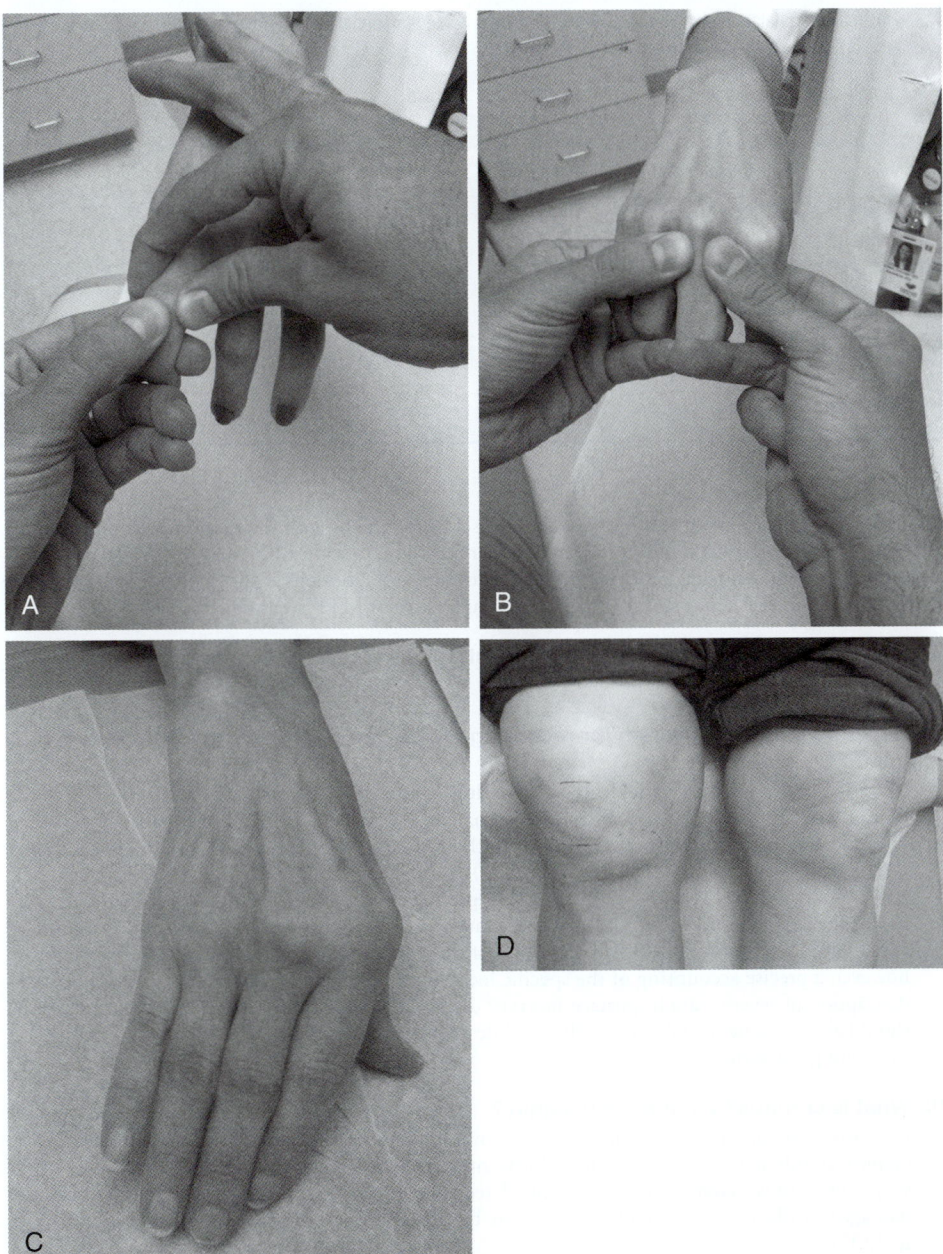

Fig. 5.1 (A) Four-finger technique for detection of synovitis in proximal interphalangeal joint of a normal individual. (B) Dorsal two-finger technique in metacarpophalangeal (MCP) joint. (C) Visual inspection suggests swelling at the second and third MCP as evidenced by loss of the valley between metacarpal heads and lack of definition of the extensor tendons overlying those joints. (D) Asymmetric loss of the medial sulcus on the right knee, suggestive of effusion. The superior aspect of the patellar as well as the borders of Hoffa's fad pad are outlined.

TABLE 5.3 Typical Joints Comprising the Examination 'Joint Count'

Peripheral Joints	
Hand	Foot
• Distal interphalangeal	Interphalangeal
• Proximal interphalangeal	Metatarsophalangeal
• Metacarpophalangeal	Talocalcaneal (subtalar)
• Thumb carpometacarpal	Ankle
Wrist	Knee
Elbow	
Axial Joints	
Shoulder	Spine
• Glenohumeral	• Cervical
• Acromioclavicular	• Thoracic
• Sternoclavicular	• Lumbar
Hip	Temporomandibular
Sacroiliac	

of the examined joint in conjunction with dorsal ballottement with the examiner's thumb and index finger from each hand (dorsal four-finger technique). Additional clues to the detection of effusion and/or synovitis in other joints include patellar ballottement, the "bulge sign" at the knee (see Question #31), and splaying of the toes (suggestive of MTP swelling).

8. **Which joints are included in a joint count?**
   See Table 5.3.

9. **Describe the STWL system for recording the degree of arthritic involvement of a joint.**
   The STWL system records the degree of **swelling, tenderness, warmth,** and **limitation** of motion in a joint based on a quantitative estimate of severity. A score of 0 (normal), 1 (mild), 2 (moderate), or 3 (severe) can be assigned to the S, T, and W categories. Limitation of motion is scored as 0 (normal), 1 (25% loss of motion), 2 (50% loss), 3 (75% loss), or 4 (ankylosis), or range of motion (ROM) can be recorded in degrees. For example, Rt. 2nd MCP S2T2W1L2 means the right second MCP joint has moderate synovitis, moderate tenderness, mild warmth, and a 50% loss of normal ROM. Formal use of this system is not common in every day practice; however, a precise accounting of the specific location of tender and swollen joints, as well as a description of severity, are important facets of disease monitoring. In addition, the examiner should also evaluate for joint instability and describe deformities such as swan-neck, ulnar deviation, and genu varum.

10. **What is crepitus? What does it signify?**
    Crepitus is an audible or palpable "grating" sensation felt during joint motion. The **fine** crepitus of inflamed synovium is of uniform intensity and perceptible only with a stethoscope. In contrast, **coarse** crepitus is easily detected, of variable intensity, and transmitted from damaged cartilage and/or bone. Crepitus may be elicited by compressing a joint throughout its ROM.

11. **In the examination of an arthritic hand, what features enable you to differentiate rheumatoid arthritis from osteoarthritis?**
    See Table 5.4.

TABLE 5.4 Examination Findings in Rheumatoid Arthritis and Osteoarthritis

FEATURE	RHEUMATOID ARTHRITIS	OSTEOARTHRITIS[a]
Symmetry	Yes	Occasional
Synovitis	Yes	Rarely[b]
Nodules	Yes	No
Digital infarcts	Seldom	No
Bony hypertrophy	No	Yes
Joint Involvement		
Distal interphalangeal	No	Heberden's nodes
Proximal interphalangeal	Yes	Bouchard's nodes
Metacarpophalangeal	Yes	No[c]
Thumb carpometacarpal	No	Yes
Wrist	Yes	No[d]
Deformities	Swan neck	Distal interphalangeal or proximal interphalangeal angulation
	Boutonniere	
	Subluxation	
	Ulnar drift	

[a]Osteoarthritis may occur secondary to any inflammatory arthritis.
[b]Synovitis can occur in inflammatory erosive osteoarthritis.
[c]Osteoarthritis of the index and middle finger metacarpophalangeal joints may be a feature of hemochromatosis or calcium pyrophosphate deposition disease.
[d]Osteoarthritis of the wrist may occur secondary to trauma or crystalline arthritis.

12. How do you determine if joint pain is originating from intraarticular or extraarticular structures?

"Stressing" a joint (and its accompanying intraarticular structures) is easily accomplished by gentle passive ROM of the joint by the examiner. In contrast, pain during attempted active ROM (performed by the patient) against a joint held immobile by the examiner suggests pathology in the surrounding tendons. Local tenderness by direct palpation of periarticular structures such as a bursa or tendon may also indicate that the origin of pain is extraarticular.

13. How do tender points and trigger points differ?

See Table 5.5.

14. Define photosensitivity and photophobia.

Photosensitivity refers to the development of a **rash following <30 minutes of sun exposure** (typically ultraviolet-B light). This feature is noted among 30% to 60% of patients with cutaneous lupus (discoid or subacute cutaneous lupus), systemic lupus erythematosus, and dermatomyositis. Photophobia indicates **ocular sensitivity** to light and can be found in patients with uveitis and other ocular conditions.

15. What rheumatic disorders, other than rheumatoid arthritis, may exhibit subcutaneous nodules?

Systemic lupus erythematosus	Multicentric reticulohistiocytosis
Rheumatic fever	Sarcoidosis
Tophaceous gout	Vasculitis
Juvenile idiopathic arthritis	Panniculitis
Systemic sclerosis (calcinosis)	Lupus profundus
Erythema nodosum	

TABLE 5.5 Clinical Features of Tender Points and Trigger Points

FEATURE	TENDER POINT	TRIGGER POINT
Disorder	Fibromyalgia	Myofascial pain syndrome
Distribution	Widespread	Regional
Abnormal tissue	No	±
Tenderness	Focal	Focal
Referred pain	No	Yes

16. What historical or physical features are essential for the diagnosis of Raynaud phenomenon?

Raynaud phenomenon is a reversible, vasospastic disorder characterized by transient, stress-induced (e.g., cold temperature) ischemia of the digits, nose-tip, and/or ears. As a result of vasospastic alterations in blood flow, a triphasic color response is usually observed. The initial color is **white** (ischemic pallor), then **blue** (congestive cyanosis), and finally **red** (reactive hyperemia). The diagnosis of Raynaud phenomenon best correlates with the initial "dead-white" pallor of ischemia. It should primarily involve the fingers and not the entire hand. History and exam should also evaluate for the presence of digital ulcerations or infarcts (primary Raynaud phenomenon in isolation should never cause such findings).

17. Describe the examination of a patient with suspected median nerve entrapment of the wrist (carpal tunnel syndrome [CTS]).

Thenar atrophy is a reliable sign of CTS but occurs only as a consequence of chronic disease with damage to the motor nerve. Acute or subacute CTS symptoms are typically sensory (the median nerve supplies sensory innervation to the palmar surface of the thumb, index finger, middle finger, and radial half of the ring finger). Its symptoms may be reproduced by provocative tests. **Tinel's test** is best performed with the wrist in extension. The full width of the transverse carpal ligament is then percussed using a broad-headed, reflex hammer or the examiner's long finger. In contrast, **Phalen's test** is performed by gently positioning the wrist at full volar flexion for 60 seconds. Nerve conduction velocity studies are useful in confirming the clinical diagnosis of CTS. Conditions such as CTS, Raynaud, and other diseases affecting the neurovascular bundle may cause hand pain and result in referral to a rheumatologist. In contrast to arthritic etiologies, the pain is poorly localized (e.g., diffuse hand discomfort versus localization to specific joints).

18. What is Finkelstein's test?

Finkelstein's test is a useful adjunct to direct palpation in the clinical diagnosis of wrist **tenosynovitis (de Quervain's)**, involving the **abductor pollicis longus** and **extensor pollicis brevis** tendons. Performance of this maneuver can help differentiate pathology secondary to de Quervain's from conditions involving nearby structures such as osteoarthritic involvement of the carpometacarpal joint. See Chapter 61 (Regional Musculoskeletal Disorders) for a description of the maneuver and treatment recommendations.

19. What are the best maneuvers to quickly assess shoulder function?

Ask the patient to raise their hands over their head by fully abducting both shoulders with palms up (touchdown sign). From this position, ask them to clasp their fingers together behind their head while keeping their elbows back. Next to test abduction and external rotation, ask the patient to reach behind his head and touch/scratch the superior medial edge of the opposite scapula (Apley's "scratch" test). Finally, to test internal rotation and adduction, have the patient put their hands at their sides and then reach behind their back and try to touch the inferior angle of the opposite scapula. If the patient can perform these maneuvers, their shoulder function is normal.

20. In the evaluation of shoulder pain, what single maneuver can best differentiate glenohumeral joint involvement from that of the periarticular tissues?

Significant glenohumeral joint pathology can usually be excluded if the **passive external rotation** of the shoulder is unrestricted and pain-free.

21. Why is it important to know about the various provocative tests that can be done during the shoulder exam?

Periarticular structures account for 80% of shoulder pain. Hence, even in patients with known inflammatory disease, the etiology of shoulder pain may often be located outside the gleno-humeral joint. As such, an understanding of provocative maneuvers (to identify supraspinatus tendinitis, impingement syndrome, and biceps tendinitis) is important. See Chapter 61 (Regional Musculoskeletal Disorders) for further description of these tests.

22. How do you diagnose "tennis elbow" (lateral epicondylitis)?

In addition to direct palpation, tennis elbow may be diagnosed by stressing the wrist extensor muscles at their origin, the lateral epicondyle. This provocation maneuver requires the patient to form a fist and maintain the wrist in extension. The examiner then flexes the wrist against resistance, while supporting the patient's forearm. Pain arising from the lateral epicondyle confirms the diagnosis. See Chapter 61 (Regional Musculoskeletal Disorders) for additional information on the diagnosis and treatment of lateral epicondylitis.

23. When examining a swollen, inflamed elbow, how can you differentiate olecranon bursitis from true arthritis?

Differentiation may be difficult as a result of swelling, pain, and limitation of ROM (extension and flexion). Rotation of the forearm, with the elbow flexed at 90 degrees, is one maneuver that can help differentiate the two disorders. True arthritis of the elbow will inhibit pronation and supination of the radiohumeral joint, whereas in olecranon bursitis, the joint moves freely. Synovitis usually distends the normal sulcus of the ulnar groove, not over the tip of the olecranon. Full extension of the elbow exacerbates true arthritis, whereas it does not affect olecranon bursitis.

24. When a patient has true hip joint pathology, where is the pain usually reported and how is the hip joint examined?

Despite misconceptions of the lay public, true hip pain is felt in the **groin** region in 90% of cases. In contrast, pain in the lateral hip region or buttock is usually referred to from the lumbar spine or trochanteric bursa. Hip pain may occasionally radiate from the groin to the anteromedial thigh, greater trochanter, buttock, and knee. Assessment of hip mobility may help differentiate hip pathology from other causes of groin pain (e.g., adductor tendinitis). The origin of the hip joint as the source of pain can be confirmed by one of two maneuvers: reproducing the pain during passive external or internal rotation of the hip in the seated position, or rotating the lower leg while the subject is lying supine with the knee in extension using the hip joint as a pivot (log roll). ROM of the hip can best be assessed while supine by placing the hip in to flexion (with the knee flexed), whereas abduction and adduction should be assessed with the knee extended. Hip extension requires the patient to position the ipsilateral pelvis off the examining table so the lower leg can be extended posteriorly. In hip disease, the first motion lost is internal rotation.

Patrick's test (**FABER**: flexion-abduction-external rotation maneuver) is performed with the patient lying supine and the examiner **fl**exes, **ab**ducts, and **e**xternally **r**otates the patient's leg so that the foot is on top of the opposite knee (forms numeral 4). The examiner lowers the leg toward the examining table. If there is a difference between the two legs, the test indicates hip disease (groin pain) or sacroiliitis (sacroiliac joint pain).

25. What does a positive Trendelenburg's test indicate?

A positive Trendelenburg's test reveals weakness of the **gluteus medius** muscle, which may indicate hip joint pathology. The test is performed by observing the patient from behind as he or she stands on one leg. Normally, gluteus medius contraction of the ipsilateral, weight-bearing limb will elevate or allow the contralateral pelvis to remain in level. In contrast, a weakened gluteus medius muscle cannot support the contralateral pelvis, and thus it will drop. Neurogenic causes (i.e., L5 nerve root compression) of gluteus medius weakness should also be excluded, as it represents another potential etiology of a positive test.

26. Why do we examine a patient for leg-length inequality, and how is this measured?

Leg-length discrepancy is associated with several "mechanical disorders" such as chronic back pain, trochanteric bursitis, and degenerative hip disease. **True** leg-length discrepancy reflects measurable differences (congenital or acquired) of both limbs using the anterior, superior iliac spines, and medial malleoli as landmarks. **Apparent** or functional leg-length discrepancy is primarily a measure of "pelvic tilt", typically induced by scoliosis or hip contractures. This apparent inequality is determined in the supine position by measuring the distance from the umbilicus to each medial malleoli. True leg-length measurement is usually equal in disorders of apparent leg-length discrepancy. Correction of significant inequality (≥1 cm) with a simple shoe lift can be therapeutic.

27. Describe the physical findings of a patient with meralgia paresthetica.

Meralgia paresthetica (lateral femoral cutaneous nerve entrapment syndrome) results from compression of the lateral femoral cutaneous sensory nerve as it passes under the inguinal ligament medial to the anterior pelvic brim. Typical symptoms include burning dysesthesias and pain over the anterolateral thigh, unaffected by hip rotation or straight leg raise. In some patients, these symptoms may be elicited by performing **Tinel's test** at the site of entrapment. Common causes of compressive injury include obesity (pannus), pregnancy, and heavy work belts as well as noncompressive causes of nerve injury such as diabetes.

28. How do you diagnose trochanteric bursitis?

The diagnosis of trochanteric bursitis is best made by direct palpation of the soft tissues overlying the greater trochanter of the femur. Trochanteric bursa pain may also be elicited by hip abduction, flexion, and external rotation and relieved by lidocaine injection.

29. What is Ober's test?

Ober's test evaluates the iliotibial band for contracture. The patient lies on the unaffected side with the lower leg flexed at the hip and knee. The examiner abducts and extends the upper leg (affected side) with the knee flexed at 90 degrees. The examiner slowly lowers the limb with the muscles relaxed. A positive test result occurs if the affected leg does not fall back to the level of the tabletop. This indicates iliotibial band tightness, which can lead to altered gait causing low back pain, recurrent trochanteric bursitis, and lateral knee pain due to "snapping" of the iliotibial band over the lateral femoral condyle causing iliotibial bursitis.

30. When examining a swollen knee, how can you tell if it is inflamed?

In the absence of erythema, **warmth** may be the best indicator of inflammation in a swollen knee. Knee temperature, as determined by feeling with the back of your hand, is generally cooler than the quadriceps muscles or pretibial skin in normal individuals. Thus, if comparative palpation reveals the anterior knee skin to be warmer than these regions or the contralateral knee, inflammation is likely.

31. When examining a swollen knee, how can you determine if an effusion is present?

In addition to comparing the symmetry of the medial knee region with the unaffected knee, the **bulge sign** is a useful finding when evaluating minimal effusions. To perform this maneuver, the supine patient should relax the quadriceps muscle and have the supported knee flexed to 10 degrees. The examiner's palm is used to "milk" a potential effusion from the medial knee to the suprapatellar or lateral compartment. A reverse, similar maneuver is then performed on the lateral side. If rapid filling of the medial patellar fossa occurs, the bulge test is positive.

32. What is the patellofemoral compression test?

This test is used to evaluate damage (e.g., osteoarthritis) to the retropatellar surface. With the patient in the supine position and the knee in slight flexion, the examiner compresses the patella against the femoral condyles. The patient is then asked to extend the knee forcefully, thus contracting the quadriceps muscle. With quadriceps contraction, the patella will be displaced proximally against the femur. If this maneuver produces pain, the test is positive. Patients usually report that squatting or stair climbing reproduces their pain.

33. How do you differentiate prepatellar bursitis from knee arthritis?

A typical feature of acute inflammatory arthritis of the knee is loss of extension as a result of pain due to capsular stretch from the underlying effusion. In prepatellar bursitis, the swelling tends to be localized anteriorly over the patella, and pain is increased during knee flexion and direct palpation. Thus, if an inflamed knee demonstrates full extension without pain and a negative bulge sign, the disease is likely extraarticular.

34. When evaluating an unstable knee, how do you perform Lachman's test?

Lachman's test is a type of drawer test used to evaluate the integrity of the anterior cruciate ligament. It is best performed by holding the knee in 15 to 20 degrees of flexion. While stabilizing the thigh with one hand, the examiner uses the other hand to pull the tibia forward. A mild "give" or forward subluxation is suggestive of anterior cruciate laxity or tear. Congenital laxity (hypermobility) must be excluded by comparison of both knees.

35. Where is the pes anserine bursa?

The pes anserine ("goose foot") bursa is on the medial side of the knee between the aponeurosis of the hamstring's insertion and the medial collateral ligament, approximately 5 cm below the anteromedial joint line. It is a common cause of medial knee pain and is frequently mistaken for osteoarthritis of the knee. Reproduction of pain by direct palpation with the resolution of the pain after a lidocaine injection confirms the diagnosis.

36. Describe the ankle joint examination.

The ankle is a hinge joint. Palpation for synovitis is best done over the anterior (not lateral) aspect of the joint. When the ankle is at the normal position of rest (right angle between foot and leg), the ankle (tibiotalar joint) normally has 20 degrees of dorsiflexion and 45 degrees of plantar flexion. Subtalar (talocalcaneal) joint motion is tested by the examiner grasping the calcaneus with the hand and inverting (25 degrees) and everting (15 degrees) the foot while the ankle joint is held motionless. Muscular strength is assessed by the patient walking on her toes and heels.

37. List some common causes of heel pain.

- Achilles tendonitis: insertional or noninsertional. Usually due to overuse or overpronation of foot.
- Preadventitial Achilles bursitis (pump bump): usually due to rubbing from shoe wear on a calcaneus that has Haglund's deformity.
- Retrocalcaneal bursitis: inflammation of bursa between Achilles tendon and calcaneus.
- Calcaneal stress fracture.
- Plantar fasciitis: pain along medial plantar aspect of heel. Pain worse on first getting out of bed in morning with weight stretching the plantar fascia. Not due to heel spurs.

38. What type of patient usually gets posterior tibialis tendonitis?

Posterior tibialis tendonitis dysfunction occurs commonly in women aged 45 to 65 years. It is associated with flatfoot deformity, obesity, and rheumatoid arthritis. Pain and swelling occur along the medial aspect of ankle. Patients cannot stand on their toes owing to pain and/or weakness.

39. How should the foot be examined?

With shoes and socks off! The foot is usually neglected in the physical examination but can be a source of lower extremity pain. Have the patient stand and put weight on his/her feet to see if there is excessive pronation (flat feet) or a high-arched cavus deformity. Check the ROM of the MTP joints. The ROM for functional ambulation is 65 to 75 degrees of dorsiflexion for first MTP joint and 60 degrees for lesser MTP joints. Have the patient ambulate in her bare feet. Foot deformity, ankle instability, and lack of ROM of the toes (particularly the first MTP) can result in gait abnormalities that can contribute to ankle, knee, hip, and lower back pain.

40. Name and describe five types of abnormal gaits.

- **Antalgic:** the patient remains on the painful extremity for as short a time as possible during the stance phase of gait. This is known as a "gait of pain" and usually indicates pain in the knee, ankle, or foot.
- **Coxalgic:** patient with hip pain will lean toward the painful hip during the midstance phase to place the center of gravity over the hip. This lessens the stress on the hip and lessens pain.

- **Trendelenburg:** a patient with a weak gluteus medius muscle will lurch toward the involved side to place the center of gravity over the hip. This can be seen in an L5 radiculopathy. This "gait of weakness" is similar to the coxalgic gait in appearance, but it is a result of weakness and not pain.
- **Steppage:** loss of ankle dorsiflexion (foot drop) such as seen with peroneal nerve injuries will cause the patient to flex the hip excessively and bend the knee during the midswing phase so the toe does not scrape the floor. Often there is a loud slap as the foot then hits the floor at the end of the swing phase.
- **Simian:** a patient with spinal stenosis will often walk flexed forward to lessen the stenosis of the spinal canal. It is so called because it is suggestive of a gorilla walking pattern.

BIBLIOGRAPHY

American College of Rheumatology Ad Hoc Committee on Clinical Guidelines. Guidelines for the initial evaluation of the adult patient with acute musculoskeletal symptoms. *Arthritis Rheum.* 1996;39:1.

Davis JM. *History and Physical Examination of the Musculoskeletal System. Firestein and Kelley's Textbook of Rheumatology.* 12th ed. Elsevier: Philadelphia; 2025.

Mills JA. *Physical Examination of the Musculoskeletal System. Current Diagnosis and Treatment: Rheumatology.* 4th ed. McGraw-Hill: United States; 2021.

Omair MA, Keystone EC. The dorsal 4-finger technique: a novel method to examine metacarpophalangeal joints in patients with rheumatoid arthritis. *J Rheumatol.* 2018;45(3):329–334.

Robinson DB, El-Gabalawy HS. Evaluation of the patient: history and physical examination. In: Klippel JH, ed. *Primer on the Rheumatic Diseases.* 13th ed. New York: Springer; 2008:6–14.

Laboratory Evaluation

Jason R. Kolfenbach, MD

1. What is ESR and how is it measured?

The Westergren ESR is the gold standard and is a measurement of the distance in millimeters that red blood cells (RBCs) fall within a specified tube over 1 hour. ESR is an indirect measurement of inflammation based on alterations in acute-phase reactants and quantitative immunoglobulins.

2. What are acute-phase reactants?

Acute-phase reactants are a heterogeneous group of proteins (fibrinogen, haptoglobin, CRP, serum amyloid A, ferritin, alpha-1-antitrypsin, and others) synthesized in the liver as part of the acute inflammatory response. Common inciting events include infection, malignancy, trauma, tissue injury, or rheumatic disease. Interleukin-6 (IL-6), an inflammatory cytokine, is an important mediator that stimulates the production of acute-phase reactants.

3. What factors influence the ESR?

Any condition that causes either a rise in the concentration of acute-phase reactants or hypergammaglobulinemia (polyclonal or monoclonal) will cause an elevation of the ESR. The increased concentration of these proteins decreases the negative charge of RBCs, thus dissipating inter-RBC repulsive forces and leading to closer aggregation (rouleaux formation). This causes the RBCs to fall faster resulting in an elevation of the ESR. Noninflammatory conditions that can elevate the ESR (typically through an increase in plasma fibrinogen) include pregnancy, diabetes, end-stage renal disease, and heart disease. In addition, aging, anemia, female sex, and obesity can be associated with an elevated ESR. Alterations in number (polycythemia), size (microcytosis), or shape (spherocytosis, sickle cell) of erythrocytes may physically interfere with rouleaux formation and thus lower the ESR.

PEARL: A rough rule of thumb for the age-adjusted upper limit of normal for ESR (mm/hour) is: Male = age/2; Female = (age + 10)/2

4. What causes an extremely high or extremely low ESR?

- Markedly elevated ESR (>100 mm/hour)
  - Infection, bacterial (35%)
  - Connective tissue diseases: giant cell arteritis, polymyalgia rheumatica, SLE, and other vasculitides (25%)
  - Malignancy: lymphomas, myeloma, and others (15%)
  - Other causes (25%)

- Markedly low ESR (0 mm/hour)
  - Afibrinogenemia/dysfibrinogenemia
  - Agammaglobulinemia
  - Extreme polycythemia (hematocrit >65%)
  - Increased plasma viscosity

5. Is the nonautomated, 60-minute Westergren method the most commonly used technique to measure the ESR?

No. Surveys reveal that roughly two-thirds of laboratories across the globe use either modified automated measurements based on the Westergren method or alternative novel methods. Techniques based on the Westergren method utilize specialized vacuum tubes that can be filled without the need for transfer by a technician. Many of these instruments use infrared light to measure the final length of sedimentation, with results measured at 15–30 minutes depending on the instrument and then extrapolated to Westergren (60 minute) values. Alternative novel methods of ESR measurement may use centrifugation or rapid acceleration of the blood sample followed by photometric rheology to measure rouleaux formation. This latter technique uses an infrared laser to track the RBC-plasma interface at several points during sedimentation and then transforms the data on established sedimentation curves from the Westergren method. Results can be available in as little as 20 seconds to 5 minutes with some instruments. Several studies have shown that results may differ between automated ESR measurements and the traditional Westergren test, especially at higher ESR values where automated values are often falsely lower. The influence of anemia, hyperfibrinogenemia, and other factors listed in Question #3 on methods utilizing photometric rheology is uncertain.

6. Describe an approach to the evaluation of an elevated ESR.

a. Complete history and physical examination and routine screening laboratories (complete blood count, chemistries, liver enzymes, and urinalysis). Make sure that routine health care maintenance is up-to-date. Repeat ESR to ensure it is still elevated and there is no laboratory error.
b. If there is no clear association after step a, consider the following:
  - Review medical records to compare with any previously obtained ESR data to determine how long the ESR may have been elevated.
  - Check SPEP, fibrinogen, and CRP levels for evidence of acute-phase response as well as to rule out myeloma or polyclonal gammopathy.
c. If still no obvious explanation, recheck the ESR in 1–3 months. Up to 80% of patients will normalize. Follow the patient for the development of other symptoms or signs of disease if ESR remains elevated.

7. What is CRP?

CRP is a pentameric protein composed of five identical, noncovalently-linked, 23-kD subunits. It is present in trace concentrations in the plasma of all humans, and it has been highly conserved over hundreds of millions of years of evolution. Although its exact function is unknown, it shows important recognition and activation properties. Ligands recognized by CRP include phosphatidylcholine as well as other phospholipids and some histone proteins. CRP can activate the classical complement pathway; it can bind to and modulate the behavior of phagocytic cells in both proinflammatory and antiinflammatory ways. CRP is produced as an acute-phase reactant by the liver in response to IL-6 and other cytokines. Elevation occurs within 4 hours of tissue injury and peaks within 24–72 hours. In the absence of inflammatory stimuli, it falls rapidly, with a half-life of about 18 hours. A normal value is typically < 0.5–1.0 mg/dL (<5.0–10.0 mg/L) depending on the laboratory. Age, race, and obesity may affect the normal values. Table 6.1 below outlines the age and obesity-adjusted upper limit of normal for CRP. CRP is measured by immunoassay or nephelometry.

PEARL: Levels >8–10 mg/dL (>80-100 mg/L) should suggest bacterial infection, systemic vasculitis, acute polyarticular crystal disease, or widely metastatic cancer.

TABLE 6.1 Age and Obesity Adjusted Upper Limit of Normal for CRP	
Age-adjusted upper limit of normal for CRP (mg/dL)	
Male	Age/50
Female	(Age + 30)/50
Obesity-adjusted upper limit of normal for CRP (mg/dL)	
Male	1.0 + (BMI-25)/25
Female	1.0 + (BMI-25)/12.5

BMI, body mass index.

8. When should you order a CRP instead of an ESR?

Both tests measure components of the acute-phase response and are useful in measuring generalized inflammation. The ESR is affected by multiple variables; as such, an elevation of the ESR can be less specific for an inflammatory process. For example, hypergammaglobulinemia can cause a persistently elevated ESR, preventing it from becoming normal even in situations where the inflammatory response has subsided. The CRP, however, is not affected by immunoglobulin levels as it measures a specific acute-phase reactant. It rises more quickly and falls more quickly (within hours) than the ESR, which tends to remain elevated for a longer time (decreases by 50% in 1 week) after the inflammation subsides. As such, the CRP test may be preferred in situations where monitoring early response to therapy is desired, when factors influencing the ESR specifically are present (see Question #3), or when there are discordant results for the ESR and CRP that are suggestive of noninflammatory factors influencing the ESR.

9. How does the serum protein electrophoresis (SPEP) change in response to inflammation?

The SPEP directly quantifies the acute-phase response. Inflammation is followed by characteristic protein alterations that are reflected on the high-resolution electrophoresis (which separates proteins in to five distinct regions: albumin peak, α-1, α-2, β I & II regions, and gamma region). The typical pattern of SPEP for the inflammatory response includes increases in the α-2 zone most prominently (e.g., α-2 macroglobulin, haptoglobin), gamma zone (immunoglobulins), α-1 zone (e.g., α-1 antitrypsin, others) and the β-γ area (CRP). Negative acute-phase reactants are seen on the SPEP as a diminished albumin peak and β region (transferrin).

PEARL: A rough rule of thumb for normal levels (% of the total protein) of the five regions on the SPEP is: α-1 (5%); α-2 (10%); β (15%); gamma (20%); albumin (50%)

10. What is serum procalcitonin (PCT) and how should it be interpreted in the setting of an autoimmune disease?

PCT is a propeptide of calcitonin and is produced in the thyroid gland. Virtually all PCT in the thyroid is converted to calcitonin; therefore, serum levels are undetectable or very low in healthy individuals (0.05 ng/mL). In bacterial infections, PCT levels are significantly elevated. The source of production in this setting is thought to lie outside the thyroid gland, although the exact site of production and the biologic function of elevated PCT are unknown. The clinical utility of the PCT test has been most extensively studied in bacterial infections among the general population, with data suggesting a role of PCT in the decision of when to start and/or stop antibiotic therapy (common cut-off level ≥0.5 ng/mL).

The potential utility of PCT in differentiating infection from disease flare in patients with autoimmune disease has been examined in small retrospective and prospective cohort analyses. Disease activity in RA and SLE is associated with minor elevations in PCT levels, but values ≥0.5 ng/mL are more commonly seen in patients with bacterial infections. One study in SLE showed that CRP values were more sensitive and specific for infection compared to PCT. Additional studies have suggested a potential role for PCT in differentiating septic arthritis from other causes of inflammatory arthritis. Of importance, some forms of vasculitis and adult-onset Still's disease have been associated with elevated PCT in the absence of bacterial infection. Nonrheumatic conditions that have been associated with elevated PCT in the absence of infection include surgery, trauma, cardiogenic shock, pancreatitis, and some forms of cancer such as small-cell lung carcinoma.

Bacterial infections associated with a systemic inflammatory response are most commonly associated with elevated PCT levels, whereas viral infections are not associated with elevated PCT levels. Of interest, tumor necrosis factor-α (TNFα) and other cytokines have been identified as potential upregulators of PCT production. As such, there is a theoretical concern about the clinical accuracy of PCT in patients on immunosuppressive medication. Limited data suggest that steroid therapy does not impair PCT levels in patients with concurrent bacterial infection. In addition, studies have shown similar rates of positive PCT values (≥ 0.5 ng/mL) among infected patients with autoimmune disease, regardless of whether they were on biologic therapy or not. Further investigation of this area is needed.

11. How are ANAs measured?

The preferred method is the indirect immunofluorescence (IIF) technique. Permeabilized cells are fixed to a microscope slide and incubated with the patient's serum, allowing ANAs to bind to the cell nuclei. After washing, a fluorescein-labeled secondary antibody is added, which binds to the patient's antibodies (which are bound to the nucleus). Cells are visualized through a fluorescence microscope to detect nuclear fluorescence. The amount of ANAs in a patient's serum is determined by diluting the patient's serum prior to adding the serum to the fixed cells—the greater the dilution (titer) at which nuclear fluorescence is detected, the greater the amount of ANAs present in the patient's serum. Most laboratories use human epithelial type 2 (HEp-2) cells (a proliferating cell line derived from a human epithelial tumor cell) for the substrate to detect ANAs. This is because rapidly growing and dividing cells contain a larger array and higher concentration of nuclear antigens (such as Sjögren's syndrome-related antigen A [SS-A] and centromere antigens). Older testing methods for IIF used rat or mouse liver and kidney tissue as the substrate, which lowered the sensitivity for the detection of antigens such as SS-A.

Enzyme-linked immunoassay (ELISA) methods and multiplex bead assays are now commonly used by many laboratories to detect ANAs as these methods are cheaper and easier to perform. These platforms generally include an array of 8 to 10 autoantigens compared with >100 autoantigens in HEp-2 cells. Data have shown that ELISA and multiplex bead assays may be less sensitive than IIF methods. Furthermore, ELISA methods can potentially denature the purified target antigen in the solid phase assay raising the potential for false-positive results as well. As such, IIF remains the "gold standard" according to the American College of Rheumatology.

12. What is a lupus erythematosus (LE) cell?

An LE cell is a neutrophil or macrophage that has engulfed the intact nucleus of another cell. One of the earliest reports of this phenomenon was in 1948 by Hargraves and colleagues at the Mayo Clinic, on inspection of bone marrow biopsies among 25 patients with SLE. It is now understood that an LE cell represents the end result of ANAs binding to a nucleus and fixing complement, resulting in subsequent phagocytosis. LE cells have been reported in the synovial fluid as well as pleural and pericardial effusions in patients with SLE, but are uncommonly found in undisturbed peripheral blood. To identify this phenomenon in patients with suspected SLE, a specific preparation (the LE cell prep) is carried out: the peripheral blood sample is disrupted (increasing cell permeability and access to the nucleus), incubated for a period of time, and then inspected. The presence of engulfed nuclei within neutrophils or macrophages (LE cells) is considered a positive test and represents an early surrogate marker for the ANA antibodies presumed to be involved in the phagocytic process. This was the major method of measuring ANAs in the 1950s and 1960s. This test is time-consuming and relatively insensitive in detecting ANAs (70–80%) compared with IIF, and is no longer commonly performed.

13. At what point is an ANA test considered positive?

A positive ANA is arbitrarily defined as the level of ANAs that exceeds the level seen in 95% of the normal population. Each laboratory must determine the level that it considers positive, and this level may vary significantly among laboratories. In most laboratories where HEp-2 cells are used as substrate to detect an ANA, clinically significant titers are usually $\geq 1{:}160$.

14. Can a positive ANA occur in a normal healthy individual?

Yes. The frequency depends on ANA titer and patient characteristics:
- ANA 1:40: 20–30% of healthy individuals can be positive.
- ANA 1:80: 10–15% positive
- ANA 1:160: 5% positive
- ANA 1:320: 3% positive
- A healthy relative of an SLE patient: 5–25% positive (usually low titers)
- Elderly (age >70 years): up to 70% positive at ANA titer 1:40

15. Can a patient with SLE ever be ANA-negative?

Yes, but very rarely. Few patients (<1%) with active, untreated SLE will have a negative ANA.
In general, patients with SLE and a negative ANA will usually have one of the following:
- Hereditary early complement component deficiency (C2, C4). These patients usually have low-titer ANAs.
- Have antibodies only to the nuclear antigen SS-A (Ro) and are ANA-negative because:
  1. The substrate used in the fluorescent ANA test did not contain sufficient SS-A antigen to allow detection of those antibodies. While such patients are ANA-negative on rodent tissue substrates, they are almost always positive when HEp-2 substrate is used; OR
  2. The antibody is only directed against the 52 kDa SS-A/Ro protein, which is located in the cytoplasm, and not against the 60 kDa SS-A/Ro protein, which is located in the nucleus.
- A very few cases of SLE may have antibodies restricted to cytoplasmic constituents (e.g., ribosomes, ribosomal P, and others).
- A minority of SLE patients (up to 10–15%) will become ANA-negative with treatment and their disease becomes inactive.
- Rarely, SLE patients with severe proteinuria may be ANA-negative due to antibody loss in the proteinuria. ANA becomes positive with decrease in proteinuria with therapy.
- SLE patients with end-stage renal disease on chronic dialysis can become ANA-negative.
- Technical factors and the prozone effect can sometimes be responsible for a negative ANA.

16. What medical conditions are associated with a positive ANA?

See Table 6.2.

TABLE 6.2 Medical Conditions Associated with a Positive ANA

CONDITION	% ANA-POSITIVE
Systemic lupus erythematosus	99–100
Drug-induced lupus	100
Mixed connective tissue disease	100
Autoimmune liver disease (hepatitis, cholangitis)	100
Systemic sclerosis (limited and diffuse subsets)	95
Sjögren disease (SjD)	85–90
Oligoarticular juvenile idiopathic arthritis (uveitis)	70–80
Idiopathic inflammatory myositis (IIM)	40–80
Antiphospholipid antibody syndrome	40–50
Rheumatoid arthritis	30–50
Autoimmune thyroid disease (Hashimoto, Graves)	30–50
Primary pulmonary hypertension	40
Multiple sclerosis	25
Neoplasia (especially lymphoma)	15–25
Chronic infections (subacute bacterial endocarditis, tuberculosis, mononucleosis)	Varies

ANA, antinuclear antibody.

PEARL: A positive ANA in a person with a single autoimmune clinical manifestation, such as discoid lupus, Raynaud's, antiphospholipid syndrome, or idiopathic thrombocytopenic purpura, increases the risk for developing other manifestations of a connective tissue disease in the future. Similarly, the ANA also provides prognostic value for patients with oligoarticular juvenile idiopathic arthritis in regard to risk for the development of subsequent uveitis.

17. Can the ANA titer be used to follow disease activity in patients with SLE or other autoimmune diseases?

No. There is no evidence that variations in ANA titer (level) as measured by the screening ANA correlate with disease activity.

18. What is the significance of the pattern of ANA?

ANA patterns refer to the patterns of nuclear fluorescence observed under the fluorescence microscope (Fig. 6.1). Certain patterns of fluorescence are associated with certain nuclear antigens that are in turn associated with specific diseases (Table 6.3).

Patterns of staining provide a clue to the category of nuclear antigens involved and are dependent on the type of substrate used and, to a certain extent, the experience of the technician. Reliance on ANA patterns has largely been replaced by identification of specific ANAs through the ANA profile (see Question #20).

19. Is the ANA a good screening test for SLE or another autoimmune disease?

No. Simple mathematics indicates that if 5% of the US population is ANA-positive, then 16 million individuals will have a positive ANA. In contrast, the prevalence of SLE is only approximately 1/1000 (320,000 individuals with SLE in the United States). Thus, even if we presume 100% of SLE patients are ANA-positive, screening the entire population for ANA would result in many more normal individuals detected who are ANA-positive than SLE (i.e., 50 to 1). The clinical value of an ANA test is tremendously enhanced by ordering an ANA when there is a reasonable pre-test probability (i.e., clinical suspicion) of an autoimmune disease. Alternatively, a negative ANA (or 1:40 titer) makes it highly unlikely that the patient has SLE, mixed connective tissue disease (MCTD), Sjögren disease, or systemic sclerosis (high-sensitivity tests help rule out disease).

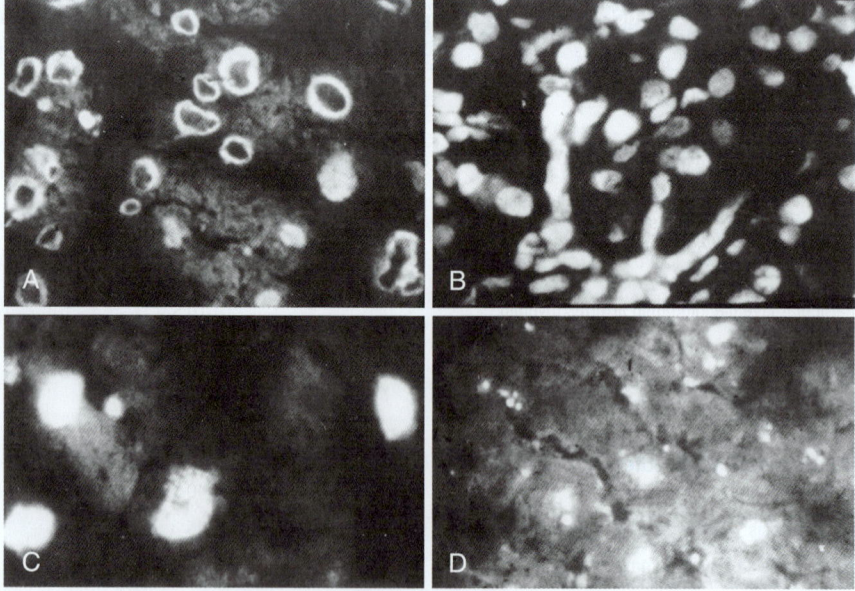

Fig. 6.1 Patterns of antinuclear antibody fluorescence. (A) Rim (peripheral); (B) homogenous (diffuse); (C) speckled; (D) nucleolar. (© 2014 American College of Rheumatology. Used with permission.)

TABLE 6.3 ANA Pattern and Associated Rheumatic Diseases

Homogenous (diffuse)	
• DNA-histone (nucleosome)	SLE, drug-induced LE, and other diseases
• Mi-2	Dermatomyositis
Rim (peripheral)	
• dsDNA	SLE
Speckled	
• SS-A (Ro)	SLE, SCLE, SjD, systemic sclerosis, and other diseases
• SS-B (La)	SLE, SjD, SCLE
• RNP	MCTD, systemic sclerosis, SLE
• Sm	SLE
• Ku	SLE, polymyositis/systemic sclerosis overlap
Nucleolar	
• Topoisomerase I (Scl-70)[a]	Systemic sclerosis (diffuse type) (20–30%)
• RNAP III[a]	Systemic sclerosis (diffuse type) (4–20%)
• Fibrillarin (U3-RNP)	Systemic sclerosis (diffuse type) (8%)
• TH/TO	Systemic sclerosis (limited type) (5%)
• PM- Scl (PM-1)	Polymyositis overlap (1%)
Centromere (kinetochore)	
• CENP	Limited scleroderma
Dense-fine speckled (DFS)	
• DFS70	Healthy population

CENP, centromere protein; *LE,* lupus erythematosus; *MCTD,* mixed connective tissue disease; *RNAP,* RNA polymerase; *RNP,* ribonuclear protein; *SCLE,* subacute cutaneous lupus erythematosus; *SLE,* systemic lupus erythematosus; *SS-A,* Sjögren's syndrome-related antigen A.
[a]Scl-70 & RNAP III have also been associated with a speckled pattern on indirect immunofluorescence.

20. Which diseases are associated with the different antibodies measured in the ANA profile?

See Table 6.4.

> **PEARL:** An ANA-positive patient with an autoimmune disease frequently may not have one of the specific autoantibodies listed in Tables 6.3 and 6.4. This is because of the 100 to 150 ANAs against specific autoantigens that have been described, only about 10 of the most common are routinely tested for.

21. In some diseases, antibodies against cytoplasmic antigens can be more helpful diagnostically than antibodies against nuclear antigens. Which diseases?

Patients with these diseases frequently lack antibodies to nuclear antigens and are, therefore, often ANA-negative. Consequently, the specific anticytoplasmic antibody should be ordered when these diseases are suspected. See Table 6.5 below.

22. Which of the antibodies measured in the ANA profile are useful to follow disease activity?

Antibodies to dsDNA often parallel disease activity in SLE. High titers of antibody to dsDNA are associated with lupus nephritis and increases in dsDNA antibody levels are frequently predictive of a flare of lupus activity. Other antibodies included in the ANA profile are markers of disease subsets but do not fluctuate with disease activity.

TABLE 6.4 ANA Profile Antibodies

	dsDNA	RNP	SM	SS-A	SS-B	CENTROMERE
Systemic lupus erythematosus	60–70%	30%	30%	40%	15%	Rare
Rheumatoid arthritis	(-)	(-)	(-)	5%	Rare	(-)
Mixed connective tissue disease	(-)	100% (high titer)	(-)	Rare	Rare	Rare
Diffuse systemic sclerosis	(-)	20% (low titer)	(-)	10–20%	Rare	5–10%
Limited systemic sclerosis	(-)	(-)	(-)	(-)	(-)	30–40%
Sjögren disease syndrome	(-)	Rare	(-)	75%	40–50%	(-)

TABLE 6.5 Autoimmune Diseases Associated With Anticytoplasmic Antibodies

DISEASE	CYTOPLASMIC ANTIGEN	FREQUENCY
Polymyositis	tRNA synthetase (anti-Jo-1, others)	20–30%
	Signal recognition particle	4%
Systemic lupus erythematosus	Ribosomal P	5–10%
Granulomatosis with polyangiitis	Serine proteinase-3 (seen only in neutrophils)	90%
Microscopic polyangiitis (+ other anti-neutrophil cytoplasmic antibody vasculitides)	Myeloperoxidase, others (seen only in neutrophils)	70%
Primary biliary cirrhosis	Mitochondria	80%

23. What is Crithidia luciliae and what is its relevance to the diagnosis of SLE?

Crithidia luciliae is a parasite that uses the housefly as its host. It contains a kinetoplast, a modi-fied mitochondria that contains a dense collection of circularized dsDNA that can be utilized as a substrate alongside patient serum for the detection of antibodies to dsDNA. The intact circular DNA is free of loose strands of ssDNA and other nuclear antigens, and is more resistant to becoming denatured than DNA in plastic ELISA wells. These attributes improve the specificity of the test (98–100%) to detect antibodies to dsDNA compared with other methods, although at a lower sensitivity (50–55%). Testing is performed by IIF, often referred to as CLIFT, *Crithidia luciliae* indirect fluorescent test. This test may be useful in situations where clinical suspicion for lupus is low but prior testing reveals low titer dsDNA antibody by other methods.

24. What syndromes are associated with antibodies to SS-A (Ro)?

Antibodies to SS-A/Ro may target one or both of two cellular proteins with different molecular weights (52 kDa and 60 kDa) and cellular locations. The 52-kDa protein is an interferon-induc-ible protein located in the cytoplasm. It functions as an E3 ubiquitin ligase that adds ubiquitin to several proteins involved in the inflammatory and immune response resulting in their acceler-ated degradation. The 60-kDa protein binds to small noncoding RNAs located in the nucleus. It functions as an RNA chaperone that binds to defective cellular and viral RNAs to hasten their degradation. Diseases associated with these antibodies include:
- SLE
- Sjögren disease (SjD)
- Subacute cutaneous lupus (a variant of lupus characterized by prominent photosensitivity and rash)

- Neonatal lupus
- Congenital heart block
- Undifferentiated connective tissue disease
- Neuromyelitis optica spectrum disorder
- Other diseases: primary biliary cirrhosis (30%), IIM-associated ILD (20%), and systemic sclerosis (10–20%)

Notably, some diseases have antibodies directed preferentially against one of the two SS-A/Ro proteins. Antibodies primarily against 52 kDa SS-A/Ro are seen in patients with IIM-associated ILD and in patients with systemic sclerosis. Patients with the other autoimmune diseases listed earlier typically have antibodies against both 52 kDa and 60 kDa SS-A/Ro proteins.

25. What is the significance of antibodies to ribonuclear protein (RNP)?

Antibodies to RNP produce a speckled pattern on immunofluorescent ANA, reflective of the focal distribution of their target; the spliceosomal snRNPs in the nucleus are involved in pre-mRNA splicing. These antibodies are seen in a number of autoimmune diseases, including SLE, systemic sclerosis, and MCTD. The presence of very high levels of anti-RNP is highly suggestive of MCTD, a syndrome of overlapping disease manifestations with features of systemic sclerosis, SLE, and polymyositis. Patients with anti-RNP antibodies are more likely to have Raynaud phenomenon, pulmonary hypertension, myositis, and esophageal dysmotility.

26. What is the significance of an ANA with a nucleolar or centromere pattern?

The patient either has systemic sclerosis or has a high risk of developing this disease. The nucleolar pattern is seen in patients with diffuse disease, limited disease with anti-TH/TO, or polymyositis overlap (anti-PM-Scl). Anticentromere antibodies are associated with limited systemic sclerosis.

27. Describe how the ANA pattern and antigen specificity are used in the diagnosis of connective tissue diseases.

See Fig. 6.2.

28. How should you evaluate an unexplained positive ANA in a patient with nonspecific arthralgias?

- History and physical examination: Listen for symptoms and look for objective signs of a connective tissue disease, particularly occult SjD.
- Obtain an ANA profile: ANA titers ≥1:160 or the presence of disease-specific autoantibodies usually indicates that the ANA is significant.
  - Consider testing for anti-DFS70 antibodies. This antibody is directed against a coactivator of nuclear transcription and is associated with healthy individuals with a positive ANA. Therefore, if this is the only autoantibody present, the patient is unlikely to have an autoimmune disease as the cause of the positive ANA. The dense-fine speckled pattern may also be reported on ANA testing by indirect immunofluorescence (IIF); this pattern is highly associated with anti-DFS70 antibody by ELISA.
- Obtain additional studies looking for evidence of immune hyperactivity and/or organ involvement:
  - Complete blood count: Look for anemia of chronic disease, neutropenia, and thrombocytopenia.
  - Liver enzymes: If elevated, consider autoimmune hepatitis.
  - Creatinine, urinalysis: look for evidence of end-organ disease which, if present, would warrant an expedited evaluation.
  - C3, C4: Look for hypocomplementemia.
  - SPEP: Look for polyclonal gammopathy.
  - RF, ESR, PTT (lupus anticoagulant).

If any of these is abnormal, the ANA may be indicative of an evolving autoimmune disease and the patient will need to be followed closely. Note that a history of Hashimoto thyroiditis or Grave disease can be associated with a positive ANA with negative specific autoantibodies.

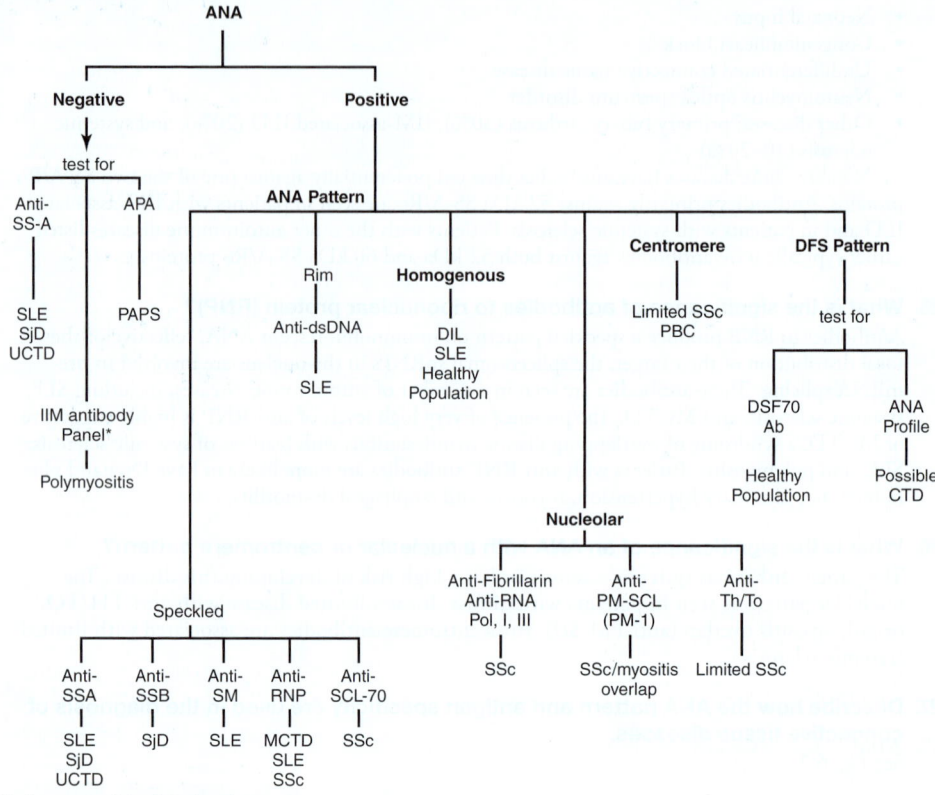

*In the appropriate clinical context
DFS = derse fine speckled
CTD = connective tissue disease

Fig. 6.2 Use of ANA pattern and antigen specific antibody testing in patients with suspected rheumatic disease. *APA*, antiphospholipid antibodies (lupus anticoagulant, anticardiolipin and beta-2 glycoprotein antibodies); *CTD*, connective tissue disease; *DFS*, dense-fine speckled; *DIL*, drug-induced lupus; *MCTD*, mixed connective tissue disease; *PAPS*, primary antiphospholipid syndrome; *RNA Pol*, RNA polymerase; *SCL-70*, topoisomerase I; *SSc*, systemic sclerosis (scleroderma); *UCTD*, undifferentiated connective tissue disease. *Consider ordering in the appropriate clinical context

29. What are RFs, and how are they measured?

Rheumatoid factor (RF) is the general term used to describe an autoantibody directed against antigenic determinants on the Fc fragment of immunoglobulin G. RF may be of any isotype: IgM, IgG, IgA, or IgE. IgM RF is the primary isotype routinely measured by clinical laboratories, using nephelometry, ELISA, and latex agglutination techniques. In RA, RF has sensitivity of 60% to 80% and specificity of 80% to 90%. RA patients who are RF-positive tend to have more aggressive joint disease and are at an increased risk to develop extraarticular manifestations. Disease activity of rheumatoid arthritis is best determined by clinical assessment and not by RF titer. Teleologically, RFs probably developed in humans as a mechanism to help remove immune complexes from circulation. Therefore, many conditions associated with chronic inflammation are also associated with RF positivity.

RF can be positive in normal individuals but usually at a low titer, with males and females affected equally. Age affects the frequency of a positive RF in normal individuals with 2–4% (20–60 years), 5% (60–70 years), and 10–25% (>70 years) positive at low titers.

30. What are the causes of a positive RF?

The common denominator for the production of RF is chronic immune stimulation. The most common diseases associated with RF production are: CHRONIC, as the mnemonic indicates:

CH	Chronic disease, especially hepatic (primary biliary cholangitis [45–70%]) and pulmonary diseases (idiopathic pulmonary fibrosis [10–50%], silicosis [30–50%], asbestosis [30%])
R	Rheumatoid arthritis, 70–85% of patients
O	Other rheumatic diseases, such as SLE (15–35%), systemic sclerosis (20–30%), MCTD (50–60%), SjD (75–95%), polymyositis (5–10%), and sarcoidosis (15%)
N	Neoplasms, especially after radiation or chemotherapy (5–25%)
I	Infections, such as HIV, mononucleosis, parasitic infections (20–90%), chronic viral infections (15–65%), hepatitis B/C (20–75%), chronic bacterial infections (subacute bacterial endocarditis [25–50%], syphilis [5–13%], and others), mycobacterial infections (tuberculosis [8%], leprosy [5–58%])
C	Cryoglobulinemia, 40–100% of patients

31. What are anti-citrullinated protein antibodies (ACPAs) and how are they tested for?

ACPAs are directed against citrulline residues on various proteins formed by post-translational deimination of arginine by the enzyme peptidylarginine deiminase. Commercial assays have been developed to identify some of these antibodies. The tests utilize a cyclic peptide substrate engineered to mimic the shape of proteins in antibody-peptide complexes. The resulting cyclic citrullinated peptide (CCP) results in higher affinity antibody binding than linear peptide substrates, thereby improving the sensitivity of the assay. These antibodies are found in patients with RA with a sensitivity similar to RF (75%) but with increased specificity (90–95%). Notably some RA patients (10%) may be negative for RF but positive for anti-CCP.

There is good evidence for an association of anti-CCP with more rapid radiologic joint damage in RA patients. The high specificity of anti-CCP antibodies helps diagnostically separate RA from other diseases, such as hepatitis C, which can present with polyarthralgias and a positive RF.

32. What is the difference between ACPA and anti-CCP antibodies?

Researchers have identified RA-related autoantibodies directed against specific citrullinated peptides in the synovium, joint fluid, and other target tissues of patients with RA. The term *ACPA* was developed as an umbrella term for this collection of antibodies directed against specific citrullinated peptides. Several potentially important joint-targeted citrullinated autoantigens, including fibrinogen, α-enolase, type II collagen, and vimentin, in RA have been discovered. The exact citrullinated proteins included in the commercially available anti-CCP test, however, are proprietary. As such, it is uncertain how much overlap exists between these assays and the joint-specific targets identified through research. ELISA-based assays using specific joint-targeted peptides have been investigated, including mutated citrullinated vimentin (anti-MCV antibody). In regard to diagnosis, research has not shown a clear role for the testing of individual ACPA assays over commercially available anti-CCP tests. Multiplex assays are currently being investigated that can allow for simultaneous testing of numerous ACPAs. Further investigation is needed to determine if such platforms may improve the sensitivity for the detection of ACPAs in RA patients who are seronegative for RF and anti-CCP.

33. What are ANCAs?

ANCAs are antibodies directed against specific antigens present in the cytoplasm of neutrophils. There are three different types of IIF staining patterns for ANCAs using ethanol-fixed neutrophils as substrate:

- **C-ANCA pattern:** diffuse cytoplasmic staining on immunofluorescence. The most common antibodies causing this pattern are directed against serine PR3. Less commonly, the target antigen is bactericidal/permeability-increasing protein or others.
- **P-ANCA pattern:** perinuclear staining pattern around the nucleus. The most important antibody causing this pattern is directed against MPO. Other antigen targets include elastase, cathepsin G, lactoferrin, lysozyme, and azurocidin.
- **Atypical ANCA pattern:** snow-drift staining pattern around nucleus, with patchy cytoplasmic staining as well, often confused with the P-ANCA pattern. Usually seen in patients with inflammatory bowel disease, connective tissue diseases, or autoimmune hepatitis.

34. Which diseases are associated with ANCAs?

Patients who are ANCA-positive should have ELISA testing for specific antibodies directed against PR3 and MPO, which are the most relevant autoantibodies associated with an underlying systemic necrotizing vasculitis. Other disease associations with C-ANCA and P-ANCA are typically negative for anti-PR3 and anti-MPO antibodies:

- **C-ANCA (PR3-positive):** Granulomatosis with polyangiitis, microscopic polyangiitis (usually P-ANCA), eosinophilic granulomatosis with polyangiitis (rare)
- **P-ANCA (MPO-positive):** Microscopic polyangiitis, eosinophilic granulomatosis with polyangiitis, pauci-immune glomerulonephritis (renal-limited vasculitis), Goodpasture's disease, drug-induced syndromes (hydralazine, propylthiouracil, minocycline, others)
- **P-ANCA (MPO-negative):** Autoimmune gastrointestinal disorders (ulcerative colitis, primary sclerosing cholangitis, autoimmune hepatitis), rheumatic diseases (RA, SLE, many others), cystic fibrosis, HIV infection, certain other acute and chronic infectious or neoplastic diseases (rare)
- **Anti-HNE:** Antibodies against human neutrophil elastase are commonly seen in ANCA-positive disease associated with cocaine. The ANCA staining pattern is often atypical or perinuclear, but can be cytoplasmic or have multiple patterns.

> **PEARL:** If C-ANCA is not against PR3, or P-ANCA is not against MPO, look for causes other than vasculitis for the positive ANCA.

35. Do ANCA titers fluctuate with disease activity?

This is controversial. There is some evidence among patients with granulomatosis with polyangiitis (who are PR3-positive), especially those treated with rituximab, that rising titers of C-ANCA or PR3 can correlate with disease activity. In addition, in patients treated with rituximab who subsequently become C-ANCA/PR3-negative, absence of antibody coupled with undetectable peripheral B-cell counts is associated with a low risk of flare. However, patients with stable or negative ANCA titers have been known to flare, while those with rising titers may not, indicating that changes in ANCA titers need to be coupled with clinical assessment to inform decisions on subsequent therapy. There is little evidence that P-ANCA titers fluctuate with disease activity.

36. What are the causes of decreased circulating complement components?

Serum complement may be decreased as a result of:
1. Decreased production, owing to either a hereditary deficiency or liver disease (complement components are synthesized in the liver).
2. Increased consumption (proteolysis) as a result of complement activation. A major cause of complement consumption is increased levels of circulating immune complexes, which activate the classical complement pathway.

37. What clinical conditions are associated with hereditary complement deficiencies?

See Table 6.6.

TABLE 6.6 Conditions Associated with Hereditary Complement Deficiencies

COMPLEMENT COMPONENTS	DISEASE
Early (C1, C2, C4)	SLE-like disease Glomerulonephritis
Mid (C3, C4)	Recurrent pyogenic infections SLE-like disease
Terminal (C5–C9)	Recurrent infections (especially gonococci and meningococci)
Regulatory proteins	HAE (C1INH), aHUS (Factor H, Factor I, MCP), AMD (Factor H, Factor I), PNH (CD55/DAF & CD59)

aHUS, atypical hemolytic uremic syndrome; *AMD,* age-related macular degeneration; *C1INH,* C1-esterase inhibitor; *DAF,* decay-accelerating factor; *HAE,* hereditary angioedema; *MCP,* membrane cofactor protein; *PNH,* paroxysmal nocturnal hemoglobinuria; *SLE,* systemic lupus erythematosus.

38. Can a patient with active inflammation involving circulating immune complexes have a normal complement level?

Yes. The serum level of complement components represents a balance between consumption and production. Complement components are acute-phase reactants, so their production by the liver increases with inflammatory states. If increased production keeps pace with consumption, the result will be a normal level of complement. Clinically, this means that while a decreased level of complement (C3, C4) is confirmatory evidence for complement consumption, normal complement levels cannot exclude complement consumption.

39. What diseases are associated with decreased levels of complement (not hereditary deficiency)?

- Rheumatic diseases
  - SLE
  - Systemic vasculitis (especially polyarteritis nodosa, urticarial vasculitis)
  - Cryoglobulinemia (types II and III)
  - RA with extraarticular manifestations (rare)
- Infectious diseases
  - Subacute bacterial endocarditis
  - Bacterial sepsis (pneumococcal, gram-negative)
  - Viremias (especially hepatitis B)
  - Parasitemias
- Glomerulonephritis
  - Post-streptococcal
  - Membranoproliferative

40. What complement components should one order?

- Complement components (**C3** and **C4**): measured by nephelometry. Low levels of both C3 and C4 indicate classic complement pathway activation usually by immune complexes. Alternative complement pathway activation is indicated by low levels of C3 with normal C4. A normal C3 but low C4 suggests heterozygous C4 deficiency or low-level complement pathway activation.
- **CH50** (total hemolytic complement assay): the test name describes how the measurement is carried out, by assessing the ability of serum complement to hemolyze sheep RBCs that have been sensitized with rabbit IgM. Only in the presence of all nine complement components will the antibody activate complement, form the membrane attack complex, and lead to cell lysis. As such, it is a good screen for complement deficiency. A CH50 level of 0 or "unmeasurable" is suggestive of a hereditary homozygous complement deficiency and should prompt testing for individual complement levels (C2 is the most common homozygous deficiency, followed by C4 and C1q). It is not a good disease activity marker as in active inflammation its level can be either low, normal, or high, reflecting the end result of balance between production and consumption of the complement components.

41. How do you separate iron deficiency anemia (IDA) from anemia of chronic disease (ACD) in a patient with a chronic inflammatory disease like RA?

In patients with uncomplicated IDA, measurement of iron status with serum level of iron (low), percent iron saturation (low), total iron-binding capacity (TIBC; high), and ferritin (low) are adequate. However, in patients with inflammatory disease, TIBC can be elevated and ferritin can be normal as a result of the acute-phase response. Thus, to separate IDA from ACD, the gold standard is a bone marrow biopsy. However, studies have shown that serum ferritin >100 ng/mL excludes iron deficiency in patients with an active inflammatory disease as indicated by an elevated ESR/CRP. Likewise, serum ferritin <50–60 ng/mL, particularly when associated with an elevated serum transferrin receptor level, is highly specific for IDA in patients with RA.

42. Other than an elevated ESR, CRP, and ACD, what additional tests suggest systemic inflammation?

Patients with a systemic inflammatory disease such as vasculitis frequently have a reactive thrombocytosis, mild elevation of hepatic alkaline phosphatase, and low albumin. The low albumin is due to hepatic synthesis of acute-phase reactants at the expense of albumin.

43. What is the Vectra® test? What is the 14-3-3η (eta) test?

The **Vectra**® test is a multibiomarker assay that can be measured in patients with RA as a disease activity assessment tool. This test measures 12 immune, endothelial, bone, cartilage, and metabolic protein biomarkers (VCAM-1, EGF, VEGF-A, IL-6, TNF-RI, MMP-1, MMP-3, YKL-40, leptin, resistin, SAA, CRP) that are involved in the underlying biology of RA. Serum concentrations of the biomarkers are integrated into a proprietary algorithm that generates a single score from 1 to 100 that classifies disease activity as high (>45), moderate (30–44), or low (1–29). Studies report a good correlation with clinical disease activity measures (disease activity score 28 or DAS28, clinical disease activity index or CDAI, and simplified disease activity index or SDAI). The test may be used as an adjunctive measure of disease activity in specific patients, but data do not suggest a role for routine use in all patients alongside traditional clinical markers of disease activity.

PEARL: Studies have shown that test results may be influenced by tocilizumab independent of disease activity. Tocilizumab results in elevation of serum IL-6 levels, resulting in higher Vectra® scores and loss of correlation with other clinical disease activity measures.

The **14-3-3η (eta) protein** is one of seven isoforms of the 14-3-3 protein family, which are ubiquitous intracellular chaperones that regulate communication pathways involved in inflammation. Patients with RA and erosive psoriatic arthritis have high levels of this protein in the synovial fluid. The protein is thought to be secreted by synovial fibroblasts and synovial macrophages. Recent studies have demonstrated an association between elevated serum levels and subsequent evolution from undifferentiated arthritis to RA and/or erosive arthritis. This protein can be quantified in the serum through a commercially available ELISA test. Of note, elevated serum levels can be seen in a small percentage of healthy patients (15%), while established RA patients under good control can have normal values.

It is uncertain whether these two testing platforms offer additional benefits beyond traditional clinical disease activity measurements (CDAI, DAS28) or markers of disease presence (RF, CCP, CRP). Further investigation is needed.

BIBLIOGRAPHY

Andersson M, Cronstein, B. Acute phase reactants. *Firestein and Kelley's Textbook of Rheumatology*. 12th ed. Elsevier: Philadelphia; 2024:907–919.

Buhaescu I, Yood RA. Serum procalcitonin in systemic autoimmune diseases—where are we now? *Semin Arthritis Rheum*. 2010;40(2):176–183.

Bultink IEM, Lems WF, Vande Stadt RJ. Ferritin and serum transferrin receptor predict iron deficiency in anemic patients with rheumatoid arthritis. *Arthritis Rheum*. 2001;44:979–981.

Curtis JR, van der Helm-van Mil AH, Knevel R, et al. Validation of a novel multi-biomarker test to assess rheumatoid arthritis disease activity. *Arthritis Care Res*. 2012;64:1794–1803.

Darrah E, Rosen A, Andrade F. Autoantibodies in RA. *Firestein and Kelley's Textbook of Rheumatology*. 12th ed. Elsevier: Philadelphia; 2024:890–906.

Fussner LA, Hummel AM, Schroeder DR, et al. Factors determining the clinical utility of serial measurements of antineutrophil cytoplasmic antibodies targeting proteinase 3. *Arthritis Rheumatol*. 2016;68:1700–1710.

Kratz A, Plebani M. ICSH recommendations for modified and alternnate methods measuring the erythrocyte sedimentation rate. *Int J Lab Hem*. 2017;39:448–457.

Miller A, Green M, Robinson B. Simple rule for calculating a normal erythrocyte sedimentation rate. *Br Med J*. 1983;286:266.

Peng SL, Craft JE. Anti-nuclear antibodies. *Firestein and Kelley's Textbook of Rheumatology*. 12th ed. Elsevier: Philadelphia; 2024:875–889.

Serio I, Arnaud L. Can procalcitonin be used to distinguish between disease flare and infection in patients with systemic lupus erythematosus: a systematic literature review. *Clin Rheumatol*. 2014;33:1209–1215.

Shaikh MM, Hermans LE. Is serum procalcitonin measurement a useful addition to a rheumatologist's repertoire? A review of its diagnostic role in systemic inflammatory diseases and joint infections. *Rheumatology (Oxford)*. 2015;54(2):231–240.

Shmerling RH. Diagnostic tests for rheumatic disease: clinical utility revisited. *So Med J*. 2005;98:704.

Steen VD. Autoantibodies in systemic sclerosis. *Semin Arthritis Rheum*. 2005;35:35–42.

Wener MH, Daum PR, McQuillan GM. The influence of age, sex, and race on the upper reference limit of serum C-reactive protein concentration. *J Rheumatol*. 2000;27:2351–2359.

Arthrocentesis, Synovial Fluid Analysis, and Synovial Biopsy

Sterling G. West, MD and Liudmila Kastsianok, MD

CHAPTER 7

 KEY POINTS

1. Aspirate any monoarticular inflammatory arthritis.
2. The synovial fluid analysis should be viewed as a liquid biopsy of the joint.
3. The most important tests to send synovial fluid for are cell count, crystal examination, Gram stain, and culture.
4. The synovial fluid analysis can determine if the arthritis is noninflammatory, inflammatory, hemarthrosis, crystalline, or infectious.
5. Synovial biopsy is critical to help establish a diagnosis in a patient with a chronic monoarticular inflammatory arthritis.

1. When should arthrocentesis be performed?

Undoubtedly, the single most important reason to perform arthrocentesis is to check for joint infection. Timely identification and treatment of a patient with septic arthritis is of paramount importance to a favorable clinical outcome. Furthermore, arthrocentesis is generally indicated to gain diagnostic information through synovial fluid analysis in the patient with a monoarticular or polyarticular arthropathy of unclear etiology characterized by joint pain and swelling.

2. When is arthrocentesis contraindicated?

When the clinical indication for obtaining synovial fluid is strong, such as in the patient with suspected septic arthritis, there is no absolute contraindication to joint aspiration. Relative contraindications include **bleeding diatheses,** such as hemophilia, anticoagulation therapy, or severe thrombocytopenia; however, these conditions can be frequently treated or reversed before arthrocentesis. **Cellulitis** overlying a swollen joint can make the approach to the joint space difficult, but this rarely precludes the ability to perform the procedure. **Bacteremia** confers a small risk to seeding a joint with microorganisms during the arthrocentesis.

3. How safe is arthrocentesis in patients on warfarin (Coumadin)? Direct oral anticoagulants (DOACs)?

Although hemarthrosis has been reported following joint aspiration in anticoagulated patients, it appears to be uncommon. A previous study found no hemorrhagic complications in patients on Coumadin with an international normalized ratio of <4.5. Using the smallest needle necessary for the procedure and applying prolonged pressure following the arthrocentesis are recommended. The bleeding risk in patients taking warfarin with INR 2–3 is 0.2% or lower. There is no need to withhold DOACs before doing an arthrocentesis.

4. What techniques should be used when performing an arthrocentesis of the knee to rule out a septic joint?

The procedure should be performed using an **aseptic technique.** A topical antiseptic should be applied to the area. Nonsterile gloves should always be worn as part of universal precautions. Sterile gloves should be used if palpation of the area is foreseen after antiseptic preparation and before placement of the needle. A 25-gauge needle should be used to administer a local anesthetic (e.g., 1% lidocaine without epinephrine). The aspiration itself should be performed using an 18-, 20-, or 21-gauge, 1.5-inch needle, when possible, and a 10-mL to 30-mL syringe. Aspiration techniques for other individual joints are described elsewhere. Ultrasonography can be a useful bedside tool for guiding needle placement for aspiration.

5. What precautions should be taken if the patient is "allergic" to povidone–iodine, lidocaine, or latex?

- Patients with topical iodine reactions can have their skin cleansed with chlorhexidine or pHisoHex followed by an alcohol pad.
- True "caine" allergy is extremely rare. Many of the symptoms that occur during dental procedures are due to the epinephrine or preservatives (parabens) in the lidocaine (Xylocaine) and not an IgE-mediated reaction. To be absolutely sure, skin testing and subcutaneous incremental challenge would have to be done. This is usually not practical; therefore, options include numbing the area with a skin refrigerant (ethyl chloride) only or using a local anesthetic from the benzoic acid ester group that does not cross-react with lidocaine, such as chloroprocaine (Nesacaine). Note that a patient with a procaine (Novocain) reaction can use lidocaine (Xylocaine).
- Most latex allergies are minor local reactions. However, some patients can have a severe latex allergy. In these patients, arthrocentesis must be performed using latex-free gloves and syringes. The rubber stopper on the top of the lidocaine must be removed because sticking a needle through this can result in latex protein being introduced into the lidocaine.

6. What are the potential complications of arthrocentesis?

- Infection (risk <1 in 10,000)
- Bleeding/hemarthrosis
- Vasovagal syncope
- Pain
- Cartilage injury or nerve damage.

7. Where does normal synovial fluid come from?

Synovial fluid is a selective transudate of plasma. Large molecules such as clotting factors are excluded, and therefore normal synovial fluid does not clot spontaneously. Synovial fluid is viscous like an egg white (synovial is derived from *ovum*, Latin for egg) due to hyaluronic acid produced by fibroblast-derived type B synoviocytes and contributes to the lubricating function of the fluid. With inflammation, cells with their degradative enzymes enter the joint cavity breaking down the hyaluronans causing the synovial fluid to become less viscous. In addition, clotting factors gain entry causing the synovial fluid to clot spontaneously.

8. What studies should be performed for synovial fluid analysis?

Visual inspection commenting on synovial fluid clarity and color should be performed. Because the single most important determination of synovial fluid analysis is for the presence of infection, **Gram stain** and **culture** should be performed on samples from joints with even relatively low suspicion for infection. Determining **total leukocyte count** and **differential** helps in differentiating between noninflammatory and inflammatory joint conditions. Lastly, **polarized microscopy** should be performed to look for the presence of pathological crystals. Chemistry determinations, such as glucose and total protein, are unlikely to yield helpful information beyond that obtained by previous studies; therefore, they should not be routinely ordered. Normal synovial fluid glucose is within 20 mg/dL of the serum value unless inflammation or infection is present. Normal synovial fluid protein averages around 2 g/dL (33% of the serum total protein) and increases with inflammation. Lactate dehydrogenase, uric acid, pH, electrolytes, and immunological studies are of no value and should not be ordered. New techniques to detect indolent infections including PCR using organism-specific primers or amplifying bacterial 16S ribosomal sequences may be useful but are less sensitive on synovial fluid than synovial tissue. Synovial fluid alpha-defensin levels are elevated in >95% of periprosthetic joint infections.

9. What if no synovial fluid is obtained (a "dry tap")?

Even if no fluid is aspirated into the syringe, frequently one or two drops of fluid and/or blood can be found within the needle and its hub. This amount is sufficient for culture, in which case the syringe with a capped needle should be submitted to the microbiology laboratory. If one extra drop can be spared, it can be placed on a microscope slide with a coverslip for estimated cell count (1 white blood cell [WBC]/40 × objective = 500 WBCs) and polarized microscopy. When microscopy is completed, the coverslip can be removed, and the specimen may then serve as a smear for Gram stain. The specimen remaining on the coverslip may be an adequate smear on which to perform a Wright stain, allowing determination of leukocyte differential. Thus, two drops of fluid can yield the same important diagnostic information as that obtained from a larger specimen, with the exception of a leukocyte count. The lesson to be learned from this is that when a "dry tap" is encountered, the needle and syringe should not be reflexively discarded.

10. What are some causes of "dry taps"?

Inability to obtain synovial fluid from a joint with an obvious effusion can be because of
- Synovial fluid is too thick to aspirate through the lumen of a needle.
- Obstruction of the needle lumen with debris such as rice bodies (infarcted pieces of synovium in synovial fluid) or thick fibrin.
- Chronically inflamed synovium can undergo fat replacement and become markedly thickened (lipoma arborescens), so that the needle never makes it into the effusion.
- In the knee, a medial plica or medial fat pad (especially in obese patients) may block the needle. In this case, aspirate from the lateral aspect of the knee.
- Poor technique and not getting into the joint with a needle. Ultrasonography for needle placement can avoid this cause of a dry tap.

11. Within what time frame should synovial fluid analysis occur?

Synovial fluid should be analyzed as soon as possible after the fluid is drawn. If it is delayed for >6 hours, results may be spuriously altered. Problems that can arise include:
- Decrease in leukocyte count (due to cell disruption).
- Decrease in number of crystals (primarily calcium pyrophosphate dihydrate [CPPD]).
- Appearance of artifactual crystals.

12. How may synovial fluid WBC count be estimated by "wet drop" examination?

When microscopy is performed, the synovial fluid WBC count can be easily estimated. The finding of two or fewer WBCs per high-power field (40 × high dry objective) confidently suggests a noninflammatory fluid (<2000 WBCs/mm^3). If greater than four WBCs per high-power field are seen, there is a significant risk that the synovial fluid is inflammatory, and formal determination of the WBC count should be ordered. The rule of thumb is that one WBC seen at 40 × objective estimates 500 cells in total WBC count. For example, if you observe 10 WBCs in a 40 × field, the estimated cell count would be 5000/mm^3.

13. Describe the classification based on synovial fluid analysis.

Synovial fluid classification is given in Table 7.1.

14. Name some causes of noninflammatory (group 1) joint effusions.

Osteoarthritis, joint trauma, mechanical derangement, pigmented villonodular synovitis, prosthetic wear, and avascular necrosis.

TABLE 7.1 Synovial Fluid Classification

		Total White Blood Cells	
FLUID TYPE	**APPEARANCE**	**COUNT/mm³**	**% POLYMORPHONUCLEAR CELLS**
Normal	Clear, viscous, pale yellow	0–200	<10
Group 1 (noninflammatory)	Clear to slightly turbid	200–2000	<20
Group 2 (inflammatory)	Slightly turbid	2000–50,000	20–75
Group 3 (pyarthrosis)	Turbid to very turbid	>50,000–100,000	>75

BOX 7.1 Rheumatic Disorders With Group 2 (Inflammatory) Synovial Fluid

Rheumatoid arthritis	Polyarteritis nodosa
Gout	Familial Mediterranean fever
Pseudogout	Sarcoidosis
Psoriatic arthritis	Infectious arthritis
Ankylosing spondylitis	Viral (hepatitis B, rubella, HIV, parvovirus, others)
Reactive arthritis	Bacterial (gonococci)
Juvenile idiopathic arthritis	Fungal
Rheumatic fever	Mycobacterial
Systemic lupus erythematosus	Spirochetal (Lyme disease, syphilis)
Polymyalgia rheumatic	Subacute bacterial endocarditis
Giant cell arteritis	Palindromic rheumatism
Granulomatosis with polyangiitis	
Hypersensitivity vasculitis	

---

15. Group 2 (inflammatory) synovial fluid is typical for which rheumatic disorders?

Typical rheumatic disorders for group 2 (inflammatory) synovial fluid are given in Box 7.1.

16. Other than joint sepsis, which conditions are associated with a group 3 fluid (pyarthrosis)?

When a group 3 fluid is discovered, septic arthritis must be assumed until proven otherwise by synovial fluid culture. A few disorders may cause noninfectious pyarthrosis, sometimes referred to as joint **pseudosepsis.**
- Crystal: gout more commonly than pseudogout.
- Reactive arthritis.
- Rheumatoid arthritis.

17. How does the synovial fluid WBC differential help in diagnosing an inflammatory arthritis?

- Neutrophil predominance: most inflammatory synovial fluids. Septic arthritis and crystalline arthropathies have >90–95% polymorphonuclear cells (PMNs).
  - Ragocytes are neutrophils that have ingested immune complexes: consider rheumatoid arthritis, septic arthritis, and crystalline arthritides where ragocytes account for more than 50–70% of all nucleated cells in the synovial fluid.
- Lymphocyte predominance (>70%): consider systemic lupus erythematosus and mycobacterial infections.
- Macrophage predominance (>80%): consider spondyloarthropathies, "Milwaukee shoulder."
  - Lipid-laden macrophages: traumatic, pancreatic disease.
- Monocyte predominance (>80%): consider viral arthritis, serum sickness, and spondyloarthropathies.
- Eosinophil predominance: hypereosinophilia syndrome, parasitic arthritides, arthrography (dye), therapeutic radiation, metastatic adenocarcinoma, idiopathic.
- Mast cells present: consider spondyloarthropathies and systemic mastocytosis.

18. List some causes of hemarthrosis (see Chapter 48: Arthropathies Associated With Hematologic Diseases).

- Trauma
- Bleeding diatheses
- Tumors
- Pigmented villonodular synovitis
- Hemangiomas
- Scurvy
- Iatrogenic (post procedure)
- Arteriovenous fistula
- Intense inflammatory disease
- Charcot's joint

PEARL: Fat/lipid droplets (look like bubbles) in bloody synovial fluid (may have tomato soup appearance) should suggest subchondral fracture if the joint has been traumatized or avascular necrosis.

TABLE 7.2 Comparison of Polarized Light Microscopic Findings of Synovial Fluid From a Joint With Gout and a Joint With Pseudogout

	GOUT	PSEUDOGOUT
Crystal	Urate	Calcium pyrophosphate dihydrate
Shape	Needle	Rhomboid or rectangular
Birefringence	Negative	Positive
Color of crystals parallel to axis of red-plate compensator	Yellow	Blue

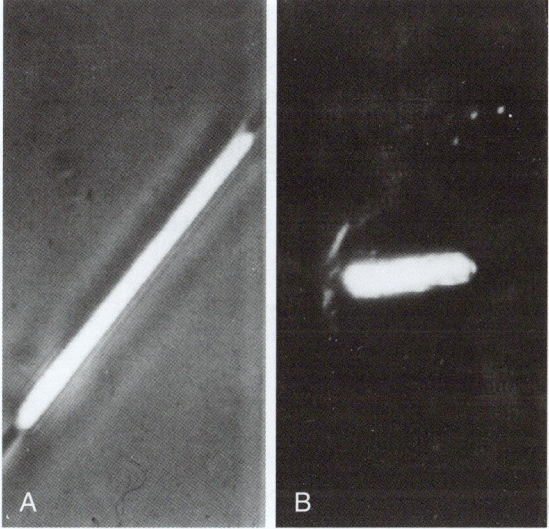

Fig. 7.1 (A) Urate crystal of gout, showing needle shape. (B) Calcium pyrophosphate dihydrate crystal of pseudogout, showing rhomboid shape.

19. Compare the polarized light microscopic findings of synovial fluid from a joint with gout and one with pseudogout.

A comparison of polarized light microscopic findings of synovial fluid from a joint with gout and pseudogout is given in Table 7.2.

PEARL: For the crystal color, use the mnemonic **ABC** (alignment, blue, calcium). If the crystal aligned with the red-plate compensator is blue, it is CPPD. Urate crystals are the opposite, being yellow when parallel to the compensator. Crystals within WBCs are more indicative of crystalline arthropathy than free-floating crystals. Note that hydroxyapatite crystals are too small to see with polarized light (Fig. 7.1).

20. Are there any "tricks" to increase the yield of finding uric acid crystals in a patient who clinically has gout?

Occasionally, you may encounter a patient who clinically has gout, but you cannot find crystals on synovial fluid examination. Some "tricks" that have been tried are to centrifuge the fluid and examine the centrifugate for crystals (especially helpful for CPPD crystals). Another trick is to cool the fluid in the refrigerator, although this usually does not work. Finally, putting fluid on a microscope slide and allowing it to dry for 2 to 3 hours may allow overhydrated uric acid crystals to dehydrate and be drawn toward each other to form spherules that are easier to see.

21. What special stains can be done on the cytocentrifuge preparation to help establish the diagnosis?

- Wright stain.

  Lupus erythematosus cell: PMNs with ingested homogeneous nuclear material.

  Reiter's cell: large macrophage with ingested PMNs (cytophagocytic mononuclear cells).

  Hydroxyapatite crystals in PMNs.

  Charcot–Leyden crystals in eosinophils.
- Alizarin Red S: stains calcium crystals (hydroxyapatite and CPPD).
- Oil Red O/Sudan Black: stains for fat globules.
- Congo Red: stains amyloid fragments.

22. What are the indications to perform a synovial biopsy?

The main indication for a synovial biopsy is chronic (>6–8 weeks), nontraumatic, inflammatory (synovial fluid white blood cell count >2000 cells/mm^3) arthritis limited to one or a few joints in which the diagnosis has not been made by history, physical examination, laboratory studies, or synovial fluid analysis with culture (including both fungi and mycobacteria). The most important diagnosis to rule out is septic arthritis. PCR testing for bacterial and fungal infections is more accurate using synovial tissue than synovial fluid.

Synovial biopsies are also important for research purposes to assess the pathophysiology of various arthritides and response to various treatments.

23. What diseases can be diagnosed with a synovial biopsy?

- Chronic infections
  - Fungal arthritis
  - Mycobacterial arthritis including leprosy
  - Spirochetal arthritis (Lyme disease, syphilis)
  - Whipple's disease
  - Chlamydia
  - Parasitic arthritis
- Other systemic diseases
  - Plant thorns and foreign body
  - Camptodactyly-arthropathy-coxa vara-pericarditis syndrome
  - Chronic sarcoidosis
  - Erdheim-Chester disease
- Infiltrative/deposition diseases*
  - Multicentric reticulohistiocytosis
  - Amyloidosis
  - Pancreatic fat necrosis
  - Ochronosis
  - Hemochromatosis
  - Crystal-induced arthritis
- Tumors
  - Pigmented villonodular synovitis
  - Synovial osteochondromatosis
  - Synovial cell sarcoma
  - Leukemia/lymphoma
  - Metastatic disease to the joint
  - Synovial hemangioma
  - Lipoma arborescent
- Notably, up to 65% of chronic monoarticular arthritides (usually the knee) remain undiagnosed even after a synovial biopsy and analysis.

24. Does a synovial biopsy help in the diagnosis of a systemic connective tissue disease such as rheumatoid arthritis (RA)?

No. Although a synovial biopsy in a patient with RA may be compatible with the diagnosis, it is not pathognomonic. Clearly, spondyloarthropathies can produce synovial biopsies that look very much like those obtained from patients with RA although prominent plasma cell infiltration suggests RA. In the future, synovial biopsies with histological and molecular analysis may better predict what biological therapy a patient is most likely to respond to.

25. How can synovial tissue be obtained and what are the advantages and disadvantages of each method?

An ultrasound-guided forceps biopsy has advantages/disadvantages similar to a needle biopsy but can indirectly visualize the best site to biopsy, which lessens sampling error.

	Advantages	*Disadvantages*
Closed needle biopsy	Least expensive Least traumatic One skin incision	Small biopsy specimens Sampling error
Ultrasound-guided: needle or portal + forceps Needle arthroscopic biopsy	Less sampling error Minimally invasive Direct visualization	Small biopsy specimens Two skin incisions Moderately expensive
Arthroscopic biopsy	Direct visualization Large biopsy specimen	Expensive Invasive

26. Which joints can be biopsied?

Any joint can be biopsied depending on the technique and instrumentation chosen. Usually, large joints, most commonly the knee, are biopsied. Smaller joints can be biopsied also but require a special needle.

27. How many specimens must be obtained to minimize sampling error?

Taking six to eight specimens from multiple locations in the joint being biopsied reduces sampling error and leads to biopsy specimen variability of <10%. Using an ultrasound to guide biopsy sites can increase the yield.

28. What is the complication rate for obtaining a synovial biopsy by arthroscopy? What about ultrasound-guided synovial biopsy (UGSB)?

The total complication rate for arthroscopy by a needle or large bore method is similar—15/1000 arthroscopies. This includes temporary joint swelling in 10%, hemarthrosis in 0.9%, deep vein thrombosis in 0.2%, and joint infection in 0.1% of cases.

The complication rate for UGSB ranges from 1.5–11.2%. Most complications are minor and self-limiting (e.g., presyncope, mild arthralgia, minor bleeding, and transient nerve block). Major complications are reported infrequently (up to 0.24%), such as nerve injury, tendon limitation, and instrument failure.

BIBLIOGRAPHY

Ahmed I, Gertner E. Safety of arthrocentesis and joint injection in patients receiving anticoagulation at therapeutic levels. *Am J Med*. 2012;125:265–269.

Clayburne G, Daniel DG, Schumacher HR. Estimated synovial fluid leukocyte numbers on wet drop preparations as a potential substitute for actual leukocyte counts. *J Rheumatol*. 1992;19:60.

El-Gabalawy HS, Tanner S. Synovial fluid analysis, synovial biopsy, and synovial pathology. In: Firestein GS, Budd RS, Gabriel SE, Koretzky GA, McInnes IB, O'Dell JR, eds. *Firestein and Kelley's Textbook of Rheumatology*. 11th ed. Philadelphia: Elsevier; 2021:841–858.

Gatter RA, Andrews RP, Cooley DA, et al. American College of Rheumatology guidelines for performing office synovial fluid examinations. *J Clin Rheumatol*. 1995;1:194–200.

Humby F, Romao VC, Manzo A, et al. A multicenter retrospective analysis evaluating performance of synovial biopsy techniques in patients with inflammatory arthritis. *Arthritis Rheumatol*. 2018;70:702–710.

Ingegnoli F, Coletto LA, Scotti I, et al. The crucial questions on synovial biopsy: when, why, what, where, and how? *Front Med*. 2021;8:705382.

Kerolus G, Clayburne G, Schumacher HR. Is it mandatory to examine synovial fluids promptly after arthrocentesis? *Arthritis Rheum*. 1989;32:271.

Lee YS, Koo KH, Kim HJ, et al. Synovial fluid biomarkers for the diagnosis of periprosthetic joint infection: a systematic review and meta-analysis. *J Bone Joint Surg*. 2017;99:2077–2084.

Roberts WN, Hayes CW, Breitbach SA, et al. Dry taps and what to do about them: a pictorial essay on failed arthrocentesis of the knee. *Am J Med*. 1996;100:461.

Saraiva F. Ultrasound-guided synovial biopsy: a review. *Front Med*. 2021;8:632224.

Yui J, Preskill C, Greenlund L. Arthrocentesis and Joint injection in patients receiving direct oral anticoagulants. *Mayo Clin Proc*. 2017;92:1223–1226.

CHAPTER 8

Radiographic and Imaging Modalities

Colin Strickland, MD and Mary Elizabeth Buchanan, MD

 KEY POINTS

1. Inflammatory arthritis causes periarticular osteopenia, marginal erosions, and uniform joint space narrowing.
2. Noninflammatory, degenerative arthritis causes sclerosis, osteophytes, nonuniform joint space narrowing, and cyst formation.
3. Chronic tophaceous gout typically causes erosions with a sclerotic margin and overhanging edge in peripheral small joints.
4. Sacroiliitis, best seen on a modified anteroposterior Ferguson view of the sacrum, is the radiologic hallmark of inflammatory axial arthropathy.

1. Is there a pattern approach to interpreting a plain radiograph for arthritis?

In assessing a skeletal radiograph, a pattern approach using the mnemonic **ABCDES** can be very helpful.

A —Alignment: Rheumatoid arthritis (RA) and systemic lupus erythematosus (SLE) are characterized by deformities, such as ulnar deviation at metacarpophalangeal (MCP) joints.
—Ankylosis: Seronegative spondyloarthropathies frequently cause ankylosis. Prior surgical arthrodesis or infection are additional causes.

B —Bone mineralization: Periarticular osteopenia is typical of RA or infection and is rare in crystalline arthropathy, seronegative spondyloarthropathies, and osteoarthritis (OA).
—Bone formation: Reactive bone formation (periostitis) is the hallmark of seronegative spondyloarthropathies. Osteophytosis is seen in OA and calcium pyrophosphate deposition disease (CPPD) and can be present in any end-stage arthritis.

C —Calcifications: Soft tissue calcific densities may be seen in gouty tophi, SLE, or scleroderma. Cartilage calcification is typical of CPPD.
—Cartilage space: Symmetric and uniform cartilage loss results in radiographic joint space narrowing that is typical of inflammatory disease. Focal or nonuniform joint space loss in the area of maximal stress in weight-bearing joints is the hallmark of OA.

D —Distribution of joints: Symmetric distribution of affected joints suggests an inflammatory arthropathy such as RA, whereas OA commonly results in asymmetric joint involvement. Specific sites of involvement may facilitate the differentiation of arthritides. Distal interphalangeal joint involvement, for example, is common in OA and psoriatic arthritis.
—Deformities: Swan neck or boutonniere deformities of the hands are typical of RA.

E —Erosions: In addition to their presence or absence, the character of erosions may be diagnostic, as with overhanging edges and sclerotic margins in gout. Marginal erosions are more suggestive of an inflammatory arthropathy such as RA.

S —Soft tissue and nails: Look for distribution of soft tissue swelling, nail hypertrophy in psoriatic arthritis, and sclerodactyly in scleroderma.
—Speed of development of changes: Septic arthritis will rapidly destroy the affected joint.

> **PEARL:** When obtaining radiographs on patients with arthritis, always order weight-bearing radiographs to evaluate joint space narrowing in lower extremity joints (hip, knee, ankles).

2. Describe the radiographic features of inflammatory arthritis (synovial-based diseases).

1. Soft tissue swelling
2. Periarticular osteopenia
3. Uniform loss of cartilage (diffuse joint space narrowing best seen in weight-bearing joints)
4. Bony erosion in "bare" areas

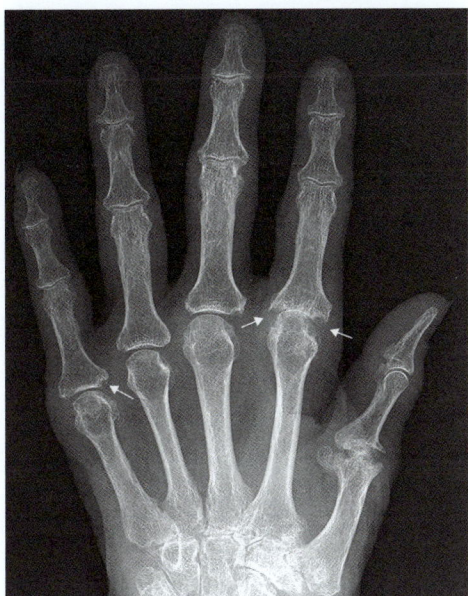

Fig. 8.1 Radiograph of a hand showing marginal erosions (arrows) and subtle periarticular osteopenia indicative of inflammatory arthropathy.

Synovial inflammation causes soft tissue swelling. The inflammation also results in hyperemia, which, coupled with the inflammatory mediators released (such as prostaglandin E2), causes periarticular (juxtaarticular) osteopenia. With chronicity, inflammatory arthritis may lead to more diffuse demineralization (due to disuse and other factors) of the joints due to pain. As the inflammation leads to synovial hypertrophy and pannus formation, the pannus erodes into the bone. These erosions occur first in the marginal "bare areas" where synovium abuts bone that does not possess protective cartilage (Fig. 8.1). The pannus ultimately extends over the cartilaginous surface and/or erodes through the bone to the undersurface of the cartilage. Cartilage destruction results either by enzymatic action of the inflamed synovium and/or by interference with normal cartilage nutrition. Owing to its generalized nature, this cartilage destruction is radiographically seen as uniform or symmetric, diffuse joint space narrowing observed best in weight-bearing joints. It is important to remember that some findings of degenerative arthritis may be superimposed on those of an inflammatory nature, particularly in long-standing cases.

3. What is the "bare area"? Why do the earliest erosions begin here?

In synovial articulations, hyaline articular cartilage covers the ends of both articulating bones. The articular capsule envelops the joint cavity and is composed of an outer fibrous capsule and a thin inner synovial membrane. The synovial membrane typically does not extend over cartilaginous surfaces but lines the nonarticular portion of the synovial joint and also covers the intracapsular bone surfaces that are not covered by cartilage. These unprotected bony areas occur at the peripheral aspect of the joint and are referred to as "bare areas" (Fig. 8.2).

In these areas, the bone does not have a protective cartilage covering. Consequently, the inflamed synovial pannus, which occurs in inflammatory arthritides such as RA, comes in direct contact with bone, resulting in marginal erosions. These "bare areas" are where you should look for the earliest evidence of erosions. Specialized views including the Norgaard view (ball-catcher's view) of the hands are optimal for demonstrating the earliest erosive changes in an inflammatory peripheral arthritis, whereas the anteroposterior Ferguson view of the sacroiliac joints demonstrates the earliest changes in an inflammatory axial arthropathy. With progression of disease, the pannus proliferates to cover the cartilage surfaces, resulting in cartilage destruction (radiographically apparent as joint space narrowing) and more diffuse bony erosions.

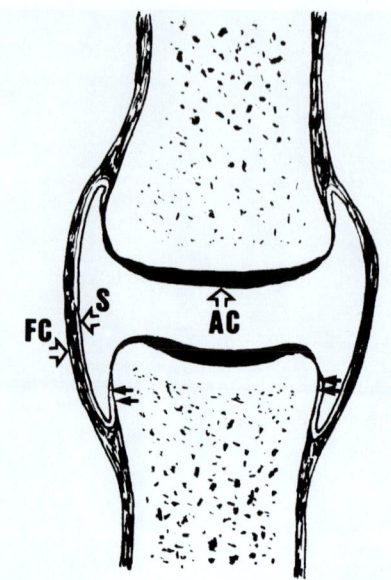

Fig. 8.2 Diagram of a typical synovial joint. Small black arrows indicate the "bare areas" where bone is exposed to synovium without overlying cartilage. *AC,* articular cartilage; *FC,* fibrous capsule; *S,* synovium.

4. List the rheumatic disease categories that typically cause radiographic features of inflammatory arthritis.

- RA (adult and juvenile)
- Seronegative spondyloarthropathies
- Septic arthritis
- Connective tissue diseases

5. Describe the radiographic features of noninflammatory, degenerative arthritis (cartilage-based diseases).

1. Sclerosis/osteophytes
2. Nonuniform loss of cartilage (focal joint space narrowing in area of maximal stress in weight-bearing joints)
3. Cysts/geodes

The causes of degenerative arthritis are multifactorial. However, the primary problem and end result is **cartilage degeneration.** As the cartilage degenerates, the joint space narrows. However, in contrast to uniform, diffuse narrowing seen with inflammatory arthritides, the noninflammatory, degenerative arthritides tend to have nonuniform, focal joint space narrowing, being most pronounced in the area of the joint where stresses are more concentrated (e.g., superolateral aspect of hip, medial compartment of the knee; Fig. 8.3).

Following cartilage loss, subchondral bone becomes sclerotic or eburnated owing to trabecular compression and reactive bone deposition. With denudation of cartilage, synovial fluid can be forced into underlying bone, forming subchondral cysts or geodes with sclerotic margins. As an attempted reparative process, the remaining cartilage undergoes endochondral ossification to develop osteophytes. Such osteophytes commonly occur first at margins or non-stressed aspects of the joint (e.g., medial and lateral aspects of the distal femur and proximal tibia of the knee).

6. List the rheumatic disease categories that typically cause radiographic features of noninflammatory arthritis.

- Degenerative joint disease (e.g., primary OA and secondary causes of OA, such as post-traumatic arthritis, congenital bone diseases, and others).

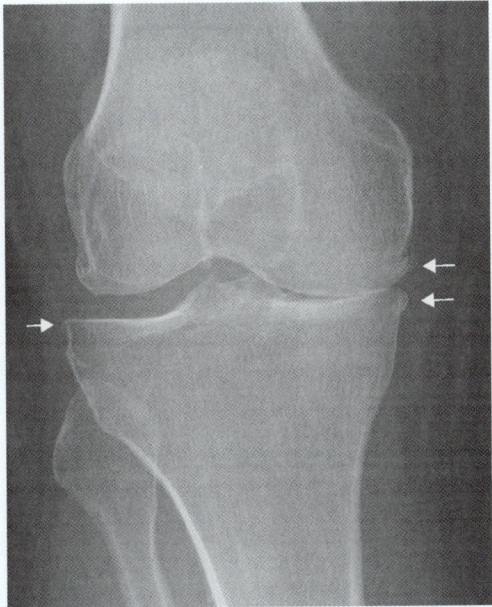

Fig. 8.3 Knee radiograph demonstrating osteophytes (arrows) as well as asymmetric medial joint space narrowing consistent with degenerative osteoarthrosis.

- Metabolic or endocrine diseases (e.g., CPPD, ochronosis, acromegaly) may demonstrate findings best characterized as degenerative though the distribution or specific features (such as extensive chondrocalcinosis in CPPD) may allow for more definitive characterization.

7. What are the typical sites of joint involvement in primary (idiopathic) OA compared with secondary causes of noninflammatory, degenerative arthritis?

Primary (idiopathic) OA can cause noninflammatory, degenerative arthritic changes in the following joints:
- Hands
  - DIPs
  - Proximal interphalangeal joints (PIPs)
  - First carpometacarpal joint (CMC) of thumb
- Acromioclavicular joint of shoulder
- Cervical, thoracic, and lumbosacral spine
- Hips
  - Subchondral cysts (Egger's cysts) in superior acetabulum are characteristic
- Knees
  - Patellofemoral, medial, and lateral compartments
- Feet
  - First metatarsophalangeal joint (MTP)

Secondary causes of degenerative arthritis can result in noninflammatory, degenerative changes in any joint (not just those for primary disease). Consequently, if a patient has degenerative changes in any of the following joints, you must consider secondary causes of OA:
- Hands
  - MCPs (Fig. 8.4)
- Wrist
- Elbow
- Glenohumeral joint of shoulder (can be involved in primary OA also)
- Ankle
- Feet, other than the first MTP

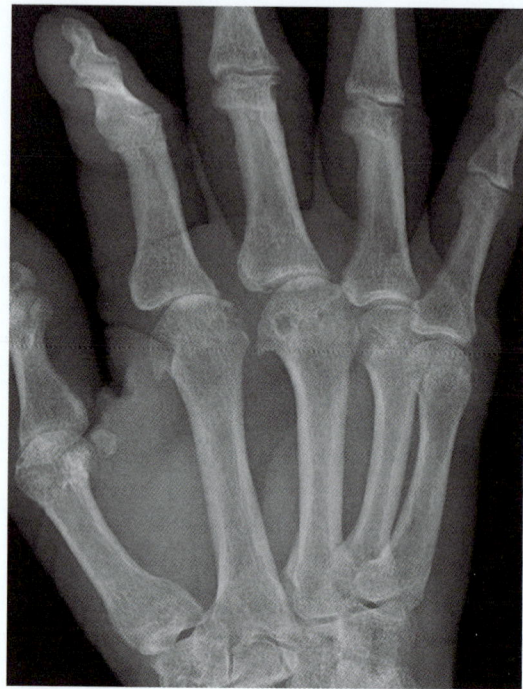

Fig. 8.4 Hand radiograph with joint space narrowing and hook osteophyte formation at the index and long finger metacarpal heads. This pattern is suggestive of pyrophosphate arthropathy or hemochromatosis.

If the degenerative changes involve only one joint, consider traumatic arthritis. If multiple joints are involved, consider a metabolic or endocrine disorder that has caused the cartilage to degenerate in several joints. Note that the end stage of an underlying inflammatory arthritis that has destroyed the cartilage can result in degenerative changes superimposed on the inflammatory radiographic features.

8. Describe the radiographic features of chronic gouty arthritis.
- Erosions with sclerotic margins and an overhanging edge (Fig. 8.5). These are caused by tophaceous deposits in the synovium slowly expanding into bone. The bone reacts and forms a sclerotic margin around the erosion.
- Relative preservation of joint space until late in disease.
- Relative lack of periarticular osteopenia for the degree of erosion seen.
- Nodules in soft tissue (i.e., tophi) near involved joints. Unlike rheumatoid nodules, tophi can become calcified.

9. What other diseases can give radiographic features similar to those of chronic gouty arthritis?
- Mycobacterial and some chronic fungal infections
- Diffuse tenosynovial giant cell tumor (formerly called pigmented villonodular synovitis or PVNS)
- Amyloidosis
- Multicentric reticulohistiocytosis (MRH)
- Synovial osteochondromatosis

10. Compare the radiographic features of inflammatory and noninflammatory spinal arthritis.
Inflammatory spinal arthritis is typically related to either infection or seronegative spondyloarthropathy. Hematogenous spread of infection usually results in **osteomyelitis** originating near

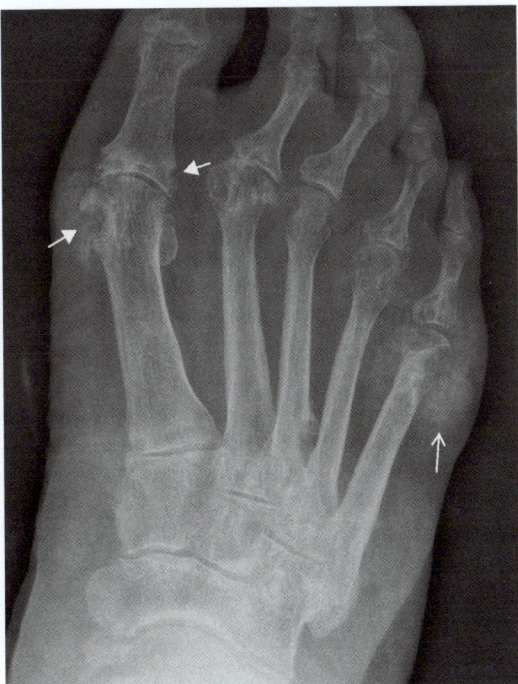

Fig. 8.5 Foot radiograph with large gouty erosions at the first metatarsal head. Note the characteristic overhanging edge (arrow) and the preservation of the metatarsophalangeal joint space. There are also gouty tophi adjacent to the first, fourth, and fifth metatarsophalangeal joints.

the endplate regions with subsequent spread to the intervertebral disc. The typical radiographic appearance of osteomyelitis is disc space narrowing with poorly defined cortical endplates and destruction of the adjacent vertebrae (Fig. 8.6). Although this appearance is highly suggestive of infection, other inflammatory arthropathies, such as RA (cervical spine), seronegative spondyloarthropathies, and CPPD, can rarely give a similar appearance.

Ankylosing spondylitis (AS) is associated with squared anterior vertebral bodies with sclerotic anterior corners, syndesmophytes (ossification of the annulus fibrosus), discovertebral erosions (Andersson lesions), and vertebral and facet joint fusion (Fig. 8.6). Psoriatic or chronic reactive arthritis may cause spinal changes similar to AS; however, more typical is the presence of large bulky nonmarginal paravertebral ossifications near the thoracolumbar junction. Radiographic sacroiliitis will also be present in spondyloarthropathy patients who have inflammatory spinal disease (see *Chapters* 33–36).

Noninflammatory lumbar arthritis is characterized by disc space narrowing and vacuum phenomenon, endplate proliferation, and bony sclerosis in the absence of sacroiliitis (Fig. 8.6; Table 8.1, Table 8.2). Degenerative diseases of the vertebral column can affect cartilaginous joints (discovertebral junction), synovial joints such as facet joints, or ligaments (enthesopathy). Typically, degeneration of the disc results in cartilage fissuring, with subsequent diminution in height and vacuum phenomenon (gas within the disc) and ultimately, bony sclerosis (intervertebral osteochondrosis). Endplate bony proliferation (spondylosis deformans) is generally believed to be initiated by annulus fibrosus disruption. Ligamentous degeneration also occurs; ligamentum flavum hypertrophy may contribute to spinal stenosis, whereas ossification of the anterior longitudinal ligament is characteristic of diffuse idiopathic skeletal hyperostosis (DISH) (see Chapter 80).

11. What is the difference between an osteophyte and a syndesmophyte?
See Table 8.2.

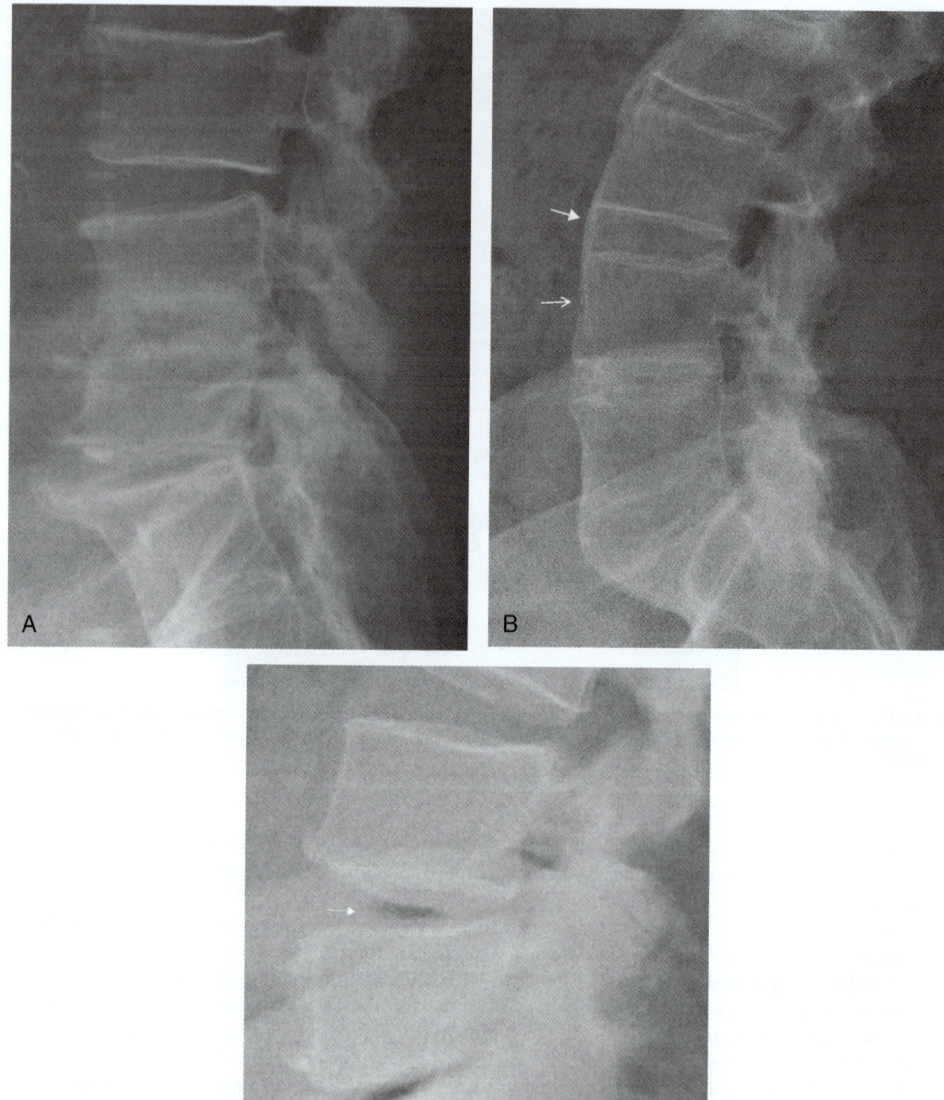

Fig. 8.6 (A) Lateral lumbar spine radiograph demonstrating endplate erosions and irregular sclerosis consistent with discitis/osteomyelitis. (B) Lateral lumbar spine radiograph demonstrating thin syndesmophytes (arrow) and squaring of the vertebral bodies (thin arrow) in this patient with ankylosing spondylitis. (C) Lateral lumbar spine radiograph demonstrating bony endplate proliferation and vacuum disc phenomenon (*arrows*) indicating disc degeneration.

TABLE 8.1 Radiographic Features of Inflammatory Versus Noninflammatory Spinal Arthritis

	INFLAMMATORY		NONINFLAMMATORY
	Infection	**Spondyloarthropathy**	
Sacroiliac joints	Unilateral erosions	Erosions	Normal
Vertebral bodies	Irregular, eroded endplates	Squaring ± erosions	Sclerosis
Disc space	Narrowed	Variable	Narrowed, vacuum
	One site	Multiple sites	Multiple sites
Syndesmophytes	–	+	–
Osteophytes	–	–	+
Osteopenia	+	+	–
Soft tissue mass	+	–	–

TABLE 8.2 Comparing Osteophyte and Syndesmophyte Features

	OSTEOPHYTE	**SYNDESMOPHYTE**
Disease association	Osteoarthritis	Spondyloarthropathy[a]
Vertebral involvement	Cervical Lumbar	Cervical and lower thoracic Lumbar
Vertebral orientation	Horizontal	Vertical
Pathogenesis	Endochondral ossification calcification "Bony spurs"	Outer annulus fibrosus "Vertebral bridging"
Complications	Radiculopathy	Ankylosis
	Vertebrobasilar ischemia	"Bamboo spine" Fracture

[a]Includes axial spondyloarthropathy (ankylosing spondylitis), psoriatic arthritis, chronic reactive arthritis, and enteropathic arthritis.

12. What rheumatic disease categories typically have unique radiographic features and are difficult to categorize using the inflammatory, noninflammatory, or gout-like patterns of radiographic changes?
- Collagen vascular disease (e.g., scleroderma, SLE)
- Endocrine arthropathies (e.g., hyperparathyroidism, acromegaly, hyperthyroidism)
- Miscellaneous (sickle cell disease, hemophilia, Paget disease, avascular necrosis, Charcot joints, sarcoidosis, hypertrophic osteoarthropathy)

13. List the most common diseases associated with the following radiographic changes seen in the hands.
- **Extensive arthritis of multiple DIP joints**
  - Primary OA
  - Psoriatic arthritis
  - Multicentric reticulohistiocytosis (MRH)
- **Thumb CMC joint arthritis**
  - Primary OA
- **Index and long finger MCP joint arthritis**
  - Hemochromatosis: hook-like osteophytes involving all the MCPs
  - CPPD: involves primarily index and long finger MCPs.
  - Acromegaly (initially widened joint spaces, later osteoarthritic changes)
  - RA or psoriatic arthritis if erosive changes
- **Arthritis mutilans of the hands (or feet)**

- Psoriatic arthritis
- RA
- Chronic gouty arthritis
- MRH

14. **Outline the approach to the radiographic diagnosis of a patient with peripheral arthritis** (See Fig. 8.7).

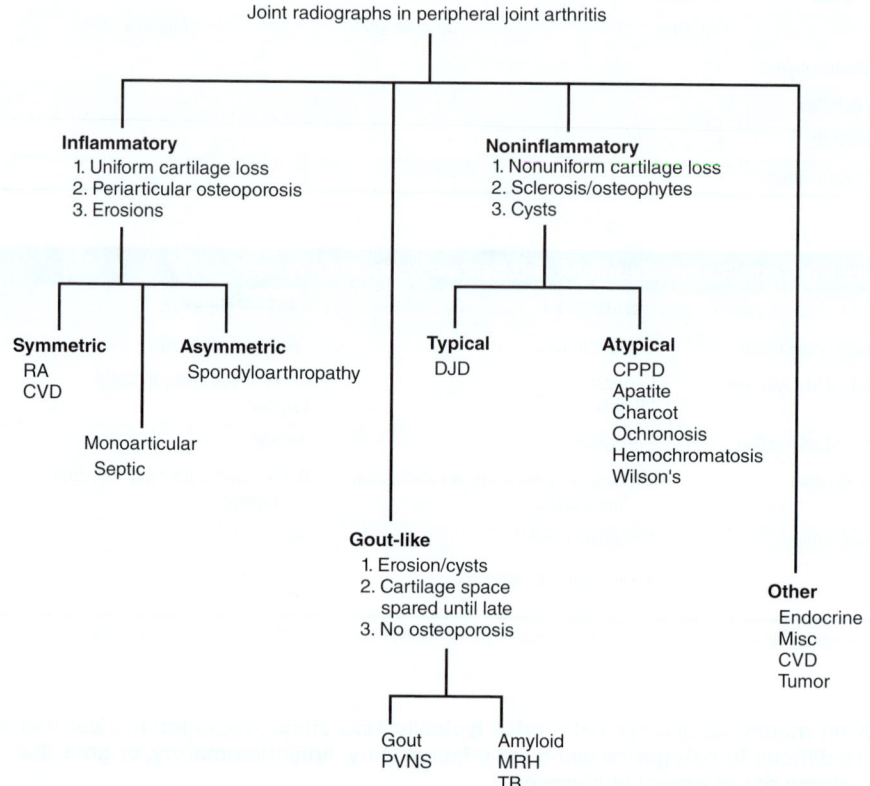

Fig. 8.7 Approach to radiographic diagnosis in patient with peripheral arthritis. *CPPD,* calcium pyrophosphate deposition disease; *CVD,* collagen vascular disease; *DJD,* degenerative joint disease (osteoarthrosis); *MRH,* multicentric reticulohistiocytosis; *PVNS,* pigmented villonodular synovitis; *TB,* tuberculosis.

15. **List the most common diseases associated with the following radiographic changes seen in the upper extremity and shoulder.**

Radioulnar joint arthritis
   RA
   Juvenile idiopathic arthritis (JIA)
   CPPD
Swan neck and/or ulnar deviation deformities
   RA if erosive changes and nonreversible deformities
   SLE if nonerosive with reversible deformities
Elbow nodules in soft tissue
   RA
   Tophaceous gout (particularly if contains calcific density deposits)
   Scleroderma-associated calcium deposits

Distal clavicle resorption
  Post-traumatic osteolysis
  RA
  Hyperparathyroidism

16. **Outline an approach to the radiographic diagnosis of a patient with arthritis of the spine** (See Figure 8.8).

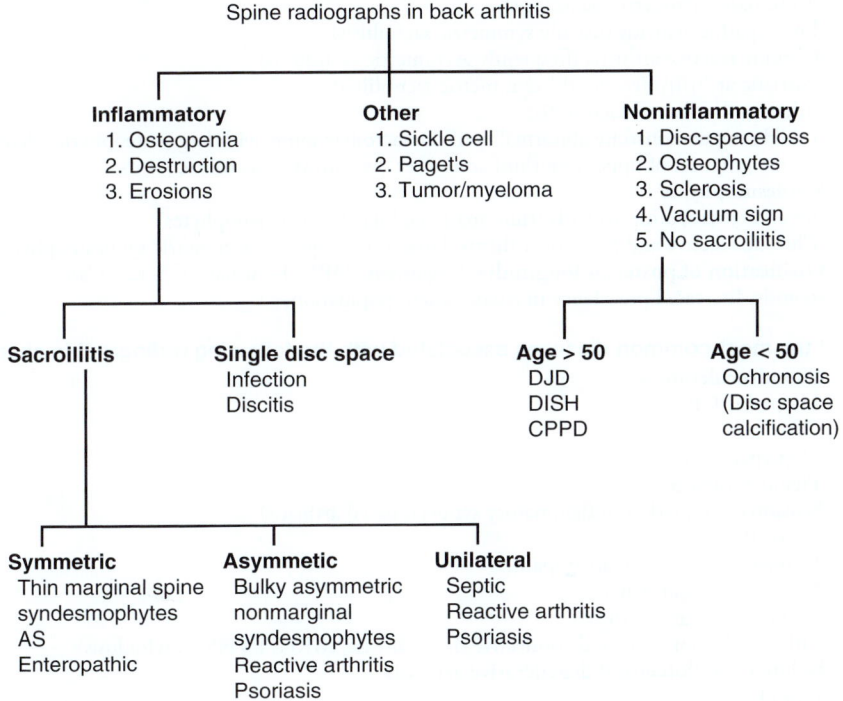

Fig. 8.8 Approach to radiographic diagnosis in patient with arthritis involving the spine. *AS,* ankylosing spondylitis; *DISH,* diffuse idiopathic skeletal hyperostosis.

17. **List the most common diseases associated with the following radiographic changes seen in the feet.**
    - **Destructive arthritis of the great-toe interphalangeal joint**
      Chronic reactive arthritis
      Psoriatic arthritis
      Gout and RA, less commonly
    - **Destructive arthritis at great-toe MTP joint**
      RA
      Chronic gouty arthritis
      Chronic reactive and psoriatic arthritis, less commonly
      Primary OA if noninflammatory productive changes predominate
    - **MTP joint erosive arthritis**
      Chronic reactive or psoriatic if asymmetric distribution
      RA if a symmetric distribution
    - **Calcaneal spurs**
      Traction spurs (noninflammatory)—blunted spur with well-corticated margin
      Seronegative spondyloarthropathies (inflammatory spurs)—pointed spur with poorly corticated margin and/or erosions

18. List the most common diseases associated with the following radiographic changes seen in the spine.
- **Vacuum disc sign**
  Disc degeneration
- **Disc space calcification at multiple levels**
  Ochronosis if the patient is young (<30 years)
  CPPD and others
- **Sacroiliitis**
  AS (usually symmetric sacroiliitis)
  Enteropathic arthritis (usually symmetric sacroiliitis)
  Chronic reactive arthritis (frequently asymmetric sacroiliitis)
  Psoriatic arthritis (frequently asymmetric sacroiliitis)
  Infection (unilateral sacroiliitis)
  DISH may demonstrate abnormality of the sacroiliac joints with large osteophytic sclerosis at the junction of upper one-third and lower two-thirds of sacroiliac joints
- **Syndesmophytes**
  AS and enteropathic arthritis (thin, marginal bilateral syndesmophytes)
  Chronic reactive and psoriatic arthritis (large, nonmarginal, asymmetric syndesmophytes)
- **Ossification of posterior longitudinal ligament (OPLL)**—usually C3–C4. Can cause spinal stenosis. Increased prevalence in Asian patient population.

19. List the most common diseases associated with the following radiographic changes.
- **Chondrocalcinosis**
  Idiopathic CPPD
  OA
  Hyperparathyroidism
  Hemochromatosis
- **Erosions** (hallmark of inflammatory synovial-based arthritis)
  RA or JIA
  Seronegative spondyloarthropathies
  Chronic gouty arthritis
  Septic (infectious) arthritis
  Others (SLE rarely, mixed connective tissue disease, MRH, PVNS, amyloidosis)
- **Isolated patellofemoral degenerative arthritis**
  CPPD

20. Give the characteristic radiographic features of the different arthritides.
- **RA: Symmetric, erosive arthritis,** uniform joint space narrowing (especially weight-bearing joints). The most common sites are small joints of hands and feet (MCPs, PIPs, wrists, MTPs) and the cervical spine. Soft tissue nodules that do not calcify. Swan neck deformities and ulnar deviation.
- **JIA:** Periarticular osteoporosis, but joint space narrowing and erosions are typically absent until late. Periosteal reaction and **bony fusion** (carpus, facets in cervical spine) may distinguish it from RA. Overgrowth of bone at the margins of a joint suggests JIA.
- **AS: Bilateral, symmetric sacroiliitis** with ankylosis. **Bilateral, thin, marginal** syndesmophytes in the spine may cause spinal fusion (bamboo spine). Peripheral arthropathy affects large axial joints (shoulders, hips).
- **Chronic reactive arthritis** (formerly Reiter's syndrome): Can be bilateral or **unilateral, asymmetric sacroiliitis.** Peripherally, there is a predilection for **lower extremities** (especially the interphalangeal joint of the great toe), with erosions and fluffy periostitis. Enthesopathy with erosions and calcifications at tendon insertions into the calcaneus. Frequently, asymmetric joint involvement. **Large, asymmetric, nonmarginal** (jug-handle) bridging syndesmophytes.
- **Psoriatic arthritis:** Axial arthropathy similar to chronic reactive arthritis. Peripherally, it has an upper extremity predilection; DIP or PIP fusion. "Pencil-in-cup" deformity. Enthesopathy and periostitis. Erosions of several joints of a single digit (MCP, PIP, and DIP of one finger).

Frequently, asymmetric joint involvement. Acroosteolysis. Jug-handle (chunky) bridging syndesmophytes in the spine.

- **Gout: Erosions with overhanging edges and sclerotic margins.** Preserved joint space. Soft tissue tophi that can contain calcium.
- **CPPD:** Osteoarthritic changes at sites atypical for DJD (MCPs, elbow, radiocarpal, ankle, shoulder).
- **Osteoarthrosis (OA):** Nonuniform joint space narrowing, sclerosis, **osteophytosis,** cysts. The most common sites include the DIPs, PIPs, thumb CMC, knees, hips, acromioclavicular joint, first MTP, and spine.
- **Neuropathic joint (Charcot arthropathy):** Destruction, disorganization, density (i.e., sclerosis), debris, dislocation **(the five Ds).**
- **SLE:** Reversible swan neck and ulnar deviation deformity and subluxation, but absence of erosions.
- **Scleroderma:** Tapered, atrophic soft tissues **(sclerodactyly)** with soft tissue calcifications. Acroosteolysis of terminal phalanges.
- **Hemochromatosis:** Chondrocalcinosis. **Degenerative changes at MCPs** with "hook-like" spurs. Cystic changes of the radiocarpal joint of the wrist.
- **Ochronosis: Vertebral disc calcification,** chondrocalcinosis, OA in multiple joints (especially the spine) at a young age.
- **Acromegaly:** Widened joint and disc spaces. Large spurs at bases of distal phalanges (spade phalanges).
- **Hyperparathyroidism: Subperiosteal resorption** at the radial side of middle phalanges. Soft tissue calcifications, chondrocalcinosis, **"salt and pepper" skull,** ligament and tendon ruptures.
- **Avascular necrosis: Crescent sign** of subchondral sclerosis and lucency. Hips and shoulders are most commonly affected.
- **Hypertrophic osteoarthropathy (periosteal reaction):** Intrathoracic pathology such as primary lung cancer. Less likely causes include thyroid acropachy, voriconazole treatment, or pachydermoperiostosis. Other causes of periosteal reaction include venous stasis and infection.

21. **What are TR and TE time parameters and how do they relate to magnetic resonance imaging (MRI)?**

    MRI functions by submitting the tissue to a strong magnetic field and then disturbing that magnetization in tissue by using radiofrequency (RF) pulses. The return of an RF signal from the tissue is then detected and used to construct an image. TR is the time of repetition parameter or the time between 90° RF pulses. TE is the time to echo or the time between 90° pulse and the time when the signal from the tissue is recorded. Modulation of TR and TE parameters determines how much T1 and T2 weighting any given image displays (Table 8.3). TR and TE also determine how long a sequence takes to acquire (from seconds to minutes) and how much heating of the tissue occurs.

TABLE 8.3 General Imaging Appearance of Tissues on T1- and T2-Weighted Sequences

STRUCTURE	T1 INTENSITY	T2 INTENSITY
Fat, fatty marrow	High	High
Hyaline cartilage	Intermediate	Intermediate
Muscle	Intermediate	Intermediate
Fluid, edema	Low	High
Neoplasm	Low	High
Cortical bone	Very low	Very low
Tendon, ligaments	Very low	Very low

High signal appears white on magnetic resonance imaging; low signal appears black on magnetic resonance imaging.

22. What is the difference between T1- and T2-weighted images on MRI?

T1- or T2-weighting typically refers to spin-echo MR sequences. **T1-weighted images** are short TR (300–1000 ms) and short TE (10–30 ms) and provide excellent anatomic detail. In contrast, **T2-weighted images** are long TR (1800–2500 ms) and long TE (40–90 ms), sensitive for detecting fluid and edema. An intermediate-weighted sequence or **proton density** sequence combines T1 and T2 weighting by having a long TR (>T1) and short TE (<T2). This technique has some advantages of both T1 and T2-weighted sequences and is commonly used in musculoskeletal imaging.

Two other sequences commonly used are gradient echo and short tau (T1) inversion recovery (STIR). **Gradient echo** sequences can be T1, T2, and proton density-weighted and permit very rapid acquisition with thin-section, high-resolution images. **STIR** is a fat-suppression technique that is very sensitive in the detection of fluid or edema. These images greatly aid in the detection of subtle marrow and soft tissue disease, such as muscle tears, but have relatively poor spatial resolution.

Gadolinium is a paramagnetic element used as a contrast agent in MRI. It adds to the cost of MRI but depicts areas of increased blood flow on T1-weighted images, which is helpful in the detection of early erosions and in distinguishing between effusion and synovial inflammation. Gadolinium should generally be avoided in patients with significant renal insufficiency (creatinine clearance < 30 cc/minute) due to the risk of nephrogenic systemic fibrosis.

23. Describe the appearances of the various tissues on T1- and T2-weighted MR images.

See Table 8.3.

24. In which clinical situations is a computed tomography (CT) scan superior to MRI and vice versa?

Radiographs should be obtained before a CT scan or MRI when evaluating musculoskeletal disorders. Radiographs depict subtle calcifications and collections of gas that may be very difficult to detect with MRI alone. CT scan is useful mainly to detect and characterize bony abnormalities but requires higher radiation exposure than radiography. It is used occasionally when MRI is contraindicated (e.g., pacemaker). MRI utilizes nonionizing radiation and can demonstrate subtle soft tissue and bony changes before they become radiographically apparent.

- **CT scan indications:**
  Acute trauma (complex fractures)
  Tarsal coalition
  Intraarticular osteocartilaginous loose bodies
- **MRI scan indications:** See Table 8.4

25. What is a dual-energy CT (DECT) scan?

DECT scan is a CT scanner that has two x-ray tubes capable of producing different energies (80 kV and 140 kV). Image reconstruction algorithms detect uric acid deposits based on their lower attenuation of x-rays than calcium (bone). By color coding the different attenuation values (uric acid versus calcium), the uric acid deposits can be demonstrated in addition to bone. Findings of urate by DECT have been adopted as a diagnostic criterion for the diagnosis of gout.

26. What imaging features are typically seen in infections of bones or joint spaces?

TABLE 8.4 Indications for MRI Scan	
Cervical spine disease or instability	Osteomyelitis
Spinal stenosis or disc disease	Soft tissue tumors or skeletal muscle pathology
Internal derangement of the knee	Tenosynovial giant cell tumor (PVNS)
Rotator cuff tears and tendinosis	Inflammatory sacroiliitis
Avascular necrosis	Synovitis and tenosynovitis

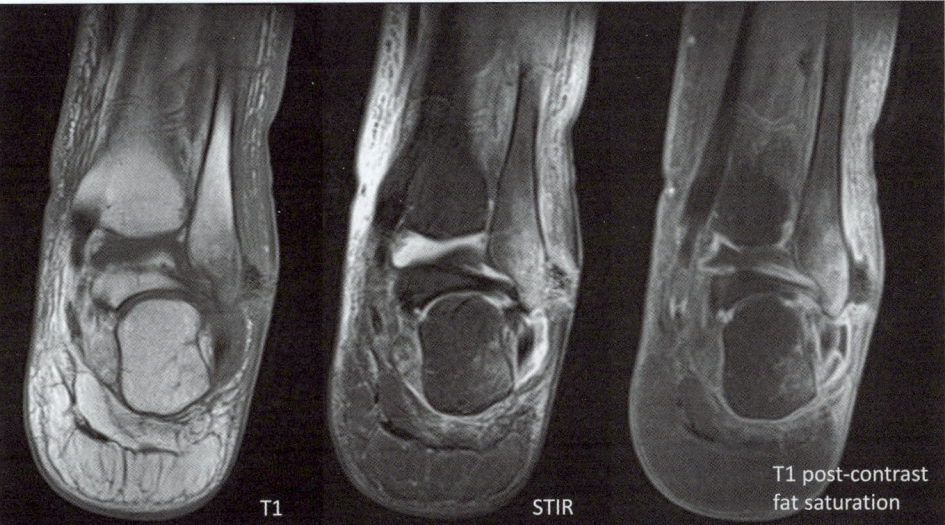

Fig. 8.9 MRI images in the coronal plane of a patient with osteomyelitis of the distal fibula. Note the overlying ulcer. T1-weighted images demonstrate decreased signal intensity of marrow at the site of infection. STIR images show increased fluid signal within bone and surrounding soft tissue. Post-contrast T1-weighted images with fat saturation demonstrate enhancement within the region of acute infection.

In acute osteomyelitis, the earliest radiographic abnormality is **soft tissue swelling** with obliteration of normal tissue planes. Hyperemia results in osteopenia, and bone destruction or periostitis may not be visualized for 7–14 days. MRI is much more sensitive for detection of early osteomyelitis. MRI is particularly helpful in defining the full extent of osteomyelitis, particularly when amputation is a therapeutic option (Fig. 8.9). Intravenous contrast is not necessary for the diagnosis of osteomyelitis. However, it is generally recommended because it increases diagnostic sensitivity for concomitant soft tissue abnormalities such as abscesses, fistulas, and vascular complications. Osteomyelitis may be associated with **Brodie's abscess,** usually in the metaphysis of tubular bones in skeletally immature patients (i.e., children). A well-marginated **lucent defect** (commonly elongated) is seen surrounded by a thick band of sclerosis. With chronic osteomyelitis, radiodense spicules of necrotic bone, referred to as **sequestra,** may be seen within the lucent defect.

27. What are some of the potential uses of ultrasound in the evaluation of musculoskeletal conditions?

Ultrasound is well suited to detect abnormalities of superficial structures. High-frequency linear transducers offer high spatial resolution.

Potential indications include:

- **Tendon pathology:** Tears and inflammation in tendons such as the posterior tibial tendon, Achilles tendon, shoulder, or finger tendons are well demonstrated. Fluid in the tendon sheath is also well visualized. Flexor tenosynovitis may be an early predictor for persistent RA development.
- **Enthesitis:** Can detect inflammatory enthesitis in peripheral areas.
- **Soft tissue masses:** Ultrasound can be used to confidently diagnose several benign superficial soft tissue masses including lipomas, epidermal inclusion cysts, and ganglion cysts. Non-radiopaque foreign bodies are often invisible on radiographs but are well demonstrated by ultrasound.
- **Joint and bursal inflammation:** Synovitis and effusions of superficial joints are well demonstrated. Can show "double contour" sign in gouty arthritis patients and hyperechoic chondral deposits in chondrocalcinosis. Can be used to predict the evolution of RA and to follow disease activity and structural progression.
- **Guide articular and periarticular aspiration and/or injections.**

- **Parotid and submandibular glands:** Can detect changes compatible with Sjögren's syndrome.
- **Nerve entrapment:** Diagnose median nerve, ulnar nerve, and posterior tibial nerve entrapment. Pitfalls of ultrasound imaging include:
- **Operator dependence:** The accuracy of ultrasound is highly affected by the training level and experience of the user. Certain structures such as the metacarpal head may demonstrate a normal defect that simulates an erosion. Radiographs are needed for comparison and confirmation.
- **Deep central portions of joints are obscured:** Cartilage and meniscal injuries are usually not visible.

28. What role does nuclear medicine have in musculoskeletal imaging?

- **Bone scintigraphy** (bone scan) is routinely performed with 99mTc-labeled diphosphonates, which are adsorbed onto the surface of the bone proportional to the local osteoblastic activity and skeletal vascularity. Bone scans are therefore sensitive in detecting bone abnormalities but somewhat nonspecific as a tumor, trauma, infection, or other pathology can all cause increased tracer uptake. Bone scintigraphy is the screening examination of choice for the evaluation of bony metastatic disease and Paget disease, as it images the entire skeleton. Bone scans commonly detect metastatic disease or osteomyelitis while plain radiographs are still normal, as up to 50% of bone must be decalcified for radiographic detection of tumor or infection versus a tiny fraction for bone scan. Bone scintigraphy can also detect stress fractures earlier than radiographs. In arthritis, MRI and ultrasonography have replaced bone scintigraphy. Other common indications for bone scanning are in the evaluation of chronic regional pain syndrome or metabolic bone disease.
- **Single-photon emission CT** allows increased sensitivity and specificity when assessing spinal pathology. It is frequently combined with conventional CT scanning to map an abnormality on bone scan to an exact anatomic site (facet joint, pars intra-articularis, or vertebral body)
- **Positron emission tomography (PET)** typically uses ^{18}F-Fluorodeoxyglucose which goes to the sites of increased glucose utilization to map metabolically active bone and soft tissue, providing precise anatomic localization of lesions. PET scans have been used in the diagnosis and monitoring of large vessel vasculitis, osteomyelitis, and sarcoidosis. It is most commonly used in oncologic imaging for both diagnosis and monitoring of treatment.

29. What is a three-phase bone scan?

A three-phase bone scan evaluates blood flow to a particular area of the musculoskeletal system during the first few minutes of imaging and then soft tissue uptake (20–30 minutes following injection). A delayed third phase is acquired 2 to 4 hours later. Areas of increased blood flow will have increased activity in the first two phases of imaging, while areas of bony remodeling will have increased uptake and thus activity in the third (delayed imaging) phase (Table 8.5). Bone scans are highly sensitive to abnormalities of bone (including fracture, infection, tumor, and arthritis) but are nonspecific. The entire skeleton may be imaged, thus making the technique useful in the detection of metastatic lesions.

30. What is the role of arthrography in the evaluation of musculoskeletal problems?

Arthrography is infrequently performed and involves injection of contrast (direct arthrography) into a joint followed by CT or MRI imaging. Historically, detection of small lesions such as glenohumeral labral tears or acute cartilage injuries required arthrography, but modern imaging equipment has decreased the need for the procedure as soft tissue contrast and spatial resolution

TABLE 8.5 Scintigraphic Activity on Three-Phase Bone Scan for Infection

	CELLULITIS	SYNOVITIS	OSTEOMYELITIS[a]
First phase	+	+	+
Second phase	+	+	+
Third phase	−	−	+

[a]During the third phase, tracer uptake for osteomyelitis is more localized on one side of the joint, whereas synovitis is more diffuse.

TABLE 8.6 Average Ionizing Radiation Exposure for Radiologic Procedures

- Mammography—0.5 mSv
- Chest x-ray—0.02 mSv
- HRCT chest—0.98 mSv
- Lumbar spine x-ray—1.25 mSv
- Bone scan—6.3 mSv
- Upper gastrointestinal series—6 mSv
- Barium enema—8 mSv (with fluoroscopy)
- Dual-energy x-ray absorptiometry (DEXA)—0.001 mSv
- Head CT scan—2 mSv
- Ultrasound—0
- MRI—0
- PET/CT scan—25 mSv

TABLE 8.7 Relative Costs of Radiographic Procedures Used in Musculoskeletal Imaging

Plain radiograph	$300	DEXA scan	$200
Ultrasound	$400	CT scan	$1500
Arthrography	$450	MRI scan	$2000–2500
Bone scan	$1100	PET scan	$3500–5000

have improved. Fluoroscopic or ultrasound-guided aspiration, however, remains commonly performed when possible septic arthritis is a clinical concern.

31. What is the radiation exposure to an individual undergoing one of these imaging studies?

The conversion for radiation units is as follows:
- 1 Sievert (Sv) = 1 Gray (Gy) = 100 Rem = 100 Rad
  The average background radiation exposure a person is exposed to is:
- Natural background = 3.1 mSv/year
- Flight from New York to Los Angeles = 0.030 mSv
  The average ionizing radiation exposure for radiologic procedures: See Table 8.6

32. What are the relative costs of the radiographic procedures used in musculoskeletal imaging of a specific joint (e.g., the shoulder)?

See Table 8.7

BIBLIOGRAPHY

Brower AC, Flemming DJ, eds. *Arthritis in Black and White*. 3rd ed. Philadelphia, PW: Saunders; 2012.
Di Matteo A, Mankia K, Azukizawa M, Wakefield RJ. The role of musculoskeletal ultrasound in the rheumatoid arthritis continuum. *Curr Rheumatol Rep*. 2020;22:41–53.
He L, Delzell P, Schils J. Comparison of MRI findings after musculoskeletal ultrasound: an opportunity to reduce redundant imaging. *J Am Coll Radiol*. 2018;15:1116–1119.
Hendrick RE, Dodd GD, Fullerton GD, Hendee WR, Borgstede JP, Larke F. The University of Colorado Radiology Adult Dose-Risk Smartcard. *J Am Coll Radiol*. 2012;9:290–292.
Jacobson JA. *Fundamentals of Musculoskeletal Ultrasound*. 3rd ed. Philadelphia, PW: Elsevier; 2018.
McAlindon T, Kisson E, Nazarian L, et al. American College of Rheumatology report on reasonable use of musculoskeletal ultrasonography in rheumatology clinical practice. *Arthritis Care Res*. 2012;64:1625–1640.
Mettler FA, Guiberteau MJ. *Essentials of Nuclear Medicine and Molecular Imaging*. 7th ed. Philadelphia, PA: Elsevier; 2018.
Neogi T, Jansen TL, Dalbeth N, et al. 2015 Gout classification criteria: an American College of Rheumatology/European League Against Rheumatism collaborative initiative. *Ann Rheum Dis*. 2015;74:1789–1798.
Pierce JL, Perry MT, Wessell DE, et al. ACR appropriateness criteria® suspected osteomyelitis, septic arthritis, or soft tissue infection (excluding spine and diabetic foot): 2022 update. *J Am Coll Radiol*. 2022;19:S473–S487.
Resnick DL et al., eds. *Bone and Joint Imaging*. 4th ed. Philadelphia, PA: Elsevier; 2024.
Troum OM, Pimienta O, Olech E. Magnetic resonance imaging applications in early rheumatoid arthritis diagnosis and management. *Rheum Dis Clin North Am*. 2012;38:277–297.
Zufferey P, Rebell C, Benaim C, Ziswiler HR, Dumusc A, So A. Ultrasound can be useful to predict an evolution towards rheumatoid arthritis in patients with inflammatory polyarthralgia without anticitrullinated antibodies. *Joint Bone Spine*. 2017;84:299–303.

CHAPTER 9

Electromyography and Nerve Conduction Studies

Dianna Quan, MD and Stacy Dixon, MD, PhD

⟫ KEY POINTS

1. Nerve conduction studies (NCS) and needle electromyography (EMG) are the most useful diagnostic tests in determining the presence, type, severity, and chronicity of a suspected neuromuscular disorder.
2. Although the information collected during NCS and needle EMG testing is more objective and quantitative than that obtained by a standard clinical examination, there are many important technical factors that contribute to the collection of accurate data. Selection of a reputable or accredited laboratory and an experienced electrodiagnostic consultant will help ensure the most accurate data and reliable interpretation.
3. Sensory NCS are the most useful way to distinguish preganglionic (radiculopathy) from postganglionic (peripheral neuropathy or plexopathy) processes that cause numbness.
4. NCS can help distinguish between demyelinating and axonal neuropathies. Demyelinating neuropathies have moderate to severe slowing of the nerve conduction velocities with relatively preserved compound muscle action potential (CMAP)/sensory nerve action potential (SNAP) amplitudes. Axonal neuropathies have reduced CMAP/SNAP amplitudes with relatively preserved conduction velocities.
5. On EMG, the motor unit action potentials (MUAPs) in neurogenic disorders have characteristic large amplitudes with long durations and reduced recruitment. The MUAPs in myopathic disorders have small amplitudes with short durations and early recruitment.

1. What is an EMG?

It is a term used in two ways:
- As a general description of the combination of NCS and needle EMG testing.
- More specifically, to describe the needle electrode recording performed to assess the function of motor units.

2. What is an NCS?

NCS may be performed on either sensory or motor nerves. From the skin surface, a brief electrical stimulus is applied to the nerve of interest, and the evoked electrical signal is recorded distally from another point in the nerve in the case of a sensory nerve, or from the innervated muscle in the case of a motor nerve; the evoked responses are known as SNAP or CMAP, respectively. Characteristics of the evoked action potentials such as amplitude, onset and/or peak latency, and conduction velocity provide information about the axon and myelin components of the tested nerve.

3. Name some other types of electrodiagnostic tests.

- **Repetitive stimulation studies** are utilized for the evaluation of the neuromuscular junction (e.g., in myasthenia gravis).
- **Somatosensory evoked potentials** are used to evaluate conduction within the spinal cord and brain.
- Other, less frequently used tests include **single-fiber EMG, motor-evoked potentials,** and **nerve root stimulation.**

4. What is a motor unit?

A motor unit includes the **motor neuron** found within the anterior horn of the spinal cord, its **axon,** the **neuromuscular junction,** and the associated **muscle fibers** supplied by the axon. The electrodiagnostic physician can utilize a combination of needle EMG, NCS, repetitive stimulation, and other electrophysiologic tests to assess the individual components of the motor unit.

5. What are the clinical indications for ordering an EMG?

An EMG should be ordered to determine the localization and severity of a suspected neuromuscular disorder. The NCS and needle EMG are almost always performed together in reputable laboratories. Testing can distinguish between neurogenic (nerve or neuron-related), myopathic (muscle-related), and neuromuscular junction disorders. In neurogenic conditions, testing can often distinguish between disorders primarily affecting myelin (i.e., demyelinating neuropathies) and axonal or neuronal disorders. An EMG is generally not useful in the assessment of brain or spinal cord disease. In order to get the most useful information from the test, the requesting physician should indicate his or her clinical question or concern as specifically as possible. It is not usually necessary to request particular procedures (e.g., NCS, repetitive stimulation, needle EMG) as a qualified electrodiagnostic consultant can decide what is needed to answer the clinical question.

6. What are some common disorders of nerve?

Functionally, the peripheral nervous system starts in the vicinity of the spinal neural foramen where the sensory and motor fibers join. At its most proximal level, peripheral nervous system injury in the form of **radiculopathy** is caused by an injury to a nerve root due to structural disease (e.g., herniated disc or trauma), inflammation, or other causes. **Plexus involvement** by disease or injury may occur in the upper (brachial plexus) or lower extremity (lumbar or lumbosacral plexopathy).

Peripheral nerve conditions can be acquired or genetically mediated. Examples of genetic conditions include the hereditary sensory and motor neuropathies (e.g., Charcot–Marie–Tooth disease). Acquired peripheral neuropathies can stem from conditions such as diabetes, toxins (medications or other exogenous substances), inflammatory disorders, or metabolic disturbances.

Focal neural entrapment can be seen in carpal tunnel syndrome (CTS), cubital tunnel syndrome, or tarsal tunnel syndrome, and a few others.

7. Describe three main types of nerve injury.

Nerves sustain a gradient of injury, which was originally defined by Seddon:
1. **Neurapraxia** is the functional loss of conduction without anatomic change of the axon, usually due to focal demyelination. With remyelination, conduction returns to normal.
2. In **axonotmesis,** the axonal continuity is lost. With its loss, Wallerian degeneration occurs in the distal segment. Recovery, which is frequently incomplete, occurs as a result of axonal regrowth at a rate of 1–3 mm/day in otherwise healthy individuals.
3. **Neurotmesis** results from the separation of the entire nerve, including its supporting connective tissue. Regeneration frequently does not occur. Nerves with this degree of trauma may need surgical attention for recovery to occur.

8. Do these types of nerve injuries occur together?

Neurapraxia and axonotmesis commonly occur as a result of the same injury. When compression is relieved from the involved segment of the nerve, two periods of healing typically occur. One is relatively immediate, from hours to weeks, as the neurapraxia resolves. A second period of healing, from weeks to months, may occur as a result of axonal regrowth.

9. What is an innervation ratio?

For each motor axon, there are a variable number of associated muscle fibers. Depending on the specific requirement of control, the ratio may be quite low or extremely high. The innervation ratio of the extraocular muscles is typically 1:3, owing to the fine control required for binocular vision. Conversely, the innervation ratio of the gastrocnemius can be as high as 1:2000, since most movements involving the plantar flexors of the ankle are relatively large motions requiring more force than accuracy.

10. What are some common disorders of muscle?

Muscle disease can be acquired or genetically mediated. Acquired muscle diseases such as inflammatory myopathies are most often proximal and symmetrical in distribution. A notable exception is inclusion body myositis, which has a predilection for the quadriceps and finger flexors and may be quite asymmetrical. Genetic myopathies or muscular dystrophies may also demonstrate specific patterns of muscle group involvement that may aid in diagnosis. In general, the degree of clinical weakness in a particular muscle correlates well with the severity of the findings on needle EMG examination.

11. Why is temperature recorded during the course of an electrodiagnostic examination?

Nerve conduction velocities drop by 1.5 to 2.5 m/s per 1°C reduction in both sensory and motor nerves. These changes can be significant. Failure to warm the limb to a standard temperature, usually 30°C for the leg and 32°C for the arm, can result in false-positive studies, leading to a misdiagnosis.

12. Is nerve conduction velocity the same throughout the length of a nerve?

Nerve conduction velocities vary among nerves and along their lengths. Normally, proximal nerve conduction is faster than distal nerve conduction because of the increased temperature and larger diameter of the proximal nerve segments. For example, median nerve conduction velocity from wrist to palm should be faster than from palm to finger.

13. How is the sensory portion of the peripheral nervous system tested?

Sensory NCS are the primary means to test the integrity of the sensory nerves. The amplitude of the SNAP, its point of onset (onset latency), and its peak latency can be compared with standardized normal values and with those from the opposite extremity. Sensory NCS are only abnormal in lesions distal to the dorsal root ganglia where sensory neurons reside. Abnormal SNAPs can be an important way of distinguishing between peripheral neuropathies or plexopathies and radiculopathies. In the latter, SNAPs are usually normal even when a patient complains of numbness. Using the complementary information obtained from motor NCS and needle EMG examination, an electromyographer can further localize the lesion to a particular spinal nerve root, the portion of the plexus, or a particular peripheral nerve.

14. How do motor NCS differ from sensory NCS?

Motor responses are measured in millivolts (mV) whereas sensory responses are measured in microvolts (μV). Characteristics of the CMAP such as latency, amplitude, and duration are measured at each site of stimulation. Unlike the SNAP, the motor nerve conduction velocity cannot be calculated from a single stimulation site. The latency of the motor nerve includes not only transit time along the motor axon but also the time it takes the response to transmit through the neuromuscular junction (NMJ) and depolarize the muscle. Therefore, to accurately calculate the conduction velocity of a motor nerve, two points of stimulation are required. The conduction velocity can be calculated for the segment between the points of stimulation.

15. What is the F-wave? How is it clinically useful?

The F-wave is a delayed motor potential recorded by stimulating a motor nerve in the distal extremity. As the electrical impulse travels backward along the nerve to the spinal cord, a small population of anterior horn cells is stimulated, resulting in small motor action potentials that can be recorded from the associated muscle. Abnormal F-waves can indicate proximal nerve diseases such as radiculopathy or plexopathy. Prolonged or absent F-waves are also early findings in Guillain–Barré syndrome and other demyelinating nerve disorders.

16. Describe the components of a needle EMG evaluation.

Insertional/spontaneous activity: An EMG needle inserted into a normal muscle should evoke brief electrical discharges of muscle fibers. Increased or prolonged electrical activity may indicate abnormalities of the muscle fibers or the nerves supplying them. Fibrillations, positive sharp waves, and complex repetitive discharges are electrical signals that represent abnormal spontaneous firing of muscle fibers due to nerve or muscle damage. There should be no spontaneous activity in a healthy relaxed muscle.

   Motor unit analysis: When a patient slightly contracts a muscle, MUAPs can be recorded. The parameters of interest include the amplitude, duration, number of phases, and firing pattern of the MUAPs. Assessment of these parameters occurs in real time and is generally subjective. The quality of the interpretation depends on the skill and experience of the electromyographer, techni-cal recording conditions, and patient cooperation.

Recruitment: When a patient contracts a muscle more forcefully, a large number of MUAPs can be recorded. How "full" this pattern of MUAPs is reflects the underlying health of the motor units and the ability of the patient to "recruit" available motor units. In myopathic conditions, recruitment may be "early" because myopathic motor units generate less force than healthy ones. In neurogenic conditions, recruitment may be reduced as a result of axon or neuron loss.

17. How do fasciculations, fibrillations, and positive sharp waves differ on needle EMG recording?

A **fasciculation** potential is an involuntary firing of an entire motor unit, that is, a single motor neuron and all its innervated muscle fibers. This is seen as a large electrical spike on the needle EMG recording of a relaxed muscle. It is sometimes clinically visible in the patient as a brief, irregular twitch of the muscle. This can often be seen in normal individuals; however, if in excess, it may be a sign of a motor nerve or motor neuron disorder.

A **fibrillation** potential is an involuntary contraction of a single muscle fiber that usually indi-cates denervation or muscle damage. Unlike a fasciculation, a fibrillation usually does not cause clinically visible muscle movement.

Positive sharp wave potentials are similar to fibrillation potentials in that they represent abnormal muscle fiber firing from nerve or muscle damage. They are identified by their initial positive deflection from the baseline as opposed to the initial negative deflection of a fibrillation potential.

18. How do normal EMG findings compare with the findings seen in a denervated muscle (neurogenic disorder)?

Note that fibrillations and positive sharp waves are not seen in acutely denervated muscles until 7 to 14 days after the onset of axonal degeneration. Full reinnervation of denervated muscle, resulting in large, polyphasic MUAPs, may take 3 to 4 months or more. In patients with rein-nervation after nerve injury, muscles may be clinically strong and yet be very abnormal on needle EMG testing. See Table 9.1.

19. How do normal EMG findings compare with those seen in a myopathic disorder?

The weaker a patient with myopathy is, the more likely the needle EMG findings will be abnormal. In patients with very mild weakness or those with steroid myopathy, the needle EMG recording may appear normal. See Table 9.2.

TABLE 9.1 Electromyography Findings for Normal and Denervated Muscles

ELECTROMYOGRAPHY FINDINGS	NORMAL	ACUTE DENERVATION	CHRONIC DENERVATION/ REINNERVATION
Spontaneous activity	None	Fibrillations, positive sharp waves	None
Motor unit action potential morphology	Normal	Normal	Large amplitude, long dura-tion, variable increased polyphasia
Recruitment	Normal or full recruitment	Reduced recruitment	Reduced recruitment

TABLE 9.2 Electromyography Findings for Normal Muscle and Myopathic Disorders

ELECTROMYOGRAPHY FINDINGS	NORMAL MUSCLE	MYOPATHY
Spontaneous activity	None	Variable fibrillations, positive sharp waves
Motor unit action potential morphology	Normal	Small amplitude, short duration, increased polyphasia
Recruitment	Normal	Early recruitment

20. How can a demyelinating peripheral neuropathy and an axonal peripheral neuropathy be differentiated by NCS and needle EMG?

Axonal loss and demyelination rarely occur in strict isolation, but some electrodiagnostic features may indicate relatively more damage to myelin versus axons. The features of **demyelinating neuropathies** include moderate to severe slowing of conduction velocity, temporal dispersion of evoked sensory or motor action potentials, conduction block, and prolonged distal latencies. **Axonal neuropathies** show milder slowing of nerve conduction, with generally low sensory and motor amplitudes on NCS. The needle EMG shows denervation abnormalities early in axonal neuropathies and only later in demyelinating neuropathies when axons are secondarily affected.

21. Which systemic diseases cause a predominantly demyelinating peripheral neuropathy? An axonal peripheral neuropathy?

In most rheumatologic conditions wherein neuropathy is present, the axons are primarily affected, though myelin is rarely completely normal. Demyelination may predominate in a few disorders, such as acute inflammatory demyelinating polyneuropathy (Guillain–Barré syndrome), chronic inflammatory demyelinating polyneuropathy, multifocal motor neuropathy, anti-myelin-associated glycoprotein antibody syndrome, other paraproteinemias, and some hereditary neuropathies. Drug-induced peripheral neuropathy (DIPN) can be caused by many different medications and is typically a length-dependent axonal sensorimotor polyneuropathy. However, some medications such as tumor necrosis factor-α (TNF-α) inhibitors can cause demyelinating peripheral neuropathies.

22. How is EMG/NCS used in diagnosing CTS? What is ulnar nerve entrapment at the elbow (cubital tunnel syndrome)?

CTS or compressive median neuropathy at the wrist is the most common entrapment neuropathy, affecting 1% of the population. CTS may show segmental nerve conduction slowing across the wrist. SNAP latencies of the median nerve are delayed most often, but with increasing severity, motor latencies can be affected. Denervation of the thenar muscles seen on needle EMG indicates moderate to severe CTS. Clinical correlation is recommended for mild CTS as sometimes NCS/EMG studies are normal despite classic symptoms of hand pain/numbness in a median nerve distribution.

In cubital tunnel syndrome, the ulnar nerve is compressed at the elbow resulting in motor or sensory nerve conduction slowing. Needle EMG examination may identify denervation in the ulnar-innervated muscles of the hand and forearm. The ulnar nerve can also be compressed at the wrist.

23. List a few nerve abnormalities that can be differentiated by EMG/NCS from common peripheral nerve syndromes.

See Table 9.3.

TABLE 9.3 Nerve Abnormalities and Possible Differential Diagnoses

PERIPHERAL NERVE SYNDROME	DIFFERENTIAL DIAGNOSIS
Carpal tunnel syndrome	C6–C7 radiculopathy Other areas of median nerve entrapment
Ulnar entrapment at the elbow	C8 radiculopathy Brachial plexus lesion
Radial nerve palsy	C7 radiculopathy
Suprascapular nerve lesion	C5–C6 radiculopathy
Peroneal nerve palsy	L4–L5 radiculopathy
Femoral nerve lesion	L3–L4 radiculopathy

BIBLIOGRAPHY

Aminoff MJ. *Electrodiagnosis in Clinical Neurology.* 6th ed. London: Elsevier Saunders; 2012.

Dumitru D. *Electrodiagnostic Medicine.* 2nd ed. Philadelphia: Hanley & Belfus; 2001.

Kimura J. *Electrodiagnosis in Diseases of Nerve and Muscle: Principles and Practice.* 4th ed. New York: Oxford University Press; 2013.

Jones MR, Urits I, Wolf J, et al. Drug-induced peripheral neuropathy: a narrative review. *Curr Clin Pharmacol.* 2020;15(1):38–48.

Preston DC, Shapiro BE. *Electromyography and Neuromuscular Disorders: Clinical-Electrophysiologic-Ultrasound Correlations.* 4th ed. Philadelphia: Elsevier; 2020.

CHAPTER 10

Approach for Patients With Monoarticular Arthritis Symptoms

Jason R. Kolfenbach, MD

> **KEY POINTS**
>
> 1. Most common diagnoses in acute monoarticular arthritis: crystalline, septic, osteoarthritis, trauma.
> 2. Most important diagnostic test in acute monoarticular arthritis: synovial fluid analysis and culture.
> 3. Most important diagnoses to rule out in chronic monoarticular arthritis: indolent infection and tumor.
> 4. Best diagnostic tests in chronic monoarticular arthritis: synovial fluid analysis, radiograph, magnetic resonance imaging (MRI), arthroscopy with synovial biopsy and culture.

1. What conditions can be mistaken for a monoarticular process?

Several common inflammatory processes occur in the soft tissues around, but not in, the joints. These conditions can be painful and may mimic arthritis. Examples include rotator cuff tendinitis of the shoulder, olecranon bursitis of the elbow, and prepatellar bursitis of the knee. It is important to distinguish these disorders from true joint diseases because their management is often quite different from that of monoarticular arthritis. Careful history and physical examination usually allow correct identification of the affected region (see Chapter 61: Regional Musculoskeletal Disorders).

2. List the diseases that commonly present with monoarticular arthritis.

See Box 10.1.

BOX 10.1 Diseases That Commonly Present With Acute Monoarticular Arthritis

Septic	Other
Bacterial	Osteoarthritis
Mycobacterial	Juvenile idiopathic arthritis
Lyme disease	Coagulopathy
Fungal	Avascular necrosis of bone
Crystal deposition diseases	Foreign-body synovitis
Gout	Pigmented villonodular synovitis
Calcium pyrophosphate dihydrate deposition disease	Palindromic rheumatism
Hydroxyapatite deposition disease	Lipoma arborescens
Calcium oxalate deposition disease	Synovial osteochondromatosis
Traumatic	Synovioma/sarcoma/metastatic disease
Fracture	Neuropathic (Charcot joint)
Internal derangement	
Hemarthrosis	

---

3. What polyarticular diseases occasionally present with a monoarticular onset?

Rheumatoid arthritis	Reactive arthritis
Juvenile idiopathic arthritis	Psoriatic arthritis
Viral arthritis	Enteropathic arthritis
Sarcoid arthritis	Whipple's disease

4. What is the most critical diagnosis to consider in the patient with monoarticular symptoms?

Joint infection, which represents a rheumatologic emergency, is the most critical diagnosis to consider and must be diagnosed quickly and managed aggressively. Bacterial infections, especially those due to Gram-positive organisms, can destroy the joint cartilage within a few days. Prompt and proper treatment of the septic joint will usually leave it without permanent structural damage. Additionally, as the septic joint is usually the result of the hematogenous spread of infection from another body site, early recognition of the joint process allows more timely diagnosis and treatment of the primary infection. When evaluating a patient with acute monoarticular arthritis, a good rule of thumb is to assume that the joint is infected until proven otherwise ("aspirate, or litigate!").

5. **What six questions should you ask when obtaining a history from a patient with monoarticular arthritis?**
   a. What is the timing of onset?
      - seconds to minutes: consider internal derangement, loose body, fracture/trauma.
      - several hours to 2 days: consider infection, crystal diseases, inflammatory arthritis syndromes, and palindromic rheumatism.
      - insidiously over weeks: consider indolent infections, osteoarthritis, inflammatory arthritis syndromes, and tumors.
   b. Is there a history of intravenous drug use or recent infection of any kind? Consider infection.
   c. Has the patient ever experienced prior episodes of acute joint pain and swelling? Consider crystal diseases most commonly, as well as other inflammatory arthritis syndromes.
   d. Has the patient had symptoms such as a skin rash, low back pain, diarrhea, urethral discharge, ocular inflammation/irritation, or mouth sores? Consider spondyloarthritis such as reactive arthritis, psoriatic arthritis, enteropathic arthritis, or axial spondyloarthritis.
   e. Is there a history of a bleeding diathesis or use of anticoagulants? Consider hemarthrosis.
   f. Has the patient been treated with a prolonged course of glucocorticoids? Consider infection, avascular necrosis, and fragility fracture.

6. **Is the age of the patient useful in the differential diagnosis?**
   Patient age is extremely useful in differential diagnosis. With the exception of infection (which occurs in all age groups), some joint diseases presenting as monoarticular arthritis are more likely to occur at certain ages.
   - In children, consider congenital dysplasia of the hip, slipped capital femoral epiphysis, transient synovitis of the hip, Legg–Calvé–Perthes disease, or a monoarticular presentation of juvenile idiopathic arthritis.
   - In young adults, consider axial and peripheral spondyloarthritis, rheumatoid arthritis, or internal derangement of the joint. A septic joint in this age group is often due to gonococcal infection.
   - Older adults are more likely to have crystalline arthritis, osteoarthritis, osteonecrosis, or internal derangement of the joint. A septic joint is less likely due to gonococcal organisms compared to younger patients.

7. **Is fever a useful sign?**
   Yes, but it can be misleading. Fever is often present in infectious arthritis, but it may be absent. Fever, however, can also be a feature of acute attacks of gout and pseudogout, rheumatoid arthritis, juvenile idiopathic arthritis, sarcoidosis, and reactive arthritis. Many clinicians have been fooled by a gout attack masquerading as cellulitis or a septic joint.

8. **What are the most likely diagnoses in hospitalized patients who develop acute monoarticular arthritis following admission for another medical or surgical disease?**
   Acute gout, pseudogout, and infection are by far the most common causes of acute monoarticular arthritis in this setting. These patients are often middle-aged or elderly, which is the primary age range for crystalline arthropathies. In addition, they often have hospitalization-related risk factors known to provoke gout or pseudogout attacks; for example, trauma, surgery, hemorrhage, infection, or medical stress such as renal failure, myocardial infarction, and stroke. Clinicians must be especially careful to exclude infection in such hospitalized patients.

9. **What are the two most common etiologies for acute (non-traumatic) monoarticular arthritis overall?**
   Crystalline arthritis represents 80% of all cases of acute monoarticular arthritis, with infectious etiologies representing 15% of cases.

10. What is the single most useful diagnostic study in the initial evaluation of monoarticular arthritis?

Synovial fluid analysis.

11. List the most common indications for arthrocentesis and synovial fluid analysis.

- **Suspicion of infection:** As little as 2 mL of fluid is sufficient for Gram stain, culture, and white blood cell (WBC) count and differential.
- **Suspicion of crystal-induced arthritis:** The sensitivity of polarizing microscopy in identifying birefringent crystals approaches 90% in acute gout and 70% in acute pseudogout.
- **Suspicion of hemarthrosis:** Bloody joint fluid is characteristic of traumatic arthritis, clotting disorder, and rare conditions such as pigmented villonodular synovitis (PVNS) and hydroxyapatite crystalline arthropathy.
- **Differentiating inflammatory from noninflammatory arthritis:** The degree of elevation of synovial fluid WBC count is useful in narrowing the list of possible diagnoses (see also Chapter 7: Arthrocentesis, Synovial Fluid Analysis, and Synovial Biopsy).

12. What other diagnostic studies are useful in the initial evaluation of monoarticular arthritis?

- Radiograph of the joint: Although frequently normal, the radiograph may disclose important information. It may diagnose unsuspected fracture, osteonecrosis, osteoarthritis, or juxtaarticular bone tumor. The presence of chondrocalcinosis, a radiologic feature of calcium pyrophosphate dihydrate deposition (CPPD) disease, increases suspicion for a pseudogout attack. Tumor, chronic fungal or mycobacterial infection, and other indolent destructive processes may be revealed. A contralateral joint radiograph for comparison may be useful, especially in children.
- Complete blood count: Leukocytosis supports the possibility of infection.

13. What other diagnostic studies are useful in selected patients in the initial evaluation of monoarticular arthritis?

- Cultures of blood, urine, or other possible primary sites of infection: mandatory when a septic joint is being considered.
- Serum prothrombin and partial thromboplastin time: useful if the patient is receiving anticoagulation or if a coagulation disorder is suspected.
- Erythrocyte sedimentation rate or C-reactive protein: although results are often nonspecific, significant elevation may suggest an inflammatory process.
- Serum uric acid levels: notoriously unreliable in making or excluding the diagnosis of gout. These may be spuriously elevated in acute inflammatory conditions or acutely diminished in a true gout attack.
- Serologic tests for antinuclear antibodies (ANAs) and rheumatoid factor: these tests are rarely if ever indicated in the initial evaluation of acute monoarticular arthritis. However, the ANA may be positive in the oligoarticular form of juvenile idiopathic arthritis.

14. If infection cannot be adequately ruled out by initial diagnostic studies, what should you do?

The patient should be hospitalized and treated presumptively for a septic joint until culture results become available. This is usually indicated in the patient with synovial fluid findings suggesting a highly inflammatory process (synovial fluid WBC count >50,000/mm^3) but with a negative synovial fluid Gram stain and no obvious primary source of infection. To lessen the confusion regarding response to therapy, antiinflammatory drugs should be withheld during this period.

15. A diagnosis is always established by the end of the first week of onset of acute monoarticular arthritis. Is that correct?

No. Many patients defy initial attempts at diagnosis despite appropriate evaluation. A few achieve spontaneous remission, leaving the physician frustrated about the diagnosis but relieved. Many patients, however, continue to have symptoms.

TABLE 10.1 Inflammatory and Noninflammatory Causes of Chronic Monoarticular Arthritis

INFLAMMATORY	NONINFLAMMATORY
Mycobacterial infection	Osteoarthritis
Fungal infection	Internal derangement of the knee
Lyme arthritis	Avascular necrosis of bone
Monoarticular presentation of rheumatoid arthritis	Pigmented villonodular synovitis
Seronegative spondyloarthritis	Lipoma arborescens
Sarcoid arthritis	Neuropathic (Charcot joint)
Foreign-body synovitis	Synovial chondromatosis
	Synovioma

16. The initial evaluation is unrevealing and the arthritis persists. What should be done?

If the initial evaluation was carefully accomplished, a period of watchful waiting is often useful at this time. As noted previously, some processes will resolve spontaneously. Others become polyarticular, and the differential diagnosis will change to reflect the new joint involvement. New findings, such as the skin rash of psoriasis, occasionally emerge to aid in diagnosis. In a small number of patients, monoarticular arthritis persists, and further evaluation for chronic monoarticular arthritis must be undertaken.

17. What is the definition of chronic monoarticular arthritis? Why is it useful to consider this as a category separate from acute monoarticular arthritis?

Chronic monoarticular arthritis can be arbitrarily defined as **symptoms persisting within a single joint for >6 weeks**. The differential diagnosis shifts away from some important and common causes of acute arthritis, such as pyogenic infection and acute crystal deposition diseases. In patients with an inflammatory synovial fluid, the likelihood of chronic inflammatory syndromes, such as mycobacterial or fungal septic arthritis, or an axial or peripheral spondyloarthritis, increases. In patients with a noninflammatory process, a structural abnormality or internal derangement is a possibility.

18. Name the most likely causes of chronic monoarticular arthritis.

Table 10.1 lists the most likely causes of chronic monoarticular arthritis.

19. What six questions should you ask when obtaining a history from a patient with chronic monoarticular arthritis?

a. Is there a history of tuberculosis or a positive tuberculin skin test/interferon-gamma release assay? Consider mycobacterial disease.

b. Has the patient had unique environmental exposures: (1) Is the patient a farmer, gardener, or floral worker? Consider sporotrichosis; (2) Was the patient exposed to contaminated water sources, such as a home aquarium? Consider mycobacterium marinum.

c. If the knee is involved, has the joint been damaged in the past? Does it ever "lock" in flexion? Consider internal derangement and osteoarthritis.

d. Has the patient ever experienced previous acute attacks of joint pain and swelling that resolved spontaneously in any joint? Consider inflammatory joint syndromes.

e. Has the patient recently been treated with a prolonged course of corticosteroids for any reason? Consider osteonecrosis of bone.

f. Has the patient had symptoms such as a skin rash, low back pain, diarrhea, urethritis, or uveitis? Consider spondyloarthritis.

20. What physical findings are useful in the differential diagnosis of chronic monoarticular arthritis?

- Extraarticular features of the spondyloarthritis family, such as skin rashes (psoriasis, keratoderma blennorrhagicum), oral ulcers, urethral discharge, conjunctivitis, uveitis
- Erythema nodosum, a feature of sarcoidosis and inflammatory bowel syndrome
- A positive McMurray maneuver in the knee examination, suggesting internal derangement

21. In evaluating chronic monoarticular arthritis, what initial studies should be obtained?

- Radiograph of the joint: Radiographs are often revealing in chronic arthritis. Chronic infections by mycobacteria and fungi often cause radiographically detectable abnormalities. Osteoarthritis, avascular necrosis of bone, and other causes of noninflammatory chronic arthritis also have characteristic radiographic appearances. Radiographs of the contralateral joint for comparison may be helpful.
- Synovial fluid analysis, when possible: This analysis is useful in dividing possible causes of the joint process into two broad diagnostic categories—inflammatory and noninflammatory arthritis. A bloody synovial effusion points to PVNS, hydroxyapatite arthritis, synovial chondromatosis, synovial sarcoma, or neuropathic joint. Additional causes of a hemarthrosis can be seen in Chapter 48 (Arthropathies Associated With Hematologic Diseases, Box 48.1). Cultures of synovial fluid may demonstrate mycobacterial or fungal infection.

22. In evaluating chronic monoarticular arthritis, what additional studies are indicated in *selected patients*?

- Erythrocyte sedimentation rate or C-reactive protein: Although results are often nonspecific, significant elevation may suggest an inflammatory process.
- Radiograph of sacroiliac joints: This may demonstrate asymptomatic sacroiliitis, especially in young patients presenting with chronic monoarticular arthritis as an initial manifestation of axial spondyloarthritis.
- Chest radiograph: To detect evidence of prior mycobacterial disease or pulmonary sarcoidosis.
- Skin test reaction to tuberculin or interferon-gamma release assay: A negative test is useful in excluding mycobacterial infection.
- Serologic tests for Lyme disease (*Borrelia burgdorferi*), rheumatoid factor, anti-cyclic citrullinated peptide antibody, ANA, and human leukocyte antigen B27.

These additional studies are most helpful in suspected inflammatory etiologies of chronic monoarticular arthritis, as well as those patients without a definitive etiology after initial joint aspiration and radiograph of the affected joint.

23. Are other diagnostic studies useful in the evaluation of chronic monoarticular arthritis?

- **Arthroscopy:** Arthroscopy allows direct visualization of many important articular structures and provides the opportunity for synovial biopsy in large and medium-sized joints. It is particularly useful for diagnosing internal derangement of the knee.
- **Synovial biopsy:** Microscopic evaluation with culture of synovial tissue is useful in the diagnosis of benign and malignant tumor, fungal and mycobacterial infections, and foreign-body synovitis.
- **MRI of the joint:** Useful in diagnosing avascular necrosis of bone, internal derangement of the knee, PVNS, osteomyelitis, and destruction of periarticular bone.
- **Universal primer:** Synovial fluid can be tested for bacteria, fungi, and mycobacterial infections that cannot be grown in culture. 16S rRNA sequencing employs a gene encoding small subunit ribosomal RNA. This rRNA sequence contains conserved regions common to microbial organisms as well as divergent sequences unique to each microbial species. When a small piece of this sequence is used as a primer in a polymerase chain reaction (PCR) assay, it acts as a universal primer for nonselective amplification of microbial DNA in the patient's synovial fluid. Once the DNA has been amplified, the PCR product is then stained with ethidium bromide and visualized by electrophoresis on an agarose gel. If microbial DNA is identified, it can then be directly sequenced to identify the species. Bacterial, fungal, and mycobacterial organisms can be detected with this testing, but not viral organisms.

24. How often is a specific diagnosis made in patients with chronic monoarticular arthritis?

Appropriate evaluation yields a diagnosis in approximately two-thirds of patients. Fortunately, the most serious and treatable diseases yield to diagnosis if a carefully reasoned clinical approach is taken.

BIBLIOGRAPHY

American College of Rheumatology Ad Hoc Committee on Clinical Guidelines. Guidelines for the initial evaluation of the adult patient with acute musculoskeletal symptoms. *Arthritis Rheum*. 1996;39:1–8.

Deane K, West SG. Differential diagnosis of monoarticular arthritis. In: Wortmann R, ed. *Crystal-Induced Arthropathies*. New York: Taylor & Francis Group; 2006:135–156.

Singh N, Vogelgesang SA. Monoarticular arthritis. *Med Clin N Am*. 2017;101:607–613.

Van Vollenhoven R. *Evaluation of Monoarticular and Polyarticular Arthritis. Kelley and Firestein's Textbook of Rheumatology*. 11th Ed. Philadelphia, PA: Elsevier; 2021:663–677.

CHAPTER 11

Approach for Patients With Polyarticular Arthritis Symptoms

Jason R. Kolfenbach, MD

The patient's history and physical examination are the cake. Lab and x-ray are the frosting. You've got to bake the cake before you reach for the frosting.

—George V. (Geordie) Lawry

Imparted to the author as a 2nd year medical student at the University of Iowa in 2002.

» KEY POINTS

1. History and physical examination, not laboratory testing, are the most important components of the initial diagnostic process.
2. The two most common causes of polyarthritis are osteoarthritis (OA) and rheumatoid arthritis (RA).
3. Extraarticular features, such as the malar rash of systemic lupus erythematosus (SLE), are often the keys to diagnosing polyarticular syndromes.
4. Laboratory tests are most useful to confirm the diagnosis based on your history and physical examination.

---

1. What are the most important tools that the clinician can use on a patient with polyarticular arthritis symptoms?

A careful history and physical examination. Isolated laboratory results or imaging studies provide definitive answers in only a few instances. Tests are often most useful in confirming the suspected diagnosis or in providing prognostic information. When confronted with a patient with polyarticular symptoms, an inexperienced clinician often will slight the most important elements of evaluation, the history and physical examination, opting instead for "shotgun" laboratory testing. Although tests such as rheumatoid factor (RF), uric acid, antistreptolysin O titers, and antinuclear antibodies may be indicated in many instances, the history and physical examination will reveal the majority of the information required for diagnosis.

2. How are the many diseases causing polyarticular symptoms classified?

No single classification scheme can be used to differentiate a wide variety of diseases presenting with polyarticular symptoms. In most instances, the clinician uses several variables in combination to reduce the number of diagnostic possibilities. These variables include:
- acuteness of onset of the process
- degree of inflammation of the joints
- temporal pattern of joint involvement
- distribution of joint involvement
- age and sex of the patient
- extraarticular features

3. Which diseases commonly present with acute polyarticular symptoms?

See Table 11.1

4. Which diseases commonly present with chronic (persisting >6 weeks) polyarticular symptoms?

See Box 11.1

TABLE 11.1 Diseases With Acute Polyarthritis Symptoms

INFECTION	OTHER INFLAMMATORY
Gonococcal	Rheumatoid arthritis
Meningococcal	Polyarticular and systemic juvenile idiopathic arthritis
Lyme	Acute sarcoid arthritis
Acute rheumatic fever	Systemic lupus erythematosus
Infective endocarditis	Reactive arthritis
Viral (esp. rubella, hepatitis B and C, parvovirus, Epstein–Barr, HIV)	Psoriatic arthritis Polyarticular gout

BOX 11.1 Diseases With Chronic Polyarticular Arthritis Symptoms

Inflammatory
    Rheumatoid arthritis
    Systemic lupus erythematosus
    Polyarticular gout
    Juvenile idiopathic arthritis
    Systemic sclerosis
    Chronic CPP crystal inflammatory arthritis (*pseudo-RA*)
    Psoriatic arthritis
    Polymyalgia rheumatica
    Vasculitis
    Reactive arthritis
    Enteropathic arthritis
    Sarcoid arthritis
Noninflammatory
    Osteoarthritis
    Osteoarthritis with CPPD (*pseudo-OA*)
    Fibromyalgia
    Hemochromatosis
    Benign hypermobility syndrome

PEARL: Despite a long list of diseases causing polyarthritis, over 75% of patients with inflammatory arthritis will have RA (30%), crystalline arthritis, psoriatic arthritis, reactive arthritis, or sarcoidosis. The vast majority with noninflammatory polyarthritis will have OA.

5. How do polyarthritis, polyarthralgia, and diffuse aches and pains differ?

Polyarthritis is definite inflammation (swelling, tenderness, warmth) of more than four joints demonstrated by physical examination. A patient with two to four involved joints is said to have pauci- or oligoarticular arthritis. Patients presenting with polyarthritis should be evaluated for a variety of etiologies in the acute (see Question 3) and chronic setting (see Question 4).

Polyarthralgia is defined as pain in more than four joints without demonstrable inflammation by physical examination. The chronic noninflammatory arthritides commonly present with polyarthralgia.

Diffuse aches and pains are poorly localized symptoms originating in the joints, bones, muscles, or other soft tissues. The joint examination does not reveal inflammation. Polymyalgia rheumatica, fibromyalgia, SLE, polymyositis, and hypothyroidism commonly present with these symptoms.

6. **Describe the three characteristic temporal patterns of joint involvement in polyarthritis**
   a. Migratory pattern: Symptoms are present in certain joints for a few days and then remit, only to reappear in other joints. Rheumatic fever, early gonococcal arthritis, early Lyme disease, Whipple's disease, and acute childhood leukemia are examples.
   b. Additive pattern: Symptoms begin in some joints and persist, with subsequent involvement of other joints. This pattern is common in RA, SLE, and other polyarticular syndromes.
   c. Intermittent pattern: This pattern is typified by repetitive attacks of acute polyarthritis with remission between attacks. A prolonged observation may be necessary to establish this phenomenon. Crystalline arthropathy is the most common category causing this pattern of arthritis. Psoriatic arthritis, reactive arthritis, palindromic rheumatism, familial Mediterranean fever, and Whipple's disease may present in this manner as well. RA, remitting seronegative symmetrical synovitis with pitting edema (RS3PE), SLE, sarcoidosis, and Still's disease can also present episodically early in their disease course.

7. **How is the distribution of joint involvement helpful in the differential diagnosis of polyarthritis?**
   Different diseases characteristically affect different joints. Knowledge of typical joints involved in each disease is a cornerstone of diagnosis in polyarthritis. In practice, knowledge of which joints are spared in each form of arthritis is also quite useful. See Table 11.2.

8. **Name the two most common causes of chronic polyarthritis.**
   a. OA: The prevalence of OA rises steeply with age. About 10% to 20% of people aged 40 years have evidence of OA, and 75% of women aged >65 years have OA. This very high prevalence makes OA the single most likely diagnosis in older patients complaining of polyarticular pain who have noninflammatory signs and symptoms.
   b. RA: The prevalence of RA in the United States is approximately 0.5–1%, making it one of the most common causes of chronic inflammatory polyarthritis.

9. **What are the most likely diagnoses in women aged 25 to 50 years who present with chronic oligoarticular or polyarticular symptoms?**
   Benign hypermobility syndrome, fibromyalgia, OA, RA, SLE, and spondyloarthritis (psoriatic arthritis, reactive arthritis, IBD-associated arthritis, and axial spondyloarthritis).

TABLE 11.2 Distribution of Joint Involvement in Polyarthritis

DISEASE	JOINTS COMMONLY INVOLVED	JOINTS COMMONLY SPARED
Gonococcal arthritis	Knee, wrist, ankle, hand IP	Axial
Lyme arthritis	Knee, shoulder, wrist, elbow	Axial
Rheumatoid arthritis	Wrist, MCP, PIP, elbow, glenohumeral, cervical spine, hip, knee, ankle, tarsal, MTP	DIP, thoracolumbar spine
Osteoarthritis	First CMC, DIP, PIP, cervical spine, thoracolumbar spine, hip, knee, first MTP, toe IP	MCP, wrist, elbow, glenohumeral, ankle, tarsal
Reactive arthritis	Knee, ankle, tarsal, MTP, first toe IP, elbow, axial	
Psoriatic arthritis	Knee, ankle, MTP, first toe IP, wrist, MCP, hand IP, axial	
Enteropathic arthritis	Knee, ankle, elbow, shoulder, MCP, PIP, wrist, axial	
Polyarticular gout	First MTP, tarsal, subtalar, ankle, knee	Axial
CPPD disease	Knee, wrist, shoulder, ankle, MCP, hand IP, hip, elbow	Axial
Sarcoid arthritis	Ankle, knee	
Hemochromatosis	MCP, wrist, ankle, knee, hip, feet, shoulder	

CMC, carpometacarpal; *CPPD*, calcium pyrophosphate dihydrate deposition; *DIP*, distal interphalangeal; *IP*, interphalangeal; *MCP*, metacarpophalangeal; *MTP*, metatarsophalangeal; *PIP*, proximal interphalangeal.

10. **What are the most likely diagnoses in men aged 25 to 50 years who present with chronic oligoarticular or polyarticular symptoms?**

Spondyloarthritis, gonococcal arthritis, hemochromatosis, OA, and RA.

11. **What are the most likely diagnoses in patients aged over 50 years presenting with chronic polyarticular symptoms?**

OA, RA, calcium pyrophosphate dihydrate deposition (CPPD) disease, polymyalgia rheumatica, and paraneoplastic polyarthritis.

12. **What is morning stiffness? How is it useful in sorting out the causes of polyarticular symptoms?**

Morning stiffness refers to the amount of time it takes for patients with polyarthritis to "limber up" after arising in the morning. It is useful in differentiating inflammatory from noninflammatory arthritis. In inflammatory arthritis, morning stiffness lasts for >1 hour. In untreated RA, it averages 3.5 hours and tends to parallel the degree of joint inflammation. In contrast, noninflammatory processes, such as OA, may produce transient morning stiffness that lasts for <15 minutes.

13. **List possible causes of fever and polyarthritis**

Infectious arthritis: septic arthritis, bacterial endocarditis, Lyme disease, viral arthritis
Reactive arthritis: enteric infections, genitourinary infections
Systemic rheumatic diseases: RA*, SLE*, Still's disease, systemic vasculitis
Crystal-induced arthritis: gout, pseudogout
Miscellaneous diseases: malignancy, familial Mediterranean fever, rheumatic fever, idiopathic inflammatory myositis (IIM), sarcoidosis, Behcet's disease, inflammatory bowel disease, IgA vasculitis, Kawasaki's disease, erythema nodosum, erythema multiforme, Sweet syndrome, Whipple's disease, relapsing polychondritis

---

*Note that fever, as a disease manifestation of RA and SLE, is uncommon. In such patients, especially in the presence of immunosuppressive medications, fever should be presumed secondary to infection until proven otherwise.

14. **Define tenosynovitis. How is its presence useful in the differential diagnosis of polyarticular symptoms?**

Tenosynovitis is inflammation of the synovial-lined sheaths surrounding tendons in the wrists, hands, ankles, and feet. Physical examination usually reveals tenderness and swelling along the track of the involved tendon between the joints. It is a characteristic feature of RA, gout, reactive arthritis, psoriatic arthritis, gonococcal arthritis, and tuberculous and fungal arthritis. It is distinctly uncommon in other causes of polyarticular disease.

15. **List skin lesions that can be useful in the diagnosis of acute or chronic polyarthritis.**
    - Erythema chronicum migrans (Lyme arthritis)
    - Erythema nodosum (sarcoid arthritis, enteric arthritis)
    - Psoriatic plaques (psoriatic arthritis)
    - Keratoderma blennorrhagicum (reactive arthritis)
    - Erythema marginatum (acute rheumatic fever)
    - Palpable purpura (vasculitis)
    - Livedo reticularis (vasculitis, antiphospholipid antibody syndrome)
    - Vesiculopustular lesions or hemorrhagic papules (gonococcal arthritis)
    - Butterfly rash, discoid lupus, or photosensitive rash (SLE)
    - Thickening of the skin, digital pitting/ulcers, telangiectasias (systemic sclerosis)
    - Heliotrope rash on eyelids, upper chest, and extensor aspects of joints (dermatomyositis)
    - Gottron's papules overlying the extensor aspects of the metacarpophalangeal and interphalangeal joints of the hands (dermatomyositis)
    - Gray/brown skin hyperpigmentation (hemochromatosis)
    - Periungual nodules (multicentric reticulohistiocytosis)

16. **Which rheumatic diseases should be considered in a patient with Raynaud's phenomenon and polyarticular symptoms?**
    - Mixed connective tissue disease (prevalence of Raynaud's >90%)
    - Systemic sclerosis (prevalence >90%)
    - SLE (prevalence of 20%)
    - IIM (prevalence of 20%–40%)
    - Vasculitis (variable prevalence, depending on the particular syndrome)

17. **What other systemic features are seen in diseases causing polyarthritis?**
    (See Table 11.3)

18. **Which tests are most useful in evaluating a patient with chronic polyarticular symptoms?**
    Complete blood count, creatinine, urinalysis, liver-associated enzymes, erythrocyte sedimentation rate or C-reactive protein, antinuclear antibody (ANA), RF, anti-cyclic citrullinated peptide antibody, and radiographs. In some patients, consider serum uric acid, thyroid-stimulating hormone, iron studies, human leukocyte antigen-B27, and synovial fluid analysis.

19. **What is the significance of a positive ANA in a patient with chronic polyarticular symptoms?**
    A patient with polyarthralgia or polyarthritis who has a significantly elevated ANA titer (≥1:320) has an elevated risk of one of the following diseases: SLE (including drug-induced lupus), RA, Sjögren's disease, IIM, systemic sclerosis, or mixed connective tissue disease. The history and physical examination should be directed toward the clinical findings commonly seen in these diseases. A careful medication history may reveal that the patient has received drugs that can cause drug-induced lupus (see Chapter 16: Drug-Induced Lupus). An absence of objective findings on exam, coupled with lack of end-organ dysfunction through laboratory evaluation, is reassuring evidence against a rheumatic etiology. It is important to note that a positive ANA is a feature of several other chronic diseases other than those listed earlier and can also be found in normal healthy individuals, although usually in low titer (see also Chapter 6: Laboratory Evaluation).

20. **Why should an RF not be ordered in the evaluation of patients with acute polyarticular symptoms?**
    RF has a low sensitivity and specificity for RA in patients with acute polyarticular symptoms. Serum RF may be positive in acute infectious syndromes caused by hepatitis B, Epstein–Barr, influenza, and other viruses, but disappears as the viral syndrome resolves. In addition, while the sensitivity of RF approaches 75% to 85% among patients with established RA, it may be found in only 50% to 70% of patients upon initial evaluation (see also Chapter 6: Laboratory Evaluation). When RF testing is used in patients with chronic polyarthritis, documented on exam (joint swelling), the diagnostic utility is significantly improved.

21. **Which chronic polyarticular diseases are most likely to be associated with low serum complement levels?**
    SLE and some of the vasculitis syndromes. Low serum complement levels (C3, C4, and total hemolytic complement) usually suggest the presence of an immune complex disease. In SLE, cryoglobulinemia (especially hepatitis C), and some diseases associated with vasculitis (infective endocarditis, urticarial vasculitis), immune complexes may activate the complement cascade, resulting in consumption of individual complement components. In many instances, the liver is unable to produce these components as rapidly as they are consumed, resulting in a fall in serum levels.

22. **When should arthrocentesis for synovial fluid analysis be considered in the evaluation of polyarthritis?**
    When the diagnosis has not been established and joint fluid can be obtained. Both of these requirements need to be met. For example, a patient with obvious OA established by history, physical examination, and radiographs does not require a diagnostic aspiration in an uncomplicated knee effusion. If it can be obtained, synovial fluid analysis can be useful in the diagnosis of

TABLE 11.3 Extraarticular Organ Involvement in Polyarticular Rheumatic Diseases

DISEASE	LUNG	PLEURA	PERICARDIUM	HEART MUSCLE	HEART VALVE	KIDNEY	GI TRACT	LIVER
Acute rheumatic fever		•	•	•	•			
Viral arthritis								•
Bacterial endocarditis					•	•		
RA	•	•	•	•	•			
SLE	•	•	•	•	•	•		
Systemic sclerosis	•	•	•	•		•	•	•
Idiopathic inflammatory myositis	•	•	•	•				
Reactive arthritis					•		•	
Enteropathic arthritis							•	•
Polyarticular gout						•		
Sarcoid arthritis	•			•		•		•
Vasculitis	•							
Hemochromatosis				•				•

bacterial joint infection and crystal-induced arthritis. Even if a specific diagnosis is not forthcoming, synovial fluid analysis reduces the list of diagnostic possibilities by categorizing the process as either inflammatory or noninflammatory.

23. Should radiographs of affected joints always be obtained?

Not always. As a general rule, patients with new-onset acute polyarticular arthritis will not benefit from joint radiographs. Radiographs are more valuable when evaluating chronic arthritis that has been relatively long-standing. OA, chronic RA, psoriatic arthritis, gout, CPPD disease, systemic sclerosis, and sarcoidosis all have specific appearances on radiographs that are very useful in diagnosis. However, it should be remembered that OA is so common it may coexist with other arthritis syndromes, and radiographic changes may be a mixture of both types of arthritis in a given patient.

24. Why should the rheumatologist consider a Zen-like approach to the evaluation of chronic polyarthritis?

Many chronic polyarticular diseases may require months or years to diagnose; therefore, tremendous patience is often required. This prolonged but often necessary period of observation is frustrating to many patients (and providers) who hope for a more immediate diagnosis. Zen philosophy is based on the idea that life can be difficult and the primary source of personal discontent is an individual's longing for things to be different. Contentment lies in the acceptance of the complexities of life and the ability to let go of this desire and longing. Clinicians and trainees who desire clearly defined diagnoses at presentation may be more content in fields where fractures and acute coronary syndrome are commonplace. In contrast, the characteristics of chronic polyarticular diseases require an extraordinary degree of patience and a long-term perspective, in that:

- Many present insidiously with few objective findings for prolonged times.
- Many initially masquerade as other diseases before finally settling into their usual pattern.
- Characteristic laboratory abnormalities may require months or years to develop.
- Joint symptoms may precede the extraarticular features of the disease by months or years.
- Joint radiographs may not show characteristic changes of arthritis for months or years.

As Sir William Osler famously said, "Medicine is a science of uncertainty and an art of probability." He was likely thinking of rheumatology when he made this observation.

BIBLIOGRAPHY

van Vollenhoven RF. *Evaluation of Monoarticular and Polyarticular Arthritis. Kelley and Firestein's Textbook of Rheumatology.* 11th ed. Philadelphia, PA: Elsevier; 2021:663–677.

West S. Polyarticular joint disease. In: Klippel JH, Stone JH, Crofford LJ, White PH, eds. *Primer on the Rheumatic Diseases.* 13th ed. Atlanta: Springer Arthritis Foundation; 2008:47–57.

Approach to the Patient With Neuromuscular Symptoms

Matthew S. West, MD

 KEY POINTS

1. Localization of a patient's neuromuscular symptoms is paramount in evaluation and diagnosis.
2. Myopathies tend to be more proximal and symmetric in location.
3. Peripheral neuropathies are often distal and symmetric, whereas lesions of the nerve root, plexus, and mononeuritis multiplex are asymmetric.
4. Small fiber neuropathy causes pain, dysesthesia, allodynia, and autonomic dysfunction.
5. The statin drugs are the most common cause of drug-induced myopathy and usually present with myalgia.
6. "Young adult stroke" should raise diagnostic suspicion for a rheumatic cause.

1. **Discuss the relationship between rheumatic diseases and neuromuscular disease.**

   Many primary rheumatic diseases, such as systemic lupus erythematosus, Sjögren's syndrome, rheumatoid arthritis, and systemic vasculitis, are frequently complicated by the peripheral nervous system or myopathic disease. Rheumatic diseases can affect any part of the peripheral nervous system through different mechanisms. For example, chronic synovitis, joint contractures, and deformities seen in rheumatoid arthritis can lead to muscle atrophy, weakness, and nerve compression. Other rheumatic diseases such as polymyositis are dominated by immune-mediated inflammation of the muscle, though the differential diagnosis of myopathy is quite broad. Neuromuscular manifestations of rheumatic diseases may present as early and dominant findings or as late complications of well-established diseases. There may also be complications of therapy for rheumatic diseases, as with the use of glucocorticoids.

2. **What are the cardinal symptoms of neuromuscular lesions?**

   Weakness, alteration in sensation, and/or **pain** are the most common symptoms reported by patients. Weakness should be differentiated from fatigue and malaise. Fatigue differs from weakness in that fatigue is a loss of strength with activity that recovers with rest. Malaise is a subjective feeling of weakness without objective findings.

3. **Many patients complain of weakness. What is the best way to determine the cause of weakness in a given patient?**

   The first step is to exclude **systemic causes** of fatigue or weakness, such as cardiopulmonary disease, anemia, hypothyroidism, malignancy, sleep apnea, or depression. Many of these patients have malaise rather than weakness, and their examination usually fails to reveal true muscle weakness if they give their best effort. The carefully directed history and physical examination, combined with focused laboratory testing, are usually effective in eliminating these causes of weakness (Box 12.1).

BOX 12.1 Common Systemic Causes of Weakness or Fatigue

Cardiopulmonary disease
Hypo- or hyperthyroidism
Malignancy
Anemia
Sleep apnea
Depression
Chronic infection
Poor physical conditioning
Chronic inflammatory disease

---

4. Once systemic causes of weakness have been excluded, what is the next step?

The neuromuscular causes of weakness should be considered. A useful method of categorizing neuromuscular diseases is by their customary level of anatomic involvement, beginning with the spinal cord and proceeding distally through nerve roots, peripheral nerves, neuromuscular junctions, and muscles (Box 12.2).

5. Many patients complain of pain. What historical features are most useful in the differential diagnosis of pain?

Acute pure spinal cord lesions are typically not painful, although occasionally painful extensor or flexor muscle spasms will occur. Nerve root compression commonly produces pain and paresthesia in the affected nerve distribution (e.g., sciatica). Peripheral nerve disease is often manifested by numbness and paresthesia; weakness can be seen when motor nerves are involved (e.g., Guillain–Barré syndrome). Neuromuscular junction lesions are not painful.

Myopathies may or may not be painful. In sorting them out, the following concepts are useful:
- Inflammatory myopathies are usually dominated by weakness, not pain. The exception to this rule is when the inflammatory myopathy has a fulminant onset, when pain may be a dominant feature.
- Muscle pain on exertion is suggestive of vascular insufficiency or diseases of muscle metabolism.

6. How does the distribution of weakness, numbness, or pain aid in differentiating neurogenic from muscular lesions?

Myopathies tend to cause proximal and symmetrical (bilateral) weakness and/or pain involving the shoulder girdle and hip girdle. If present, pain may be reported as aching or cramping.

Neuromuscular junction involvement presents with weakness involving ocular, bulbar, and proximal muscles without numbness or pain.

Peripheral neuropathies most commonly cause distal (hands and feet) numbness, weakness, and/or pain. Length dependence is an essential component for large fiber neuropathy and affects deep tendon reflexes and vibratory sensation. Small fiber neuropathy is non-length dependent and can affect proximal regions, be patchy, and affect the autonomic nervous system.

Nerve root compression causes asymmetric weakness and pain that may be either proximal or distal, depending on the level of the involved nerve root.

Spinal cord lesions usually are associated with a distinct sensory level around the trunk or abdomen if above the lumbar spine. Distal spastic weakness, often with impairment of bowel and bladder sphincter function, is also a feature of spinal cord disease.

BOX 12.2 Diseases Affecting Neuromuscular Structures by Level of Anatomic Involvement

SPINAL CORD	NERVE ROOT	PERIPHERAL NERVE	NEUROMUSCULAR JUNCTION	MUSCLE
Amyotrophic lateral sclerosis	Herniated nucleus pulposus	Vasculitis	Myasthenia gravis Lambert-Eaton Syndrome	Inflammatory myopathy
Transverse myelitis		Guillain–Barré syndrome		Hypothyroidism
Vasculitis	Cervical spondylosis	Collagen vascular diseases		Hyperthyroidism
Collagen vascular diseases	Lumbar spondylosis	Nerve compression		Muscular dystrophy
Cervical spondylosis		Amyloidosis		Glucocorticoid use
Lumbar spondylosis				Vasculitis
				Collagen vascular diseases

7. **How does the temporal pattern of weakness or pain aid in diagnosis?**
   - **Abrupt onset** of weakness is more characteristic of Guillain–Barré syndrome, poliomyelitis, vasculitic neuropathy, and hypokalemic periodic paralysis.
   - **Intermittent** weakness may occur with myasthenia gravis, the rare cause of metabolic myopathy, and hypokalemic periodic paralysis.
   - **Gradual onset** of weakness or pain is typical of most muscle diseases, including inflammatory myopathies, muscular dystrophies, and endocrine myopathies, as well as most neuropathies. It may also occur with myasthenia gravis.

8. **What is meant by fatigability? How is it useful in diagnosing neuromuscular disease?**
   Fatigability is defined as progressive weakness of muscle with repetitive use, followed by recovery of strength after a brief period of rest. It is a classic finding in myasthenia gravis often involving eye movements, eyelids (ptosis), and proximal upper extremity muscle groups. Lambert–Eaton myasthenic syndrome is often the reverse of myasthenia gravis, where there is a paradoxical increase in muscle strength observed with repetitive muscle contraction.

9. **How does the family history aid in diagnosis?**
   Many of the muscular dystrophy syndromes have strong patterns of inheritance (Table 12.1).

10. **Name three hormones whose deficiency or excess is associated with myopathy.**
    Thyroxine (hypothyroidism or hyperthyroidism)
    Cortisol (Addison's disease or Cushing's disease)
    Parathyroid hormone (hypoparathyroidism or hyperparathyroidism)

11. **Which drugs are most commonly responsible for neuromuscular symptoms?**
    Glucocorticoids, Chloroquine, Alcohol, D-Penicillamine, Statins, Emetine, Hydroxychloroquine, Colchicine, Cocaine, Fibrates, Zidovudine, Amiodarone, Interferon α, Antifungals, chemotherapeutic agents (e.g., vinca alkaloids, others), antibiotics (e.g., isoniazid, others), nucleoside reverse transcriptase inhibitors (e.g., d4T)

12. **What toxins should be sought in the evaluation of neuromuscular symptoms?**
    - **Organophosphates:** These are used in pesticides, petroleum additives, and modifiers of plastic. Their toxicity affects peripheral nerves and the neuromuscular junction leading to flaccid weakness, depressed deep tendon reflexes, and pupillary dilation. Signs of cholinergic excess (e.g., salivation, lacrimation, others) should be present.
    - **Lead:** Lead toxicity can result in encephalopathy and psychiatric problems (children), abdominal pain, and peripheral neuropathy appearing in the hands before the feet (adults).
    - **Thallium:** This toxin is used in rodenticides and industrial processes. Patients present with sensory and autonomic neuropathy. Alopecia usually develops at the onset of symptoms.
    - **Arsenic, mercury** (electrical and chemical industry): Arsenic, mercury, and industrial solvents containing aliphatic compounds can also cause neuromuscular symptoms.

TABLE 12.1 Muscular Dystrophy Syndromes Inheritance Patterns	
Duchenne muscular dystrophy	X-linked recessive
Becker muscular dystrophy	X-linked recessive
Limb-girdle muscular dystrophies	Autosomal recessive or dominant
Facioscapulohumeral muscular dystrophy	Autosomal dominant
Myotonic dystrophy	Autosomal dominant
Proximal myotonic myopathy	Autosomal dominant

13. What are the key elements of the physical examination in the evaluation of neuromuscular symptoms?

See Table 12.2.

TABLE 12.2 Key Elements of Physical Examination	
SYSTEM	**EXAMINE FOR**
General	Cardiopulmonary disease, infection, thyroid disease, malignancy
Joints	Synovitis, deformities, contractures
Muscles	Muscle bulk, tenderness, weakness, fasciculations
Neurologic	Sensory abnormalities, deep tendon reflexes, weakness

14. What is Gowers' sign?

A patient attempts to rise from a seated position by climbing up his legs with his hands. It is seen in patients with proximal lower extremity muscular weakness due to myopathy.

15. How is muscle weakness graded by the physical examiner?

The most commonly accepted scale is the Medical Research Council Grading System. Because there is a wide range of muscle strength between grades 5 and 4, it is common to assign intermediate values such as 5– or 4+ to many muscle groups in the examination (Table 12.3).

TABLE 12.3 Manual Grading of Muscle Strength	
GRADE	**DEGREE OF STRENGTH**
5	Normal strength
4	Muscle contraction possible against gravity plus some examiner resistance.
3	Muscle contraction possible against gravity only.
2	Muscle contraction possible only with gravity removed.
1	Flicker of muscle contraction observed but without movement of extremity.
0	No contraction

16. How are deep tendon reflexes graded by the physical examiner?

See Table 12.4.

TABLE 12.4 Grading of Deep Tendon Reflexes	
GRADE	**STRENGTH OF CONTRACTION**
4	Clonus
3	Exaggerated
2	Normal
1	Present but depressed
0	Absent

17. How can alterations in deep tendon reflexes aid in differentiation of neuromuscular diseases?

- Spinal cord lesions (above L1 to L2) and upper motor neuron disease usually produce exaggerated deep tendon reflexes and pathologic extensor plantar reflexes. Of note, acute spinal cord lesions can occasionally lead to depressed or absent reflexes initially (i.e., spinal shock).

- Nerve root and peripheral nerve lesions usually produce depressed or absent reflexes. Small fiber neuropathies often have normal reflexes.
- Primary muscle diseases do not usually present with altered deep tendon reflexes. Late in the disease process, however, substantial muscle atrophy may cause reduction or loss of the reflex.
- Hyperthyroidism produces exaggerated tendon reflexes.
- Hypothyroidism produces depressed deep tendon reflexes with a slow relaxation phase.
- Many people aged over 60 years experience natural loss of their ankle reflexes.

18. **Which screening laboratory tests can evaluate for systemic causes of neuromuscular symptoms?**

See Box 12.3.

BOX 12.3 Screening Tests for Neuromuscular Diseases

Complete blood count
Serum electrolytes, calcium, magnesium, phosphorus
Serum muscle enzymes
Erythrocyte sedimentation rate
C-reactive protein
Serum liver enzyme tests
Serum renal function tests
Serum 25-hydroxyvitamin D level
Thyroid function tests
Chest radiograph
Electrocardiogram

---

19. **Which serum enzymes are elevated in muscle disease?**

See Table 12.5.

TABLE 12.5 Clinical Utility of Serum Muscle Enzymes

SERUM ENZYME	CLINICAL UTILITY
Creatine kinase	Most sensitive and specific for muscle disease
Aldolase	Elevated in muscle, liver, and erythrocyte diseases
Lactic dehydrogenase	Elevated in muscle, liver, erythrocyte, and other diseases
Aspartate aminotransferase	Most specific for inflammatory muscle disease

20. **What are other causes of elevation of serum creatine kinase (CK) besides myopathy?**

Intramuscular injections
Muscle crush injuries
Recent strenuous exercise
Myocardial infarction
Race of individual (Healthy African–Americans may have significantly higher CK levels than the "normal" values derived from the entire population. Notably, their CK is always less than 1000 IU/L and their aldolase will be normal.)

21. **Are additional specific tests useful in the evaluation of neuromuscular symptoms?**

See Table 12.6.

TABLE 12.6 Additional Diagnostic Tests in Neuromuscular Disease Evaluation

SPECIFIC TEST	SUSPECTED DISEASE PROCESSES
Serum myositis-specific antibodies Serum anti-synthetase antibodies	Inflammatory myopathy+/– cancer Inflammatory myositis +/– interstitial lung dz
Serum antinuclear antibodies Serum myositis-associated antibodies	Inflammatory myopathy, vasculitis, neuropathy Inflammatory myositis with rheumatic dz
Serum rheumatoid factor	Inflammatory myopathy, vasculitis
Serum complement assay	Inflammatory myopathy, vasculitis
Serum cryoglobulins	Vasculitis
Hepatitis B surface antigen and hepatitis C Ab	Vasculitis
Anti-neutrophil cytoplasmic antibodies	Vasculitis
Acetylcholine receptor antibodies	Myasthenia gravis
Serum parathyroid hormone	Parathyroid disease
Electromyography and nerve conduction tests	Disease of nerve roots, peripheral nerves, or myopathies
Muscle biopsy	Inflammatory or metabolic myopathies, vasculitis
Skin biopsy	Small fiber neuropathy, vasculitis
Nerve biopsy	Vasculitis
Magnetic resonance scan	Spinal cord, nerve root, and myopathic processes

22. What is mononeuritis multiplex?

Mononeuritis multiplex is a pattern of motor and sensory involvement of multiple individual peripheral nerves; it is a classic neurologic presentation of systemic vasculitis. First, one peripheral nerve becomes involved (usually with burning dysesthesias), followed by other individual nerves, often with motor dysfunction as well. The patchy nature of nerve involvement reflects the patchy vasculitis of the vasa nervorum, which is the underlying cause of the neuropathy. Mononeuritis multiplex can also be present in diabetes mellitus, sarcoidosis, lead neuropathy, and Wartenberg's migratory sensory neuritis.

23. What is small fiber neuropathy?

Small fiber neuropathy is due to destruction of the lightly myelinated A-delta and unmyelinated C fibers including nociceptors and autonomic fibers. Patients can present with a variety of symptoms including pain, dysesthesias, allodynia, and autonomic dysfunction (e.g., sweating, urination, bowel function). Symptoms can be distal, proximal, bilateral, and patchy and do not follow a particular sensory nerve distribution. Patients have normal strength, reflexes, proprioception, and vibratory sense but reduced thermal and pinprick sensation on testing. Nerve conduction velocities are normal. The etiology of small fiber neuropathy can be idiopathic (50%) or due to metabolic diseases (e.g., diabetes, others), immune diseases (e.g., Sjogren's, SLE, sarcoidosis, others), fibromyalgia (controversial), toxic (e.g., chemotherapeutics, alcohol, others), infections (e.g., Lyme, HIV, COVID, others), or heredity (e.g. Fabry's, others) causes. Diagnosis is confirmed via punch biopsy of the skin showing reduced intra-epidermal nerve fiber density, especially when less than the fifth percentile. Treatment is symptomatic, including anti-epileptics (e.g., pregabalin, others), antidepressants (tricyclics, SNRIs), and tramadol.

24. What are the most common causes of proximal shoulder girdle and hip girdle aches, pains, and/or weakness? How are they differentiated?

Six diseases are responsible for >90% of diffuse, proximal aches or weakness (Table 12.7). The first step is to decide the dominant clinical finding—pain or weakness. To determine if true weakness is present, the examiner should ask the patient to ignore any pain that may occur during muscle strength testing so that a true measure of muscle strength can be determined. Often patients can provide a brief full-strength effort and then giveaway when pain is the predominant cause. Although patients with fibromyalgia syndrome and polymyalgia rheumatica may complain of weakness in addition to pain, they are not truly weak on physical examination.

TABLE 12.7 Common Causes of Proximal Muscle Pain and/or Weakness

DISEASE	PAIN	WEAKNESS	ERYTHROCYTE SEDIMENTATION RATE	SERUM CREATINE KINASE	SERUM THYROXINE (T4)
Fibromyalgia	Yes	No	Normal	Normal	Normal
Polymyalgia rheumatica	Yes	No	Marked elevation	Normal	Normal
Polymyositis	Usually none	Yes	Usually	Elevated Normal	Normal
Corticosteroid myopathy	No	Yes	Normal	Normal	Normal
Hyperthyroidism	No	Yes	Normal	Normal	Elevated
Hypothyroidism	Yes	Yes	Normal	Elevated	Depressed

25. What are critical illness polyneuropathy (CIP) and critical illness myopathy (CIM)?

Intensive care unit (ICU)-acquired weakness is a group of neuromuscular disorders commonly affecting patients with critical illnesses. CIP is most likely to occur in patients with severe sepsis, multiple organ dysfunction, and those receiving prolonged mechanical ventilation (26% to 65% of patients on ventilators for >5 to 7 days). Manifestations include limb muscle weakness, reduced or absent deep tendon reflexes, loss of distal sensation, and respiratory insufficiency due to phrenic nerve involvement. CIM most commonly occurs in patients who have received intravenous glucocorticoids in the ICU setting. Patients have severe muscle weakness, preserved reflexes/sensation, and difficulty weaning off a ventilator. Half of the patients have an elevated CK. Clinical presentation, serum CK levels, electrodiagnostic testing, and muscle biopsy findings can separate patients with CIP from those with CIM; however, it is not uncommon for both conditions to coexist in the same individual. Treatment is supportive care, limiting the use of glucocorticoids and paralytics, and nutritional support. Patients usually take weeks to months to recover their strength.

26. What is the diagnostic significance of young adult stroke? What rheumatic syndromes should be considered in the differential diagnosis of cerebrovascular disease?

Most cerebrovascular diseases occur in patients aged over 50 years as a result of long-standing hypertension, atherosclerosis, and cardiac emboli. When ischemic cerebrovascular disease occurs in patients aged <50 years, the possibility of several rheumatic syndromes should be especially considered: (Box 12.4)

BOX 12.4 Rheumatologic Causes of Stroke in Young Patients

Systemic lupus erythematosus
Antiphospholipid antibody syndrome
Takayasu's arteritis
Isolated angiitis of the central nervous system
Polyarteritis nodosa
Granulomatosis with polyangiitis (Wegener's)

BIBLIOGRAPHY

Alshekhlee A, Kaminksi HJ, Ruff RL. Neuromuscular manifestations of endocrine disorders. *Neurol Clin.* 2002;20:35–58.
Christopher-Stine L, Stojan G. Metabolic, drug-induced, and other noninflammatory myopathies. In: Hochberg MC, Gravallese EM, Smolen JS, van der Heijde D, Weinblatt E, Weisman MH, eds. *Rheumatology.* 8th ed. Philadelphia: Elsevier;2023:1395–1403.

Dalakas MC. Muscle biopsy findings in inflammatory myopathies. *Rheum Dis Clin North Am.* 2002;28:779–798.

Goglin SE, Imboden JB, eds. Neurologic manifestations of rheumatic diseases. *Rheum Dis Clin.* 2017; 43 (4):xiii-xiv.

Halilu F, Christopher-Stine L. Myositis-specific antibodies: overview and clinical utilization. *Rheumatol Immunol Res.* 2022;3:1–10.

Hermans G, van den Berghe G. Clinical review: intensive care unit acquired weakness. *Crit Care.* 2015;19:274.

Jones MR, Urits I, Wolf J, et al. Drug-induced peripheral neuropathy: a narrative review. *Curr Clin Pharmacol.* 2020;15:38–48.

Neal RC, Ferdinand KC, Ycas J, Miller E. Relationship of ethnic origin, gender, and age to blood creatine kinase levels. *Am J Med.* 2009;122:73–78.

Nirmalananthan N, Holton JL, Hanna MG. Is it really myositis? A consideration of the differential diagnosis. *Curr Opin Rheumatol.* 2004;16:684–691.

Rodolico C, Bonanno C, Pugliese A, et al. Endocrine myopathies: clinical and histopathological features of the major forms. *Acta Myol.* 2020;39:130–135.

Saperstein DS. Small fiber neuropathy. *Neurol Clin.* 2020;38:607–618.

Schulze M, Kötter I, Ernemann U, et al. MRI findings in inflammatory muscle diseases and their noninflammatory mimics. *AJR.* 2009;192:1708–1716.

Toledano M. Neurologic manifestations of rheumatologic disease. *Continuum.* 2023;29:734–762.

CHAPTER 13

Perioperative Management of Patients With Rheumatic Diseases

Kevin D. Deane, MD, PhD and Kim Nguyen Tyler, MD

---

1. Why is it important for rheumatic disease patients to be evaluated perioperatively?

Patients with rheumatic diseases can have unique problems because of their underlying rheumatic disease, complications of medical therapy including immunosuppression, and limitations in functional status. The perioperative evaluation can identify factors that may contribute to surgical risk so that appropriate action can be taken to reduce the risk of complications.

2. List the essential items to review in the perioperative evaluation of a patient with a rheumatic disease.

A comprehensive evaluation should include consideration of the "ABCDE'S":

A —adjust medications
B —bacterial prophylaxis
C —cervical spine disease, cardiovascular (CV) risk
D —DVT prophylaxis
E —evaluate extent and activity of disease; maximize disease control
S —stress-dose steroid coverage (see Questions 13–15)

3. How are patients with rheumatic diseases "cleared" for surgery?

The term "clearance" was used at a time when the goal of the preoperative assessment was to roughly divide patients into those able to tolerate surgery ("cleared") and those unable to tolerate surgery. The term is largely historical, as patients are uncommonly excluded from consideration for an operative procedure solely on the basis of their underlying medical conditions. However, patients with rheumatic diseases may be at increased risk for perioperative complications due to a variety of factors. A more appropriate goal of the preoperative assessment is to optimize safety and improve outcomes through risk stratification and address potential perioperative problems to minimize their potential adverse effects.

4. List four important issues to address in the preoperative history and physical examination of patients with rheumatic diseases.

A. **Medication management:** patients with inflammatory rheumatic diseases may be on medications that increase their chance of developing perioperative complications such as infections or poor wound healing. A guideline published by the American College of Rheumatology and the American Association of Hip and Knee Surgeons (ACR/AAHKS) that was updated in 2022 helps with the management of these medications (see Questions 22 and 23).

B. **CV risk:** patients with inflammatory rheumatic disease have an increased risk of CV events. Many are elderly and/or physically impaired; therefore, determining CV risk may be more difficult because of physical inactivity. In the absence of specific recommendations for patients with rheumatic disease, it is prudent to at minimum follow guidelines for the general population set forth by the American Heart Association/American College of Cardiology. These guidelines do not recommend advanced cardiac evaluation (such as a pharmacologic stress test) in patients requiring emergency surgery; in elective surgeries, the risk of the surgery and patient-specific risk categories are taken into account to determine whether additional cardiac testing is necessary.

- Patients with active cardiac disease (unstable coronary artery disease, decompensated heart failure, hemodynamically significant valvular disease, high-grade arrhythmias) typically require pharmacologic stress testing regardless of the risk of surgery.
- Low-risk surgical procedures (dental surgery, ocular surgery, inguinal repair) do not typically warrant additional evaluation regardless of patient-specific risk factors.
- Moderate-risk surgical procedures (e.g., joint arthroscopy) do not typically warrant additional evaluation for low-risk patients who can be defined as having no more than one of the following: history of ischemic heart disease, history of heart failure, history of cerebrovascular disease, current diabetes requiring insulin treatment, serum creatinine >2.0 mg/dL.
- Moderate-risk surgical procedures in higher-risk patients, especially those with low functional status, may require pharmacologic stress testing and a preoperative cardiology evaluation. Low functional status in this setting is commonly defined as an inability to complete four metabolic equivalents (METs) or the equivalent of climbing one set of stairs.
- High-risk surgical procedures (vascular surgery, intrathoracic, or intraabdominal surgery), especially in patients with low functional status, may require pharmacologic stress testing and a preoperative evaluation by cardiology.

C. **Cervical spine disease:** patients with RA and other forms of inflammatory arthritis may have C1-C2 disease that could damage the spinal cord during intubation; as such, preoperative evaluation of the cervical spine may be indicated. See Questions 8 and 9 for more information.

D. **Occult infections:** patients should be examined for cavities and/or signs of dental abscess, pharyngitis, and skin infection (look at the feet); testing should be performed for cystitis in symptomatic patients as well, as all may serve as sources of infection for total joint arthroplasties. Patients with an enlarged prostate are at increased risk of catheter-induced postoperative urinary tract infections.

5. **What laboratory tests are routinely required for patients with rheumatic diseases scheduled for elective surgery?**

There is no consensus on preoperative screening evaluations. Specific clinical scenarios such as patients on anticoagulation or certain disease-modifying antirheumatic drugs (DMARDs) may justify a selected set of laboratory and imaging evaluations. Table 13.1 outlines potential preoperative evaluations for patients with rheumatic disease.

6. **Are patients with rheumatic diseases at increased risk for perioperative complications compared with other patients?**

Patients with rheumatic diseases may have a higher incidence of postoperative wound infections and impaired wound healing than nonrheumatic patients, usually because of medications used

TABLE 13.1 Potential Preoperative Evaluations

TEST	CONSIDER IN A PATIENT WITH
Liver function tests	Use of: Nonsteroidal anti-inflammatory drug, methotrexate, leflunomide, IL-6 inhibitor, JAK inhibitor use
Prothrombin time/partial thromboplastin time	Liver disease or bleeding disorder Antiphospholipid antibody syndrome
Chest imaging (may include standard x-ray or other imaging such as computed tomography)	Acute pulmonary symptoms, abnormal examination Pulmonary and/or cardiovascular disease Thoracic surgery
Pulmonary function tests	Same as chest imaging
Cervical spine x-ray (flexion and extension views)	Rheumatoid arthritis, juvenile idiopathic arthritis, axial spondyloarthritis

to treat their disease. Accelerated CV disease may be seen in patients with chronic inflammatory diseases such as RA, systemic lupus erythematosus (SLE), and psoriasis/psoriatic arthritis due to disease activity or medications. In addition, these groups may have higher rates of asymptomatic CV disease than nonrheumatic populations. As such, CV risk assessment should be performed in all patients with inflammatory rheumatic disease (see Question 4).

7. Should patients with active synovitis undergo elective surgery?

Usually, they should not. Patients with active synovitis may have significant pain in the postoperative period from their arthritis that impairs functional status, impedes progress with rehabilitation, and prolongs hospitalization. Patients with active synovial disease and its consequent disability should have the inflammation controlled as much as possible prior to elective surgical procedures. If a patient does have active disease in the perioperative period and systemic corticosteroids or DMARDs are inadvisable, intraarticular corticosteroids may be considered. Notably, intraarticular steroids in a joint that is being considered for arthroplasty or other surgery may lead some orthopedic surgeons to delay surgery; as such, it is important to consult with the orthopedic surgeon before injecting a joint that is being considered for surgery.

8. Why is it important to evaluate patients with RA for cervical spine disease before surgery?

Although cervical spine disease in RA has decreased in frequency, instability of the cervical spine may still be present in patients with RA. In particular, cervical spine **atlantoaxial subluxation** can occur secondary to inflammation and weakening of the transverse ligament that holds the odontoid process of C2 against the anterior arch of C1. Manipulation of the neck during intubation and transport of the patient, especially extreme flexion or extension, can cause compression of the spinal cord by the odontoid process. Most anesthesiologists advocate for preoperative flexion and extension C-spine radiographs for RA patients with the following risk factors (C-SPINE), as significant cervical spine disease may be asymptomatic:

C —corticosteroid use

S —seropositive RA

P —peripheral joint destruction

I —involvement of cervical nerves (paresthesia, neck pain, weakness)

N —nodules (rheumatoid)

E —established disease (present >10 years)

In addition, patients with axial involvement from spondyloarthritis and juvenile onset inflammatory arthritis may also have C1-C2 disease, and preoperative evaluation of the cervical spine in these individuals should be considered.

9. How is atlantoaxial (C1–C2) instability diagnosed? How is it managed?

Instability of C1 to C2 is diagnosed when the interval between the odontoid process and the anterior arch of the atlas is >3 mm on lateral flexion and extension radiographs (Fig. 13.1). This indicates that the transverse ligament has been compromised. When the interval exceeds 7 to 8 mm, it is likely that the alar ligaments are compromised as well, significantly increasing the risk of spinal cord compromise.

Patients with symptoms attributable to C1 to C2 instability should have surgical stabilization performed prior to elective surgery. Patients with asymptomatic or mild disease may be considered for intubation with fiberoptic assistance, or respiration with a laryngeal mask to minimize the extremes of motion associated with routine intubation.

10. What is cricoarytenoid (CA) disease? How can it impact anesthetic complications?

The CA joint is a true diarthrodial articulation. As such, it may be a target for the same destructive changes that can occur in other small joints in patients with RA. The degree of CA disease correlates with peripheral joint disease. Symptoms of CA involvement include tracheal pain, dysphonia, stridor, dyspnea, and dysarthria. Some patients may have minor symptoms related to synovitis, but over time develop fibrous replacement of the normal cartilage and ankylosis across the joint space. CA disease may be clinically silent, and involvement in some patients may be identified following unsuccessful attempts at endotracheal intubation by standard techniques. This can result in trauma to the adducted vocal cords, with subsequent edema, inflammation, and airway obstruction.

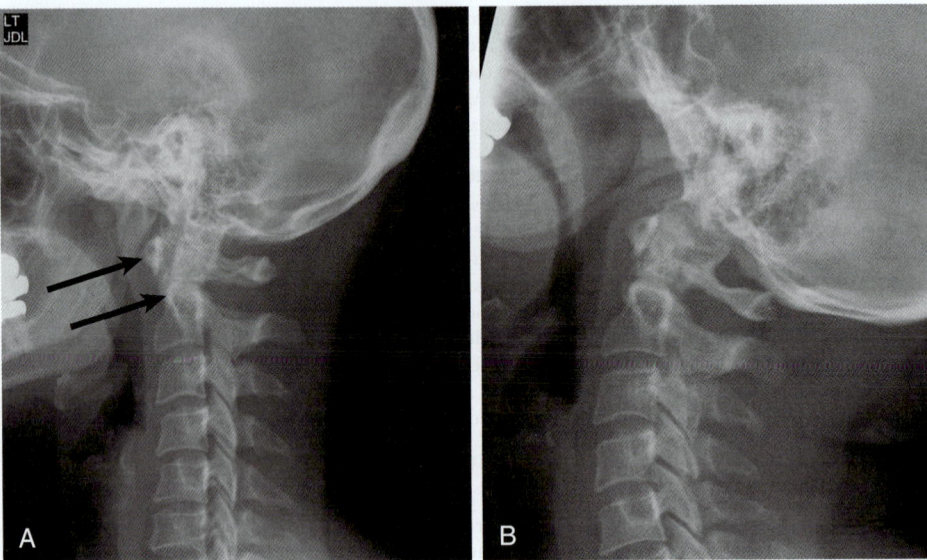

Fig. 13.1 Atlantoaxial instability. Arrows show separation of the odontoid process of C2 from the anterior arch of C1 (6 mm) in a patient with severe rheumatoid arthritis. (A) Lateral (neutral position) view. (B) Extension view.

Perioperative fiberoptic laryngoscopy is recommended for all patients with symptoms of CA disease. Treatment includes systemic or locally injected corticosteroids. Intubation under fiberoptic guidance is also recommended during surgery. Patients with severe CA disease should be considered for elective tracheostomy if the vocal cords are found to be chronically adducted.

11. Should aspirin (ASA) and nonsteroidal anti-inflammatory (NSAIDs) drugs be discontinued preoperatively in rheumatic disease patients?

Patients treated with ASA and acetylsalicylate-containing medications may be at risk for increased surgical bleeding because these drugs impair platelet aggregation for the life of the platelet (7–10 days). ASA should be discontinued 7 to 10 days before most planned surgeries. However, ASA may reduce the risk of perioperative vascular events and should be continued in patients taking it for secondary prevention of CV events and through certain vascular surgeries (cardiac artery bypass graft surgery, carotid endarterectomy). Consulting with the surgeon on their preferences for NSAID use prior to the procedure may be indicated.

Traditional NSAIDs may also decrease platelet aggregation; however, unlike ASA, NSAID binding to the COX-1 site in platelets is reversible and declines with discontinuation of the medicine. NSAIDs have also been associated with more frequent episodes of gastrointestinal bleeding when given perioperatively. To reduce risk of bleeding, one could consider holding these medications preoperatively for approximately four half-lives of the drug to allow return of normal platelet function and may be restarted 2 to 3 days postoperatively provided the patient is stable. Recently, there has been an increased push for the use of NSAIDs for post-operative pain, in particular to avoid opiate use. However, due to concern regarding the CV risk of NSAIDs, they should be used cautiously in the postoperative period, especially in patients at increased risk for CV events. Alternative medications for pain/inflammation may be preferred during this time and include acetaminophen or judicious use of tramadol or narcotic analgesics. Salsalate is a nonacetylated salicylate that does not affect the prostaglandin synthesis pathway. As such, it does not affect platelet function and may be considered in this setting.

PEARL: Ask about nonprescription drugs and supplements. Many rheumatic disease patients may take complementary and alternative medicine therapies that can affect platelet function (e.g., turmeric, ginkgo, ginger, Artri King) or interact with anesthesia.

12. How does the normal adrenal gland respond to surgery?

In a baseline state, the adrenal gland secretes the equivalent of 20 to 30 mg of cortisol (e.g., hydrocortisone; equivalent to 5–7.5 mg prednisone) per day, but with major stress or general anesthesia, it may increase 10-fold up to 200 to 300 mg of cortisol (50–75 mg of prednisone) per day. Cortisol levels typically peak within 24 hours of the time of surgical incision and return to normal after 72 hours if no other factors contribute to perioperative stress.

13. What causes exogenous corticosteroid-related perioperative adrenal insufficiency?

The administration of exogenous corticosteroids can interfere with the normal function of the hypothalamic–pituitary–adrenal (HPA) axis and blunt endogenous cortisol excretion. With stress, the adrenal output blunted by exogenous corticosteroids may become inadequate to support physiologic demands, which include vascular tone and maintenance of blood pressure. The following patients are at risk for corticosteroid-related adrenal insufficiency:
- Patients with features of Cushing's syndrome (e.g., moon facies, buffalo hump).
- Patients on a prednisone dose (or equivalent of another corticosteroid) of: ≥20 mg daily for ≥3 weeks.

If there is any concern about whether clinically significant adrenal insufficiency may occur, an adrenal stimulation test may be performed or the patient should receive stress-dose steroids empirically. Patients who become adrenally insufficient during stress (infection, trauma) usually become hypotensive (systolic <90 mmHg) in spite of fluid resuscitation. These patients should be placed on intravenous (IV) hydrocortisone 100 mg every 8 hours with subsequent tapering once the stress resolves. Tapering is best achieved by lowering the dose and not the frequency (i.e., every 8 hours) of hydrocortisone.

14. How can patients at risk of adrenal insufficiency be tested preoperatively?

The cosyntropin stimulation test evaluates the ability of the adrenal gland to respond to stress. After the baseline cortisol level has been obtained, 250 μg of cosyntropin (an adrenocorticotropic hormone [ACTH] analog) is injected IV or intramuscularly, and the cortisol level is measured after 30 and 60 minutes. Patients with a normal HPA axis should typically be able to double their baseline cortisol level in response to stress (cosyntropin), but those with an already high basal level may not be able to do so. As such, current recommendations are to use the peak cortisol measurement (highest value tested among baseline, 30-minute, and 60-minute post cosyntropin) rather than measurements of cortisol level change. If any value is >18 μg/dL, adrenal insufficiency is ruled out.

15. How should steroids be dosed in the perioperative period and are stress-dose steroids needed for all individuals who are taking or who have received recent steroids?

Data suggest that most patients on low-dose corticosteroids do not require perioperative stress-dosing, especially if the patient is undergoing a minor procedure and is monitored closely in the perioperative period. The 2022 ACR/AAHKS guidelines on perioperative management for elective total knee or hip arthroplasty recommend that the current daily dose of steroid be continued throughout the operative period, without routine supraphysiologic dosing. There have been several studies reporting that the risk of symptomatic adrenal insufficiency in the post-operative period is low, whereas the potential risks from stress dose steroids (poor wound healing, infection, hyperglycemia, etc.) are higher. For major surgery or in the setting of anticipated physiologic stress (e.g., serious infections or trauma), some providers may elect to provide perioperative stress-dose steroids due to the potential life-threatening complications of adrenal insufficiency. In this setting, treatment is often given empirically without formal testing. Of note, the anesthetic agent, etomidate, may interfere with adrenal corticosteroid synthesis; as such, if this agent is used for anesthesia, stress-dose steroids should be considered regardless of the level of surgical risk.

In patients receiving stress-dose steroids, tapering back to the baseline corticosteroid dose should occur within 48 to 72 hours if possible to avoid increased risk of infection and/or problems with wound healing. Elaborate tapering schedules are not required unless postoperative complications prolong stress after surgery. In general, patients on oral steroids preoperatively may typically resume their normal daily dose once stable postoperatively and tolerate oral medications.

TABLE 13.2 Perioperative Regimens for Stress-Dose Corticosteroid Administration

LEVEL OF SURGICAL STRESS	SURGICAL PROCEDURE	STRESS-DOSE STEROIDS
Superficial procedure	Skin biopsy	Continue daily dose of corticosteroids
Minor	Procedures under local anesthesia and <1 hour Colonoscopy, cataract surgery, carpal tunnel release, tenosynovectomy, knee arthroscopy Most minor oral, podiatry/orthopedic foot procedures (hammer toe correction, toe fusion)	Continue daily dose of corticosteroids
Moderate	Unilateral total joint replacement Complex foot reconstruction Lower extremity vascular surgery Uncomplicated appendectomy Gallbladder removal	Consider continuing preoperative daily oral dose. *If stress dose steroids needed:* Hydrocortisone 50mg IV intraoperatively in OR, then 25mg IV every 8 hours for 24 hours. On the second postoperative day, resume preoperative daily dosing regimen (IV dosing may be considered if oral intake is not tolerated)
Major	Multiple trauma Colon resection, bilateral joint replacement, revision arthroplasty, multiple-level spinal fusion Any surgery requiring cardiopulmonary bypass	Hydrocortisone 100mg IV on call to OR or early intraoperatively, then 50mg IV every 8 hours for 24 hours, then resume the preoperative daily dose on the second postoperative day (may be oral if tolerating oral intake, or IV)

IV, Intravenous; *OR*, operating room.
Caveats:
(1) Patients must be monitored carefully for signs of adrenal insufficiency (hypotension) in the perioperative period and stress dosing may need to be adjusted.
(2) If postoperative hypotension develops, patients should be assessed for etiologies other than adrenal insufficiency including volume depletion, cardiovascular disease, pulmonary embolus, and infection.

Hydrocortisone is considered the corticosteroid of choice for stress-dose regimens because it has a rapid onset of action compared with other agents. There is clinical variation in the literature regarding the dose and duration of stress-dose steroid regimens; Table 13.2 outlines one reasonable approach.

16. Name the two most common organisms to infect a prosthetic joint at the time of surgery.
- Coagulase-negative staphylococci (may be difficult to identify due to slow or minimal growth and because it may initially be considered a skin contaminant).
- Staphylococcus aureus.

17. What is the standard antibiotic prophylaxis for prosthetic joint surgery?
The goal of perioperative antibiotics is to reduce organism burden and prevent postoperative infection. For joint replacement surgery, cefazolin is typically used with the first dose given immediately preoperatively and continued for 24 hours postoperatively. Vancomycin or clindamycin may be used in patients who are allergic to penicillin. There are no data to support the use of prophylactic antibiotics for >24 hours postoperatively. Other measures to reduce postoperative infection include skin cleansing preoperatively with agents such as chlorhexidine, and smoking cessation.

18. Should patients who have prosthetic joints be prescribed antibiotic prophylaxis prior to undergoing dental procedures (controversial)?
There is no strong clinical data to support the utility of routine antibiotic prophylaxis during dental procedures in low-risk patients with prosthetic joints. As such, the American Academy of Orthopedic Surgeons (AAOS), in conjunction with the American Dental Association (ADA)

TABLE 13.3 High-Risk Populations With Prosthetic Joints That May Require Antibiotic Prophylaxis Prior to Dental Procedures

Severe immunocompromised states (e.g., AIDS, cancer patients with febrile neutropenia, rheumatoid arthritis patients on biologic DMARDs or prednisone >10 mg daily)[a]
Known diabetes, especially if poorly controlled
History of prosthetic joint infection requiring an operation
Arthroplasty within the last year
Dental procedures with manipulation of gingival tissue, the periapical region of teeth, or perforation of oral mucosa[b]

DMARD, Disease-modifying antirheumatic drug.
[a]The American Academy of Orthopedic Surgeons and the American Dental Association guideline consider methotrexate and hydroxychloroquine as non-immunocompromising agents and make no specific mention of other nonbiologic DMARDs.
[b]Of importance, *less invasive procedures (routine dental cleaning, etc.) do not mandate antibiotic prophylaxis* regardless of other patient-specific risk factors.

and with input from the Infectious Disease Society of America, suggests that clinicians consider discontinuing the practice of routine antibiotic prophylaxis in low-risk populations. However, this recommendation is based on low-level evidence and may not be applicable to high-risk groups. The AAOS-ADA clinical practice guideline recognizes certain clinical scenarios that may confer an increased risk of infection and justify consideration of prophylactic antibiotics (Table 13.3). The AAOS has an online risk assessment tool that clinicians can use to enter these risk factors for specific patients and aid in decision-making (website address at the end of this chapter). Importantly, final decisions on the use of antibiotic prophylaxis should be made in consultation with the dental and orthopedic services.

Antibiotics prescribed for these selected patients may provide benefit without excess risk. In the absence of good data, the following agents may be rational choices: amoxicillin, cephalexin, or azithromycin (for the penicillin-allergic patient), all dosed once orally 1 hour before the procedure. Antibiotic prophylaxis is not necessary for patients with small joint (e.g., metacarpophalangeal joint) replacements, pins, plates, or screws.

19. Should patients with antiphospholipid antibodies (APLs) be given antibiotic prophylaxis prior to dental, urologic, and gastrointestinal procedures?

Patients with APLs may have underlying valvular disease that could theoretically predispose them to endocarditis following procedures known to cause transient bacteremia. Nonetheless, data have not supported a role for antibiotic prophylaxis for the majority of patients with valvular heart disease, and only a subset of patients with the following conditions should routinely receive antibiotics:

- Prosthetic valves and/or prosthetic materials used for valve repair (e.g., annuloplasty rings, prosthetic material used in repair of congenital heart defects).
- History of infective endocarditis.
- History of cardiac transplant with valve regurgitation.
- Unrepaired cyanotic congenital heart defects.

It is important to note that even among these high-risk groups, prophylactic antibiotics are not recommended for low-risk dental procedures such as routine cleaning and are reserved for procedures which manipulate gingival tissue, the periapical area of teeth or perforate the oral mucosa. Current guidelines do not outline formal recommendations for patients with APLs and known valvular abnormalities, and clinical data regarding antibiotic prophylaxis in this group are limited. As such, clinical judgment should be used regarding this decision and should take into consideration the risk of infection overall in patients with rheumatic conditions on immunosuppression.

20. How should agents used to treat/prevent osteoporosis be used around dental procedures?

Medication-related osteonecrosis of the jaw (MRONJ) has been associated with dental procedures in individuals who are being treated with medications to treat/prevent osteoporosis (prevalence <0.05%; see Chapter 87: Bone Strengthening Agents). Most cases are in individuals using bisphosphonates (BPs); however, cases have been reported in individuals using denosumab as well. There are only rare cases reported in individuals using agents such as estrogens, teriparatide, abaloparatide, raloxifene, romosozumab and calcitonin.

To reduce the risk of MRONJ, preventative measures are recommended that include regular cleanings, control of caries and infections, minimizing corticosteroid use, smoking cessation, and minimizing bone injury during invasive dental procedures. Pre- and post-operative use of antibiotics and antimicrobial mouth rinses have been shown to be helpful for prevention of MRONJ in limited studies. While temporary discontinuation of BPs prior to invasive dental procedures is sometimes seen in practice, there are no data to support this strategy nor in delaying dental treatment in those already on antiresorptive therapy. The American Dental Association last released guidance on this topic in 2011. No formal recommendations were made for or against withholding BPs in this setting, but a recommendation was made to not withhold invasive dental procedures in patients currently on bisphosphonates for osteoporosis given the very low risk of MRONJ and higher risk of dental complications from delayed intervention. Similarly, the American Association of Oral and Maxillofacial Surgeons position paper on this topic was updated in 2022. Previous versions of this position statement suggested withholding BPs in longer-term users (>4 years). Given the lack of evidence directly supporting this strategy, no formal recommendation on withholding BPs was made in the 2022 update. Information on the ADA website for this topic, and references for both guidelines is included at the end of this chapter.

Of importance, special consideration must be made not to delay the administration of denosumab due to the risk of worsening bone mineral density and increased risk for fracture with its delayed administration.

21. What are the options for DVT prophylaxis in patients undergoing joint replacement procedures?

DVT risk varies with the procedure, with hip replacement being higher risk than knee replacement (note: surgical repair of a hip fracture has higher risk than routine hip replacement). There are several groups that have published guidelines in this area (e.g. American College of Chest Physicians [ACCP], American Academy of Orthopedic Surgeons [AAOS] and American Society for Hematology [ASH]) and there is some variance in recommendations; furthermore, guidelines in this area are changing as new therapies are developed. Because of the variability of recommendations, a good rule is to consult with the surgical team for latest recommendations; however, the following are options for DVT prophylaxis:

- Full anticoagulation with a directly acting oral anticoagulant (DOAC) (e.g., dabigatran, rivaroxaban) or low molecular weight heparin (LMWH) beginning immediately after surgery and continuing for 10–14 days, and potentially up to 35 days in high-risk individuals. High-risk may be defined as those with a personal or family history of venous thromboembolism, active cancer, known hypercoaguable state, anticipated prolonged immobility and medical co-morbidities such as obesity. The ACCP guidelines also suggest that fondaparinux may be used; aspirin is also recommended in low-risk individuals although data supporting its efficacy are limited.
- Heparin (unfractionated) or warfarin may be used although they require more intensive monitoring, and in the case of warfarin, it is necessary to bridge to adequate anticoagulation effect (usually 5 days) with LMWH or unfractionated heparin.
- Other approaches to reduce risk of DVT include early mobilization and use of pneumatic compression devices, worn on the lower extremities at all times starting the morning of surgery, until the patient is ambulatory or discharged. Compression stockings only offer minimal protection against DVT, and the effectiveness of this approach as single therapy has not been determined in patients with rheumatic disease (many of whom are at elevated risk of clot).
- Most recommendations are against prophylactic use of an inferior vena cava filter.

22. Should the dosing of conventional synthetic DMARDs (csDMARDs) and targeted synthetic DMARDs (tsDMARDs) be altered prior to elective surgery?

The choice to continue or stop DMARDs perioperatively depends on the underlying disease and disease activity, type of surgery, and type of DMARD. Minimizing the risk for infection and poor wound healing should be balanced against the risk of disease flare. Unfortunately, there is no strong evidence-based guidance for management of DMARDS in all situations, and shared decision making between the patient, rheumatologist and surgeon is critically important. However, the 2022 ACR/AAHKS guidelines for patients undergoing total knee arthroplasty (TKA) and total hip arthroplasty (THA) provide guidance that while focused on joint replacements, may be extrapolated to other types of surgeries.

For non-SLE rheumatic diseases, the guidelines recommend continuing csDMARDs, including methotrexate, sulfasalazine, hydroxychloroquine, leflunomide, doxycycline, and tsDMARD apremilast throughout the perioperative period. The tsDMARDs tofacitinib, baricitinib, and upadicitinib should be stopped 3 days prior to surgery and restarted post-operatively once there are no signs of infection, good wound healing, and removal of sutures (typically 2 weeks). In SLE, the choice to continue csDMARDs perioperatively depends on disease severity. For example, in patients with severe SLE (see Table 13.4 for definitions of disease severity), it is recommended to continue agents such as mycophenolate mofetil, azathioprine, cyclosporine, tacrolimus and voclosporin throughout the operative period to maintain disease control. This is in contrast to patients with non-severe SLE where these medications are recommended to be temporarily held 1 week prior to surgery. See Table 13.4 for additional details.

Of note, careful consideration must also be made regarding perioperative issues that may affect metabolism and/or clearance of DMARDs including renal or hepatic insufficiency, anticoagulation, or antibiotics.

23. What about the use of biologic DMARDs (bDMARDs) in the perioperative period for elective procedures?

For non-SLE rheumatic diseases, as well as non-severe SLE, it is generally recommended to plan for surgery at the end of the dosing cycle plus 1 week for each specific bDMARD. The bDMARD should be restarted once there are signs of good wound healing, no signs of infection, and sutures/staples have been removed; this is typically approximately 14 days after surgery.

Those with severe SLE should continue belimumab and anifrolumab through surgery without interruption (planning for surgery at the end of a dosing cycle), with the goal of maintaining disease control. Patients with severe SLE on rituximab should plan for surgery in the last month of the dosing cycle (typically in month 5 or 6 for patients receiving this medication every 6 months).

Regarding rituximab, one should be aware of potential hypogammaglobulinemia in those patients who have received repeated cycles of this medication. Although specific guidelines are not available, one could consider replacing immunoglobulin (Ig) G if levels are low (typically <300 mg/dL, or <500 mg/dL if there are recurrent infections).

24. What about management of antirheumatic therapy around surgeries other than TKA and THA?

There are limited data regarding perioperative use of DMARDs for surgeries other than elective TKAs and THAs, and recommendations are predominantly based on expert opinion. In addition to careful shared decision making, a reasonable approach could be to apply the guidelines for TKA and THAs. Alternatively, for surgeries that involve opening the abdomen or chest, a reasonable approach is to stop csDMARDs and tsDMARDs 1 week prior to surgery, if possible, and resume 1–2 weeks after surgery in the absence of wound healing complications or infection. For bDMARDs, if possible, the surgery should occur at the end of the dosing cycle plus one week and resume once there are signs of good wound healing, no evidence of infection, and all sutures/staples are removed (typically approximately 14 days after surgery).

25. A patient with RA is found to have a swollen, warm, and tender knee on postoperative day 4 after a cholecystectomy. Should the patient have an arthrocentesis performed?

Yes. An acutely inflamed joint postoperatively should always be aspirated to exclude a septic joint. Do not assume that the symptoms are due to a flare of RA, especially if the involved joint seems inflamed out of proportion to the rest of the patient's disease activity (a "red, hot joint" is not typical of inflammatory arthritis due to autoimmune disease). Keep in mind that patients with RA may have "pseudoseptic arthritis," where synovial fluid white blood cell count is >50,000/mm^3, mimicking infection. This arthritic manifestation may be due to rebound autoimmune-mediated inflammation in a patient whose immunosuppression has been held perioperatively.

TABLE 13.4 Perioperative Management of Conventional Synthetic and Targeted Synthetic Disease-Modifying Antirheumatic Drugs[a]

DMARD	PERIOPERATIVE RECOMMENDATION[B, C]
Patients with RA, SpA (including PsA), JIA	
Methotrexate, hydroxychloroquine, sulfasalazine, leflunomide, doxycycline	Continue through the perioperative period
Apremilast	Continue through the perioperative period
Prednisone	Continue daily dosing through the perioperative period; for most patients, stress dosing is not necessary for knee and hip replacements
Tofacitinib, baricitinib, upadicitinib	Withhold for 3 days prior to surgery Resume ~2 weeks post-op
Biologics, including rituximab	Withhold surgery until after the next dose is due. Resume ~2 weeks post-op
Patients with SLE **Severe organ manifestations (e.g., nephritis, CNS lupus, severe hemolytic anemia, cardiopulmonary disease, vasculitis, etc.) requiring ongoing induction or maintenance treatment**	
Mycophenolate mofetil, azathioprine, cyclosporine, tacrolimus, voclosporin, anifrolumab and belimumab[d]	Continue through the perioperative period
Rituximab	Consider surgery in the last month of the dosing cycle (typically month 5 or 6)
Patients with SLE **Nonsevere manifestations**	
Mycophenolate mofetil, azathioprine, cyclosporine, tacrolimus (and potentially voclosporin)	Withhold 1 week prior to surgery Resume ~2 weeks post-op
Belimumab, rituximab (and potentially anifrolumab)	Perform surgery at end of dosing cycle Resume ~2 weeks post-op
Corticosteroids	Continue the daily dosing throughout the perioperative period; for most patients, stress-dosing is not indicated for knee and hip replacements

DMARD, Disease-modifying antirheumatic drug; *RA,* rheumatoid arthritis; *SpA,* spondyloarthritis; *PsA,* psoriatic arthritis; *JIA,* juvenile idiopathic arthritis; *SLE,* systemic lupus erythematosus.

[a]Adapted from Goodman SM, Springer BD, Chen AF, et al. 2022 American College of Rheumatology/American Association of Hip and Knee Surgeons Guideline for the Perioperative Management of Antirheumatic Medication in Patients with Rheumatic Diseases Undergoing Elective Total Hip or Total Knee Arthroplasty. *Arthritis Care Res.* 2022;74(9):1399–1408.

[b]These recommendations are adapted from guidelines for total knee and hip replacement. They may be applicable to other forms of surgery; however, there is limited evidence-based data supporting their use in specific conditions.

[c]Medications should be resumed postoperatively once the patient is doing well (wound without infection and healing well, patient taking oral medications, no new renal/hepatic insufficiency); for joint replacement surgery, this typically is ~14 days post-operatively.

[d]Cyclophosphamide is not included in these recommendations but patients on this agent should be considered to wait for elective surgery until the course of therapy is completed.

26. **A patient with chronic tophaceous gout develops acute onset left knee pain and swelling postoperatively. Aspiration reveals negatively birefringent, needle-shaped crystals. Can you be certain of the diagnosis of acute gouty arthritis?**

Not yet. In patients with chronic gout, uric acid crystals can be seen on synovial fluid aspirated from an asymptomatic joint—in this case, the presence of crystals is not diagnostic of an acute gout flare. Sepsis and gout can occur simultaneously, so evaluation for infection (Gram stain and culture) is mandatory.

27. What predisposes patients to perioperative gout attacks?
- Dehydration.
- Increased uric acid production as a result of adenosine triphosphate breakdown (energy utilization) during surgery.
- Medicines (diuretics, heparin, low dose aspirin, cyclosporine).
- Minor trauma to the joint during surgery and transport.
- Infections.
- Hyperalimentation.
- Perioperative cessation of medications used to manage gout (allopurinol, febuxostat, pegloticase, colchicine, and probenecid).
- Preoperative serum uric acid levels ≥9 mg/dL.

PEARL: Some of the risk factors for gout flare including dehydration, trauma and metabolic derangements may also lead to flares of calcium pyrophosphate deposition disease (CPPD). In particular, manipulation of the head and neck may lead to a flare of CPPD around C1-C2 (the "crowned dens syndrome").

---

28. What are the options for treating patients with acute gouty arthritis postoperatively if they are unable to take oral agents?
- Indomethacin or another NSAID per nasogastric tube or suppositories per rectum. These agents may be contraindicated if the patient is at risk for surgical bleeding or gastric ulcer disease, and in the setting of known CVD or renal insufficiency. Intramuscular ketorolac 30 to 60 mg is another option if NSAID use is appropriate.
- Triamcinolone acetonide 40 to 60 mg/day intramuscularly for one to two doses. This may be the safest option in many cases.
- Methylprednisolone 20–60 mg IV daily for several days, and then replace with oral prednisone, tapering when appropriate.
- Corticosteroid preparation injected into the joint (if you are sure it is not infected).
- IL-1 inhibitors are conditionally recommended in the ACR 2020 Guideline for Gout Management for those patients who don't respond or are intolerant to other anti-inflammatory therapies. IL-1 inhibitor therapies include anakinra 100mg subcutaneously daily until resolution of flare, which typically takes 3–5 days (most cost effective of the IL-1 inhibitors). Another option is canakinumab 150mg subcutaneously given as a single dose or rilonacept 320mg subcutaneously given as a single dose.
- Corticotropin gel 40 to 80 units subcutaneous injection daily every 24 to 72 hours (uncommonly used because of cost).

29. What special considerations should be made in the perioperative management of patients with antiphospholipid syndrome?
It is essential to minimize the amount of time without anticoagulation and avoid the use of vitamin K, which can complicate the resumption of therapeutic warfarin use. Another important concept is to minimize all aspects of Virchow's triad (hypercoagulability, stasis, and endothelial injury). Examples of this include using external pneumatic compression devices in the operating room and postoperatively, setting the blood pressure cuffs to inflate less frequently, avoiding tourniquets, encouraging ambulation as soon as possible after surgery and limiting intravascular line placement and removing them as soon as they are no longer needed. Importantly, once anticoagulation is resumed with warfarin, patients will need a bridge with LMWH until they are fully anticoagulated, which is typically up to 5 days after resumption of warfarin, even if the INR is in the therapeutic range earlier than that.

30. What is the perioperative approach to those patients who are APL-positive without a history of blood clots (controversial)?
The concern is that surgery and its postoperative issues may tip a person with a potential predisposition to clot into a hypercoagulable state where a clinically apparent clot develops. There is a general consensus to apply standard perioperative DVT prophylaxis approaches that are used in

general populations; however, there is controversy on whether to continue prophylactic anticoagulation after discharge and regarding duration of therapy. Some experts advocate for the continuation of prophylactic doses of LMWHs or therapeutic warfarin for 1 to 6 weeks postoperatively (including patients in the postpartum period).

31. What other disease-specific precautions should be considered in rheumatic diseases other than RA?

- **Sjögren's disease:** use lubricating gel and artificial tears during anesthesia to prevent corneal abrasion. Do not give pilocarpine preoperatively to avoid bronchospasm and bradycardia. Minimize the use of anticholinergic drugs during the perioperative period. Dryness may increase the risk of pneumonia.
- **Juvenile idiopathic arthritis:** micrognathia may make intubation difficult. Cervical spine instability can occur.
- **Ankylosing spondylitis:** cervical spine immobility may make intubation difficult. Restrictive chest excursion may increase the risk of pneumonia. Heterotopic ossification can complicate THA.
- **Psoriatic arthritis:** skin disease can flare at the surgical site (Koebner phenomenon).
- **Active vasculitis:** arterial punctures or devices (e.g., arterial line for blood pressure monitoring) can lead to vasospasm and increased risk for vascular occlusion.
- **SLE:** treat with IVIG if the patient has severe thrombocytopenia and needs emergency surgery. There is increased CV risk.
- **Raynaud syndrome:** finger sticks for glucose or other monitoring may lead to wounds that are difficult to heal; oxygen saturation monitors may not be accurate in Raynaud's and therefore, other sites (e.g., forehead, earlobe) for monitoring may be considered.
- **Systemic sclerosis:** poor venous access at sites of thickened skin; difficult intubation if decreased oral aperture (less than 4 cm incisor to incisor; consider fiberoptic intubation); risk of aspiration increased (esophageal dysmotility); postoperative ileus increased; arterial vasospasm increased in all organs including heart and kidneys; increased risk of scleroderma renal crisis in hypovolemic conditions. Increased risk of adverse outcome in patients with pulmonary hypertension. Increased cardiac arrhythmia risk.

BIBLIOGRAPHY

Coursin DB, Wood KE. Corticosteroid supplementation for adrenal insufficiency. *JAMA*. 2002;287(2):236–240.

Falck-Ytter Y, Francis CW, Johanson NA, et al. Prevention of VTE in orthopedic surgery patients: antithrombotic therapy and prevention of thrombosis, 9th ed: American College of Chest Physicians Evidence-Based Clinical practice guidelines. *Chest*. 2012;141(suppl 2):e278S–e325S.

Ferguson LD, Sattar N, McInnes IB. Managing cardiovascular risk in patients with rheumatic disease. *Rheum Dis Clin North Am*. 2022;48(2):429–444.

FitzGerald J, Dalbeth N, Mikuls T, et al. 2020 American College of Rheumatology guidelines for the management of gout. *Arthritis Care Res*. 2020;72(6):744–760.

Goodman SM, Springer B, Chen A, et al. 2022 American College of Rheumatology/American Association of Hip and Knee Surgeons guideline for the perioperative management of antirheumatic medication in patients with rheumatic diseases undergoing elective total hip or total knee arthroplasty. *Arthritis Care Res*. 2022;74(9):1399–1408.

Hellstein JW, Adler RA, Edwards B, et al. Managing the care of patients receiving antiresorptive therapy for prevention and treatment of osteoporosis: executive summary of recommendations from the American Dental Association Council on Scientific Affairs. *J Am Dent Assoc*. 2011;142(11):1243–1251.

Krause ML, Matteson EL. Perioperative management of the patient with rheumatoid arthritis. *World J Orthop*. 2014;5(3):283–291.

MacKenzie CR, Goodman SM. Stress dose steroids: myths and perioperative medicine. *Curr Rheumatol Rep*. 2016;18(7):47.

Mallory GW, Halasz SR, Clarke MJ. Advances in the treatment of cervical rheumatoid: less surgery and less morbidity. *World J Orthop*. 2014;5(3):292–303.

Quinn RH, Murray JN, Pezold R, et al. The American Academy of Orthopaedic Surgeons appropriate use criteria for the management of patients with orthopaedic implants undergoing dental procedures. *J Bone Joint Surg Am*. 2017;99(2):161–163.

Ruggiero SL, Dodson TB, Aghaloo T, Carlson ER, Ward BB, Kademani D. American Association of Oral and Maxillofacial Surgeons' position paper on medication-related osteonecrosis of the jaws –2022 update. *J Oral Maxillofac Surg*. 2022;80(5):920–943.

Saunders KH, Erkan D, Lockshin MD. Perioperative management of antiphospholipid antibody-positive patients. *Curr Rheumatol Rep*. 2014;16(7):426.

Shahi A, Parvizi J. Prevention of periprosthetic joint infection. *Arch Bone Jt Surg*. 2015;3(2):72–81.

FURTHER READING

AAOS Appropriate Use Criteria for consideration of antibiotic prophylaxis in patients with prosthetic joints undergoing dental procedures: http://www.orthoguidelines.org/go/auc/default.cfm?auc_id=224995&actionxm=Terms.

ADA Guidelines for Consideration of Antibiotic Prophylaxis in patients with cardiac valvular conditions undergoing dental procedures: https://www.ada.org/en/member-center/oral-health-topics/antibiotic-prophylaxis#.W24kj2H-v6g.email.

ADA Statement on Osteoporosis Medications and MRONJ: https://www.ada.org/resources/ada-library/oral-health-topics/osteoporosis-medications

CHAPTER 14

Rheumatoid Arthritis

Kristen Demoruelle, MD, PhD and Timothy M. Wilson, MD

> ## KEY POINTS
>
> 1. Rheumatoid arthritis (RA) is the most common chronic inflammatory arthritis.
> 2. Synovitis of the small joints of the hands (metacarpophalangeal joints [MCPs], proximal interphalangeal joints [PIPs]) and wrists is the classic initial pattern.
> 3. RA patients with extraarticular manifestations are usually seropositive.
> 4. Early and aggressive therapy should target low disease activity for optimal outcomes.
> 5. RA patients have accelerated atherosclerosis warranting aggressive risk factor modification.

1. What is RA?

RA is a chronic, systemic, inflammatory disorder of joints that is characterized by its pattern of joint involvement, and in the majority of cases, serum elevations of autoantibodies that include (among others) rheumatoid factor (RF) and antibodies to citrullinated protein/peptide antigens (ACPA). The primary site of pathology is the synovium of the joints. The synovial tissue becomes inflamed and proliferates, forming **pannus** that invades bone, cartilage, and ligaments and leads to damage and deformities. Extraarticular manifestations such as lung disease may accompany the joint disease, but arthritis represents the major manifestation.

2. What is the etiology and pathogenesis of RA?

The exact cause of RA remains unknown, but it is likely multifactorial, with genetic (human leucocyte antigen [HLA] genes and others) and environmental factors (smoking, silica, and others) playing important roles. Autoantibodies (RF, ACPAs) can be found in the blood several years before the development of joint inflammation during a phase of RA development called "preclinical RA." The preclinical period of RA suggests that the initiating events in RA may occur outside of the joints (Fig. 14.1). These initiating events may take place at mucosal surfaces and involve a complex interaction between the genes and environment, as well as the innate and adaptive immune systems. Over time, systemic autoimmunity can transition to clinical symptoms and joint inflammation at which time an individual may meet classification criteria for RA.

Genetic factors: The major histocompatibility complex (MHC) region coding for certain HLA-DR genes accounts for a large proportion of the known genetic risk for RA. The susceptibility to RA is mainly associated with the third hypervariable region of DRβ chains from amino acids 70 to 74 (referred to as the **shared epitope;** so named because this unique amino acid sequence can be found on numerous DR4 and DR1 alleles that are enriched in RA populations). In addition, over 100 genetic loci outside the MHC have been associated with an increased risk of developing RA; each of these increases the odds of developing RA by only 1.2–2-fold, although this varies among ethnicities. Polymorphisms of PTPN22, TRAF1-C5, STAT4, TNFAIP3, and PADI4 are well established. Epigenetic factors (histone modification, DNA methylation) are also likely to be important.

In addition to population-based genetic studies, twin studies show that the concordance rate for RA is 12% to 15% in monozygotic twins and 2% to 3% in fraternal twins. This is in comparison with the rate of RA in the general population of ~0.5% to 1% and suggests that familial factors (genetics and/or shared environmental risk) account for a substantial portion of an individual's susceptibility to RA. It is important to keep in mind that 80% to 90% of all RA is sporadic, that is, occurring in individuals with no family history of RA.

Environmental factors: Smoking is the best-characterized environmental risk factor for RA. It is more strongly associated with ACPA-positive (1.9-fold) compared with ACPA-negative (1.3-fold) RA. Cigarette exposure in the setting of two shared epitope alleles can increase the odds for ACPA-positive RA by 21-fold. The smoking-associated risk of RA is dose-dependent

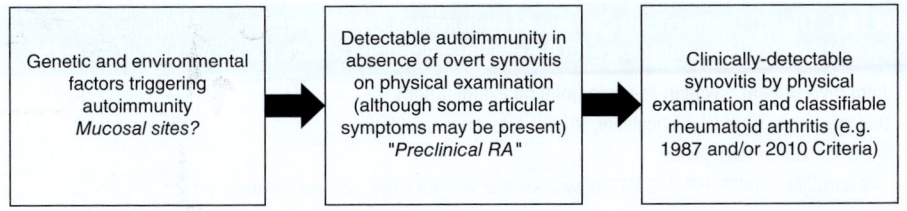

Fig. 14.1 Model of the natural history of rheumatoid arthritis (RA) development. In this model, genetic and environmental factors lead to triggering of autoimmunity that can be detectable initially in the absence of synovitis. Over time this progresses to overt synovitis and classifiable RA. The period in which there are detectable biomarkers in absence of synovitis can be termed "Preclinical RA."

(2-fold for >20 pack years) and persists for 10 to 20 years after a person quits smoking. Other inhaled factors (e.g., silica dust, air pollution) have also been associated with RA. While the exact role that they may play in the development of RA is uncertain, **bacteria** in the microbiomes of mucosal sites (e.g., mouth, lung, gut) may also contribute to RA development. For example, *Porphyromonos gingivalis* (an organism associated with periodontitis) can express peptidylarginine deiminase (PAD) enzymes that can citrullinate resident proteins through the posttranslational modification of arginine to citrulline. Studies have also found that RA patients have repeated breaches in the oral mucosa that release citrullinated oral bacteria into circulation which can be targeted by ACPA. *Prevotella copri* (*P. copri*) is expanded in the stool of patients with RA, and antibody responses to *P. copri*-derived peptides are found in a portion of individuals with RA and at risk for RA. Also, a strain of the stool bacteria *subdoligranulum* (*S. dido*) was found to be targeted by monoclonal autoantibodies from individuals with and at risk for RA, and can trigger arthritis when gavaged in germ-free mice. **Viruses** (Epstein–Barr virus [EBV], parvovirus B19) have been associated with RA as well. The exact role of microbial organisms in the initiation and propagation of RA-related autoimmunity is unknown, and this remains an active area of research.

Autoantibodies: Multiple autoantibody systems are implicated in RA pathogenesis, including RF and anti-modified protein antibodies (AMPAs). AMPAs can include antibodies to citrullinated, carbamylated (homocitrulline), and acetylated proteins. These neoantigens cause a heightened immune response when presented to the immune system by HLA-DR molecules containing the shared epitope. ACPAs and anticarbamylated antibodies can bind citrullinated and carbamylated proteins locally or form immune complexes that can deposit in the tissue, thereby directly playing a role in disease pathogenesis. While ACPAs have been linked to inflammation and more severe RA, some ACPA have also been linked to anti-inflammatory properties.

Initiation of clinical disease: The mechanism of initiation of clinical synovitis is unknown. It is hypothesized that ACPAs could target citrullinated proteins in the joint. In addition, certain immune complexes that include ACPAs and RF can deposit in synovial postcapillary venules inciting inflammation through complement activation. Tissue inflammation can increase vascular permeability with the influx of more inflammatory cells (e.g., neutrophils, CD8 T cells) and antibodies (including ACPAs). Inflammation can upregulate PAD enzymes and myeloperoxidase causing citrullination and carbamylation, respectively, of synovial proteins and cartilage proteins. Binding of ACPAs can lead to osteoclastogenesis, chondrocyte damage, and release of degraded collagen and proteoglycan neoepitopes from cartilage. In addition, neutrophils can release neutrophil extracellular traps that can drive local inflammation, and carbamylated proteins on NETs can drive local osteoclastogenesis.

Perpetuation of clinical disease: RA is thought to be perpetuated by activation of the adaptive immune system, with the innate immune system and self-antigens acting as a persistent adjuvant. For example, neoepitopes created by synovial inflammation and cartilage injury can be taken up by an influx of dendritic cells into the synovium. Dendritic cells from a genetically predisposed host will more efficiently present the neoantigens to T lymphocytes in the synovial tissue and draining lymph nodes. Epitope spreading may occur, with a break in tolerance and an immune response directed toward native antigens. T-cells, macrophages, synovial fibroblasts, and B cells may be activated in different combinations to produce proinflammatory cytokines that perpetuate chronic synovitis and tissue destruction. Activation of local osteoclasts can facilitate the development of bony erosions.

BOX 14.1 The 2010 American College of Rheumatology (ACR)/European Alliance of Associations for Rheumatology (EULAR) Classification Criteria for Rheumatoid Arthritis

1. Joint involvement (swollen or tender joint on examination)	(0–5 points max)
• One medium to large joint (shoulders, elbows, hips, knees, ankles)	0
• 2–10 medium to large joints	1
• 1–3 small joints (MCP, PIP, 2–5 MTP, or wrist with or without large joint involvement)	2
• 4–10 small joints (with or without large joint involvement)	3
• >10 joints (at least one small joint involved)	5
2. Serology	(0–3 points max)
• Negative RF and negative ACPA	0
• Low positive RF or low positive ACPA (≤3 times the normal upper limit)	2
• High positive RF or high positive ACPA (>3 times the normal upper limit)	3
3. Acute-phase reactants	(0–1 point max)
• Normal CRP and normal ESR	0
• Abnormal CRP or abnormal ESR	1
4. Duration of symptoms	(0–1 point max)
• <6 weeks	0
• ≥6 weeks	1

To apply these criteria, the patient must have at least one joint swollen with inflammatory arthritis on clinical examination that is not explained by another disease. Magnetic resonance imaging/ultrasound may be used to confirm clinical findings.
ACPA, anticitrullinated protein antibody; *CRP*, C-reactive protein; *ESR*, erythrocyte sedimentation rate; *MCP*, metacarpophalangeal joint; *MTP*, metatarsophalangeal joint; *PIP*, proximal interphalangeal joint; *RF*, rheumatoid factor.
From Aletaha D, Neogi T, Silman AJ, et al. 2010 Rheumatoid arthritis classification criteria: an American College of Rheumatology/European League Against Rheumatism collaborative initiative. *Ann Rheum Dis.* 2010;69:1580–1588.

Prevention of clinical disease: Smoking cessation is the only modifiable risk factor demonstrated to reduce RA risk. In addition, clinical trials are underway in the United States and Europe to determine whether intervention with immune-modulating therapies can prevent the onset of joint disease in individuals who are at a high risk of developing RA in the future. To date, abatacept is the only intervention that has demonstrated the potential to reduce the incidence of RA in a subset of high-risk individuals.

3. **Discuss the 2010 American College of Rheumatology (ACR)/European Alliance of Associations for Rheumatology (EULAR) criteria for the classification of RA (Box 14.1).**
With the knowledge that early, effective treatment of RA improves long-term outcomes, the 2010 ACR/EULAR classification criteria for RA were designed to identify individuals with RA at an earlier stage of disease compared with the 1987 ACR RA classification criteria. The criteria demonstrate 82% sensitivity and 61% specificity for RA when compared with control subjects with non-RA rheumatic disease. While these criteria can be a guide, the purpose of classification is to define a homogenous population for study purposes. Ultimately, the diagnosis of RA is established clinically by the rheumatologist.

4. **What other diseases should be excluded prior to making the diagnosis of RA?**
COMMON DISEASES

Seronegative spondyloarthritis, calcium pyrophosphate deposition disease, connective tissue diseases (systemic lupus erythematosus [SLE], scleroderma, polymyositis, vasculitis, mixed connective tissue disease, polymyalgia rheumatica), osteoarthritis (OA), viral infection (EBV, HIV, hepatitis B, parvovirus, rubella, hepatitis C, chikungunya), polyarticular gout, fibromyalgia, reactive arthritis.

UNCOMMON DISEASES:

Hypothyroidism, relapsing polychondritis, subacute bacterial endocarditis, rheumatic fever, hemochromatosis, sarcoidosis, hypertrophic osteoarthropathy, Lyme disease, hyperlipoproteinemias (types II, IV), amyloid arthropathy, hemoglobinopathies (sickle cell disease), malignancy and paraneoplastic syndrome, and Behçet's disease.

RARE DISEASES:

Familial Mediterranean fever, Whipple's disease, multicentric reticulohistiocytosis, angioimmunoblastic lymphadenopathy, remitting seronegative symmetrical synovitis with pitting edema (RS3PE), and SAPHO—synovitis, acne, pustulosis, hyperostosis, and osteitis.

PEARL: A clinician should consider a diagnosis *other than* RA particularly in patients who have an asymmetric arthritis, migrating pattern, predominantly large-joint arthritis, distal interphalangeal (DIP) joint involvement, rashes, back disease, renal disease, leukopenia, or hypocomplementemia.

5. Discuss the epidemiologic characteristics of RA.

- Race/ethnicity—worldwide, all races. Native Americans (Algonquian and Pima Indians) have higher prevalence.
- Sex distribution—females > males 2–3:1.
- Age—the average age of onset of RA in women is 40 to 60 years, men are older.
- Occurs in about 0.5–1% of adults in the United States. The prevalence increases with age.

6. Describe the various ways in which RA can present.

a. Typical patterns of onset (90% of patients)
- **Insidious** (55–65%): Onset with arthritic symptoms of pain, swelling and stiffness, with the number of joints increasing over weeks to months.
- **Subacute** (15–20%): Similar to insidious onset but more systemic symptoms.
- **Acute** (10%): Severe onset, some have fever.

b. Variant patterns of onset (10% of patients)
- **Palindromic (episodic) pattern:** Usually involves less than five joints and resolves within several days. After an asymptomatic period, a flare in the same or another joint(s) occurs. Over time, 33% to 50% evolve into RA involving more joints persistently. Seropositive patients and those with elevated acute-phase reactants are more likely to progress to RA. The optimal treatment for individuals with "palindromic/episodic" RA is not known; however, antimalarial therapy may decrease the frequency of attacks and progression to RA.
- **Insidious onset of elderly (>65 years):** Present with severe pain and stiffness of limb girdle joints, often with diffuse swelling of hands, wrists, and forearms. May be difficult to differentiate from polymyalgia rheumatica and RS3PE.
- **Arthritis robustus:** Typically seen in men who are physically active and involved in manual labor. Patients have bulky, proliferative synovitis causing joint erosions and deformities, but the patient experiences little pain or disability.
- **Rheumatoid nodulosis:** Patients with recurrent pain/swelling in different joints, subcutaneous nodules, and subchondral bone cysts on radiographs.

7. Which joints are commonly affected in RA? (Box 14.2)

The joints most commonly involved at onset are the MCPs, PIPs, wrists, and metatarsophalangeal joints (MTPs). Larger joints generally become symptomatic after small joints. Patients may start out with only a few joints involved (oligoarticular onset) but progress to involvement of multiple joints (polyarticular) in a symmetric distribution within a few weeks to months. Of note, most of the descriptions of RA presentation were made during an era where initial diagnosis was made months to years after the onset of symptoms. As health-care systems are identifying individuals with RA earlier in the disease course through more widespread testing of autoantibodies, it may be that the joints understood to be first involved in RA will change.

Involvement of the thoracolumbar, sacroiliac, or hand DIP joints is very rare in RA and should suggest another diagnosis, such as a seronegative spondyloarthritis (sacroiliac joints), psoriatic arthritis (DIP joints) or OA (lumbar spine, DIP joints; Fig. 14.2).

BOX 14.2 The Most Common Joints Involved During the Course of Rheumatoid Arthritis

MCP	90–95%	Ankle/subtalar	50–60%
PIP	75–90%	Cervical spine (esp. C1–C2)	40–50%
Wrist	75–80%	Elbow	40–50%
Knee	60–80%	Hip	20–40%
Shoulder	50–70%	Temporomandibular	10–30%
MTP	50–60%		

MCP, metacarpophalangeal joint; *MTP*, metatarsophalangeal joint; *PIP*, proximal interphalangeal joint.

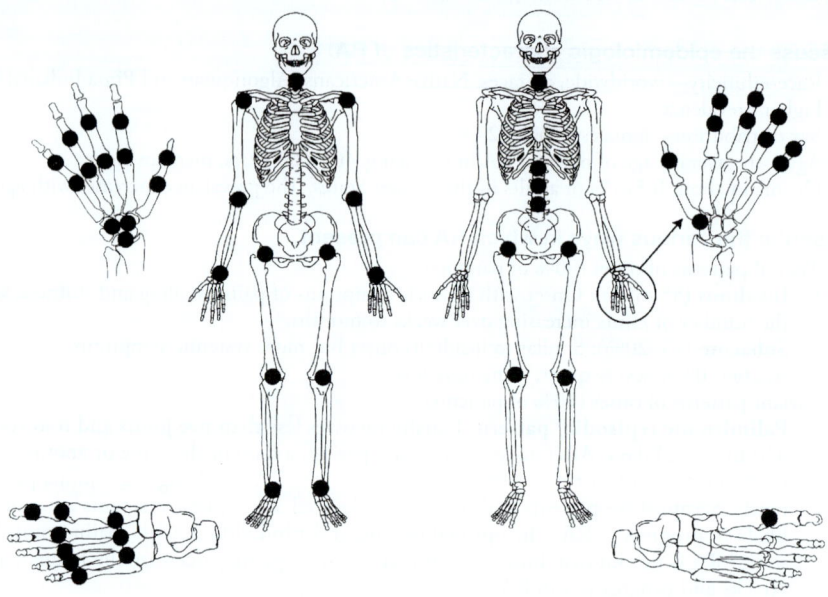

Fig. 14.2 Joint distribution of rheumatoid arthritis (RA; *left*) and osteoarthritis (OA; *right*).

8. What clinical and laboratory findings help predict whether a patient with early undifferentiated arthritis (UA) will develop RA?

Among patients with UA who do not meet the 1987 RA classification criteria, 33% will progress to RA (by 1987 criteria) over the following year, 33% will be diagnosed with another type of inflammatory arthritis, and 33% will undergo spontaneous remission. When using the newer 2010 RA classification criteria, 6% to 22% of patients with UA will progress to RA, 53% will have persistent UA, 3% will be diagnosed with another type of inflammatory arthritis, and 22% will undergo spontaneous remission. These differences likely reflect the improved sensitivity of the 2010 criteria (with a significant proportion of UA patients now classified as RA at the time of initial evaluation) as well as the mandate within the new classification criteria to rule out competing diagnoses as the cause of inflammatory arthritis before applying the criteria to a specific patient (improved specificity). Predictors of progression to RA by 2010 classification criteria include: 1) higher score on 2010 classification criteria at baseline (42% with a score of 5 will develop RA; therefore, number of involved joints, duration of symptoms, and presence of autoantibodies and elevated inflammatory markers are all important factors) and 2) grey scale synovitis on ultrasound.

9. What is pannus?

The synovium is the primary site for the inflammatory process in RA. The inflammatory infiltrate consists of mononuclear cells, primarily CD4+ T lymphocytes (30–50% of cells), as well as activated macrophages, B cells (5% of cells), plasma cells (some making RF and ACPA), and dendritic cells that can lead to an organizational structure that resembles a lymph node. Notably unlike the synovial fluid, few, if any, polymorphonuclear leukocytes (PMNs) are found in the synovium. The inflammatory cytokine milieu causes the synovial lining cells (macrophage-like and fibroblast-like synoviocytes) to proliferate. The inflamed synovium becomes thickened, boggy, and edematous and develops villous projections. This proliferative synovium is called **pannus** and it is capable of invading bone and cartilage, causing destruction of the joint. One of the most important cells in the pannus contributing to cartilage destruction is the fibroblast-like synovio-cyte, which has tumor-like characteristics capable of tissue invasion.

10. What are the common deformities of the hand in RA (Fig. 14.3)?

Fusiform swelling—synovitis of PIP joints, causing them to appear spindle-shaped.

Boutonnière deformity—flexion of the PIP and hyperextension of the DIP joint caused by weakening of the central slip of the extensor tendon and a palmar displacement of the lateral bands. This deformity resembles a knuckle being pushed through a buttonhole.

Swan-neck deformity—results from contraction of the flexors (intrinsic muscles) of the MCPs, resulting in flexion contracture of the MCP joint, hyperextension of PIP, and flexion of the DIP joint.

Ulnar deviation of fingers—with subluxation of MCP joints. This results from weakening of the extensor carpi ulnaris and ulnar collateral ligament at the wrist, leading to radial displacement of the distal carpal row and a corresponding slip of the finger extensor tendons (to the ulnar side) at the MCP joints, contributing to the characteristic appearance.

Hitchhiker thumb—hyperextension of IP joint with flexion of MCP and exaggerated adduction of first metacarpus. Causes inability to pinch. Also referred to as a "Z-deformity."

"Piano key" ulnar head—secondary to destruction of ulnar collateral ligament leading to a float-ing ulnar styloid.

11. Does RA affect the feet?

In some patients, the feet may be the first manifestation of RA, although this can be difficult to recognize because synovitis in the MTPs is difficult to assess. The "MTP" squeeze test, where the forefoot is squeezed by the examiners' hand, may provide a clue to synovitis if there is tenderness in any of the MTPs with this maneuver. In addition, over 33% of patients develop significant foot deformities during the course of RA. The most common deformity is **claw toe** or **hammer toe.** This is caused by inflammation of the MTP joints leading to subluxation of the metatarsal heads. When this problem occurs, the patient has difficulty fitting his or her toes into the shoe because the tops of the toes rub on the shoe box, resulting in callous or ulcer formation. Additionally, because the soft tissue pad that normally sits underneath the metatarsal heads is displaced, the heads of the metatarsal bones are no longer cushioned and become very painful to walk on, fre-quently resulting in calluses on the inferior surface of the foot. Patients commonly complain that it feels as though they are walking on pebbles or stones. Arthritic involvement of the tarsal joints and subtalar joints can result in flattening of the arch of the foot and hindfoot valgus deformity.

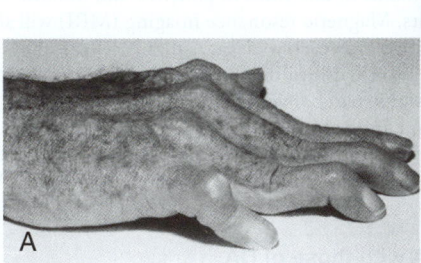
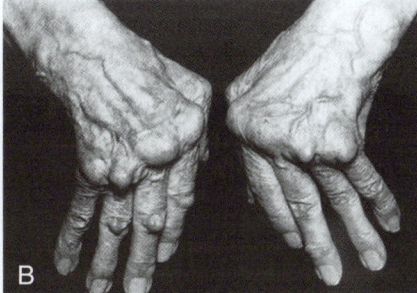

Fig. 14.3 (A) Swan neck (second to fourth fingers) and boutonnière (fifth finger) deformities. (B) Ulnar deviation of fingers (note rheuma-toid nodules). (© 2014 American College of Rheumatology. Used with permission.)

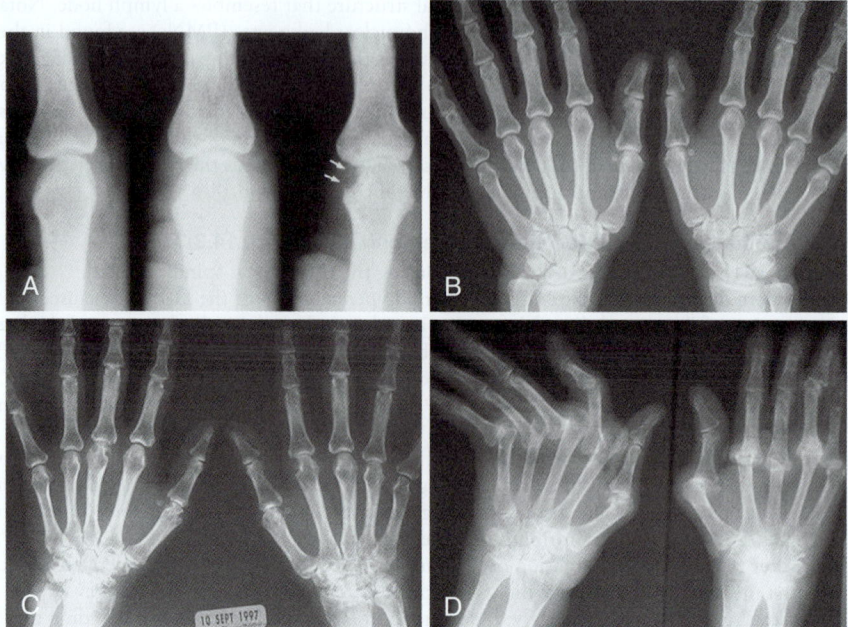

Fig. 14.4 (A) Progressive marginal erosions (*arrows*) of a metacarpophalangeal (MCP) joint. (B) Early rheumatoid arthritis (RA) with symmetrical joint space narrowing and juxtaarticular osteoporosis. (C) The same patient, 5 years later, with significant marginal erosions and severe wrist involvement. (D) Severe RA with destruction of MCP joints, subluxation of MCP joints (*left*) leading to ulnar deviation, and marked wrist involvement. (A, Copyright 2018 American College of Rheumatology. Used with permission.)

12. Describe the radiographic features of RA.

The mnemonic **ABCDE'S** is a convenient way to remember these:

A—Alignment, abnormal; no ankylosis

B—Bones—periarticular (juxtaarticular) osteopenia; no periostitis or osteophytes

C—Cartilage—uniform (symmetric) joint space loss in weight-bearing joints; no cartilage or soft tissue calcification

D—Deformities (swan-neck, ulnar deviation, boutonnière) with symmetrical distribution

E—Erosions, marginal

S—Soft-tissue swelling; nodules without calcification.

The radiographic changes in RA take months to develop. Juxtaarticular osteopenia is seen early in the course of the disease, followed later by more diffuse osteopenia. Joint erosions typically occur at the margins of small joints. Later, joint space narrowing and deformities develop. The earliest erosions occur in the hands (2, 3, 5 MCPs) before the feet in one-third of patients with erosive disease; the feet (1, 5 MTPs) before the hands in one-third of patients; and in both hands and feet at the same time in one-third of patients. Magnetic resonance imaging (MRI) will show 40% more erosions than conventional radiography. However, a caveat is that MRI can show MCP and/or wrist erosions or synovitis in 2% and 9% of healthy individuals, respectively. Musculoskeletal ultrasound can also show more erosions than conventional radiography, but can also be present in 0% to 18% of healthy individuals. Larger erosions (>2 mm), especially at the 2nd and 5th MCP, 5th MTP, and distal ulna, were most specific for RA (>85%). Ultrasound-detected tenosynovitis and erosions can also predict future RA development in individuals with ACPA positivity. See Fig. 14.4.

13. Compare the radiographic features of RA with those of OA.

See Table 14.1.

TABLE 14.1 Radiographs in Rheumatoid Arthritis and Osteoarthritis

	RHEUMATOID ARTHRITIS	OSTEOARTHRITIS
Sclerosis	±	++++
Osteophytes	±	++++
Osteopenia	+++	0
Symmetry	+++	+
Marginal/periarticular erosions	+++	0
Cysts	++	++
Narrowing	+++	+++

14. What are the typical features of the synovial fluid in RA?

The synovial fluid is inflammatory, with white blood cell (WBC) counts typically between 5000 and 50,000/mm³. Rarely, synovial fluid WBC count can exceed 100,000/mm³ (pseudoseptic) but infection must always be ruled out. Generally, the differential shows a predominance (>50%) of PMNs. The protein level is elevated, and the glucose level may be lower than serum values (40–60% of serum glucose). There are no crystals in the fluid, and cultures are negative. Unfortunately, there are no specific findings in the synovial fluid that allow a definitive diagnosis of RA.

15. How is the cervical spine involved in RA?

Historically, the cervical spine is involved in 30% to 50% of RA patients, with C1–C2 the most commonly involved level. Fortunately, the rates of significant cervical spinal disease in RA are decreasing with modern therapy. Arthritic involvement of the cervical spine can lead to instability with potential impingement of the spinal cord; thus it is important for the clinician to consider obtaining radiographs of the cervical spine in both flexion and extension before surgical procedures requiring intubation. It is important to note that cervical spine disease often parallels peripheral joint disease. The earliest and most frequent symptom of subluxation is pain radiating to the occiput. Pain, neurologic involvement, and death are the main concerns with subluxation. The patterns of cervical spine involvement include:

- **C1–C2 subluxation** (60–65% cases) can result in **anterior** (most common), **lateral** (rotary), and **posterior** (least common) atlantoaxial subluxation. Anterior subluxation at C1–C2 results in a widening of the gap between the arch of C1 and the odontoid of C2 (>3 mm). This is caused by synovial proliferation around the articulation of the odontoid process with the anterior arch of C1, leading to stretching and rupture of the transverse and alar ligaments, which keep the odontoid in contact with the arch of C1. The risk of spinal cord compression is greatest when the anterior atlantoodontoid interval is ≥9 mm, or the posterior atlantoodontoid interval is ≤14 mm. (Fig 14.5)
- **C1–C2 impaction** (20–25% cases; sometimes referred to as superior migration of the odontoid) is the next most common form of cervical spine disease in RA. Destruction is between the occipitoatlantal and atlantoaxial joint articulations between C1 and C2, causing a cephalad movement of the odontoid into the foramen magnum, which may impinge on the brainstem. Overall, it has the worst prognosis neurologically, especially when the odontoid is ≥5 mm above Ranawat's line.
- **Subaxial involvement** (10%–15% cases) is the least common and typically involves C2–C3 and C3–C4 facets and intervertebral disks. This can lead to "stair-stepping" with one vertebrae subluxing forward on the lower vertebrae. Translation of more than 3.5 mm of one vertebra on the other is usually clinically relevant. Subaxial disease usually occurs later than other forms of cervical involvement.

16. What are the typical laboratory findings in RA patients?

- **Complete blood count:** Anemia of chronic disease and thrombocytosis correlate with active disease. The WBC count and the differential should be normal unless the patient has Felty's syndrome or another disease.

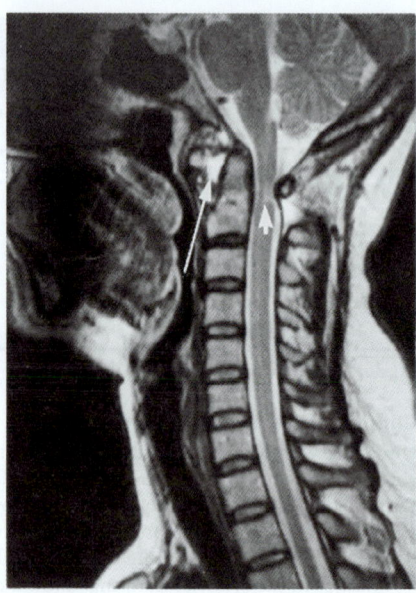

Fig. 14.5 Magnetic resonance imaging of the cervical spine demonstrating pannus formation of the C1–C2 articulation (*long arrow*) and impingement of the odontoid on the spinal cord (*arrow*).

- **Chemistries:** Normal renal, hepatic, and uric acid tests. Albumin may be low in active disease because it is a negative acute-phase reactant.
- **Urinalysis:** Normal.
- **Erythrocyte sedimentation rate (ESR):** Usually elevated. Can be normal in patients with early, limited disease. ESR can be elevated as a result of inflammation and hypergammaglobulinemia.
- **C-reactive protein (CRP):** Usually elevated. May be more ideal than ESR in following disease activity because it is not influenced by hypergammaglobulinemia.
- **RF:** Positive in 60% to 80%, with a specificity of 80% to 86% for RA. RF positivity is associated with extraarticular manifestations including subcutaneous nodules. Note that several diseases with arthritis can have a positive RF such as hepatitis C (40–75%), SLE (20%), Sjögren's disease (SjD, 70%), tuberculosis (60%), and subacute bacterial endocarditis (45–68%).
- **ACPA:** The most common clinically available ACPA is the anti-cyclic citrullinated peptide (anti-CCP) assay. Several versions of anti-CCP testing are available, with sensitivities ranging from 57% to 67% and specificity ranging from 93% to 99%. Anti-CCP is positive in 10% to 15% of RF-negative RA patients. Both RF and anti-CCP are associated with disease severity, erosions, and increased mortality. Higher titer antibodies (in the case of ACPA and RF) have a higher specificity for RA. However, antibody titers do not correlate with disease activity, so serial testing is unnecessary.
- **Antinuclear antibodies (ANAs):** Positive in 30% to 50%. Not typically directed against any specific antigens (e.g., SS-A, SS-B, ribonucleoprotein, Smith, double-stranded DNA).
- **Anti-neutrophil cytoplasmic antibodies:** Usually negative. If positive, it should not have specificity against proteinase 3 or myeloperoxidase.
- **Complement (C3, C4):** Normal or elevated. If it is low, consider a disease other than RA.
- **Novel autoantibodies:** There are several autoantibodies in testing and development that may be of significance to RA diagnosis, management, and disease severity. These include antibodies to carbamylated proteins, PAD enzymes, and others.
- **Novel inflammatory panels:** There are a growing number of inflammatory markers such as cytokines, chemokines, adipokines, and other products of joint inflammation which are being evaluated in the diagnosis and management of RA (see Chapter 6: Laboratory Evaluation).

17. List some of the extraarticular manifestations of RA.

General	Cardiac
Fever	Pericarditis
Lymphadenopathy	Myocarditis
Weight loss (including RA cachexia)	Coronary vasculitis
Fatigue	Nodules on valves
Dermatologic	**Neuromuscular**
Palmar erythema	Entrapment neuropathy
Subcutaneous nodules	Peripheral neuropathy
Vasculitis	Mononeuritis multiplex
Neutrophilic dermatoses	
Ocular	**Hematologic**
Episcleritis	Felty's syndrome
Scleritis	Large granular lymphocyte syndrome
Choroid and retinal nodules	Lymphomas
Pulmonary	**Others**
Pleuritis	Sjögren's disease
Nodules	Amyloidosis
Interstitial lung disease	Osteoporosis
Obstructive lung disease (including asthma, COPD, bronchiolitis and bronchiectasis)	Atherosclerosis

18. Which patients with RA are most likely to get extraarticular manifestations?

Patients who are RF or ACPA positive, HLA-DR4 positive, and males are more likely to have extraarticular manifestations. RF positivity may be more strongly associated with extraarticular manifestations than ACPA positivity, but both have been associated. It is important for clinicians to rule out other causes such as infection, malignancy, and medications, before ascribing an extraarticular manifestation to RA, especially if the patient is RF-negative.

19. How commonly do fever and lymphadenopathy occur in RA patients as a result of their rheumatic disease?

They are uncommon and generally seen only in those patients with severely active disease. Infection and lymphoreticular malignancy should always be considered in an RA patient with these symptoms.

20. What are rheumatoid nodules? Where are they found?

Rheumatoid nodules are subcutaneous nodules that have the characteristic histology of a central area of fibrinoid necrosis surrounded by a zone of palisades of elongated histiocytes and a peripheral layer of cellular connective tissue. Historically, they occur in 20% to 35% of RA patients, typically those who are RF-positive and have severe disease. They tend to occur on the extensor surface of the forearms, in the olecranon bursa, over joints, and over pressure points such as sacrum, occiput, and heel. They frequently develop and enlarge when the patient's RA is active and may resolve when disease activity is controlled. Methotrexate can rarely be associated with increased nodulosis in some RA patients, even when the disease is well controlled. Nodules caused by methotrexate tend to present as multiple small nodules on the finger pads.

21. Which diseases should be considered in a patient with subcutaneous nodules and arthritis?

RA, xanthoma, gout (tophi), SLE (rare), amyloidosis, rheumatic fever (rare), sarcoidosis, multicentric reticulohistiocytosis, and leprosy.

22. Which cutaneous disorder can cause lesions that pathologically are similar to rheumatoid nodules?

Granuloma annulare lesions have been called "benign" rheumatoid nodules and can look somewhat similar to RA nodules on histopathology. Patients with granuloma annulare do not have arthritis and are RF-negative. These lesions are more common in childhood.

23. What are the ocular manifestations of RA?

Both episcleritis and scleritis can occur in less than 1% of RA patients. If scleral inflammation persists, scleral thinning and scleromalacia perforans can occur. Peripheral ulcerative keratitis (PUK) and corneal melt are rare but severe and blinding manifestations and typically require aggressive immunotherapy. Sicca symptoms of dry eyes frequently accompany coexistent SjD. Uveitis in any form is uncommon in RA and if present should warrant evaluation of an alternate diagnosis or overlapping rheumatic disease.

24. Discuss the pulmonary manifestations of RA.

- **Pleural disease:** Pleurisy and pleural effusions (often unilateral) occur commonly in RA but are symptomatic in <5%. They can occasionally be the first manifestations of RA. Pleural effusions are characterized as cellular exudates with high protein and lactate dehydrogenase levels, a low glucose level (resulting from a defect in the transport of glucose across the pleura), and frequently a low pH (masquerading as an infection). Tuberculosis must be ruled out in patients at risk.
- **Nodules:** Rheumatoid nodules in the lung may be solitary or multiple and can cavitate or resolve spontaneously. **Caplan's syndrome** involves multiple nodules occurring in the lungs of RA patients who are coal miners (a pneumoconiosis in the setting of RA). In patients at risk (smokers), lung cancer needs to be ruled out.
- **Interstitial lung disease (ILD):** ILD occurs commonly in RA patients but is symptomatic and progressive in <10%. RA-ILD is more common in males and smokers. The strongest risk factor for developing ILD in RA is the presence of a polymorphism in the *MUC5B* gene. In RA, the **usual interstitial pneumonia (UIP)** pattern of ILD is most common, which is in contrast to the nonspecific interstitial pneumonia (NSIP) pattern that is most common in other connective tissue disease associated-ILDs. Fibrosis primarily involves the lower lobes. In rare cases, ILD can antedate the onset of arthritis.
- **Organizing pneumonia (OP):** Can be secondary to RA or disease-modifying antirheumatic drugs (DMARDs). OP is less common, but more responsive to corticosteroid therapy, than RA-associated bronchiolitis obliterans (BO), UIP, or NSIP.
- **Airways disease:** Airways disease in RA can range from mild disease that may only be seen on imaging to an emphysema-like disease with more significant airway obstruction. In addition, bronchiectasis may be seen. The most severe form of airways disease is **BO,** also called **constrictive bronchiolitis.** Patients have subacute onset of dyspnea (weeks), a hyperinflated chest x-ray, and small airway obstruction on pulmonary function tests. This condition can be rapidly fatal. Smoking may play some role in all of these airway findings. Finally, upper airway disease may be seen in the form of **cricoarytenoid disease** that can mimic tracheal stenosis.

25. What are the clinical consequences of the cardiac manifestations of RA?

Pericarditis	Pain (1% of rheumatoid arthritis patients)
	Tamponade (rare)
	Constriction (uncommon)
Nodules	Conduction abnormalities
	Valvular problems
Coronary arteritis	Myocardial infarction
Myocarditis	Congestive heart failure

26. Which types of vasculitis occur in RA patients?

Vasculitis most commonly occurs in RA patients with longstanding, poorly treated disease, significant joint involvement, high-titer RF, and nodules. Thankfully, the incidence of RA-associated vasculitis has decreased substantially in the past 25 years. The types of vasculitis are:

- **Leukocytoclastic vasculitis**—usually presents as palpable purpura and results from inflammation of postcapillary venules.
- **Small arteriolar vasculitis**—presents as small infarcts of digital pulp/nailfolds (rarely gangrene) and frequently is associated with a mild distal sensory neuropathy caused by vasculitis of the vasa nervorum.
- **Medium-vessel vasculitis**—can resemble polyarteritis nodosa with visceral arteritis, mononeuritis multiplex, and livedo reticularis.

27. What three findings make up the classic triad of Felty's syndrome?

Felty's syndrome is (1) **RA** in combination with (2) **splenomegaly** and (3) **leukopenia.** Felty's syndrome is seen in 1% of RA patients who have RF, subcutaneous nodules, and other extraarticular manifestations. Most (>90%) of patients are HLA-DR4 positive and RF positive. The leukopenia is generally a neutropenia (<2000/mm^3); thrombocytopenia may occur. The major complications of Felty's syndrome include bacterial infections (20-fold increase compared with other RA patients) and chronic non-healing ulcers. Severe bacterial infections correlate with neutrophil counts of <1000/mm^3. Patients with Felty's syndrome also have a 13-fold increased risk of developing non-Hodgkin's lymphoma, and a subset of patients may have large granular lymphocyte syndrome (Question #28 below). Some patients develop nodular regenerative hyperplasia of the liver with portal hypertension and varices that can bleed.

Treatment is the same as that for RA patients with joint disease and can include use of methotrexate or other DMARD therapy. With control of the RA, leukopenia may improve. Granulocyte colony-stimulating factor (G-CSF) has been used and shown effective at increasing WBC counts and decreasing infections in some patients (neutrophils <1000/mm^3). However, G-CSF can be associated with increased arthritis and vasculitis in some Felty's syndrome patients when the WBC count is raised. Splenectomy is reserved for patients with severe, recurrent bacterial infections or patients with chronic nonhealing leg ulcers who are not responsive or tolerant to drug therapy. Unfortunately, neutropenia recurs in 25% of patients who undergo splenectomy.

28. What other clinical problems occur with increased frequency in RA patients?

Atherosclerosis—Patients with RA develop atherosclerosis 10 years earlier than those without RA who have the same traditional cardiovascular (CV) risk factors. Traditional CV risk factors underestimate risk in patients with RA, which is estimated to be 1.5-fold higher than the general population. In addition to modifying traditional risk factors (hypertension, hyperlipidemia, obesity, and tobacco use), control of RA disease activity is recommended to reduce CV disease risk in patients with RA.

SjD—Approximately 20% to 30% of RA patients develop associated sicca with dry eyes and dry mouth. These patients often do not have anti-SS-A or anti-SS-B antibodies. RA patients who have systemic features of SjD and fulfill classification criteria for that diagnosis are now called RA with associated SjD (formerly called secondary SjD).

Amyloidosis—RA patients rarely develop amyloid A-associated amyloidosis. This occurs in longstanding, poorly controlled RA and usually presents as nephrotic syndrome.

Osteoporosis—seen in many RA patients and is related to disease activity, immobility, and medications. Insufficiency fractures of the spine, sacrum, and other areas are common in longstanding disease.

Entrapment neuropathy—median nerve (carpal tunnel), posterior tibial nerve (tarsal tunnel), ulnar nerve (cubital tunnel), and posterior interosseous branch of the radial nerve are most commonly involved.

Laryngeal manifestations—cricoarytenoid arthritis can present as pain, dysphagia, hoarseness, and rarely, stridor.

Ossicles of ear—tinnitus and decreased hearing.

Renal and gastrointestinal involvement—rare. Abnormalities are typically attributable to nonsteroidal antiinflammatory drugs (NSAIDs) causing renal insufficiency or gastric ulcers with hemorrhage.

Large granular lymphocyte (LGL) syndrome—a syndrome of neutropenia, splenomegaly, susceptibility to infections, and LGLs bearing CD2, 3, 8, 16, and 57 surface phenotypes in the peripheral blood smear (although a bone marrow biopsy is often required to confirm the diagnosis). These cells have enhanced natural killer and antibody-dependent cell-mediated cytotoxicity activity. It is now recognized that when this syndrome occurs in RA patients, it is a subset of Felty's syndrome. Approximately a third of Felty's syndrome patients have significant clonal expansions of these cells on their peripheral smear.

29. Are patients with RA at increased risk for joint infections?

Unfortunately, yes. Joint infections tend to occur in damaged joints, and RA patients may have many of these. Patients are also at increased risk secondary to immunosuppressive medication. Any time an RA patient presents with one or two joints that are swollen, red, and hot, out of proportion to the other joints, the clinician should suspect infection. In addition, following joint replacement surgeries, an infected artificial joint is a constant concern. The most common infecting organism is *Staphylococcus aureus,* although coagulase-negative *Staphylococcus* species may cause indolent joint infections and should be considered in postoperative patients with inflammatory joint findings in the operated-upon joint.

30. Do any markers help predict if an RA patient will have severe disease and a poor prognosis?

Long disease duration prior to treatment, RF and ACPA positivity, and poor functional status (health assessment questionnaire score >1) at presentation are the best predictors of subsequent disability and joint damage. Other factors include:

- Generalized polyarthritis involving both small and large joints (>13 total joints)
- Extraarticular disease, especially nodules and vasculitis
- Persistently elevated ESR or CRP
- ANA positivity (if also RF positive)
- Radiographic erosions within 2 years of disease onset
- HLA-DR4 genetic marker
- Lower educational attainment.

31. What are the most important goals for the treatment of RA?

- **Treat early:** the best results are seen when RA patients are started on therapy within 3–6 months of synovitis onset. This goal may be difficult to reach because of delay in presentation to primary care, delay in referral to rheumatology, and delays between referral and first visit with the rheumatologist.
- **Treat to a target:** aim for low disease activity or remission.

32. What instruments are used to measure RA disease activity?

There are several validated instruments that can be used to measure disease activity. Each uses various combinations of tender (TJC) and swollen joint count (SJC), patient global assessment of disease (PtGA), physician global assessment of disease (PhGA), patient pain, CRP or ESR, and the multidimensional health assessment questionnaire (MDHAQ). The most important thing is that disease activity is measured; the type of instrument used is of less importance. The instruments commonly used are shown in Table 14.2.

Disease activity score in 28 joints (DAS28): calculate using the DAS calculator (www.das-score.nl). Components: TJC (0–28), SJC (0–28), ESR, PtGA (0–10).

Simplified disease activity index (SDAI): TJC (0–28) + SJC (0–28) + PtGA (0–10) + PhGA (0–10) + CRP (mg/dL)

Clinical disease activity index (CDAI): TJC (0–28) + SJC (0–28) + PtGA (0–10) + PhGA (0–10)

Routine assessment of patient index data (RAPID): MDHAQ (0–10) + patient pain (0–10) + PtGA (0–10)

There are a growing number of studies supporting biomarker assessment (cytokine and chemokine panels) and/or imaging studies such as ultrasound (assessment for power Doppler signal to the joints and/or evidence of gray scale synovitis) as useful tools in determining disease activity. The exact role of these instruments in routine clinical practice remains to be determined.

TABLE 14.2 Classification of Disease Activity

INSTRUMENT (SCORE RANGE)	REMISSION	LOW DISEASE ACTIVITY	MODERATE DISEASE ACTIVITY	SEVERE DISEASE ACTIVITY
DAS28 (0–9.4)	≤2.6	≤3.2	>3.2 to ≤5.1	>5.1
SDAI (0–86)	≤3.3	≤11	>11 to ≤26	>26
CDAI (0–76)	≤2.8	≤10	>10 to ≤22	>22
RAPID3 (0–30)	≤1	<6	≥6 to ≤12	>12

CDAI, clinical disease activity index; *DAS28,* disease activity score in 28 joints; *RAPID3,* routine assessment of patient index data; *SDAI,* simplified disease activity index.

33. Discuss the management principles for the initial treatment of RA.

Current strategies include early aggressive treatment with one or more conventional synthetic DMARDs (csDMARDs; see Chapter 83: DMARDs: Conventional Synthetic and Targeted Synthetic Agents) and/or biologic DMARDs (bDMARDs; see Chapter 84: DMARDs: Biologic Agents), in addition to symptomatic therapy with NSAIDs, low-dose prednisone, physical therapy (see Chapter 88: Rehabilitative Techniques), occupational therapy, rest, and patient education. Methotrexate is commonly considered a first-line treatment and can induce low disease activity as monotherapy in about 30% of patients. Therapy should be advanced in patients who fail to reach low disease activity or remission with an adequate dose (15–25 mg/week) of methotrexate after 3 to 6 months. In this situation, therapy may consist of addition of csDMARDs to methotrexate or addition of a bDMARD or targeted synthetic DMARD (tsDMARD, such as a Janus Kinase inhibitor [JAKi]) to methotrexate. In the former approach, sulfasalazine and hydroxychloroquine may be added to methotrexate (commonly referred to as triple therapy). Patients intolerant to methotrexate may have leflunomide or, less commonly, azathioprine substituted. Patients who are adherent to triple therapy achieve low disease activity in 40% to 50% of cases without an increase in medication toxicity. Options for bDMARDs and tsDMARDs include tumor necrosis factor-α inhibitors, interleukin-6 inhibitors (tocilizumab or sarilumab), anti-CD20 agents (rituximab), JAKis (tofacitinib, upadacitinib, or baracitinib), IL-1 receptor antagonist (anakinra) or selective costimulation modulator agents (abatacept). These therapies can be and are often used in conjunction with methotrexate or another csDMARD. Patients on their first bDMARD can achieve low disease activity in 40% to 50% of cases. RA patients who fail to respond to an initial biologic agent should be switched to another biologic agent with a different mode of action. Rituximab can be helpful in both seropositive and seronegative diseases, but efficacy is better in seropositive RA patients. Short-term corticosteroids for more immediate relief of joint pain at the time of diagnosis may be considered, but several guidelines (including the 2021 American College of Rheumatology RA Guidelines) recommend against longer-term use.

Precision medicine is a major area of research in RA. One of the goals of this field is to determine in advance which drug will work best in individual patients in order to avoid costly and ineffective therapies, and improve the time to disease control for individual patients. Approaches may include blood tests for inflammatory or autoimmune biomarkers, genetic testing (including gene expression profiles and genes related to drug metabolism), and potentially synovial biopsy to further characterize the immunologic drivers in individual patients. Precision medicine holds the promise of improved patient outcomes and lower cost of care (through elimination of a trial-and-error approach).

While biologic therapies have greatly improved the treatment of the articular manifestations of RA, there is ongoing research focusing on how to most effectively treat extra-articular manifestations such as ILD. Mycophenolate mofetil and rituximab are often used as lung-targeted therapies in the setting of RA-ILD, although the former is thought to be less effective in treating articular disease. The antifibrotic medication nintedanib is approved in progressive fibrotic RA-ILD.

Special attention should be given to preventative therapies in all RA patients including immunizations (flu, pneumonia, zoster, COVID-19), CV disease (smoking cessation, blood pressure control, lipid management, weight loss as appropriate), and osteoporosis (calcium, vitamin D, and other targeted therapy such as antiresorptives).

34. Can use of DMARDs in preclinical RA prevent the development of RA?

Several clinical trials in the US and Europe have investigated whether using csDMARDs or bDMARDs prior to the onset of RA (defined by synovitis on clinical examination) in individuals at increased risk for future RA (based on serum ACPA positivity +/– arthralgias +/– ultrasound or MRI evidence of synovitis) could potentially prevent progression to RA. These studies have investigated methotrexate, hydroxychloroquine, rituximab, and abatacept. While some interventions have delayed RA, only abatacept has demonstrated a potential to prevent RA in a subset of individuals.

35. What is the long-term prognosis for RA patients?

RA is clearly a disease that can shorten survival and produce significant disability, especially before the use of modern therapeutic approaches that include early and more aggressive use of csDMARDs, bDMARDs, and tsDMARDs. Historically, RA was found to shorten the life span of patients by roughly 5 to 10 years. Many studies over the past decade, however, have demonstrated that RA mortality is improving and near that of non-RA populations in many countries (although rates are not quite equal yet). In addition, aggressive DMARD/biologic therapy appears to reduce disability (30%) and the need for joint replacement surgery (50%).

Some patients who are treated aggressively very early following the onset of synovitis (<3 months) may enter a state of prolonged disease remission (deep remission) and may be able to have therapy decreased or potentially withdrawn. Most studies that have investigated this area have focused on decreasing drug regimens rather than complete cessation of DMARD therapy (e.g., drug-free remission). Spacing of bDMARDs rather than sudden discontinuation is recommended. Success with reducing medication regimens is more likely when attempted early in the course of RA (disease duration <2 years) and in seronegative patients.

36. What causes the increased mortality in RA patients?

- **CV:** One of the leading causes of death in patients with RA; frequency is increased by 1.5 to 2-fold over the general population.
- **Infections:** Pneumonia is especially common in patients with RA. Historically, fatal infections are increased fivefold over the general population.
- **Cancer and lymphoproliferative malignancies:** Lymphoma and leukemia are increased two- to threefold. Lung cancer is increased by 1.5- to 3.5-fold. Melanoma may be increased. Other solid tumors do not appear to be increased in RA.
- **Lung disease:** When ILD is present, it is associated with a threefold increase in mortality, and this is more pronounced in those with a UIP pattern.
- **Others:** Include renal disease as a result of amyloidosis, gastrointestinal hemorrhage resulting from NSAIDs, and RA complications. With the treatments available today, fewer deaths are attributable to RA complications such as vasculitis and atlantoaxial subluxation.

37. What is seronegative RA?

It is a term to identify patients with RA who are RF and ACPA-negative. Although called seronegative, some of these patients have a positive ANA (without antibodies against any specific antigen) or antibodies to carbamylated proteins or PAD enzymes. In general, RA patients who are seronegative have a better prognosis, fewer extraarticular manifestations, and better survival. Additionally, a number of these patients over time will, in fact, be found to have some other disease. Thus, when dealing with seronegative RA patients, the clinician should always look for the possibility of psoriatic arthritis, lupus, calcium pyrophosphate crystal deposition disease, gout, hemochromatosis or another form of arthritis other than RA.

38. What is the RS3PE syndrome?

A syndrome characterized by an acute, severe onset of symmetrical synovitis of the small joints of the hands, wrists, and flexor tendon sheaths, accompanied by pitting edema of the dorsum of the hand ("boxing-glove" hand). Other joints may be involved. This syndrome affects mostly elderly (mean age, 70 years) white men (male/female ratio, 4:1). All patients are RF negative. Symptoms do not respond to NSAIDs but are very sensitive to low-dose prednisone and hydroxychloroquine. Bony erosions do not occur. The disease predictably remits in <36 months and, unlike RA, does not recur after withdrawal of medications. Severe pitting edema at the hands has also been reported in polymyalgia rheumatica and as a paraneoplastic syndrome. Because of this association with cancer, patients with this syndrome should be carefully evaluated for underlying malignancy.

ACKNOWLEDGMENTS

The authors would like to thank Drs. Sterling West, James O'Dell, Jennifer Elliott, Annemarie Whiddon, and Kevin Deane for their contributions to this chapter in the previous editions.

BIBLIOGRAPHY

Aletaha D, Neogi T, Silman AJ, et al. 2010 rheumatoid arthritis classification criteria: an American College of Rheumatology/European League Against Rheumatism collaborative initiative. *Arthritis Rheum.* 2010;62(9):2569–2581.

Anderson J, Caplan L, Yazdany J, et al. Rheumatoid arthritis disease activity measures: American College of Rheumatology recommendations for use in clinical practice. *Arthritis Care Res (Hoboken)*. 2012;64(5):640–647.

Dadoun S, Zeboulon-Ktorza N, Combescure C, et al. Mortality in rheumatoid arthritis over the last fifty years: systematic review and meta-analysis. *Joint Bone Spine*. 2013;80(1):29–33.

Deane KD, Demoruelle MK, Kelmenson LB, Kuhn KA, Norris JM, Holers VM. Genetic and environmental risk factors for rheumatoid arthritis. *Best Pract Res Clin Rheumatol*. 2017;31(1):3–18.

Deane KD, Striebich CC, Holers VM. Editorial: prevention of rheumatoid arthritis: now is the time, but how to proceed? *Arthritis Rheumatol*. 2017;69(5):873–877.

Dekkers JS, Verheul MK, Stoop JN, et al. Breach of autoreactive B cell tolerance by post-translationally modified proteins. *Ann Rheum Dis*. 2017;76(8):1449–1457.

Firestein GS. Pathogenesis of rheumatoid arthritis: the intersection of genetics and epigenetics. *Trans Am Clin Climatol Assoc*. 2018;129:171–182.

Fraenkel L, Bathon JM, England BR, et al. 2021 American College of Rheumatology guideline for the treatment of rheumatoid arthritis. *Arthritis Care Res*. 2021;73(7):924–939.

Holers VM, Demoruelle MK, Kuhn KA, et al. Rheumatoid arthritis and the mucosal origins hypothesis: protection turns to destruction. *Nat Rev Rheumatol*. 2018;14(9):542–557.

Humby FC, Al Balushi F, Lliso G, Cauli A, Pitzalis C. Can synovial pathobiology integrate with current clinical and imaging prediction models to achieve personalized health care in rheumatoid arthritis? *Front Med (Lausanne)*. 2017;4:41.

Jeka S, Dura M, Zuchowski P, Zwierko B, Waszczak-Jeka M. The role of ultrasonography in the diagnostic criteria for rheumatoid arthritis and monitoring its therapeutic efficacy. *Adv Clin Exp Med*. 2018;27(9):1303–1307.

Mackey RH, Kuller LH, Moreland LW. Update on cardiovascular disease risk in patients with rheumatic diseases. *Rheum Dis Clin North Am*. 2018;44(3):475–487.

Smolen JS, Aletaha D, Barton A, et al. Rheumatoid arthritis. *Nat Rev Dis Primers*. 2018;4:18001.

Wijbrandts CA, Tak PP. Prediction of response to targeted treatment in rheumatoid arthritis. *Mayo Clin Proc*. 2017;92(7):1129–1143.

FURTHER READING

www.rheumatology.org including the 'Rheum2Learn' modules and Clinical Practice Guidelines

CHAPTER 15

Systemic Lupus Erythematosus

Jeffrey Shen, MD and Lisa Criscione-Schreiber, MD, MEd

The wolf, I'm afraid is tearing up the place.
—Flannery O'Connor, July 5, 1964

KEY POINTS

1. Systemic Lupus Erythematosus (SLE) is a chronic autoimmune disease that can affect multiple organs and systems. SLE is characterized by dysregulation of both innate and adaptive immunity with extensive autoantibody production that causes immune complex-mediated inflammation and, untreated, damage to affected organs.
2. All people with SLE should be treated with hydroxychloroquine. Additional immunomodulatory therapies should be tailored to organ and system-specific disease manifestations.
3. Active SLE manifests with objective findings on physical examination, laboratory, or imaging studies. It is important to understand typical SLE presentations to accurately attribute symptoms and signs to active SLE.

PART 1: INTRODUCTION TO LUPUS

1. What is Systemic Lupus Erythematosus (SLE)?

SLE is a chronic, systemic autoimmune disorder characterized by multiple immune system abnormalities. The presence of detectable serum autoantibodies is a defining feature. The development of SLE appears to result from a confluence of genetic predisposition and environmental triggers.

SLE is clinically heterogeneous, which can make it challenging to recognize early, especially since no single test can confirm the diagnosis. People with SLE may accumulate clinical manifestations over time. SLE sometimes overlaps with other rheumatologic conditions such as rheumatoid arthritis or myositis, which may complicate the diagnostic process. SLE is incurable with current treatments, but in most cases can be effectively managed through immune system modulation to prevent irreversible organ damage. Individuals with SLE usually require lifelong therapy.

2. What is the pathogenesis of SLE?

The immunologic basis of SLE is complex and has not been fully elucidated, though improved understanding has led to more effective treatments. Nearly every aspect of the described immune system has been found to be abnormal in some studied individuals with SLE or in animal models.

Defective clearance of apoptotic cells plays a central role in the development of autoimmunity. When apoptotic cells are not cleared effectively, necrotic centers develop, exposing nucleic debris such as DNA or RNA to the immune system. Protein-bound nucleic acids (self-DNA or self-RNA) are the antigens recognized by SLE autoantibodies (anti-dsDNA or anti-Sm respectively). Antigen-autoantibody complexes can deposit in organs triggering inflammation and damage, either directly through immune complex deposition, or as a result of immune system activation in response to deposited immune complexes. Lupus nephritis is a classic example of injury initiated by immune complex deposition.

Dysregulation in self-tolerance can lead to the emergence of autoreactive B- and T-cell lymphocytes. Extrafollicular autoreactive B-cell populations are expanded in SLE and constitute a major source of autoantibodies. Factors including B-cell activating factor (BAFF, also known as B-lymphocyte stimulator or BLyS) promote the survival of these autoreactive B cells. This disease mechanism is targeted through the biologic therapy belimumab, which is an anti-BAFF monoclonal antibody.

Persistent nucleic debris containing DNA or RNA from defective apoptotic clearance can also bind to Toll-like receptors (TLR). In the normal immune system, TLRs recognize foreign (e.g. viral and other microbial) nucleic acids. In SLE, when TLR7 and TLR9 in plasmacytoid dendritic cells (pDCs) bind apoptotic RNA and DNA, respectively, type-1 interferon (IFN) is released. While virus/microbial-induced inflammation causes temporary interferon-mediated inflammation, in SLE, the IFN1 pathway-related genes are persistently active in pDCs and other innate immune system cells. This is known as the interferon signature, and modulating this pathway of lupus pathogenesis has been a target for therapy; anifrolumab is a monoclonal antibody that binds to the type 1 interferon receptor, preventing activation. In addition, when endogenous and exogenous nucleic acid ligands are recognized by B-cell receptors (BCRs) and internalized into B cells, they bind TLR7 or TLR9 to activate related signaling pathways and thus govern the proliferation and differentiation of B cells. TLR7 hyperresponsiveness in B cells is a significant contributor to the pathogenesis of SLE, mediating germinal center and extrafollicular B-cell responses to promote the expansion of antibody-secreting plasma cells and accelerate disease progression. TLR 9 binding results in increased conversion of B cells to plasma cells and less conversion of B cells to Bregs. TLR9 binding is also important for production of anti-dsDNA antibodies. Notably, hydroxychloroquine interferes with TLR7 and TLR9 signaling in endosomes. Drugs to block TLR7 activation are in development.

Overall, we do not fully understand what causes SLE or how it leads to each of its many disease manifestations. Ongoing research efforts continue to explore the intricate pathophysiologic mechanisms of SLE.

3. Who gets SLE?

SLE predominantly affects young women, with significantly higher prevalence (3-4x) among Black/African-American, Asian, and Hispanic individuals. As SLE typically develops at a young to middle age, elderly individuals who present with new-onset SLE should be evaluated for drug-induced SLE or underlying malignancy.

Most cases of SLE occur sporadically. Genetic predisposition is important, and studies have shown that family members of a person with SLE have an increased risk for developing the illness, though an identical twin of an individual with SLE has a less than 50% chance of developing SLE. In exceptional cases, young patients with monogenic disorders of the innate immune system may develop SLE. These conditions include those with mutations leading to defective complement function (c1q, c2, or c4 deficiency), dysregulation in interferon pathway (TREX), and hyperactive Toll-like receptor signaling (TLR7 gain-of-function). These rare instances underscore the critical role of innate immune system dysfunction in the pathogenesis of lupus, highlighting that the disease is not solely caused by pathogenic autoantibodies.

4. How is SLE diagnosed?

SLE is a clinical diagnosis, as no tests exist that can singlehandedly diagnose lupus. While specific diagnostic criteria for SLE have not been established, classification criteria have been developed and are continually refined (see Table 15.1), which can aid in the diagnostic process. The distinction between diagnostic and classification criteria is that diagnostic criteria are devised to identify patients with a condition and should have an optimal balance of specificity and sensitivity. Classification criteria are needed for research purposes and were developed to capture a subset of patients with homogenous enough features to provide clarity when interpreting research study results. If patients included in research studies had features that varied too much, confounding factors could make study results difficult to interpret. The manifestations included as classification criteria are largely distinguishing features commonly seen in SLE and uncommonly seen in other rheumatic illnesses. Serositis and lupus nephritis are two such examples. Features like Raynaud phenomenon, lymphadenopathy, or anti-SSA (Ro) antibodies are seen in multiple autoimmune diseases, so are not included in SLE classification criteria since they are commonly seen in, but not specific for SLE. In clinical practice, classification criteria can serve as a diagnostic aid to assist in recognizing individuals with usual manifestations of lupus but can potentially miss patients with atypical presentations.

5. What is the role of a positive antinuclear antibody (ANA) in the diagnosis of SLE?

Greater than 98% of patients with SLE demonstrate elevated serum levels of ANA, which is a hallmark of the disease. For research purposes, a positive ANA is required to classify an individual as having SLE. This test, however, is not specific for SLE. Only a small percentage (5%) of people

TABLE 15.1 Systemic Lupus International Collaborating Clinics Classification Criteria for Systemic Lupus Erythematosus (2019)

CLINICAL DOMAINS AND CRITERIA	WEIGHT	IMMUNOLOGY DOMAINS AND CRITERIA	WEIGHT
Constitutional		**Antiphospholipid antibodies**	
Fever	2	Positive anti-cardiolipin	2
Hematologic		Positive anti-beta-2-glycoprotien	2
Leukopenia	3	Positive lupus anticoagulant	2
Thrombocytopenia	4	**Complement Proteins**	
Autoimmune hemolysis	4	Low C3 or Low C4	3
Neuropsychiatric		Low C3 and Low C4	4
Delirium	2	**SLE-Specific Antibodies**	
Psychosis	3	Anti-dsDNA	6
Seizure	5	Anti-smith	6
Mucocutaneous			
Non-scarring alopecia	2		
Oral ulcers	2		
Subacute cutaneous OR discoid lupus	4		
Acute cutaneous lupus	6		
Serosal			
Pleural or pericardial effusion	5		
Acute pericarditis	6		
Musculoskeletal			
Joint involvement	6		
Renal			
Proteinuria of >0.5 g/24h	4		
Renal biopsy with Class II or V nephritis	8		
Renal biopsy with Class III or IV nephritis	10		

To be classified as having SLE, an individual must first have documentation of an ANA at a titer of ≥1:80 at least once. After that criterion has been fulfilled, if an individual displays a collection of the manifestations below totaling ≥10, they can be classified as having SLE. Importantly, a criterion can only be counted if there is not a more likely explanation than SLE for that finding. The criteria do not need to be met simultaneously but can be additive.

with a positive ANA will develop SLE. Some people with a positive ANA will have other autoimmune diseases such as scleroderma, hypothyroidism, or autoimmune hepatitis.

A high titer positive ANA is not always clinically significant, as not all ANAs are pathogenic. Meeting the classification criteria for SLE requires an ANA titer of greater than or equal to 1:80.

A person who is ANA-negative is extremely unlikely to have or develop SLE. In the past, less sensitive ANA assays sometimes did not detect positive anti-SSA/Ro (52 kD and 60 kD) antibodies as a positive ANA even though they (SSA and SSB autoantibodies) recognize nuclear antigens. This situation is rarely seen today.

It is of practical importance to recognize that there are different laboratory assays for ANA including indirect immunofluorescence (IFA) and ELISA, among other methods. Individual laboratories may not only use different assays but may report ANA results differently in terms of which titers are reported and the threshold for ANA positivity. Furthermore, different IFA kits have been shown to vary widely in reporting ANA positivity. Therefore, in certain settings it may be reasonable to repeat an ANA test that has previously been negative. However, once a patient has had a positive ANA, re-testing is unlikely to add useful clinical information.

6. How should individuals exhibiting some clinical features of SLE but not meeting the classification criteria for SLE be considered?

Many conditions can present similarly to SLE, and these should be considered in patients with only one or two features of SLE, especially if the ANA is negative (see secret #5, Chapter 1). Hypothyroidism, dermatomyositis, and drug-induced lupus can mimic certain manifestations of SLE and can present with a positive ANA. Some patients early in the course of SLE may not yet meet classification criteria until additional manifestations arise.

If after careful clinical review, no alternative diagnosis is likely, individuals who meet some classification criteria for SLE can be classified as having **undifferentiated connective tissue disease**, or the illness may be called "incomplete lupus erythematosus". Incomplete lupus erythematosus is a term usually used to describe individuals who meet fewer than four classification criteria for SLE, and are thought to either a) have early SLE disease and will likely later develop the manifestations needed to fulfill classification criteria for SLE, or b) have a collection of signs that are consistent with a diagnosis of SLE (e.g. positive ANA, leukopenia, inflammatory arthritis, fever, Raynaud's phenomenon, and lymphadenopathy).

7. How does one classify patients who meet criteria for SLE and also manifest features of another autoimmune disease?

Some people meet classification criteria for more than one rheumatic disease. Individuals with SLE and characteristics of other autoimmune diseases may be described as having an overlap syndrome. Most commonly, people will have SLE and also meet classification criteria for Sjogren syndrome with sicca symptoms and a positive anti-SSA (Ro) autoantibody. In certain situations, another name is used to describe an overlap syndrome. The overlap syndrome when a patient meets criteria for SLE along with scleroderma and myositis is called mixed connective tissue disease (MCTD). Patients with MCTD have antibodies to RNP, which is an ANA. The nomenclature of overlap syndromes can be a source of great confusion to both rheumatologists and non-rheumatologists.

8. What are some of the major clinical associations of the autoantibodies most commonly seen in SLE? See Table 15.2.

TABLE 15.2 Autoantibodies in Systemic Lupus Erythematosus and Some of Their Clinical Associations

TARGET	CLINICAL ASSOCIATIONS	FREQUENCY (%)
dsDNA	Diagnosis specificity for SLE. Occasional correlation with disease activity (especially lupus nephritis)	50–70
Histones (H1, H2A, H2B, H3, H4)	SLE and drug-induced lupus	70–100
Sm (SnRNP* core proteins B, B', D, E)	High diagnostic specificity for SLE. No correlation with disease activity	20–30
U1-RNP* (SnRNP specific proteins A, C, 70-kDa)	SLE and mixed connective tissue disease (MCTD)	30–35
Ro/SS-A (60-kDa and 52-kDa proteins) La/SS-B (48-kDa protein)	Neonatal lupus (especially if anti-52-kDa) Photosensitivity, Sjogren's disease and sicca symptoms, SLE.	30 15
Anti-Cardiolipin Anti-Beta-2-glycoprotein Lupus anticoagulant	Antiphospholipid syndrome	30–50
Anti-ribosomal P	Diffuse NPSLE, hepatitis	12–16

SnRNP, small nuclear ribonucleoprotein; *SLE*, systemic lupus erythematosus; *NPSLE*, neuropsychiatric lupus erythematosus.

9. Are there forms of lupus besides systemic lupus erythematosus?

The term "lupus" is often used interchangeably with systemic lupus erythematosus (SLE). However, "lupus" is also used to describe several other conditions:

1. **Cutaneous lupus**, such as discoid lupus, often occurs without systemic symptoms. Patients may not know whether they have systemic or isolated cutaneous lupus, and some may have been told they have a diagnosis of "lupus" by a physician. In these cases, a comprehensive evaluation should be performed to distinguish between these diagnoses prior to labeling the illness as either SLE or cutaneous lupus.

2. **Drug-induced lupus** is used to describe a condition similar to SLE in reaction to a drug. Common shared features include constitutional symptoms, arthralgia, myalgia, and cutaneous lupus. Internal organ involvement such as pericarditis, nephritis, or neuropsychiatric disease is very rare in drug-induced lupus. Dermatological manifestations are the same as those observed in SLE or isolated cutaneous lupus. Skin biopsy cannot differentiate whether a rash is due to SLE or drug-induced cutaneous lupus; each exhibits identical features of vacuolar interface dermatitis with dermal mucin deposition. Unlike other drug reactions where the presence of an eosinophilic infiltrate may indicate a medication reaction, biopsies of rashes from drug-induced lupus typically do not show an eosinophilic infiltrate. Patients with drug-induced lupus typically have resolution of symptoms within several weeks to a few months of discontinuing the offending drug, but sometimes anti-inflammatory pharmacotherapy is required. Hydralazine, procainamide, and quinidine are classically associated with drug-induced lupus. Proton pump inhibitors are an increasingly recognized cause of drug-induced lupus due to their widespread use.

3. **Neonatal lupus** is a condition that can affect babies born to women with antibodies to SSA (Anti-Ro) and SSB (Anti-La). The neonatal lupus syndrome can include a lupus rash that resolves spontaneously within three months of life, or it can lead to severe complications when it affects the neonatal cardiac conduction system, resulting in congenital heart block. Women harboring these autoantibodies should be treated with hydroxychloroquine before and during pregnancy to mitigate the risk of neonatal lupus.

4. **Lupus pernio** is a misnomer, as this facial rash is actually a cutaneous manifestation of sarcoidosis. Lupus pernio is not seen in SLE or cutaneous lupus. Lupus pernio is different from pernio, which is a term that is confusingly sometimes used to indicate chilblain lupus. Chilblain lupus is also not SLE, but a separate cutaneous vascular entity that affects the extremities, causing purple/red, tender papules on fingertips and the tips of toes. In contrast to lupus pernio, chilblain lesions can occur in people with SLE or can manifest in individuals without any known autoimmune disease. To minimize confusion, it is advisable to refrain from using the terms "pernio" or "lupus pernio" and instead employ "cutaneous sarcoidosis," "cutaneous lupus," or "chilblains" when referring to these distinct clinical entities.

10. What is the importance of identifying each patient's manifestations of SLE?

People with SLE may have various disease manifestations, each of which requires consideration regarding the specific treatment approach. Hydroxychloroquine (or chloroquine) is the only medication that is indicated for every person with SLE. Beyond its efficacy in addressing specific manifestations, research indicates that it can reduce SLE disease activity, reduce lupus flares, and confer a mortality benefit. Additional site and organ-specific manifestations may respond more completely to some medications than others, as will be discussed below.

A recently developed conceptual model categorizes SLE manifestations into type 1 and type 2 lupus. This terminology considers inflammatory manifestations and organ complications of SLE that improve with immunosuppressive medications to be type 1 lupus. Symptoms such as fatigue, brain fog, and chronic widespread pain are termed type 2 lupus in this model. While type 2 symptoms are more subjective, these are the symptoms that individuals with SLE find most debilitating and are associated more strongly with poor quality of life and disability. Unfortunately, symptoms considered under the type 2 umbrella generally respond poorly to immunosuppressive therapy and can persist even when type 1 lupus activity is well controlled.

Regardless of how a provider describes these symptoms, it is important to acknowledge with patients that many symptoms of SLE do not improve with immunosuppressive therapy. Rather, these symptoms are currently addressed with nonpharmacologic interventions including routine cardiovascular exercise, sleep hygiene, physical therapy and cognitive therapies. Pharmacologic measures that can be trialed include tricyclic antidepressants, muscle relaxants, and selective serotonin-norepinephrine reuptake inhibitors.

11. Can lupus be cured?

There is no cure for SLE currently and people with this chronic condition require lifelong therapy. In contrast, individuals with drug-induced lupus may be cured after removal of the offending drug. Management of SLE is focused on treating specific disease manifestations and balancing treatment with potential adverse effects of therapies. Researchers are investigating several novel approaches including bone marrow transplant and CAR T-cell therapy as potentially curative treatments for SLE. Hematopoietic stem cell transplant has been an investigational therapy for severe and refractory cases of SLE. In some studies with relatively short follow up, some individuals experienced complete remission of their disease while others had partial improvement. There are case reports of individuals with refractory and severe SLE responding to autologous CD19 CAR T cells. In these few cases, a single infusion of CAR T cells led to the eradication of detectable SLE-specific autoantibodies and clinical remission for several years.

While these findings are promising, the absence of rigorous studies involving larger patient cohorts prevents extrapolation of these results to the broader SLE population and it is too early to categorize SLE as curable.

PART 2: CLINICAL FEATURES & DIAGNOSTIC CONSIDERATIONS

12. What are some general challenges in the diagnosis of SLE?

The diagnosis of SLE can be straightforward. For example, an individual with classic manifestations of SLE like a malar rash and inflammatory arthritis with a positive ANA and other laboratory features consistent with SLE such as anti-dsDNA, leukopenia and hypocomplementemia clearly meets classification criteria for SLE. As described above (see question #4), the lupus classification criteria are designed to include homogeneous disease groups in studies, and not to capture patients with rare manifestations or early disease.

The diagnosis of SLE can be challenging because people may experience symptoms that are theoretically consistent with SLE. Healthcare providers who are less experienced in examining individuals with SLE may not fully appreciate the nuances of objective manifestations. For example, while oral and nasal ulcers are part of the classification criteria for SLE, aphthous ulcers are extremely common. However, oral ulcers in lupus are generally painless, and tend to occur on the tongue or on the hard palate. These locations are different from typical aphthae, which tend to occur along the gum line, inner lips, and buccal mucosa. Additionally, many providers and patients have a difficult time differentiating arthralgia (joint pain) from arthritis, which is joint pain with objective swelling and inflammation inside joints. To meet this specific classification criterion, an individual must display objective evidence of inflammatory arthritis. Additionally, photosensitivity as pertains to lupus means a person develops a rash in response to sun exposure that is visible, palpable, symptomatic, and lasts at least a day or more.

As mentioned previously (question #5), while ANAs are detectable in many individuals, with a prevalence that increases with age, only 5% of people with a positive ANA develop SLE. Providers may be unaware of this distinction.

Many people experience chronic symptoms such as fatigue, widespread pain, mood disturbance, and cognitive dysfunction. Fibromyalgia syndrome is a disorder characterized by widespread pain and somatic symptoms, but this condition does not cause physical examination or laboratory abnormalities. An individual with a normal physical examination, normal blood counts and inflammatory markers, and a positive ANA likely has fibromyalgia syndrome with a positive ANA. While some such individuals may go on to develop SLE, most do not.

People ultimately diagnosed with SLE may develop manifestations and meet classification criteria for other autoimmune disorders before being diagnosed with SLE. Such illnesses commonly include rheumatoid arthritis (RA, usually seronegative) and Sjogren's syndrome. Rheumatoid arthritis and lupus arthritis can look identical early in the disease course, but a person initially diagnosed with RA may later develop other objective findings consistent with SLE. Similarly, Sjogren's syndrome is the most frequently overlapping autoimmune disease with SLE; many individuals with SLE have positive anti-SSA(Ro) antibodies and sicca symptoms.

In short, SLE is characterized by objective evidence of inflammation both on physical examination and in laboratory studies. Relying solely on symptoms should be avoided when diagnosing SLE. Disease mimics such as viral infections or drug-induced SLE should be considered and excluded. If uncertainty remains, patients can be monitored, and empiric initiation of hydroxy-chloroquine can be considered.

13. Is routine screening indicated for any manifestations of SLE that may not be easily recognized by patients?

Lupus nephritis

Especially in early stages, lupus nephritis may be asymptomatic. Glomerular damage leads to impaired filtration and proteinuria. The early signs of proteinuria such as bubbly urine or pedal edema may be ignored or mis-attributed by affected individuals. Routine urinalysis at least 1-2 times annually, more frequently if lupus is active, to detect hematuria, proteinuria, or pyuria followed by microscopy to identify the presence of red blood cells or their casts can help identify lupus nephritis early.

Hematologic disease

Cytopenias including leukopenia, anemia, and thrombocytopenia do not typically cause symptoms until they are severe. Therefore, routine CBC monitoring is indicated. Patients with significant anemia (symptomatic or requiring transfusions) or who develop acute drop in hemoglobin levels should be evaluated for hemolysis with a peripheral blood smear, and serum tests for indirect bilirubin, reticulocyte count, haptoglobin, and lactate dehydrogenase.

Although nonspecific, symmetric lymphadenopathy is a common feature of SLE that can be missed if a lymph node exam is not performed. However, in patients with bulky or asymmetric lymphadenopathy and B symptoms (fever, night sweats, unintentional weight loss), lymphoma and other lymphoproliferative diseases should be considered in the differential diagnosis.

Autoantibodies

Antiphospholipid syndrome (APS) is another common overlap syndrome among people with SLE. As APS leads to arterial and venous thromboses, it carries a high morbidity. Patients may not realize that a previous miscarriage or blood clot in the distant past is worth mentioning due to this association. Therefore, taking a detailed clotting and pregnancy history and screening for APS autoantibodies (anti-cardiolipin, anti-beta-2-glycoprotein, lupus anticoagulant assay) can help identify this syndrome. Additionally, all women with SLE who are considering pregnancy should be screened for APS antibodies as these pregnancies have high rates of fetal loss without anticoagulant therapy. Women considering pregnancy should also be screened for anti-SSA(Ro) and SSB(La) antibodies, as these antibodies can cause neonatal lupus (See Question #9).

Mucocutaneous disease

Oral ulcers in SLE tend to be painless and affect the roof of the mouth. Even with large ulcers, patients may not notice pain, but could mention painless bleeding after eating or brushing teeth. An oral exam is an important part of the routine evaluation of lupus.

14. What are the most common constitutional manifestations seen in SLE?

Constitutional symptoms including fatigue, fever, arthralgia, myalgia, unintentional weight loss, headaches, generalized weakness, and malaise are all common in SLE. Frequently these occur with other objective findings on exam (lymphadenopathy, malar rash, inflammatory arthritis) or laboratory testing (cytopenia, presence of SLE autoantibodies) that are more specific for SLE.

Although constitutional symptoms are commonly seen in SLE, they are not specific for a diagnosis of SLE and may occur in numerous other conditions mimicking SLE such as viral infections or lymphoma.

15. How and when should patients with fever of unknown origin be evaluated for SLE?

Fever of unknown origin (FUO) was classically defined as a fever (temperature of 100.4°F (38°C)) that persists for three weeks and is of unknown cause despite extensive workup. By this definition, SLE was described as a rare cause for FUO (5% or less).

Current definitions for FUO require a temperature of 101°F on two separate occasions during an illness lasting at least three weeks, occurring in a non-immunosuppressed patient. Standard FUO evaluation includes routine investigations for typical and common atypical infections as well as malignancies. If a patient has undergone standard evaluation over 3 weeks and no etiology is found, they can be labeled as having FUO. Since SLE, rheumatoid arthritis, giant cell arteritis, and other conditions can cause FUO, inflammatory markers, ANA, and RF are part of the recommended FUO evaluation. If a patient has FUO and negative ANA, investigations should be focused on conditions other than SLE. The presence of a positive ANA suggests that evaluation for SLE or other autoimmune diseases could be revealing. Investigations for a rheumatologic cause of an FUO should include a physical exam, especially looking for subtle manifestations of disease, and targeted laboratory investigation to assess for SLE. See question #13 for some manifestations that may be overlooked.

What if a patient with FUO tests positive for autoantibodies (such as anti-dsDNA, SSA) and has nonspecific signs that may be attributable to SLE but also a number of other conditions (e.g. generalized lymphadenopathy and other constitutional symptoms)? Such individuals may be monitored for development of other signs of SLE, or if other causes are ruled out, a clinician may diagnose early or incomplete SLE or undifferentiated connective tissue disease, depending on the situation. Hydroxychloroquine may be started empirically with a low to moderate-dose steroid taper to manage fever.

Major mimics of SLE that cause fever of unknown origin and may include detectable autoantibodies include viral infections (human immunodeficiency virus, hepatitis B/C, parvovirus, Epstein-Barr virus), drug-induced SLE, lymphoma, and culture-negative endocarditis. Remember that, like SLE, endocarditis and serum sickness are immune-complex mediated diseases that can cause fever, rash, synovitis, glomerulonephritis, and hypocomplementemia. Reasonable diagnostic considerations include an infectious workup, echocardiogram, lymph node examination with consideration of excisional lymph node biopsy (core or needle is inadequate to identify lymphoma), and careful medication history review.

16. What are the musculoskeletal features of SLE?

Arthralgia and myalgia

Joint and muscle pain are common in SLE and can be attributed to a combination of inflammation, immune system dysfunction, and other factors. Sometimes arthralgia and myalgia are part of an SLE flare and subside once the flare is resolved. Such symptoms can be managed with supportive care and nonsteroidal pain relievers. Physical examination will differentiate muscle and joint pain from inflammatory arthritis and myositis, which warrants a separate approach to evaluation and management.

Arthralgia and/or myalgia are common complaints that can have many etiologies including metabolic (hypothyroidism), mechanical (bursitis, deconditioning, repetitive injury), fibromyalgia, or osteoarthritis, which will not improve with SLE-directed treatment.

Inflammatory arthritis

SLE inflammatory arthritis typically involves the small joints of the hands and feet but can affect any joint. Synovitis (painful, tender swelling of joints) is common, though generally the swelling is not as prominent as that seen in rheumatoid arthritis. In some patients with SLE, chronic inflammation and repeated episodes of synovitis in the small joints, particularly those of the hands, may lead to deformities known as **Jaccoud arthropathy** (Fig. 15.1). This condition is characterized by swan-neck deformities, ulnar deviation of fingers, and hyperextension at the metacarpophalangeal joints. SLE does not typically cause erosive arthritis. Hand deformities in SLE are classically reversible when the joints are passively maneuvered, while those in rheumatoid and other erosive arthritides tend to become fixed such that the joints cannot be moved back into normal conformation.

Myositis

Inflammatory muscle disease can occur in individuals with SLE. Typically, lupus myositis presents with proximal muscle weakness, sometimes with pain. Occasionally dermatomyositis overlaps with lupus and affected individuals develop cutaneous features of dermatomyositis, muscle weakness/pain, and interstitial lung disease. The pathophysiology of myositis in SLE is not completely understood, and there are no characteristic features in the muscle biopsy to reliably differentiate lupus myositis from dermatomyositis. As the skin biopsy in both SLE and dermatomyositis can show interface dermatitis with increased dermal mucin, these conditions cannot be differentiated by biopsy of muscle or skin but tend to be differentiated based on the distribution of the rash, the presence or absence of characteristic autoantibodies, and other objective signs of SLE. Direct immunofluorescence (DIF) on skin biopsy of rashes shows more intense IgG and other immune reactants at the dermal-epidermal junction in SLE than dermatomyositis.

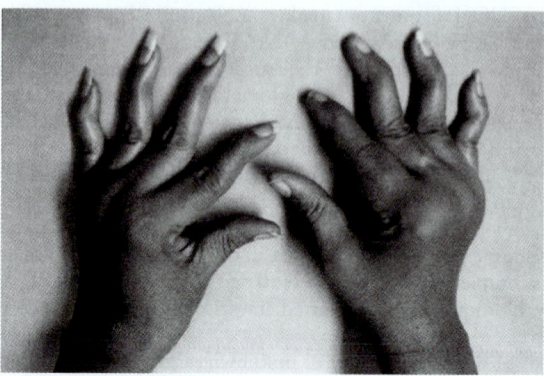

Fig. 15.1 Jaccoud arthropathy: Swan-neck deformities which are reversible.

17. Which mucocutaneous disease features are suggestive of SLE?

Oral Ulcers

The classically painless oral ulcers of SLE can be easily overlooked by patients or physicians without careful examination of the oral cavity. As described previously (Question #12), oral ulcers are common in the general population, and people with SLE can develop usual aphthae or oral ulcers from herpes simplex virus.

Alopecia

Alopecia is very common in SLE and can have different presentations and causes. Telogen effluvium is a common occurrence in any metabolic disease and people with SLE may describe this as hair falling out more easily than before. SLE can cause diffuse alopecia and has a specific predilection for causing temporal and occipital hair loss or breakage. Lupus can also cause patchy alopecia. Such alopecia can occur with or without discoid lesions. Non-discoid patches of hair loss may be overlooked by patients due to their location.

Rashes

Rashes in lupus are subclassified as acute, subacute, and chronic cutaneous lupus. In this section, we will describe some of the common forms of cutaneous lupus.

Acute Cutaneous Lupus

The classic malar rash and bullous lupus are two forms of acute cutaneous lupus. The term malar rash describes an erythematous photosensitive rash on the face in a butterfly distribution (see Fig. 15.2). Classically this rash spares the nasolabial folds, which helps distinguish it from rosacea, another photosensitive skin condition that causes a butterfly-distribution facial rash.

Subacute Cutaneous Lupus (SCLE)

SCLE lesions generally start as erythematous macules or papules in sun-exposed areas that develop into scaly, pruritic plaques frequently with hypopigmented centers. Several medications can cause SCLE (e.g. thiazides, calcium channel blockers, others). SCLE lesions resemble those of psoriasis, but generally with less scale (see Fig. 15.3). SCLE lesions resolve without scarring but frequently leave hyperpigmentation, hypopigmented areas that mimic vitiligo, or telangiectasias in previously involved areas. A skin biopsy of SCLE lesions will show lymphocytic infiltration at the dermal-epidermal junction (interface dermatitis), frequently with increased dermal mucin.

Chronic Cutaneous Lupus

CLE or discoid lupus most frequently occurs in isolation, without systemic signs of lupus. Discoid lesions are characteristically photosensitive, round, erythematous patches that can occur on any sun exposed skin, including the scalp where it will cause loss of hair in the affected area. As lesions expand, central areas lose pigmentation while the leading edge becomes hyperpigmented, giving the lesion a well-defined appearance (see Fig. 15.4). Without adequate treatment, lesions may permanently scar with loss of pigmentation, skin atrophy, and irreversible alopecia. Biopsy of discoid lesions will show interface dermatitis, along with periadnexal inflammation, follicular

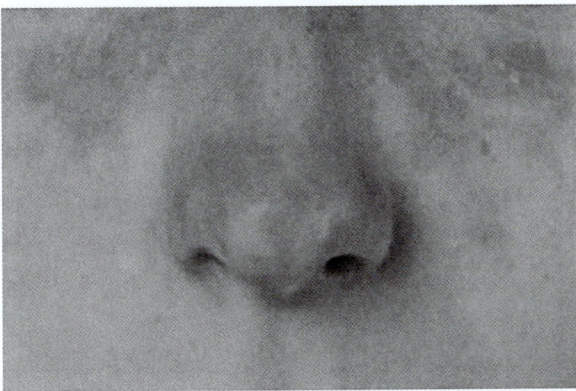

Fig. 15.2 Malar Rash: Typical photosensitive butterfly-distribution symmetric rash on face, notably sparing the nasolabial folds.

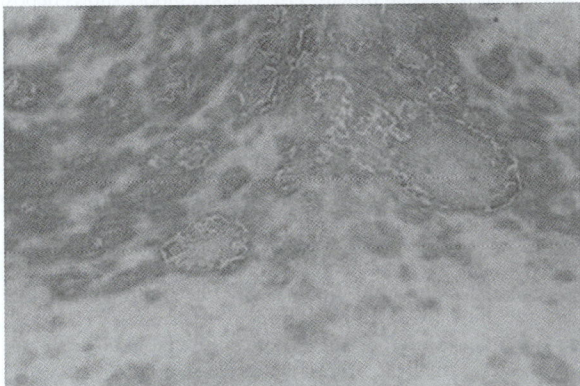

Fig. 15.3 Subacute Cutaneous Lupus: Annular coalescing lesions of subacute cutaneous lupus.

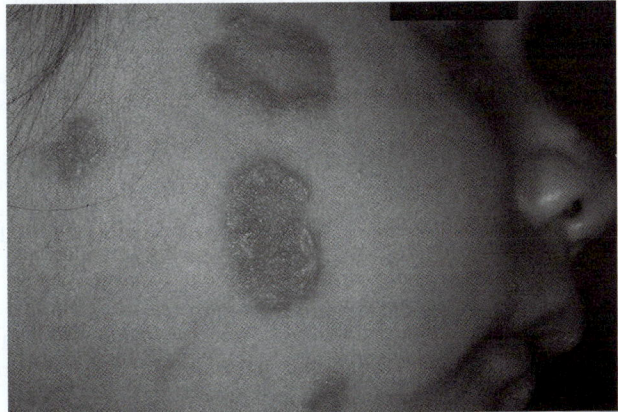

Fig. 15.4 Discoid Lupus Plaques: Classic annular red-to-purple inflammatory plaques. Note that the center is hypopigmented, and the border is brightly erythematous, elevated, and well defined.

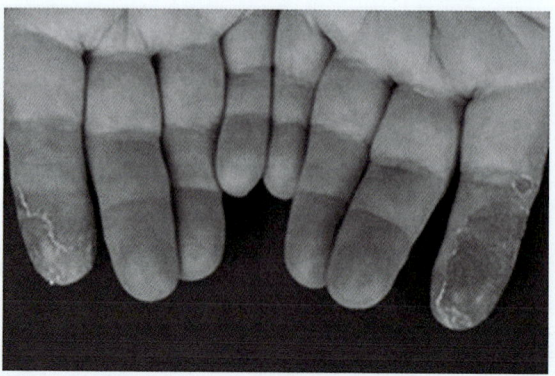

Fig. 15.5 Chilblain Lupus Erythematosus. Erythematous plaques on the acral extremities.

plugging, and often extensive dermal mucin. DIF on skin biopsy shows deposition of IgG and other immune reactants at the dermal-epidermal junction.

18. What are some less common cutaneous lupus lesions?

Lupus profundus

This form of chronic cutaneous lupus describes a lobular panniculitis that appears as painful plaques or nodules with induration. When these lesions resolve they leave areas of fat atrophy resulting in "dents" in the skin. Lupus profundus occasionally affects the breast and causes calcifications that can mimic mastitis or breast cancer.

Chilblain lupus

This form of chronic cutaneous lupus presents as tender red to blue lesions on the acral extremities, (fingers, toes, nose, ears) triggered by cold exposure (see Fig. 15.5). Chilblain lupus is often referred to as pernio. It is important to not confuse pernio (which may occur in lupus) with lupus pernio (which is actually a form of cutaneous sarcoidosis and not seen in SLE, see Question #9).

Bullous lupus erythematosus

This form of acute cutaneous lupus presents as a blistering eruption and is thought to be mediated by autoantibodies to type VII collagen. Histology will show a neutrophilic dermatosis underneath bulla at the dermal-epidermal junction. Direct immunofluorescence will frequently show linear IgG deposition at the dermal-epidermal junction. This linear IgG deposition is known as the "lupus band." The lupus band has been identified in both normal appearing and affected sun-exposed skin of individuals with all types of lupus rashes. While this IgG deposition is fairly specific for lupus skin rashes, it is less sensitive for identifying cutaneous lupus. Therefore, the finding of a lupus band in a skin biopsy from a person with a rash can help confirm a diagnosis of cutaneous lupus, but lack of linear IgG deposition does not rule out lupus. Bullous lupus rashes can occur anywhere on the skin or mucosal surfaces and can present as small vesicles up to larger bullae. On skin biopsy, bullous lesions are characterized by a subepidermal blistering with a neutrophilic infiltrate in the dermis.

19. What are the major ways for SLE to affect the kidneys?

Lupus nephritis (LN) is divided into six pathologic classes. See Tables 15.3 and 15.4 for lupus nephritis classification and definitions of activity and chronicity in lupus nephritis. It is important to differentiate between LN classes since management differs.

In addition to LN, people with lupus may develop other kidney diseases such as tubulointerstitial nephritis, podocytopathy, thrombotic microangiopathies due to anti-phospholipid syndrome, thrombotic thrombocytopenic purpura, or complement-mediated atypical hemolytic uremic syndromes. All these rare renal complications are managed differently. A high index of suspicion should be kept for thrombotic microangiopathies (TMA) in any lupus patient with new decline in renal function, since TMA is a life-threatening condition requiring urgent treatment,

TABLE 15.3 International Society of Nephrology and the Renal Pathology Society Classification of Renal Biopsies

CLASS	CLINICAL MANIFESTATIONS	HISTOLOGY DESCRIPTION	LIGHT MICROSCOPY	EM OR IF
I/Minimal mesangial	None	Mesangial immune deposits by IF +/– EM	Normal	
II/Mesangial proliferative	Microscopic hematuria +/– proteinuria; rare HTN	Mesangial hypercellularity or mesangial matrix expansion; few subepithelial/ subendothelial deposits by IF or EM		
III/Focal A = active lesions C = chronic lesions	Hematuria and proteinuria +/– HTN, decreased GFR, or nephrotic syndrome	<50% of glomeruli affected; IF almost uniformly involved; EM-immune deposits +/– mesangial area and in subendothelial space	Segmental proliferation wire loops Note areas of cellular hyperproliferation and areas that are spared	Note mesangial deposits
IV/Diffuse IV-S = segmental IV-G = global A = active lesions C = chronic lesions	Hematuria, proteinuria (frequently nephrotic), cellular casts, and generally decreased GFR; HTN is common; Hypocomplementemia and elevated dsDNA also seen frequently	>50% involvement of glomeruli; generalized hypercellularity of mesangial and endothelial cells; IF-full house pattern, extensive deposition; EM-immune complexes in both subendothelial and subepithelial distributions	Note hypercellularity of mesangial area and early formation of a crescent	Subendothelial deposits Note dark areas proximal to the basement membrane which visually look like thickened loops on LM
V/Membranous	Extensive proteinuria with minimal hematuria or renal function abnormalities	Granular global or segmental subepithelial immune deposits by IF or EM	Note thickened capillary loops without proliferation within the mesangial areas	Subepithelial deposits. Note dark areas distal to the basement membrane
VI/Advanced sclerosing	Chronic kidney disease	>90% global glomerulosclerosis thought 2/2 lupus nephritis; no activity		

EM, electron microscopy; *GFR,* glomerular filtration rate; *HTN,* hypertension; *IF,* immunofluorescence.

TABLE 15.4 Pathologic Features of Chronicity and Activity in Lupus Nephritis

CHRONICITY	ACTIVITY
Glomerular sclerosis	Cellular proliferation
Fibrous crescents	Fibrinoid necrosis
Fibrous adhesions	Cellular crescents
Interstitial fibrosis	Hyaline thrombi

and requires close collaboration with nephrologists and hematologists for optimal care. Of note, two APOL1 risk alleles are present in about 13% of African Americans. The APOL1 risk alleles cause a type of focal segmental glomerulosclerosis (FSGS) now termed APOL1 nephropathy. This condition presents with proteinuria and can be differentiated from lupus nephritis by kidney biopsy. APOL1 nephropathy can overlap with lupus nephritis.

20. What is the role of laboratory testing and biopsy in the diagnosis of lupus nephritis?

Because lupus nephritis causes high morbidity and recommended treatments vary depending on the class of lupus nephritis, renal biopsy is an important part of the diagnostic workup. **See** Table 15.3 **for classification of lupus nephritis by biopsy.**

Lupus nephritis can be detected by urinalysis, urine microscopy, and 24-hour urine protein assessment. Urinalysis and microscopy can identify blood components, casts, and protein in the urine. The ratio of measured protein to creatinine in a spot urine sample can estimate the number of grams of proteinuria in 24 hours, but this measurement varies based on several factors and is convenient but not as accurate as a 24-hour urine protein measurement. Creatinine should be obtained to assess for renal function. Cystatin C values must be interpreted with caution in lupus nephritis, as levels may increase with inflammation.

Immune complexes activate the complement cascade and fix complement, which can decrease serum levels of complement proteins C3 and C4 in patients with active lupus nephritis. When this occurs, complements may be used as a disease biomarker for lupus nephritis activity. Anti-dsDNA antibodies are thought to be pathogenic in lupus nephritis; in individuals with anti-dsDNA positivity and lupus nephritis, the titers of anti-dsDNA often correlate with disease activity.

21. What are the hematologic manifestations of SLE?

Cytopenia

All hematopoietic cell lines may be reduced in SLE including red cells, white cells, and platelets. These can occur in isolation or in combination with each other. In patients with SLE who have cytopenia, the differential diagnosis should also include medication toxicity (especially with immunosuppressants such as mycophenolate, azathioprine, or cyclophosphamide), and bone marrow suppression due to infection in the appropriate clinical context.

Anemia

Anemia is a common hematologic manifestation in SLE and has several potential etiologies. As SLE often affects young women, heavy menstrual bleeding is a common cause of iron deficiency anemia. SLE is an inflammatory disease and thus can lead to anemia of inflammation, previously called anemia of chronic disease. Anemia of inflammation occurs when there is decreased circulating iron for hematopoiesis, mediated by elevation of hepcidin and suppression of ferroportin, the iron transporter. Another important mechanism for anemia in SLE is hemolysis. Clinicians should assess for hemolysis in individuals with SLE through evaluation of a blood smear and laboratory studies including reticulocyte count, haptoglobin and lactate dehydrogenase. The finding of a newly elevated mean corpuscular volume (MCV) may suggest active hemolysis since reticulocytes are large and can falsely elevate the MCV. Hemolytic anemia in SLE may arise from conditions such as warm autoimmune hemolytic anemia (95% Coombs' test positive) or thrombotic microangiopathy.

Leukopenia

Leukopenia is another common hematologic finding in SLE. Lupus leukopenia is most commonly due to lymphopenia detected on a complete blood count differential. However, the lymphopenia in SLE is usually not associated with opportunistic infections. Sometimes individuals with SLE develop neutropenia, which is often mediated by anti-granulocyte antibodies (not anti-nuclear cytoplasmic antibodies [ANCA] which are a laboratory hallmark of small-vessel vasculitis).

Thrombocytopenia

Decreased platelet counts in SLE closely resemble immune-mediated thrombocytopenia (ITP). The underlying mechanism is believed to involve anti-platelet antibodies, including anti-glycoprotein antibodies. Thrombocytopenia can also be a manifestation of APS, TTP, or TMA which can also occur in SLE patients.

Macrophage Activation Syndrome (MAS)

This is one of the most critical and potentially life-threatening hematologic complications of SLE. MAS results when dysregulation of the innate immune system leads to uncontrolled inflammation with severe clinical manifestations. It is sometimes triggered by an infection (e.g., EBV). MAS typically presents with high fever, pancytopenia, liver dysfunction, and coagulopathy. These symptoms are indicative of systemic inflammation and organ involvement. Serum ferritin levels are an important diagnostic marker of MAS, with significant elevation often exceeding 10,000 ng/mL. This extreme elevation is a distinctive feature of MAS and highlights the intensity of the systemic inflammatory response.

22. What is lupus serositis?

Lupus serositis refers to inflammation of the membranes that line some of the internal organs in the body (pericarditis, pleuritis, or peritonitis) due to lupus. Lupus serositis is generally very painful, characterized by exudative effusions (pericardial effusion, pleural effusion, or ascites). Lupus pleuritis and pericarditis are much more common than lupus peritonitis. Lupus serositis must be differentiated from effusions in these areas, which can be non-inflammatory and related to hypoalbuminemia, heart failure, cirrhosis, or other mechanisms.

23. What layers of the heart can be inflamed in SLE?

SLE can cause pericarditis, myocarditis, and endocarditis. Lupus pericarditis is managed similarly to other forms of lupus serositis. Rarely, lupus pericardial effusions can develop rapidly and cause life-threatening cardiac tamponade. This is a rheumatologic emergency.

The differential diagnosis of pleuritic chest pain in lupus includes lupus pericarditis, viral pericarditis, lupus pleuritis, infectious pneumonia, pulmonary embolism (such as from anti-phospholipid syndrome), and in rare cases viral or lupus myocarditis. Classically individuals with lupus pericarditis will describe chest pain that is worse when recumbent and improves with leaning forward.

When lupus affects the endocardium, small non-infective vegetations can form on the valves, most commonly on the mitral and aortic valves. These non-infective vegetations consist of fibrin, platelets, and other immune cells. This presentation is also called **Libman-Sacks endocarditis**, which is commonly associated with antiphospholipid syndrome.

24. What are pulmonary manifestations of SLE?

Pleural inflammation or pleuritis is a common pulmonary manifestation of SLE. When there is isolated pleural inflammation, or the inflammation has not yet caused accumulation of a detectable effusion, patients describe pain with inspiration, also called pleurisy. Individuals with SLE may develop exudative, inflammatory pleural effusions with or without pain.

Shrinking lung syndrome is a rare manifestation of SLE. Typical symptoms include pleuritic chest pain and dyspnea. Pulmonary function testing shows progressive decrease in lung volumes with absence of pathology on chest imaging. Chest diaphragms may be elevated and inspiratory pressure is decreased.

Sometimes SLE affects the pulmonary parenchyma or causes interstitial disease. In such cases, one should be alert for other signs of an overlap syndrome with myositis or scleroderma, both of which are associated with non-specific interstitial pneumonia (NSIP).

Another rare and severe manifestation of lupus is diffuse alveolar hemorrhage. In this condition, pulmonary capillaritis results in bleeding into the lung parenchyma, leading to profound hypoxemia and blood loss. The occurrence of a sudden drop in hemoglobin level along with new pulmonary infiltrates on chest imaging (classically sparing the sub-pleural space) suggests the possibility of diffuse alveolar hemorrhage. In such cases, emergent diagnostic bronchoscopy will reveal lavage fluid that becomes increasingly hemorrhagic with each successive bronchoalveolar lavage aliquot from the same location.

Pulmonary emboli can result from antiphospholipid syndrome or as a complication of Libman-Sacks endocarditis. Diffuse alveolar hemorrhage can also occur in this context. Finally, sometimes individuals with SLE develop pulmonary arterial hypertension (PAH). This can be an isolated manifestation, or secondary to advanced ILD with scarring.

25. What diagnostic considerations are important when evaluating neuropsychiatric lupus (NPSLE)?

Neuropsychiatric lupus (NPSLE), also referred to as CNS lupus, can be the initial lupus presentation and is a potentially deadly complication of lupus with several different clinical presentations. Symptoms suggesting severe NPSLE include psychosis, catatonia, seizures, encephalopathy, and focal deficits (from infarctions). The three neuropsychiatric presentations that are included as criteria for SLE include delirium, psychosis, and seizure. Individuals who present with seizures, delirium, or psychosis generally have diffuse brain involvement, and these manifestations represent the condition that was previously termed "lupus cerebritis" or "lupus psychosis." Evaluation of NPSLE should include serum anti-ribosomal P antibodies (diffuse NPSLE), antiphospholipid antibodies (stroke, chorea, seizures), and a lumbar puncture with cerebrospinal fluid sent for cell count and differential, protein, glucose, cultures, oligoclonal bands, IgG index, and antineuronal antibodies. Typically, the cerebrospinal fluid in NPSLE is characterized by lymphocytic predominance. Neuroimaging with MRI may show infarcts and white matter disease which correspond to small vessel vasculopathy. Autopsy studies have suggested that the smallest vessels, which are affected by inflammation and complement mediated immune complex deposition, are not visible on high resolution brain MRI or formal angiogram. This makes the diagnosis of NPSLE challenging and may explain why in some cases the brain MRI may be normal in individuals with active disease.

Many individuals with SLE complain of mild cognitive impairment, commonly described as "brain fog." This manifestation generally does not respond to aggressive immunosuppressive therapy and is not part of SLE classification criteria. While frequently a consequence of SLE, additional evaluation of these symptoms should also include consideration of sleep disturbance, depression or anxiety, and other conditions that can negatively impact concentration and may be amenable to other therapeutic interventions.

26. How does transverse myelitis from SLE present?

Transverse myelitis (TM) is a rare central nervous system complication of SLE. If not treated quickly, it can produce irreversible paralysis or other neurologic deficits, so it is important for the astute clinician to quickly recognize this rare complication of lupus. Affected individuals usually experience acute-onset numbness, tingling and weakness in the extremities, difficulty with balance, and loss of bowel/bladder control. Vague pain or sensory complaints localizing to a limb, abdomen, or back may occur due to referred pain and can be diagnostically confusing. Diagnosis requires a high index of suspicion and MRI imaging of the spine. Patients with longitudinally extensive (3 or more vertebral bodies) TM should be tested for anti-aquaporin-4 (neuromyelitis optica) antibodies. Patients frequently have anti-SSA/Ro antibodies. CSF examination often shows inflammation but may be nonspecific or even normal. TM may also occur at a less extensive level (1-2 vertebral bodies in length) due to spinal cord infarction from vasculitis or clot due to antiphospholipid syndrome. Regardless of etiology, one must inquire about urinary incontinence as patients may be reticent to mention this symptom. Since it can present with vague discomfort and paresthesia, many patients with transverse myelitis may not recognize the urgency of being evaluated and treated.

27. In what ways can the gastrointestinal tract be involved in SLE?

- Esophageal dysmotility: Usually involves upper third of esophagus in patients with SLE myositis, common in overlap syndromes.
- Pancreatitis: Usually due to gallstones, alcohol, or hypertriglyceridemia. Can be due to medications (azathioprine [AZA]). If due to SLE, the patient will have diffusely active disease.
- Serositis: Only occurs in patients with active systemic disease. Rare to get frank ascites. Need to R/O infection.
- Mesenteric vasculitis: Likely associated with active disease. Will see bowel wall edema and sometimes fat-stranding on computed tomography of abdomen.

- Hepatitis: usually a result of medications or other non-lupus etiology (e.g. viral, alcohol, NASH, etc.). Hepatitis due to lupus is associated with increased disease activity and anti-ribosomal P antibodies. Patients do not have anti-smooth muscle, anti-liver-kidney microsome, or antimitochondrial antibodies unless there is a rare overlap with autoimmune hepatitis or primary biliary cirrhosis.
- Intestinal pseudo-obstruction: Rare manifestation with obstruction picture but without identifiable mechanical or obstructive causes. Can present with abdominal pain, vomiting, diarrhea and/or constipation, abdominal distension, and weight loss along with an x-ray suggestive of obstruction.
- Protein-losing enteropathy (PLE): Consider in patients with severely low albumin but no proteinuria. Most patients have chronic diarrhea and edema from low serum proteins. Diagnosis is made by measuring fecal alpha-1 antitryspin or transferrin. Stool should not have these proteins unless there is a PLE.

PEARL: A gastrointestinal manifestation (serositis, vasculitis, hepatitis, and pancreatitis) is unlikely to be due to SLE unless the patient has evidence of active SLE in other organs and abnormal serologies.

PART 3: GENERAL MANAGEMENT PRINCIPLES AND PROGNOSIS

28. What medications are used to treat SLE?

Every person with SLE should take hydroxychloroquine (unless they have a known hypersensitivity or allergy to it) due to its many proven benefits in this illness. Hydroxychloroquine is an antimalarial drug that is effective for managing many of the manifestations of SLE. Though the exact mechanisms that make hydroxychloroquine effective in SLE are still under investigation, it is known to be immunomodulatory, seeming to improve some of the immune system aberrations that characterize SLE without suppressing response to infections. To avoid retinal toxicity, long-term hydroxychloroquine dosing should be maintained below 5 mg/kg/day using actual body weight, and at or below 400 mg daily. Checking Glucose-6-Phosphate Dehydrogenase (G6PD) levels is not necessary prior to initiating treatment with hydroxychloroquine. While there are no specific recommendations for dose reduction in the setting of renal disease, one can monitor whole blood levels of hydroxychloroquine for dose adjustment. Therapeutic whole blood level is 750-1200 ng/mL. Hydroxychloroquine is generally well tolerated; the most common side effect is gastrointestinal upset. Rarely, individuals may experience troublesome neuropsychological reactions such as sleep disturbance, nightmares and others that may preclude use. Additionally, it can cause prolonged QTc, and monitoring should be considered when needed in combination with other potentially QTc prolonging medications. Allergic rashes from hydroxychloroquine can take weeks to resolve related to this medication's long elimination half-life, and acute generalized exanthematous pustulosis (AGEP) is a very serious and fortunately rare idiosyncratic reaction that precludes future use of the drug. While hydroxychloroquine and some treatments such as corticosteroids can treat many different inflammatory manifestations, other pharmacotherapies including both biologic and non-biologic agents are more suitable for targeting certain manifestations. Table 15.5 lists the different steroid sparing medications frequently used in the management of SLE. Recently, obinutuzumab (type II anti-CD20 monoclonal antibody) has been shown in a clinical trial to be effective for the treatment of lupus nephritis. CAR T-cell therapy targeting CD19 on B cells (see Chapter 85) has been shown in small case series to be effective against treatment-resistant SLE. Neither are FDA-approved therapies for SLE and both are expensive.

29. How is inflammatory arthritis due to SLE managed?

Initial treatment of inflammatory arthritis with NSAIDs is frequently effective and can be prescribed as long as there are no contraindications. If used long-term, renal function monitoring is indicated. In most cases, NSAIDs should be avoided in individuals with active lupus nephritis. Hydroxychloroquine is very effective for arthritis in SLE, though takes time to be effective and NSAIDs or a short course of low to moderate dose prednisone can be effective initial management of inflammatory arthritis in SLE.

TABLE 15.5 Mechanisms of Systemic Lupus Erythematosus Treatments

MEDICATION	MECHANISM OF ACTION	ONSET
Glucocorticoids	Block NF-kB lowering inflammatory proteins and cytokines. Induce anti-inflammatory protein expression	Quick (days)
Hydroxychloroquine	Multiple, including inhibiting IFN-1 production through endosomal toll-like receptor inhibition, decreased NET formation	Slow (months)
Mycophenolate mofetil	Depletes guanosine in lymphocytes	Slow (months)
Azathioprine	Purine metabolite antagonist	Slow (months)
Voclosporin, Tacrolimus, Cyclosporine	Calcineurin inhibitors	Slow (weeks)
Cyclophosphamide	Alkylating agent	Slow (weeks to months)
Rituximab	Monoclonal antibody to CD20 (found on B cells)	Slow (weeks to months)
Belimumab	Monoclonal antibody to B-cell activating factor (BAFF or BLyS)	Slow (weeks to months)
Anifrolumab	Monoclonal antibody to subunit 1 of the type I interferon receptor	Slow (weeks to months)

In some individuals SLE causes chronic inflammatory arthritis despite treatment with hydroxychloroquine and NSAIDs. If repeated depot corticosteroids or tapering courses are required to manage inflammatory arthritis, disease modifying anti-rheumatic drugs (DMARDs) are employed to avoid the long-term adverse effects of prednisone. Methotrexate, used at doses similar to those in rheumatoid arthritis, is effective for inflammatory arthritis in many people with SLE. This medication is renally excreted and should be avoided in any individuals with abnormal renal function. Methotrexate is not dialyzable and even one dose in a patient with end stage renal disease can lead to profound pancytopenia, mucositis, and severe opportunistic infections. Leflunomide is metabolized in the liver and can also be used to manage lupus inflammatory arthritis. Azathioprine has also been effective for lupus arthritis. Biologic agents such as belimumab, anifrolumab, and rituximab are also utilized to manage lupus inflammatory arthritis.

30. How are mucocutaneous manifestations of SLE managed?

Mucosal Ulcers

Oral ulcers are common and may not be directly due to SLE. Oral ulcers from SLE are frequently painless, may not be noticed, and generally respond to medications for other manifestations of SLE, including hydroxychloroquine. If needed for painful ulcers, addition of topical steroids can reduce inflammation and topical anesthetics can be used as needed for pain relief.

Rash

Ultraviolet light can trigger cutaneous and other flares of lupus. Everyone with cutaneous lupus should be counseled to use daily photoprotection including sunscreen (applied every 2 hr when in sun) of at least SPF30 strength and photoprotective apparel. See question #38 for additional information.

Subacute cutaneous lupus and discoid lupus

In addition to photoprotection and hydroxychloroquine (which generally requires six weeks to six months to have full efficacy), topical steroids or topical calcineurin inhibitors (tacrolimus or pimecrolimus) are employed. Topical steroids should be used in a time-limited fashion, as long-term use leads to skin atrophy. Employing lower potency topical steroids on the face or close to the eyes except occasional considerations to prevent scarring in severe facial discoid lupus. Intralesional corticosteroid injections by a dermatologist are sometimes used for lesions resistant to topical treatments. Many patients experience widespread or refractory skin disease requiring additional oral therapy. Occasionally chloroquine is used (never in combination with hydroxychloroquine), and quinacrine may be used as additive therapy in some individuals. For cutaneous lupus refractory to the above interventions, oral DMARDs such as methotrexate, azathioprine, or mycophenolate can be used. Biologic DMARDS are also effective, particularly anifrolumab or belimumab.

31. How is lupus nephritis managed?

Therapy of lupus nephritis (LN) depends on the pathologic class and must incorporate important considerations such as pregnancy planning and fertility, medication adherence, and access to care. All individuals with lupus nephritis should be treated with hydroxychloroquine (HCQ) with monitoring of whole blood levels.

Class I lupus nephritis does not necessarily require immunosuppression but should be monitored closely over time. Class II lupus nephritis is generally treated with a tapering dose of steroids over several weeks. The primary pharmacotherapies used for induction therapy of classes III, IV, and V lupus include cyclophosphamide and mycophenolate, along with high, then tapering doses of glucocorticoids. Mycophenolate mofetil (MMF) is generally considered to be first-line therapy for lupus nephritis and clinical trial data support its use as induction and maintenance therapy for lupus nephritis. Medication adherence with MMF can be a challenge due to a high pill burden and side effects. Proton pump inhibitors can interfere with MMF absorption. Long-term data also support using intravenous cyclophosphamide-based regimens as induction therapy for lupus nephritis. Cyclophosphamide (CYC) is generally given either using what is termed "the NIH protocol," with monthly infusions of cyclophosphamide for 6 months, or the "Euro-lupus protocol" (i.e., 500 mg every 2 weeks for six doses) with a lower cumulative dose of cyclophosphamide over 12 weeks. These regimens were shown in the Euro-Lupus Nephritis Trial (ELNT) to be roughly equivalent in short-term remission induction and long-term renal outcomes for class III/IV lupus nephritis. Recent trials have led to routine addition of belimumab, a monoclonal antibody that neutralizes soluble B-cell activating factor (BAFF), or voclosporin, a calcineurin inhibitor to lupus nephritis therapy to improve response rates in lupus nephritis. Belimumab is effective for managing many manifestations of SLE and is given either as a weekly subcutaneous injection (initial dosing is increased in lupus nephritis) or as a monthly intravenous infusion (after an initial loading regimen). Voclosporin offers lower risk of hypertension and nephrotoxicity than the other calcineurin inhibitors tacrolimus and cyclosporine and does not require monitoring of drug levels. It is particularly effective for proteinuria. Obinutuzumab (type II anti-CD20 monoclonal antibody) has shown in a clinical trial to be an effective therapy for lupus nephritis but is not yet FDA approved for that indication.

Recently, the ACR updated guidelines for treatment of lupus nephritis as follows: 1) All SLE patients (pts) should be treated with HCQ and all pts with proteinuria (>0.5 g/g) should receive renin-angiotensin-aldosterone inhibitors, 2) All pts with LN should receive pulse IV glucocorticoids at 250-1000 mg/d for 1-3 days followed by oral prednisone < 0.5 mg/kg up to 40 mg/d with taper to target dose >5 mg/d by 6 months, 3) All pts with class III/IV/V LN should begin with triple therapy including glucocorticoids (GC) plus MMF plus either belimumab (if significant extrarenal manifestations) or voclosporin or other calcineurin inhibitor (if proteinuria > 3 g/g or class V LN). Pts unable to tolerate MMF can be treated with GC plus belimumab plus CYC (Euro-lupus protocol preferred). CYC with a calcineurin inhibitor has never been studied so was not recommended, 4) Therapy should be for 3-5 years and patient monitored for proteinuria every 3 months until complete renal response and then monitored every 3-6 months, 5) Pts with LN and end-stage kidney disease should proceed to early transplant over long-term dialysis. Complete serologic remission is not required to undergo kidney transplant.

32. How are hematologic complications of SLE managed?

Cytopenia

Asymptomatic mild anemia (not requiring transfusion), leukopenia, lymphopenia, and thrombocytopenia do not require immediate treatment. Often these manifestations may subside with hydroxychloroquine, and frequently respond to other pharmacotherapies for SLE.

Hemolytic anemia may require collaboration with hematology specialists. Warm autoimmune hemolytic anemia frequently improves with glucocorticoids and rituximab, with mycophenolate often used for maintenance therapy. Microangiopathic hemolytic anemias such as complement mediated thrombotic microangiopathy and thrombotic thrombocytopenic purpura may require immunosuppressives, plasmapheresis, anti-complement (e.g. eculizumab), or intravenous immunoglobulin.

Mild leukopenia may not require any change in treatment and may intermittently occur in individuals with SLE. Severe leukopenia or neutropenia are uncommon in SLE; when this occurs, a search for other causes such as bone marrow suppression from medications, infections, or a malignant condition should be considered.

Symptomatic or severe lupus thrombocytopenia is treated similarly to immune thrombocytopenia purpura (ITP) with glucocorticoids. Additional steroid-sparing agents frequently used include intravenous immunoglobulin (IVIG), mycophenolate, or rituximab.

Macrophage Activation Syndrome

Individuals affected by macrophage activation syndrome in lupus require initial treatment with high dose corticosteroids, often intravenously, with daily monitoring of laboratory parameters to determine the need for additional therapy. The IL-1 antagonist anakinra is frequently used to effectively manage this condition. IL-6R antagonists such as tocilizumab can be added to steroids for further dampening of immune system hyperactivation. Coordinated effort with hematology specialists may benefit patients. MAS is also called hemophagocytic lymphohistiocytosis (HLH), which can also occur in individuals without an underlying autoimmune disease; in such cases, it is managed differently, with chemotherapeutic agents.

33. How is lupus serositis managed?

Pleuritis usually improves with non-steroidal anti-inflammatory drugs (NSAIDs) and supportive care. On occasion, functionally limiting pain continues despite the use of these conservative measures, and intramuscular depot glucocorticoids or a moderate-dose steroid taper can be helpful. Colchicine is an additional steroid-sparing agent with some efficacy in lupus-associated pericarditis. Pericarditis also responds to NSAIDS and can also be treated with intramuscular depot glucocorticoids or a moderate-dose steroid taper. Individuals with large pericardial effusions with tamponade physiology may require therapeutic pericardiocentesis along with high dose glucocorticoids. Such cases may require additional disease-modifying therapy.

34. How is neuropsychiatric lupus (NPSLE) managed?

Due to the rarity and heterogeneity of NPSLE, there is no clinical trial data to guide management which is largely empiric, and at best based on case series level evidence. Severe manifestations of neuropsychiatric lupus are generally treated with high-dose glucocorticoids with a prolonged taper, and often with cyclophosphamide or rituximab. There is no evidence to support a specific cyclophosphamide regimen for NPSLE. All patients who present with NPSLE should be evaluated for anti-phospholipid syndrome which may warrant the addition of anticoagulation. This is especially important when individuals present with stroke or spinal cord infarcts. Seizures are one of the criteria-meeting manifestations of NPSLE. Individuals with seizures must be managed with

TABLE 15.6 Systemic Lupus Erythematosus Disease Activity and Damage Scores

MEASURE	EXAMPLE	USE
Disease activity	SLEDAI SLEDAI-2K SELENA-SLEDAI SRI LLDAS BILAG/BICLA DORIS PGA	Mostly used in studies to enroll subjects with active SLE and to assess change in activity with an intervention
Damage scores	SLICC damage index (SDI) BILD (patient-reported measure)	To quantitate damage incurred through longstanding SLE activity. Assessed damage includes cardiovascular disease and stroke, glucocorticoid-induced osteoporosis, diabetes, impaired renal function, cancer

BILAG, British Isles Lupus Assessment Group; *BICLA*, BILAG-based Composite Lupus Assessment; *BILD*, brief index of lupus damage; *DORIS*, Definition of Remission in SLE; *LLDAS*, Lupus Low Disease Activity State; *PGA*, Physician Global Assessment; *SELENA*, Safety of Estrogens in Lupus Erythematosus National Assessment trial; *SLEDAI*, systemic lupus erythematosus disease activity index; *SLICC*, Systemic Lupus International Collaborating Clinics; *SRI*, Systemic Lupus Erythematosus Responder Index.

a combination of aggressive anti-inflammatory therapy along with standard anti-seizure measures. Similarly, a person with psychosis from NPSLE (previously classically termed "lupus cerebritis") is managed with anti-psychotic pharmacotherapies along with immunosuppressive therapy to manage the CNS inflammation. Transverse myelitis from lupus is also aggressively managed with cyclophosphamide or other aggressive DMARD regimens and can be reversible. Again, symptoms such as spasticity or neuropathic findings can be managed with adjunctive therapies.

35. What disease activity and damage indices are used in SLE?

In lupus, disease burden can be measured by disease activity or damage. The disease activity measures give an assessment of the degree of active inflammation, whereas the damage scores give an idea of the downstream effects of the disease or therapies. These are used more in clinical trials than clinical practice. However, a good rule of thumb is a patient who spends 50% of the time in low disease activity while on low dose prednisone ($\leq$ 5mg/d) and stable immunosuppressants has 50% less damage accrued compared to someone who does not achieve low disease activity. The validated disease activity and damage scoring systems are outlined in Table 15.6.

36. Why is it important to discuss future pregnancy planning with biological women with SLE?

It is important to partner with women and to ascertain their hopes and plans regarding childbearing, as becoming a parent is a very strong drive in many individuals. Unfortunately, misinformation abounds regarding SLE and pregnancy, ranging from the belief that women with SLE lose fertility, to beliefs that women must try to conceive early on in the disease before it gets worse, or beliefs that doctors will tell them they should not become pregnant and therefore they feel reluctant to share their true intentions or plans.

To ensure the healthiest possible outcome for both mother and baby, it is very important to plan childbearing during a time when lupus activity is well controlled. Controlled lupus is defined as, ideally, stable disease while an individual is taking hydroxychloroquine, has not required treatment with steroids over 5 mg/day prednisone equivalent for the 6 months preceding conception, and with urine protein below 500 mg/24 hours.

The American College of Rheumatology 2020 Guideline for the Management of Reproductive Health in Rheumatic and Musculoskeletal Diseases provides useful guidance for management. Women with SLE contemplating pregnancy should have an anti-Ro (SSA) antibody checked along with screening for antiphospholipid antibodies. The presence of anti-Ro antibodies does not preclude pregnancy but isassociated with the development of neonatal lupus including congenital cardiac conduction abnormalities. Therefore, pregnant women who are anti-Ro positive require enhanced screening through fetal echocardiograms during the second trimester of pregnancy. All women with SLE should be treated with low-dose aspirin during pregnancy, but antiphospholipid antibody syndrome must be identified, as it requires anticoagulation throughout pregnancy.

One should frequently ascertain patient desires regarding childbearing because some medications for SLE are contraindicated during pregnancy. Every woman of childbearing age should be reassured that hydroxychloroquine is safe and associated with improved pregnancy outcomes among women with SLE. Hydroxychloroquine has not been associated with eye problems in neonates or children born to women who have taken this medication during pregnancy. Several medications used to treat lupus are known teratogens. Mycophenolate mofetil causes birth defects in about 25% of pregnancies exposed to this medication in utero, primarily abnormalities of the face and ears. Methotrexate is an abortifacient and has been reported to cause birth defects. Cyclophosphamide can also cause birth defects. While leflunomide has an FDA category X warning, it has not been found to increase the chance of birth defects in exposed pregnancies, but nonetheless, with this potential risk women should be counseled to not attempt conception while taking leflunomide and if they conceive while taking it, a cholestyramine wash-out should be undertaken. Importantly, women of childbearing age should all be encouraged to take a prenatal vitamin daily since the increased folic acid intake lowers the incidence of neural tube defects in the infant. Azathioprine is the preferred non-biologic DMARD to manage active lupus during pregnancy. There are insufficient data regarding the use of biologic DMARDs for SLE during pregnancy and decisions must be individualized in consultation with maternal fetal medicine experts and reproductive rheumatologists.

Women with SLE can have successful pregnancies and it is important to ascertain pregnancy desire at every visit, and then to partner with women to ensure that they have the safest pregnancies possible with SLE.

37. What are some patient-specific barriers to optimally managing SLE?

SLE frequently has its onset during the teen and early adult years, the time when most individuals complete their education and establish their careers. Being struck with a severe, multi-system illness during this time of life can derail patients' plans for developing financial security and independence. While many of these individuals can qualify (in the US) for state or federally sponsored health care coverage, people with SLE may also experience limited availability of reliable transportation to medical care. In addition, many hospitals lack rheumatologists on staff to perform inpatient consultation for individuals with life- or organ-threatening manifestations of lupus. Thus, patients may suffer from delayed diagnosis and potentially inadequate or inappropriate management of rare or severe lupus manifestations. The increasing incorporation of telemedicine into routine medical care and adoption of technology-enhanced learning through ECHO programs has the potential to improve access to care.

In the United States, cultural barriers to care exist. Care received in racially incongruent patient/provider pairs can be associated with worse outcomes than seen in same-race pairs, possibly related to lack of trust. Additionally, cultural and religious beliefs surrounding medications and illness can impact adherence with recommended therapy. Patients may be influenced by family or friends encouraging them to not take medications for SLE. It is important to ask about these beliefs that may impact care.

Limited health literacy and numeracy are significant barriers to care in lupus. Management of severe SLE is complicated, with patients often being prescribed several medications in simultaneously tapering and increasing doses. Managing variable doses of medications is challenging. It is very important to provide very clear instructions to individuals with SLE, and where possible, to involve allied health professionals to review medication doses, administration, and help manage side effects. Health literacy is important for patients to be able to partner in informed decisions about health care. There is much information and misinformation about SLE available to patients through the internet; distinguishing reliable medical information requires health care literacy.

Finally, medication adherence has been studied extensively in SLE. Adherence rates among individuals with SLE average from 30%– 50%. The challenges to adherence are myriad and include misunderstanding about prescribed dosages and administration, beliefs about the utility and potential side effects of medications, cultural influences as described above, navigating pharmacy locations and benefits (since biologic medications may be dispensed through specialty pharmacies remote from local pharmacies), and especially, medication costs. Though individual medications for SLE may be relatively affordable, when individuals are prescribed several medications to manage lupus (e.g. hydroxychloroquine, steroids, an immunosuppressive, anti-hypertensives, medications to manage side effects such as prophylactic antibiotics and bisphosphonates), costs and complexity add up quickly. These costs are incurred by individuals, who may not have financial stability due to the age at diagnosis as mentioned above and can combine with other factors to make care for lupus challenging.

38. What are the most frequent adverse effects of SLE therapy?

Perhaps the most concerning adverse effects of SLE therapy are related to the use of daily systemic glucocorticoids. It has been shown that much of the damage related to lupus is from the indiscriminate and frequent use of steroids as opposed to damage from the disease itself. Long-term use of corticosteroids to manage lupus and lupus flares can lead to obesity, hyperglycemia and diabetes mellitus, cataracts, central serous retinopathy, and osteopenia. Therefore, care should be taken to limit high dose steroids to short-term therapy for potentially life- or organ-threatening manifestations, and to use conventional or biologic DMARDs to manage more significant manifestations of SLE.

Hydroxychloroquine raises concern due to the association with retinal deposits of the medication that, if not detected, can lead to visual effects including blindness. However, more recent guidelines recommend limiting this dose to 5 mg/kg/day (max dose 400 mg/d) or less which is associated with a lower chance of ocular toxicity. In addition, current ocular toxicity monitoring includes highly sensitive tests such as OCT and MERG testing which can detect any abnormalities extremely early so appropriate action (e.g. stopping the medication or intensified monitoring) can be undertaken.

Many of the adverse effects of SLE therapy are related to their immunosuppressive nature. DMARDs that impact T-cell function can make individuals susceptible to viral infections such as reactivation of varicella in shingles or severe infections with COVID or influenza. Therefore, one should encourage annual influenza and COVID vaccination for all individuals with SLE taking immunosuppressive therapies, and prescription for Shingrix (inactivated varicella) vaccination series should be considered even for individuals under 50 due to the high risk of virus reactivation. HPV vaccine should be given to those at risk.

Other medications used to manage SLE can make individuals susceptible to different kinds of infections, depending on how they impact the immune system. Eculizumab, which inhibits complement, makes individuals susceptible to invasive infection with encapsulated organisms (e.g. meningococcemia).

Anti-B-cell therapies such as belimumab and rituximab (RTX) can make individuals more susceptible to infections (e.g. progressive multifocal leukoencephalopathy due to JC virus in patients on RTX).

Cyclophosphamide is an alkylating agent used to treat some severe manifestations of SLE such as central nervous system involvement and lupus nephritis. When used at higher doses (e.g. NIH protocol: $750 - 1000$ mg/m^2 IV monthly) one must be alert to the possibility of hemorrhagic cystitis caused by a metabolite (acrolein) of cyclophosphamide that is toxic to bladder cells. Mesna is used to prophylactically prevent hemorrhagic cystitis. In addition, cyclophosphamide may be titrated to achieve leukopenia and immunosuppression, which can leave treated individuals susceptible to severe and atypical infections including fungal infections. The EuroLupus protocol (500 mg IV every 2 weeks x 6 doses) is less likely to cause these problems.

39. What lifestyle modifications can help in the management of SLE?

Patients often ask what they can do besides taking medications to help manage SLE. Rashes are a major SLE manifestation. These rashes are frequently photosensitive, meaning they arise and worsen with exposure to UV light. Most people do not use photoprotection daily, and when they do, they often apply inadequate amounts. Patients should be encouraged to apply sunscreen of at least SPF 30 every single day, even in winter and even if they do not plan to venture outdoors, as most windows do not fully block UV light. One study did demonstrate decreased flares with sunscreen containing avobenzone and padimate O. Additionally, wearing hats and sun-protective clothing, especially those labeled with SPF protection or "sun sleeves" kept in the car, can prove useful and easy to use correctly. Vitamin D supplementation is important to maintain 25OH vitamin D levels ≥30-40 ng/mL.

Many individuals with SLE experience chronic pain, fatigue, and other troublesome somatic symptoms along with sleep disturbance, cognitive difficulties and "brain fog." Such symptoms can be classified as Type 2 lupus (see question #10), and many individuals with SLE additionally meet diagnostic criteria for fibromyalgia syndrome. These symptoms, which can be present outside of detectable physical examination, laboratory or other signs of active inflammation, are generally treated using the same principles employed to manage chronic somatic symptoms. Such interventions include gradual adoption of an exercise program, attention to sleep hygiene and other healthful living behaviors. Medications shown to improve fibromyalgia symptoms can be directed toward these symptoms as well, including selective norepinephrine reuptake inhibitors (SNRIs). Additionally, cognitive behavioral therapy (CBT) and other non-pharmacologic interventions can assist individuals in learning to self-manage troublesome symptoms and the psychological impact of living with an unpredictable and frequently severe disease.

Finally, individuals with SLE are at increased risk (10x) for developing cardiovascular disease due to ongoing inflammation and some of the comorbid conditions that can come with long-term use of systemic steroids (e.g. obesity, diabetes). Therefore, adopting healthy lifestyle modifications such as following a heart-healthy diet, engaging in regular cardiovascular exercise, and smoking cessation are all important for individuals with SLE. Patients with hyperlipidemia and/or hypertension (goal <120–130/80) who do not respond to lifestyle modifications should receive appropriate therapy with medications.

40. What is the prognosis for SLE patients?

With improvement in therapy, the 5-year survival rate is ≥90% and 10-year is ≥85%–90% in developed countries. However, the overall standardized mortality ratio remains 2–5x higher than a healthy age-matched population. Younger age, non-white race, male sex, smoking, antiphospholipid antibodies, and inability to achieve lupus low disease activity as well as several social determinants are associated with higher mortality. Previous studies reported that SLE patients were more likely to die of disease activity or infection within the first 5 years of disease onset and die of atherosclerotic disease and malignancy after 5 years. With better use of immunosuppressive therapies and faster tapering of glucocorticoids, infection causes fewer deaths than in the past. The most common causes of death and morbidity are:

- **Active SLE:** accounts for 20%–35% of deaths particularly during the first 5 years of disease. Lupus nephritis, NPSLE, vasculitis, and pneumonitis are the most lethal.
- **Infection:** accounts for 10%–20% of all deaths. All microbial infections are increased. For each increase of prednisone by 10mg/d, the risk of infection increases up to 11-fold.
- **Cardiovascular disease:** accounts for 25%–40% of deaths and is the most common cause of death in SLE patients in Western countries. An increased risk of cardiovascular events (coronary artery, cerebrovascular, peripheral vascular disease) occurs throughout the disease course.
- **Malignancy:** accounts for 10%–30% of deaths and occur throughout the disease course. Hematologic malignancies [especially non-Hodgkin's lymphoma (SIR 3–5)] and possibly HPV-associated cervical cancer are particularly increased possibly due to use of immunosuppressive medications. Squamous cell skin cancer can arise in discoid lesions.

SLE and its therapy causes multiple morbidities. Up to 30%–50% will develop organ damage during the first 5 years with 10%–20% developing end-stage renal disease during their disease course. Neuropsychiatric deficits, cardiovascular disease, and disfiguring skin lesions are also common. Glucocorticoids contribute to osteoporosis even at low doses. Osteonecrosis occurs in up to 40%–50% of patients. Prednisone at doses ≥20 mg/d for over a month puts patients at increased risk for osteonecrosis.

41. Can glucocorticoids or immunosuppressive medications be tapered or stopped in SLE patients?

This is controversial. However, there are some unofficial guidelines to consider:

- Patients with severe life or organ-threatening manifestations at baseline or during their disease course are more likely to flare with stopping glucocorticoids or immuno-suppressive medications.
- Patients who reach complete clinical and serologic remission on therapy are less likely to flare than patients who only reach lupus low disease activity state (LLDAS). Notably, only 10% of SLE patients ever achieve complete remission.
  - Patients should be in remission or LLDAS on prednisone 5 mg/d (and stable immunosuppressives) for 24 months if history of severe disease (e.g. nephritis, NPSLE) or 12 months if non-severe disease (e.g. arthritis, rash) before attempting to taper off prednisone while continuing immunosuppressives and hydroxychloroquine. Prednisone taper from 5 mg/d to off is over 6 and preferably 12 months.
  - Patients should remain in remission or LLDAS off prednisone for 12 months (hx non-severe SLE) to 24 months (hx severe SLE) before attempting to taper off any immunosuppressives. Hydroxychloroquine should be continued.
  - Patients need close follow-up/monitoring during tapering and resume medications if signs of flare.
- Hydroxychloroquine should not be stopped (unless drug toxicity develops) to lessen chance of an SLE flare when tapering other medications.
  - Since hydroxychloroquine retinal toxicity is a concern with prolonged use (especially if ≥ 10 years of use and/or ≥ 100 grams total cumulative dose) many physicians lower maintenance dose (e.g. 400 mg qd to 200 mg qd).
- Shared decision making: risk of flare with medication tapering/discontinuation should be discussed with patient.

BIBLIOGRAPHY

Alharbi S. Gastrointestinal manifestations in patients with systemic lupus erythematosus. *Open Access Rheumatol.* 2022;14:243–253.

Aringer M, Costenbader KH, Daikh DI, et al. 2019 EULAR/ACR classification criteria for systemic lupus erythematosus. *Arthritis Rheumatol.* 2019;71(9):1400–1412.

Bengtsson AA, Ronnblom L. Systemic lupus erythematosus: still a challenge for physicians. *J Int Med.* 2017;281:52–64.

Bertsias GK, Tektonidou M, Amoura Z, et al. Joint European League Against Rheumatism and European Renal Association-European Dialysis and Transplant Association (EULAR/ERA-EDTA) recommendations for the management of adult and paediatric lupus nephritis. *Ann Rheum Di.* 2012;71:1771–1782.

Carter EE, Barr SG, Clarke AE. The global burden of SLE: prevalence, health disparities, and socioeconomic impact. *Nature Rev.* 2016;12:605–620.

Cho J, Shen L, Huq M, et al. Impact of low disease activity, remission, and complete remission on flares following tapering of corticosteroids and immunosuppressive therapy in patients with SLE: a multinational, prospective cohort study. *Lancer Rheumatol.* 2023;5:584–593.

Collins E, Gilkeson G. Hematopoetic and mesenchymal stem cell transplantation in the treatment of refractory systemic lupus erythematosus–where are we now? *Clin Immunol.* 2013;148:328–334.

Crow MK. Etiology and pathogenesis of SLE. In: Firestein GS, Budd RC, Gabriel SE et al., eds. *Kelley's Textbook of Rheumatology.* 11th ed. Philadelphia, PA: Elsevier; 2021:1398–1412.

Dima A, Jurcut C, Chasset F, et al. Hydroxychloroquine in systemic lupus erythematosus: overview of current knowledge. *Ther Adv Musculoskelet Dis.* 2022;14. 1759720 × 211073001.

Fanouriakis A, Kostopoulou M, Andersen J, et al. EULAR recommendations for the management of systemic lupus erythematosus: 2023 update. *Ann Rheumatic Dis.* 2024;83:15–29.

Golder V, Hoi A. Systemic lupus erythematosus: an update. *Med J Austr.* 2017;206:215–220.

Grossman JM. Lupus arthritis. *Best Pract Res Clin Rheumatol.* 2009;23:495–506.

Hanly JG, Su L, Urowitz MB, et al. A longitudinal analysis of outcomes of lupus nephritis in an international inception cohort using a multistate model approach. *Arthritis Rheumatol.* 2016;68:1932–1944.

Hanly JG, Urowitz MB, Gordon C, et al. Neuropsychiatric events in systemic lupus erythematosus: a longitudinal analysis of outcomes in an international inception cohort using a multistate model approach. *Ann Rheum Dis.* 2020;79:356–362.

Hepburn AL, Narat S, Mason JC. The management of peripheral blood cytopenias in systemic lupus erythematosus. *Rheumatology (Oxford).* 2010;49:2243–2254.

Kidney Disease: Improving Global Outcomes (KDIGO) Lupus Nephritis Work Group. KDIGO 2024 clinical practice guideline for the management of lupus nephritis. *Kidney Int.* 2024;105:S1–S69.

Lionaki S, Skalioti C, Boletis JN. Kidney transplantation in patients with systemic lupus erythematosus. *World J Transplant.* 2014;4:176–182.

Mackensen A, Muller F, Mougiakakos D, et al. Anti-CD19 CAR T cell therapy for refractory systemic lupus erythematosus. *Nature Med.* 2022;28:2124–3132.

Mahieu MA, Strand V, Simon LS, et al. A critical review of clinical trials in systemic lupus erythematosus. *Lupus.* 2016;25:1122–1140.

Petri M, Kim MY, Kalunian KC, et al. Combined oral contraceptives in women with systemic lupus erythematosus. *N Engl J Med.* 2005;353:2550–2558.

Pisetsky DS, Clowse MEB, Criscione-Schreiber LG, et al. A novel system to categorize the symptoms of systemic erythematosus. *Arthritis Care Res.* 2019;71(6):735–741.

Rovin BH, Ayoub IM, Chan TM, et al. Executive summary of the KDIGO 2024 clinical practice guideline for the management of lupus nephritis. *Kidney Int.* 2024;105:31–34.

Sun K, Eudy AM, Criscione-Schreiber LG, et al. Racial disparities in medication adherence between African American and Caucasian patients with systemic lupus erythematosus and their associated factors. *ACR Open Rheumatol.* 2020;2(7):430–437.

Tektonidou MG, Lewandowski LB, Hu J, et al. Survival in adults and children with systemic lupus erythematosus. *Ann Rheum Dis.* 2017;76:2009–2016.

Tsang-A-Sjoe MWP, Bultink IEM. Systemic lupus erythematosus: a review of synthetic drugs. *Expert Opin Pharmacother.* 2015;16:2793–2806.

Tseng CE, Buyon JP, Kim M, et al. The effect of moderate-dose corticosteroids in preventing severe flares in patients with serologically active, but clinically stable, systemic lupus erythematosus: findings of a prospective, randomized, double-blind, placebo-controlled trial. *Arthritis Rheum.* 2006;54:3623–3632.

Tsokos GC, Lo MS, Costa Reis P, Sullivan KE. New insights into the immunopathogenesis of systemic lupus erythematosus. *Nat Rev Rheumatol.* 2016;12:716–730.

Wallace DJ, Hahn BH, eds. *Dubois' Lupus Erythematosus.and Related Syndromes.* 10th ed. Philadelphia, PA: Elsevier; 2024.

Weening JJ, D'Agati VD, Schwartz MM, et al. Renal Pathology Society Working Group on the Classification of Lupus, N. The classification of glomerulonephritis in systemic lupus erythematosus revisited. *Kidney Int.* 2004;65:521–530.

Yu F, Haas M, Glassock R, Zhao MH. Redefining lupus nephritis: clinical implications of pathophysiologic subtypes. *Nat Rev Nephrol.* 2017;13:483–495.

Yurkovich M, Vostretsova K, Chen W, Avina-Subeta J. Overall and cause specific mortality in patients with systemic lupus erythematosus: a meta-analysis of observational studies. *Arthritis Care Res.* 2014;66:608–616.

Further Reading

www.lupus.org.

www.lupuspregnancy.

CHAPTER 16

Drug-induced Lupus Erythematosus

Christopher C. Striebich, MD, PhD

1. What is DILE and who gets it?

DILE is a lupus-like illness that occurs in some individuals after exposure to a causative drug for a few weeks to more than a year. There are over 100 drugs with various chemical structures from more than 10 drug categories that have been implicated in causing DILE.

Unlike idiopathic systemic lupus erythematosus (SLE), systemic DILE occurs more commonly in Caucasians and older individuals (>age 50 years), reflecting the group of patients most likely to take these medications. It affects both males and females equally. Exceptions to this are DILE caused by minocycline and terbinafine that occurs mostly in young women and drug-induced SCLE that occurs mostly in older women. Although uncommon, DILE has been reported in children.

2. Describe the classification of DILE.

Similar to idiopathic SLE, DILE can be classified into three major forms:

- **Systemic DILE:** patients present with arthralgia, myalgia, serositis, and constitutional symptoms after taking a drug for at least a month. Overall symptoms tend to be less severe than idiopathic SLE. Patients typically have a positive antinuclear antibody (ANA) but may only have one other clinical criterion for lupus. It affects both males and females equally.
- **Drug-induced SCLE:** predominant skin involvement (papulosquamous more than annular) similar to idiopathic SCLE. Usually with photosensitivity and can be associated with other cutaneous lesions (e.g., vasculitis and bullous lesions). It affects older females predominantly. It usually occurs 1 to 5 months after initiating therapy with the offending medication. Drug-induced SCLE should be suspected in anyone who develops SCLE after the age of 50 years.
- **Chronic cutaneous DILE:** discoid lupus skin lesions. This is a rare form of DILE and usually occurs in patients treated with fluorouracil compounds.

3. Name 10 drugs definitely associated with ANA production and manifestations of systemic DILE. What is the risk of developing DILE with each?

See Table 16.1.

4. What are the clinical manifestations of systemic DILE, and how do they differ from those of idiopathic SLE?

Patients with systemic DILE can develop a variety of signs and symptoms that typically come on abruptly. Similar to SLE, these include fever and/or other constitutional symptoms (50%), arthritis/arthralgias (80–95%), myalgias, serositis (50% with procainamide, 25% with quinidine, unusual with others), hepatomegaly (5–25%), and erythematous papular rashes (20%). Discoid lesions and malar erythema (2%) are uncommon. Some patients may develop pulmonary infiltrates (e.g., procainamide). More severe manifestations of SLE, such as cytopenias, nephritis,

TABLE 16.1 Drugs Definitely Associated With ANA Production and Manifestations of Systemic DILE

HIGH (>5%)	MODERATE	LOW (<1–2%)
Procainamide (15–20%)	Quinidine	Isoniazid
Hydralazine (5–10%)		Methyldopa
		Chlorpromazine
		Minocycline (5/10,000 patients)
		Anti-tumor necrosis factor-α agents (2/1000 patients)
		D-penicillamine
		Interferon-α

and central nervous system (CNS) involvement, are very rare in DILE, as is the presence of anti-double-stranded DNA (anti-dsDNA) antibodies and hypocomplementemia. One exception is that anti-tumor necrosis factor (TNF) agents and interferon-α (IFNα) can induce anti-dsDNA antibodies and hypocomplementemia in patients who develop systemic DILE caused by these medications.

5. **List other drugs for which there is more than anecdotal evidence for causing DILE.**
   Various drugs have been associated with causing DILE and can be categorized as follows:
   - **Definite:** procainamide, hydralazine, quinidine, isoniazid, minocycline, anti-TNFα agents, IFNα, D-penicillamine, methyldopa, and chlorpromazine. Some lists also include carbamazepine, levodopa, and practolol which have a low risk of causing DILE.
   - **Probable:** anticonvulsants (mephenytoin, phenytoin, carbamazepine, ethosuximide), antithyroid drugs [propylthiouracil (PTU), methimazole], beta-adrenergic blocking agents, sulfasalazine, antimicrobials (sulfonamides, nitrofurantoin), lithium, captopril, docetaxel, hydrochlorothiazide, glyburide, amiodarone, levodopa, terbinafine, ticlopidine, immune checkpoint inhibitors, and IFNγ. DILE has also been reported in patients receiving rifampin or rifabutin for treatment of a mycobacterial infection, particularly if they also are receiving clarithromycin or ciprofloxacin. This suggests that altered metabolism of rifampin/rifabutin by these medications induced the DILE.
   - **Possible:** statins, valproate, gemfibrozil, griseofulvin, lamotrigine, valproate, others.
   - There are over 40 other drugs that have been reported to cause DILE or SCLE in isolated case reports.

6. **How do the clinical manifestations of procainamide-induced lupus differ from those of hydralazine-induced lupus?**
   Patients with DILE caused by procainamide or hydralazine commonly have arthralgias/arthritis, myalgias, and fever but rarely manifest severe lupus nephritis or CNS involvement. Patients with procainamide-induced disease are more likely to have pleuritis and/or pericarditis, whereas patients with hydralazine-induced disease are more likely to have rashes.

7. **Which autoantibodies are most commonly seen in DILE? How do these compare with the autoantibodies seen in idiopathic SLE?**
   - **ANA:** as in SLE, almost all patients with DILE will have a positive ANA; however, the spectrum of ANAs in DILE is much more limited than that seen in SLE. Notably, offending drugs are more likely to cause a positive ANA than symptomatic DILE. For example, procainamide causes a positive ANA in 90% of patients on the drug for over 2 years, but only 20% develop DILE.
   - **Antihistone antibodies:** these are the most common autoantibodies in DILE but frequency and specificity vary between drugs. Most patients (95%) with symptomatic drug-induced disease due to procainamide, hydralazine, chlorpromazine, and quinidine demonstrate elevated levels of IgG antihistone antibodies. Alternatively, patients who develop DILE due to minocycline, PTU, TNFα antagonists, and statins have antihistone antibodies in fewer than

20% (minocycline) to 60% (TNFα antagonists) of patients. Note that antibodies to histones are not specific to DILE and are present in 50% to 80% of patients with idiopathic SLE.

- **Other autoantibodies against nuclear antigens:** antibodies to dsDNA are highly specific for idiopathic SLE and rarely found in DILE, with the exception of DILE due to anti-TNFα agents or IFNα. Antibodies to Sm, RNP, Ro/SS-A, and La/SS-B are common in idiopathic SLE but are unusual or do not persist in DILE. Anti-Ro/SS-A antibodies are present in over 80% of patients with drug-induced SCLE lesions.
- **Antiphospholipid antibodies:** can be seen in both systemic DILE and idiopathic SLE. In systemic DILE, they occur most commonly with three drugs (chlorpromazine, procainamide, and quinidine), tend to be IgM, and are rarely associated with thrombosis.

8. Is testing for antihistone antibodies clinically useful to distinguish systemic DILE from idiopathic SLE in a patient taking either procainamide or hydralazine?

Testing for antihistone antibodies can occasionally be useful in situations in which the diagnosis of DILE is being considered. As discussed, nearly all patients (95%) with symptomatic procainamide- or hydralazine-induced lupus demonstrate elevated serum levels of IgG antihistone antibodies. Thus, a negative test would make this diagnosis unlikely. However, a positive test for antihistone antibodies has much less diagnostic value because 50% to 80% of patients with active idiopathic SLE also have a positive test. Furthermore, some patients taking either procainamide or hydralazine will have a positive test but not have symptoms of a lupus-like disease. Asymptomatic patients tend to have IgM and not IgG antihistone antibodies. In most cases in which DILE is being considered, performing an ANA test and if positive (usually in a homogenous pattern), taking the patient off the offending agent may be the most cost-effective approach to the situation.

9. Contrast the type of antihistone antibodies found in systemic DILE versus idiopathic SLE.

In certain specialized research laboratories, the specificity of antihistone antibodies for individual histones (i.e., H1, H2A, H2B, H3, and H4), histone complexes, or intrahistone epitopes can be distinguished. Overall, antihistone antibodies in DILE tend to be much more focused on certain histone complexes than those in idiopathic SLE. For example, in procainamide-induced lupus (and most other causes of DILE), the onset of symptomatic disease has been associated with the production of IgG antibodies to the H2A–H2B–DNA complex. Although this complex is also a target in about 15% of patients with SLE, autoantibodies in idiopathic SLE are frequently directed to other individual histones (H1 and H2B) and other histone complexes. In hydralazine-induced disease, the major target is the H3–H4 complex. In contrast to procainamide-induced lupus and SLE, autoantibodies induced by hydralazine appear to be directed more to determinants hidden within the chromatin rather than exposed on the surface.

10. Are antineutrophil cytoplasmic antibodies (ANCAs) ever seen in systemic DILE?

Up to 80% to 85% of patients with minocycline-induced lupus can have a positive perinuclear ANCA (pANCA) with or without specificity for myeloperoxidase (anti-MPO). PTU and hydralazine can both cause DILE with an associated pANCA. However, both PTU and hydralazine therapy can also cause a positive pANCA usually with anti-MPO specificity that is associated with a more severe pauci-immune vasculitis with necrotizing glomerulonephritis and possible pulmonary involvement (see Chapter 28: Antineutrophil Cytoplasmic Antibody-Associated Vasculitis). Notably, 15% to 20% of idiopathic SLE patients can have a positive ANCA.

11. What percentage of patients taking procainamide, hydralazine, isoniazid, or anti-TNFα therapy develop a positive ANA? What percentage of patients develop systemic DILE?

Nearly 75% of patients receiving procainamide therapy will develop a positive ANA test within the first year of treatment, and over 90% develop a positive ANA by 2 years, yet only 20% develop DILE. In contrast, 15% to 50% of patients taking hydralazine will demonstrate a positive test after a year of drug therapy with 5% to 10% developing DILE, especially if they are slow acetylators. Up to 20% of patients on isoniazid develop a positive ANA, but few develop symptoms of DILE. Finally, between 13% and 83% of patients on anti-TNFα therapy develop a positive ANA (most commonly infliximab), but few (<1%) develop DILE. Therefore, it is important to note that many more patients will demonstrate a positive ANA test than develop DILE, and the presence of a positive ANA test without symptoms is not a valid reason for stopping the medication.

12. What are the characteristic clinical features of minocycline-induced lupus?

There have been multiple cases of DILE affecting young individuals (females > males, ages 14 to 31 years) after an average of 30 months (range, 6–72) of minocycline use for acne in doses of 50 to 200 mg/day. All patients have arthritis/arthralgias and most have a positive ANA (92%). Fever (38%), rash (20% to 30%), pleuritis/pneumonitis (10%), hepatitis (50% with elevated liver-associated enzymes), and anticardiolipin antibodies (33%) can be seen. Interestingly, only 10% to 15% have antihistone antibodies, but 67% to 85% have a positive pANCA with or without anti-MPO specificity.

13. Therapeutic use of IFNα and inhibitors of anti-TNFα have been associated with the development of SLE. How are these cases similar to classic DILE and how do they differ?

As in other causes of DILE, autoimmunity due to the use of biologic therapies is more likely to cause the formation of lupus-associated autoantibodies than systemic DILE. In contrast to classic DILE, the formation of anti-dsDNA antibodies is commonly seen. Patients taking IFNα are more likely to develop typical lupus manifestations such as oral ulcers, alopecia, and nephritis and frequently require corticosteroids or other lupus therapies to treat the disease. Anti-TNF agents (most commonly infliximab or etanercept) cause ANAs in 13% to 83% of patients and anti-DNA antibodies in 3% to 32% of patients, but symptomatic DILE occurs in only 2 out of 1000 patients and resolves within 5 half-lives of stopping the drug. Patients with TNFα antagonist-induced lupus syndrome typically have arthralgias but are more likely to have rash, hematologic abnormalities (leukopenia, thrombocytopenia), anti-dsDNA antibodies, and hypocomplementemia and less likely to have antihistone antibodies (60%) than most other medications causing systemic DILE.

14. What drugs have been associated with causing drug-induced SCLE?

Hydrochlorothiazide, calcium channel blockers (e.g., diltiazem), angiotensin-converting enzyme inhibitors, proton pump inhibitors (PPI), terbinafine, anti-TNFα agents, statins, leflunomide, diclofenac, bupropion, acebutolol, and various agents to treat malignancies (e.g., docetaxel, hydroxyurea, anti-PD-1 and anti-PD-L1 inhibitors, and others) are among the drugs that have been reported to cause SCLE. In addition to having a positive ANA, these patients frequently (80%) also have a positive anti-SSA (Ro) antibody, and thus more closely resemble idiopathic SCLE. However, the cutaneous eruption in drug-induced SCLE is more widespread in distribution and may be bullous or vasculitic. In addition, the anti-SSA(Ro) antibody will disappear in 75% of patients with drug-induced SCLE after the drug is stopped and the rash is resolved. With the widespread use of many of these medications, drug-induced SCLE is becoming increasingly common and should be considered in any patient taking one of these medications, *particularly if they develop SCLE after the age of 50 years.*

15. What drugs have been associated with causing chronic cutaneous DILE?

Chronic cutaneous DILE presenting with discoid lesions is very rare. It is usually triggered by fluorouracil compounds or their modern derivatives such as capecitabine.

16. Do similar genetic factors predispose patients to develop DILE and SLE?

The genetic risk factors in DILE and idiopathic SLE appear to be quite separate. The major risk for procainamide- or hydralazine-induced lupus appears to be acetylator phenotype. Metabolism of these drugs involves the hepatic enzyme N-acetyl transferase, which catalyzes the acetylation of amine or hydrazine groups. The rate at which this reaction takes place is under genetic control. Approximately 50% of the US white population are fast acetylators, with the rest being slow acetylators. The slow acetylators, when treated with procainamide or hydralazine, develop ANAs earlier and at higher titers and are more likely to develop symptomatic disease than fast acetylators. Despite its chemical similarity to procainamide and its similar drug action, N-acetylprocainamide has not been associated with drug-induced ANA production or DILE.

In idiopathic SLE, acetylator phenotype does not appear to be involved in genetic susceptibility. Instead, human leukocyte antigen (HLA) class II genes, complement deficiencies, and multiple other genes are important in the complex genetic basis of SLE (see Chapter 15: Systemic Lupus Erythematosus). HLA-DR4 and null gene for C4 may contribute to the risk of developing hydralazine-induced DILE.

17. What hypotheses have been proposed for pathogenetic mechanisms causing DILE?

- **Genetic:** slow acetylator status (see Question #16).
- **Epigenetic:** procainamide and hydralazine can decrease T-cell DNA methylation leading to overexpression of LFA-1 that induces autoreactivity.
- **Adaptive immunity:** drug-induced changes in T-cell signaling and function.
  - Small molecule drugs can act as haptens or agonists for drug-specific T cells.
- **Innate immunity:** activated neutrophils
  - Procainamide is oxidized by activated neutrophils resulting in production of the toxic metabolite, procainamide hydroxylamine, which can cause direct cytotoxicity. Several other drugs causing DILE can also undergo biotransformation similar to procainamide resulting in the generation of toxic metabolites.
  - Activated neutrophils can release MPO and reactive oxygen species, which can cause direct cytotoxicity.
  - Some drugs causing DILE can trigger neutrophil extracellular trap (NET) formation leading to nuclear autoantigen exposure that can stimulate autoreactive T and B cells.

18. Is the use of drugs (e.g., procainamide) associated with DILE contraindicated in patients with SLE? Can they exacerbate disease activity?

The population at risk for developing systemic DILE is very different compared with that developing idiopathic SLE. There is no evidence that drugs capable of causing systemic DILE will change or worsen disease activity in a patient with idiopathic SLE. However, if an alternative drug is available, it may be prudent to use it so that there would not be any confusion if the SLE patient has a disease flare in the future. This is especially true for minocycline, which should be avoided if possible. Additionally, in patients with SCLE who get worsening rash, it is advisable to eliminate medications (e.g., PPI) that can cause drug-induced SCLE, if at all possible.

19. What is the treatment of DILE?

The first and most important intervention is to discontinue the offending drug. Nonsteroidal anti-inflammatory drugs will often help control the symptoms such as arthralgias, as the disease gradually resolves after the drug is stopped. Patients with more severe signs and symptoms, especially those with pericarditis or pleuritis, often require a short course of corticosteroids to control their disease. In more prolonged cases, antimalarials can be used. More toxic agents, such as azathioprine or cyclophosphamide, are almost never required in the treatment of DILE; however, they may be needed in drug-induced ANCA vasculitis. Overall, the prognosis of DILE is good and symptoms resolve with stopping the offending drug. Notably, the positive ANA may persist for a prolonged time (>1 year) even after symptoms resolve.

BIBLIOGRAPHY

Arnaud L, Mertz P, Gavand PE, et al. Drug-induced systemic lupus: revisiting the ever-changing spectrum of the disease using the WHO pharmacovigilance database. *Ann Rheum Dis.* 2019;78:504–508.

Bataille P, Lebrun-Vignes B, Tubach F, et al. Proton pump inhibitors associated with drug-induced lupus erythematosus. *JAMA Dermatol.* 2022;158:1208–1210.

Dlott JS, Roubey RA. Drug-induced lupus anticoagulant and antiphospholipid antibodies. *Curr Rheumatol Rep.* 2012;14:71–78.

Laurinaviciene R, Sandholdt LH, Bygum A. Drug-induced cutaneous lupus erythematosus: 88 new cases. *Eur J Dermatol.* 2017;27:28–33.

Michaelis TC, Sontheimer RD, Lowe GC. An update in drug-induced subacute cutaneous lupus erythematosus. *Dermatol Online J.* 2017;23:1–10.

Murphy G. Drug-induced lupus erythematosus. In: Wallace DJ, Hahn BH, Askanase A et al, eds. *Dubois' Lupus Erythematosus and Related Syndromes.* 10th ed. Philadelphia, PA: Elsevier; 2025:407–412.

Rubin R. Drug-induced lupus. *Expert Opin Drug Saf.* 2015;14:361–378.

Sawalha AH. Editorial: the innate and adaptive immune response are both involved in drug-induced autoimmunity. *Arthritis Rheumatol.* 2018;70:330–333.

Shovman O, Tamar S, Amital H, et al. Diverse patterns of anti-TNF-α-induced lupus: case series and review of the literature. *Clin Rheumatol.* 2018;37:563–568.

Vaglio A, Grayson PC, Fenaroli P, et al. Drug-induced lupus: traditional and new concepts. *Autoimmun Rev.* 2018;17:912–918.

FURTHER READING

https://medlineplus.gov/ency/article/000446.htm.
https://resources.lupus.org/entry/about-drug-induced-lupus.

Systemic Sclerosis

Melissa Griffith, MD

1. What is SSc?

SSc, commonly referred to as scleroderma, is a rare and potentially devastating systemic auto-immune disease characterized by vasculopathy and organ fibrosis. Almost all patients with scleroderma have skin thickening ("sclero" = thick, "derma" = skin), Raynaud phenomenon, and esophageal reflux or dysmotility. ILD and pulmonary arterial hypertension are the leading causes of scleroderma-related death.

2. Describe the classification scheme of scleroderma.

It is crucial to distinguish the localized forms of scleroderma (see Chapter 18: Scleroderma Mimics) from the generalized (systemic) forms (Fig. 17.1).

- **Localized scleroderma:** dermal fibrosis without internal organ involvement. The two types of localized scleroderma are:
  1. **Morphea:** single or multiple plaques, commonly on the trunk.
  2. **Linear scleroderma:** bands of skin thickening commonly located on the legs or arms, but sometimes on the face (*en coup de sabre*) that typically follow a linear path.
- **Generalized scleroderma = SSc.**
  1. **Limited cutaneous SSc (lcSSc, limited scleroderma):** Patients with lcSSc have skin thickening limited to the neck, face, or distal to the elbows and knees. Patients with lcSSc may not come to clinical attention until many years after symptom onset. Patients often describe long-standing Raynaud phenomenon and gastroesophageal reflux disease (GERD) and may have telangiectasia, skin calcifications (calcinosis), and digital edema or sclerodactyly as their only skin manifestations. Among those with lcSSc, the presence of **anti-Scl-70 (anti-topoisomerase) antibody** is associated with a high risk for the development of progressive ILD, and the presence of **anticentromere antibody (ACA)** carries the highest risk for PAH. Renal crisis is exceedingly rare in lcSSc. Limited scleroderma is not "mild" scleroderma, as the "limited" descriptor refers only to limited skin involvement and not internal organ manifestations. Patients with lcSSc still have life-threatening disease, often driven by pulmonary, cardiac, or gastrointestinal (GI) involvement (Fig. 17.2).
  2. **Diffuse scleroderma (dcSSc):** Patients with dcSSc have skin thickening that extends proximal to the elbows or knees or with truncal involvement. In contrast to lcSSc, patients with dcSSc usually present relatively abruptly. Common presenting symptoms include puffy hands, Raynaud phenomenon, arthritis, carpal tunnel symptoms (due to surrounding edema or inflammation), fatigue, and rapidly progressive skin thickening. These patients often have the onset of Raynaud phenomenon within a year of developing SSc. Patients with dcSSc are at a higher risk for progressive ILD and can also develop PAH.

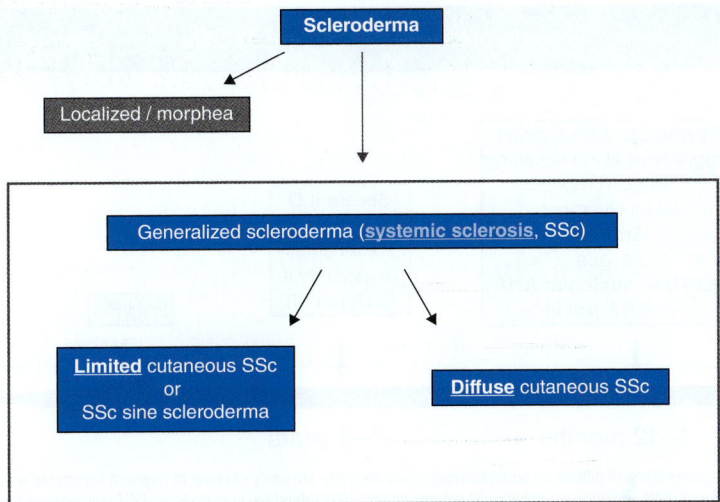

Fig. 17.1 Classification scheme of scleroderma.

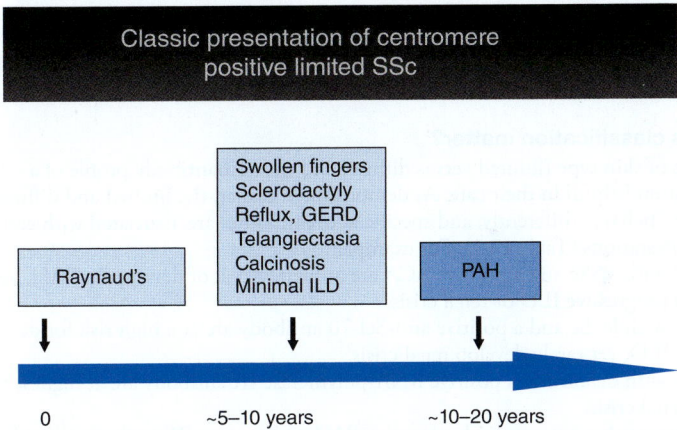

Fig. 17.2 *GERD*, gastroesophageal reflux disease; *ILD*, interstitial lung disease; *PAH*, pulmonary arterial hypertension; *SSc*, systemic sclerosis.

Patients with diffuse skin thickening and a positive **RNA polymerase III antibody** are at highest risk of developing SRC (Fig. 17.3).

3. **Systemic sclerosis sine scleroderma (ssSSc):** Patients with internal manifestations of SSc *along with a scleroderma-specific antibody* (such as a nucleolar-pattern antinuclear antibody [ANA], ACA, anti-Scl-70 antibody, or anti-RNA polymerase III antibody), but without evidence of skin thickening, are described as having ssSSc. Some experts consider this a subset of lcSSc, given that some patients early in the disease course may develop subsequent cutaneous involvement. Nonetheless, a distinct population will lack cutaneous features over time and fall within this category of SSc. Examples of ssSSc include:
   - Raynaud phenomenon, digital edema, ILD, and a positive anti-Scl-70 antibody
   - Raynaud phenomenon, GERD, PAH, and a positive ACA

3. What is CREST?

CREST refers to patients with SSc who have clinical manifestations of **c**alcinosis, **R**aynaud phenomenon, **e**sophageal dysmotility, **s**clerodactyly, and **t**elangiectasia. The term is somewhat outdated and often misleading as it may give the wrong impression that it is distinct from SSc or represents a mutually exclusive category of SSc (patients with lcSSc, and to a lesser degree dcSSc,

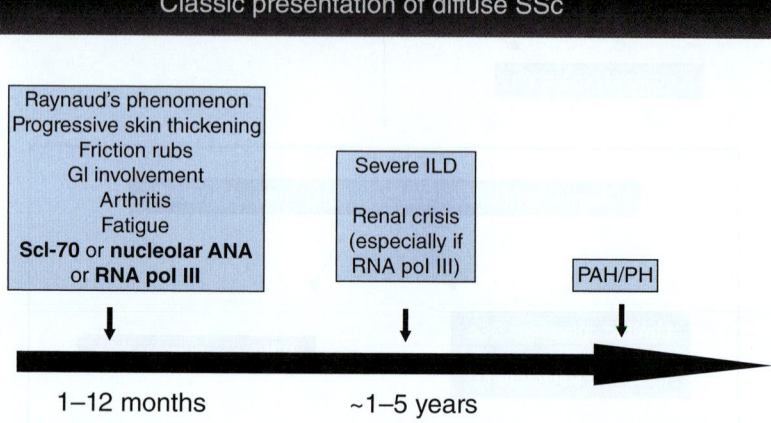

Fig. 17.3 Classic presentation of diffuse systemic sclerosis. Note the close proximity of onset of Raynaud symptoms with skin thickening and/or finger puffiness. *ANA*, antinuclear antibody; *GI*, gastrointestinal; *ILD*, interstitial lung disease; *PAH*, pulmonary arterial hypertension; *PH*, pulmonary hypertension.

can both have some or all of these clinical manifestations). It is preferable to categorize patients with SSc into one of three subgroups (lcSSc, dcSSc, ssSSc), with clear documentation of clinical manifestations and autoantibody status.

4. Why does classification matter?

Knowledge of skin type (limited versus diffuse) and the autoantibody profile of a scleroderma patient is often helpful in their care. As demonstrated earlier, the limited and diffuse scleroderma phenotypes "behave" differently, and specific autoantibodies are associated with certain internal organ manifestations (Table 17.1). For example:

- Patients with lcSSc and a positive ACA are at highest risk of developing PAH, yet rarely develop progressive ILD or renal crisis.
- Patients with lcSSc and a positive anti-Scl-70 antibody are at a high risk for developing progressive ILD, yet rarely develop renal crisis.
- Patients with dcSSc and a positive RNA-polymerase III antibody are at highest risk of developing renal crisis.
- Data suggest that patients with a positive RNA polymerase III antibody are at higher risk for malignancy, highlighting the importance of age-appropriate cancer screening in SSc patients with this autoantibody.

TABLE 17.1 Predominant Features Associated With SSc-Specific Autoantibodies

	ACA[a]	TH/TO	U1-RNP (MCTD)	PMSCL	U3-RNP (FIBRILLARIN)	SCL-70 (TOPOISOMERASE I)	RNA POL III[b]
SSc subset (% pts)	Limited (50–90%)	Limited (4–16%)	Limited (100% MCTD)	Limited (3%)	Diffuse (7%)	Diffuse (20–30%)	Diffuse (25%)
Lungs	PAH	ILD + PAH	PAH ILD	ILD Myositis	ILD + PAH	ILD	-
Kidneys	-	-	-	-	SRC	SRC	SRC

[a]ACA antibody positive patients should be screened for primary biliary cirrhosis with antimitochondrial antibody test and LFTs
[b]RNA polymerase III antibody positive patients are also at higher risk for malignancy
From Steen VD. Autoantibodies in systemic sclerosis. *Semin Arthritis Rheum.* 2005;35(1):35–42.
ACA, anticentromere antibody; *ILD*, interstitial lung disease; *MCTD*, mixed connective tissue disease; *PAH*, pulmonary arterial hypertension; *SRC*, scleroderma renal crisis.

5. What are the current American College of Rheumatology (ACR)/European Alliance of Associations for Rheumatology (EULAR) classification criteria for SSc?

Items	Sub-items	Weight
Skin thickening of fingers of both hands extending proximal to metacarpophalangeal (MCP) joints		9
Skin thickening of fingers (only count the highest score)	Puffy fingers	2
	Whole finger, distal to MCP	4
Fingertip lesions (only count the highest score)	Digital tip ulcers	2
	Pitting scars	3
Telangiectasia		2
Abnormal nailfold capillaries		2
Pulmonary arterial hypertension and/or interstitial lung disease		2
Raynaud phenomenon		3
Scleroderma-related antibodies (any of anti-centromere, anti-topoisomerase I [anti-ScL 70], anti-RNA polymerase III)		3
Patients with a total score of ≥9 are classified as having definite systemic sclerosis (sensitivity 91%, specificity 92%)		

Other potential causes of skin thickening must be excluded prior to application of these criteria to a specific patient (see Chapter 18: Scleroderma Mimics).
From Hoogen F, Khanna D, Fransen J, et al. 2013 Classification criteria for systemic sclerosis. Arthritis Rheum. 2013;65:2737-2747.

6. Who gets SSc?

SSc is most commonly seen in women (F:M = 4:1) aged 35 to 64 years. It occurs at a younger age in African–American women than in European–American women. While men are less likely to get SSc, men with SSc have increased mortality rates at 5 and 10 years compared to women. Choctaw Native Americans residing in Oklahoma have the highest reported disease prevalence in the United States.

7. What is the cause of SSc?

Unknown. The etiology of SSc may involve a complex interplay among a genetically susceptible host, sex-related factors, and environmental triggers. Pathophysiological mechanisms that may play a role in disease development include endothelial disruption, platelet activation, fibroblast proliferation, fetal microchimerism, and increased transforming growth factor-β. Some environmental factors, particularly silica dust, have been associated with an increased risk of SSc.

8. Are there effective treatments for SSc?

It depends on which aspect of SSc is considered. Effective therapies exist for SSc-associated GERD, SRC, ILD, and PAH. Raynaud's phenomenon often responds to vasodilator therapy (see Chapter 73: Raynaud phenomenon). However, there remain large unmet needs with regard to managing the fibrotic aspects of the disease (especially skin thickening and progressive lung fibrosis), as well as SSc-associated calcinosis and GI dysmotility. Strategies for the management of these manifestations, including the more challenging forms of involvement, will be discussed in this chapter.

9. What are the indications for immunosuppressive therapy in SSc?

Immunosuppression in SSc is typically reserved for those with progressive skin thickening, progressive ILD, inflammatory myopathy, or inflammatory arthritis. As such, many patients with SSc do not require immunosuppressive/immunomodulatory therapy. For example, patients with centromere-positive lcSSc often may not require immunosuppression as their features tend to be more vascular in nature along with GI involvement.

10. What are the chief causes of mortality in SSc?

With the introduction and success of ACE-inhibitor therapy in the management of SRC more than 30 years ago, the chief cause of SSc-associated mortality has dramatically shifted from renal disease to lung and heart disease. A EUSTAR database study (~6000 SSc patients) found that among SSc-related deaths, 35% were attributed to ILD, 26% to PAH, 26% to cardiac causes (mainly heart failure and arrhythmias), and only 4% to renal disease. The leading causes of non-SSc-related death included infections (33%), malignancies (31%), and cardiovascular causes (29%).

11. Compare and contrast organ system involvement in diffuse and limited SSc.

See Table 17.2.

TABLE 17.2 Organ System Involvement in Diffuse and Limited Systemic Sclerosis

ORGAN SYSTEM INVOLVEMENT	DIFFUSE (%)	LIMITED (%)
Skin thickening	100	95
Telangiectasias	30	80
Calcinosis	5	45
Raynaud phenomenon	85–95	95
Arthralgias or arthritis	80	60
Tendon friction rubs	65	5
Myopathy	20	10
Esophageal hypomotility	75	75
Pulmonary fibrosis	35–60	25–35
Congestive heart failure	10	1
Renal crisis	15	1

12. How is the skin affected in SSc?

The hallmark of scleroderma is thickened skin, thought to be due to the excessive production of normal type I collagen by a subset of fibroblasts along with the accumulation of glycosaminoglycan and fibronectin in the extracellular matrix. There is loss of sweat glands and hair in the areas of tight skin. Although patients may seem to have areas of clinically involved and uninvolved skin, immunohistochemistry and other analytic techniques have demonstrated that all skin tends to be abnormal. Skin thickening begins on the fingers and hands in virtually all cases of SSc. When skin thickening begins elsewhere, morphea, eosinophilic fasciitis, or another scleroderma mimic (see Chapter 18: Scleroderma Mimics) should be considered. The progression of skin tightening can be quite variable among patients. The **modified Rodnan skin score (mRSS)** is used clinically and in clinical trials to quantify skin involvement. The score is calculated by assessing 17 areas on the body. Each area is graded from 0 (no involvement) to 3 (severe involvement), for total possible score of 51. Skin scores over 15 to 20 and rapid progression (within first year) indicate more severe skin thickening. Most patients' skin, with no therapy, softens or atrophies over 3 to 10 years (Fig. 17.4).

13. Does skin disease uniformly predict internal organ involvement?

Not necessarily. Retrospective cohorts and evidence from randomized controlled trials have demonstrated an association between the degree of skin thickening (by mRSS) and subsequent progression of lung disease and overall survival. In addition, SRC is typically seen in patients with early dcSSc and only rarely encountered in lcSSc. Nonetheless, an individual patient can manifest signs of internal organ involvement in the absence of skin disease (ssSSc) or can develop progressive internal organ involvement in the setting of established, stable skin disease. In contrast, a patient with severely thickened skin may have little or no internal organ involvement. Given the potential disconnect between categories of SSc (lcSSc, dcSSc, ssSSc) and internal organ involvement, autoantibody phenotyping and careful assessment for internal organ involvement are required in all patients with SSc.

14. How is skin thickening treated?

Based on limited data, therapeutic options for skin thickening primarily include **mycophenolate mofetil** (MMF), **methotrexate,** and **rituximab. Cyclophosphamide** (CYC) has shown benefit for skin tightening as a secondary measure in randomized controlled trials for SSc-ILD, but it is uncommonly used (at least as first-line therapy) due to its side-effect profile. Tocilizumab failed to show statistical benefit for cutaneous involvement in a phase 3 study, but is still included as

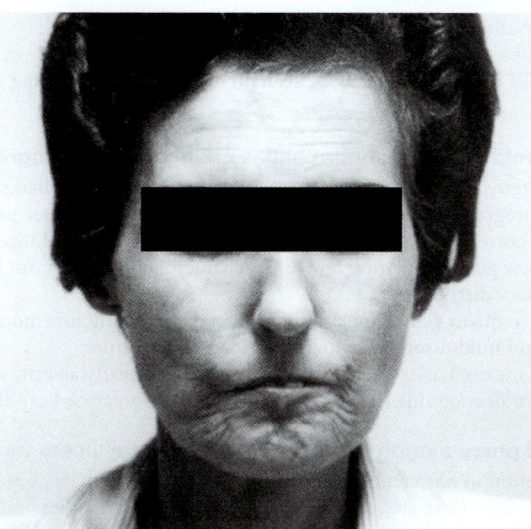

Fig. 17.4 Scleroderma patient demonstrating tightened facial skin. Note exaggerated radial furrowing about the lips (tobacco pouch sign).

a potential treatment option in the 2024 EULAR guidelines for SSc. Numerous small series and anecdotal evidence suggest that there is a possible role for high-dose intravenous immunoglobulin (2 g/kg per month). Clinical trials are ongoing to study novel agents in the treatment of scleroderma.

Data from clinical trials of autologous hematopoietic stem cell transplantation (HSCT) demonstrate that this modality can be effective for skin thickening as well. Given significant treatment-related morbidity and mortality, this treatment should only be considered for the more severe or refractory cases that have failed conventional therapy. More recently, the effectiveness of CAR-T therapy in SSc is being studied. UVA light therapy may also have a role in localized or limited SSc in the first 3 years of disease. Short-term, low-dose prednisone (<15 mg/day) and benzodiazepines can provide relief for the pruritus associated with the *acute phase* of skin thickening and may supplement conservative management with topical emollients (alcohol free), oatmeal baths, use of lukewarm (rather than hot) showers or baths, and avoidance of scratching (scratch-itch cycle). Symptoms of pruritus may also be relieved with agents such as gabapentin or pregabalin; in recalcitrant disease, low-dose naltrexone may be considered based on limited reports in the literature.

15. What is Raynaud phenomenon?

Raynaud phenomenon, frequently the first symptom of SSc, is an episodic, self-limited, and reversible vasomotor disturbance manifested as color changes bilaterally in the fingers, toes, and sometimes ears, nose, tongue, and lips. The color changes are **pallor, cyanosis** and then **erythema** (white, blue, and then red) that occur sequentially in response to environmental cold, emotional stress, or spontaneously. There does not need to be a three-color change to diagnose Raynaud phenomenon; episodic pallor or cyanosis that reverses to erythema or normal skin color may be all that is seen, especially in patients of color. Patients may describe symptoms of numbness, tingling, or pain on recovery. (see Chapter 73: Raynaud Phenomenon).

16. In a patient with new-onset Raynaud phenomenon, what findings would suggest early SSc?

- Positive SSc-specific autoantibody (e.g., nucleolar-staining ANA, ACA, anti-Scl-70, Pm-Scl, or RNA polymerase III antibody).
- Nailfold capillary abnormalities such as capillary drop-out and/or dilatation (see Chapter 73: Raynaud Phenomenon).
- Tendon friction rubs.

- Digital edema/puffy hands.
- Digital infarctions or ulcerations.
- Dilated, patulous esophagus, as may be seen on cross-sectional imaging (esophageal hypomotility).

17. How do the nailfold capillary abnormalities change as SSc progresses?

There are three patterns of microvascular changes seen on nailfold capillaroscopy (NFC) as patients with SSc progress. Monitoring of NFC may help identify disease progression, as loss of capillary density is correlated with the development of PAH and digital ulcers:

- Early pattern: few giant capillaries, few capillary microhemorrhages, no loss of capillaries, and preserved capillary distribution.
- Active pattern: frequent giant capillaries, frequent capillary microhemorrhages, moderate loss of capillaries, and mild disorganization of capillary architecture.
- Late pattern: giant capillaries and microhemorrhages are nearly absent, severe loss of capillaries, capillary ramification due to neoangiogenesis and disorganized capillaries.

18. How is Raynaud phenomenon treated? How are digital ulcers treated?

Raynaud phenomenon in SSc can be a challenge to effectively manage, but not all patients require specific medical therapy. Here are some general management principles:

- **First, keep hands and body warm.** Many patients always carry gloves. When going to cold places, patients may bring rechargeable heat packs or exothermic reaction bags (chemical heat packs), which can be obtained at sporting goods, hardware, and other stores. Repeated soaking in warm water sometimes helps. Newer heated gloves, socks, vests and jackets are growing in popularity with patients.
- Cigarette smoking exacerbates Raynaud phenomenon and should be avoided.
- Various prescription vasodilators can be used in the treatment of secondary Raynaud phenomenon associated with SSc, including **calcium-channel blockers** (first-line therapy), angiotensin-receptor blockers, topical nitrates, phosphodiesterase type-5 inhibitors (PDE5i; sildenafil), and prostacyclin analogs. In addition, endothelin receptor antagonists (ERAs) may be helpful in some patients (see Chapter 73: Raynaud phenomenon for examples of common dosing regimens and approach to treatment strategies).
- Antiplatelet therapy, anticoagulation, statin medications, and fluoxetine have all been used (with some benefit) in the treatment of Raynaud's (see Chapter 73: Raynaud Phenomenon).
- Digital ulcers occur in 30% to 40% of patients. All the therapies listed earlier have been used to accelerate healing and prevent recurrence, with varying levels of success. Bosentan has been shown to reduce the likelihood of new digital ulcer formation.
- For cases of digit-threatening ischemia, intravenous prostacyclin can be instituted.
- Alternative modalities that can be tried in refractory cases include local botox or nerve block injections, digital sympathectomy, and hyperbaric oxygen treatment to expedite digital ulcer healing.

19. Why is baseline cardiopulmonary testing important in patients with scleroderma and what testing is recommended?

The leading causes of death in SSc are lung and heart disease. All patients with SSc require initial cardiopulmonary assessments and longitudinal surveillance for development of lung or heart involvement, as data suggest better outcomes in patients with earlier-stage disease. Baseline testing includes:

- Thoracic high-resolution computed tomography (HRCT) scan (Fig. 17.5). Chest x-ray is inadequate.
- Complete pulmonary function tests (PFTs; lung volumes, spirometry, and diffusing capacity for carbon monoxide [DLco])
- Echocardiography (Fig. 17.6)
- Six-minute walk testing to assess for oxygen desaturation (best to use a forehead probe as finger pulse-oximetry can be unreliable due to Raynaud phenomenon)
- Electrocardiogram (EKG) to screen for conduction system abnormalities. Ambulatory EKG monitoring (Holter monitor) has been shown to be more sensitive than a resting 12-lead EKG, and in one study, it was helpful in identifying patients at risk for sudden cardiac death (e.g., population who may benefit from implantable cardiac defibrillator placement).

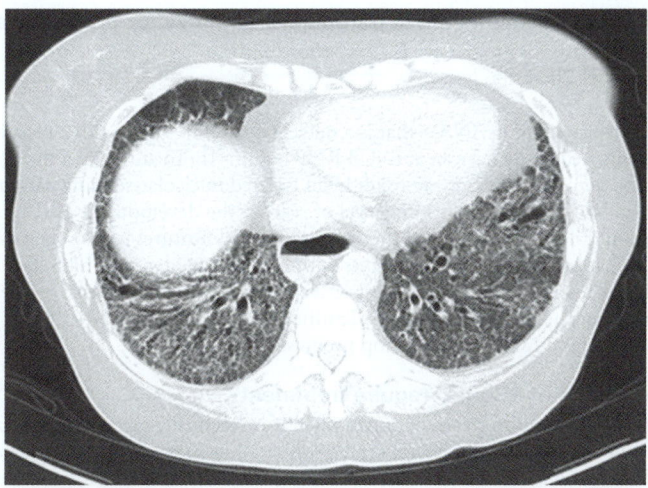

Fig. 17.5 High-resolution computed tomography image with bibasilar fibrotic interstitial lung disease characteristic of systemic sclerosis. Note also the dilated, fluid-filled esophagus.

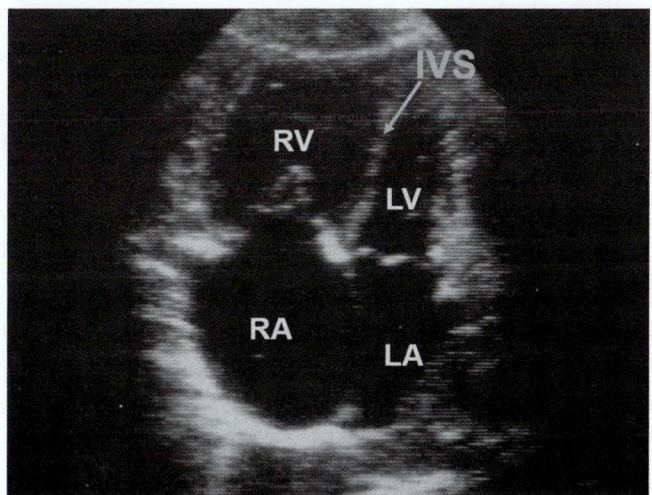

Fig. 17.6 Echocardiographic features of pulmonary arterial hypertension: dilated right atrium, dilated right ventricle, flattening of the interventricular septum. *IVS,* interventricular septum; *LA,* left atrium; *LV,* left ventricle; *RA,* right atrium; *RV,* right ventricle.

20. What types of lung disease do SSc patients get?

ILD and PAH are the two most common types of lung involvement identified in SSc and are the leading causes of SSc-associated mortality. Airways or pleural disease is rare in SSc.

21. What is the most common ILD pattern seen in SSc?

Fibrotic nonspecific interstitial pneumonia (NSIP), identified in about two-thirds of biopsied cases, followed by usual interstitial pneumonia (UIP), identified in about one-third of cases, are by far the two most common ILD patterns in SSc.

22. Which scleroderma patients are at particularly high risk for progressive ILD?

Patients at highest risk for progressive ILD are those with:

- Positive anti-Scl-70 antibody
- dcSSc
- Isolated nucleolar-staining ANA—that is a nucleolar-staining ANA with a negative anti-Scl-70. These patients frequently have an anti–U3 RNP or anti-Th/To antibody. Pm-Scl antibody is a less common autoantibody but can result in an isolated nucleolar-staining pattern as well.

  However, all SSc patients are at some level of risk for the development of ILD, and therefore, monitoring should not be restricted to those with high-risk features only. When assessed by thoracic HRCT, approximately 75% patients with SSc have evidence of bibasilar ILD. Clinically significant ILD (presence of symptoms, restrictive defect on PFT, or extensive disease by HRCT) warranting immunosuppressive therapy is identified in approximately 20–30% of patients. Patients with a positive ACA rarely develop progressive ILD.

23. Does the presence of SSc-ILD require treatment?

Not necessarily. ILD requires treatment only when it is "clinically significant" or *progressive* in nature. The ILD evaluation includes assessment of breathlessness, determining extent of disease by thoracic HRCT, complete PFTs (lung volumes, spirometry, and DLco) and assessment for oxygen desaturation with exercise (6-minute walk test). Research has shown that greater extent of involvement on HRCT (>20–50% of lung affected) is associated with an increased risk of progressive ILD (≥10% drop in forced vital capacity [FVC]) as well as a more robust response to therapy with cyclophosphamide.

24. How are PFTs and thoracic HRCT scan useful in the evaluation of patients with SSc?

Serial FVC and DLco allow for objective quantification of ventilatory capacity and gas exchange, respectively. These parameters are useful in assessing the degree of respiratory impairment due to ILD and may provide clues about coexistent PAH as well (based on disproportionate or isolated reduction in the DLco). They are especially helpful when trying to assess for disease progression and response to therapy. Patients who decline ≥10% of predicted FVC or ≥15% of predicted DLco are considered to have *progressive disease* by PFT. In patients with SSc-ILD, pulmonary physiology is a stronger predictor of survival than underlying histopathologic pattern (FVC < 70%: 5-year survival 60–65%).

Important information relevant to SSc-ILD can also be obtained by HRCT imaging. ILD presence (HRCT is more sensitive for detection of ILD than baseline PFTs), pattern, and extent of involvement can be assessed by HRCT. Disease progression can also be monitored on serial scanning. Patients with >20% of their lung affected by ILD on HRCT have a poor prognosis (5-year survival 60%).

25. When should a patient with SSc-ILD undergo surgical lung biopsy?

A surgical lung biopsy is rarely indicated in SSc-ILD. However, in patients with an atypical pattern of lung injury on CT scan or with compelling alternative explanations for ILD (e.g., concerns for hypersensitivity pneumonitis), biopsy may be considered following consultation with pulmonology and CT surgery (preferably in a SSc or pulmonary fibrosis center). NSIP and UIP are the most common types of ILD encountered in SSc, and histopathology has not been shown to impact prognosis in patients with these ILD patterns. As such, surgical lung biopsy is not typically indicated when HRCT is consistent with either pattern.

26. What are the therapeutic options for progressive SSc-ILD?

- **Mycophenolate mofetil (MMF)** is often considered first-line therapy for patients with progressive SSc-ILD. MMF use is associated with modest improvements in FVC, degree of fibrosis on HRCT, health-related quality of life, and mRSS. In Scleroderma Lung Study II, treatment with MMF for 2 years was as effective as treatment with oral CYC for 1 year. The lower toxicity profile of MMF makes it a more favorable option in general, and its use in this setting has largely supplanted CYC as first-line therapy.

- **Tocilizumab** is FDA-approved for ILD in early SSc (60 months or less). While it did not significantly impact skin endpoints, it did demonstrate stabilization of FVC in comparison to placebo.
- **Rituximab (RTX)** can be used in the setting of progressive CTD-ILD, including SSc-ILD, based on several recent trials
- **Cyclophosphamide (CYC)** can be given by monthly intravenous route or as daily oral therapy. It is associated with modest improvements in FVC and degree of fibrosis on HRCT.
- Treatment with **autologous HSCT** may have beneficial effects on the ILD component of SSc. It is typically reserved for those with dcSSc who have failed conventional therapies. Similarly, trials of CAR-T therapy in SSc are ongoing.
- **Nintedanib**, a tyrosine kinase inhibitor, may be used as a second-line monotherapy or as an adjunct to immunosuppressive treatment for SSc-ILD. Nintedanib is also approved for use in other progressive fibrosing forms of ILD. Pirfenidone, another anti-fibrotic agent, was studied in SLS III but failed to show benefit (the study was unfortunately underpowered due to the Covid-19 pandemic).
- Corticosteroids are not indicated for the treatment of SSc-ILD
- In refractory cases, azathioprine, or calcineurin antagonists (cyclosporine or tacrolimus) may be considered.
- Lung transplantation is reserved for patients with progressive disease despite conventional therapies. SSc patients have increased mortality following lung transplantation compared to patients with other forms of ILD, but similar outcomes to transplants in the setting of non-SSc-related PAH. Particular attention should be paid to GI disease in the setting of SSc, which can lead to early transplant failure.

27. What is the role of stem cell transplant in the therapy of SSc?

Autologous HSCT is an effective therapy for skin thickening and ILD in patients with dcSSc and can favorably impact long-term survival. However, this approach is associated with 3% to 10% risk of treatment-related mortality. Two multicenter trials have been published regarding treatment response of autologous HSCT compared with CYC for severe dcSSc. The European trial (ASTIS) showed that those treated with HSCT had improved event-free survival and decreased mortality at a median follow-up of approximately 6 years. Clinically meaningful improvements in objective and patient-reported outcome measures were observed at 2 years. However, there was significant treatment-related mortality (10.1%) during the first year as well as more severe adverse events during the first 2 years of follow-up. In the North American trial (SCOT), event-free survival at 54 months was seen in 79% of the transplantation group and 50% of the CYC group. At 72 months, Kaplan–Meier estimates of event-free survival (74% versus 47%) and overall survival (86% versus 51%) also favored transplantation. Treatment-related mortality in the transplantation group was 3% at 54 months and 6% at 72 months, as compared with 0% in the CYC group.

In light of these data, experts recommend that HSCT should be considered in patients with early dcSSc (within 5 years of disease onset) with mild-to-moderate internal organ involvement, and should generally be restricted to patients who have failed to improve or have worsened on conventional immunosuppressive agents. In addition, active smokers should be excluded based on evidence of increased mortality risk. Patients with severe internal organ involvement are commonly ineligible for HSCT due to the higher risk associated with therapy in this setting. Cardiopulmonary involvement specifically is associated with higher mortality in HSCT; invasive and noninvasive testing is required to evaluate for primary cardiac or pulmonary involvement, pericardial disease, or pulmonary hypertension (PH). Studies such as PFTs, HRCT, transthoracic echocardiogram, cardiac magnetic resonance imaging (MRI), and commonly right heart catheterization (RHC) are recommended before consideration of HSCT.

28. Discuss the frequency of PAH and its impact on survival in SSc.

The prevalence of RHC-confirmed SSc-PAH is estimated to be 10% to 15%. The presence of PAH in a scleroderma patient has a devastating impact on survival. Prior to the availability of PAH-specific therapies, the 5-year survival was 10% for SSc patients with PAH compared with 80% for SSc patients without PAH. The presence of advanced disease (functional class III-IV) portends a particularly poor outcome. Over the past 15 years, multiple PAH-specific therapies have become available, and their implementation has led to clinical improvement and an overall improved prognosis in patients with SSc-PAH compared with historical controls.

29. How is PH classified?

The current classification scheme divides PH into five distinct clinical groups:
Group 1: PAH
Group 2: PH associated with left heart disease
Group 3: PH associated with chronic hypoxia (e.g., PH associated with ILD)
Group 4: Chronic thromboembolic-associated PH
Group 5: PH with unclear or multifactorial mechanisms (e.g., sarcoidosis)

30. What types of PH are seen in SSc?

Patients with SSc most often have PAH (Group 1), but can also have other types, particularly PH due to left heart disease (Group 2) or PH-ILD (Group 3). Because PAH-specific therapies are typically only approved for patients with PAH (Group 1), distinguishing whether a patient has PAH or an alternative category is very important (of note, inhaled treprostinil is approved for Group 3 PH as well; see Question 35).

A diagnosis of PAH *absolutely* requires cardiac hemodynamic assessment via RHC. The definition of PAH was recently redefined by a mean pulmonary artery pressure >20 mmHg, pulmonary capillary wedge pressure (PCWP) of ≤15 mmHg, and pulmonary vascular resistance of >2 Wood units. In PH due to left heart disease, the elevated pulmonary pressures are a result of either systolic or diastolic dysfunction and confirmed by an increased PCWP >15mmHg on RHC. With PH-ILD, the elevated pulmonary pressures are considered to be a result of chronic hypoxia secondary to underlying lung disease. It is often a challenge to determine the degree of ILD necessary to cause secondary PH.

31. What are the presenting symptoms and signs of PAH?

Dyspnea and fatigue are the two most common symptoms of PAH; yet, both are ubiquitous and unreliable among patients with scleroderma. Patients often underreport such symptoms, and providers have a difficult time reliably quantifying their severity or progression. It is important for all scleroderma patients to undergo PAH screening, *including patients who do not report dyspnea.*

There are few signs of early PAH on physical examination, but several important exam findings suggest advanced PAH (i.e., features of right heart dysfunction including lower extremity edema, the murmur of tricuspid regurgitation, jugular venous distension, hepatomegaly, and right ventricular heave).

32. List some risk factors for PAH in SSc.

- lcSSc (especially long-standing disease).
- Duration of Raynaud's (longer duration = higher risk).
- ACA.
- Isolated nucleolar-pattern ANA.
- Extensive telangiectasia.
- DLco <60% in the absence of extensive ILD or other cause of low DLco (e.g., emphysema, as described in some SSc patients with combined pulmonary fibrosis & emphysema).
- FVC%/DLco% ratio > 1.6 (meaning a disproportionately low DLco).

33. What specific clinical, echocardiographic, PFT, and biomarker findings suggest PAH in a patient with SSc?

Features associated with the presence of PAH in SSc are outlined in Table 17.3.

- The best predictor for the development of PAH in scleroderma is **declining DLco.** The DLco is usually very low (<50% predicted) at the time of diagnosis of SSc-PAH, and this is generally in the absence of significant ILD.
- All scleroderma patients should have a baseline set of complete PFTs including DLco, and these should be repeated yearly in most patients. Restrictive physiology (i.e., reductions in total lung capacity or FVC) is seen with ILD, while disproportionate reductions in the DLco are more commonly seen with PAH. A disproportionate decline in the DLco relative to the FVC, as demonstrated by FVC%/DLco% ratio > 1.6, is a strong predictor of PAH development.

TABLE 17.3 Features Associated With the Presence of Pulmonary Hypertension in Systemic Sclerosis

SYMPTOMS	RECENT-ONSET EXERTIONAL DYSPNEA
Physical examination findings	Evidence of right heart compromise (e.g., lower extremity edema, the murmur of tricuspid regurgitation, jugular venous distension, hepatomegaly, or right ventricular heave)
Echocardiographic findings	Right ventricular systolic pressure > 40 mmHg Tricuspid regurgitation jet > 2.8 m/s Right ventricular dilation/hypokinesis Right atrial dilation Pericardial effusion
Pulmonary function test parameters	DLco% < 60% in absence of extensive interstitial lung disease or other cause (e.g., emphysema) FVC%/DLco% >1.6
Other features	Elevated BNP or NT-proBNP Unexplained oxygen desaturation with exercise

BNP, B-type natriuretic peptide; *DLco,* diffusing capacity for carbon monoxide; *FVC,* forced vital capacity; *NT-proBNP,* N-terminal-pro-B-type natriuretic peptide.
From Fischer A, Bull TM, Steen VD. A practical approach to screening for scleroderma-associated pulmonary arterial hypertension. *Arthritis Care Res (Hoboken).* 2012; 64(3):303–310.

- For those at high risk for ILD progression (e.g., those with a positive anti-Scl-70 or isolated nucleolar-ANA), one may choose to obtain PFTs even more frequently. A 6-minute walk test can identify exercise intolerance and hypoxemia, but it is not useful as a screening tool for SSc-PAH because it is neither specific nor sensitive for PAH.
- Baseline echocardiogram is recommended in all SSc patients and should be repeated yearly in most patients. It is reasonable in lower-risk patients (e.g., DLco >70% and stable longitudinally and/or patients with excellent aerobic exercise capacity without symptoms) to reduce the frequency of echocardiography to every 2 years. There are a variety of algorithms that can be used to estimate the probability of PAH and potentially reduce the utilization of echocardiogram and other high-cost testing (ESC/ERS guidelines, the DETECT and ASIG algorithms).
- Features on echocardiography that suggest the presence of PH include: right atrial dilation, right ventricular dilation, right ventricular dysfunction, flattening of the interventricular septum, pericardial effusion, or elevated estimated right ventricular systolic pressure (RVSP). Notably, there are significant limitations to its role as a screening tool for SSc-PAH. Echocardiographic views of the right side of the heart can be limited by technical issues (body habitus, etc.) and up to 15% of patients do not have a visible tricuspid regurgitation jet, thereby not allowing for RVSP estimation.

Elevated B-type natriuretic peptide (BNP) and N-terminal-pro-BNP (NT-proBNP) are surrogate biomarkers for myocardial disease and are frequently elevated in patients with SSc-PAH. They may be useful as an adjunctive component of SSc-PAH screening, with a caveat that early patients without significant right heart failure will have normal values. Both proteins reflect generalized cardiac dysfunction (including left heart failure) and are not specific for PAH. However, recent data do suggest that among those with SSc-PAH, high-levels of BNP or NT-proBNP are associated with a worse prognosis.

34. What is the gold-standard test for confirming PAH?

RHC is the gold-standard test for the diagnosis of PH and is absolutely required to confirm the diagnosis of PAH. It has an overall complication rate of 1.1%, mainly related to venous access problems. If any patient with scleroderma has unexplained dyspnea with an echocardiogram showing an estimated RVSP >40 mmHg or evidence of right ventricular dilatation or hypokinesis, RHC should be strongly considered. As mentioned earlier, RVSP is not always reliable or available, so the practitioner often needs to consider other factors to decide whether or not to proceed with RHC. RHC should also be strongly considered in a scleroderma patient with risk

TABLE 17.4 Decision Algorithm for Screening and Performing a Right Heart Catheterization in Scleroderma

	LOW RISK	MILD RISK	MODERATE RISK	HIGH RISK
Dyspnea, or Raynaud duration > 8 years, positive anti-centromere or isolated nucleolar-ANA	No	Yes	Yes	Yes
DLco (without extensive emphysema or ILD)	>70%	>70%	<70%	<60%
FVC%/DLco%	<1.6	<1.6	>1.6	>1.6
RVSP[a]	<35 mmHg	<35 mmHg	>35 mmHg	>40 mmHg
Next step	Repeat PFTs annually, Repeat echo in 2–3 years	Repeat PFTs annually, Repeat echo annually	Consider repeat echo in 3–6 months or proceed to RHC	Proceed to RHC

[a]The presence of echocardiographic features of right ventricular hypokinesis or dilatation or an increased BNP or NT-proBNP in a dyspneic scleroderma patient should lead to RHC irrespective of the estimated RVSP.

ANA, antinuclear antibody; *BNP,* B-type natriuretic peptide; *DLco,* diffusing capacity for carbon monoxide; *FVC,* forced vital capacity; *ILD,* interstitial lung disease; *NT-proBNP,* N-terminal-pro-B-type natriuretic peptide; *PFT,* pulmonary function test; *RHC,* right heart catheterization; *RVSP,* right ventricular systolic pressure.

From Fischer A, Bull TM, Steen VD. A practical approach to screening for scleroderma-associated pulmonary arterial hypertension. *Arthritis Care Res (Hoboken).* 2012; 64(3):303–310.

factors for PAH, particularly those with a disproportionately low DLco of <60% or FVC%/DLco% ratio >1.6. Other common scenarios that may prompt an evaluation with RHC (even in the setting of a normal estimated RVSP) include: unexplained dyspnea, findings of right heart compromise on physical examination, oxygen desaturation on exercise, right heart abnormalities on echocardiogram, an elevated BNP, or NT-proBNP. An echocardiogram with an estimated RVSP < 40 mmHg, without any other PAH-suggestive features, should reassure the practitioner that the pulmonary artery pressures are normal.

As part of the standard RHC procedure, acute vasodilator testing via catheter-infused adenosine, nitric oxide, or prostacyclin may be performed. Although current guidelines recommend that patients with idiopathic PAH undergo vasoreactivity testing as part of their initial RHC, no such consensus exists for SSc-PAH. Because vasoreactivity is so uncommon in scleroderma, the lack of its availability as part of the RHC should not preclude performing RHC (Table 17.4).

35. Are there effective PAH therapies?

Yes. Conventional therapy for PAH typically includes treatment with **calcium channel blockers,** fluid/volume control (diuretics, fluid restriction, low-salt diet), and supplemental oxygen. Chronic anticoagulation with warfarin was classically administered as an adjunctive therapy for idiopathic PAH, but is not recommended in SSc-associated PAH due to the increased risk of bleeding relative to idiopathic PAH patients and unclear benefit in this population.

The development of PAH-specific therapies has resulted in improved survival for patients with SSc-associated PAH. These agents may be used as monotherapy, or commonly in combination with one another. There are multiple categories of PAH-specific therapies, each representing a novel pathophysiologic pathway: **prostacyclins** (inhaled [ilioprost, treprostinil], subcutaneous or intravenous [epoprostenol, treprostinil], oral selexipag), **oral endothelin receptor antagonists** (bosentan, ambrisentan, macitentan), **transforming growth factor-beta receptor modulation/ activin receptor ligand trap (sotatercept), calcium channel blockers** (nifedipine, amlodipine, and diltiazem), and **nitric oxide potentiators** (oral phosphodiesterase-type 5 inhibitors [sildenafil, tadalafil] or guanylate cyclase stimulator [riociguat]). The AMBITION trial demonstrated that initial combination therapy with an endothelin receptor antagonist (ambrisentan) and a phosphodiesterase-type 5 inhibitor (tadalafil) was associated with less clinical deterioration than treatment with either agent alone, without an increase in the side-effect profile. As a result, 2024

EULAR guidelines say to consider combination PDE5i and ERA as first-line treatment in SSc-PAH. In addition, inhaled treprostinil has recently been approved for group 3 PH (PH due to lung disease). The presence of multiple available therapies (including the routine implementation of combination therapy) has made the management of SSc-PAH increasingly more complex, and collaboration with PAH-treating providers is recommended.

36. What types of heart diseases occur with SSc?

Myocardial, pericardial, or **conduction system disease** are all potential cardiac complications associated with SSc. **Diastolic dysfunction** is one of the more common cardiac manifestations of SSc and can lead to PH due to left heart disease. **Cardiomyopathy** associated with SSc can be difficult to distinguish from ischemic cardiomyopathy; cardiac MRI may be useful in this regard as patients with SSc-cardiomyopathy typically have evidence of an infiltrative or fibrotic process. SSc-cardiomyopathy may be more commonly seen in African–Americans, those with diffuse skin involvement and RNA polymerase III antibody positivity. **Pericardial effusions** are almost always asymptomatic, are associated with the presence of PH, and do not require specific intervention. Symptomatic, inflammatory **pericarditis** is rare and may be treated with nonsteroidal anti-inflammatory drugs, low-dose corticosteroids, or colchicine. Cardiovascular disease including coronary artery disease is increased in SSc (hazard ratio 3.2). In general, cardiac disease in SSc is associated with a poor prognosis, accounting for 26% of all SSc-related deaths and 29% of non–SSc-related deaths.

37. What is scleroderma renal crisis (SRC)?

SRC, one of the most feared complications of SSc, may present as acute renal crisis after sustained hypertension and less commonly as normotensive renal failure. SRC occurs in up to 5% of the entire SSc population and in 5% to 20% of patients with dcSSc. Patients with early diffuse skin thickening, especially patients with RNA polymerase III antibody positivity, are at highest risk for SRC and vigilant surveillance is indicated. Renal crisis may be the presenting manifestation of SSc and can sometimes precede skin thickening. Renal crisis typically occurs early in the course of the disease, with a mean onset of 3.2 years, and more often in the fall and winter months. Serologically, the presence of **RNA polymerase III antibody** conveys a higher risk of SRC (antibody present in approximately 50% of cases of SRC, but <20% of SSc overall).

SRC typically presents with an abrupt onset of arterial hypertension (>150/90; although 10% are normotensive), appearance of grade III (flame-shaped hemorrhages and/or cotton-wool exudates) or grade IV (papilledema) retinopathy, and the rapid deterioration of renal function (within a month). Pericardial effusion is frequently present. Abnormal laboratory tests include elevated renal function tests, proteinuria, consumptive thrombocytopenia, microangiopathic hemolysis (**schistocytes; 50%**), elevated renin levels (twice the upper limit of normal or greater), and normal or only mildly decreased ADAMTS 13 levels (>20% of normal). This latter test may be important given the similar clinical presentation of thrombotic thrombocytopenic purpura/hemolytic uremic syndrome and SRC. In addition, a subset of patients with SSc may suffer acute renal failure secondary to an antineutrophil cytoplasmic antibody (ANCA)-associated glomerulonephritis, another potential mimicker of SRC. However, these patients do not typically present with the hemolytic manifestations of SRC, hypertension does not predominate to the same degree, and they can be distinguished by laboratory evaluation (red blood cell casts, ANCA antibody) and biopsy.

Approximately 50% of patients who develop SRC will require dialysis, but nearly half of these patients will be able to discontinue dialysis after 3 to 18 months on ACE inhibitor therapy. Five-year mortality is still significant and ranges from 20% to 40% in the literature.

38. Which therapeutic intervention has helped avoid renal failure in patients with SSc?

The use of **ACE inhibitors** has dramatically changed the outcome of renal involvement in SSc. Captopril and enalapril are the most studied ACE inhibitors in scleroderma, but probably any of the ACE inhibitors are effective. Angiotensin II receptor antagonists have not been proven effective in treating SRC.

39. Should ACE inhibitors be used prophylactically in patients with SSc to prevent SRC?

There is no data to support prophylactic ACE inhibitor therapy in patients with SSc. In addition, some data suggest that patients on an ACE inhibitor at the time of diagnosis of SRC may have a worse prognosis. Routine use of ACE inhibitors may prevent early identification of SRC in some patients by modulating hypertension as an early sign of SRC.

40. What are some risk factors for SRC?

- Early diffuse scleroderma (first 1–4 years after diagnosis).
- Tendon friction rubs.
- Corticosteroid (prednisone > 20 mg/day or prolonged low dose) or cyclosporine use.
- Anti-RNA polymerase III antibody (50–60%).

Patients with risk factors for SRC should receive counseling regarding routine home blood pressure monitoring (daily or every other day) and be monitored closely with frequent follow-up evaluations and laboratory assessments for microangiopathic hemolytic anemia, thrombocytopenia, and renal dysfunction.

41. How is SRC treated? What are poor prognostic signs?

Patients with SRC should be hospitalized. They should be put on a short-acting ACE inhibitor with the goal of decreasing systolic blood pressure by 20 mmHg within the first 24 hours. Hypotension should be avoided. The ACE inhibitor should be maximized to normalize the blood pressure. Up to 30% of patients will have continued blood pressure elevation on ACE inhibitors. These patients should have calcium channel blockers added as second-line therapy, followed by angiotensin-receptor blockers. The use of endothelin receptor antagonists, prostacyclin, and eculizumab has been described in the literature for resistant cases. Poor prognostic factors include: (1) male gender, (2) initial creatinine > 3 mg/dL, (3) normotensive at onset, and (4) cardiac involvement with myocarditis or arrhythmias. Approximately 50% to 60% patients will require dialysis within the first 24 months, with half of those recovering enough renal function to stop dialysis. Therefore, ACE inhibitor therapy should be continued indefinitely even in patients who have progressed to dialysis, and kidney transplantation should be delayed at least 24 months.

42. What are the GI manifestations of SSc?

Upper GI tract: GERD (heartburn), hypomotility, dysphagia, nausea, stricture formation, risk of Barrett's esophagus (10–15%), gastric antral vascular ectasia (GAVE). Cough due to aspiration is a common symptom associated with GERD. Calcium channel blockers used to treat Raynaud can make GERD worse. Reflux severity has been associated with increased radiographic change and extent of fibrosis in SSc-ILD.

Lower GI tract: Hypomotility, bloating, nausea, small intestinal bacterial overgrowth (manifested by fluctuating constipation and diarrhea), malabsorption, intestinal pseudo-obstruction, pneumatosis coli, loss of rectal sphincter tone with resultant fecal incontinence, and rectal prolapse. Calcium channel blockers used to treat Raynaud phenomenon can make constipation worse.

43. Discuss the pathophysiologic progression of GI involvement in SSc.

Although no longitudinal studies have been performed to document the anatomic progression in the GI system, there is good circumstantial evidence to suggest an orderly series of steps leading to progressive dysfunction. First, there is neural dysfunction thought to be due to arteriolar changes of the vasa nervorum leading to dysmotility. Second, there is smooth muscle atrophy. Third, there is fibrosis of the smooth muscle.

44. How are upper GI tract manifestations assessed in patients with SSc?

- Esophageal dysmotility may be documented by manometry, barium esophagram, or by a routine upper GI series with barium swallow.
- A dilated, patulous esophagus is a frequent incidental finding noted on thoracic computed tomography scans of patients with SSc.
- Endoscopy is used to assess reflux esophagitis, candidiasis, Barrett's esophagus, and strictures of the lower esophageal area. Patients who develop Barrett's esophagitis are at risk for developing adenocarcinoma and will need surveillance endoscopies every 1 to 2 years depending on the presence of dysplasia.

45. How is esophageal dysmotility treated in SSc patients?

Treatment is designed to decrease complications of acid reflux, such as esophagitis, stricture, or nocturnal aspiration of stomach contents. The head of the bed should be elevated 4 to 6 inches through the use of foam wedges, custom mattresses, or placement of stable blocks underneath the box springs; adding more pillows to sleep on may only make matters worse by decreasing stomach area. The patient should not eat for 2 to 3 hours prior to bedtime. The acid content in the stomach should be decreased in the evening with antacids, H2 blockers, or proton pump inhibitors. Motility agents such as metoclopramide (5–10 mg) or erythromycin (motilin receptor agonist; 250 mg) before meals may be helpful early in the disease, but often become ineffective later in the course due to tachyphylaxis and eventual GI smooth muscle fibrosis. Domperidone can be an effective pro motility agent, but it is no longer available in the United States and requires a prescription through an international pharmacy. Erythromycin and domperidone **can cause a prolonged QT interval.** A recent case study described success with a gastric per-oral endoscopic pyloromyotomy (GPOEM) procedure in SSc patients with refractory gastroparesis; additional research is needed to determine the safety and clinical utility in this setting. Endoscopic injection of botox into the pyloric sphincter has been used for resistant cases of GERD as well. For more refractory cases of GI dysmotility, injectable octreotide may be considered. Of note, extreme caution should be exercised before consideration of a Nissen fundoplication for the treatment of GERD in a patient with SSc (due to the heightened risk of dysphagia in patients with dysmotility). Preoperative manometry is mandatory, and less invasive procedures should be considered (partial wrap, or Toupet fundoplication; use of laparoscopically placed magnetized beads, the *LINX* procedure; transoral incisionless fundoplication, or TIF procedure).

46. What is a "watermelon stomach"?

Watermelon stomach is a descriptive term for GAVE and is the result of extensive and prominent telangiectasia involving the gastric mucosal surface. This can be a cause of chronic iron deficiency anemia and acute upper GI bleeding in scleroderma. Laser treatment or argon plasma coagulation are effective treatments for GAVE.

47. Patients with SSc may have small and large bowel involvement. What symptoms and signs do these patients have?

Involvement of the **small intestine** (17–57% patients) and colon (10–50% patients) is common. The major manifestations are due to diminished peristalsis with resulting stasis and dilatation. The diminished peristalsis can lead to bacterial overgrowth (33–40% of patients; positive hydrogen breath test, high folate, $\geq 10^5$ organisms/mL of jejunal fluid). Later, malabsorption can be a major problem (low albumin, low B6/B12/folate/25-OH Vit D, high fecal fat, low D-xylose absorption test, low β carotene, high international normalized ratio due to low vitamin K). Patients may report abdominal distention and pain due to dilated bowel, obstructive symptoms from intestinal pseudo-obstruction, or diarrhea from bacterial overgrowth or malabsorption. If the malabsorption becomes severe, the patient may have signs of vitamin deficiencies or electrolyte abnormalities.

Patients with **large bowel** involvement affecting the anorectum can suffer from debilitating fecal incontinence. This may be due to a neuropathy more than sphincter atrophy/fibrosis. Atrophy and thinning of the muscular wall in the colon can lead to "wide mouth" diverticulae. It should be emphasized that barium studies are relatively contraindicated in SSc patients with poor GI motility owing to the risk of barium impaction. Rectal prolapse has also been reported.

48. How are small and large bowel problems managed in these patients?

Intestinal dysmotility/constipation
- Stimulation of gut motility with domperidone, metoclopramide, or erythromycin (30 minutes before meals). It is important to note that data for prokinetic agents outside of short-term use for gastric motility is extremely limited.
- Newer secretory agents, as well as colonic motility agents (e.g. prucalopride), for constipation may also be used.
- Injectable octreotide may help in severe or refractory cases.

- Fiber may help colonic dysmotility. Some patients may experience symptoms of bloating, but dietary fiber intake through 100% whole grain products, fruits, and vegetables is generally safe and recommended.
- Maintaining exercise may help move food through the digestive tract.

Diarrhea

- Diarrhea is commonly treated initially as if it were due to bacterial overgrowth. An antibiotic is given that can partially decrease the gut flora, such as rifaximin (550 mg thrice a day [TID]), ciprofloxacin (500 mg twice a day [BID]), amoxicillin-clavulanic acid (875 mg BID), or metronidazole (500 mg TID) for 10 days. In most cases, this stops the diarrhea. In patients with relapse, cyclic (rotating) antibiotic courses can be used.
- Agents that slow intestinal motility, such as paregoric or loperamide, should be avoided.
- If diarrhea persists, an infectious and malabsorption work-up should be pursued. Most patients with malabsorption can be treated with supplemental vitamins, minerals, and predigested liquid food supplements. A rare patient will need total parenteral nutrition.
- Dietary modification (for symptoms of bloating, alternating diarrhea, and constipation): patients may consider removing specific food that may be more difficult to digest (e.g., gluten and lactose). A food diary may allow patients to identify specific triggers. Some patient advocacy groups suggest a low FODMAP (fermentable, oligosaccharides, disaccharides, monosaccharides, and polyols) diet. Additional online data can be found at the end of this chapter. Despite the potential merits of eliminating some "problem foods," patients should be advised to exercise caution with dietary restriction given the increased risk of malnutrition in SSc and the fact that many patients can be severely underweight. Consultation with a dietician should be considered.

Rectal involvement

- Fecal incontinence is treated with biofeedback, sacral nerve stimulation (limited data on tibial nerve stimulation), and/or surgical repair.
- Rectal prolapse includes management of constipation and possibly surgical correction.

49. What is calcinosis?

Calcinosis consists of cutaneous deposits of basic calcium phosphate that characteristically occur in the hands (especially over the proximal interphalangeal joints and fingertips), periarticular tissue, and over bony prominences (especially the extensor surface of the elbows and knees), but can occur virtually anywhere on the body. The deposits of calcium are firm, irregular, and generally nontender, ranging in diameter from 1 mm to several centimeters. They can become inflamed, infected, or ulcerated and may discharge a chalky white material. Calcinosis can be persistent for years. It is extremely difficult to treat, and no therapy is consistently successful. Therapies that have been used with little supporting data include warfarin (in an attempt to inhibit the vitamin K-dependent Gla matrix protein), teracyclines, and diltiazem. Case reports of topical sodium thiosulfate have been described in patients with calcinosis cutis in the setting of systemic lupus erythematosus, dermatomyositis, and SSc, but clinical trials and even case series of significant size are lacking. Intravenous bisphosphonate use has been used with some success for calcinosis secondary to juvenile dermatomyositis, and intravenous and intralesional sodium thiosulfate has been described in case reports of SSc as well (of note, thiosulfate can bind to any calcium salt, hence bone mineral density should be monitored if this medicine is used chronically for any length of time). More recently, tofacitinib use has shown promise in dermatomyositis associated calcinosis; additional research in the setting of SSc is needed. Surgical resection should be considered a last resort option, and deposits can reoccur.

50. What are telangiectasia?

Telangiectasia are dilated venules, capillaries, and arterioles. In SSc they tend to be matte telangiectasia, which are oval or polygonal macules 2 to 7 mm in diameter found on the hands, face, lips, and oral mucosa. They are seen more commonly with limited SSc. Telangiectasia are usually harmless but can be a cosmetic problem. They may disappear spontaneously over time. Laser therapy has been used to remove them with some success, but commonly they will return. When they occur in the GI mucosa (called "watermelon stomach" or GAVE), they can bleed, leading to iron deficiency anemia.

51. Describe the bone and articular involvement in SSc.

Bone involvement is usually demonstrated by resorption of bone. Acrosclerosis with osteolysis is common. Resorption of ribs, mandible, acromion, radius, and ulna has been reported. Arthralgias and morning stiffness are relatively common, but erosive arthritis is rare. Hand deformities and ankylosis are seen, but these are usually attributed to the tethering effects of skin thickening instead of joint involvement. Tendon sheaths can become inflamed and fibrinous, mimicking arthritis. Tendon friction rubs can be palpated typically over the wrists, ankles, and knees and are found primarily in patients with diffuse SSc (50–65%). Friction rubs are due to fibrin deposition in the tenosynovial sheath and/or increased thickness of the tendon retinacula.

52. Discuss the three types of muscle abnormalities seen in SSc.

1. Mild proximal weakness due to a noninflammatory benign myopathy. On histology, this myopathy looks normal or shows a type 2 muscle fiber atrophy. This pattern of fiber loss is seen with inactivity and corticosteroid use. The muscle enzymes are typically normal.
2. Mild elevation of muscles enzymes with waxing and waning of symptoms. Muscle biopsy reveals interstitial fibrosis and fiber atrophy. Minimal inflammatory cell infiltration is noted. Not typically treated with corticosteroids.
3. Inflammatory myopathy with elevated muscle enzymes (as seen with polymyositis). These patients are considered to have an overlap syndrome, and many fit the definition of mixed connective tissue disease. The myositis is treated with immunosuppressive therapy.

ACKNOWLEDGMENTS

The author and editors would like to thank Dr. Aryeh Fischer for his contribution to this chapter in the previous edition.

BIBLIOGRAPHY

Bernstein EJ, Peterson ER, Sell JL, et al. Survival of adults with systemic sclerosis following lung transplantation: a nationwide cohort study. *Arthritis Rheumatol.* 2015;67(5):1314–1322.

Brown ZR, Nikpour M. Screening for pulmonary arterial hypertension in systemic sclerosis: Now or never!. *Eur J Rheumatol.* 2020;7(suppl 3):S187–S192.

Christmann RB, Wells AU, Capelozzi VL, et al. Gastroesophageal reflux incites interstitial lung disease in systemic sclerosis: radiologic, histopathologic, and treatment evidence. *Semin Arthritis Rheum.* 2010;40:241–249.

Coghlan JG, Denton CP, Grünig E, et al. Evidence-based detection of pulmonary arterial hypertension in systemic sclerosis: the DETECT study. *Ann Rheum Dis.* 2014;73(7):1340–1349.

Connolly KL, Griffith JL, McEvoy M, et al. Ultraviolet A1 phototherapy beyond morphea: experience in 83 patients. *Photodermatol Photoimmunol Photomed.* 2015;31:289–295.

Davuluri S, Lood C, Chung L. Calcinosis in systemic sclerosis. *Curr Opin Rheumatol.* 2022;34(6):319–327.

Del Galdo F, Lescoat A, Conaghan PG, et al. EULAR recommendations for the treatment of systemic sclerosis: 2023 update. *Ann Rheum Dis.* 2025;84(1):29–40.

Domsic RT, Medsger TA. Autoantibodies and their role in scleroderma clinical care. *Curr Treat Options in Rheum.* 2016;2:239–251.

Fernández-Codina A, et al. Cardiac involvement in systemic sclerosis: differences between clinical subsets and influence on survival. *Rheumatol Int.* 2017;37(1):75–84.

Galiè N, Barberà JA, Frost A, et al. Initial use of ambrisentan plus tadalafil in pulmonary arterial hypertension. *N Engl J Med.* 2015;373:834–844.

Gonzalez J-M, Granel B, Barthet M, et al. G-POEM may be an optional treatment for refractory gastroparesis in systemic sclerosis. *Scand J Gastroenterol.* 2020;55:777–779.

Gyger G, Baron M. Gastrointestinal manifestations of scleroderma: recent progress in evaluation, pathogenesis, and management. *Curr Rheumatol Rep.* 2012;14:22–29.

van den Hoogen F, Khanna D, Fransen J, et al. 2013 Classification criteria for systemic sclerosis. *Arthritis Rheum.* 2013;65:2737–2747.

Hughes M, Pauling JD, Armstrong-James L, et al. Gender-related differences in systemic sclerosis. *Autoimmun Rev.* 2020;19(4).

Humbert M, Kovacs G, Hoeper MM, et al. ESC/ERS Scientific Document Group. 2022 ESC/ERS guidelines for the diagnosis and treatment of pulmonary hypertension. *Eur Heart J.* 2022;43(38):3618–3731.

Jaeger VK, Wirz EG, Allanore Y, et al. Incidences and risk factors of organ manifestations in the early course of systemic sclerosis: a longitudinal Eustar study. *PLOS One.* 2016;11:e0163894.

Jordan S, Distler JH, Maurer B, et al. Effects and safety of rituximab in systemic sclerosis: an analysis from the European Scleroderma Trial and Research (EUSTAR) group. *Ann Rheum Dis.* 2015;74(6):1188–1194.

Kowal-Bielecka O, Fransen J, Avouac J, et al. Update of EULAR recommendations for the treatment of systemic sclerosis. *Ann Rheum Dis.* 2017;76:1327–1339.

Lin CY, Chen HA, Chang TW, et al. Association of systemic sclerosis with incident clinically evident heart failure. *Arthritis Care Res (Hoboken).* 2023;75(7):1452–1461.

Maher TM, et al. Rituximab versus intravenous cyclophosphamide in patients with connective tissue disease-associated interstitial lung disease in the UK (RECITAL). *Lancet Respir Med.* 2023;11(1):45–54.

Mankikian J, et al. Rituximab and mycophenolate mofetil combination in patients with interstitial lung disease (EVER-ILD): a double-blind, randomised, placebo-controlled trial. *Eur Respir J.* 2023;61(6):2202071.

Roth MD, Tseng CH, Clements PJ, et al. Predicting treatment outcomes and responder subsets in scleroderma-related interstitial lung disease. *Arthritis Rheum.* 2011;63(9):2797–2808.

Steen VD, Medsger TA. Changes in causes of death in systemic sclerosis, 1972-2002. *Ann Rheum Dis.* 2007;66(7):940–944.

Sullivan KM, Goldmuntz EA, Keyes-Elstein L, et al. Myeloablative autologous stem-cell transplantation for severe scleroderma. *N Engl J Med.* 2018;378(1):35–47.

Tashkin DP, Roth MD, Clements PJ, et al. Mycophenolate mofetil versus oral cyclophosphamide in scleroderma-related interstitial lung disease (SLS II): a randomized controlled, double-blind, parallel group trial. *Lancet Respir Med.* 2016;4(9):708–719.

Tucker AE, Perin J, Volkmann ER, et al. Associations between patterns of esophageal dysmotility and extra-intestinal features in patients with systemic sclerosis. *Arthritis Care Res (Hoboken).* 2022.

Tyndall AJ, et al. Causes and risk factors for death in systemic sclerosis: a study from the EULAR Scleroderma Trials and Research (EUSTAR) database. *Ann Rheum Dis.* 2010;69(10):1809–1815.

Rangarajan V, Matiasz R, Freed BH. Cardiac complications of systemic sclerosis and management: recent progress. *Curr Opin Rheumatol.* 2017;29(6):574–584.

Scleroderma Lung Study III. NCT03221257. Available at: https://clinical-trials.gov/ct2/show/NCT03221257.

Volkmann ER, McMahan ZH, Smith V, et al. Risk of malnutrition in patients with systemic sclerosis-associated interstitial lung disease treated with nintedanib. *Arthritis Care Res (Hoboken).* 2023;75(8):1690–1697.

Volkmann ER, Tashkin DP, Leng M, et al. Association of Symptoms of Gastroesophageal Reflux, Esophageal Dilation, and Progression of Systemic Sclerosis-Related Interstitial Lung Disease. *Arthritis Care Res (Hoboken).* 2022. doi:10.1002/acr.25070.

Waxman A, et al. Inhaled treprostinil in pulmonary hypertension due to interstitial lung disease. *N Engl J Med.* 2021;384(4):325–334.

FURTHER READINGS

Eating Well with Scleroderma (Scleroderma Foundation): https://scleroderma.org/resources-center (search for Digestive under Topics).

Scleroderma Foundation: www.scleroderma.org.

Patient-centered Scleroderma Self-Management Recommendations: https://www.sruk.co.uk/about-us/news/6-tips-self-management https://www.aad.org/public/diseases/a-z/scleroderma-self-care.

Scleroderma Mimics

Laura K. Hummers, MD, ScM

---

1. Mimics of scleroderma are often distinguishable from systemic sclerosis (SSc) based on the distribution and quality of skin changes.
2. Scleredema and scleromyxedema both cause mucinous deposition in the skin and may be associated with monoclonal gammopathies.
3. Eosinophilia may be absent during clinical presentation of eosinophilic fasciitis (EF).
4. Outbreaks of scleroderma mimics have occurred in association with specific exposures.
5. Biopsy of thickened skin requires special consideration including a request for specific stains for mucin and/or full-thickness biopsy to include deeper tissue structures.

---

1. **What clinical characteristics help distinguish scleroderma mimics from systemic sclerosis?**

   Scleroderma mimics often (but not always) have following characteristics:
   - Lack of Raynaud phenomenon (present in nearly all patients with scleroderma)
   - Lack of nailfold capillary abnormalities including dilatation and dropout
   - Lack of positive antinuclear/scleroderma-specific antibodies (present in 90–95% of SSc)
   - An atypical skin distribution relative to systemic sclerosis (mimics often spare fingers but include the back)
   - Lack of characteristic organ involvement associated with SSc (e.g., dysphagia/patulous esophagus, interstitial lung disease, cutaneous telangiectasia)

2. **List some of the diseases and potential exposures associated with skin abnormalities that may mimic the cutaneous sclerosis seen in SSc (see Box 18.1).**

BOX 18.1 Medical Conditions and Exposures Associated With Cutaneous Sclerosis

Disease mimics
- Localized scleroderma
  - Morphea/generalized morphea
  - Deep or pansclerotic morphea
  - Linear scleroderma (extremity or *en coup de sabre*)
- Scleredema
- Scleromyxedema
- Eosinophilic fasciitis
- Chronic graft-versus-host disease (cGVHD)
- POEMS syndrome—polyneuropathy, organomegaly, endocrinopathy, monoclonal gammopathy, and skin changes
- Pachydermoperiostitis
- Lichen sclerosis et atrophicus
- Metabolic diseases
  - Diabetic cheiroarthropathy (see Chapter 47: Endocrine-Associated Arthropathies)
  - Hypothyroidism (myxedema)
  - Porphyria cutanea tarda
  - Phenylketonuria
- Systemic amyloidosis
- Lipodermatosclerosis
- Genetic disorders (e.g., Werner syndrome)

Medication/treatment/toxin-related
- L-tryptophan (eosinophilia-myalgia syndrome [EMS])
- Aniline-denatured rapeseed oil (toxic oil syndrome)

Continued

BOX 18.1 Medical Conditions and Exposures Associated With Cutaneous Sclerosis—cont'd

- Gadolinium (nephrogenic systemic fibrosis; NSF)
- Immune Checkpoint Inhibitors
- Bleomycin
- Pentazocine
- Carbidopa
- Melphalan
- Docetaxel (taxotere)
- Post-radiation fibrosis

Occupational exposure
- Vinyl chloride
- Silica
- Pesticides (malathion, diniconozole)
- Organic solvents (benzene, toluene, and others)
- Epoxy resins

Recognition of the various causes of cutaneous sclerosis is especially important in the evaluation of a patient who lacks some of the key features of SSc (see Question 1), particularly the Raynaud phenomenon and sclerodactyly. In such patients, consideration should be given to the list of conditions associated with skin thickening outlined in Box 18.1, with consideration for skin biopsy if the diagnosis remains unclear. Several of the more common conditions rheumatologists encounter that mimic SSc (localized scleroderma, scleredema, scleromyxedema, eosinophilic fasciitis, and several medication/toxin-induced syndromes) will be discussed.

LOCALIZED SCLERODERMA

3. How is localized scleroderma different than the limited cutaneous form of SSc?

Localized scleroderma is a distinct clinical entity from SSc (see Chapter 17: Systemic Sclerosis). It is a local fibrosing condition that lacks systemic organ involvement, and as such should not be considered part of the spectrum of SSc. Confusion among patients and providers often arises because of the similar terminology of limited cutaneous SSc (often referred to as limited scleroderma) and localized scleroderma. Localized forms of scleroderma include single plaque morphea, generalized morphea, and linear scleroderma and are distinguished by lack of systemic disease features. The distribution of skin disease is often distinct and presents as single or multiple plaques of thickened skin or as a "streak" of thickened skin on an extremity or on the face (*en coup de sabre*). Notably, skin biopsy changes in localized scleroderma are indistinguishable from systemic sclerosis.

4. Do patients with morphea commonly evolve into SSc?

No. A rheumatologic evaluation is helpful in patients with cutaneous sclerosis to identify signs of SSc or other systemic diseases associated with skin thickening (see Question 2). If the clinical evaluation suggests morphea, focus can then be directed toward therapies to help the localized fibrotic disease and reassurance given to the patient regarding the absence of SSc. Rare case reports detailing a transition from morphea to SSc exist (more commonly in pediatric literature), but there are no data to suggest that this occurs more commonly than the incidence rate of SSc in the general population.

5. What are the clinical features of the different subtypes of morphea?

Several different classification systems exist for morphea. In general, these diseases can be categorized as (1) circumscribed (plaque-variant), (2) generalized (multiple plaques), (3) deep, and (4) linear (in an extremity or *en coup de sabre* in the face/scalp). Morphea is more common in children than adults. The etiology is unclear, but various infectious agents, trauma, and medications have been postulated. Skin involvement is common in the truncal region and can be seen in the breasts and extremities as well but typically spares the hands and fingers. It is not associated with Raynaud phenomenon and does not affect internal organs, which distinguishes it from SSc.

Some patients with localized scleroderma may also overlap with eosinophilic fasciitis (see below). Clinical features often differ by disease category:

- **Circumscribed (superficial or deep):** most frequent subtype; comprises most cases of adults with morphea. It typically presents as a well-circumscribed lesion surrounded by an erythematous border. Later, the central portion may become indurated and sclerotic. The lesions can be shiny and may lack hair and exocrine glands similar to SSc.
- **Generalized:** defined as four or more lesions (>3 cm in size) that involve two or more anatomic sites. Lesions are often symmetrical and may coalesce over time.
  - **Pansclerotic:** Disabling pansclerotic morphea is a subtype of the generalized morphea category. This rare subtype occurs in childhood and can be rapidly progressive, involving deeper structures to the level of the bone and resulting in skin necrosis, open ulcers, muscle atrophy, and joint contracture. It is associated with an elevated risk of cutaneous squamous-cell carcinoma.
- **Deep:** morphea lesions that extend beyond epidermis and dermis, potentially including layers of fat, fascia, and muscle. Often symmetric; located on the extremities. More common in childhood.
- **Linear**: most common category among children. May affect a unilateral limb or less commonly the scalp and face (*en coup de sabre;* most commonly in the region between the eyebrow and the hairline). Linear scleroderma can extend beyond the skin to fascia, muscle, and bone leading to tissue atrophy. Not associated with Raynaud phenomenon or internal organ involvement, but some patients have arthritis (10–15%). Neurologic symptoms and ocular disease (including uveitis) can occur in the *en coup de sabre* form and may overlap with the Parry–Romberg syndrome (see Question 7).

6. Which treatment options can be considered in patients with morphea?

Not all patients with morphea require pharmacologic intervention and it is important to note that morphea lesions typically are self-limited. It is important to first assess whether lesions are active (early or changing with findings such as an erythematous border) as these are most responsive to therapy. Chronic lesions may not require medications but may benefit from referrals to physical therapy and/or occupational therapy (if contractures or other functional impairments are present) or plastic surgery (for injection of fillers, autologous fat transfers, or other restorative procedures). Patients are commonly under the care of a dermatologist, but a rheumatologist may be asked to co-manage when systemic therapies are considered.

Topical therapies, intralesional steroids, and phototherapy can be used as initial treatment in patients with superficial diseases that do not extend beyond the dermis. Oral prednisone may be considered in patients with generalized and deep forms of morphea (particularly if EF overlaps) as well as those with linear disease (especially if concern for potential contracture or growth limitation) or circumscribed forms that progress despite topical approaches. Methotrexate and mycophenolate mofetil have the best data among immunosuppressive medications and are often used as steroid-sparing agents (these medications are also often used as first-line therapy). Additional medications have less supporting data.

7. What is Parry–Romberg syndrome and what is its potential relation to linear scleroderma?

Parry–Romberg syndrome is the term given to progressive hemifacial atrophy. It typically affects children and adolescents, with tissue atrophy involving layers that can extend from the skin down to subcutaneous fat, muscle, and bone. Skin fibrosis may be absent among many patients with progressive hemifacial atrophy, but up to 40% have concurrent linear scleroderma (*en coup de sabre* variant), thus raising speculation that the two conditions may represent a spectrum of the same disease. This is a controversial area, as data are limited. The two conditions share a similar age of onset, can be associated with similar neurologic and ophthalmologic sequelae, and coexist in 40% of patients with hemifacial atrophy. Furthermore, there are case reports of patients with *en coup de sabre* progressing to hemifacial atrophy, and 30% to 40% of patients with Parry–Romberg syndrome will have findings of localized scleroderma outside the face. Despite these commonalities, the majority of patients with Parry–Romberg syndrome have no history of cutaneous sclerosis, and the extent of atrophy often extends to the maxillary, oral, and mandibular areas (sites less commonly involved by *en coup de sabre*).

SCLEREDEMA AND SCLEROMYXEDEMA

8. What is scleredema?

Scleredema is characterized by firm, nonpitting skin edema that typically begins on the neck and upper back and spreads to the shoulders and trunk. The face and extremities (typically upper) can also be involved. The hands and feet are usually spared. The onset of skin involvement can be abrupt. Skin biopsy typically shows normal epidermis but thickened dermis with broad bands of collagen that appear separated on histology due to mucin deposition between the collagen bundles. There are three subtypes of scleredema based on the underlying cause:

- **Type I:** scleredema adultorum (scleredema of Buschke) and scleredema neonatorum follow an infection or febrile illness, with resolution typically occurring over months. Female predominance (2:1) with age of onset commonly <20 years.
- **Type II:** scleredema with no preceding febrile illness and a slow, progressive course. There is a female predominance (2:1). Frequently associated with paraproteinemia (most commonly IgG, IgA). Progression to multiple myeloma has been reported in 25% to 45% of patients.
- **Type III:** scleredema diabeticorum occurs in association with poorly controlled diabetes mellitus (type I or II). There is a male predominance (10:1), and prevalence of 2% to 10% has been reported among patients with diabetes.

Although there is no consistently effective therapy, Type I scleredema may be mild and self-limiting, and therefore treatment may not be necessary. In patients with protracted courses with symptomatic lesions and/or functional impairment, ultraviolet A1 (UVA1) phototherapy has been effective in case reports and represents the first-line therapy. Additional agents that have been tried in scleredema with variable success include cyclosporine, methotrexate, and tamoxifen. Diabetes-related (Type III) scleredema may improve with better blood sugar control.

9. What is scleromyxedema?

Scleromyxedema (papular mucinosis) is characterized by a wide-spread eruption of small (2–3 mm), nonpruritic, waxy papules on the face, neck, upper trunk, distal forearms, and dorsal surface of the hands (sparing the palms). Patients characteristically have skin changes around the forehead and ears, and involvement of these areas should prompt consideration for this condition. However, otherwise, it is a distribution that is nearly identical to systemic sclerosis and in some areas (like the fingers) may be very difficult to distinguish from systemic sclerosis. The disease is also systemic and is associated with near-universal presence of monoclonal gammopathy (IgG, both lambda and kappa). Thyroid studies should be normal. The typical age of onset is 30 to 80 years, and men and women are affected equally. Skin biopsies reveal a normal epidermis, a perivascular mononuclear cell infiltrate, mucin deposition in the papillary dermis, fibroblast proliferation, and fibrosis. Extracutaneous disease can be common and also may overlap with scleroderma including joint and muscle disease, Raynaud phenomenon, and dysphagia. A severe form of neurologic involvement known as dermato-neuro syndrome consists of global CNS disturbance that may progress to seizures and coma. Of interest, the etiology of extracutaneous disease is uncertain and cannot be solely explained by excessive mucin deposition in target organs.

10. What therapy options exist for scleromyxedema?

Historically, therapies used in multiple myeloma (melphalan, cyclophosphamide) have been described with variable success in scleromyxedema, but also come with the risk of significant side effects. However, many case series have described the successful use of intravenous immunoglobulin (IVIG). Given its favorable side-effect profile in comparison with other myeloma treatment regimens, IVIG should be considered for initial therapy. Successful treatment often requires maintenance IVIG, as relapses off therapy are common. Corticosteroids and thalidomide use have also been described in case reports with some success.

EOSINOPHILIC FASCIITIS (DIFFUSE FASCIITIS WITH EOSINOPHILIA)

11. What causes eosinophilic fasciitis?

EF was first described in 1974 by Dr. Lawrence Shulman and has been called Shulman's disease. No association with ingestion of chemicals has been convincingly demonstrated. Strenuous physical exertion may precede its onset in up to 40% of patients. Notably, two similar conditions,

EMS in the United States and toxic oil syndrome in Spain have been related to toxic exposures (L-tryptophan and aniline-denatured rapeseed oil, respectively; see Question #20). Some cases of eosinophilic fasciitis have been associated with malignant and nonmalignant hematologic conditions, and there are multiple case reports of EF described after the use of immune checkpoint inhibitors.

12. Who is most commonly affected by EF?

The mean age of onset is 40 to 50 years, with a slight male predominance. EF has been more commonly reported among Caucasians. Patients with morphea may often have a component of eosinophilic fasciitis

13. What are the clinical manifestations of EF?

Disease onset is usually sudden and begins with edema and pain in the affected area, most commonly in the **extremities**. EF often spares the fingers, hands, and feet. However, in those with an EF–morphea overlap, the feet are often characteristically involved. The examination of the skin often reveals a "woody," firm texture that is deep to the dermis (a distinguishing feature from SSc), with an orange-peel appearance *(peau d'orange)*. The **groove sign** is an indentation caused by tethering of the dermis to the fascial and muscular tissue layers along the tract of superficial veins, and is best seen with elevation of the extremity. Although the induration often remains confined to the extremities, it may variably affect areas of the trunk. Inflammatory and fibrotic disease extends to the muscle and can result in a low-grade myositis with mild CPK elevation. Contractures and restricted range of motion of the digits and extremities may occur as a consequence of fascial involvement and tethering. Sclerodactyly and nail fold capillary abnormalities do not occur.

14. What laboratory and radiographic abnormalities usually occur in patients with EF?

Peripheral eosinophilia is present in 80% of untreated patients. An elevated erythrocyte sedimentation rate, high C-reactive protein, and polyclonal hypergammaglobulinemia may also be present. Aldolase is sometimes characteristically elevated. Magnetic resonance imaging (MRI) shows fascial thickening and enhancement of the fascia with gadolinium.

It is important to note that as many as 20% of patients with EF do not have peripheral eosinophilia, and other lab tests are nonspecific. As such, the diagnosis of EF is a clinical diagnosis based on characteristic skin findings and MRI. Biopsy is obtained if the diagnosis is unclear, but requires a full-thickness biopsy (skin to fascia). Biopsy may or may not demonstrate eosinophilic infiltration (usually it will not if the patient has been treated with steroids; see Question #17). Approximately 30% of patients with EF may have overlap with morphea.

15. Is eosinophilia uniformly present throughout the course of an EF patient's illness?

No. Eosinophilia is often present only during the early stages of the patient's illness and tends to decline later. The degree of eosinophilia does not closely parallel disease activity and resolves quickly with corticosteroid therapy, so it is very often not appreciated.

16. Is there any reason to expect hematologic abnormalities to be associated with EF?

Hematologic problems have been appreciated in 10% to 15% of patients with EF. Those described in a small number of patients include immune-mediated hemolytic anemia and thrombocytopenia, aplastic anemia, myelodysplasia, and lymphoproliferative diseases (multiple myeloma, lymphoma). These complications may occur at any time during the course of EF and do not correlate with the severity of disease.

17. How is the diagnosis of EF confirmed histologically?

In the right clinical context, with typical exam findings and fasciitis demonstrated by MRI, a surgical biopsy may not be required. But when the diagnosis is unclear, a full-thickness surgical skin biopsy of an involved area is required. The biopsy should include skin, subcutis, fascia, and muscle. Although inflammation and fibrosis are generally found in all layers (except for the epidermis which is normal), they are usually most intense in the subcutis and fascia. The inflammatory infiltrate consists of abundant lymphocytes, plasma cells, and histiocytes. Eosinophilic infiltration can be seen, especially early in the disease process, but is variably present and often absent if the patient has received any corticosteroids.

18. Describe the course of illness in patients with EF.

If untreated, fascial inflammation may lead to joint contractures in the affected areas. In addition, the skin that is initially indurated will frequently become bound down and develop a *peau d'orange* appearance. In some patients, the illness is self-limited with spontaneous improvement. Occasionally, complete remission can occur even after ≥2 years. Young age at onset and trunk involvement are poor prognostic signs, and many patients may have some mild residual joint restriction even with effective therapy.

19. Are any therapies effective in patients with EF?

High-dose prednisone (40–60 mg/day) often results in marked and rapid improvement in eosinophilia and gradual improvement in the fasciitis and contractures in more than 70% of treated patients. Given the potential morbidity associated with treatment delay and the improved clinical response with therapy initiation in the edematous phase of disease, clinicians should aim for early initiation of corticosteroids followed by a gradual taper over 12 to 18 months. Some patients may be refractory to prednisone therapy and require early initiation of immunosuppressive therapy, particularly if there is an overlap with morphea. Methotrexate and mycophenolate mofetil are most often used for treatment-resistant cases. Physical therapy to minimize flexion contractures is important. Strenuous physical exercise should be avoided.

EXPOSURE/TOXIN-RELATED SCLERODERMA MIMICS

20. What outbreaks of scleroderma-like diseases have occurred in the past?

There have been at least three outbreaks of a scleroderma-like illness that have occurred in the past, raising the possibility of similar outbreaks in the future. One outbreak was termed *toxic oil syndrome* and was caused by exposure to aniline-denatured rapeseed oil in Spain in 1981. This syndrome was characterized by an acute febrile illness with eosinophilia, myalgia, rash, and pulmonary edema/infiltrates, followed by skin fibrosis, joint contractures, and subsequent disability. The second outbreak was eosinophilia-myalgia syndrome, and was linked to tainted L-tryptophan that was sold as a supplement in the United States for insomnia. This syndrome was characterized by induration and thickness of the skin of the extremities, myalgias, and eosinophilia. More recently, nephrogenic systemic fibrosis (NSF; also called nephrogenic fibrosing dermopathy) was a syndrome that was causally linked to specific gadolinium-contrast agents administered during MRI scans. While not technically an outbreak, the syndrome occurred over the course of more than a decade, and then abruptly ended following system-wide changes in gadolinium administration and the development of newer contrast agents. This syndrome was characterized by indurated plaques of hyperpigmented, thickened skin. In addition, involvement of subcutaneous structures was common, resulting in severe joint contractures and disability. NSF typically occurred in patients with severe renal impairment (GFR commonly <15mL/min) at the time of the exposure. Due to modifications in the types of gadolinium used for MRI, this disease has largely vanished.

21. What is the typical course and presentation of a patient with NSF?

NSF typically presents within 2 to 4 weeks of an at-risk patient receiving gadolinium-containing contrast during MRI. Cutaneous features first involved lower extremities and then extended proximally, with predominant extremity involvement. The face and fingers were usually spared. The skin could often develop a *peau d'orange* appearance and "cobblestone" texture over the upper arms, back, and thighs. Flexion deformities of fingers, elbows, and knees were commonly disabling. Fibrosis of any visceral organ could occur. Raynaud phenomenon was not reported. Immunosuppressive therapy was largely ineffective, but physical therapy was initiated to help with contractures. Potential beneficial therapies described included UVA phototherapy, extracorporeal photopheresis, and renal transplantation.

CHRONIC GRAFT-VERSUS-HOST DISEASE

22. How common is cutaneous sclerosis among patients suffering from cGVHD?

Among patients receiving an allogeneic bone marrow transplant, 70% will develop cGVHD. Cutaneous sclerosis can be seen in 15% of patients suffering from cGVHD. Sites of skin involvement include the trunk and extremities, which differentiate it from SSc. Autoantibodies against Scl70, PM-Scl, and ANCA have been reported, but it is distinguished from primary autoimmune disorders by the recent history of the patient having undergone allogeneic bone marrow transplantation as well as absence of features commonly seen in rheumatic diseases associated with those autoantibodies.

23. What treatment options exist for patients with cGVHD with cutaneous sclerosis?

Prednisone and cyclosporine have been described in the initial management of cGVHD. Additional therapies with anecdotal evidence include phototherapy, extracorporeal photopheresis, sirolimus, imatinib, thalidomide, and rituximab. Prevention strategies aimed at reducing the risk of cGVHD include the use of antithymocyte globulin in the pretransplant period as well as cyclosporine, IVIG, and rituximab in the posttransplant period.

24. Has scleroderma or scleroderma-like disorders been described in association with immune checkpoint inhibitor (ICI) therapy?

Yes. Cases of systemic-sclerosis-like disease have been reported in patients with malignancies treated with immune checkpoint inhibitors (ICI). This appears to be much less frequent than other rheumatic disease manifestations reported after ICI. Cases in the literature describe atypical cutaneous involvement (lack of classic SSc progression, which typically starts at the digits and extends proximally), with less frequent findings of Raynaud phenomenon, as well as ANA and scleroderma-specific antibodies. Both morphea and eosinophilic fasciitis have been reported after ICI use as well.

ACKNOWLEDGMENT

The author would like to thank Drs. Puja Chitkara, Gregory Dennis, Aryeh Fischer, and Jason Kolfenbach for their contributions to this chapter in prior editions.

BIBLIOGRAPHY

Farooqi S, Mumtaz A, Arif A, et al. The clinical manifestations and efficacy of different treatments used for nephrogenic systemic fibrosis: a systematic review. *Int J Nephrol Renovasc Dis.* 2023;16:17–30.

Ferreli C, Gasparini G. Cutaneous manifestations of scleroderma and scleroderma-like disorders: a comprehensive review. *Clinic Rev Allerg Immunol.* 2017;53:306–336.

Jacobe H. Pathogenesis, clinical manifestations, and diagnosis of morphea (localized scleroderma) in adults. UpToDate; 2024.

Knobler R, Geroldinger-Simić M, Kreuter A, et al. Consensus statement on the diagnosis and treatment of sclerosing diseases of the skin, part 2: scleromyxoedema and scleroedema. *J Eur Acad Dermatol Venereol.* 2024;38(7):1281–1299.

Lipsker D, Cosnes Bessis A. Prospective evaluation of frequency of signs of systemic sclerosis in 76 patients with morphea. *Clin Exp Rheumatol.* 2015;33(4 suppl 91):S23–S25.

Macklin M, Yadav S, Jan R, et al. Checkpoint inhibitor-associated scleroderma and scleroderma mimics. *Pharmaceuticals (Basel).* 2023;16(2):259.

Mango RL, Bugdayli K, Crowson CS, et al. Baseline characteristics and long-term outcomes of eosinophilic fasciitis in 89 patients seen at a single center over 20 years. *Int J Rheum Dis.* 2020;23(2):233–239.

Mazori DR, Femia AN, Vleugels RA. Eosinophilic fasciitis: an updated review on diagnosis and treatment. *Curr Rheumatol Rep.* 2017;19:74–86.

Morgan N, Hummers L. Scleroderma mimickers. *Curr Treatm Opt Rheumatol.* 2016;2(1):69–84.

Orteu CH, Ong VH, Denton CP. Scleroderma mimics—clinical features and management. *Best Pract Res Clin Rheumatol.* 2020;34(1):101489.

Rongioletti F, Merlo G, Cinotti E, et al. Scleromyxedema: a multicenter study of characteristics, comorbidities, course and therapy in 30 patients. *J Am Acad Derm.* 2013;69:66–72.

Woolen SA, Shankar PR, Gagnier JJ, et al. Risk of nephrogenic systemic fibrosis in patients with stage 4 or 5 chronic kidney disease receiving a Group II gadolinium-based contrast agent: a systematic review and meta-analysis. *JAMA Intern Med.* 2020;180(2):223–230.

Yaqub A, Chung L. Localized cutaneous fibrosing disorders. *Rheum Dis Clin N Am.* 2013;39:347–364.

CHAPTER 19

Idiopathic Inflammatory Myopathies

Timothy Kaniecki, MD and Lisa Christopher-Stine, MD, MPH

⟫ KEY POINTS

1. Idiopathic inflammatory myopathies (IIM) are a group of heterogeneous inflammatory muscle diseases that can be further subgrouped into distinct clinical entities based on clinical presentation and myositis-specific antibody (MSA) profile. MSAs are predictive of extramuscular disease manifestations, treatment response, and prognosis.
2. Apart from inclusion body myositis (IBM), the muscle involvement of IIMs can be characterized by proximal muscle weakness, elevated serum muscle enzymes, abnormal electromyography, and abnormal muscle biopsy.
3. Antisynthetase syndrome (ASyS) is more commonly associated with interstitial lung disease (ILD), inflammatory arthritis, mechanic's hand changes, and Raynaud phenomenon. Muscle disease may be hypomyopathic or amyopathic.
4. IBM should be considered in patients aged over 50 years with both proximal and distal muscle weakness, myopathic and neuropathic features on electromyography, and poor response to immunosuppressive therapy.
5. Cancer screening is essential in all patients with adult-onset IIM, with advanced screening tools recommended for patients with high-risk phenotypes, such as positivity for anti-TIF-1γ or anti-NXP2.

1. What are the idiopathic inflammatory myopathies (IIMs)?

IIMs are a heterogeneous group of inflammatory disorders classically characterized by proximal muscle weakness, but can have additional systemic organ involvement including the skin, joints, lungs, heart, and gastrointestinal tract. These can be further characterized by myositis-specific antibodies (MSA) and myositis-associated antibodies (MAA); MSAs possess strong clinical phenotype associations and can be useful in predicting clinical manifestations, treatment response, and prognosis.

2. How are the idiopathic inflammatory myopathies (IIMs) sub-grouped?

Many classification systems have been devised for IIM, although none are universally agreed upon. Subgroups have classically been characterized by unique clinical features (muscle, skin, age of onset, etc.) although in recent years has broadened to include MSAs and histology/pathogenesis. This is an evolving field. Notable subgroups include:
- Adult-onset dermatomyositis (DM)
  - DM
  - Clinically amyopathic DM (CADM)
- Antisynthetase syndrome (ASyS)
- Immune-mediated necrotizing myopathy (IMNM)
- Overlap myositis (myositis associated with other connective tissue diseases)
- Juvenile-onset DM (JDM)
- Adult-onset polymyositis (PM)
- Inclusion body myositis (IBM)

Some classification systems add the following to the earlier list of inflammatory diseases of the muscle:
- Myositis associated with eosinophilia
- Focal myositis
- Giant cell myositis

3. What are the epidemiologic features of IIM?

- Variance of terminology used, heterogeneity of clinical presentation, and ongoing evolution of classification criteria in IIM are persistent obstacles to case identification for epidemiological studies.
- IIMs remain a rare disease group, with incidence estimated to range from 0.1 to 2 per 100,000 person-years, and prevalence ranging from 2 to 33 per 100,000.

- Incidence of adult-onset IIM increases with age, with a peak at 50 years for most subgroups (the exception being IBM, with peak incidence trending later to the early 60s).
- The female-to-male ratio is 2–3:1 for DM/PM; for overlap myositis, this increases to 8–10:1. In JDM the female-to-male ratio is closer to 1:1. Only IBM has a male predominance, reported to be 0.5–1:1.
- Ethnic and regional variance has been described but not fully characterized.

4. List the serum markers of skeletal muscle damage.

Serum markers for muscle damage include creatine phosphokinase (CPK), aldolase, myoglobin, aspartate aminotransferase (AST), alanine aminotransferase (ALT), and lactate dehydrogenase (LDH).

5. Outline the Bohan and Peter criteria for diagnosing DM/PM.

In 1975, Bohan and Peter proposed the first set of clinical and laboratory criteria to be used to diagnose DM and PM. While knowledge of IIMs has since expanded and more modern classification and diagnostic schema have taken advantage of this broadened understanding of histopathology, MSAs, and emerging clinical phenotypes, the simplicity of the Bohan and Peter criteria still makes them clinically useful. However, it should be noted that these criteria lack specificity, as these criteria may capture genetic muscle diseases, and can miss IBM.

- *Proximal motor weakness*: insidious-onset, progressive symmetric muscle weakness of the limb-girdle and anterior neck flexor muscles.
  - Other striated muscle groups such as the pharyngeal and upper esophageal muscles can be involved, leading to dysphagia and/or dysphonia. Patients are at higher risk for aspiration pneumonia and reduced nutritional intake.
  - Myocardial involvement is uncommon but can be associated with certain MSA phenotypes.
  - Pain is typically absent or minimal unless there is a significant fasciitis component.
  - IMNM is associated with more rapidly progressive muscle weakness.
  - Ocular and facial motor weakness is strikingly unusual and should make one consider alternative diagnoses, such as neuromuscular junction disorders or genetic myopathies.
- *Elevated serum muscle enzymes*: CPK is elevated in almost all patients at some point during active disease; aldolase, myoglobin, AST, ALT, and LDH are typically elevated as well. Myoglobinuria can be seen in active disease, although this rarely causes clinical rhabdomyolysis.
  - The combination of elevated CPK, aldolase, AST, and CPK muscle/brain (M/B) fraction >2–3% of total CPK is highly characteristic of an inflammatory myopathy. Notably, some IIM patients have an elevated aldolase but normal CPK (patients with this muscle enzyme pattern reportedly are more likely to have an associated cancer).
- *Characteristic electromyography (EMG)*: typically demonstrates an irritable myopathy, characterized by short and small polyphasic motor units, fibrillations, positive sharp waves, insertional irritability, and high-frequency repetitive discharges. It has good sensitivity (85%) but low specificity (33%).
  - Isolated IIM disease should not demonstrate abnormalities on simultaneous nerve conduction studies (NCS) unless there is a coexisting neuropathy. Neuropathic disease can lead to subsequent myopathic abnormalities on EMG, although an irritable myopathy is not typically seen. IBM does have an association with peripheral neuropathy.
- *Characteristic muscle biopsy*: muscle biopsy should be performed in most cases to confirm the suspected diagnosis. The histologic pattern can be helpful both diagnostically and prognostically (Fig. 19.1).
- *Characteristic cutaneous features*: skin biopsy shows interface dermatitis, usually with mucin, similar to that of systemic lupus erythematosus (SLE). The presence or lack of rash delineates DM from PM, respectively.

In patients without rash, a diagnosis of PM is defined as: definite (meeting four of the four other criteria), probable (meeting three of the four criteria), and possible (meeting two of the four criteria). In patients with rash, a diagnosis of DM was defined as: definite (meeting three of the four other criteria), probable (meeting two of the four criteria), and possible (meeting one of the four criteria).

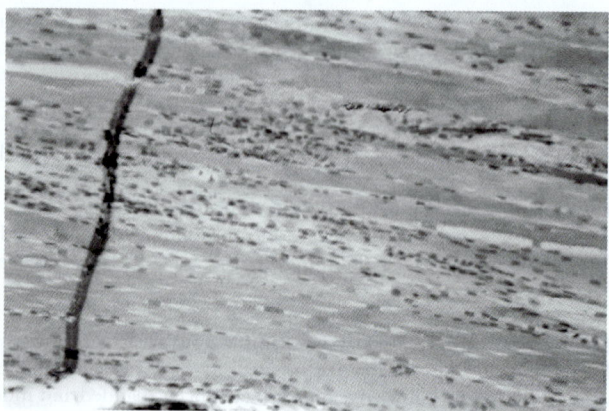

Fig. 19.1 Muscle biopsy demonstrating inflammatory infiltrate and muscle fiber necrosis in a patient with polymyositis.

6. What are other clinical features and diagnostic tests used to help support a diagnosis of IIM?

- *MSAs and MAAs*: identify clinical subsets among the major categories of IIM. Patients with IIM will only have one MSA, since they are mutually exclusive. However, MSAs and MAAs can coexist, particularly the anti-Sjogren's syndrome–related antigen A (SSA/Ro 52kD).
- *Muscle magnetic resonance imaging (MRI)*: areas of inflamed muscle demonstrate increased signal on T2-weighted images with fat suppression (short tau inversion recovery [STIR] images) but not on T1-weighted images, denoting areas of edema/inflammation (Fig. 19.2). Sensitivity is high, ranging from 96% to 100%; however, these findings are not specific and can be seen in a wide range of muscular and neurologic conditions. In chronic disease, MRI can also show fatty degeneration on T1-weighted images, which is unlikely to improve with immunosuppressive medications.
- *Extra-muscular and extra-cutaneous organ involvement*: the presence of features such as Raynaud phenomenon, inflammatory arthritis, interstitial lung disease (ILD), or constitutional symptoms (fever, night sweats, weight loss) may be useful in formulating a diagnosis of IIM, particularly within certain MSA subgroups. The range of organ involvement can have implications for treatment decisions.

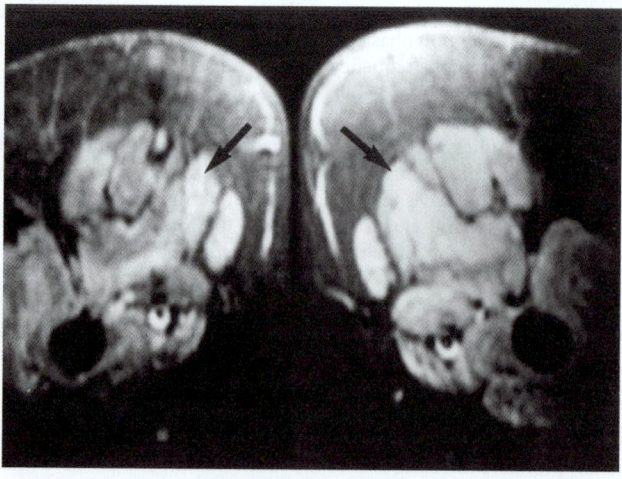

Fig. 19.2 Magnetic resonance imaging scan of a patient with polymyositis. T2-weighted images demonstrate increased signal intensity of affected muscle tissue (*arrows*).

7. Describe the dermatologic manifestations of DM.

- *Heliotrope rash (≤50% of DM patients):* purple to erythematous rash affecting the eyelids, malar region, forehead, and nasolabial folds (note that the eyelids and nasolabial folds are typically spared in the rash of acute cutaneous SLE). There can be associated orbital edema; the upper eyelids are most commonly affected. The tip of the nose is typically spared.
- *Gottron's papules (60–80% of DM patients):* purple to erythematous macules or papules on the dorsal and lateral surfaces of the hands and fingers, extending linearly along the extensor tendon sheaths, most pronounced over the metacarpophalangeal and interphalangeal joints. There can be associated skin desquamation. This can also occur over the extensor surfaces of the wrists, elbows, and knees (referred to in this instance as Gottron's sign).
- *V-sign rash:* confluent macular erythematous rash over the anterior chest and neck.
- *Shawl-sign rash:* erythematous macular rash over the shoulders and proximal arms.
- *Holster-sign rash:* erythematous rash over the lateral aspect of the proximal thighs.
- *Nailfold abnormalities:* periungual erythema, cuticular overgrowth, and/or dilated capillary loops with hemorrhagic infarcts. This can occur independently of the presence of Raynaud phenomenon.
- *Scalp involvement:* atrophic, erythematous, and scaly plaques. This can often be confused with seborrheic dermatitis or scalp psoriasis. Lesions are often pruritic.
- *Photosensitivity:* common with the rashes mentioned above.
- *Subcutaneous calcification:* seen most commonly in JDM but can occur in adult-onset disease; can be very extensive. Calcinosis located on extensor surfaces or pressure points may be prone to ulceration, leading to difficult-to-heal chronic ulcers.
- *Poikiloderma:* hypo- or hyperpigmentation of the skin, associated with telangiectasia and atrophy, can be representative of chronic skin damage. This more commonly affects regions of high UV light exposure (upper chest, upper back, upper extremities).

PEARL: a patient with proximal muscle weakness, elevated muscle enzymes, and the characteristic rash of DM rarely needs a muscle biopsy to confirm the diagnosis.

8. What conditions may mimic the cutaneous features of DM?

The interface dermatitis seen on DM skin biopsy is indistinguishable from that of acute cutaneous SLE. Other disorders that may clinically mimic cutaneous DM include trichinosis, allergic contact dermatitis, and drug reactions (the most common being hydroxyurea, penicillamine, diclofenac, and anti-tumor necrosis factor agents).

9. What measures can be taken to maximize muscle biopsy yield?

- Biopsy a muscle that is clearly weak, but not severely so.
- Biopsy the muscle contralateral to the one that is abnormal by EMG (i.e., perform neurodiagnostic studies unilaterally, and biopsy the contralateral side based on EMG results). Do not biopsy a muscle that has undergone recent (<2–4 weeks) EMG evaluation to avoid spurious results from EMG artifact.
- Do not biopsy a muscle within 3 months of an episode of rhabdomyolysis.
- MRI scan of the muscle can also be helpful to direct the location of muscle biopsy.

10. List the characteristic clinical features of adult-onset DM.

- Both muscle and cutaneous disease can independently present as the first manifestation of DM, or can present concurrently.
- Muscle involvement: 70% of cases have elevated serum muscle enzymes (see Question 4); with the remainder of cases classified as CADM (normal serum muscle enzymes) or hypomyopathic DM (normal CPK, but elevated aldolase and/or abnormal muscle MRI).
- MSAs are found in 50–70% of cases and help identify clinical subsets.
- Muscle pathology: perivascular and perimysial inflammatory cell infiltrate consisting of lymphocytes (CD4+ T cells and B cells), macrophages, and plamacytoid dendritic cells, with perifascicular MHC-I expression and membrane attack complex (MAC) complement deposition on small blood vessels, with reduced capillary numbers. Over 50% have perifascicular atrophy.

11. Describe the MSAs associated with adult-onset DM and their associated clinical phenotypes.

- *Anti-Mi-2 (nucleosome remodeling deacetylase complex)*: In 4–20% of cases, classic DM pheno-type with high CPK levels, muscle weakness, and characteristic cutaneous involvement. No association with malignancy or ILD. Generally responsive to treatment with a good prognosis, although relapses are common. Associated with positive antinuclear antibody (ANA) with a speckled pattern. The MSA targets the chromodomain helicase DNA-binding protein, which is part of the nucleosome remodeling deacetylase complex that participates in the remodeling of chromatin by deacetylating histones.

- *Anti-MDA-5 (melanoma differentiation-associated gene 5)*: 13–30% of cases overall, with a stronger incidence in Asian DM patients (10–50%). Associated with cutaneous disease with or without ulcerations, distinct palmar papules, arthritis, fevers, and ILD (which can be rapidly progressive). Classically thought of as CADM, however mild muscle disease or hypo-myopathic DM can occur. ANA is typically negative but can show a cytoplasmic pattern. This MSA targets the MDA-5 protein which is a cytoplasmic RNA helicase that has an important role in the innate immune system response during RNA viral infections. Recent cohort studies have supported the separation of anti-MDA-5 DM cases into three distinct clinical phenotype clusters, which continue to be further defined.
  - A rapidly-progressive ILD cluster, associated with minimal cutaneous and muscle disease, but markedly elevated inflammatory markers and high-titer anti-Ro52 antibodies. The prognosis is poor and aggressive treatment is typically warranted. More common in patients of Asian background.
  - An arthralgia/arthritis cluster, associated with milder ILD but more prominent cutaneous and articular disease. Anti-Ro52 antibodies and Raynaud phenomenon can also be seen, with less significant inflammatory marker elevation. Prognosis is improved relative to the rapidly-progressive ILD cluster.
  - An ulcerative cutaneous disease cluster, associated with severe cutaneous disease compli-cated by ulcerations, can have more significant muscle disease, but minimal ILD. Male sex and the presence of Raynaud phenomenon appear to be protective. Best prognosis of the three clusters.

- *Anti-TIF-1γ (transcriptional intermediator factor 1, also described as p155/140)*: 10%-20% of cases, are associated with relatively mild muscle disease (although dysphagia is common and can be severe), and generally more extensive cutaneous disease. A well-demarcated, erythematous ovoid patch on the posterior hard palate is a diagnostic clue seen in up to 40% of patients. More extensive periorbital edema has also been noted. In adult-onset DM, there is a strong association with malignancy; the sensitivity for diagnosing cancer-associated DM is 78%, with a specificity of 89% (positive and negative predictive values of 58% and 95%, respectively). ANA is positive with a speckled pattern. This MSA targets the TIF-1γ protein, which belongs to a family of TIF-1 proteins that are interferon-responsive and play both posi-tive and negative roles in carcinogenesis, including regulation of the tumor suppressor p53.

- *Anti-NXP2 (nuclear matrix protein 2, previously known as MJ or p140)*: 3–24% of cases, are associated with prominent muscle disease but only modest cutaneous disease. More specific features can include involvement of the finger extensor muscles, as well as peripheral subcu-taneous edema. May have fingertip ulcerations, and subcutaneous calcifications are common. In adult-onset disease, this is associated with underlying malignancy. ANA is positive with a speckled or nuclear multiple dots pattern.

- *Anti-SAE (small ubiquitin-like modifier-1 activating enzyme, also known as SUMO)*: <10% of cases, cutaneous disease usually precedes muscle disease and is more severe. Dysphagia is com-mon and there may be a component of mild ILD. An association with malignancy, particu-larly in Asian populations, has been reported. ANA is positive with a speckled pattern.

12. What is clinically amyotrophic DM (CADM)? What is DM sine dermatitis?

- Occasionally, the cutaneous manifestations of DM occur in the absence of clinically apparent muscle involvement, referred to as CADM. Perhaps half or more of such patients will develop muscle disease over time, but a significant proportion manifest with skin-limited disease. This form can be associated with malignancy (such as in anti-TIF-1γ and NXP2). Other patients will still develop extra-muscular manifestations like ILD (such as anti-MDA-5).

- In rare cases, patients can present with an IIM that on muscle biopsy looks like DM (see Question 10) but has no skin manifestations. This is referred to as DM sine dermatitis. These patients can have characteristic DM MSAs.

13. List the characteristic clinical features of ASyS

- *Muscle disease*: when present, myositis usually manifests first. CPK values typically range 5 to10 times above the upper limit of normal.
    - Muscle pathology: scattered perimysial infiltrate of CD68+, CD4+, and CD8+ cells, with an edematous or fragmented perimysium that stains with alkaline phosphatase, with or without perifascicular myofiber necrosis. Perifascicular MHC-I expression is seen, but minimal complement deposition. HLA-DRβ1*0301 is more common in these patients.
- *Cutaneous disease:* cracking and fissuring of the skin of the finger pads (radial side) and plantar feet are common, labeled as **mechanic's hands** and **hiker's feet**, respectively. Some patients may have a DM-like rash, although this is less common.
- *Lung disease*: ILD is the most frequent manifestation of ASyS, which is chronic and commonly progressive. The most common pattern is nonspecific interstitial pneumonia (NSIP) with a bibasilar lobe predominance.
- *Other manifestations*: fevers, arthralgias/arthritis, and Raynaud phenomenon can also occur with all MSA subtypes. There is a rare association with malignancy in older patients.
- *Antisynthetase antibodies*: MSAs that bind to and inhibit aminoacyl-tRNA synthetases, which normally facilitate amino acid binding to its cognate tRNA. These can be used to identify distinct clinical subsets. ANA is positive with a cytoplasmic speckled pattern. Concurrent anti-Ro52 positivity is associated with worse disease.

14. Describe the MSAs associated with ASyS and their associated clinical phenotypes.

- *Anti-Jo-1 (histidyl tRNA synthetase)*: the most common MSA for ASyS, seen in 15–30% of IIM cases, and typically presents with a triad of myositis, ILD, and arthritis. Prognosis relative to other ASyS antibodies is better; however, this may be attributable to earlier diagnosis rates given symptomatic arthritis.
- *Anti-PL-7 (threonyl tRNA synthetase)*: 5-10% of cases, with ILD as the most common manifestation; this can be an isolated finding. Myositis and arthritis are less common, and when present typically occur later in the disease course. Association with pericardial effusion and pericarditis has been described.
- *Anti-PL-12 (alanyl tRNA synthetase)*: <5% of cases, associated with a more severe form of ILD, and is typically isolated. More commonly seen in black women. Pulmonary hypertension has been described, although whether this manifestation is a consequence of progressive ILD versus an isolated primary phenomenon is not fully characterized at this time.
- *Anti-EJ (glycyl tRNA synthetase)*: <2% of cases, ILD is the initial presenting symptom, with later-onset myositis. Arthritis can occur but is less common.
- *Anti-OJ (isoleucyl tRNA synthetase)*: <2% of cases, typically presents with isolated ILD, however, when present the myositis is typically more severe, demonstrating higher CPK levels and increased muscle necrosis on biopsy.
- Other anti-tRNA synthetases (Ha, Zo, KS, Mas, lysyl, Ly, valyl) have been described in a few patients.

15. List the characteristic clinical features of immune-mediated necrotizing myopathy (IMNM).

- *Muscle disease*: the most predominant feature, characterized by more rapid-onset progressive proximal muscle weakness (typically presenting acutely to sub-acutely), with marked CPK elevations (>10-50 times the upper limit of normal), and myalgias.
    - *Muscle pathology*: prominent scattered necrosis of muscle fibers with varying stages of myophagocytosis and regeneration, endomysial fibrosis, and proliferation. Inflammatory infiltrate is uncommon, but if seen is typically composed of paucilymphocytic macrophages. MHC-I staining is diffuse but can be very faint. Complement deposition is sarcolemmal or on small blood vessels. There is a strong association with HLA-DRB1*11:01, particularly with anti-HMGCR antibodies.

PEARL: while characteristic, necrosis on muscle biopsy is not specific for IMNM and can be seen less commonly in other IIM subgroups, including DM and ASyS.

- *Other manifestations*: ILD and cardiac involvement can be seen in cases with positive anti-SRP; rash and arthritis are not typically seen. IMNM is rarely associated with malignancy, HIV infection, or other overlap connective tissue disease.
- MSAs are found in 80% of cases. These antibody titers have been found to correlate with levels of disease activity, suggesting a direct pathologic role.

16. Describe the MSAs associated with IMNM and their associated clinical phenotypes.

- *Anti-SRP (signal recognition particle)*: 5–15% of IIM cases, tend to have the more severe phenotype within IMNM. Severe muscle disease is typically very acute and can be associated with significant muscle pain (due to fiber necrosis) and severe muscle atrophy. Associated dysphagia, myocarditis, ILD, and inflammatory arthritis have been described. ANA may be positive with a cytoplasmic speckled pattern. This MSA targets a 54-kDA protein in a RNA complex involved with intracytoplasmic protein translocation.
- *Anti-HMGCR (3-hydroxyl-3methylglutaryl-coenzyme reductase; 200/100 kDa)*: 6–10% of cases, typically present as severe isolated muscle disease. Scapular winging has been described in rare cases. Prior statin exposure is seen in 15–65% of cases, and confirmation of the diagnosis warrants lifelong avoidance of this medication class (natural statin-like compounds in foods should also be avoided, like those found in red yeast rice and certain mushrooms). ANA is typically negative. This MSA targets the HMGCR enzyme, which converts HMG-CoA to mevalonic acid as a part of the cholesterol synthesis pathway.

PEARL: anti-HMGCR positivity can discriminate direct statin muscle toxicity from IIM; the former diagnosis may allow for a retrial of an alternative medication within the statin family.

17. List the characteristic clinical features of adult-onset PM.

- The discovery and characterization of other IIM subgroups and MSAs have led to an overall reduced prevalence of PM, with most patients now being classified as ASyS, IMNM, CADM, IBM, or genetic muscle disease.
- *Muscle involvement*: presents with proximal muscle weakness and elevated serum muscle enzymes.
- *Muscle pathology*: inflammatory infiltrate is endomysial with T cells surrounding non-necrotic muscle fibers; degeneration, necrosis, and regeneration are seen. There is a diffuse distribution of MHC-I expression and no rimmed vacuoles.

18. What are some MAAs associated with CTD-overlap myositis?

- The most common overlap is myositis associated with systemic sclerosis. MAAs seen include anti-PM-Scl, U1-RNP (ribonucleoprotein), Ku, and U3-RNP.
- Other CTDs such as SLE, Sjogren's Syndrome, and mixed connective tissue disease (MCTD) can also be seen in overlap myositis. MAAs seen include anti-U1-RNP, SSA/Ro (52kD), and SSB/La.

19. List the characteristic clinical features of IBM.

- *Muscle disease*: characterized by insidious asymmetrical weakness that is painless and involves both the proximal and distal muscle groups, frequently including the quadriceps and long finger flexors. Axial involvement can lead to bent forward posture of the spine. Dysphagia is seen in >50% of cases. Muscle atrophy is prominent and can lead to a predisposition to falls. Muscle disease progression is the slowest amongst the IIMs with active muscle involvement, with decline occurring over several years on average.
  - Serum CPK values may be mildly elevated or normalized; almost always <1000 U/L.
  - EMG can show both myopathic and neuropathic changes.

- *Muscle pathology*: endomysial inflammatory infiltrate (primarily CD8+ T-cells) surrounding and/or invading non-necrotic muscle fibers, with a diffuse distribution of MHC-I expression. The key finding of **rimmed vacuoles** within myofibers may be missing in 20–40% of biopsies. Red ragged and cytochrome oxidase-negative fibers may also be seen.
- *Extra-muscular organ involvement*: can be associated with other CTDs, particularly Sjogren's syndrome. Otherwise, IBM is typically isolated to the skeletal muscles.
- *MAA*: anti-cN-1A (cytosolic 5'-nucleotidase 1A) can be positive in patients with IBM (4–21% of cases). This MAA is also associated with primary Sjogren's Syndrome and SLE. When not associated with an overlapping CTD, the ANA is typically negative.

20. How does IBM differ from other IIMs?

Incidence increases with age, with IBM being the most common IIM above 50 years. IBM is the only IIM more common in males. The pattern of muscle involvement, with the involvement of distal muscle groups and frequently asymmetric initial presentation, distinguishes IBM from other IIMs. Patients may endorse difficulties with fine motor tasks, axial maneuvers (such as turning over in bed), and intermittent falls, which are not typical for other IIMs. Response to immunosuppressive therapies is poor.

21. How does juvenile-onset IIM differ from adult-onset IIM (see Chapter 69)?

95% of cases can be classified as JDM; 65% have a corresponding MSA. Unlike adult-onset DM, there is no increased malignancy risk. There is a higher prevalence of calcinosis and gastrointestinal infarcts. ASyS and IMNM are rare but have been described. Genetic muscle diseases such as muscular dystrophies should be ruled out.

22. Is there an association between IIM and underlying neoplastic disease?

An increased risk for associated malignancy has been well-described for IIM, although this risk correlates with specific MSA profiles. In general, the incidence of malignancy in DM ranges from 5.5–42%, with a 4.66-fold increased risk relative to the general population. This is sometimes referred to as having cancer-associated myositis. Malignancy is present typically at myositis onset or within the first year (68%), and almost always occurs within 3 years of myositis onset. Risk increases with age, particularly if disease onset is >40 years. The most commonly reported malignancies are typically hematologic or lymphatic in origin, followed by adenocarcinomas (lung, ovary, breast, pancreas, stomach, colon, nasopharyngeal, cervical, and prostate).

23. What MSAs are associated with malignancy?

Anti-TIF-1γ and NXP2 have the strongest association with malignancy when seen in adult-onset DM; notably these specific antibody-malignancy associations have not been seen in JDM. A weaker association with malignancy and anti-SAE, Mi-2, MDA5, and HMGCR has been described. Notably, both anti-SRP and the antisynthetase antibodies have a negative association with malignancy.

PEARL: Ulcerative skin lesions in adult-onset DM patients are highly associated with an underlying malignancy.

---

24. How should patients with high-risk MSAs be screened for malignancy?

The International Myositis Assessment and Clinical Studies Group (IMACS) recently published evidence-based guidelines for malignancy screening in IIM. Their recommendations involve risk-stratification of patients based on positive risk factors for malignancy (such as certain autoantibody profiles described in Question 23, later age of disease onset, dysphagia, and persistently high disease activity despite immunosuppression) and negative risk factors (lower risk autoantibodies, presence of Raynaud phenomenon, inflammatory arthritis, or ILD). All patients, regardless of risk factors, should at baseline continue age- and sex-appropriate cancer screenings as directed by their regional/national guiding body.

Enhanced cancer screenings are recommended for "high-risk" disease phenotypes, which include full-body CT scan (neck, thorax, abdomen, and pelvis), cervical cancer screening,

TABLE 19.1 Differential Diagnosis of Myopathies

NEUROMUSCULAR DISORDERS	INFECTIOUS MYOSITIS
Muscular dystrophies (e.g., Duchenne's) Neuromuscular junction disorders (e.g., myasthenia gravis, Eaton–Lambert syndrome) Denervating conditions (e.g., amyotrophic lateral sclerosis)	Bacterial (*Staphylococcus, Streptococcus, Borrelia burgdorferi*) Viral (e.g., HIV, adenovirus, influenza) Parasitic (e.g., *Toxoplasma, Trichinella, Taenia*)
Endocrine disorders Hypothyroidism (may see CK as high as 3000) Hyperthyroidism Acromegaly Cushing's disease Addison's disease **Miscellaneous** Sarcoidosis Other rheumatic disorders (e.g., polymyalgia rheumatica, fibromyalgia syndrome, inflammatory arthritides, vasculitis) Carcinomatous neuromyopathy Organ failure (uremia, liver failure) Amyloidosis Acute rhabdomyolysis	**Metabolic myopathies** Glycogen storage diseases (e.g., McArdle's or myophosphorylase deficiency, acid maltase deficiency) Abnormalities of lipid metabolism (e.g., carnitine deficiency, carnitine palmitoyl transferase deficiency) Mitochondrial myopathies Nutritional disorders (malabsorption, vitamin D and E deficiencies) Electrolyte disorders (hypocalcemia and hypercalcemia, hypokalemia, hypophosphatemia) **Drug- and toxin-induced myopathies** Statins, interferon-α, d-penicillamine, colchicine, amiodarone, antimalarials, ZDV/AZT (zidovudine), alcohol, glucocorticoids, cocaine, antifungals, anti-tumor necrosis factor inhibitors

mammography, pelvic or transvaginal ultrasound (for ovarian cancer), fecal occult blood testing, and serum tumor markers [specifically, prostate-specific antigen (PSA) and CA-125]. This should be done in addition to "standard-risk" screenings, which include evaluation of blood counts, liver and renal function panels, inflammatory markers, urinalysis, plain chest radiograph, and serum immunoglobulins (with serum protein electrophoresis and free light chains). An additional conditional recommendation was made for 18F-FDG PET-CT body scan in "high-risk" patients without malignancy detected by the aforementioned screening tests, particularly patients with a positive Anti-TIF-1γ.

25. When should patients with IIM complete cancer screenings?

All screening tests should be pursued at the time of diagnosis, regardless of underlying risk factors. For high-risk patients, the IMACS recommends repeating the "standard-risk" screening tests annually for three years (see Question 24), in addition to the complete initial screening at diagnosis.

26. What conditions should be considered in the differential diagnosis of inflammatory myopathies?

See Table 19.1 for full differential diagnosis. It is crucial to rule out other treatable causes of muscle weakness that may be confused with IIM. All patients should be screened for drugs and infections that may affect the muscles. Endocrinopathies such as thyroid disease, hypothalamic-pituitary-adrenal axis dysfunction, and calcium dysregulation should be evaluated. Features that are atypical for IIM and should prompt evaluation for other etiologies of muscle weakness include slow onset of symptoms over years (aside from IBM), severe muscle cramping associated with exercise, facial/ocular muscle weakness, early-onset respiratory or distal muscle weakness, additional neurologic symptoms, and lack of other extra-muscular manifestations in a patient with negative MSA evaluation (i.e. no rash, ILD, Raynaud, etc.). A family history of muscle disease should also prompt evaluation for genetic myopathies. Finally, an elevated CPK (<1000 U/L) with a normal aldolase in an asymptomatic black patient is usually a normal variant.

27. What is the approach to the treatment of IIM?

- Treatment of IIM is complex and multifaceted, with therapeutic decisions based on a combination of disease severity, MSA/MAA profile, specific organ involvement, and co-morbidities. There presently are no comprehensive consensus-driven guidelines, due to lack of robust clinical trials and heterogeneity of the disease.
- *Corticosteroids*: these remain the mainstay of initial therapy as clinical studies have demonstrated these agents improve serum muscle enzyme levels and muscle strength; however, chronic and/or singular use of steroids should be avoided, since monotherapy is associated with high flare rates and low remission rates, and chronic use is associated with many adverse events. Conventional dosing in practice typically ranges from 0.5 to 1.0 mg/kg of prednisone equivalent daily, followed by a prolonged taper over several months. Pulse IV steroids are sometimes considered in patients were severe disease manifestations (such as rapidly-progressive ILD).
  - *Repository Corticotrophin Injection (RCI)*: a combination of ACTH and other pro-opiomelanocortin peptide injection that targets melanocortin receptors through steroid-dependent and steroid-independent mechanisms, it has been shown to improve DM/PM disease activity in small, short-term observational and open-label studies. It is FDA approved and has a lower side effect profile but lacks randomized controlled trial data and is expensive. This medication is not available outside of the United States and is very expensive.
- *Traditional immunosuppressive agents*: methotrexate (MTX, up to 25 mg/wk orally or subcutaneously) or azathioprine (AZA, up to 2–3 mg/kg/day) are frequently used in combination with corticosteroids as first-line therapy. There has been increased use of mycophenolate mofetil (MMF, up to 1000–1500 mg twice daily) or calcineurin inhibitors (such as cyclosporine and tacrolimus) in recent years, particularly in patients with concurrent ILD. These agents can take several months to reach full therapeutic effect. Cyclophosphamide is rarely used, typically reserved for severe cases with rapidly progressive ILD or vasculitis. Combination immunosuppressive agents are sometimes used in refractory cases.
- *Intravenous Immunoglobulin (IVIG)*: an anti-inflammatory and immuno-modulatory therapy used for the treatment of dermatomyositis. Octagam brand IVIG is the first IVIG formulation FDA-approved, following a positive randomized control clinical trial. Dosed at 2 g/kg/month in a divided dose (over 2–5 days), it typically requires up to six months to achieve full therapeutic benefit. It is helpful in treating muscle, skin, and lung disease. While it has the benefit of not being immunosuppressive, side effect profile includes increased risk for thromboembolic events, acute kidney injury, and aseptic meningitis.
- *Rituximab*: a biologic CD20+ B cell-depleting agent that has demonstrated safety and efficacy in patients with refractory disease; while a large randomized clinical trial failed to meet its primary endpoint, a majority of patients showed clinical improvement in muscle and skin disease, as well as corticosteroid dose reduction. It also has been increasingly used in myositis-associated ILD. Typical dosing is an initial 1000 mg on days 1 and 15, followed by repeat dosing every 6 months.

> **PEARL:** rituximab has been shown to be of significant clinical benefit in anti-SRP IMNM, in which serology titers appear to correlate with disease activity.

- *Exercise and physical therapy*: strength training and rehabilitation should begin early in the treatment course and should be advocated for in all patients with IIM. This has been shown to improve functioning and quality of life.
- Many other immunosuppressive agents are currently under investigation, including abatacept, anifrolumab, apremilast, tocilizumab, and tofacitinib.

28. How do you separate steroid myopathy from persistent IIM disease activity?

Patients with IIM that initially responded to corticosteroids may later complain of weakness while maintained on these drugs, particularly when at a dose of >20 mg/day prednisone equivalent. Steroid myopathy is a process of type IIb muscle fiber atrophy and does not cause an elevated CPK or aldolase. Muscle MRI with STIR images may be helpful in distinguishing active inflammation from atrophy.

ACKNOWLEDGMENT

The authors would like to thank Sterling G. West, MD, for his contributions to this chapter in the previous edition.

BIBLIOGRAPHY

Abel A, Lazaro E, Ralazamahaleo M, et al. Phenotypic profiles among 72 caucasian and afro-caribbean patients with antisynthetase syndrome involving anti-PL7 or anti-PL12 autoantibodies. *Eur J Intern Med.* 2023;115:104–113.

Aggarwal R, Charles-Schoeman C, Schessl J, et al. Trial of intravenous immune globulin in dermatomyositis. *N Engl J Med.* 2022;387:1264–1278.

Alexanderson H, Boström C. Exercise therapy in patients with idiopathic inflammatory myopathies and systemic lupus erythematosus—a systematic literature review. *Best Pract Res Clin Rheumatol.* 2020;34:101547.

Allenbach Y, Benveniste O, Stenzel W, Boyer O. Immune-mediated necrotizing myopathy: clinical features and pathogenesis. *Nat Rev Rheumatol.* 2020;16:689–701.

Allenbach Y, Mammen AL, Benveniste O, Stenzel W. Immune-Mediated Necrotizing Myopathies Working Group. 224th ENMC international workshop: Clinico-sero-pathological classification of immune-mediated necrotizing myopathies. Zandvoort, the Netherlands, 14–16 October 2016. *Neuromuscul Disord.* 2018;28:87–99.

Allenbach Y, Uzunhan Y, Toquet S, et al. Different phenotypes in dermatomyositis associated with anti-MDA5 antibody: study of 121 cases. *Neurology.* 2020;95:e70–e78.

Bohan A, Peter JB. Polymyositis and dermatomyositis (first of two parts). *N Engl J Med.* 1975;292:344–347.

Bohan A, Peter JB. Polymyositis and dermatomyositis (second of two parts). *N Engl J Med.* 1975;292:403–407.

Cavagna L, Trallero-Araguás E, Meloni F, et al. Influence of antisynthetase antibodies specificities on antisynthetase syndrome clinical spectrum time course. *J Clin Med.* 2019;8(11):2013.

Chandra T, Aggarwal R. Clinical trials and novel therapeutics in dermatomyositis. *Expert Opin Emerg Drugs.* 2020;25:213–228.

Cox JT, Gullotti DM, Mecoli CA, et al. "Hiker's feet': a novel cutaneous finding in the inflammatory myopathies. *Clin Rheumatol.* 2017;36(7):1683–1686. doi:10.1007/s10067-017-3598-5.

Goyal NA. Inclusion body myositis. *Continuum (Minneap Minn).* 2022;28:1663–1677.

Khoo T, Lilleker JB, Thong BY, Leclair V, Lamb JA, Chinoy H. Epidemiology of the idiopathic inflammatory myopathies. *Nat Rev Rheumatol.* 2023;19:695–712.

Lundberg IE, Fujimoto M, Vencovsky J, et al. Idiopathic inflammatory myopathies. *Nat Rev Dis Primers.* 2021;7:86.

Lundberg IE, Tjärnlund A, Bottai M, et al. 2017 European League Against Rheumatism/American College of Rheumatology classification criteria for adult and juvenile idiopathic inflammatory myopathies and their major subgroups. *Ann Rheum Dis.* 2017;76:1955–1964.

Mainetti C, Terziroli Beretta-Piccoli B, Selmi C. Cutaneous manifestations of dermatomyositis: a comprehensive review. *Clin Rev Allergy Immunol.* 2017;53:337–356.

Marco JL, Collins BF. Clinical manifestations and treatment of antisynthetase syndrome. *Best Pract Res Clin Rheumatol.* 2020;34:101503.

Marzęcka M, Niemczyk A, Rudnicka L. Autoantibody markers of increased risk of malignancy in patients with dermatomyositis. *Clin Rev Allergy Immunol.* 2022;63:289–296.

Oldroyd AGS, Callen JP, Chinoy H, et al. International guideline for idiopathic inflammatory myopathy-associated cancer screening: an international myositis assessment and clinical studies group (IMACS) initiative. *Nat Rev Rheumatol.* 2023;19:805–817.

Pinal-Fernandez I, Casciola-Rosen LA, Christopher-Stine L, Corse AM, Mammen AL. The prevalence of individual histopathologic features varies according to autoantibody status in muscle biopsies from patients with dermatomyositis. *J Rheumatol.* 2015;42:1448–1454.

Rosow LK, Amato AA. The role of electrodiagnostic testing, imaging, and muscle biopsy in the investigation of muscle disease. *Continuum (Minneap Minn).* 2016;22:1787–1802.

Sasaki H, Kohsaka H. Current diagnosis and treatment of polymyositis and dermatomyositis. *Mod Rheumatol.* 2018;28:913–921.

Trallero-Araguás E, Rodrigo-Pendás JÁ, Selva-O'Callaghan A, et al. Usefulness of anti-p155 autoantibody for diagnosing cancer-associated dermatomyositis: a systematic review and meta-analysis. *Arthritis Rheum.* 2012;64:523–532.

Xu L, You H, Wang L, et al. Identification of three different phenotypes in anti-melanoma differentiation-associated gene 5 antibody-positive dermatomyositis patients: implications for prediction of rapidly progressive interstitial lung disease. *Arthritis Rheumatol.* 2023;75:609–619.

CHAPTER 20

Mixed Connective Tissue Disease, Overlap Syndromes, and Undifferentiated Connective Tissue Disease

Nathaniel J. Harris, MD, PhD and David L. Leverenz, MD, MEd

 KEY POINTS

1. Mixed connective tissue disease (MCTD) may present with manifestations seen in systemic lupus erythematosus (SLE), systemic sclerosis (SSc), and idiopathic inflammatory myopathies (IIM) and is associated with high-titer speckled antinuclear antibodies (ANAs) and uridine-rich ribonucleoprotein (U1-RNP) antibodies.
2. The absence of Raynaud phenomenon or a high titer U1-RNP should suggest a disease other than MCTD.
3. Pulmonary arterial hypertension (PAH) and interstitial lung disease (ILD) are major causes of mortality in patients with MCTD.
4. Roughly 25% of patients presenting with features of a rheumatologic disease do not fulfill criteria for a defined disorder.
5. Approximately 25% of patients with undifferentiated connective tissue disease (UCTD) evolve into a more specific diagnosis over time.

1. **What is the difference between MCTD, overlap syndrome, and UCTD?**
   - **MCTD:** first described by Sharp et al. in 1972, MCTD refers to a specific overlap syndrome characterized by a combination of manifestations seen in SLE, SSc, and idiopathic inflammatory myopathies (see Fig. 20.1). The autoantibody pattern is a high-titer, speckled ANA, and

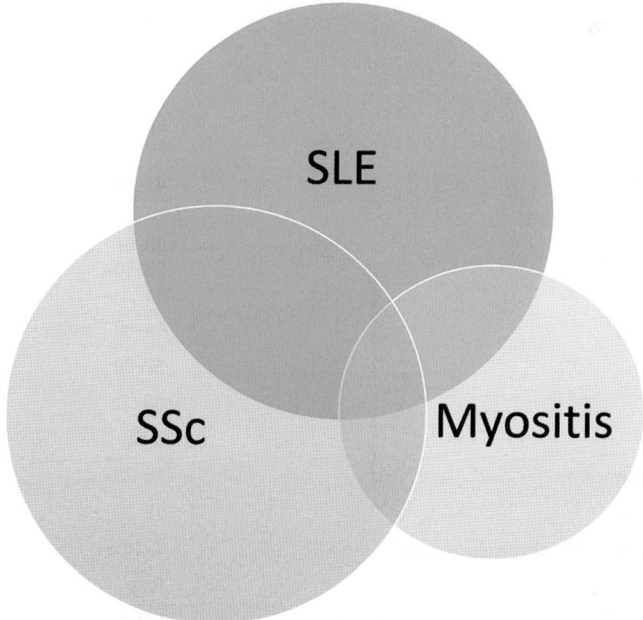

Fig. 20.1 The Clinical Spectrum of MCTD. MCTD presents with manifestations seen in SLE, SSc, and idiopathic inflammatory myopathies.

high-titer U1-RNP antibody. These patients often lack other specific autoantibodies such as anti-Sm, anti-ds DNA, and anti-centromere. MCTD is 15 times more common in women than in men. The mean age at diagnosis is 37 years, with a range of 4 to 80 years. There is no apparent racial or ethnic predisposition.

- **Overlap syndrome:** these patients have features of more than one of the six classic systemic autoimmune rheumatic diseases (SLE, SSc, polymyositis [PM], dermatomyositis, rheumatoid arthritis [RA], and Sjogren disease [SjD]). In this scenario, patients will commonly meet classification criteria for both rheumatic conditions. Some overlap syndromes, like certain myositis overlap syndromes, have specific autoantibody associations.
- **UCTD:** refers to a situation in which a patient has clinical features of one or more of the systemic autoimmune rheumatic diseases, but does not meet criteria for any one specific diagnosis. Most descriptions of UCTD include ANA positivity as a requirement for classification. Over time, ~25% of patients with UCTD will develop additional clinical features that will allow a specific disease diagnosis, whereas the majority will remain undifferentiated.

MIXED CONNECTIVE TISSUE DISEASE

2. What are the early clinical manifestations of MCTD, and how do they change over time?

The onset of MCTD is characterized by features of SSc, SLE, and/or IIM, usually evolving over time (Table 20.1). The most common manifestations at disease onset are Raynaud phenomenon, which is present in nearly all patients with MCTD, and a characteristic type of joint involvement in which the hands are diffusely swollen with puffy fingers (~70% of patients). Over time, joint involvement can result in deformities that resemble Jaccoud's arthropathy; a few patients develop erosive, destructive arthritis. Sclerodermatous skin changes can occur at disease onset or evolve over time. Esophageal dysmotility is common at disease onset. Many patients have myositis with elevated muscle enzymes and/or proximal muscle weakness; however, myositis is not required

TABLE 20.1 Clinical Features of Patients With Mixed Connective Tissue Disease

CLINICAL MANIFESTATION	FREQUENCY (%) AT DIAGNOSIS
Arthritis/arthralgia	50–100
Jaccoud arthropathy	30
Erosions	20
Swollen hands and puffy fingers	54–86
Raynaud phenomenon	50–99
Nailfold capillary changes	50
Esophageal dysmotility	43–88
Mucocutaneous lesions	
Sclerodermatous changes	33–67
Skin rash	38–50
Mouth sores	45
Myositis	14–60
Lymphadenopathy	39–50
Fever	33
Serositis	6–30
Hepatosplenomegaly	15–25
Trigeminal neuralgia	15
Renal disease (membranous glomerulonephritis)	7–10%
Myocarditis	Rare
Hypertensive crisis	Rare
Aseptic meningitis	Rare

for patients to be diagnosed with MCTD. The absence of severe central nervous system (CNS) disease is a hallmark of MCTD, and if present, may suggest an alternative diagnosis.

Over time, some manifestations of MCTD tend to become less severe and less frequent. In particular, inflammatory features including arthralgias, arthritis, myositis, serositis, fever, lymphadenopathy, hepatomegaly, and splenomegaly become less common. Persistent problems are most often those associated with SSc, such as sclerodactyly, Raynaud phenomenon, esophageal dysmotility, interstitial lung disease, and pulmonary arterial hypertension (PAH).

3. What are the common gastrointestinal (GI) manifestations of MCTD?

The most common GI manifestations are similar to those of scleroderma: upper and lower esophageal sphincter hypotension with gastroesophageal reflux leading to heartburn/dyspepsia, esophageal dysmotility, and/or stricture with dysphagia. Esophageal function is abnormal in up to 85% of patients, although it may be asymptomatic. Small bowel and colonic disease is less common in MCTD than in scleroderma. Other less common GI complications include intestinal vasculitis, acute pancreatitis, and chronic active hepatitis.

4. What are the pulmonary manifestations of MCTD, and how are they managed?

Involvement of the lung parenchyma with interstitial lung disease (ILD) is common (as high as 75%) in MCTD, although many patients are asymptomatic. Management involves identifying the specific abnormalities and directing therapy appropriately. Medications such as azathioprine, mycophenolate mofetil, rituximab, or cyclophosphamide may be used to treat ILD with an inflammatory component. Up to 25% will develop severe pulmonary fibrosis. Aspiration secondary to esophageal disease may also contribute to pulmonary disease. PAH is a major cause of morbidity and mortality in patients with MCTD. It usually is due to bland intimal proliferation and medial hypertrophy of pulmonary arterioles. Patients with nailfold capillary abnormalities similar to those seen in scleroderma are most at risk. See Table 20.2 for a listing of the typical pulmonary manifestations of MCTD and their relative frequencies.

5. What are the typical laboratory findings in a patient with MCTD?

Anemia is usually that of chronic disease. Coombs' positivity is detected in up to 60% of patients, although overt hemolytic anemia is uncommon. Thrombocytopenia was initially reported to be uncommon, but it has been noted in up to 60% of patients in recent cohorts. The sedimentation rate is usually elevated due to hypergammaglobulinemia. Antibodies against nuclear antigens other than U1-RNP such as Ro, La, Sm, and dsDNA were reported to be uncommon in early studies of MCTD; however, these antibodies are reported more frequently in recent cohorts. Antiphospholipid antibodies have been reported in up to one-quarter of patients (Table 20.3).

TABLE 20.2 Pulmonary Manifestations of Mixed Connective Tissue Disease	
SYMPTOMS	
Dyspnea	15–20%
Chest pain and tightness	7%
Cough	5%
Chest X-ray Findings	
Interstitial changes/NSIP	15–66%
Small pleural effusions	5–10%
High-Resolution Computed Tomography Scan Findings	
ILD/nonspecific interstitial pneumonia	15–66%
Pulmonary Function Studies	
Restrictive pattern	69%
Decreased carbon monoxide diffusion	66%
Pulmonary hypertension	23–30%

TABLE 20.3 Laboratory Findings in Patients With Mixed Connective Tissue Disease

ABNORMALITY	FREQUENCY (%)
ANA	100
Anti-U1-RNP	100
Anti-Ro	34
Anti-dsDNA	32
Anti-Sm	7
APS antibodies	4–26
Rheumatoid factor	50
Hypocomplementemia	2
Anemia	19–75
Leukopenia/lymphopenia	57–75
Thrombocytopenia	7–63
Hypergammaglobulinemia	80

6. What is U1-RNP?

Patients with MCTD appear to mount an antigen-driven immune response directed against U1-RNP, especially against an immunodominant epitope on the 70-kD polypeptide. U1-RNP is a uridine-rich small nuclear ribonucleoprotein (snRNP) that consists of U1-RNA and U1-specific polypeptides 70 kD, A, and C. U1-RNP is one of the spliceosomal snRNP complexes (U1, U2, U4/U6, U5, and others) whose function is to assist in splicing pre-messenger RNA to mature spliced RNA. Patients with MCTD form high titers of antibodies against U1-RNP, particularly U1-70kD and U1-RNA, but also polypeptides A and C, producing a high-titer ANA with a speckled pattern. One hypothesis is that a genetically predisposed (i.e., HLA-DR4) individual mounts a specific immune response against a microbial antigen (for example, cytomegalovirus glycoprotein) that cross-reacts with U1-70kD peptide, which has been modified during cellular apoptosis. Anti-U1-RNP antibodies can be present in other autoimmune diseases such as SLE and SSc, but typically in lower titers. U2-RNP has been implicated in immune-mediated myositis and is included on some myomarker panels, and U3-RNP has been implicated in the development and severity of SSc.

7. Is MCTD a milder disease than SLE or SSc?

The initial description by Sharp et al. of MCTD noted mild disease, lacking pulmonary, renal and severe CNS involvement, with good response to therapy including low-dose corticosteroids. The prognosis was thought to be better than SLE or SSc. However, subsequent studies have demonstrated that MCTD may have a worse prognosis compared to SLE, due to pulmonary hypertension and (to a lesser extent) renal vasculopathy similar to that seen in scleroderma renal crisis. Pulmonary hypertension is the primary disease-associated cause of death in MCTD. In addition, recent longitudinal cohorts describe renal and CNS involvement in 10% and 20% of MCTD patients, respectively. In general, the reported frequency of many features of MCTD has changed over time, potentially due to lack of consensus classification criteria.

8. What is the course and prognosis of MCTD?

Over a 10-year period, most patients are still classified as MCTD across cohorts. However, some patients evolve into a different connective tissue disease in 5 to 10 years. There is a low incidence of life-threatening renal and neurologic disease in MCTD, but up to 20% of patients had neurologic involvement in some cohorts. The major risk of mortality results from progressive PAH and its cardiac sequelae.

As a general rule, the SLE-like features of arthritis and pleurisy are treated with NSAIDs, antimalarials, low-dose prednisone (<20 mg/day), methotrexate, and other DMARDs. Inflammatory myositis is treated with high doses of prednisone (60 mg/day) and sometimes methotrexate, azathioprine, or mycophenolate. SSc-like features of Raynaud phenomenon, dysphagia, and reflux esophagitis are treated as in SSc (Chapter 17: Systemic Sclerosis). Serious end-organ involvement such as myocarditis or ILD may require aggressive treatment with corticosteroids alongside cyclophosphamide, rituximab, and/or mycophenolate. Some evidence suggests that PAH secondary to MCTD or SLE (but not SSc) may benefit from immunosuppressive medication such as cyclophosphamide (controversial given limited data, and should not replace standard therapy for PAH). Standard approaches to the diagnosis and management of PAH are outlined in Chapter 17: Systemic Sclerosis.

9. What is the utility of diagnosing, or labeling, a patient with MCTD?

MCTD as a distinct clinical entity has long been controversial. There have been at least four classification schemes, and no diagnostic criteria are formally accepted. There is substantial variation in clinical features at diagnosis and follow-up across cohorts, and U1-RNP, which was initially hailed as a promising diagnostic feature, is present in many other diseases, particularly SLE. While treatment is ultimately directed at the manifestations of rheumatic disease in patients with MCTD, there is likely some benefit to the label if for no other reason than it prompts clinicians to screen for serious organ involvement including PAH, ILD, and scleroderma renal crisis.

OVERLAP SYNDROMES

10. What is the most common disease in overlap syndromes, and with which other diseases is it associated?

SjD is the most common disease in overlap syndrome and is seen with RA, SLE, SSc, PM, MCTD, primary biliary cholangitis (PBC), necrotizing vasculitis, autoimmune thyroiditis, chronic active hepatitis, mixed cryoglobulinemia, and hypergammaglobulinemic purpura.

11. What other overlap syndromes are seen?

Other overlap syndromes not associated with high-titer anti-U1-RNP antibodies are:
- SLE is associated with inflammatory myopathy in 4% to 16% of cases.
- SLE can be associated with RA ("Rhupus") with positive rheumatoid factor, nodules, and erosive polyarthritis. This overlap is relatively uncommon, and the diagnosis should not be made simply because of a positive ANA in a patient with RA, nor in patients with lupus with inflammatory arthritis but without rheumatoid factor/cyclic citrullinated peptide positivity and/or erosive disease.
- SSc can be associated with myositis. One specific overlap is characterized by antibody to PM-Scl, a complex of 16 polypeptides located at the site of ribosomal assembly in the nucleolus (hence patients with PM-Scl antibody commonly have a nucleolar pattern ANA on immunofluorescent antibody assay).
- Limited SSc can be associated with PBC. Limited SSc precedes PBC by an average of 14 years. Antimitochrondrial antibodies can be seen in 18% to 27% of limited SSc patients. Many also have SjD.
- SSc can be associated with antineutrophil cytoplasmic antibody (ANCA)-associated vasculitis (perinuclear ANCA/anti-myeloperoxidase).
- Myositis overlap syndromes: antisynthetase antibody syndromes (see Chapter 19: Idiopathic Inflammatory Myopathies).

UNDIFFERENTIATED CONNECTIVE TISSUE DISEASE

12. What is UCTD?

UCTD is a term used to describe patients with signs and/or symptoms suggestive of a rheumatic disease but not meeting diagnostic or classification criteria for a defined connective tissue disease (CTD). The concept of UCTD was first introduced in 1980. To date, there remains no widely accepted classification or diagnostic criteria for UCTD. Though definitions vary, most proposed criteria require patients to have a positive ANA (or other autoantibody) in addition to suggestive symptoms.

13. How common is UCTD?

Roughly 25% of patients presenting to rheumatologists may not fulfill the criteria for a defined connective tissue disease at the time of presentation. The majority of patients with UCTD are female (80–95%) with disease onset during the fourth decade (30–40 years).

14. How often do patients with UCTD progress to a more defined rheumatic disease?

Approximately 25% of patients with UCTD evolve into a defined systemic rheumatic disease, typically within the first 5–6 years of symptom onset. In contrast, about 75% of patients with UCTD remain stable for many years with no significant change in symptoms. These two groups of UCTD patients are sometimes referred to as evolving and stable UCTD (eUCTD and sUCTD, respectively). Among the eUCTD patients, the most common rheumatic diseases that patients evolve into are SLE (~25%), RA (~25%), SjD (~20%), SSc (~10%), and MCTD (~10%) (Fig. 20.2).

15. What are the most common clinical and serologic characteristics of UCTD?

The most frequent clinical manifestations of UCTD (affecting >25% of patients) are Raynaud's, arthralgia/arthritis, and sicca symptoms. Other common symptoms (affecting 2–25% of patients) include cytopenias, myalgia/muscle weakness, photosensitivity, alopecia, telangiectasias, oral ulcers, esophageal dysmotility, serositis, and peripheral neuropathy. Occasionally, patients with UCTD will develop interstitial lung disease, at which point they may be categorized as having interstitial pneumonia with autoimmune features (IPAF). It is rare for patients with UCTD to develop other major organ involvement such as kidney or CNS disease. From a serologic perspective, most patients in reported cohorts of UCTD are ANA-positive; however, this reflects the fact that most proposed criteria for UCTD mandate the presence of an ANA. The next most commonly seen autoantibodies in UCTD are anti-Ro/SSA (13–35%) and low-titer RNP antibodies (6–29%).

16. Are there clinical features that predict the future development of a defined rheumatic disease?

Certain combinations of features are predictive for the development of a defined CTD:
- Fever, serositis, photosensitivity, discoid lupus, and/or positive anti-dsDNA, anti-Sm, anti-cardiolipin, or multiple antibody specificities—SLE.

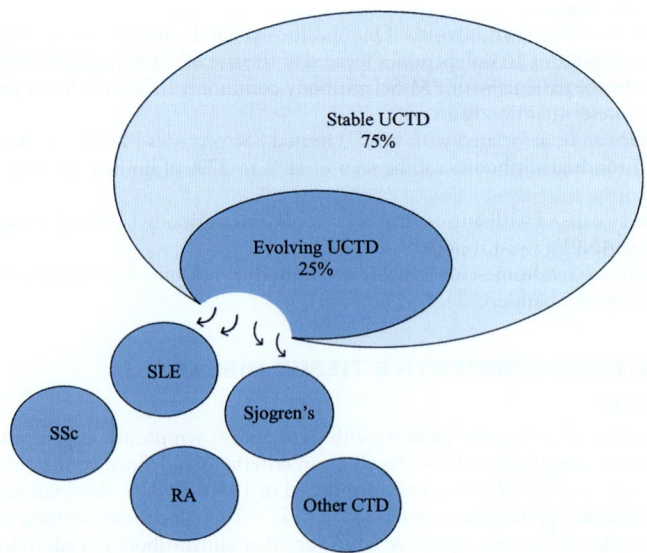

Fig. 20.2 **The Clinical Spectrum of UCTD.** Approximately 25% of patients with UCTD evolve into a more clearly defined rheumatic disease over the first several years of illness. This is termed "evolving UCTD". The most common rheumatic diseases that patients evolve into are SLE, SSc, SjD, and RA.

- Raynaud phenomenon, abnormal nailfold capillaries, sclerodactyly, and nucleolar ANA—SSc.
- Xerostomia and anti-SSA antibodies—SjD.
- RNP antibody—MCTD.

17. What is the difference between UCTD and incomplete lupus erythematosus (ILE)?

In 1989, the term *incomplete lupus erythematosus* (ILE) was proposed to describe patients with features of SLE but lacking enough clinical manifestations to meet full classification criteria for this disease. As such, ILE can be considered to be a subset of the UCTD spectrum. Other commonly used terms for ILE include "early lupus" and "possible lupus."

18. Can hydroxychloroquine or other interventions prevent the progression of UCTD to a more defined rheumatic disease?

There is limited evidence that in patients with ILE, hydroxychloroquine might delay the onset of SLE. It is not known if hydroxychloroquine or other treatments have any impact on the natural history of the broader category of UCTD.

ACKNOWLEDGMENT

The authors wish to thank Drs. Vance Bray and the late Richard Brasington for their contributions to this chapter in the previous editions.

BIBLIOGRAPHY

Alves MR, Isenberg DA. Mixed connective tissue disease: a condition in search of an identity. *Coin Exp Med.* 2020;20:159–166.

Benyamine A. Quantification of antifibrillarin (anti-U3 RNP) antibodies: a new insight for patients with systemic sclerosis. *Diagnostics.* 2021;11(6):1064.

Cappelli S, Bellando Randone S, Martinovic D, et al. "To be or not to be", ten years after: evidence for mixed connective tissue disease as a distinct entity. *Semin Arthritis Rheum.* 2012;41:589–598.

Fischer A, Antoniou KM, Brown KK, et al. An Official European Respiratory Society/American Thoracic Society research statement: interstitial pneumonia with autoimmune features. *Eur Respir J.* 2015;46(4):976–987.

Furst D, Grossman J. Mixed connective tissue disease. *Rheum Dis Clinics North Am.* 2005;31(3):411–574.

Greer JM, Panush RS. Incomplete lupus erythematosus. *Arch Intern Med.* 1989;149(11):2473–2476.

Hajas A, Szodoray P, Nakken B, et al. Clinical course, prognosis, and causes of death in mixed connective tissue disease. *J Rheumatol.* 2013;40(7):1134–1142.

Hassoun PM. Pulmonary arterial hypertension complicating connective tissue diseases. *Semin Respir Crit Care Med.* 2009;30:429.

Hoffman RW, Maldonado ME. Immune pathogenesis of mixed connective tissue disease: a short analytical review. *Clin Immunol.* 2008;128:8.

James JA, Kim-Howard XR, Bruner BF, et al. Hydroxychloroquine sulfate treatment is associated with later onset of systemic lupus erythematosus. *Lupus.* 2007;16(6):401–409.

Lambers WM, Westra J, Bootsma H, et al. From incomplete to complete systemic lupus erythematosus; a review of the predictive serological immune markers. *Semin Arthritis Rheum.* 2021;51(1):43–48.

LeRoy EC, Maricq HR, Kahaleh MB. Undifferentiated connective tissue syndromes. *Arthritis Rheum.* 1980;23(3):341–343.

Mosca M, Tani C, Talarico R, Bombardieri S. Undifferentiated connective tissue diseases (UCTD): simplified systemic autoimmune disease. *Autoimmun Rev.* 2011;10:256–258.

Rodriguez-Reyna TS, Alarcon-Segovia D. Overlap syndromes in the context of shared autoimmunity. *Autoimmunity.* 2005;38:219.

Rubio J, Kyttaris VC. Undifferentiated connective tissue disease: comprehensive review. *Curr Rheumatol Rep.* 2023 May;25(5):98–106.

Sharp GC, Irvin WS, Tan EM, et al. Mixed connective tissue disease—an apparently distinct rheumatic disease syndrome associated with a specific antibody to an extractable nuclear antigen (ENA). *Am J Med.* 1972;52:148–159.

Venables PJW. Mixed connective tissue disease. *Lupus.* 2006;15(3):117.

Sjögren Disease

Sara S. McCoy, MD, PhD

1. Who was Sjögren, and what is his disease?

Henrich Sjögren was born in 1899 in Stockholm and received his MD from the Karolinska Institute in 1927. His description of **keratoconjunctivitis sicca (KCS)** and arthritis serves as the basis for Sjögren disease (SjD). SjD has also been known as Mikulicz disease (lacrimal and salivary gland enlargement now associated with a multitude of diseases such as sarcoidosis, lymphoma, tuberculosis, and IgG4 disease, among others), Gougerot syndrome, sicca syndrome, and autoimmune exocrinopathy. SjD refers to a slowly progressive, autoimmune disease that primarily affects exocrine organs (e.g., lacrimal and salivary glands). Focal lymphocytic infiltration of these organs is a hallmark and contributes to reduced lacrimal and salivary flow.

2. What is the difference between primary and associated SjD?

- **Primary SjD** is diagnosed in a patient with KCS as well as systemic autoimmunity characteristic of SjD, and in the absence of a concurrent rheumatic condition. Primary SjD is immunogenetically associated with HLA-DRB1*0301 and DRB1*1501 and serologically associated with antibodies to Ro/SSA.
- **Associated SjD** (SjD in association with another systemic autoimmune disease) is diagnosed in the presence of another rheumatic condition, most frequently rheumatoid arthritis (RA). The immunogenetic and serologic findings typically include those of the accompanying disease (e.g., HLA-DR4-positive if associated with RA). Patients with associated SjD should fulfill the classification criteria of each condition, a scenario commonly referred to as an overlap syndrome (see Chapter 20). Extraglandular features including parotid enlargement, lymphadenopathy, and lymphoma are more common in primary SjD. The 2016 ACR/European League Against Rheumatism [EULAR]) Classification Criteria define primary but do not address associated SjD separately.

3. Who typically develops SjD?

Primary SjD affects 0.01% to 4% of the population depending on criteria used. It predominantly affects females (female: male = 9:1), with bimodal peaks in incidence in the 20s to 30s and after 50 years of age, most frequently occurring in the perimenopausal time period. It is less frequent in children; however, identification of pediatric SjD is complicated by the fact that glandular dysfunction (tear and saliva production) is less severe than in adults. In addition, pediatric patients present with parotitis or arthralgias more frequently than adults. Symptoms progress relatively slowly and there is frequently a delay of 5 to 10 years between symptom onset and diagnosis, though this delay is shrinking. SjD occurs in 10–30% of patients with RA, 5–20% of patients with SLE, and to a lesser extent in other rheumatic diseases. Of interest, many of the older studies describing the prevalence of SjD in RA utilized the 2002 American-European Consensus Group criteria for secondary SjD, where neither SS-A antibody nor positive focus score was required for classification.

TABLE 21.1 Clinical Manifestations of Primary Sjögren's Disease	
SICCA SYMPTOMS	**PREVALENCE (%)**
Xerophthalmia	90–95
Xerostomia	90–95
Dyspareunia	40–60
Parotid gland enlargement	40–60
Extraglandular features	
Arthralgias/arthritis	45–60
Raynaud's phenomenon	13–33
Esophageal dysfunction	30–35
Autoimmune thyroid disease	14–33
Lymphadenopathy	15–20
Lung involvement	10–20
Kidney involvement	5–10
Liver involvement	5–10
Cutaneous vasculitis	5–10
Lymphoma	5–10
Peripheral neuropathy	2–5
Central nervous system disease	1–2
Myositis	1–2

4. What are the clinical manifestations of primary SjD?

Manifestations can be divided into glandular and extraglandular organ involvement, the latter of which is seen in 40–60% of patients and may precede the development of KCS (Table 21.1). Common extraglandular sites of involvement include the articular, pulmonary, and peripheral nervous systems.

5. What is the underlying pathogenesis of primary SjD?

The mechanisms driving SjD are complex and not fully elucidated. There are accumulating data regarding disease pathobiology, and several theories regarding disease initiation have been described. Many hypothetical models begin in a genetically predisposed host who is exposed to an inflammatory stimulus such as a viral infection, initiating disease onset. In one such model, intracellular antigens such as Ro/SS-A form a complex with human small noncoding Y RNA (hYRNA). During apoptosis, these complexes accumulate in apoptotic blebs and present themselves for recognition by SS-A antibody. The immune complexes in turn lead to downstream stimulation of dendritic cell TLRs and B-cells, subsequently leading to an interferon response and immune activation.

Local tissue inflammation may also drive lymphocyte-epithelial crosstalk, wherein epithelial cells function as antigen presenting cells capable of activating CD4+ T cells. Furthermore, epithelial cells can promote lymphocyte chemotaxis through chemokine production. Finally, epithelial cells may promote B-cell activation through cytokine production. In mild disease, the infiltrating lymphocytes are primarily CD4+ T cells; in more severe disease, B cells are predominant. The cellular infiltrate also contains CD8+ T cells, plasma cells, dendritic cells, and macrophages.

Several mechanisms have been proposed to link tissue inflammation to the resultant dryness characteristic of SjD:

a. Dysregulation of acinar cells, the primary producers of saliva.
b. Autoantibodies to muscarinic 3 receptors antagonize parasympathetic neurotransmitter-induced saliva production.

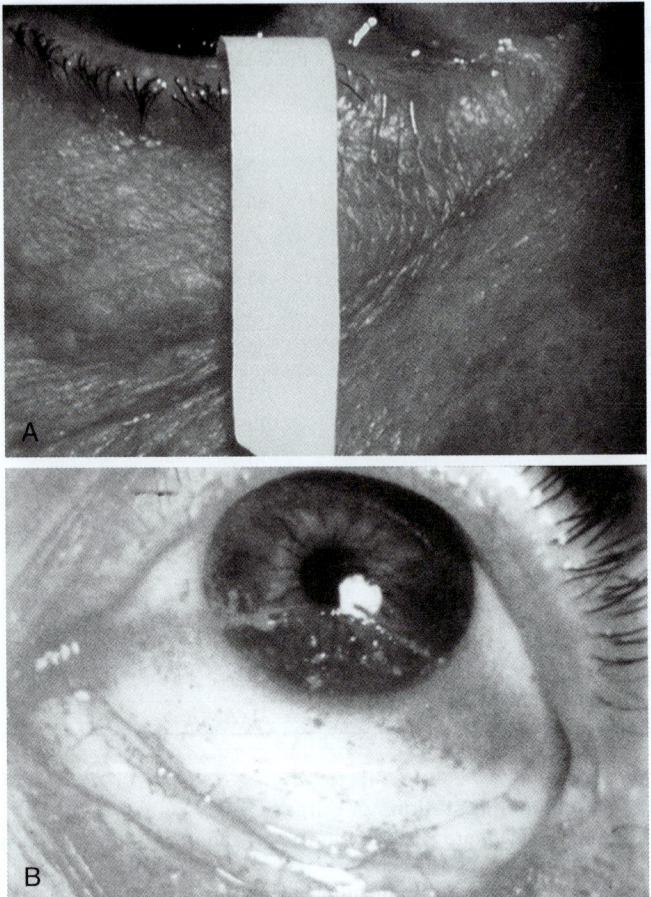

Fig. 21.1 (A) Schirmer's test demonstrating decreased tear production. (B) Rose Bengal test with increased dye uptake in areas of devitalized epithelium. (Copyright 2014 American College of Rheumatology. Used with permission.)

    c. MicroRNAs secreted from infiltrating T cells impair the secretory signaling cascade.

    d. Decreased aquaporin expression on acinar cells in SjD, as well as diminished responsiveness to muscarinic stimulation, compared to healthy individuals. This ultimately results in reduced water transportation from acinar cells.

6. What are the most common ocular symptoms of primary SjD?

Dry eyes in SjD, also known as **xerophthalmia** or **KCS,** results from a deficient aqueous layer of tear film, which normally comprises 90% of tear volume. Symptoms include a foreign body or gritty sensation; painful, burning, itchy, or red eyes; blurred vision, and/or photophobia. Symptoms worsen as the day progresses as a result of evaporation of ocular moisture. Notably, some of the eye pain is due to central nervous system input as topical anesthetics do not eliminate the pain completely. This pattern contrasts with blepharitis, a low-grade inflammation of the meibomian glands, in which crusting and discomfort are most pronounced in the morning. KCS can lead to infections, corneal ulceration, and rarely vision loss. Screening for dry eye involves several simple validated questions: (1) "Do you have a recurrent sensation of sand or gravel in the eyes?" (2) "Have you had daily, persistent, troublesome dry eyes for more than three months?" (3) "Do you use tear substitutes more than three times daily?"

7. **What tests are used to document dry eyes in a patient with suspected primary SjD?**

The three most common tests for dry eyes include the **Schirmer's test,** ocular surface staining **(OSS)**, and tear break-up time **(TBUT)**. For the **Schirmer's test,** a piece of filter paper is placed under the inferior eyelid without anesthesia and the amount of wetness is measured (Fig. 21.1A). Normal wetting is >15 mm in 5 minutes, whereas <5 mm meets one of the classification criterion for SjD. There is a 15% false-positive and false-negative rate with Schirmer's testing.

The remaining tests are performed by an ophthalmologist using a slit-lamp examination. **OSS** is performed using a sequential examination with **fluorescein dye** for the cornea, followed by **lissamine green dye** to assess the conjunctiva. Fluorescein dye targets areas of cellular disruption (indicating dryness severe enough to cause corneal epithelial injury), whereas lissamine green dye stains conjunctival epithelial surfaces that have been damaged or devitalized. Staining uptake is typically maximal along the palpebral fissure, where maximum exposure to the environment and evaporation of tears occurs. The OSS is the sum of a 0–6 score for fluorescein staining of the cornea and a 0–3 score for lissamine green staining in the nasal and temporal bulbar conjunctiva, respectively (total score 0–12). An OSS ≥5 in at least one eye meets one of the classification criteria for SjD. **TBUT** measures disruption in tear film and indicates an abnormal mucus layer if the tear film is ≤10 seconds. These tests have largely replaced the **Rose Bengal** stain, which is used less commonly due to toxic effects on corneal epithelial cells (Fig. 21.1B).

8. **What are the common symptoms of dry mouth?**

Normal saliva production is 1 to 1.5 L/day. Dry mouth symptoms, known as **xerostomia,** occur when the salivary flow rate decreases to <50% of the basal flow rate. It may result in a variety of problems including:
- Burning sensation.
- Change in taste (metallic, salty, bitter).
- Difficulty swallowing.
- Disturbed sleep (due to dry mouth and/or nocturia).
- Gastroesophageal reflux symptoms (due to lack of saliva buffer).
- Increase in dental caries, cracked teeth, loose fillings.
- "Lipstick sign" (adherence of patient's lipstick onto front teeth).
- Predisposition to oral candidiasis (atrophic variant, which presents as an erythematous tongue or presentation as angular cheilitis).
- Problems wearing dentures.

Validated screening questions for dry mouth in SjD include: (1) "Have you had a daily feeling of dry mouth for more than 3 months?" (2) "Have you had recurrent or persistently swollen salivary glands as an adult?" (3) "Do you frequently drink liquids to aid in swallowing dry foods?"

9. **What methods determine salivary gland involvement in SjD?**

Sialometry (sensitivity 56%, specificity 81%) can be used to quantitate saliva production. An unstimulated whole salivary flow rate of ≤0.1 mL/minute meets criterion for xerostomia. **Scintigraphy** (sensitivity 75%, specificity 78%) utilizes the uptake and secretion of Tc-99m pertechnetate following intravenous injection to quantify salivary flow rate. **Sialography** is used to outline the salivary duct anatomy but may predispose to pain, infection, or duct rupture. Both **magnetic resonance imaging** (MRI; sensitivity 81%, specificity 93%) and **ultrasonography** (sensitivity 69%, specificity 92%) can detect parenchymal heterogeneity. Salivary gland ultrasound is increasingly used in clinic for diagnostic and prognostic purposes.

Minor salivary gland (MSG) biopsy (sensitivity 80%, specificity 82%) is the gold standard for SjD diagnosis in anti-SSA antibody negative individuals (Fig. 21.2). An incisional biopsy through the lower labial mucosa yielding 5 to 10 minor glands is adequate for assessment (a minimum of 8 mm^2). An area of ≥50 lymphocytes surrounded by normal tissue is defined as a focus, with a focus score (FS) of ≥1 foci/4 mm^2 supporting a diagnosis of SjD. The procedure may be complicated by persistent lip numbness in up to 6% of patients. The findings in the MSG biopsy generally parallel involvement of major glands; therefore, biopsy of multiple salivary glands is generally not necessary for diagnostic purposes.

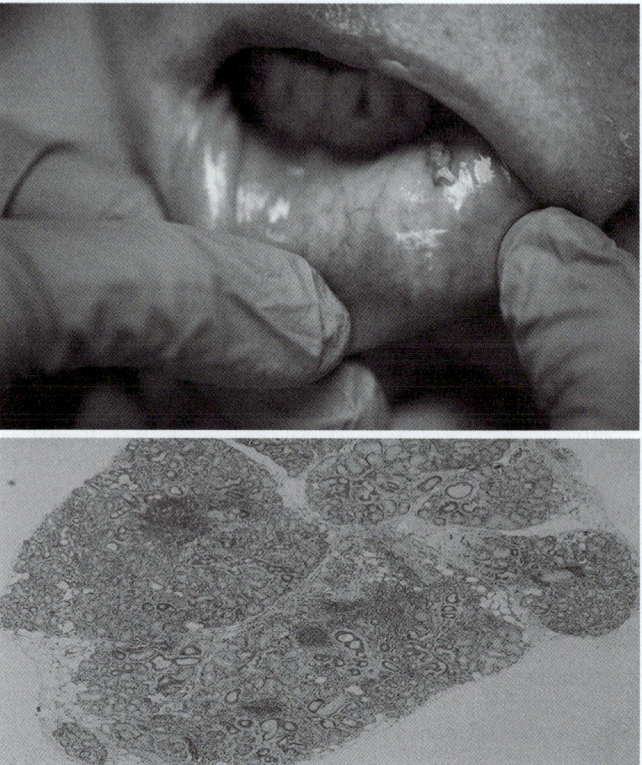

Fig. 21.2 Minor salivary gland biopsy with histopathology demonstrating mononuclear cell infiltration and partial destruction of the salivary gland.

10. What are other causes of dry eyes and dry mouth besides primary SjD?

Medications
- Antihistamines
- Benzodiazepines
- Clonidine
- Diuretics
- Tricyclic antidepressants
- Immune checkpoint inhibitors

Conditions
- Amyloidosis
- Blepharitis
- Cystic fibrosis
- Dehydration
- Diabetes mellitus (uncontrolled)
- Graft-versus-host disease
- Granulomatous diseases (sarcoid, tuberculosis, leprosy)
- Hepatitis C infection
- HIV/AIDS
- IgG4-related disease
- Mucus membrane pemphigoid
- Psychogenic causes (fear, depression)
- Viral infections (especially mumps)
- Vitamin A deficiency

Others
- Age-related sicca syndrome
- Congenitally absent or malformed glands (rare; lacrimoauriculodentodigital syndrome)
- Contact lens irritation
- History of radiation to the head and neck

11. What are other causes of salivary gland enlargement besides primary SjD? See Table 21.2.

TABLE 21.2 Differential Diagnosis of Salivary Gland Enlargement		
Usually unilateral		
Bacterial infection	Chronic sialadenitis	Lymphoma
Obstruction	Primary salivary gland neoplasms	
Usually bilateral (asymmetric)		
Granulomatous diseases	HIV/Diffuse infiltrative lymphocytosis syndrome (see Chapter 41: HIV-Associated Rheumatic Syndromes)	IgG4-related disease (may be massive)
Recurrent parotitis of childhood	Viruses (mumps, cytomegalovirus, influenzae, coxsackie A)	
Bilateral (symmetric)		
Acromegaly	Alcoholism	Anorexia/bulimia
Chronic pancreatitis	Diabetes mellitus	Gonadal hypofunction
Hepatitis cirrhosis	Hyperlipoproteinemia	Idiopathic

12. What other exocrine glands can be involved in primary SjD?
Patients can have dry upper airways leading to nonallergic rhinitis, sinusitis, and bleeding. In addition, involvement of the larynx (hoarseness), trachea (dry cough), vagina (dyspareunia), gastrointestinal (GI) tract (dysphagia; constipation), and skin (xerosis; pruritis) can be seen.

13. Describe the arthritis of primary SjD.
The distribution of arthritis in SjD is similar to that of RA. Symmetric arthralgias and/or arthritis of the wrists, metacarpophalangeal, and proximal interphalangeal joints, frequently associated with morning stiffness and fatigue, is characteristic. In contrast to RA, Sjögren's arthritis is nonerosive and tends to be mild. Anti-citrullinated protein antibodies may be seen in 8% to 10% of patients with primary SjD and may predict a more severe joint phenotype or progression to RA.

14. Describe the clinical characteristics of other extraglandular manifestations of primary SjD.
- **Lung manifestations:** include xerotrachea/xerobronchitis, nonspecific interstitial pneumonitis, lymphocytic interstitial pneumonitis, usual interstitial pneumonitis, bronchiolitis (constrictive), and bronchial-associated lymphoid tissue lymphoma. Due to thick secretions and recurrent pneumonias, patients can develop bronchiectasis. Among patients with interstitial pneumonia with autoimmune features (IPAF), SjD was the most common final diagnosis.

PEARL: Consider SjD in any patient with sicca and unexplained lung disease.

- **Renal disease:** includes type I distal renal tubular acidosis (10%) that rarely can lead to severe potassium wasting and muscle paralysis, tubular interstitial nephritis (<5%), glomerulonephritis, and nephrogenic diabetes insipidus

- **GI:** includes a higher prevalence of celiac disease (both diseases share similar genetics of HLA-DRB1*0301 and HLA-DQB1*0201). Suspect in patients with diarrhea and vitamin D deficiency. Primary biliary cholangitis (5%), autoimmune hepatitis, and recurrent pancreatitis (<5%) have also been described.
- **Vasculitis:** cutaneous vasculitis (palpable purpura) is most common, whereas necrotizing vasculitis (similar to polyarteritis nodosa) or cryoglobulinemia in the absence of hepatitis C is infrequent.

15. How is the nervous system affected by primary SjD?

- **Central nervous system:** includes focal and diffuse patterns of involvement that may lead to multiple sclerosis–like brain lesions, sensory/motor deficits, seizures, encephalopathy, or cognitive impairment. Longitudinally extensive transverse myelitis (LETM; ≥4 vertebral segments) and optic neuritis have been described in patients with SjD alongside serum anti-aquaporin-4 antibodies, representing an overlap with neuromyelitis optica. Pulse-dose corticosteroids in addition to rituximab represent induction therapy, followed by maintenance immunosuppression with mycophenolate mofetil, azathioprine or rituximab. Any patient presenting with LETM and/or optic neuritis should have occult SjD ruled out.
- **Peripheral nervous system:** peripheral neuropathy can be motor (mononeuritis multiplex), pure sensory, or sensorimotor. Patients with burning paresthesias and pain, but normal nerve conduction velocities, may have a **small fiber neuropathy.** Up to 50% of patients with a small fiber neuropathy have findings of dysautonomia as well. These patients have selective loss of pinprick and temperature sensation (small fibers) while having normal vibratory sensation and deep tendon reflexes (large fibers). Small fiber neuropathy is diagnosed by a skin biopsy showing a reduction in epidermal nerve fibers. The initial mainstay of treatment is conservative and includes medications to reduce neuropathic pain (gabapentin, pregabalin, topical lidocaine, or capsaicin) as well as counseling on patient self-management strategies (similar to the treatment approach for widespread pain in fibromyalgia). Rarely, in patients with severe or rapidly progressive symptoms despite conservative therapy, limited data suggest that SjD-related small fiber neuropathy and/or dysautonomia may respond to intravenous immunoglobulin therapy. Rarely, patients with SjD may develop a sensory ataxic neuronopathy (sensory ganglionopathy) with features such as ataxia, areflexia, and painful paraesthesias. Adie's pupil, tachycardia, hypo/anhidrosis, and orthostatic hypotension have been reported in some patients with SjD-associated ganglionopathy as well. Disease course with this manifestation may be severe, and treatment with high-dose corticosteroids and immunosuppressive medications such as mycophenolate mofetil is indicated.

16. What are the risks of pregnancy in SjD?

Pregnant women who are positive for anti-SSA and/or anti-SSB have an increased risk of delivering a fetus with neonatal lupus or congenital heart block due to transplacental passage of these antibodies. This risk to the fetus is present in the setting of SS-A and/or SS-B positivity regardless of whether the mother has SjD, systemic lupus erythematosus, or is without clinical features of a rheumatic disease. Antimalarial use in anti-SSA positive patients during pregnancy may decrease the risk of congenital heart block in the offspring (see Chapter 78: Rheumatic Disease and the Pregnant Patient).

17. What are the typical laboratory findings in patients with primary SjD?

ANA	85–90%
Elevated erythrocyte sedimentation rate	80–90%
Hypergammaglobulinemia	80%
Anti-SSA/Ro antibody	50–70%
Rheumatoid factor (RF)	50–60%
Anti-SSB/La antibody	33–50%
Anemia of chronic disease	25%
Leukopenia	10–20%
Thrombocytopenia	8%

PEARL: Anti-SSB antibody alone (in absence of anti-SSA) does not provide additional diagnostic support for SjD. A suspected SjD patient who is anti-SSA antibody negative requires a minor salivary gland biopsy for diagnosis.

18. What other antibodies have been described in SjD?
Anti-SSA antibody may precede the diagnosis of SjD by up to two decades. A subset of SjD patients (5%), who may or may not have overlap with systemic sclerosis, have anti-centromere antibodies. These patients appear to be at higher risk for extraglandular disease, including Raynaud phenomenon and lymphoma. Anti-SSB antibody is no longer considered helpful to diagnose SjD, but patients who are positive for both anti-SSA and SSB have a higher prevalence of extraglandular organ involvement.

19. What is the risk of cancer in patients with SjD?
There is a 5- to 14-fold greater risk of developing lymphoma in SjD compared with age-matched controls, with a lifetime frequency of lymphoma of 5% to 10%. Lymphomas are usually non-Hodgkin's B-cell lymphomas (NHL) and occur at a median of 8 years following a diagnosis of SjD. Extranodal marginal zone B-cell lymphoma (also known as mucosa-associated lymphoid tissue) is the predominant subtype of NHL seen in SjD, but diffuse large B-cell and nodal marginal zone lymphomas can also occur.

20. What are risk factors for lymphoma development in SjD?
The list of risk factors continues to grow. Risk factors (highest to lowest) include cryoglobuline-mia, focus score, and disease activity (as measured by a EULAR SS Disease Activity Index >5). Other clinical risk factors include parotid enlargement, lymphadenopathy, Raynaud phenom-enon, splenomegaly, palpable purpura, glomerulonephritis, peripheral neuropathy, and disease duration (>10 years). Laboratory and histologic features associated with lymphoma include monoclonal gammopathy (IgM kappa most common), loss of a previously positive RF, leukope-nia, cryoglobulinemia, low C4 or C3, and the presence of germinal centers or high FS ($\geq$3) on the initial MSG biopsy.

Experts recommend blood tests (complete blood count, protein electrophoresis, RF, C3 and C4, and possibly cryoglobulins) every 1 to 2 years to monitor risk. If lymphoma is suspected, the evaluation should proceed with imaging (e.g., MRI or positron emission tomography) and tissue biopsy to confirm diagnosis.

21. What are the ACR/EULAR classification criteria for primary SjD?
The 2016 ACR/EULAR classification criteria were created to identify a uniform population of SjD patients suitable for research studies. Criteria were derived from the 2002 AECG and 2012 ACR criteria. The 2016 criteria have a sensitivity of 96% and specificity of 95% for SjD. A patient is considered to have primary SjD if they have at least one symptom of ocular or oral dry-ness and have a score of $\geq$4 points out of 9 from the following items:
- Labial salivary gland biopsy with lymphocytic sialadenitis and a FS $\geq$1 foci/4 mm^2 (3 points).
- Anti-SSA/Ro positive (3 points).
- OSS $\geq$5 (or van Bijsterveld score $\geq$4) in at least one eye (1 point).
- Schirmer's test $\leq$ 5 mm/5 minutes in at least one eye (1 point).
- Unstimulated whole salivary flow rate $\leq$0.1 mL/minute (1 point).

22. How is the xerophthalmia of SjD treated?
The Sjögren Foundation has published clinical practice guidelines for the management of oral, ocular, and systemic manifestations in SjD. Treatment of dry eye varies if there is concurrent meibomian gland disease and options include:
- **Modify the environment:** Reduce caffeine intake and smoking. Limit time at computer, turn off ceiling fans, and consider using a humidifier. Consider using specialized eyewear (sometimes referred to as moisture chamber glasses) that has foam or another liner on the frame to fill the gap between the frame of the glasses and the face, reducing air movement and enclosing the eye. "Grilling goggles" or "onion goggles" are similar products that look more

like sunglasses than goggles, which may be more acceptable to patients. Eliminate offending medications (see Question 10).

- **Eye drops:**
  - Preservative-free artificial tears (Refresh, TheraTears, Soothe, Systane) are generally less irritating and should be used if patients use topical tears four or more times a day.
  - Topical corticosteroids for moderate-severe disease.
  - Cyclosporine (Restasis 1 drop BID) or lifitegrast (Xiidra 1 drop BID) for moderate-severe disease. Patients should be warned that cyclosporine can initially sting and may take 4 to 12 weeks to reach full effect.
  - Autologous tears may be used for severe ocular surface disease.
- **Lubricant ointments** (Refresh PM, Lacrilube) are available and are typically used during the night.
- **Punctal occlusion** is performed by an ophthalmologist and delays tear clearance. Temporary plugs (silicone, collagen) are generally inserted before permanent obstruction is considered.
- **Scleral contact lenses** with a moisture reservoir can also be used but are costly.
- **If blepharitis is contributing to symptoms:** warm compresses, avoid local irritants (mascara), topical azithromycin, and rarely systemic antibiotics (doxycycline).

23. Describe the management for nonocular sicca symptoms in SjD.

Vaginal dryness is treated with topical lubricants. Dry skin usually improves with lotions, creams, and emollients with urea/lactate. The complications of xerostomia are best prevented by regular dental visits and daily use of fluoridated toothpaste and/or mouthwash and flossing. Other approaches to relieving xerostomia include:

- Sugar-free (not just sugarless) or xylitol-containing gum, lozenges, or candies (Xylimelts) may stimulate salivary flow.
- Avoidance of oral irritants (alcohol, coffee, nicotine) and highly acidic beverages (cola; herbal tea) that lower oral pH and accelerate cavity formation.
- Regular water ingestion.
- Oil pulling, whereby a half teaspoon of cold-pressed virgin coconut oil (or other cooking oil) is swished in the mouth.
- Removal of nasal polyps to limit mouth breathing.
- Use of wetting agents. Biotene OralBalance and BioXtra have been compared in a head-to-head clinical trial. Both treatments were effective, but patients rated the BioXtra products as more pleasant to use and more effective at relieving the perception of dry mouth. Other treatments include nonfluoride remineralization agents (NeutraSal), and saliva substitutes (Salivart, Xero-lube) as well as systemically administered secretagogues (pilocarpine, cevimeline).
- Oral candidiasis is best treated with oral application of nystatin elixir or clotrimazole troches. Topical drugs may be preferred because with significant salivary hypofunction, systemically administered antifungal drugs may not reach the mouth in therapeutically adequate amounts. Dentures must be removed while the mouth is being treated and may also need to be treated in order to prevent recurrence.

24. How do the cholinergic drugs help in dryness?

Patients with SjD have significant dryness, yet unstimulated salivary flow does not correlate with inflammatory lymphocytic infiltrate. Furthermore, by definition, most foci of lymphocytic infiltrates are surrounded by grossly normal epithelial cells. Consequently, the residual functioning tissue can be stimulated to produce more tears and saliva by the use of oral secretagogues.

Pilocarpine (Salagen up to 5 mg QID) and cevimeline (Evoxac up to 30 mg TID) are equally effective compared with placebo. Cevimeline has a longer half-life (4 hours versus 1.5 hours) and higher specificity for the M3 receptor on lacrimal and salivary glands, resulting in less flushing and diaphoresis. Patients with narrow-angle glaucoma, asthma, or those on beta blockers should avoid these drugs or be monitored closely. Common side effects are sweating, flushing, and GI disturbances (worse with cevimeline).

25. How are the other manifestations of SjD managed?

Fatigue is a common symptom that may be difficult to alleviate. It is important to rule out hypothyroidism, obstructive sleep apnea, fibromyalgia, and other common fatigue-associated comorbidities, as these conditions have therapies that may result in symptom relief. Exercise and sleep hygiene remain the mainstays of therapy for fatigue. If coexisting fibromyalgia is present, it is best to avoid tricyclic antidepressants that may aggravate dryness. Arthritis generally responds to nonsteroidal antiinflammatory drugs, antimalarials, and low doses of prednisone (≤5 mg), after which the treatment course is similar to that of RA. Severe extraglandular disease may require higher doses of systemic corticosteroids, azathioprine, mycophenylate mofetil, methotrexate, or cyclophosphamide. Based on case series, rituximab may be beneficial for severe extraglandular manifestations (e.g., vasculitis), but clinical trial data do not support its use for dryness and fatigue. The combination of hydroxychloroquine and leflunomide successfully reduced the EULAR SS disease activity index compared to placebo in a small, randomized controlled trial. Multiple phase II trials have achieved their primary endpoints for drugs targeting T- and B-cell interactions, B-cell activating factor (BAFF), APRIL, Bruton's tyrosine kinase, and interleukin 2, among others; however, phase III studies are needed to confirm the initial findings. Lymphoma should be treated in consultation with an oncologist and based on the type and stage.

ACKNOWLEDGMENT

The author and editors would like to thank Dr. Lindsay Kelmenson for her contribution to this chapter in the previous edition.

BIBLIOGRAPHY

Alani H, Henty JR, Thompson NL, Jury E, Ciurtin C. Systematic review and meta-analysis of the epidemiology of polyautoimmunity in Sjögren's syndrome (secondary Sjögren's syndrome) focusing on autoimmune rheumatic diseases. *Scand J Rheumatol.* 2018;47(2):141–154.

Antero DC, Parra AGM, Miyazaki FH, Gehlen M, Skare TL. Secondary Sjögren's syndrome and disease activity of rheumatoid arthritis. *Rev Assoc Med Bras.* 2011;57:319–322. doi:10.1590/S0104-42302011000300015.

Baer AN, McAdams DeMarco M, Shiboski SC, et al. The SSB-positive/SSA-negative antibody profile is not associated with key phenotypic features of Sjögren's syndrome. *Ann Rheum Dis.* 2015;74(8):1557–1561.

Basiaga ML, Stern SM, Mehta JJ, et al. Childhood Sjögren syndrome: features of an international cohort and application of the 2016 ACR/EULAR classification criteria. *Rheumatology (Oxford).* 2021;60(7):3144–3155.

Carsons SE, Vivino FB, Parke A, et al. Treatment guidelines for rheumatologic manifestations of Sjögren's Syndrome: use of biologic agents, management of fatigue, and inflammatory musculoskeletal pain. *Arthritis Care Res (Hoboken).* 2017;69(4):517–527.

Chatzis LG, Stergiou IE, Goules AV, et al. Clinical picture, outcome and predictive factors of lymphoma in primary Sjögren's syndrome: results from a harmonized dataset (1981–2021). *Rheumatology (Oxford).* 2022;61(9):3576–3585.

D'Agostino C, Elkashty OA, Chivasso C, Perret J, Tran SD, Delporte C. Insight into salivary gland aquaporins. *Cells.* 2020;9(6):1–23.

Fisher BA, Jonsson R, Daniels T, et al. Standardisation of labial salivary gland histopathology in clinical trials in primary Sjögren's syndrome. *Ann Rheum Dis.* 2017;76(7):1161–1168.

Fox RI, Fox CM, McCoy SS. Emerging treatment for Sjögren's disease: a review of recent phase II and III trials. *Expert Opin Emerg Drugs.* 2023;28(2):107–120.

Fujita M, Igarashi T, Kurai T, Sakane M, Yoshino S, Takahashi H. Correlation between dry eye and rheumatoid arthritis activity. *Am J Ophthalmol.* 2005;140(5):808–813. doi:10.1016/j.ajo.2005.05.025.

Harrold LR, Shan Y, Rebello S, et al. Prevalence of Sjögren's syndrome associated with rheumatoid arthritis in the USA: an observational study from the Corrona registry. *Clin Rheumatol.* 2020;39(6):1899–1905.

He J, Ding Y, Feng M, et al. Characteristics of Sjogren's syndrome in rheumatoid arthritis. *Rheumatology.* 2013;52(6):1084–1089. doi:10.1093/rheumatology/kes374.

La Rocca G, Ferro F, Sambataro G, et al. Primary-Sjögren's-syndrome-related interstitial lung disease: a clinical review discussing current controversies. *J Clin Med.* 2023;12(10):1–16.

Maehara T, Moriyama M, Hayashida JN, et al. Selective localization of T helper subsets in labial salivary glands from primary Sjögren's syndrome patients. *Clin Exp Immunol.* 2012;169(2):89–99.

Mariette X, Criswell LA. Primary Sjögren's syndrome. *N Engl J Med.* 2018;378(10):931–939.

Qin B, Wang J, Yang Z, et al. Epidemiology of primary Sjögren's syndrome: a systematic review and meta-analysis. *Ann Rheum Dis.* 2015;74(11):1983–1989.

Ramos-Casals M, Brito-Zerón P, Seror R, et al. Characterization of systemic disease in primary Sjögren's syndrome: EULAR-SS Task Force recommendations for articular, cutaneous, pulmonary and renal involvements. *Rheumatology (Oxford).* 2015;54(12):2230–2238.

Ramos-Casals M, Brito-Zerón P, Solans R, et al. Systemic involvement in primary Sjogren's syndrome evaluated by the EULAR-SS disease activity index: analysis of 921 Spanish patients (GEAS-SS Registry). *Rheumatology (Oxford).* 2014;53(2):321–331.

Seror R, Theander E, Brun JG, et al. Validation of EULAR primary Sjogren's syndrome disease activity (ESSDAI) and patient indexes (ESSPRI). *Ann Rheum Dis*. 2015;74(5):859–866.

Shahdad SA, Taylor C, Barclay SC, Steen IN, Preshaw PM. A double-blind, crossover study of Biotène Oralbalance and BioXtra systems as salivary substitutes in patients with post-radiotherapy xerostomia. *Eur J Cancer Care (Engl)*. 2005;14(4):319–326.

Shiboski CH, Shiboski SC, Seror R, et al. 2016 American College of Rheumatology/European League against rheumatism classification criteria for primary Sjögren's syndrome: a consensus and data-driven methodology involving three international patient cohorts. *Arthritis Rheumatol*. 2017;69(1):35–45.

van der Heijden EH, Blokland SA, Hillen M, et al. Leflunomide-hydroxychloroquine combination therapy in patients with primary Sjogren's syndrome (RepurpSS-1): a placebo-controlled, double-blinded, randomized clinical trial. *Lancet Rheumatol*. 2020;2(5):e260–e269.

van Nimwegen JF, Mossel E, Delli K, et al. Incorporation of salivary gland ultrasonography into the American College of Rheumatology/European League against rheumatism criteria for primary Sjögren's syndrome. *Arthritis Care Res (Hoboken)*. 2020;72(4):583–590.

Verstappen GM, Pringle S, Bootsma H, Kroese FGM. Epithelial-immune cell interplay in primary Sjögren syndrome salivary gland pathogenesis. *Nat Rev Rheumatol*. 2021;17(6):333–348.

Vitali C, Bombardieri S, Moutsopoulos HM, et al. Preliminary criteria for the classification of Sjögren's syndrome. Results of a prospective concerted action supported by the European Community. *Arthritis Rheum*. 1993;36(3):340–347.

FURTHER READING

http://www.sjogrens.org.

CHAPTER 22

Antiphospholipid Syndrome

Doruk Erkan, MD, MPH and Sterling G. West, MD

Every person who has a thrombosis has a hypercoagulable state.

—The First Law of Hematology

 KEY POINTS

1. Not every "positive" antiphospholipid antibody (aPL) result is "clinically relevant"; aPL results should be assessed based on the type, isotype, titer, persistency, and the number of positive aPL tests.
2. Antiphospholipid syndrome diagnosis should rely on the careful assessment of clinical manifestations (including potential other/concomitant causes of each manifestation) and aPL profile.
3. Antiphospholipid antibody-related clinical manifestations include moderate-to-large vessel thrombosis, microvascular disease (e.g., diffuse alveolar hemorrhage, pregnancy morbidity), and non-thrombotic manifestations (e.g., thrombocytopenia).
4. Risk stratification and elimination of other thrombosis risk factors are critical in the long-term management of aPL-positive patients with or without a history of thrombosis.
5. Our recommendation is: (1) low-dose aspirin (LDA) for primary thrombosis prevention in patients with additional cardiovascular disease (CVD) risk factors; and (2) moderate intensity (international normalized ratio: 2–3) anticoagulation (with LDA in patients with additional CVD risk factors) for secondary thrombosis prevention.
6. First-line therapy for catastrophic antiphospholipid syndrome (APS) is the combination of anticoagulation, glucocorticoids, and plasmapheresis and/or intravenous immunoglobulin.

1. What is antiphospholipid syndrome?

Antiphospholipid syndrome (APS) is a systemic autoimmune disorder with thrombotic (venous, arterial, microvascular), non-thrombotic (e.g., thrombocytopenia, cardiac valve disease), and obstetric (e.g., severe pre-eclampsia) clinical manifestations developing in patients with persistent antiphospholipid antibodies (aPL).

2. What are antiphospholipid antibodies?

Antiphospholipid antibodies are a heterogeneous group of antibodies that bind to plasma proteins with an affinity for phospholipid surfaces. Most of these plasma proteins, for example β_2-glycoprotein-I (β_2GPI) or prothrombin, are involved in coagulation.

3. What is the pathogenesis of antiphospholipid syndrome?

The primary target of aPL is β_2GPI (apolipoprotein H). This is a phospholipid-binding plasma protein that exists in the blood in a circular conformation, contains five domains, belongs to the complement control protein superfamily, and binds through its fifth domain to anionic phospholipid membranes and receptors. After binding, it undergoes a conformational change to an open "hockey stick" conformation. With this change, it becomes antigenic by exposing hidden epitopes in the first domain. In addition, the clustering of these molecules provides a high antigenic density. The pathogenic anti-β_2GPI antibodies (aβ_2GPI) bind to an epitope in the first domain of the β_2GPI molecule. This binding results in a proinflammatory and prothrombotic state including (Fig. 22.1):

- Upregulation of the expression of prothrombotic endothelial cell adhesion molecules for example e-selectin, tissue factor
- Inhibition of nitric oxide synthetase production
- Promotion of coagulation by increasing expression of glycoprotein IIb/IIIa (fibrinogen receptor) on platelets and interfering with binding of other phospholipid-binding proteins (e.g., thrombomodulin, annexins) with anticoagulant activity, resulting in the suppression of tissue factor pathway inhibitor activity, decrease in activated protein C activity, and less fibrinolysis

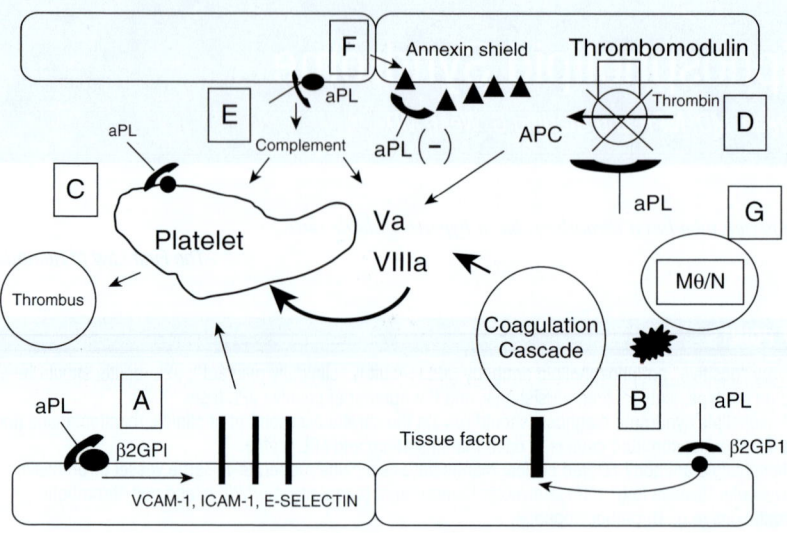

Fig. 22.1 Prothrombotic pathogenesis of the antiphospholipid syndrome. (A) Complex binding with upregulation of adhesion molecules on endothelium. (B) Complex binding with release of tissue factor activating coagulation cascade. (C) Complex binding with platelet activation and release of procoagulant factors. (D) Inhibition of thrombomodulin binding resulting in less activation of protein C. (E) Complex binding with complement activation and influx of inflammatory cells. (F) Complex binding inhibiting binding of annexin anticoagulant shield. (G) Activation of monocytes (MΘ) and neutrophils (N) with release of microparticles and neutrophil extracellular traps with tissue factor.

- Activation of neutrophils with the release of tissue factor and neutrophil extracellular traps
- Activation of monocytes with the release of microparticles containing tissue factor
- Activation of platelets with secretion of platelet factor-4 (procoagulant) and thromboxane A2 (increases platelet aggregation)
- Activation of the mammalian target of rapamycin (mTOR) pathway leading to endothelial cell proliferation
- Activation of complement, which can also lead to recruitment and activation of neutrophils, monocytes, and platelets

PEARL: Given that half of aPL-positive patients have a venous thromboembolism (VTE) and/or a cardiovascular (CVD) risk factor at the time of thrombosis, the two-hit hypothesis postulates that aPL are necessary but not sufficient to cause thrombosis, and proposes that aPL plus another prothrombotic factor (e.g. smoking, oral contraceptives, infection, surgery, others) are both necessary to "tip" the clotting cascade toward thrombosis.

4. How are antiphospholipid antibodies measured?

The common tests to detect aPL include lupus anticoagulant, anticardiolipin antibody (aCL), and $a\beta_2$GPI:

- **Lupus anticoagulant** test is a three-step functional coagulation assay. A phospholipid-dependent screening assay is performed first (generally activated Partial Thromboplastin Time [aPTT] and Diluted Russell Viper Venom Time [DRVVT]), and if prolonged, normal plasma is added in a 1:1 mix as a second step. If aPL is present, unlike a coagulation factor deficiency, the mixing study does not correct the prolonged screening assay. However, during the third confirmatory step, addition of excess phospholipid does correct the prolonged screening test. Given that aPTT is one of the screening tests used in LA assay, approximately half of patients with positive LA test have a prolonged aPTT; however, a normal aPTT does not exclude LA positivity.

- **Anticardiolipin antibodies** and **aβ₂GPI** are generally measured by an enzyme-linked immunosorbent assay (ELISA) test for immunoglobulin G (IgG), IgM, and IgA isotypes (isolated IgA positivity is extremely rare and the thrombogenic potential is not well-proven).

PEARLS: Be aware of (1) nonstandardized LA test reporting methods; (2) inaccurate LA test results in anticoagulated patients, especially if the international normalized ratio is >3; (3) the poor agreement among laboratories regarding aPL testing, especially for low-moderate level aCL/aβ₂GPI; and (4) non-ELISA automated systems used in some laboratories to test aCL/aβ₂GPI with different reference ranges compared to ELISA, and unknown "moderate" and "high" positivity thresholds.

5. How are antiphospholipid antibody test results Interpreted?

In the setting of relevant aPL-related clinical manifestation, the confidence in APS diagnosis increases with certain aPL profiles such as (1) triple aPL-positivity (LA, aCL, and aβ₂GPI), compared to double or single aPL-positivity; (2) LA test positivity in a non-anticoagulated sample, compared to positivity in an anticoagulated sample; (3) IgG aCL/aβ₂GPI positivity, compared to isolated IgM aCL/aβ₂GPI positivity; (4) moderate-to-high positive levels of aCL/aβ₂GPI (≥40 ELISA Units), compared to low positive levels of aCL/aβ₂GPI (above normal range but < 40 ELISA Units); and (5) persistent aPL positivity (on at least two occasions 12 weeks apart), compared to one-time aPL-positivity.

PEARL: Not every "positive" aPL result is "clinically relevant"; aPL results should be assessed based on the type, isotype, titer, persistency, and the number of positive aPL tests.

6. How do antiphospholipid antibodies affect prothrombin time (PT)?

Prothrombin time should not be affected by aPL. A prolonged PT might indicate prothrombin (factor II) deficiency, which can be caused by hereditary factor II deficiency, liver disease, vitamin K deficiency, or anticoagulation with warfarin. In addition, acquired factor II deficiency due to autoantibodies against factor II can rarely occur, commonly in lupus anticoagulant (LA)-positive lupus patients. It is important to detect factor II deficiency because this deficiency can be associated with excessive bleeding (LA-hypoprothrombinemia syndrome) rather than hypercoagulability. In an aPL-positive patient, if both aPTT and PT are prolonged, a prothrombin level should be measured to exclude factor II deficiency.

PEARL: It is not possible to predict when bleeding will occur in LA-positive patients with antibodies against factor II, even with an elevated PT; when bleeding occurs, the first line treatment is corticosteroids.

7. How can antiphospholipid antibodies be detected in an anticoagulated patient?

Measurement of aCL and aβ₂GPI are not affected by anticoagulation and can be reliably measured in a patient on heparin or warfarin. However, coagulation tests to detect lupus anticoagulant (LA) are affected by heparin, warfarin, and direct oral anticoagulants (DOACs).
- For unfractionated and low-molecular-weight heparin–receiving patients, plasma can be treated with heparinase to remove the heparin before the coagulation test.
- For warfarin-receiving patients, it is the PT that is primarily affected, and the aPTT is usually not prolonged. Thus, prolongation of aPTT in a patient on warfarin is still suggestive but not confirmative of the presence of LA. Although controversial and not always accurate, because warfarin depletes vitamin K–dependent factors, a 1:1 mix of the patient's plasma with normal plasma should correct the factor deficiencies induced by warfarin.
- For DOAC-receiving patients, LA test should not be ordered. If a test for LA clinically needs to be done, discuss with hematology how to safely take the patient off the DOAC for at least 48 hours prior to performing the LA test. Alert the laboratory that the patient has been on a DOAC, as it may use a DOAC adsorbent on the plasma prior to LA testing.

PEARLS: Despite the measures above, false-positive or false-negative LA results can occur in heparin- or warfarin-receiving patients; thus, results should be interpreted carefully. Lupus anticoagulant results are more likely to be accurate when the international normalized ratio is relatively low (INR<1.5–2.0) in warfarin-treated patients. Although further studies are needed to better define the diagnostic value of anti-phosphatidylserine/prothrombin antibodies (aPS/PT), including defining the relevance of different isotypes and levels, aPS/PT can be considered in selected aCL/aβ$_2$GPI-negative anticoagulated patients to clarify the LA status, since it is highly correlated with a true-positive LA.

8. How should heparinization be monitored in patients who already have a prolonged aPTT due to antiphospholipid antibodies?

In patients who are heparinized, heparin levels can be monitored directly to give an indication of anticoagulant effect by measuring the anti–factor Xa level. Alternatively, thrombin time (which measures the clotting system distal to the effects of aPL) can be used as an indicator of heparinization. In a patient on warfarin, the PT/international normalized ratio (INR) is not usually affected by aPL and can be used to monitor the adequacy of anticoagulation.

9. What is the value of a false-positive Venereal Disease Research Laboratory (VDRL) test?

The VDRL test measures agglutination (flocculation) of lipid particles that contain cholesterol and the negatively charged phospholipid cardiolipin. Antiphospholipid antibodies bind to the cardiolipin in these particles and cause flocculation, indistinguishable from that seen in patients with syphilis. A false-positive VDRL may be a clue for aPL-positivity, but in and of itself it is not a good way to screen for aPL. A false-positive VDRL or rapid plasma reagin (RPR) is seen in, at most, 50% of patients with aPL and, as such, is not recommended as an additional laboratory test in assessing an individual with suspected APS. Patients with only a false-positive VDRL and no aPL are not at increased risk for thrombosis or fetal loss.

10. What are the causes of antiphospholipid antibodies positivity?

Positive aPL can be associated with chronic immune stimulation. The primary conditions can be remembered by the mnemonic **MAIN:**

M—Medications, most commonly phenothiazines (chlorpromazine), procainamide, quinidine, hydralazine, phenytoin, α-interferon, interleukin-2, or tumor necrosis factor-α inhibitors

A—Autoimmune diseases such as SLE (20–30%), rheumatoid arthritis, dermatomyositis, Sjögren's syndrome, or systemic sclerosis

I—Infectious diseases: acute infections (bacteria, viral, especially herpes) or chronic infections (hepatitis C, HIV) (usually, transient IgM aCL without thrombosis risk).

N—Neoplasms, most commonly lymphoma.

11. When should a physician suspect antiphospholipid syndrome?

- Unexplained (recurrent) arterial thrombosis especially at a young age (<age 50)
- Unprovoked (recurrent) venous thrombosis especially at a young age (<age 50)
- Both arterial and venous thrombotic events in the same patient
- Thrombosis at unusual sites (e.g., renal, hepatic, cerebral sinuses, mesenteric, or vena cava)
- Late fetal loss, especially associated with early or severe preeclampsia, unexplained intrauterine growth restriction, or HELLP syndrome.
- False-positive syphilis tests
- Otherwise, unexplained elevated aPTT in the appropriate clinical setting
- Livedo reticularis/racemosa
- Otherwise, unexplained thrombocytopenia

12. What is the difference between disease classification and diagnosis?

Disease classification criteria aim to capture well-defined homogenous research cohorts. Given very strict and standardized definitions included in classification criteria, the goal of classification criteria is not to identify all possible patients with unusual manifestations of the disease. However, diagnostic criteria aim to identify all potential patients with a particular disease. For these reasons, classification criteria are not "diagnostic criteria," and they should not be used for therapeutic decisions.

13. Are there diagnostic criteria for antiphospholipid syndrome?

No, there are no diagnostic criteria for APS. The diagnosis of APS is a complex equation, which should be based on the aPL profile (see above), the strength of the association between aPL and the event, and the potential other causes of the event (which decrease the confidence in APS diagnosis).

14. Are there classification criteria for antiphospholipid syndrome?

Yes, there are two different classification criteria for APS. The Sapporo APS classification criteria, published in 1999 and revised in 2006, have served researchers for almost 25 years. Given the increasing number of APS clinical trials and a need for a more homogenous research cohorts, the highly specific 2023 ACR/EULAR APS classification criteria were developed, as a new tool for researchers, using rigorous methodology with multidisciplinary international input. The hierarchically clustered, weighted, and risk-stratified new criteria can be summarized in (Table 22.1):

TABLE 22.1 Summary of 2023 ACR/EULAR Antiphospholipid Syndrome (APS) Classification Criteria (please refer to the original publication or the online calculator for details and definitions; patients accumulating at least three points each from laboratory and clinical domains are classified as having APS)

Entry Criteria

At least one clinical criterion listed below (domains 1–6) <u>plus</u> positive antiphospholipid antibody (aPL) test (lupus anticoagulant test, or moderate-to-high titers of anticardiolipin or anti-β_2-glycoprotein-I antibodies [IgG or IgM]) within 3 years of the clinical criterion

Clinical Domains and Criteria:	Weight
Domain 1. Macrovascular (Venous Thromboembolism [VTE])	
• VTE with a high VTE risk profile	1
• VTE without a high VTE risk profile	3
Domain 2. Macrovascular (Arterial Thrombosis [AT])	
• AT with a high CVD risk profile	2
• AT without a high CVD risk profile	4
Domain 3. Microvascular[a]	
• Suspected	2
• Established	3
Domain 4. Obstetric	
• Three or more consecutive pre-fetal (<10w) and/or early fetal (10w 0d–15w 6d) deaths	1
• Fetal death (16w 0d – 33w 6d) in the absence of pre-eclampsia (PEC) with severe features or placental insufficiency (PI) with severe features	1
• PEC with severe features (<34w 0d) <u>or</u> PI with severe features (<34w 0d) with/without fetal death	3
• PEC with severe features (<34w 0d) <u>and</u> PI with severe features (<34w 0d) with/without fetal death	4
Domain 5. Cardiac Valve	
• Thickening	2
• Vegetation	4
Domain 6. Hematology	
• Thrombocytopenia (lowest 20–130 × 10^9/L)	2
Laboratory (aPL) Domains and Criteria	**Weight**
Domain 7. aPL test by coagulation-based functional assay (lupus anticoagulant test [LA])	
• Positive LA (single – one time)	1
• Positive LA (persistent)	5

Continued

TABLE 22.1 Summary of 2023 ACR/EULAR Antiphospholipid Syndrome (APS) Classification Criteria (please refer to the original publication or the online calculator for details and definitions; patients accumulating at least three points each from laboratory and clinical domains are classified as having APS)—cont'd

Domain 8. aPL test by solid phase assay (anti-cardiolipin antibody [aCL] ELISA and/or anti-β_2-glycoprotein-I antibody [aβ_2GPI] ELISA [persistent])[b]

• Moderate-high positive (IgM) (aCL and/or aβ_2GPI)	1
• Moderate positive (IgG) (aCL and/or aβ_2GPI)	4
• High positive (IgG) (aCL or aβ_2GPI)	5
• High positive (IgG) (aCL and aβ_2GPI)	7

[a]**Suspected:** Livedo racemosa, livedoid vasculopathy lesions by exam, or acute/chronic aPL-nephropathy by physical examination and/or laboratory, or pulmonary hemorrhage by symptoms and imaging; **Established:** Livedoid vasculopathy by pathology; acute/chronic aPl-nephropathy by pathology; pulmonary hemorrhage by bronchoalveolar lavage or pathology; myocardial disease by imaging or pathology; or adrenal hemorrhage by imaging or pathology.
[b]**Moderate** (40–79U) and **high** (≥80U) level aCL/aβ_2GPI are based on enzyme-linked immunosorbent assays (ELISA)

15. What are some of the other potential antiphospholipid antibody-related clinical manifestations that are not included in the 2023 ACR/EULAR APS criteria?

- Neurologic: Migraine, chorea, and seizures (controversial), cognitive dysfunction, white matter changes
- Dermatologic: Livedo reticularis
- Hematologic: Autoimmune hemolytic anemia (Coombs positive)
- Skeletal: Avascular necrosis (controversial)

16. What is microvascular antiphospholipid syndrome (MAPS)?

Microvascular APS refers to microangiopathy, microvascular thrombosis, and/or vasculopathy that can occur in aPL-positive patients. Patients with classic APS typically have clots predominantly in medium or larger vessels. However, it has become increasingly recognized that small vessels in the visceral organs may develop endothelial proliferation with or without clot leading to clinical manifestations resulting from ischemia and microinfarcts (e.g., livedoid vasculopathy with skin necrosis, cerebral microinfarcts with cognitive dysfunction, alveolar hemorrhage, chronic vaso-occlusive lesions with renal insufficiency [aPL-nephropathy], or ischemic cardiomyopathy).

In some of these patients, profound endothelial injury occurs in these microvessels, leading to a systemic thrombotic microangiopathy (TMA) with microangiopathic hemolytic anemia (schistocytes, high lactate dehydrogenase levels), thrombocytopenia, and organ involvement (usually kidney but other organs can be involved too) due to thrombosis of multiple small vessels. In patients with catastrophic antiphospholipid syndrome (CAPS), MAPS with/without systemic TMA predominates over the moderate-to-large vessel thrombosis typical of classic APS.

17. What is catastrophic antiphospholipid syndrome (CAPS)?

Catastrophic antiphospholipid syndrome (APS) occurs in less than 1% of patients with APS. Although rare, it is the initial presentation of APS in 50% of patients who develop CAPS. Potential triggers for CAPS development are infection, minor or major surgical procedures, pregnancy, and lupus flares. Definite CAPS classification (for research purposes) is based on having three or more organs involved simultaneously within 1 week, accompanied by histology showing predominately small vessel thrombosis in a patient with persistent aPL. In a clinical setting, it is critical to suspect and treat CAPS early as many patients presenting with multi-organ involvement will not have a clear "definite CAPS" presentation.

The most common presenting manifestations in CAPS patients are cardiopulmonary (25%) with acute respiratory failure from hemorrhage (11%), central nervous system manifestations (22%), renal insufficiency (14%), and cutaneous disease (10%). As the disease progresses, these organs are involved over 60% of the time. Thrombocytopenia occurs in two-thirds and hemolytic anemia in one-third of patients. In those who develop systemic thrombotic microangiopathy (TMA), differential diagnosis includes thrombotic thrombocytopenia purpura (TTP), hemolytic uremic syndrome (HUS), malignant hypertension, and disseminated intravascular coagulation;

TABLE 22.2 Summary for Key Findings That May Be Helpful in Differentiating Catastrophic Antiphospholipid Syndrome From Other Systemic Thrombotic Microangiopathies (please note that these conditions can sometimes overlap)

	CAPS	TTP	HUS	HELLP SYNDROME	MALIGNANT HTN	ACUTE DIC
Fever	—	30%	—	—	—	—
Thrombosis	Diffuse	CNS 66% Renal 50%	Renal 100%	Liver 100%	CNS Renal	None
Thrombocytopenia	++ 60%	+++ < 20,000	++ >20,000	++ > 20,000	+	++/+++
Hemolytic anemia Schistocytes	+ 33%	+++ >3–5%	+++ >3–5%	++ >1–2%	+/– Few	+/++ Few
PT/PTT	N/High[a]	N/N	N/N	N/N	N/N	High/High
Fibrinogen/FDPs	N/N	NI/High	N/High	N/High	N/N	Low/High
Others	+ aPL	Low (5%) ADAMTS13; very high LDH (>1000)	High C5b-C9; very high LDH (>1000)	High LAEs and LDH (>600); preeclampsia 80%	Severe HBP 100%	Low factors V and VIII

aPL, antiphospholipid antibodies; *CAPS*, catastrophic antiphospholipid syndrome; *CNS*, central nervous system; *DIC*, disseminated intravascular coagulation; *HTN*, hypertension; *FDP*, fibrin degradation products; *HUS*, hemolytic uremic syndrome; *LAE*, liver enzymes; *LDH*, lactate dehydrogenase; *N*, normal; *PT*, prothrombin time; *PTT*, partial thromboplastin time; *TTP*, thrombotic thrombocytopenia purpura.
[a]PTT high if lupus anticoagulant present.

these conditions, all under the umbrella of systemic TMA, can sometimes overlap with CAPS. In aPL-positive pregnant patients, HELLP syndrome can eventually develop into CAPS (Table 22.2).

18. Is it possible to diagnose antiphospholipid syndrome based on clinical suspicion but negative antiphospholipid antibodies?

Given that thrombosis, pregnancy morbidity, and non-thrombotic manifestations that can occur in aPL-positive patients have a broad differential diagnosis, antiphospholipid syndrome should not be diagnosed without positive antiphospholipid antibodies (aPL). The diagnostic role of non-criteria aPL tests [e.g. anti-phosphatidylserine/prothrombin antibodies (aPS/PT)] still requires further studies but rarely may be the only aPL positive in an APS patient.

19. What is the primary thrombosis prevention strategy in persistently antiphospholipid antibody-positive patients (prevention of the first thrombosis)?

- Risk stratification, aPL profile assessment, and treatment or elimination of other thrombosis risk factors, for example smoking, hyperlipidemia, hypertension, diabetes mellitus, immobilization, or birth control pills, are critical.
- Concomitant systemic autoimmune diseases should be managed aggressively. Hydroxychloroquine (HCQ) may reduce thrombotic risk in SLE patients with aPL.
- All patients with clinically relevant aPL profiles should receive prophylactic heparin treatment (~6–8 weeks, or until they are back to their normal daily activities) to prevent clots when undergoing high-risk procedures (e.g., surgery, postpartum) even if they have no previous history of clot. They should also get compression stockings and early ambulation.
- The protective effect of low-dose aspirin is not supported by prospective or randomized controlled studies; a meta-analysis demonstrated low-dose aspirin may decrease the risk of first thrombosis in aPL-positive patients; however, no significant risk reduction was observed when considering only prospective studies or those with the best methodological quality.

- In patients with clinically relevant aPL profiles, we recommend low-dose aspirin for those with SLE or additional cardiovascular disease risk factors. Statins may also lower thrombotic risk in patients with hyperlipidemia.

PEARLS: The risk of a first thrombotic event in, persistently aPL-positive patient is between 0% and 5% per year depending on the number of risk factors including aPL-profile (see Question 5 above) and concomitant risk factors. Independent risks for thrombosis based on prospective observational studies include age, male sex, hypertension, diabetes, smoking, systemic autoimmune diseases, and combined venous thrombosis risk factors.

20. What is the secondary thrombosis prevention strategy in persistently antiphospholipid antibody-positive patients with history of venous thromboembolism (prevention of the subsequent thrombosis)?

- Risk stratification, aPL profile assessment, and treatment or elimination of other thrombosis risk factors, e.g., smoking, hyperlipidemia, hypertension, diabetes mellitus, immobilization, or birth control pills, are critical.
- Concomitant systemic autoimmune diseases should be managed aggressively. HCQ in SLE patients.
- Two prospective trials demonstrated that moderate-intensity warfarin therapy (INR: 2–3), compared to high-intensity one (INR: 3–4), is sufficient to prevent further venous clots. Because the risk of recurrent thrombosis without therapy is relatively high, despite the lack of risk-stratified studies, most individuals will require lifelong anticoagulation.
- Our approach for secondary thrombosis prevention in APS patients with venous thrombo-embolism is warfarin with a target INR of 2.5 to 3, adding low-dose aspirin if patients have additional cardiovascular disease risk factors.

21. What is the secondary thrombosis prevention strategy in persistently antiphospholipid antibody-positive patients with history of arterial thrombosis (prevention of the subsequent thrombosis)?

- Risk stratification, aPL profile assessment, and treatment or elimination of other thrombosis risk factors, e.g., smoking, hyperlipidemia, hypertension, diabetes mellitus, immobilization, or birth control pills, are critical.
- Thrombolytic therapy as per expert guidelines.
- Transthoracic echocardiogram with bubble study to rule out patent foramen ovale, and a transesophageal echocardiogram to rule out valvular lesions and an intramural clot.
- Treatment during first 48 hours: low-dose ASA (81 mg daily) and prophylactic-dose LMWH. In case of a large stroke, ASA can be continued for 2 weeks without full anticoagulation to lessen the chance of bleeding into the damaged area of the brain.
- Warfarin remains the cornerstone for long-term secondary thrombosis prevention in APS patients with a target international normalized ratio (INR) of 2–3. Despite retrospective cohort studies demonstrating that high-intensity (INR 3–4) anticoagulation is more effective than moderate-intensity one (INR 2–3), two prospective RCTs of moderate- versus high-intensity warfarin did not show any difference between the treatment groups in the prevention of recurrent thrombosis. Since the number of APS patients with arterial events was relatively low in these two RCTs, high-intensity anticoagulation is still preferred by some centers.
- Our approach for secondary thrombosis prevention in APS patients with arterial thrombosis is warfarin with a target INR of 2.5 to 3, adding low-dose aspirin if patients have additional cardiovascular disease risk factors. In patients with no cardioembolic stroke, low-risk aPL profile, and/or a high-bleeding risk, treatment with only the combination of antiplatelet agents (e.g., low-dose aspirin + clopidogrel) can be considered. If use clopidogrel, make sure patient doesn't have a CYP2C19 loss-of-function genetic variant hindering its effectiveness or use ticagrelor.

22. What is the secondary thrombosis prevention strategy in persistently antiphospholipid antibody-positive patients with history of recurrent thrombosis while receiving anticoagulation?

If an antiphospholipid syndrome (APS) patient has new thrombosis while on anticoagulation, it is imperative to establish that the patient was adequately anticoagulated at the time of the recurrent thrombosis. The APS patient on warfarin should have an INR of 2 to 3 and a confirmed chromogenic factor X level of ≤20%. If the patient is adequately anticoagulated and had a venous clot, then anticoagulation should be increased to an INR of 3 to 4 or the patient switched to LMWH if the INR is difficult to maintain in a therapeutic range consistently. If the patient has an arterial clot, then the INR can be increased to 3 to 4, and/or low-dose ASA or clopidogrel can be added.

If the APS patient clots while receiving LMWH, an anti–factor Xa level should be checked to ensure it is in the therapeutic range. If the patient is therapeutic but has a venous clot and is on once-a-day enoxaparin, then using twice-a-day dosing may be helpful. Some recommend high-intensity LMWH by increasing the dose by 25–33% and following anti–factor Xa levels. If the patient has an arterial clot, then low-dose ASA can be added. If the patient is already on ASA, they can be switched to clopidogrel (after genetic testing) or use it in combination with ASA. Patients who clinically fail LMWH or develop heparin-induced thrombocytopenia (HIT) should be switched to fondaparinux.

Hydroxychloroquine and statins are potential add-on treatments for patients who have recurrent thrombosis despite therapeutic-dose anticoagulation with or without antiplatelet agents. Hydroxychloroquine has an antithrombotic effect based on platelet inhibition and protecting the annexin V anticoagulant shield from disruption by preventing anti-aPL-β2GPI complexes from binding to phospholipid membranes. Statins have immunomodulatory and anti-inflammatory properties that suppress aβ_2GPI-mediated endothelial activation. Both medications, in theory, may be beneficial in an APS patient refractory to treatment despite lack of clinical outcome studies.

PEARLS: Based on different studies, 10–30% of APS patients may develop recurrent thrombosis despite anticoagulation; the risk may vary based on aPL profile (see Question 5 above), additional thrombosis risk factors, concomitant use of antiplatelet agents, and the length of follow-up. Arterial thromboses are more likely than venous thromboses to be recurrent while on anticoagulation. Patients treated with LMWH should have intermittent platelet counts to rule out development of HIT (risk 0.2%).

23. Is it possible to stop anticoagulation in antiphospholipid syndrome patients with history of thrombosis?

Patients who had a provoked venous thrombosis due to a reversible risk factor (e.g., surgery, cast, estrogen therapy, pregnancy, immobilization) and a low-risk aPL profile may be considered for withdrawal of anticoagulation if thrombosis has resolved on imaging and D-dimer is normal (controversial—further studies are needed). Stopping anticoagulation is not recommended in APS patients with history of arterial thrombosis, pending further risk-stratified studies.

24. What are direct oral anticoagulants (DOACs) and what is their role in persistently antiphospholipid antibody–positive patients with history of thrombosis?

Direct oral anticoagulants are non–vitamin K antagonist oral anticoagulants that bind directly to specific clotting factors. Dabigatran is a factor IIa inhibitor, whereas rivaroxaban, apixaban, and edoxaban are factor Xa inhibitors. They have a rapid onset of action and a relatively short half-life. They should not be used in patients with a CrCl <30 mL/min.

Direct oral anticoagulants are currently not recommended for secondary thrombosis prevention in APS. Based on APS clinical trials comparing DOACs to warfarin as well as expert recommendations, DOACs should be avoided in APS patients with arterial thrombosis, triple aPL-positive patients, and in patients with recurrent thrombosis while on standard intensity warfarin. In triple aPL-positive thrombotic APS patients, if the patient is already on DOAC following the first VTE, then switching to vitamin K antagonists is recommended. If a patient declines the switch, close clinical surveillance while on DOAC is important, which also includes the magnetic resonance imaging of the brain for ischemic lesions.

PEARLS: A concern is that due to the short half-life of DOACs, APS patients will be at risk for a clot if they miss one dose. Patients on DOACs will have a false-positive LA test.

25. What is the treatment strategy for catastrophic antiphospholipid syndrome?

Owing to the high mortality (30–50%) in patients who develop catastrophic APS (CAPS), every effort should be made to prevent its development (e.g., avoid triggers). Patients who develop CAPS can be treated as follows:

- First-line therapy (the combination of anticoagulation, glucocorticoids, plasmapheresis, and/or IVIG) provides the best outcomes based on the analysis of the international CAPS registry.
  - Intravenous unfractionated heparin; anticoagulation may need to be delayed or interrupted if the patient is having life-threatening hemorrhagic complications (severe pulmonary hemorrhage, intracerebral hemorrhage).
  - If platelets <15,000/μL, do not start heparin and treat with glucocorticoids and IVIG. If platelets >15,000/μL, start low-dose heparin. If platelets >50,000/μL, use full-dose heparin anticoagulation. Patients on heparin should be followed with platelet counts to make sure they don't develop HIT (risk 2.6%).
  - Methylprednisolone 500–1000 mg daily for 3 to 5 days followed by high-dose oral prednisone.
  - Plasmapheresis is done generally daily for the first 3 days; replacement fluid should be albumin and not fresh frozen plasma unless the patient also has TTP/HUS.
  - IVIG after plasmapheresis completed: 0.4 g/kg/day for 5 days; slow infusion in patients with kidney involvement. Follow renal function tests.
- Second-line therapy to consider.
  - Eculizumab in patients with systemic thrombotic microangiopathy
  - Rituximab in patients with microvascular disease
  - Cyclophosphamide and/or rituximab, especially if associated with active SLE.

26. What is the role of immunosuppression in antiphospholipid syndrome?

There is no uniform approach to the management of microvascular APS and/or non-thrombotic manifestations of aPL due to heterogeneous organ involvement, and the lack of controlled studies and strong literature supporting any treatment strategy. These patients do not respond to anticoagulation and may develop these manifestations while on therapeutic anticoagulation. Given the increasing awareness of the mechanisms involved in APS pathogenesis, immunosuppressive agents have been increasingly used in the management of patients with microvascular disease or non-thrombotic manifestations, mostly based on case reports or series. A general immunosuppression strategy for these patients can be summarized as:

- Acute aPL-nephropathy due to thrombotic microangiopathy: plasma exchange.
- Chronic aPL-nephropathy due to vaso-occlusive lesions: mycophenolate mofetil with or without rituximab, consider sirolimus for resistant cases.
- Diffuse alveolar hemorrhage: mycophenolate mofetil with or without rituximab, consider intravenous immunoglobulin (IVIG) for resistant cases.
- Livedoid vasculopathy-related skin ulcers: Rituximab as the first-line therapy; pentoxifylline, sildenafil, IVIG, hyperbaric oxygen, and anticoagulation, often in combination, as the second line.
- Immune-mediated thrombocytopenia (<20,000/mm^3): glucocorticoids with or without IVIG as the first line, traditional immunosuppressives or rituximab as the second line. Splenectomy is not preferred due to perioperative thrombosis risk.
- Immune-mediated hemolytic anemia: same as thrombocytopenia.
- Heart valve lesions: no proven therapy; anticoagulation should be considered to prevent emboli. Immunosuppression does not prevent/help heart valve lesions.

PEARLS: Glucocorticoids are generally effective in patients with microvascular APS (except livedoid vasculopathy) and/or non-thrombotic manifestations (except cardiac valve disease); however, the recurrence risk is high during glucocorticoid tapering without immunosuppressive agents.

27. Is it possible to stop immunosuppression in antiphospholipid syndrome patients?

There is no rule on the duration of anticoagulation in aPL-positive patients with microvascular disease and/or non-thrombotic manifestations. After the successful discontinuation of glucocorticoids with no disease activity, the dose of the immunosuppressive agent(s) can be tapered off over time; however, the decision should be individualized on a case-by-case basis.

28. A patient with antiphospholipid syndrome on warfarin comes in with a dangerously high International Normalized Ratio (INR). What can be done?

Most patients will not have excessive major bleeding risk unless the INR is >5. Most of the time the patient can be instructed to hold warfarin until the INR decreases to the desired range. If INR must be decreased quickly, the patient can be given 1 mg or less of vitamin K orally or IV (not SC). This will decrease the excessive anticoagulation within 12 hours without making them resistant to warfarin for several days, which happens if vitamin K is given SC. If the patient has a high INR and is severely bleeding, they need to receive fresh frozen plasma to replace coagulation factors acutely. However, this will put them at risk for clotting.

29. What is the treatment strategy for pregnant patients with history of obstetric antiphospholipid syndrome only? How about if they have a history of thrombosis?

Although additional studies are needed to determine the optimal management of patients with a history of different pregnancy morbidities (e.g., pre-fetal loss, fetal loss, placental insufficiency), a general approach for patients with obstetric APS is:

- Aspirin (81–100 mg) daily is prescribed before conception.
- Once conception has occurred, prophylactic dose heparin 7500 to 10,000 units SC twice a day or low-molecular-weight heparin (LMWH) (e.g., enoxaparin 40 mg SC daily, dalteparin 5000 units SC daily) is added and continued until at least 34 weeks of gestation. The platelet count should be monitored every 2 to 4 weeks to monitor for heparin-induced thrombocytopenia (HIT). Heparin and LMWH at higher antithrombotic doses do not work any better than prophylactic doses.
- Heparin or LMWH is stopped before delivery and then reinstituted and continued at prophylactic doses for at least 6 to 8 weeks post-delivery.
- Heparin is safe during breastfeeding.
- Coumadin is contraindicated during pregnancy owing to fetal malformations.

Antiphospholipid syndrome patients with a previous history of venous or arterial thrombosis who are on chronic coumadin and become pregnant should be switched to full therapeutic doses of LMWH and low-dose ASA throughout pregnancy. In the postpartum period, they can be switched back to warfarin, which is safe during breastfeeding.

PEARLS: For high-risk obstetric APS patients, consider (1) Factor-Xa monitoring during pregnancy and (2) hydroxychloroquine, which can decrease the risk of pregnancy morbidity based on retrospective studies.

BIBLIOGRAPHY

Aggarwal R, Ringold S, Khanna D, et al. Distinctions between diagnostic and classification criteria? *Arthritis Care Res (Hoboken).* 2015;67:891–897.

Amory CF, Levine SR, Brey RL, et al. Antiphospholipid antibodies and recurrent thrombotic events: persistence and portfolio. *Cerebrovasc Dis.* 2015;40:293–300.

Arachchillage DRJ, Laffan M. Pathogenesis and management of antiphospholipid syndrome. *Br J Haematol.* 2017;178:181–195.

Barbhaiya M, Zuily S, Naden R, et al. The 2023 ACR/EULAR antiphospholipid syndrome classification criteria. *Arthritis Rheumatol.* 2023;75:1687–1702.

Coban MT, Duarte-Garcia A, McBane RD, et al. Antiphospholipid Syndrome: role of vascular endothelial cells and implications for stratification and targeted therapeutics. *J Am Coll Cardiol.* 2017;69:2317–2330.

Cohen H, Cuadrado MJ, Erkan D, et al. 16th International Congress on Antiphospholipid Antibodies task force report on antiphospholipid syndrome treatment trends. *Lupus.* 2020;29:1571–1593.

Cohen H, Hunt BJ, Efthymiou M, et al. Rivaroxaban versus warfarin to treat patients with thrombotic antiphospholipid syndrome, with or without systemic lupus erythematosus (RAPS): a randomized, controlled, open-label, phase 2/3, non-inferiority trial. *Lancet Haematol.* 2016;3:e426–e436.

Crowther MA, Ginsberg JS, Julian J, et al. A comparison of two intensities of warfarin for the prevention of recurrent thrombosis in patients with antiphospholipid antibody syndrome. *N Engl J Med.* 2003;349:1133–1138.

DeGroot PG, Meijers JCM. β2-Glycoprotein I: evolution, structure, and function. *J Thromb Haemost.* 2011;9:1275–1284.

Devreese KMJ, de Groot PG, de Laat B, et al. Guidance from the Scientific and Standardization Committee for lupus anticoagulant/antiphospholipid antibodies of the International Society on Thrombosis and Haemostasis: update of the guidelines for lupus anticoagulant detection and interpretation. *J Thromb Haemost.* 2020;18:2828–2839.

Dlott JS, Roubey RA. Drug-induced lupus anticoagulants and antiphospholipid antibodies. *Curr Rheumatol Rep.* 2012;14:71–78.

Erkan D, Harrison MJ, Levy R, et al. Aspirin for primary thrombosis prevention in the antiphospholipid syndrome. *Arthritis Rheum.* 2007;56:2382–2391.

Erkan D, Leibowitz E, Berman J, et al. Perioperative medical management of antiphospholipid syndrome. *J Rheumatol.* 2002;29:843–849.

Erkan D, Vega J, Ramon G, et al. A pilot open-label phase II trial of rituximab for non-criteria manifestations of antiphospholipid syndrome. *Arthritis Rheum.* 2013;65:464–471.

Erkan D. Expert perspective: management of microvascular and catastrophic antiphospholipid syndrome. *Arthritis Rheumatol.* 2021;73:1780–1790.

Finazzi G, Marchioli R, Brancaccio V, et al. A randomized clinical trial of high-intensity warfarin vs. conventional antithrombotic therapy for the prevention of recurrent thrombosis in patients with antiphospholipid syndrome (WAPS). *J Thromb Haemost.* 2005;3:848–853.

Garcia D, Erkan D. Diagnosis and management of the antiphospholipid syndrome. *N Engl J Med.* 2018;378:2010–2021.

Giannakopoulos B, Krilis SA. The pathogenesis of the antiphospholipid syndrome. *N Eng J Med.* 2013;368:1033–1044.

Khairani CD, Bejjani A, Piazza G, et al. Direct oral anticoagulants vs. vitamin K antagonists in patients with antiphospholipid syndromes: meta-analysis of randomized trials. *J Am Coll Cardiol.* 2023;81:16–30.

Laskin CA, Spitzer KA, Clark CA, et al. Low molecular weight heparin and aspirin for recurrent pregnancy loss: results from the randomized, controlled HepASA Trial. *J Rheumatol.* 2009;36:279–287.

Legault K, Schunemann H, Hillis C, et al. McMaster RARE-best practices clinical practice guideline on diagnosis and management of the catastrophic antiphospholipid syndrome. *J Thromb Haemost.* 2018;16:1656–1664.

Negrini S, Pappalardo F, Murdaca G, et al. The antiphospholipid syndrome: from pathophysiology to treatment. *Clin Exp Med.* 2017;17:257–267.

Ordi-Ros J, Sáez-Comet L, Pérez-Conesa M, et al. Rivaroxaban versus vitamin K antagonist in antiphospholipid syndrome: a randomized noninferiority trial. *Ann Intern Med.* 2019;171:685–694.

Ortel TL, Erkan D, Kitchens CS. How I treat catastrophic thrombotic syndromes. *Blood.* 2015;126:1285–1293.

Pengo V, Denas G, Zoppellaro G, et al. Rivaroxaban vs warfarin in high risk patients with antiphospholipid syndrome. *Blood.* 2018;132:1365–1371.

Pham M, Orsolini G, Crowson C, Snyder M, Pruthi R, Moder K. Anti-phosphatidylserine prothrombin antibodies as a predictor of the lupus anticoagulant in an all-comer population. *J Thromb Haemost.* 2022;20:2070–2074.

Rosborough TK, Jacobsen JM, Shepherd MF. Factor X and factor II activity levels do not always agree with warfarin-treated lupus anticoagulant patients. *Blood Coagul Fibrinolysis.* 2010;21:242–244.

Schreiber K, Hunt BJ. Pregnancy and antiphospholipid antibody syndrome. *Semin Thromb Hemost.* 2016;42:780–788.

Shapira I, Andrade D, Allen SL, Salmon JE. Brief report: induction of sustained remission in recurrent catastrophic antiphospholipid syndrome via inhibition of terminal complement with eculizumab. *Arthritis Rheum.* 2012;64:2719–2723.

Unlu O, Erkan D. Catastrophic antiphospholipid syndrome: candidate therapies for a potentially lethal disease. *Annu Rev Med.* 2017;68:287–296.

Woller SC, Stevens SM, Kaplan D, et al. Apixaban compared with warfarin to prevent thrombosis in thrombotic antiphospholipid syndrome: a randomized trial. *Blood Adv.* 2022;6:1661–1670.

Yachoui R, Sehgal R, Amlani B, Goldberg JW. Antiphospholipid antibodies-associated diffuse alveolar hemorrhage. *Semin Arthritis Rheum.* 2015;44:652–657.

FURTHER READING

2023 ACR/EULAR Antiphospholipid Syndrome (APS) Classification Criteria Calculator.
https://rheumatology.org/criteria.
APS Foundation of America
www.apsfa.org
APS Alliance for Clinical Trials and International Networking
www.apsaction.org

CHAPTER 23

Adult-Onset Still's Disease

W Winn Chatham, MD

 KEY POINTS

1. Systemic autoinflammatory illness characterized by quotidian fevers, transient rashes, inflammatory polyarthritis, and neutrophilic leukocytosis. Many have odynophagia due to perichondritis of the cricothyroid cartilage.
2. No specific test is diagnostic, but a ferritin level >1000 ng/mL is common.
3. Macrophage activation syndrome (MAS) is a severe, life-threatening complication occurring in 5% to 15% of patients.
4. Nonsteroidal anti-inflammatory drugs (NSAIDs) and corticosteroids can remit manifestations in up to a third of patients.
5. Methotrexate and biologics are required to induce remission of disease flares in the majority of patients including the 33% with a chronic disease course.

1. What is adult-onset Still's disease (AOSD)?

AOSD is a nonfamilial, systemic autoinflammatory disorder phenotypically indistinguishable from systemic-onset juvenile idiopathic arthritis. It is characterized by seronegative chronic poly-arthritis/arthralgias in association with a systemic inflammatory illness including a characteristic fever, various transient rashes, and a neutrophilic leukocytosis. The disease was initially described in children in 1897 by the English pathologist, Sir George F. Still. The characteristic features of this illness were subsequently reported in adults, as detailed by Eric Bywaters in 1971.

2. How do patients with AOSD generally present?

Patients tend to be young adults (75% age <35 years) who present with a prolonged course of nonspecific signs and symptoms. Patients age up to 70 years have been reported. The most striking manifestations are severe arthralgias/arthritis, spiking high fevers, and transient rashes. A prodromal sore throat due to perichondritis of the cricothyroid cartilage can occur days to weeks before other symptoms in 70% of cases. In some patients, a history may be elicited of similar episodes of this illness during their childood. Patients often appear severely ill and have often received courses of antibiotics for presumed bacterial sepsis, although cultures are negative. In severe cases, clinical and laboratory features of cytokine storm may be present due to development of macrophage activation syndrome (MAS). As many as 5% of patients being evaluated for "fever of unknown origin" may be diagnosed eventually with Still's disease.

3. Describe the characteristic fever of AOSD

The classically described fever in AOSD typically starts suddenly and rapidly reaches ≥39°C. The fever generally occurs only once a day, usually in the late afternoon or early evening, and lasts 2 to 4 hours. The fever occurs daily for over a week and typically longer. Characteristically, the patient's temperature returns to *normal or below normal* between fever spikes. This pattern is known as a **quotidian fever**. In 20% of cases, the patient may have an additional early morning spike (**double quotidian fever**). The presence of a double quotidian fever should prompt consideration of AOSD, as well as kala-azar, mixed malarial infections, Kawasaki's disease, right-sided gonococcal or meningococcal endocarditis, and miliary tuberculosis (TB).

Patients with high fevers feel very ill when febrile but feel relatively well when their body temperature is normal. This poses a dilemma for physicians, because hospital rounds and clinic visits may not occur during the times when the patient is febrile. The fever pattern in Still's disease contrasts with the pattern seen in the setting of infection; infections generally cause a baseline elevation in body temperature in addition to episodic or erratic fever spikes. However, in up to 20% of cases of AOSD, the patient's temperature may not completely normalize between fever spikes; this is particularly likely in patients who develop MAS.

TABLE 23.1 Signs and Symptoms of Adult-Onset Still's Disease

MANIFESTATION	FREQUENCY (%)
Arthralgias	98–100
Fever (>39°C)	83–100
Myalgias	84–98
Arthritis	88–94
Sore throat	50–92
Rash	87–90
Weight loss (>10%)	19–76
Lymphadenopathy	48–74
Splenomegaly	45–55
Pleuritis	23–53
Abdominal pain	9–48
Hepatomegaly	29–44
Pericarditis	24–37
Pneumonitis	9–31

4. What are the common and uncommon signs and symptoms seen in AOSD?

The common signs and symptoms of AOSD are shown in Table 23.1. Notably, the presence of odynophagia/pharyngitis with high fever may be a distinguishing feature of AOSD from lymphoma or another neoplastic disease as the cause of a febrile illness. Unusual manifestations include alopecia, mucosal ulcers, subcutaneous nodules, necrotizing lymphadenitis (Kikuchi's disease), amyotrophy, acute liver failure, abdominal pain due to lymphadenitis, pulmonary fibrosis, pulmonary hypertension (especially in women with dyspnea), cardiac tamponade, aseptic meningitis, peripheral neuropathy, interstitial nephritis, amyloidosis, hemolytic anemia, disseminated intravascular coagulation (DIC), thrombotic thrombocytopenic purpura (TTP) (suspect in patients with schistocytes and thrombocytopenia), orbital pseudotumor, uveitis, sensorineural hearing loss, myositis (10%), and MAS (secondary hemophagocytic lymphohistiocytosis [sHLH]).

5. Describe the rash associated with AOSD.

Although the rash is said to occur in the vast majority of patients with AOSD, it is often unappreciated unless specifically sought. The characteristic appearance is that of evanescent, salmon-colored, macular or maculopapular lesions that are nonpruritic. The rash is usually seen on the trunk, arms, legs, or areas of mechanical irritation such as tight clothing (beltline). Often, it is only seen when the patient is febrile. The rash can sometimes be elicited by heat, such as that produced by applying a hot towel or taking a hot bath or shower. Koebner phenomenon (i.e., the rash can be induced by rubbing the skin) is reported in approximately 40% of patients. Atypical skin rashes and urticarial lesions have also been reported in up to 14% of patients. Skin biopsies and immunofluorescent studies are nondiagnostic, showing dermal edema and a perivascular mononuclear cell infiltrate. Purpuric lesions with thrombocytopenia should suggest an associated hematologic complication that could be life-threatening such as MAS.

6. Describe the arthritis associated with AOSD.

The arthritis associated with AOSD may be overshadowed by the systemic features of the illness. It may not be present at the time of disease onset, may involve only a few joints, or be fleeting. With time, the arthritis frequently becomes polyarticular affecting both small and large joints. The joints involved in descending order include: knees, wrists (very common), ankles, elbows, proximal interphalangeal, shoulders, metacarpophalangeal, metatarsophalangeals, hips, distal

TABLE 23.2 Laboratory Findings in Adult-Onset Still's Disease

LABORATORY TEST	FREQUENCY (%)
Elevated erythrocyte sedimentation rate (>50)	96–100
Elevated C-reactive protein (often >10 × upper limit of normal)	90–100
Leukocytosis (range 12–40,000/mm^3)	71–97
Anemia	59–92
Neutrophils (≥80%)	55–88
Hypoalbuminemia	44–85
Elevated hepatic enzymes	35–85
Thrombocytosis	52–62
Ferritin >1000 ng/mL	40–70
Positive antinuclear antibodies	0–11 (should be negative)
Positive rheumatoid factor	2–8 (usually negative)

interphalangeal, sacroiliac, and temporomandibular joints. Neck pain is seen in 50% of cases. Arthrocentesis generally yields a class II inflammatory synovial fluid (mean 13,000 cells/µL), and radiographs usually reveal soft tissue swelling, effusions, and occasionally periarticular osteoporosis. Joint erosions and/or fusion of the carpal bones (40–50%), tarsal bones (20%), and cervical spine (10%) may be seen but are more common in children than adults. Destructive arthritis occurs in up to 20% to 25% of cases. Pericapitate cartilage loss is a characteristic radiographic feature in patients with a chronic articular presentation of AOSD.

7. What are the characteristic laboratory features of AOSD?

There is no diagnostic test for Still's disease. Rather, the diagnosis is one of exclusion, made in the setting of the proper clinical features and laboratory abnormalities and the absence of another explanation (such as infection or malignancy) (Table 23.2).

PEARL: Aldolase is frequently elevated, whereas creatine phosphokinase is normal. Aldolase elevation is due to liver inflammation. Procalcitonin can be elevated in AOSD even in the absence of infection.

8. What is the diagnostic significance of an elevated ferritin?

An extremely elevated serum ferritin (>1000 ng/mL) in the proper clinical setting is suggestive of Still's disease and is seen in up to 70% of patients. In the absence of MAS, values over 4000 ng/mL are seen in <50% of cases. In addition to AOSD, the differential diagnosis of fever with hyperferritinemia includes primary/familial hemophagocytic lymphohistiocytosis (fHLH), infections (HIV, TB, herpesviruses [EBV, CMV, HSV]), malignancies (colon, prostate, breast, lung, liver, and metastatic melanoma), lymphomas, liver metastasis, septic shock, catastrophic antiphospholipid antibody syndrome, and systemic lupus erythematosus (SLE), often in the setting of secondary hemophagocytic syndromes (sHLH) that can be triggered by these entities. However, unlike these other causes, the elevated ferritin in AOSD is mostly nonglycosylated (H-ferritin), with the glycosylated form (L-ferritin) being <20% of total ferritin. This pattern of ferritin (ferritin >1000 ng/mL, <20% glycosylated) has a 70% to 80% sensitivity and 84% to 93% specificity for the diagnosis of AOSD. The etiology of the elevated ferritin is postulated to be from proinflammatory cytokines (tumor necrosis factor [TNF], interleukin-6 [IL-6], IL-18, others) inducing the heme-degrading enzyme, heme oxygenase-1, on macrophages and endothelial cells causing the release of iron from heme, which stimulates ferritin synthesis. Interestingly, ferritin can then provide positive feedback by activating the nuclear factor-κB signaling pathway, leading to more proinflammatory cytokine production. Some experts recommend following ferritin levels for response to therapy.

9. What classification criteria are useful?

Several criteria have been proposed using retrospective datasets with the Yamaguchi criteria traditionally being most commonly used. Five or more criteria including two or more major criteria yield a 96% sensitivity and 92% specificity to classify a patient as having AOSD.

Yamaguchi classification criteria

Major criteria	Minor criteria
• Fever >39°C for >7 days • Arthralgias or arthritis ≥2 weeks • Characteristic rash • Leukocytosis (≥10,000/mm³ and ≥80% PMNs)	• Sore throat • Lymphadenopathy • Hepatomegaly or splenomegaly • Abnormal liver-associated enzymes • Negative RF and ANA

Exclusions: malignancy (especially lymphoma), infection (especially Epstein–Barr virus), other connective tissue diseases (especially vasculitis, SLE), Sweet's syndrome, Schnitzler syndrome, familial autoinflammatory syndromes, and drug reactions.

Subsequent criteria advocated by Fautrel et al. incorporated glycosylated ferritin <20% and maculopapular rashes without the need for incorporated exclusions. Four major criteria or three major and two minor criteria yield an 81% sensitivity and 99% specificity for AOSD.

Fautrel classification criteria

Major criteria	Minor criteria
• Fever >39°C • Arthralgias or arthritis ≥2 weeks • Transient erythema • Pharyngitis • PMN count >80% • Glycosylated ferritin <20%	• Maculopapular rash • Leukocytosis >10,000/mm³

Exclusions: none.

A more recent study based on multivariate analysis of a multi-center prospective cohort validated a point-based set of criteria. Seven or more points identified AOSD with the sensitivity of 92.5%, specificity of 93.3%, and accuracy of 92.8%, values exceeding that noted when either the Yamaguchi or Fautrel criteria were applied to the cohort.

Classification criteria

Clinical	Laboratory
• Typical rash (3 points) • Fever ≥39°C (3 points) • Pharyngitis (2 points) • Arthritis (2 points)	• Neutrophil/Lymphocyte Ratio ≥4 (2 points) • Glycosylated ferritin ≤20% (1 point)

10. Describe the suspected pathogenesis of AOSD.

An unidentified infectious or environmental trigger provides a specific danger signal (e.g., pathogen-associated and damage-associated molecular patterns) that binds to toll-like receptors on macrophages and neutrophils, leading to activation of specific inflammasomes resulting in caspase activation and overproduction of IL-1β. This cytokine can further contribute to macrophage and neutrophil activation resulting in overproduction of several other proinflammatory cytokines (IL-6, IL-8, IL-17, IL-18, TNFα, and interferon-gamma). Unidentified genetic factors may predispose a person to developing this cytokine storm. Alternatively, regulatory anti-inflammatory mechanisms (regulatory T cells, IL-10, etc) may be defective in halting the unrestrained amplification of proinflammatory cytokines.

11. How is AOSD treated?

- **Mild disease:** occurs in 25% of cases with fever, rash, and arthralgias. In these patients, higher-range dosing of NSAIDs alone can adequately control AOSD. Follow liver-associated enzymes to monitor for liver toxicity while on NSAIDs, since this is increased in AOSD. If symptoms are not controlled in 2 weeks, they are switched to moderate-dose prednisone (0.5 mg/kg/day).

- **Moderate disease:** patients who present with high fever, disabling arthritis, and mild internal organ involvement are started on high-dose prednisone (1.0 mg/kg/day) immediately. If prednisone cannot be tapered to a low dose without disease recurrence, methotrexate is added for patients with predominant articular symptoms. There is little experience using any of the other disease-modifying anti-rheumatic drugs (DMARDs) (antimalarials, azathioprine, mycophenolate mofetil, leflunomide). Sulfasalazine is often avoided owing to a high rate of intolerance and side effects.
- **Severe disease:** patients who present with life-threatening organ manifestations (liver necrosis, cardiac tamponade, MAS/ DIC) are treated with pulsed methylprednisolone followed by high-dose prednisone and early use of biologic therapy and/or calcineurin inhibitors.
- **Resistant disease (17–32% of patients):** patients who have life-threatening presentations or patients who continue to require high-dose corticosteroids (>20 mg/day) in spite of 2 months of therapy with methotrexate or another DMARD may benefit from therapy with one of the biologics. Patients with AOSD have high serum levels of TNFα, IL-1, IL-6, IL-18, and interferon-gamma. Consequently, therapy that blocks one of these cytokines including anti-TNF therapy, IL-1 inhibitors (anakinra, canakinumab, rilonacept), and IL-6 inhibitors (tocilizumab) have induced remission in 70% to 80% of AOSD patients. IL-1 inhibitors and tocilizumab are more effective than TNF inhibitors, especially for systemic manifestations. Canakinumab is the only FDA-approved biologic for AOSD. Patients with chronic articular disease and few systemic manifestations benefit most from TNF inhibitors (infliximab) and methotrexate. Rituximab, abatacept, intravenous immunoglobulin (IVIG), and stem cell transplant have been used for resistant cases. An IL-18-binding protein (tadekinig alpha) is currently in clinical trials and appears to be effective. Monoclonal antibodies against IL-18 and interferon-gamma are in clinical trials. JAK inhibitors and anti-IL-17 antibodies have been successful in case reports.

12. What is the clinical course and prognosis of Still's disease?

The course of illness generally follows one of three patterns, with approximately one-third of patients following each: self-limited single illness, intermittent flares of disease activity, or chronic Still's disease. The patients who experience a self-limited course undergo remission within 6 to 9 months. Of those with intermittent flares, two-thirds will only have one recurrence, occurring from 10 to 136 months after the original illness. A minority of patients in this group will experience multiple flares, with up to 10 flares being reported at intervals of 3 to 48 months. The recurrent episodes are generally milder than the original illness and respond to lower doses of medications. In the group that experiences a chronic course, arthritis and loss of joint range of motion become the most problematic manifestations and may result in the need for joint arthroplasty, especially of the hip. The systemic manifestations tend to become less severe.

The presence of polyarthritis or large joint (shoulder, hip) involvement and an elevated ferritin level at onset are poor prognostic signs associated with the development of chronic disease. A high fever >39.5°C is predictive of monocyclic AOSD. The 5-year survival rate in AOSD is 90% to 95%. Deaths occurring in Still's disease have been attributed to infections, liver failure, amyloidosis (2–4%), adult respiratory distress syndrome, heart failure, status epilepticus, and hematologic manifestations including DIC, TTP, and MAS/sHLH. Patients with recurrent severe flares of AOSD associated with MAS/sHLH should undergo genetic testing for perforin pathway mutations; confirmed presence of HLH-associated mutations in these patients should prompt consideration and referral for bone marrow transplantation.

13. What is MAS?

MAS is a life-threatening (20% mortality) secondary (reactive) hemophagocytic syndrome occurring in 1.7% to 19% of AOSD patients depending on the study. The pathophysiology involves dysregulation of CD8+ T lymphocytes and excessive production of cytokines resulting in abnormal activation of macrophages, a consumptive coagulopathy, and signs of multi-organ dysfunction. AOSD is one of a number of clinical disorders that can be associated with the development of MAS, common features of which include *high persistent fever* (not quotidian), *hepatosplenomegaly*, and an *extremely high ferritin* (often >10,000 ng/mL). Unlike AOSD flares without MAS in which leukocytosis and thrombocytosis are commonly seen, patients who have developed MAS rapidly develop progressive *cytopenias (≥ two of three cell lines)*, likely due to elevated levels of interferon-gamma and/or phagocytosis of hematopoietic cells by macrophages in the bone marrow and reticuloendothelial system. In addition, they develop *liver injury* (elevated amino-transferases), *fasting hypertriglyceridemia,* and a consumptive coagulopathy (DIC with elevated prothrombin time/partial thromboplastin time) causing an inappropriately *low fibrinogen level* resulting in an unexpectedly *lower sedimentation rate* for the degree of inflammation. *Soluble IL-2 receptor (CD25) levels are extremely elevated.* Although tissue biopsy is not required to diagnose MAS, *hemophagocytosis may be seen in bone marrow, lymph node, liver, or spleen biopsies.* All patients with suspected MAS should be screened by polymerase chain reaction for an active Epstein–Barr or other viral (CMV, HSV, influenza, SARS-CoV-2) infections that can initiate MAS in the presence or absence of underlying rheumatic disorders. Therapy for MAS in AOSD includes high-dose corticosteroids. Up to 50% may not respond and will require a second-line agent including cyclosporine, or biologics (IL-1, IL-6, or TNFα inhibitors). Treatment with IVIG has been reported to be efficacious, with an evolving role for INF gamma inhibitors (emapalumab) under investigation (NCT05001737). Etoposide has been used for severe refractory cases.

ACKNOWLEDGMENT

The author would like to thank Dr. Duane Pearson for his contributions to this chapter in the previous edition.

BIBLIOGRAPHY

Affleck AG, Littlewood SM. Adult-onset Still's disease with atypical cutaneous features. *J Eur Acad Dermatol Venereol.* 2005;19:360–363.

Bae CB, Jung JY, Kim HA, Suh CH. Reactive hemophagocytic syndrome in adult-onset Still disease; clinical features, predictive factors and prognosis in 21 patients. *Medicine (Baltimore).* 2015;94:e451.

Bywaters EGL. Still's disease in the adult. *Ann Rheum Dis.* 1971;30:121–133.

Chen DY, Lan HH, Hsieh TY, et al. Crico-thyroid perichondritis leading to sore throat in patients with active adult-onset Still's disease. *Ann Rheum Dis.* 2007;66:1264–1266.

Daghor-Abbaci K, Ait Hamadouche N, Makhloufi CD, et al. Proposal of a new diagnostic algorithm for adult-onset Still's disease. *Clin Rheumatol.* 2023;42:1125–1135.

De Benedetti F, Grom AA, Brogan PA, et al. Efficacy and safety of emapalumab in macrophage activation syndrome. *Ann Rheum Dis.* 2023;82:857–865.

Efthimiou P, Kontzias A, Hur P, et al. Adult-onset Still's disease in focus: clinical manifestations, diagnosis, treatment, and unmet needs in the era of targeted therapies. *Semin Arthritis Rheum.* 2021;51:858–874.

Fautrel B, LeMoël G, Saint-Marcoux B, et al. Diagnostic value of ferritin and glycosylated ferritin in adult-onset Still's disease. *J Rheumatol.* 2001;28:322–329.

Feist E, Mitrovic S, Fautrel B. Mechanisms, biomarkers, and targets for adult-onset Still's disease. *Nat Rev Rheumatol.* 2018;14:603–618.

Franchini S, Dagna L, Salvo F, et al. Efficacy of traditional and biologic agents in different clinical phenotypes of adult-onset Still's disease. *Arthritis Rheum.* 2010;62:2530–2535.

Gefraud-Valentin M, Jamilloux Y, Iwaz J, Seve P, Eliminate Y, et al. Adult-onset Still's disease. *Autoimmun Rev.* 2014;13:708–722.

Gefraud-Valentin M, Maucort-Boulch D, Hot A, et al. Adult-onset Still disease; manifestations, treatment, outcome, and prognostic factors in 57 patients. *Medicine (Baltimore).* 2014;91:93–95.

Giacomelli R, Ruscitti P, Shoenfeld Y. A comprehensive review on adult-onset Still's disease. *J Autoimmun.* 2018;93:24–36.

Junge G, Mason J, Feist E. Adult-onset Still's disease—the evidence that anti-interleukin-1 treatment is effective and well-tolerated (a comprehensive literature review). *Semin Arthritis Rheum.* 2017;47:295–302.

Kong X, Xu D, Zhang W, et al. Clinical features and prognosis in adult-onset Still's disease: a study of 104 cases. *Clin Rheumatol.* 2010;29:1015–1019.

Sfriso P, Bindoli Galozzi P. Adult-onset Still's disease: molecular pathophysiology and therapeutic advances. *Drugs.* 2018;78:1187–1195.

Tada Y, Inokuchi S, Maruyama A, et al. Are the 2016 EULAR/ACR/PRINTO classification criteria for macrophage activation syndrome applicable to patients with adult-onset Still's disease? *Rheumatol Int.* 2019;39:97–104.

Yamaguchi M, Ohta A, Tsunematsu T, et al. Preliminary criteria for classification of adult Still's disease. *J Rheumatol.* 1992;19:424–430.

CHAPTER 24

Polymyalgia Rheumatica

Tara Skorupa, MD

 KEY POINTS

1. Patients with polymyalgia rheumatica (PMR) present with severe pain and stiffness in the proximal limbs without objective weakness, with a high erythrocyte sedimentation rate (ESR) and/or C-reactive protein (CRP).
2. PMR may precede or coincide with the diagnosis of giant cell arteritis (GCA) in a significant number of patients.
3. Patients should respond dramatically within a week of initiation of 15–20 mg/day of prednisone.
4. The presence of fever, failure to respond to prednisone, and/or persistently high ESR/CRP on therapy suggest(s) the need for further evaluation to rule out GCA or another diagnosis (e.g., malignancy or infection).
5. Relapses of PMR are common with tapering of prednisone, but anti-IL-6 therapy is an effective treatment for some patients with relapsing or refractory disease.

1. How does "ESCAPE" describe the clinical features of PMR?

In PMR, it's hard to ESCAPE prednisone.
E = Elderly individuals
S = Stiffness in the AM
C = Constitutional symptoms
A = Arteritis (GCA)
P = Proximal pain bilaterally (classically, shoulder and hip girdle)
E = ESR/CRP Elevated

2. Where did the term PMR originate?

The name PMR was first published by Barber in 1957 in a report of 12 patients with proximal myalgias.

3. Define PMR.

PMR is an inflammatory disorder of older individuals characterized by pain and stiffness in the shoulders, upper arms, neck, hips, and/or thighs, in the absence of objective weakness. Constitutional symptoms are common (33–50%). The core manifestations include:

- Patient age ≥50 years
- Bilateral shoulder girdle aching
- Bilateral hip pain and/or limited range of motion
- Morning stiffness >45 minutes
- ESR >40 mm/hour and/or elevated CRP
- Absence of rheumatoid factor (RF) and anti-cyclic citrullinated peptide (CCP) antibodies
- Rapid response to corticosteroids (prednisone 15–20 mg daily) within a week
- Exclusion of other diagnoses except GCA (see Question 16)

4. Who is affected by PMR?

PMR is the second most common inflammatory rheumatic disease (after rheumatoid arthritis [RA]), with a lifetime risk of 2.4% for women and 1.7% for men. PMR rarely affects those aged <50 years, and most patients are aged >60 years, with peak incidence between 70 and 80 years. Women are affected two to three times more often than men. PMR, like GCA, most frequently affects individuals of Northern European ancestry and is less common in Black, Hispanic, Asian, and Native American individuals.

5. What is the etiopathogenesis of PMR?

The cause of PMR is not well understood, but the epidemiology of the disease provides clues to its potential etiology. The higher prevalence in certain populations has suggested both a genetic predisposition (association with HLA-DRB1 has been reported) and a potential environmental influence. Based on the often sudden onset of symptoms, an infectious etiology has been proposed, but a consistent trigger has not been identified. The pathogenesis of PMR is thought to involve an interplay between the innate and cellular adaptive immune response in the context of aging. A hallmark of both PMR and GCA is increased production of **IL-6**, which leads to an increased Th17 response and is thought to be caused by activated dendritic cells causing CD4+ T-cell stimulation. In parallel, a decreased regulatory T-cell (Treg) response may be at least partially related to age-related dysregulation of Treg homeostasis. PMR on its own tends to lack the prominent interferon-γ (IFN-γ) response of GCA. Without IFN-γ to stimulate macrophages, the arterial inflammation characteristic of GCA does not develop. Interestingly, a PMR-like illness has been reported after immune checkpoint inhibitor therapy for cancer treatment. There have also been rare cases of PMR after influenza or COVID-19 vaccine, though this is typically self-limited and should not discourage individuals from getting vaccinated.

6. Describe the typical history in PMR.

- Patients typically present with severe achy pain and stiffness, involving more than one site (shoulders, neck, and/or pelvic girdle) symmetrically. Onset may be subacute or insidious (over 2–3 months) but in many cases is more sudden. Symptoms may also start unilaterally and then progress to symmetric involvement within a few weeks.
- The shoulder girdle is the first area affected in 70–95% of patients. The neck and pelvic girdle are involved in 50–70%. A single area may be the predominant source of pain.
- The pain and stiffness can last for hours in the mornings, limiting the patient's mobility. Symptoms generally improve over the course of the day but can re-worsen after a prolonged period of immobility ("gelling phenomenon"). Nocturnal pain may awaken the patient from sleep.
- Patients may perceive muscle weakness in addition to the pain and stiffness. However, early in disease and before initiation of treatment, this actually represents guarding as opposed to neuromuscular dysfunction, which can be proven by careful neurologic exam. Similarly, a patient's reported difficulty reaching overhead or climbing stairs may be in fact due to limitation in range of motion, not true weakness.
- About 40% of patients have constitutional symptoms/signs and appear chronically ill, with anorexia, weight loss, night sweats, fatigue, depression, and low-grade fever. High fevers are unusual unless GCA is present.

7. Describe the arthritis of PMR.

The articular manifestations of PMR can vary significantly among patients, and importantly, involvement is not thought to be isolated to the joints. Patients may present with synovitis of the glenohumeral, acromioclavicular, sternoclavicular, and/or hip joints, which is generally not appreciable on exam. Though arthrocentesis is not routinely performed, synovial fluid analysis may reveal an inflammatory fluid without crystals. Proximal joint involvement is most common, but several older studies have reported more distal arthritis (usually knees or wrists) in up to 30%. When seen, this arthritis is typically nonerosive and asymmetric. Beyond true arthritis, other distal peripheral joint manifestations that have been described include an extensor tenosynovitis of the hands, a flexor tenosynovitis of the hands causing carpal tunnel syndrome, and a distal pitting edema resembling remitting, symmetric, seronegative, synovitis with pitting edema (RS3PE) syndrome.

8. What are the findings on physical examination in patients with PMR?

The patient's physical findings are less striking than the history would suggest. Patients may appear chronically ill. The neck, shoulders, hips, and thighs are often tender to the touch, and movement of affected joints worsens the pain. Active (and sometimes passive) range of motion of the shoulders and/or hips may be limited due to pain. Synovitis, if present, may be found in the knees, wrists, or sternoclavicular joints. Muscle strength testing is often confounded by the presence of pain. However, the patient's objective strength testing is expected to be normal unless disuse muscle atrophy or glucocorticoid-related muscle changes have occurred.

9. **What are the European Alliance of Associations for Rheumatology (EULAR)/
   American College of Rheumatology (ACR) classification criteria for PMR?**

   PMR remains a diagnosis of exclusion (based largely on clinical presentation, elevated inflammatory markers, and exclusion of potential mimickers), which can make it challenging to study. In
   2012, experts from the ACR and EULAR established a set of provisional **classification criteria**
   for PMR to better define PMR patient populations for the purposes of **research**. All patients are
   required to meet the entry criteria of:

   a. Age ≥50 years.
   b. Bilateral shoulder aching.
   c. Abnormal ESR and/or CRP.

   From there, a scoring system gives points for presence of morning stiffness lasting >45 minutes
   (2 points), hip pain or limited range of motion (1 point), absence of RF/CCP (2 points), and
   absence of other joint involvement (1 point). Optional ultrasound (US) criteria looking for shoulder and/or hip bursitis, tenosynovitis, and/or synovitis can yield up to an additional 2 points.
   Without US, a score ≥4 (of 6 points total) is categorized as PMR. With US, a score ≥5 (of
   8 points total) is categorized as PMR.

   With these criteria, a score ≥4 yields a sensitivity of 68% and specificity of 78% for distinguishing comparison subjects from those with PMR. The addition of ultrasound criteria only
   marginally increases specificity and slightly decreases sensitivity. These criteria are not intended for
   diagnostic purposes.

10. **Explain the source of PMR symptoms.**

    In recent years, advanced imaging studies in PMR have furthered our understanding of its underly-
    ing pathoanatomic substrate. The inflammatory shoulder and hip girdle symptoms of PMR are
    thought to be related to both synovial and musculotendinous inflammation, and there is signifi-
    cant variability of presentation among patients. MRI and ultrasound studies have demonstrated
    synovitis of the shoulders and hips, which is not typically visible on an exam. Synovial biopsies have
    also shown synovitis, with leukocyte infiltration and vascular proliferation. Ultrasound, MRI, and
    PET-CT studies have additionally allowed for visualization of bursitis (subacromial, subdeltoid,
    cervical interspinous, lumbar interspinous, trochanteric, iliopsoas), tenosynovitis, and peritendinitis
    in patients with PMR. These findings are usually proximal, but can sometimes occur more distally
    (e.g., tenosynovitis of the extensor tendons of the hands). Muscle biopsy is typically normal or
    with mild nonspecific changes. Both the musculoskeletal and constitutional symptoms of PMR are
    thought to be driven by a pro-inflammatory (chiefly IL-6) cytokine response.

11. **What is the most characteristic laboratory finding? Is it always present?**

    Elevated ESR (often >100 mm/hour) and CRP are the characteristic laboratory findings but
    are certainly not specific for PMR. PMR may sometimes (7–22%) occur with a normal or only
    mildly elevated ESR (<40 mm/hour), but in those patients the CRP is usually elevated. It has
    been reported that both ESR and CRP are normal in less than 2% of cases. In these rare patients,
    it is essential to exclude potential mimickers of PMR (see question 15).

12. **Are other laboratory abnormalities commonly encountered?**

    Lab values reflecting the systemic inflammatory process (e.g., normochromic normocytic anemia,
    thrombocytosis, increased gamma globulins) are common. Liver enzyme abnormalities may be
    seen in up to one-third of patients; an increased alkaline phosphatase level is most common.
    Renal function, urinalysis, serum creatine kinase level, antinuclear antibody (ANA), and RF and
    anti-CCP antibodies are typically normal or negative. That being said, in normal healthy older
    adults, a low-titer RF can be seen in up to 10%, and a low-titer ANA can be seen in up to 33%.

13. **How are PMR and GCA related?**

    These two disorders frequently occur together in individual patients. In fact, PMR can be seen in
    roughly half of patients with imaging or biopsy-proven GCA. It can precede, present simultane-
    ously with, or develop after the onset of clinically apparent GCA. Conversely, overt GCA occurs
    in 15–20% of patients with PMR. Notably, studies have shown subclinical vasculitis on PET,
    ultrasound, and/or biopsy in 20–30% of PMR patients without cranial or ischemic symptoms.

The clinical significance of this occult GCA in patients with PMR is unclear, and universal screening for GCA in patients with PMR is not currently recommended. Nonetheless, PMR and GCA share a number of common epidemiologic, genetic, and immunopathogenic features. The association between PMR and GCA is so strong that many have speculated that they represent a common disease spectrum as opposed to two separate entities.

14. When should a temporal artery ultrasound or biopsy be performed on a patient with PMR?

It is not necessary to pursue temporal artery ultrasound or biopsy in a patient with PMR unless the patient's symptoms or exam findings suggest the presence of GCA. Therefore, the history of a patient with suspected PMR should always include questions regarding fever, current or recent headache, jaw or tongue claudication, visual disturbance, and scalp tenderness. The arteries of the head, neck, torso, and extremities should be examined for tenderness, enlargement, bruits, and decreased pulsation, and blood pressure in both arms should be measured to assess for discrepancy. Constitutional symptoms and laboratory values in PMR and GCA can be similar and, therefore, do not distinguish between the two diagnoses. However, the failure of prednisone (20 mg/day) to significantly improve symptoms or to normalize the ESR/CRP within 1 month should raise suspicion for GCA and prompt temporal artery ultrasound (if available at your institution) or biopsy—or alternatively, should prompt investigation for an alternative diagnosis (e.g., malignancy or infection).

15. List the other conditions that should be considered in the differential diagnosis with PMR and describe how they are distinguished (Table 24.1).

TABLE 24.1 Differential Diagnosis for PMR

DIAGNOSIS	DISTINGUISHING FEATURES
Late-onset rheumatoid arthritis	See Question 16
Late-onset spondyloarthropathy	Low back pain, psoriasis, enthesitis, dactylitis, IBD symptoms; preceding reactive arthritis-related infection; abnormal sacroiliac imaging
CPPD	Prominent wrist or knee swelling; chondrocalcinosis on radiograph; calcium pyrophosphate crystals on arthrocentesis; "crowned dens" on CT C-spine
Fibromyalgia	Non-inflammatory pain; cognitive symptoms; widespread tenderness on exam; normal ESR/CRP
Inflammatory myopathy	Proximal muscle weakness, usually without pain; elevated creatine kinase; abnormal MRI thigh, electromyography, and/or muscle biopsy
Thyroid-related myopathy	Weakness > pain or stiffness; other signs/symptoms of thyroid disease; abnormal TSH
Drug-induced myopathy	Pain and weakness > stiffness; culprit medication (e.g. statin)
Malignancy (especially lymphoma, myeloma)	Clinical evidence of neoplasm. Paraneoplastic syndrome can present with symptoms mimicking PMR. There is no clear association of malignancy with PMR, however, outside a possible association with MDS.
Occult infection (TB, HIV, SBE)	Clinical suspicion of infection; cultures and serologies
Shoulder osteoarthritis, rotator cuff pathology, adhesive capsulitis	Unilateral and/or mechanical symptoms; normal ESR/CRP; physical exam findings; shoulder radiographs
Neurodegenerative disease (Parkinson's, ALS)	Stiffness and weakness with muscle atrophy > pain; normal ESR/CRP; other neurologic findings (e.g., tremor, gait disturbance, muscle fasciculations)

Adapted from Espígol-Frigolé G, Dejaco C, Mackie SL, et al. Polymyalgia rheumatica. *Lancet.* 2023;402(10411):1459–1472.
ALS, amyotrophic lateral sclerosis; *CPPD,* calcium pyrophosphate deposition disease; *CRP,* C-reactive protein; *ESR,* erythrocyte sedimentation rate; *HIV,* human immunodeficiency virus; *IBD,* inflammatory bowel disease; *MDS,* myelodysplastic syndrome; *PMR,* polymyalgia rheumatica; *SBE,* subacute bacterial endocarditis; *TB,* tuberculosis; *TSH,* thyroid-stimulating hormone.

16. How is PMR distinguished from RA specifically?

It can be difficult to distinguish PMR from new RA in older patients (late-onset RA), especially since late-onset RA can present with a PMR-like pattern of proximal joint involvement in up to 25% of patients. Features that support a diagnosis of PMR include:
- Absence of RF and anti-CCP antibodies.
- Lack of small joint synovitis (metacarpophalangeal, proximal interphalangeal, and metatarsophalangeal joints).
- Presence of peripheral extracapsular inflammation.
- Absence of erosions on radiographs.

Note that the patient's response to glucocorticoids (GCs) is not a reliable distinguishing feature. In some cases, clinical changes over time may ultimately lead to a revision of the working diagnosis from PMR to late-onset RA. For instance, if a patient develops new symmetrical small joint synovitis during prednisone taper, the diagnosis of PMR should be re-evaluated.

17. How do the ACR/EULAR guidelines recommend treating PMR?

The most recent ACR/EULAR treatment guidelines for PMR were published in 2015. In these guidelines, the expert panel recommended the following for patients with a suspected diagnosis of PMR:
- Start oral prednisone (or equivalent) at a single daily dose of 12.5 to 25 mg/day, aiming for a minimal effective dose and duration of GC. An alternative option would be intramuscular methylprednisolone every 3 weeks for less frequent administration.
- Aim to taper to 10 mg/day of prednisone within 4 to 8 weeks, but individualize the tapering plan based on clinical disease activity, laboratory markers, and GC-related adverse events.
- Once remission is achieved and prednisone dose is down to 10 mg, continue tapering by 1mg every 4 weeks. If relapse occurs during GC taper, increase prednisone back to pre-relapse dose.
- Consider early introduction of methotrexate (MTX) in individuals with high risk of relapse/prolonged therapy or GC-related adverse events.
- Do *not* use TNF-alpha inhibitors for treatment of PMR. At the time these guidelines were published, there were no recommendations regarding the use of other biologic agents. In 2023, the FDA approved sarilumab for the treatment of PMR in patients with an inadequate response to GC or whom are unable to taper GC.
- Do *not* use traditional Chinese herbal supplements for treatment of PMR.
- Consider an individualized exercise program for frail patients with PMR, aimed at preserving muscle mass/function and reducing fall risk.

18. What is the course of PMR?

PMR tends to require long courses of prednisone, and relapses are common. A 2022 meta-analysis of 21 observational studies of PMR showed that 23% of patients were able to taper off GC completely by 1 year, 49% by 2 years, and 75% by 5 years. Notably, 43% of these patients experienced at least one relapse within the first year. Possible predictors of relapse and/or prolonged GC use include the faster speed of GC taper and the presence of the HLA-DRB1*0401 allele. Female sex, older age at diagnosis, and very high ESR/CRP have been proposed as additional risk factors, though data has been conflicting on this. A recent study did not show evidence of increased mortality in patients with PMR compared to matched controls.

19. How long should prednisone be continued?

Prednisone should be tapered based on the patient's clinical response. PMR symptoms and ESR/CRP are the most reliable parameters to follow. The CRP normalizes more quickly than the ESR, which should return to the normal range within 1 month. Failure of ESR/CRP to normalize should prompt investigation for occult GCA or an alternative diagnosis. Once a patient is in clinical remission with normalization of inflammatory markers, a common strategy is to decrease the prednisone dose by 2.5 mg every 2 to 4 weeks until a dose of 10 mg/day is attained (ideally, within 4–8 weeks). Further tapering of prednisone commonly occurs by 1 mg every 4 weeks, with close clinical monitoring. During the taper, a rise of ESR/CRP in an asymptomatic patient does not necessarily justify an increase in prednisone dosage. However, the dose should not be tapered further until alternative causes for the elevated acute-phase reactant have been investigated.

Optimally, prednisone should be tapered and discontinued as quickly as possible (typically over 12 months) because GC-related side effects are common (65% of patients). Tapering GC more rapidly may be possible in a subset of patients but can increase the risk of relapse. Data from the placebo arm of several trials in PMR suggest that 20% to 30% of patients may tolerate a more rapid steroid taper over 3 to 4 months. Consideration could be given to such an approach, with the knowledge that the majority of patients would relapse and require an increase in prednisone or the addition of a steroid-sparing agent. In the event of relapse, control is often regained by only a small increase in prednisone dose, then tapering back to 1 mg above the dose at which the relapse occurred. Further tapering may be attempted at a slower rate (e.g., every 2 months) after a period of "re-captured remission." Alternatively, the addition of a steroid-sparing agent such as methotrexate or sarilumab may be considered to regain disease control, reduce the risk of relapse, and lessen overall GC burden (see Question 20 ahead).

20. What steroid-sparing disease-modifying antirheumatic drugs or biologics can be used in PMR?

MTX has shown some benefit as a steroid-sparing DMARD in the treatment of PMR. Two higher-quality randomized control trials have shown a reduction in GC dose and higher rates of remission in those receiving MTX compared to GC alone. There have been conflicting data in other studies, but notably, trials evaluating MTX in PMR have used lower dosing (7.5–10 mg weekly) than is typical in the treatment of rheumatic disease. More recently, multiple studies have demonstrated the efficacy of anti-IL-6 therapies, both tocilizumab and sarilumab, in PMR. The most consistent benefit has been described in cases of GC-resistant or relapsing disease. In the SAPHYR trial (Spiera et al., 2023), patients with GC-resistant PMR who received sarilumab had higher rates of sustained remission and lower GC doses at week 52 compared to the GC-only group. Two additional randomized controlled trials, SPARE and SEMAPHORE, showed benefit with tocilizumab in new-onset and refractory PMR, respectively (the SPARE trial had limitations including a forced taper in the placebo arm at 11 weeks, and lack of outcome data beyond week 24). The FDA approved sarilumab for use as an adjunctive treatment in PMR based on the results of the SAPHYR trial.

21. Other than medication, what should be included in the treatment plan of PMR?

- Patient education.
- Regular physician monitoring.
- Range of motion exercises, especially where muscle atrophy and/or contracture have occurred.
- Attention to GC side effects, especially osteoporosis (vitamin D and calcium supplementation, dual x-ray absorptiometry screening, and appropriate therapy for prevention or treatment of GC-induced osteoporosis), glucose intolerance, hypertension, and hyperlipidemia.
- Immunizations: high-dose flu vaccine, pneumococcal vaccine (PCV20, or Prevnar 20), updated COVID-19 booster, and recombinant zoster vaccine (Shingrix).

ACKNOWLEDGMENT

The author would like to acknowledge the contributions of Drs. Vinisha Kota and Seth Mark Berney, who were the authors of this chapter in the previous edition.

BIBLIOGRAPHY

Buttgereit F, Dejaco C, Matteson EL, et al. Polymyalgia rheumatic and giant cell arteritis: a systematic review. *JAMA.* 2016;315:2442–2458.

Coskun Benlidayi I. Why is polymyalgia rheumatica a disease of older adults? Explanations through etiology and pathogenesis: a narrative review. *Clin Rheumatol.* 2024;43(3):851–861.

Dasgupta B, Cimmino MA, Maradit-Kremers H, et al. 2012 provisional classification criteria for polymyalgia rheumatica: a European League Against Rheumatism/American College of Rheumatology collaborative initiative. *Ann Rheum Dis.* 2012;71:484–492.

Dejaco C, Singh YP, Perel P, et al. 2015 recommendations for the management of polymyalgia rheumatic: A European League Against Rheumatism/American College of Rheumatology collaborative initiative. *Ann Rheum Dis.* 2015;74:1799–1807.

Espígol-Frigolé G, Dejaco C, Mackie SL, et al. Polymyalgia rheumatica. *Lancet.* 2023;402(10411):1459–1472.

Floris A, Piga M, Chessa E, et al. Long-term glucocorticoid treatment and high relapse rate remain unresolved issues in the real-life management of polymyalgia rheumatica: a systematic literature review and meta-analysis. *Clin Rheumatol*. 2022;41(1):19–31.

Hysa E, Castagna A, Manzo C. Liver involvement in polymyalgia rheumatica and giant cell arteritis. *Reumatologia*. 2020;58(6):444–445.

Lundberg IE, Sharma A, Turesson C, et al. An update on polymyalgia rheumatica. *J Intern Med*. 2022;292(5):717–732.

Manzo C, Milchert M. Polymyalgia rheumatica with normal values of both erythrocyte sedimentation rate and C-reactive protein concentration at the time of diagnosis: a four-point guidance. *Reumatologia*. 2018;56(1):1–2.

Mekenyan L, Karalilova R, Todorov P, et al. Imaging methods in polymyalgia rheumatica: a systematic review. *Rheumatol Int*. 2023;43(5):825–840.

Ohta R, Sano C. Differentiating between Seronegative Elderly-Onset rheumatoid arthritis and polymyalgia rheumatica: a qualitative synthesis of narrative reviews. *Int J Environ Res Public Health*. 2023;20(3):1789.

Partington R, Muller S, Mallen CD, et al. Mortality among patients with polymyalgia rheumatica: a retrospective cohort study. *Arthritis Care Res (Hoboken)*. 2021;73(12):1853–1857.

Prieto-Peña D, Castañeda S, Atienza-Mateo B, et al. Predicting the risk of relapse in polymyalgia rheumatica: novel insights. *Expert Rev Clin Immunol*. 2021;17(3):225–232.

Ricordi C, Pipitone N, Marvisi C, et al. Steroid-sparing agents in polymyalgia rheumatica: how will they fit into the treatment paradigm? *Expert Rev Clin Immunol*. 2023;19(10):1195–1203.

Salvarani C, Padoan R, Iorio L, et al. Subclinical giant cell arteritis in polymyalgia rheumatica: Concurrent conditions or a common spectrum of inflammatory diseases? *Autoimmun Rev*. 2024;23(1):103415.

Spiera RF, Unizony S, Warrington KJ, et al. Sarilumab for relapse of polymyalgia rheumatica during glucocorticoid taper. *N Engl J Med*. 2023;389(14):1263–1272.

FURTHER READING

http://www.rheumatology.org/polymyalgia-rheumatica-guideline.

Approach for Patients With Suspected Vasculitis

CHAPTER 25

Brendan Antiochos, MD and Philip Seo, MD, MHS

> **≫ KEY POINTS**
>
> 1. There is no single typical presentation of vasculitis.
> 2. Vasculitis is classified by the size of the blood vessel involved: large-, medium-, or small-vessel vasculitis.
> 3. Each form of vasculitis has a characteristic clinical presentation.
> 4. Tissue biopsy or angiography may be necessary for diagnosis.
> 5. Treatment selection depends on the extent of organ involvement.

---

1. What is the definition of vasculitis? What are the consequences?

A pathologist uses the word *vasculitis* to describe inflammation of a blood vessel wall. An inflamed blood vessel may gradually lose integrity (leading to aneurysm formation) or become stenotic (leading to tissue ischemia). A rheumatologist uses the word *vasculitis* to describe the diseases that are characterized by the presence of inflamed blood vessels; these diseases are sometimes called the *systemic vasculitides*. The long-term consequences of the systemic vasculitides are the result of organ damage caused by the inflamed blood vessels and side effects of the drugs used to treat the inflammation.

2. What are the characteristic histologic features of vasculitis?

- Infiltration of the vessel wall by neutrophils, mononuclear cells, and/or giant cells.
- Fibrinoid necrosis (i.e., panmural destruction of the vessel wall; Fig. 25.1).
- Leukocytoclasis (i.e., leukocyte degranulation, sometimes described by a pathologist as "nuclear dust").
- Immune complex deposition in the vessel wall.

Perivascular infiltration (or *cuffing*) is a nonspecific histologic finding. It may be evidence of an early vasculitis, but it is also observed in a variety of disease processes. By itself, it is not diagnostic of vasculitis. Similarly, disruption of the internal elastic lamina may be seen with vasculitis but this is not a specific finding.

3. What are the immune mechanisms that can cause vasculitis?

Nearly every component of the immune system has been implicated in the pathogenesis of at least one form of vasculitis. However, there is no single immune mechanism that causes all forms of vasculitis. Some of the mechanisms that have been implicated include the following:

- **Immune complex mediated vasculitis**: Examples of immune complex-mediated vasculitis include polyarteritis nodosa (PAN), IgA-vasculitis (Henoch–Schönlein purpura), cryoglobulinemic vasculitis, and cutaneous leukocytoclastic angiitis.
- **ANCA-associated vasculitis:** Examples of ANCA-associated vasculitis include granulomatosis with polyangiitis (GPA; Wegener granulomatosis), microscopic polyangiitis (MPA), eosinophilic granulomatosis with polyangiitis (EGPA; the Churg–Strauss syndrome), and pauci-immune renal-limited vasculitis.
- **Cell-mediated vasculitis**: Examples of cell-mediated vasculitis include giant cell arteritis and Takayasu arteritis.

The immune mechanisms underlying other forms of vasculitis are less certain.

4. What is the Chapel Hill consensus conference nomenclature for the vasculitides?

Table 25.1 describes the vasculitis nomenclature agreed at the Chapel Hill consensus conference, which categorizes the systemic vasculitides based on the size of the blood vessels affected by the disease.

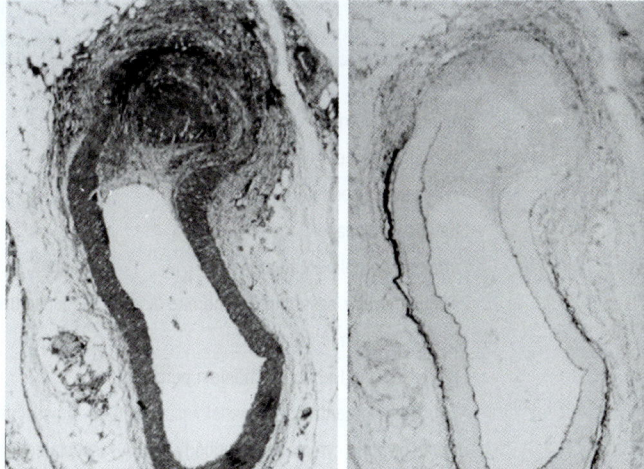

Fig. 25.1 Necrotizing vasculitis in a bowel specimen from a patient with polyarteritis nodosa. The arterial lumen is partially occluded by thrombus. The adjacent arterial wall is necrotic, resulting in destruction of the elastic laminae: *(left)* hematoxylin–eosin staining; *(right)* elastic tissue staining; lower power. (Copyright 2014 American College of Rheumatology. Used with permission).

Note: There are specific American College of Rheumatology classification criteria for many of the major types of vasculitis. These differentiate one form of vasculitis from another, rather than describing all of the manifestations of a particular form of vasculitis. These criteria cannot be used to establish a diagnosis, but may serve as a useful mnemonic to remember some of the features that are characteristic for these diseases. However, the systemic vasculitides are clinicopathologic diagnoses, and checklists are inadequate to establish (or refute) the diagnosis.

5. How should the physician approach the diagnosis of vasculitis?
  a. **Suspect the disease**. You can't diagnose what you're not looking for.
  b. **Define the extent of the disease,** by conducting a through history and physical examination, supplemented by targeted lab and radiologic tests.
  c. **Rule out vasculitis mimics,** which often include infection, malignancy, hypercoagulable states, medications, and other rheumatic diseases such as lupus.
  d. **Confirm the diagnosis**, through biopsy or angiography, when possible.

6. How does vasculitis typically present?
There is no single typical presentation of vasculitis. Vasculitis should be suspected in any constitutionally ill patient who has evidence of multisystem inflammatory disease. The clinical manifestations may suggest the size of vessel involved and the most likely vasculitis. Typical presentations are as follows:
  • **Large-vessel vasculitis:** limb claudication, bruits, asymmetric blood pressures, absence of pulses, thoracic aortic aneurysm. Temporal headache, jaw claudication, and blindness are associated with large vessel vasculitis affecting the carotid artery.
  • **Medium-vessel vasculitis:** mesenteric ischemia, cutaneous nodules, ulcers, livedo reticularis, digital gangrene, mononeuritis multiplex, renovascular hypertension, and organ infarct.
  • **Small-vessel vasculitis:** palpable purpura, painful urticaria, glomerulonephritis, alveolar hemorrhage, and scleritis.

PEARL: Headache or visual loss in the elderly (GCA), asymmetric pulses with bruits in a patient aged <30 years (Takayasu arteritis), mononeuritis multiplex (PAN), rapidly progressive pulmonary–renal syndrome (ANCA associated vasculitis), and palpable purpura (immune complex-mediated vasculitis) are the most common presentations suggesting vasculitis. Patients with systemic vasculitis feel poorly and frequently experience low-grade fever, fatigue, and weight loss.

TABLE 25.1 Vasculitis Nomenclature Agreed at the International Chapel Hill Consensus Conference

NOMENCLATURE	VASCULITIS
Large-vessel vasculitis	Takayasu arteritis
	Giant cell (temporal) arteritis
Medium-vessel vasculitis	Polyarteritis nodosa
	Kawasaki disease
Small-vessel vasculitis	Immune complex-mediated
	Antiglomerular basement membrane disease (Goodpasture syndrome)
	Cryoglobulinemic vasculitis
	IgA vasculitis (Henoch–Schönlein purpura)
	Hypocomplementemic urticarial vasculitis (anti-Clq vasculitis)
	Antineutrophil cytoplasmic antibody (ANCA)-associated (pauci-immune)
	Granulomatosis with polyangiitis (GPA)
	Microscopic polyangiitis (MPA)
	Eosinophilic granulomatosis with polyangiitis (EGPA)
Variable-vessel vasculitis[a]	Behçet disease
	Cogan syndrome
Single-organ vasculitis	Cutaneous leukocytoclastic vasculitis
	Cutaneous arteritis
	Primary central nervous system vasculitis (isolated angiitis of central nervous system)
	Isolated aortitis
	Others
Vasculitis associated with systemic disease	Lupus vasculitis
	Rheumatoid vasculitis
	Sarcoid vasculitis
	Others
Vasculitis associated with probable etiology	Hepatitis C virus-associated cryoglobulinemic vasculitis
	Hepatitis B virus-associated vasculitis
	Syphilis-associated vasculitis
	Drug-associated immune complex vasculitis (hypersensitivity vasculitis)
	Drug-associated ANCA-associated vasculitis
	Cancer-associated vasculitis
	Others

[a]Thromboangiitis obliterans (Buerger disease) was not classified at this conference but probably best fits as variable-vessel vasculitis.

7. When should the rheumatologist suspect vasculitis mimics?

Because of its protean manifestations, vasculitis can easily be confused with other diseases. Mimics of vasculitis must be excluded early in the evaluation because treatment varies dramatically, and misdiagnosis may result in morbidity and/or mortality. Vasculitis mimics should be suspected when there is:

a. A new heart murmur (infective endocarditis).
b. Necrosis of the toes (cholesterol emboli).
c. Splinter hemorrhages (infective endocarditis).
d. Prominent liver dysfunction (cryoglobulinemic vasculitis due to hepatitis C).
e. Illicit drug use (HIV; hepatitis B and C; cocaine, cannabis).
f. Prior diagnosis of neoplastic disease (paraneoplastic vasculitis)
g. History of (or risk factors for) syphilis (syphilitic aortitis)
h. History of herpes zoster or varicella infection (cerebral vasculopathy).
i. New medications, particularly if they are vasoactive (e.g., methylphenidate)
j. Isolated radiographic vascular abnormalities without inflammatory features (fibromuscular dysplasia)

8. **What disorders can mimic vasculitis?**

Any disease associated with thromboembolic phenomena can mimic a **small- or medium-vessel vasculitis**:

- These diagnoses include severe atherosclerotic disease, hypercoagulable states, and cardiac myxoma.
- Hypercoagulability due to malignancy and infective endocarditis are particularly important to consider, since they can also lead to a systemic vasculitis.
- Systemic lupus erythematosus is always worth considering, since it can affect many of the same organs impacted by a small- or medium-vessel vasculitis.
- Fibromuscular dysplasia should be considered in patients with angiographic changes affecting the carotid, renal, or mesenteric arteries in the absence of inflammation. Segmental arterial mediolysis may cause a noninflammatory vasculopathy limited to the mesentery.
- Most patients suspected of having central nervous system vasculitis actually have reversible cerebral vasoconstriction syndrome (RCVS). These diagnoses may be indistinguishable radiographically. However, RCVS is characterized by a *thunderclap* headache, and the angiographic changes resolve spontaneously after 6 to 8 weeks.

A different set of diagnoses may mimic **large vessel vasculitis**:

- Diseases affecting the connective tissues may also be associated with aortic aneurysm formation; these include Marfan's, Ehlers–Danlos, and Loeys–Dietz syndrome.
- Syphilis is an uncommon infectious cause of aortitis.
- IgG4-related diseases, lymphoma, and Erdheim–Chester disease may cause periaortitis/fibrosis, rather than true aortitis.
- Inflammatory abdominal aortic aneurysms are typically associated with severe atherosclerotic disease.

9. **What localizing clinical features suggest the different types of vasculitis?**

Table 25.2 lists features suggestive of different types of vasculitis. These features occur either before, during, or after the constitutional features and are also relatively nonspecific, with considerable overlap.

10. **What skin lesions are suggestive of vasculitis?**

- Medium-vessel vasculitis: subcutaneous nodules, "punched-out" skin ulcers, livedo reticularis/racemosa, digital gangrene.
- Small-vessel vasculitis: palpable purpura, splinter hemorrhages, hemorrhagic macules, vesiculobullous lesions, and urticaria lasting >24 hours.

Examples are shown in Fig. 25.2.

11. **Which laboratory tests are useful in the evaluation of suspected vasculitis?**

- Systemic vasculitis is associated with inflammation, which can be detected using a variety of laboratory tests:
  - The most common acute-phase reactants are the erythrocyte sedimentation rate and C-reactive protein, both of which will be elevated in patients with active vasculitis.
  - Other serologic evidence of inflammation may include anemia, thrombocytosis, hypoalbuminemia, and elevated ferritin.

TABLE 25.2 Localized Clinical Features That Suggest Different Types of Vasculitis.

SYMPTOMS	DIAGNOSIS
Jaw claudication; visual loss; palpable, thickened, tender temporal artery; or diminished temporal artery pulsation	GCA
Absent radial pulses, difficulty obtaining a blood pressure in one arm	Takayasu arteritis or large artery involvement in GCA
Sinus involvement, otitis media, scleritis	GPA or EGPA
Hypertension, renal vascular involvement	Polyarteritis nodosa or Takayasu arteritis
Asthma	EGPA
Testicular tenderness	Polyarteritis nodosa
Pulmonary–renal syndromes (hemoptysis and glomerulonephritis)	GPA and MPA SLE and Goodpasture syndrome
Palpable purpura	Cutaneous vasculitis associated with diseases causing small-vessel vasculitis

GCA, Giant cell arteritis; *GPA,* granulomatosis with polyangiitis; *MPA,* microscopic polyangiitis; *EGPA,* eosinophilic granulomatosis with polyangiitis; *SLE,* systemic lupus erythematosus.

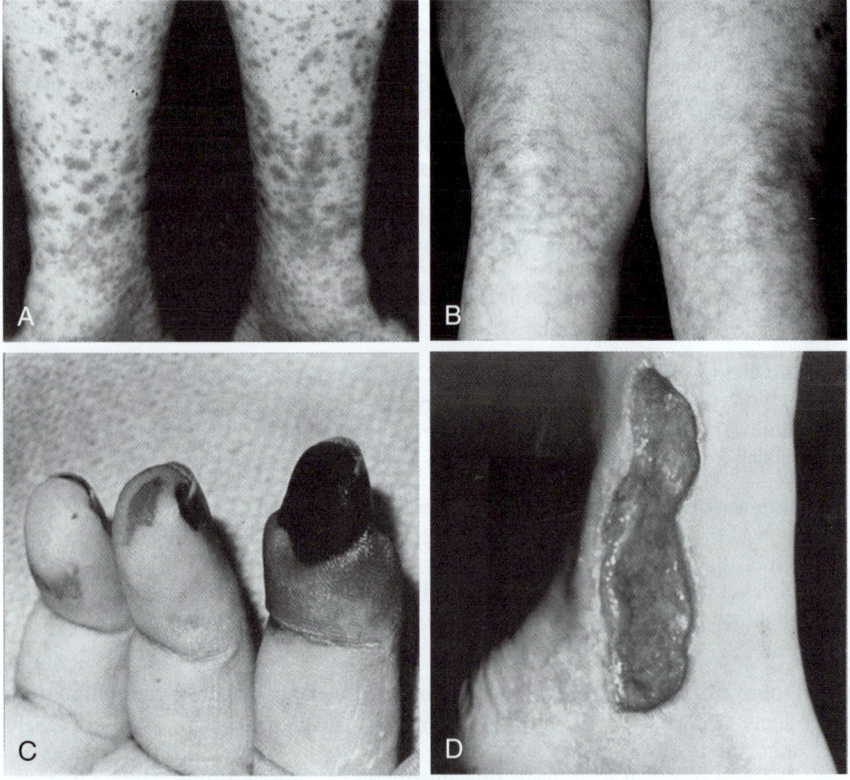

Fig. 25.2 (A) Palpable purpura. (B) Livedo reticularis. (C) Digital infarction. (D)"Punched-out" ulcer. (A, C, and D, Copyright 2014 American College of Rheumatology. Used with permission. B, From Colledge N, Walker B, Ralston S. *Davidson's Principles and Practice of Medicine.* 21st ed. Philadelphia: Churchill Livingstone; 2010, Fig. 25–37).

> **PEARL:** Note that **primary** systemic vasculitis never causes pancytopenia; patients presenting with pancytopenia should be evaluated for SLE, B-cell lymphoma, myeloma, leukemia, VEXAS syndrome, and HCV.

- Once the presence of inflammation has been confirmed, targeted testing may be used to identify evidence of specific organ dysfunction:
  - Kidney vasculitis may be first detected by examining the urine for evidence of hematuria and proteinuria. The serum creatinine does not increase until much later in the disease course.
  - Vasculitis affecting the central nervous system will demonstrate an increase in white blood cells in the cerebrospinal fluid.
  - Nerve conduction studies may confirm the presence of mononeuritis multiplex in a patient presenting with a wrist drop or a foot drop.
- Specific lab tests may be associated with specific forms of vasculitis:
  - ANCA is often present in patients with ANCA-associated vasculitis.
  - Anti-C1q antibodies are associated with urticarial vasculitis.
  - Serum cryoglobulins and rheumatoid factors are associated with cryoglobulinemic vasculitis.
  - C3/C4 are low in hypocomplementemic urticarial vasculitis and SLE. Cryoglobulinemic vasculitis is associated with a low C4 but usually a normal C3.
- Tests can also be useful to exclude vasculitis mimics:
  - Blood cultures: rule out infective endocarditis or bacteremia of another source.
  - Infectious serologies: Hepatitis B (PAN), hepatitis C (cryoglobulinemic vasculitis), HIV (any vasculitis).
  - Antiglomerular basement membrane antibody: any patient with pulmonary–renal syndrome.
  - Serum protein electrophoresis: rule out myeloma.
  - Cerebrospinal fluid studies: herpes, varicella-zoster virus (VZV DNA and anti-VZV antibody).
  - Urinary toxicology screen: rule out cocaine use.

> **PEARL:** Cocaine-associated vasculitis can be C-ANCA, P-ANCA, and/or atypical ANCA (anti–human neutrophil elastase)-positive.

Not all of these tests are ordered for all patients. The clinician must choose which test to order according to the clinical situation.

12. How might ANCAs be helpful in differentiating vasculitis?

Anti-neutrophil cytoplasmic antibodies (ANCA) may be detected using either immunofluorescence or immunoassays. When using immunofluorescence, one of three different staining patterns may be reported: peripheral, cytoplasmic, or atypical. The peripheral staining pattern is called *P-ANCA*, and corresponds to antibodies against myeloperoxidase (MPO). The cytoplasmic staining pattern is called *C-ANCA*, and corresponds to antibodies against proteinase-3 (PR3). P-ANCA/MPO-ANCA may be found with all forms of ANCA-associated vasculitis, whereas C-ANCA/PR3-ANCA is more specific for granulomatosis with polyangiitis. Notably, a small percentage of MPA and EGPA patients can be C-ANCA/PR3-ANCA positive and a small percentage of GPA patients can be P-ANCA/MPO-ANCA positive. The atypical staining pattern may be caused by several antibodies and is not associated with any form of systemic vasculitis. However, note that patients with a positive *C-ANCA* or *P-ANCA* (especially if negative for anti-PR-3 or anti-MPO) may have an inflammatory disease other than vasculitis (e.g. infections like TB, inflammatory bowel disease, others). Alternatively, patients with ANCA-associated vasculitis who are both anti-PR3 and anti-MPO positive at the same time frequently have cocaine or another drug-induced cause. Therefore, a careful history, physical examination, and evaluation are necessary to exclude other diseases and etiologies for ANCA positivity that can mimic ANCA-associated vasculitis.

13. When are hepatitis serologies helpful when vasculitis is suspected?

The presence of hepatitis B surface antigen may be found in some patients (10–25%, depending on risk factors) with PAN. Hepatitis C antibodies are often found in patients with essential mixed cryoglobulinemic vasculitis and less commonly in PAN.

14. What other diagnostic studies are commonly used in the evaluation of suspected vasculitis?

Targeted diagnostic studies are used to evaluate organs suspected of being impacted by vasculitis. Such studies may include:

- Chest radiograph.
- Lumbar puncture with cerebrospinal fluid exam (if the patient has CNS symptoms).
- Sinus radiographs or CT scans.
- Doppler ultrasound of affected artery (e.g. temporal artery in GCA)
- Angiography (if renal function is acceptable).
- EMG and NCV studies (if the patient has evidence of nerve or muscle dysfunction).
- Tissue biopsy.

15. What is the role of tissue biopsy in the diagnosis of vasculitis and in what type of vasculitis might tissue biopsy be helpful?

Tissue biopsy is the procedure of choice in the diagnosis of vasculitis. The target should be selected based on the patient's symptoms.

- In a patient suspected of having **giant cell arteritis,** temporal artery biopsy is commonly used to confirm the diagnosis.
- In a patient suspected of having **central nervous system vasculitis**, brain biopsy is the only reliable way to exclude mimics. Angiography alone is not adequate to confidently establish a diagnosis of central nervous system vasculitis.
- In any patient suspected of having **kidney vasculitis** (i.e., glomerulonephritis), a kidney biopsy should be considered. For such patients, a kidney biopsy may be useful both to confirm the diagnosis and predict the likelihood of renal recovery.
- In a patient with **skin vasculitis**, the skin is an easily accessible organ for biopsy. In addition to confirming the presence of vasculitis, direct immunofluorescence can be used to establish the type of vasculitis.
- In a patient with a lung lesion, an open lung biopsy is often required to confirm the presence of vasculitis. Fine needle biopsies of lung lesions are generally more useful to exclude other conditions (e.g., infection).
- In a patient with a **mononeuritis multiplex** affecting the lower extremity, sural nerve biopsy has a yield of 30% to 70% for confirming the presence of vasculitis if clinically involved with an abnormal NCV. Sural nerve biopsy is not useful to confirm the presence of length-dependent sensory neuropathy, which is also commonly present in patients with vasculitis.

16. If tissue biopsy is not feasible, what alternative procedures can yield a diagnosis?

Imaging may be used to demonstrate evidence of aneurysm or stenosis characteristic of large- or medium-vessel vasculitides; however, imaging studies alone are not specific for vasculitis.

- For patients suspected of having large-vessel vasculitis, magnetic resonance imaging or computed tomographic angiography may be used to look for aortic aneurysm, or stenosis of the subclavian, axillary, or carotid arteries.
- For patients suspected of having medium-vessel vasculitis, computed tomographic angiography or conventional angiography may demonstrate evidence of aneurysm or stenosis of the splanchnic arteries.
- Conventional angiography is generally used to evaluate patients suspected of having central nervous system vasculitis, or vasculitis affecting the extremities (e.g., rheumatoid vasculitis, thromboangiitis obliterans [Buerger's disease]).
- Magnetic resonance imaging lacks the resolution required to evaluate most forms of medium vessel vasculitis.

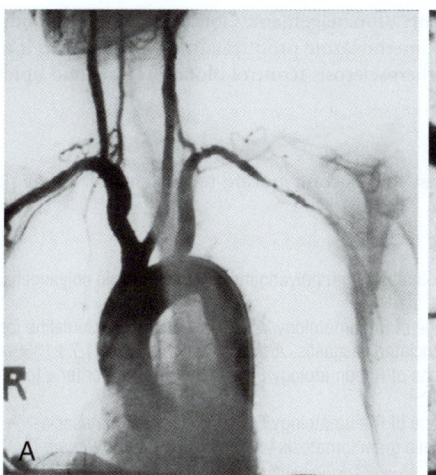 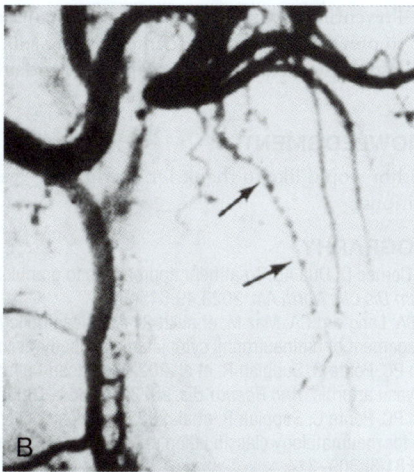

Fig. 25.3 Angiography in vasculitis. (A) Irregular tapering and narrowing of the left subclavian artery in Takayasu arteritis. (B) Typical "rosary bead" aneurysm (*arrows*) formation in a patient with isolated central nervous system.

17. List two characteristic (but not diagnostic) angiographic features of vasculitis
- Irregular tapering and concentric narrowing (Fig. 25.3).
- Aneurysms ("beading" on angiography).

18. What noninvasive tests can be used to determine vessel involvement in patients with vasculitis?
- Imaging is routinely used to evaluate patients suspected of having large- or medium-vessel vasculitis. Small caliber blood vessels cannot be visualized using standard imaging techniques.
- Conventional and computed tomography (CT) angiography are useful for imaging both medium- and large-caliber blood vessels. Conventional angiography has higher sensitivity for subtle changes.
- Magnetic resonance imaging and positron emission tomography (PET) can be used to detect inflammation in the walls of large vessels. PET has higher sensitivity for vessel wall inflammation but is often prohibitively expensive.
- Doppler ultrasound can also be used to detect evidence of vessel wall inflammation and vascular stenosis characteristic of vasculitis. However, not all vessels are accessible to ultrasound. Moreover, using ultrasound to evaluate vasculitis requires specific training that is not yet widely available in the United States.

19. Describe the general approach to the treatment of vasculitis.
- Identify and remove/treat inciting agents (e.g. medications, infection, etc).
- Clinically, we categorize most forms of vasculitis as being severe (i.e., posing an immediate threat to life or the function of a vital organ) and nonsevere disease.
- The nonsevere disease is generally treated with lower doses of glucocorticoids (e.g., prednisone 0.5 mg/kg daily) and a steroid-sparing agent, such as methotrexate or azathioprine.
- Severe disease is generally treated with high-dose glucocorticoids (e.g., prednisone 1 mg/kg daily) and more aggressive immunosuppression, such as cyclophosphamide.
- Some forms of severe vasculitis are treated with biologic therapies:
  - Giant cell arteritis is treated with tocilizumab or upadacitinib (Chapter 26)
  - Granulomatosis with polyangiitis and microscopic polyangiitis are treated with rituximab
  - Eosinophilic granulomatosis with polyangiitis is treated with mepolizumab
- Vasculitis caused by infection should focus on treating the infection first (e.g. SBE, HepB/C); some patients with severe vasculitis (e.g., glomerulonephritis) will also require a limited course of immunosuppression.

- Preventing complications is an important part of management. Consideration should be given to preventing infection (trimethoprim–sulfamethoxazole prophylaxis for *Pneumocystis* if on high-dose prednisone), osteoporosis, and atherosclerosis (control blood pressure and lipids).

ACKNOWLEDGMENT

The author would like to thank Dr. Sterling G. West for his contribution to this chapter in the previous editions.

BIBLIOGRAPHY

Berti A, Cornec D, Dua AB. Treatment approaches to granulomatosis with polyangiitis and microscopic polyangiitis. *Rheum Dis Clin North Am.* 2023;49:545–561.

Chung SA, Langford CA, Maz M, et al. 2021 American College of Rheumatology/Vasculitis Foundation Guideline for the management of antineutrophil cytoplasmic antibody-associated vasculitis. *Arthritis Rheumatol.* 2021;73:1366–1383.

Grayson PC, Ponte C, Suppiah R, et al. 2022 American College of Rheumatology/EULAR classification criteria for Takayasu arteritis. *Ann Rheum Dis.* 2022;81:1654–1660.

Grayson PC, Ponte C, Suppiah R, et al. 2022 American College of Rheumatology/European Alliance of Associations for rheumatology classification criteria for eosinophilic granulomatosis with polyangiitis. *Ann Rheum Dis.* 2022;81(3):309–314.

Jennette JC, Falk RJ, Bacon PA, et al. 2012 revised international Chapel Hill consensus conference nomenclature of vasculitides. *Arthritis Rheum.* 2013;65:1–11.

Koster MJ, Guarda M, Ghaffar U, Warrington KJ. Rheumatic masqueraders: mimics of primary vasculitis—a case-based review. *Expert Rev Clin Immunol.* 2024;20:83–95.

Koster MJ, Lasho TL, Olteanu H, et al. VEXAS syndrome: clinical, hematologic features and a practical approach to diagnosis and management. *Am J Hematol.* 2024;99:284–299.

Maz M, Chung SA, Abril A, et al. 2021 American College of Rheumatology/Vasculitis Foundation Guideline for the management of giant cell arteritis and takayasu arteritis. *Arthritis Rheumatol.* 2021;73:1349–1365.

Micheletti RG, Chiesa Fuxench Z, Craven A, et al. Cutaneous manifestations of antineutrophil cytoplasmic antibody-associated vasculitis. *Arthritis Rheumatol.* 2020;72:1741–1747.

Micheletti RG, Werth VP. Small vessel vasculitis of the skin. *Rheum Dis Clin North Amer.* 2015;41:21–32.

Moretti M, Ferro F, Baldini C, Mosca M, Talarico R. Cryoglobulinemic vasculitis: a 2023 update. *Curr Opin Rheumatol.* 2024;36:27–34.

Ozguler Y, Esatoglu SN, Hatemi G. Epidemiology of systemic vasculitis. *Curr Opin Rheumatol.* 2024;36:21–26.

Raimbeau A, Pistorius M, Goueffic Y, et al. Digital ischaemia aetiologies and mid-term follow-up: a cohort study of 323 patients. *Medicine (Baltimore).* 2021;100(20):e25659.

Ponte C, Grayson PC, Robson JC, et al. 2022 American College of Rheumatology/EULAR classification criteria for giant cell arteritis. *Ann Rheum Dis.* 2022;81:1647–1653.

Robson JC, Grayson PC, Ponte C, et al. 2022 American College of Rheumatology/European Alliance of Associations for Rheumatology classification criteria for granulomatosis with polyangiitis. *Ann Rheum Dis.* 2022;81:315–320.

Springer JM, Villa-Forte A. Vasculitis mimics and other related conditions. *Rheum Dis Clin North Am.* 2023;49(3):617–631.

Stone JH. Vasculitis: a collection of pearls and myths. *Rheum Dis Clin North Am.* 2007;33:691–739.

Suppiah R, Robson JC, Grayson PC, et al. 2022 American College of Rheumatology/European Alliance of Associations for Rheumatology classification criteria for microscopic polyangiitis. *Ann Rheum Dis.* 2022;81:321–326.

Thalen M, Gisslander K, Segelmark M, Sode J, Jayne D, Mohammad AJ. Epidemiology and clinical characteristics of biopsy-confirmed adult-onset IgA vasculitis in southern Sweden. *RMD Open.* 2024;10:e003822.

Thomas K, Vassilopoulos D. Infections and vasculitis. *Curr Opin Rheumatol.* 2017;29:17–23.

Treppo E, Quartuccio L, De Vita S. Recent updates in the diagnosis and management of cryoglobulinemic vasculitis. *Expert Rev Clin Immunol.* 2023;19:1457–1467.

Yaseen K, Nevares A, Tamaki H. A spotlight on drug-induced vasculitis. *Curr Rheumatol Rep.* 2022;24:323–336.

CHAPTER 26

Large-Vessel Vasculitis: Giant Cell Arteritis, Takayasu Arteritis, and Aortitis

Anisha B. Dua, MD, MPH

1. What are the large-vessel vasculitides?

Large vessel vasculitides cause inflammation of the aorta and its major branches. GCA and TAK are the most common phenotypes of primary large-vessel vasculitis. Other rheumatic diseases associated with aortitis include the seronegative spondyloarthropathies, relapsing polychondritis, Behçet disease, Cogan syndrome, and sarcoidosis. Infectious aortitis may be caused by several organisms. In patients without systemic symptoms who present with a thoracic aortic aneurysm, several noninflammatory genetic conditions must be ruled out.

GIANT CELL ARTERITIS

2. Is GCA known by any other names?

Yes: cranial arteritis, temporal arteritis, Horton disease, granulomatous arteritis.

3. What population does GCA primarily affect?

GCA incidence increases with age. It is nearly 10 times more common among patients in their 80s than among patients aged 50 to 60 years. GCA only affects patients aged >50 years. The disease is two to three times more common in women compared to men and is most often reported in whites of Northern European descent. GCA is the most common systemic vasculitis, with a lifetime risk of up to 0.5% to 1% in the United States.

4. How do patients with GCA present?

GCA patients may have systemic features including fevers, fatigue, and weight loss. The primary distinctions to be made are between classic symptoms attributable to **cranial involvement** (headache, scalp tenderness, jaw and/or tongue claudication, or visual symptoms such as amaurosis fugax or diplopia) and symptoms of **large-vessel involvement** (limb claudication, pulse discrepancies). Notably, some patients (15 to 20%) can present with only large-vessel/systemic symptoms (e.g., fever of unknown origin, cough, upper extremity claudication) and have none of the classic cranial GCA symptoms. Table 26.1 provides a scoring system for classification of GCA.

5. What is the relationship between GCA and polymyalgia rheumatica (PMR)?

Approximately 15-20% of patients with PMR may develop GCA, and about 50% of patients with GCA will have concurrent PMR. It is important to screen all PMR patients for signs and symptoms of GCA.

TABLE 26.1 Classification Criteria for Giant Cell Arteritis

CLASSIFICATION CRITERIA FOR GIANT CELL ARTERITIS (APPLIED AFTER DIAGNOSIS OF A MEDIUM/LARGE VESSEL VASCULITIS AND EXCLUSION OF CONDITIONS MIMICKING VASCULITIS)

Age ≥50 required at time of diagnosis

CLINICAL CRITERIA		LAB/IMAGING/BIOPSY CRITERIA	
Morning stiffness in shoulders/neck	+2	Maximum ESR ≥50 mm/hr or CRP ≥10 mg/L	+3
Sudden visual loss	+3	Positive temporal artery biopsy or halo sign on temporal artery ultrasound	+5
Jaw or tongue claudication	+2	Bilateral axillary involvement	+2
New temporal headache	+2	FDG-PET activity throughout aorta	+2
Scalp tenderness	+2		
Abnormal examination of the temporal artery	+2		

A score of ≥6 points is needed for the classification of GCA

Adapted from Ponte C, Grayson PC, Robson JC, et al. 2022 American College of Rheumatology/EULAR classification criteria for giant cell arteritis. *Ann Rheum Dis.* 2022;81(12):1647–1653.

6. What physical exam findings are most helpful in suggesting a diagnosis of GCA?

Several exam findings are somewhat specific for GCA, but most have low sensitivity. **Scalp tenderness** and **temporal artery abnormalities,** such as a reduction in the pulse, palpable tenderness, or temporal artery thickening/nodularity are helpful when present. Visual symptoms or signs (diplopia, amaurosis fugax, vision loss) are also clues that increase the likelihood of a diagnosis of GCA. Jaw and limb claudication are also symptoms that suggest a diagnosis of GCA. Due to frequent (15–20%) involvement of the aorta and its primary branches, BP and pulses should be checked in both arms to look for discrepancies (>10 mm Hg difference in systolic BP between arms) and the carotid and subclavian vessels should be auscultated for the presence of bruits.

7. What is the most common catastrophic outcome in GCA?

Visual loss occurs in 20% of patients, can be an early symptom, and is most commonly due to anterior ischemic optic neuropathy. This results from arteritis involving the **posterior ciliary branches** of the ophthalmic arteries. The blindness is abrupt and painless. Retinal and ophthalmic artery thromboses and occipital strokes are less common causes of blindness. Blindness occurs in <1% of patients after corticosteroids are begun. **In situations of threatened or impending vision loss, treatment should not be delayed for diagnostic purposes. If vision is lost in one eye and treatment is not started, vision in the other eye may be lost as soon as 1-2 weeks later.**

8. Which vessels may be affected in GCA?

Cranial involvement is the most frequently recognized and characteristic anatomic location for GCA, but other medium- or large-sized arteries can be affected. Cranial involvement of the temporal and ophthalmic arteries leads to the classic symptoms of headache and vision loss. Involvement of the vertebral and carotid blood vessels can lead to symptoms such as dizziness and stroke. Extracranial GCA usually involves the aorta and its major branches (especially the bilateral subclavian and axillary arteries) and is clinically evident in 15–20% of patients. Positron emission tomography (PET) scans show subclinical aortic inflammation in 50–80% of patients. Supradiaphragmatic aortic vessels are more commonly involved in GCA. Intracranial vessels are not involved because they lack an internal elastic lamina and vasa vasorum after entering the skull. Fig. 26.1 presents the common distribution of blood vessel involvement in GCA.

PEARL: In patients with GCA, vertebral artery abnormalities are more likely due to vasculitis than atherosclerosis.

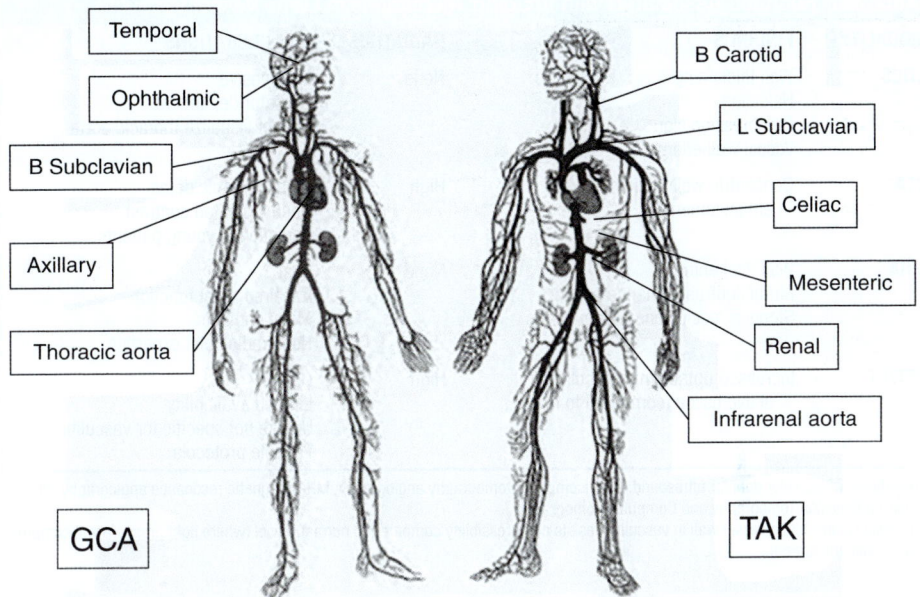

Fig. 26.1 Blood Vessel Distribution in Giant Cell Arteritis (GCA) vs Takayasu Arteritis (TAK).

9. What other catastrophic outcomes may occur in GCA patients with aortic involvement?

Aortitis can lead to aortic aneurysms and dissection. GCA patients have a 17x increased relative risk for developing thoracic aortic aneurysms and a 2.4x risk of abdominal aortic aneurysms compared with age-matched controls. Aneurysms and dissection may present with midthoracic or low back pain; these symptoms should be urgently evaluated in any GCA patient. Patients with clinical aortic involvement should be followed with magnetic resonance angiography (MRA) or computed tomography angiography (CTA) every 6 to 12 months for the development of new lesions/stenoses or the development of aneurysms. Surgery or endovascular aneurysm repair is considered when the aneurysm enlarges to >5 cm or is dissected. **All patients with suspected or newly diagnosed GCA should be screened for large vessel involvement with a noninvasive imaging modality.**

10. Describe the mortality of GCA.

The risk of death from GCA appears to be increased (3x) within the first 4 months of starting therapy. Patients typically die of vascular complications, such as stroke or myocardial infarction. After 4 months (with therapy), the mortality is similar to that of an age-matched general population except as related to aortic dissection.

11. What laboratory tests are useful for the clinical diagnosis of GCA?

The erythrocyte sedimentation rate (ESR) is the most useful laboratory test and tends to be higher in GCA than in other vasculitides. It is almost always >50 mm/hour (85–90%), typically 80 to 100 mm/hour by the Westergren method. An ESR >100 mm/hr increases the likelihood of a positive temporal artery biopsy. Although ESR is highly sensitive in GCA, specificity is poor. Other conditions that can significantly raise ESR include infections, malignancy and IVIG treatment. A minority of patients (10–15%) will have a "normal" ESR. These patients typically have fewer systemic symptoms with an ESR of 40 to 50 mm/hour accompanied by an elevated C-reactive protein (CRP). Less than 5–10% will have both an ESR < 30 mm/hr and a normal CRP.

Other nonspecific markers of systemic inflammation, including anemia, thrombocytosis, abnormal liver function tests (especially alkaline phosphatase), and an elevated CRP (frequently

TABLE 26.2 Features Associated with Imaging Techniques in Large Vessel Vasculitis

MODALITY	FINDINGS	RADIATION	CONSIDERATIONS
CDUS	Wall thickening Halo sign Compression sign* Vessel wall edema	None	Inexpensive Operator dependent Cannot visualize thoracic aorta
CTA	Concentric wall thickening with enhancement	High	High anatomic detail Need iodinated contrast Radiation in young patients
MRA	Wall thickening Mural contrast enhancement Stenosis, occlusions & aneurysms	None	Cost Impaired renal function Metal implants Need radiologist expertise
PET/CT	Increased uptake in metabolically active tissue (compared to liver)	High	Cost Limited availability Uptake not specific for vasculitis Variable protocols

Abbreviations: CDUs-color doppler ultrasound; CTA- computed tomography angiography; MRA-magnetic resonance angiography; PET/CT-Positron Emission Tomography and Computed Tomography

Compression sign*: blood vessel wall in vasculitis resists compressibility compared to normal vessel (where light pressure will compress wall and close the lumen)

to very high levels, >10 mg/dL), are commonly seen. None of these tests is diagnostic. GCA has no associated autoantibodies, such as rheumatoid factor and antinuclear antibody.

12. Is a biopsy required to make a diagnosis of GCA?

Often, but not always. Classification schemes (not used for diagnostic purposes) include a combination of clinical, laboratory, radiographic, and pathologic features (Table 26.1). In clinical care, the gold standard for diagnosis has traditionally been a temporal artery biopsy with characteristic findings; however, advances in imaging modalities allow for a diagnosis of GCA in the absence of biopsy data in some situations. Ultrasound, CTA, magnetic resonance imaging (MRI)/MRA, and fluorodeoxyglucose (FDG)-PET techniques can be used to support a diagnosis of GCA, each with different pros and cons (see Table 26.2, in addition to Questions 13 and 14 ahead).

13. What is the role of ultrasound in GCA diagnosis?

Temporal artery duplex ultrasonography is noninvasive, cost effective and can reveal homogenous arterial wall thickening (the **"halo sign"**). Ultrasound can also show stenosis or occlusion of the blood vessels and can be used to assess the subclavian, axillary, and carotid arteries in addition to the temporal artery. The sensitivity of temporal artery ultrasound ranges from ~68-87% and specificity from 81-96%. Ultrasound is highly operator dependent, so it is best performed at experienced centers. Additionally, the classic "halo" sign can disappear within a week after glucocorticoid exposure. EULAR recommendations suggest ultrasound as an initial diagnostic modality in predominantly cranial GCA, but The American College of Rheumatology/Vasculitis Foundation (ACR/VF) recommendations are to perform TA biopsy over ultrasound. Ultrasound has little role in the evaluation of aortic involvement behind the chest wall.

14. In what instances might a diagnosis be supported by radiography or nuclear medicine studies?

GCA patients presenting with aortitis and large-vessel involvement alone typically do not have cranial symptoms and have a negative temporal artery biopsy in up to 40–50% of cases. In this clinical situation, characteristic MRI/MRA, FDG-PET, or CTA findings are adequate to confirm a diagnosis of GCA. ACR/VF guidelines recommend obtaining baseline large vessel imaging in all suspected or newly diagnosed GCA patients using noninvasive imaging modalities (MRI/MRA, CT, and/or FDG-PET). High-resolution MRI may also be reasonable as an initial diagnostic study for evaluating predominantly cranial GCA if ultrasound is unavailable.

15. How should a surgeon be instructed to obtain an excisional biopsy for GCA, and how much artery should be taken?

The pulse of the temporal artery is often most easily palpable just anterior to the tragus of the ear. Biopsy in this location risks damage to the facial nerve and a preferred location targets the frontal branch of the superficial temporal artery just above the temple. Biopsies should be performed on the most symptomatic side. GCA has a propensity for skip lesions and there is shrinkage of the specimen between the OR and what is sent for pathology. The recommendation is for biopsies to be >1cm to increase the sensitivity of the test, with longer segments yielding greater sensitivity. Pathologists must review multiple segments to ensure characteristic lesions are not missed.

16. Should a biopsy be done on one or both sides?

Unilateral biopsy has a pooled sensitivity of around 80%. Additional/contralateral biopsies increase the sensitivity by 5%. The negative predictive value of bilateral negative temporal artery biopsies in a patient with cranial symptoms is 91%. The ACR/VF guidelines recommend unilateral over bilateral temporal artery biopsy which is a reasonable approach (especially in a patient with unilateral headaches or a clinically abnormal artery on the affected side). In patients with bilateral symptoms or an unclear clinical picture, performing a bilateral biopsy can increase the likelihood of confirming a diagnosis.

17. Describe the histologic features of GCA.

The classic pattern (only seen in ~50% of cases) includes transmural mononuclear or granulomatous inflammation of the media, centered on the internal elastic lamina, with multinucleated giant cells, and fragmentation of the internal elastic lamina. Arterial mural thickening and intimal hyperplasia with intraluminal thrombosis are classically described as well. Giant cells occur in only ~50% of cases. In about half of cases, a nonspecific panarteritis is seen, including mixed inflammatory infiltrates composed largely of lymphocytes (CD4+ T cells predominate) and macrophages admixed with a few eosinophils (Fig. 26.2). Neutrophils are rare. **Fibrinoid necrosis should not be seen,** and if present, would suggest an alternate diagnosis (e.g., granulomatous polyangiitis).

A few patients with GCA (5–9%) have biopsies showing only periadventitial small-vessel vasculitis (SVV) and/or vasculitis of the vasa vasorum (VVV) surrounding a noninflamed temporal artery. These patients with SVV tend to have lower ESR/CRP levels as well as less severe clinical manifestations and disease course than patients with a classic biopsy for GCA.

18. Can a pathologist diagnose GCA without observing giant cells?

Yes. Up to 50% of positive biopsies show diffuse lymphocytic infiltrate without the evidence of granulomatous inflammation or giant cells. Even after prolonged glucocorticoid therapy, healed temporal arteritis can still be diagnosed as it is characterized by intimal fibrosis, medial scarring, and eccentric destruction of the internal elastic lamina.

Importantly, fragmentation and fraying of the internal elastic lamina is a common feature of aging arteries; therefore, these features alone are not indicative of active or healed arteritis. An inflammatory cell infiltrate, even without giant cells, should be present to some degree to diagnose GCA.

19. Describe the pathogenesis of GCA.

Early in disease, following exposure to an unknown trigger, lymphocytic inflammation develops and is confined to the adventitia and external elastic lamina. In the adventitia, dendritic cells are activated to produce chemokines which attract more dendritic cells, lymphocytes, and macrophages to the area. The activated dendritic cells process and present antigens resulting in T-cell activation. Dendritic cells produce interleukin (IL)-12 and IL-18 which promote Th-1 differentiation, whereas IL-1, IL-6, and IL-21 promote Th-17 differentiation. The activated Th1 cells secrete interferon-γ, which is important in macrophage activation and granuloma formation, whereas Th17 cells produce IL-17, which is a potent proinflammatory cytokine with multiple cellular effects leading to vascular inflammation and production of matrix metalloproteinases that destroy the internal elastic lamina. Growth and angiogenic factors (vascular endothelial growth factor) provide nutritional support for the influx of T cells and macrophages to the area. Closer to the lumen, neovascularization and macrophage-produced cytokines (platelet-derived growth factor, IL-1) cause prominent intimal proliferation that leads to ischemia.

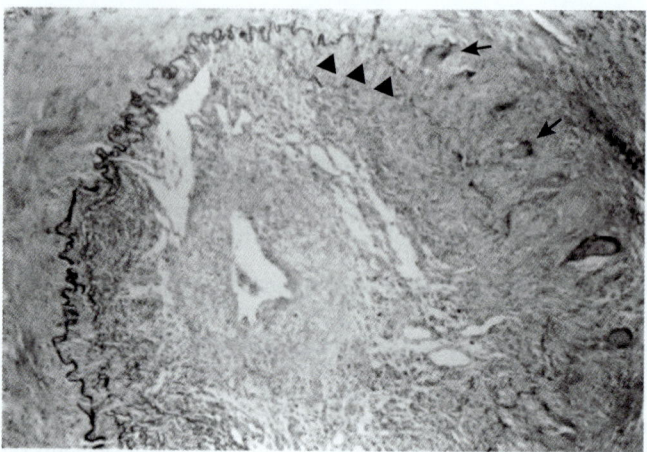

Fig. 26.2 Temporal artery biopsy in a patient with giant cell arteritis showing the disrupted internal elastic lamina (*arrowheads*) and giant cells (*arrows*).

20. Have genetic or environmental associations been described in GCA?

Yes. GCA is associated with MHC class II molecules. The majority (60%) of GCA patients express the **HLA-DRB1*04** alleles (0401 and 0404). This genotype appears to confer increased susceptibility to the disease (but is not a predictor of disease severity). Various environmental triggers have also been postulated over the years. Some infectious agents (varicella-zoster virus, mycoplasma pneumoniae, parvovirus B19, parainfluenza, Chlamydia pneumoniae) have been considered potential triggers, but conclusive evidence is lacking.

21. How is GCA initially treated?

High-dose glucocorticoids are the primary treatment modality in GCA. Initial dosing is based on consensus/expert opinion, but a reasonable initial dose for those with intact vision is prednisone 1 mg/kg daily. Those with threatened or actual vision loss at diagnosis should be treated with pulse intravenous glucocorticoids (methylprednisolone, 1 g daily × 3 days). High-dose therapy is usually sustained for about a month (or until ESR/CRP normalize), followed by a taper lasting between 6 months, and often up to 2 years or longer. The ACR/VF recommends concomitant initiation of tocilizumab along with glucocorticoids at the time of diagnosis. The use of tocilizumab has been shown to allow significant reductions in glucocorticoid load as well as the ability to achieve and sustain remission in GCA.

22. Which steroid-sparing therapies are used in GCA?

Based on randomized clinical trial data (*GiACTA*), **tocilizumab, a monoclonal antibody against IL-6 receptor, was approved by the FDA and is recommended as steroid sparing therapy in GCA.** Methotrexate has long been used as a steroid-sparing therapy in GCA, although evidence supporting its use is mixed with regard to its effectiveness. Nonetheless, methotrexate is sometimes utilized in patients with significant steroid-related side effects, diabetes, intolerance to tocilizumab, or a relapsing course with prolonged need for steroids. There is ongoing research evaluating the role of IL-17 blockade and JAK inhibition in the treatment of GCA (upadicitinib was FDA approved in GCA in 2025).

23. How is tocilizumab used in GCA?

Tocilizumab (162 mg subcutaneous weekly or 6mg/kg IV every 4 weeks) can be used as part of the initial therapy along with glucocorticoid in order to more rapidly taper prednisone and achieve sustained remission. After tapering of glucocorticoids, tocilizumab may be used alone to maintain remission. If tocilizumab is discontinued after 1 year, about half of patients will experience a relapse in their disease. Fortunately, those who relapse are generally able to regain remission with the re-initiation of tocilizumab and/or glucocorticoids. Most experts determine the length of maintenance tocilizumab therapy or weaning strategies based on the patients' clinical course, preferences, and risks for relapse.

24. Should all patients with GCA be started on aspirin?

There is some data showing that aspirin may be beneficial in preventing ischemic events in patients with vascular narrowing leading to decreased cerebral blood flow, but it is unclear whether there is benefit in those without vertebral or carotid narrowing. Aspirin should be added in patients with critical or flow-limiting involvement of the vertebral or carotid arteries, or in those with other cardiac indications.

25. Will treatment with glucocorticoids reduce the yield of a temporal artery biopsy or imaging?

Studies have shown that biopsies often show findings typical for arteritis after more than 14 days of glucocorticoid therapy, although a **biopsy should ideally be obtained within 2 weeks of starting treatment** to increase the likelihood of finding classic positive pathology. Ultrasound evidence of GCA may disappear as early as a few days after initiation of glucocorticoids (however, some patients have imaging findings that persist much longer). Ideally, fast-track clinics would allow for rapid assessment of ultrasound findings soon after the initiation of steroids in order to obtain a timely diagnosis. PET/CT imaging has a similar drop in sensitivity after ~10 days of glucocorticoid therapy. Other large vessel imaging modalities such as MRA and CTA have a decrease in sensitivity after prolonged glucocorticoid exposure as well. Ideally, all diagnostic studies should be performed as soon as possible (within 1–2 weeks) after initiation of glucocorticoids. However, despite the potential loss in sensitivity, **initiation of treatment for suspected GCA should not be withheld while awaiting the results of diagnostics (or insurance authorization for imaging) given the risk of irreversible vision loss in these patients.**

26. How is disease activity monitored in GCA?

No disease-specific biomarker is available in GCA. ESR and CRP are utilized along with clinical assessment. Changes in inflammatory markers without corresponding clinical evidence of disease activity should be monitored without escalation of therapy. Large vessel imaging should be obtained at baseline to assess for extra-cranial arterial involvement. If present, surveillance imaging should be performed periodically; however, the frequency of these assessments has not been defined. Clinical assessment should be continued long term.

TAKAYASU ARTERITIS

27. What are the other names for TAK?

Pulseless disease, aortic arch syndrome, nonspecific aortoarteritis.

28. Which patients are most typically affected by TAK?

TAK occurs most frequently in young women (8:1 female > male), peaking between the ages of 15 and 30 years. TAK occurs most commonly in Asian (Japan, China, India, Southeast Asia) women but has been reported worldwide in all racial groups.

29. How does TAK present?

A triphasic pattern of progression of disease is classically described:
- **Phase I:** pre-pulseless, 'inflammatory' period characterized by systemic complaints, such as fever, arthralgias, and weight loss, often leading to diagnostic delays.
- **Phase II:** vessel inflammation, dominated by vessel pain and tenderness.
- **Phase III:** fibrotic "burnt out" stage, when bruits and ischemia predominate.

   Patients can present in any phase or combination thereof because TAK is a chronic, recurrent disease. Up to 10% present with no symptoms, and the incidental finding of unequal pulses/BPs, bruits, or hypertension prompts further evaluation.

TABLE 26.3 Classification Criteria for Takayasu Arteritis

CLASSIFICATION CRITERIA FOR TAKAYASU ARTERITIS (APPLIED AFTER DIAGNOSIS OF A MEDIUM OR LARGE VESSEL VASCULITIS AND EXCLUSION OF CONDITIONS MIMICKING VASCULITIS)

Age ≤60 required at time of diagnosis

Evidence of vasculitis on imaging

CLINICAL CRITERIA		IMAGING CRITERIA	
Female sex	+1	One arterial territory	+1
Angina or ischemic cardiac pain	+2	Two arterial territories	+2
Arm or leg claudication	+2	Three or more arterial territories	+3
Vascular bruit	+2	Symmetric involvement of paired arteries	+1
Reduced pulse in upper extremity	+2	Abdominal aorta involvement with renal or mesenteric involvement	+3
Carotid artery abnormality	+2		
Systolic blood pressure difference in arms ≥20 mm Hg	+1		

A score of ≥5 points is needed for the classification of TAK

Adapted from Grayson PC, Ponte C, Suppiah R, et al. 2022 American College of Rheumatology/EULAR classification criteria for Takayasu arteritis. *Ann Rheum Dis.* 2022;81(12):1654–1660.

30. Describe some of the common clinical manifestations and physical exam findings of TAK.

A comprehensive vascular exam (BP, pulse, bruits) is mandatory as bruits (80%), decreased pulses (60%), and asymmetric BPs (50%) are common findings. Involvement of the subclavian and iliac arteries may lead to limb claudication. Carotid and vertebral artery involvement may lead to pre-syncope, dizziness, headache, and carotidynia (tenderness with palpation over the carotid artery). Pulmonary artery disease can occur in up to 70% of patients, with <25% having symptoms of pulmonary hypertension. Cardiac involvement with angina, myocardial infarction, heart failure, sudden death, and aortic valvular regurgitation occurs in up to 15% of patients. Renovascular hypertension can occur from the involvement of the renal arteries. Arthralgias (50%) and constitutional symptoms (40%) are common. Due to arterial stenosis, blood pressure measurements need to be obtained in all four extremities. The distribution of blood vessel involvement is shown in Fig. 26.1. Table 26.3 provides a scoring system for the classification of TAK.

31. Are there any specific laboratory tests useful for the diagnosis of TAK?

No. Nonspecific laboratory studies indicate active inflammation such as anemia of chronic disease, thrombocytosis, and an elevated ESR and CRP. The ESR does not always follow the degree of active, ongoing inflammation and may be normal in 33% to 50% of patients with active disease by arterial biopsy.

32. How is the diagnosis of TAK made?

Imaging is required to make a diagnosis of TAK. Angiography was the traditional gold standard for detecting arterial involvement in TAK; however, newer modalities are noninvasive and provide greater information about the presence or absence of active inflammation. MRA is the preferred initial modality for the diagnosis of TAK (lower radiation than other modalities), unless an endovascular intervention is anticipated. CTA, FDG-PET (Fig. 26.3), and possibly ultrasound (depending on vessel in question) are also reasonable modalities if MRA is unavailable. All are preferred over angiography. **Biopsy is not necessary to establish a diagnosis of TAK.**

33. Does the histopathologic description of TAK vary from GCA?

Yes, but not by much. The histologic appearance of TAK is a focal panarteritis very similar to GCA, including "skip lesions" and patchy involvement. Granulomatous inflammation can occur.

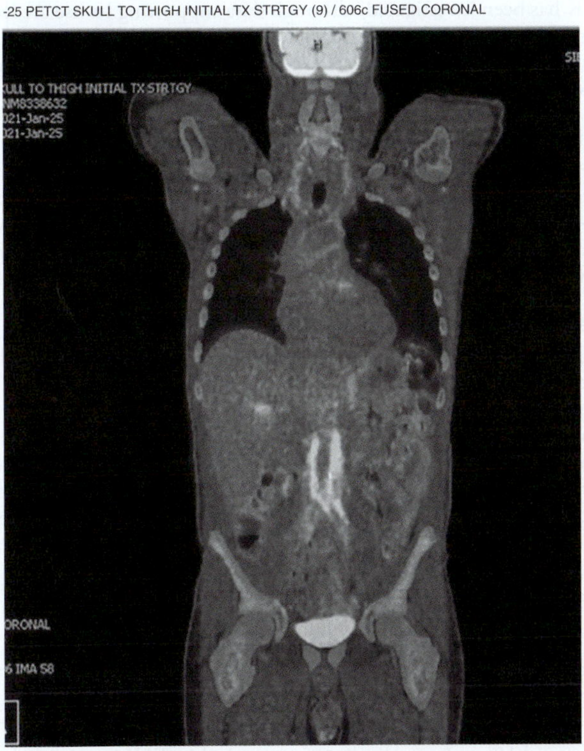
-25 PETCT SKULL TO THIGH INITIAL TX STRTGY (9) / 606c FUSED CORONAL
ULL TO THIGH INITIAL TX STRTGY
NM8338632
021-Jan-25
021-Jan-25
ORONAL
6 IMA 58

Fig. 26.3 PET scan in Takayasu arteritis showing hypermetabolic activity in the ascending thoracic aorta, infrarenal abdominal aorta, and the proximal segments of both common iliac arteries.

One point that distinguishes TAK from GCA is that the cellular infiltrate in TAK tends to localize in the adventitia and outer parts of the media (including the vasa vasorum), whereas the inflammation of GCA concentrates around the inner half of the media. Additionally, mononuclear cells in the vessel walls of TAK patients are mostly gamma-delta T lymphocytes, natural killer cells, and CD8+ T cells rather than the Th1/Th17 T-lymphocytes seen in GCA patients.

34. Is TAK a genetic disease?

Studies linking TAK to HLA class I (HLA-B52:01) and II genes have provided conflicting results and differ between ethnicities. There is no link to HLA-DRB1∗04 as is seen in GCA.

35. What is the treatment for TAK?

High-dose glucocorticoids (prednisone 1mg/kg) are the initial therapy for active inflammatory TAK, followed by long-term taper. Suggested prednisone taper after disease control is 10% of the daily dose each week. The goal is to taper off of steroids in patients who achieve remission for at least 6–12 months. Relapses are common, and about 20% of patients never achieve remission. The ACR/VF recommends initiation of another immunosuppressive agent (methotrexate, azathioprine, or a TNF inhibitor) along with glucocorticoids to decrease the risk of relapses and achieve disease control. The best evidence base and clinical experience exists for methotrexate, though the alternatives mentioned are all reasonable (taking into consideration patient age, comorbidities, and preferences).

36. Which treatments may be used in refractory TAK?

In refractory cases or relapses while on glucocorticoids or glucocorticoids with another immunomodulating agent, the addition of a TNF inhibitor is recommended. The use of tocilizumab in relapsing TAK has been investigated, although data supporting its use are less robust than in GCA. Other agents that can be considered include JAK inhibitors (baricitinib, upadacitinib, tofacitinib), and rituximab, though clinical experience and large-scale studies are lacking. Cyclophosphamide is reserved as a salvage therapy.

37. Other than immunosuppression, what else can be done to help control disease activity and comorbidities in TAK?

Blood pressure control, tobacco cessation, and lipid management are essential to reduce cardiovascular risk. Anti-platelet therapy is recommended in patients with active TAK who have flow-limiting involvement by imaging of the cranial or vertebrobasilar vessels (though should be used with caution after surgical procedures due to increased risk of bleeding).

38. How is disease activity monitored in TAK?

Unfortunately, ESR correlates with the degree of inflammation observed on a biopsied blood vessel in only about 50% of cases, so clinical assessment remains a vital tool in TAK monitoring. The role of imaging in monitoring large-vessel vasculitis inflammatory activity is an active area of research, although FDG-PET, MRI/MRA, CTA, or ultrasound may all be reasonable to confirm active disease in situations where a flare is suspected clinically (Table 26.2). The use of repeat imaging for periodic monitoring of fibrotic/structural damage is recommended, although the appropriate frequency for serial reassessment is not well determined. Given the young age of TAK patients, MRA is generally the preferred imaging modality as it avoids the radiation exposure of repeated CT studies. The presence of new vascular lesions on interval imaging should prompt strong consideration for escalation of immunosuppressive therapy.

39. Describe the long-term morbidity and mortality of TAK.

At 10 years, 50% of TAK patients suffer relapses with vascular complications. Ten to twenty percent of TAK patients suffer from strokes or TIAs. Heart failure, myocardial infarction, and ruptured aortic aneurysm are the major causes of morbidity and mortality in TAK. Despite these risks, 5-year and 10-year complication-free survival in TAK is estimated at 70% and 54% respectively. The prognosis in patients with pulmonary artery involvement is worse in those with pulmonary hypertension than those without it. The 5-year survival rates with treatment are 80% to 90%.

40. When should a vascular intervention be considered?

Angioplasty, stenting, and bypass graft surgery are sometimes indicated for symptomatic stenotic lesions that do not improve with medical therapy. Patients with TAK can develop collateral circulation bypassing the stenosis, and thus, surgical intervention may not be needed. Delaying surgical intervention until the disease is quiescent is preferred over performing the intervention while the patient has an active disease, if possible. In patients with TAK undergoing surgical intervention, the use of high-dose glucocorticoids periprocedurally is recommended if the patient has an active disease.

ISOLATED AORTITIS

41. What are potential etiologies for aortitis?

- Infection
- Idiopathic isolated aortitis
- Large vessel vasculitis (GCA and TAK)
- Other vasculitides (Polyarteritis nodosa, Behcet Disease, Cogan syndrome, IgG4-related disease, IgA vasculitis, ANCA vasculitis, cryoglobulinemia)
- Other immune mediated diseases: sarcoidosis, relapsing polychondritis, histiocytic disease (Erdheim Chester), spondyloarthritis, lupus, rheumatoid arthritis, inflammatory bowel disease, malignancy

42. What are some noninflammatory mimics of aortitis?

Fibromuscular dysplasia, vascular Ehlers-Danlos, Marfan syndrome, Loeys–Dietz syndrome, and other familial thoracic aortic aneurysm and dissection (TAAD) syndromes (see Table 26.4).

TABLE 26.4 Location of Aortic Abnormality and Associated Diseases

AREA OF INVOLVEMENT	ASCENDING AORTA (ARCH, SUBCLAVIANS, CAROTIDS)	ISOLATED DESCENDING AORTA	PULMONARY ARTERY	PERI-AORTIC INVOLVEMENT
Disease entities to consider	• Giant cell arteritis • Takayasu arteritis • Behcet disease • Familial TAAD syndromes • Marfan syndrome • Vascular Ehlers–Danlos • Loeys–Dietz syndrome	• Takayasu arteritis • Inflammatory abdominal aortic aneurysm	• Hughes-Stovin syndrome • Behcet disease	• IgG4-related disease • Lymphoma • Erdheim-Chester disease

TABLE 26.5 Histologic Patterns of Aortitis and Associated Diseases

LYMPHOPLASMACYTIC INFILTRATE	GRANULOMATOUS INFILTRATE	MIXED INFLAMMATORY PATTERN	SUPPURATIVE
IgG4-related disease (storiform fibrosis)	GCA/PMR	Relapsing polychondritis	Bacterial infection
Systemic lupus erythematosus	Takayasu arteritis	Cogan syndrome	
Ankylosing spondylitis	Sarcoidosis (noncaseating)	Behcet syndrome	
Clinically isolated aortitis	Clinically isolated aortitis (>60%)		
Syphilis	ANCA vasculitis (with necrosis)		
	Rheumatoid arthritis		
	Inflammatory bowel disease		
	Infection		

43. What are some infectious causes of aortitis?

Bacterial aortitis due to *Salmonella*, *Staphylococcus*, or *Streptococcus* usually results from bacterial seeding of an atherosclerotic plaque or aneurysmal sac via the vasa vasorum. Tuberculosis may cause aortitis from direct seeding by adjacent infected tissue or miliary spread. Aortitis is the classic cardiovascular manifestation of tertiary syphilis. Syphilitic aortitis typically involves the ascending aorta and may result in aneurysm or aortic regurgitation.

44. Describe the classification of idiopathic isolated aortitis.

Idiopathic aortitis can be approached based on the location of the aorta predominantly affected, or based on histology of surgical specimens, along with the clinical picture.
- Location: ascending aorta, isolated descending aorta, pulmonary artery involvement, peri-aortic involvement. See Table 26.4 for a list of conditions associated with aortic disease according to anatomic site.
- Histology: lymphoplasmacytic infiltrate, granulomatous, mixed inflammatory pattern, suppurative. See Table 26.5 for a list of conditions associated with aortic disease according to histologic findings.

45. What should you do if a patient has been diagnosed with clinically isolated aortitis (on imaging or biopsy)?

In cases of isolated aortitis, the entire aorta should be imaged at baseline and followed with serial imaging at regular intervals, since a significant proportion of patients have or develop abnormalities in other vascular beds. The role of immunosuppressive therapy remains unclear in patients with clinically isolated aortitis, though some clinicians will use a short course of moderate-dose prednisone tapered over a few months. Blood pressure management should be employed, especially in patients with aneurysmal disease.

ACKNOWLEDGMENT

The author wishes to acknowledge Patrick Wood, MD, who contributed to this chapter in the previous edition.

BIBLIOGRAPHY

Bilton EJ, Mollan SP. Giant cell arteritis: reviewing the advancing diagnostics and management. *Eye*. 2023;37(12):2365–2373.

Buttgereit F, Dejaco C, Matteson EL, et al. Polymyalgia rheumatica and giant cell arteritis: a systematic review. *JAMA*. 2016;315(22):2442–2458.

Comarmond C, Biard L, Lambert M, et al. Long-term outcomes and prognostic factors of complications in Takayasu arteritis: a multicenter study of 318 patients. *Circulation*. 2017;136:1114–1122.

Dejaco C, Ramiro S, Duftner C, et al. EULAR recommendations for the use of imaging in large vessel vasculitis in clinical practice. *Ann Rheum Dis*. 2018;77(5):636–643.

Gonzalez-Gay MA, Barros S, Lopez-Diaz MJ, et al. Giant cell arteritis: disease patterns of clinical presentation in a series of 240 patients. *Medicine*. 2005;84:269–276.

Grayson PC, Ponte C, Suppiah R, et al. 2022 American College of Rheumatology/EULAR classification criteria for Takayasu arteritis. *Ann Rheum Dis*. 2022;81(12):1654–1660.

Hellmich B, Agueda A, Monti S, et al. 2018 update of the EULAR recommendations for the management of large vessel vasculitis. *Ann Rheum Dis*. 2020;79(1):19–30.

Kermani TA, Byram K. Isolated aortitis: workup and management. *Rheum Dis Clin North Am*. 2023;49(3):523–543.

Mahr AD, Jover JA, Spiera RF, et al. Adjunctive methotrexate for treatment of giant cell arteritis: an individual patient data meta-analysis. *Arthritis Rheum*. 2007;56:2789–2797.

Maz M, Chung SA, Abril A, et al. 2021 American College of Rheumatology/Vasculitis Foundation guideline for the management of giant cell arteritis and takayasu arteritis. *Arthritis Rheumatol*. 2021;73(8):1349–1365.

Nakaoka Y, Isobe M, Takei S, et al. Efficacy and safety of tocilizumab in patients with refractory Takayasu arteritis: results from a randomised, double-blind, placebo-controlled, phase 3 trial in Japan (the TAKT study). *Ann Rheum Dis*. 2018;77:348–354.

Narvaez J, Bernard B, Roig-Vilaseca D, et al. Influence of previous corticosteroid therapy on temporal biopsy yield in giant cell arteritis. *Semin Arthritis Rheum*. 2007;37:13–19.

Nuenninghoff DM, Hunder GG, Christanson TJ, et al. Incidence and predictors of large artery complications in patients with giant cell arteritis: a population-based study over 50 years. *Arthritis Rheum*. 2003;48:3522–3531.

Ponte C, Grayson PC, Robson JC, et al. 2022 American College of Rheumatology/EULAR classification criteria for giant cell arteritis. *Ann Rheum Dis*. 2022;81(12):1647–1653.

Stone JH, Tuckwell K, Dimonaco S, et al. Trial of tocilizumab in giant-cell arteritis. *N Engl J Med*. 2017;377:317–328.

van der Geest KSM, Sandovici M, Brouwer E, et al. Diagnostic accuracy of symptoms, physical signs, and laboratory tests for giant cell arteritis: a systematic review and meta-analysis. *JAMA Intern Med*. 2020;180(10):1295–1304.

CHAPTER 27

Polyarteritis Nodosa, Thromboangiitis Obliterans, and Primary Central Nervous System Vasculitis

Vivek K. Murthy, MD, MSc and Sharon A. Chung, MD, MAS

 KEY POINTS

1. Polyarteritis nodosa (PAN) is a systemic inflammatory disorder producing transmural necrotizing vasculitis of the medium-sized arteries and muscular arterioles. The diagnosis should be considered in any patient with constitutional symptoms, hypertension, and signs or symptoms resulting from ischemia of the peripheral nerves, skin, and/or gastrointestinal tract.
2. PAN spares the venous system, is not associated with known autoantibodies, does not affect the lung parenchyma, and does not cause glomerulonephritis.
3. Hepatitis B virus (HBV)-associated PAN accounts for <10% of PAN cases and is treated differently than idiopathic PAN.
4. Thromboangiitis obliterans (TO) is a thrombotic vasculopathy of the peripheral circulation that is associated with tobacco use and causes limb and digital ischemia and necrosis.
5. Primary central nervous system vasculitis (PCNSV) is a rare single organ vasculitis syndrome affecting the small and medium cerebral vessels, producing encephalopathy, headaches, and focal neurological deficits from ischemic injury. A brain biopsy is often required for diagnosis.

1. What conditions affect the medium-sized arteries?

- Polyarteritis nodosa (a multi-system vasculitis syndrome)
- Kawasaki disease (see Chapter 70: Kawasaki Disease)
- Thromboangiitis obliterans, or Buerger disease (a thrombotic, inflammatory vasculopathy)
- Primary central nervous system vasculitis (a single-organ vasculitis syndrome)

2. Can vessels of other sizes be involved in medium-vessel vasculitis?

Yes, while the vascular damage in PAN most often affects the medium-sized arteries, it can also affect the smaller muscular arterioles and occasionally the capillaries. For example, palpable purpura - a classic manifestation of small-vessel vasculitis involving the capillaries - can also be seen in PAN.

POLYARTERITIS NODOSA (A MEDIUM-VESSEL VASCULITIS)

3. What is PAN?

PAN is a form of systemic vasculitis involving transmural necrotizing vasculitis of medium-sized arteries, muscular arterioles, and small arteries, which results in downstream tissue ischemia.

PAN is distinguished from the small-vessel vasculitis syndromes (e.g. ANCA-associated vasculitis, cryoglobulinemic vasculitis) because it:

1. Commonly affects the medium-sized arteries
2. Spares the capillaries, venous structures, and lung parenchyma
3. Is not associated with the presence of ANCA antibodies
4. Typically does not produce granulomatous inflammation
5. Does not cause glomerulonephritis, which is a manifestation of small-vessel vasculitis syndromes.

PAN presents with constitutional symptoms and typically affects multiple organ systems (e.g. the skin, peripheral nerves, muscles, gastrointestinal tract, kidneys, and retinal tissue). However, the lung parenchyma is virtually always spared.

4. How common is PAN?

PAN is rare. The annual incidence is estimated to be 2 to 9 cases per million people. The average age range at diagnosis is 40–60 years, though PAN can occur at any age. It affects all racial groups, and men and women are affected equally.

5. What are the clinical features of this condition?

PAN generally affects multiple organ systems. Patients may experience constitutional symptoms, such as fevers, chills, night sweats, and weight loss, along with signs and symptoms resulting from end-organ ischemia. Commonly affected organ systems include the peripheral nervous system, skin, and gastrointestinal tract. Table 27.1 outlines the major organ manifestations in PAN.

6. Are any specific laboratory tests helpful in the diagnosis of PAN?

There is no specific laboratory test to confirm a diagnosis of PAN. Laboratory studies may reveal an elevated erythrocyte sedimentation rate (ESR) and C-reactive protein (CRP), anemia of chronic disease, elevated muscle enzymes, or renal insufficiency from renal infarction or renovascular hypertension. Testing for ANA, ANCA, C3, C4, and cryoglobulins are characteristically negative or normal. Patients should be tested for human immunodeficiency virus and viral hepatitis, since these infections can cause secondary PAN syndrome.

7. How do you make the diagnosis of PAN?

PAN should be suspected in any patient with suggestive clinical features (Table 27.1). A diagnosis of PAN can be supported by compatible physical exam findings, laboratory results, and imaging findings. However, confirming a diagnosis of PAN requires supporting evidence from either a biopsy of affected tissue or from visceral angiographic studies.

8. Which tissue should be sampled to diagnose PAN?

Biopsy of an affected site is recommended over an asymptomatic site, due to higher diagnostic yield. The two most commonly biopsied sites are the skin or a peripheral sensory nerve with adjacent muscle tissue. For skin biopsies, deep punch biopsies or surgical biopsies are required to obtain subcutaneous tissue, where the medium-sized arteries reside. Nerve and muscle biopsies

TABLE 27.1 Major Organ Manifestations in PAN

ORGAN	MANIFESTATION	PREVALENCE
Renal	Renal insufficiency due to glomerular ischemia, renovascular hypertension, renal infarctions, renal arteriolar microaneurysms; *most commonly affected organ*	70%
Neurologic	Peripheral sensory, motor, or sensorimotor polyneuropathy (initially asymmetric and later evolving into a symmetric pattern) or mononeuritis multiplex; 5-10% can experience vasculitic strokes; *CNS involvement in PAN raises concern for DADA2 deficiency*	50–70%
Skin	Lower extremity predominance of involvement; livedo reticularis, ulcers, nodules, purpura, vesiculobullous eruptions; digital infarction, necrosis, and gangrene	50%
Joint	Arthralgias Arthritis	50% 20%
Muscle	Myalgia, weakness from vasculitic myositis	50–60%
Gastrointestinal tract	Mesenteric vasculitis → • abdominal pain and/or bowel angina, weight loss, malabsorption, bowel infarction or perforation, nausea, vomiting, or diarrhea • acute cholecystitis or appendicitis • pancreatic infarction and necrosis	30–35%
Other	Orchitis, retinal vasculitis	Low

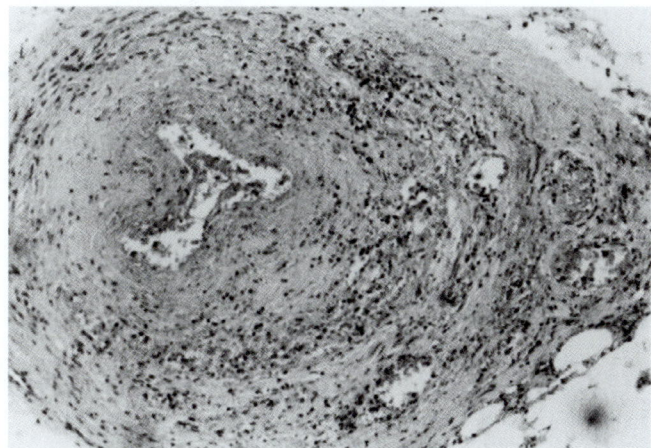

Fig. 27.1 Polyarteritis nodosa involving a medium artery.

can be performed to assess for vasculitic damage at those sites if clinically suspected. Renal biopsies are usually nondiagnostic unless an affected medium-sized artery is present in the biopsy specimen; of note, there is a risk of bleeding from renal arteriolar microaneurysms.

9. Describe the histologic features in PAN.

The pathologic lesion is a necrotizing transmural arteritis of the small and medium arteries and muscular arterioles (Fig. 27.1). Vessel involvement is often patchy and segmental. The perivascular cellular infiltrate consists of monocytes, macrophages, and neutrophils, and leukocytoclasis (fragmentation of neutrophils near disrupted blood vessels) may be seen. Granulomatous inflammation and giant cells are generally absent.

10. When do you perform angiographic studies for the diagnosis of PAN?

When clinically involved tissue is not available for biopsy (as is often the case with digital, coronary, mesenteric, or renal ischemia from medium-vessel vasculitis), angiographic studies are warranted. Conventional catheter-based angiography of the mesenteric, hepatic, and renal arteries and their branches, or of the limb arteries, is the gold-standard diagnostic test to evaluate visceral abdominal manifestations and digital ischemia. Angiography has superior resolution of medium-sized vessels compared to noninvasive imaging techniques such as computed tomography (CT) or magnetic resonance (MR) angiography.

11. Describe the angiographic findings in PAN.

In PAN, visceral angiography reveals segmental regions of vascular stenosis alternating with regions of saccular or fusiform aneurysmal dilation ("rosary bead sign"). CT and MR angiography produce lower-resolution imaging of the splanchnic arterial circulation, but may provide more information about the integrity of vessel walls. MR angiography should be considered in situations where intravenous iodinated contrast is contraindicated (Fig. 27.2).

12. List the conditions that can mimic PAN (Table 27.2).

Several conditions can mimic PAN by causing pathology in medium-sized arteries:
- **Segmental arterial mediolysis (SAM)**: a noninflammatory arteriopathy where patients present with acute pain from bleeding due to vascular rupture (e.g. acute abdominal pain due to intra-abdominal hemorrhage). CT or MR angiography typically reveals segmental regions of aneurysm and stenosis similar to those seen in PAN. Key differences in SAM include the presence of arterial dissections on arteriography and the absence of extravascular signs and symptoms, systemic inflammation, and/or a clinical prodrome.
- **Fibromuscular dysplasia (FMD)**: an idiopathic noninflammatory arteriopathy seen more commonly in young women. Affected patients develop alternating regions of vascular stenosis

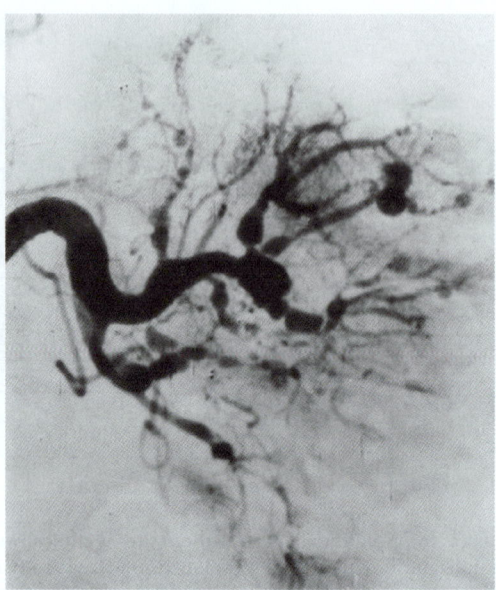

Fig. 27.2 Angiogram of a kidney in a patient with polyarteritis nodosa demonstrating multiple aneurysmal dilatations.

TABLE 27.2 Clinical Mimickers of PAN
ANCA-associated vasculitis
Cryoglobulinemic vasculitis
Vasculitis associated with RA or SLE
Drug-induced vasculitis
Antiphospholipid antibody syndrome
Buerger disease
Infective endocarditis
Human immunodeficiency virus infection
Embolism (left atrial myxoma, cholesterol emboli, cardioembolism)
Segmental arterial mediolysis
Fibromuscular dysplasia
DADA2 syndrome
VEXAS syndrome
Ehlers-Danlos, vascular subtype
Sarcoidosis

DADA2, deficiency of adenosine deaminase 2; *RA*, rheumatoid arthritis; *SLE*, systemic lupus erythematosus; *VEXAS*, vacuoles, E1 enzyme, X-linked, autoinflammatory, somatic

and dilation in the renal and cranio-cervical arteries. Manifestations depend on which vascular territory is affected (e.g. early-onset renovascular hypertension, headache or neck pain, pulsatile tinnitus, limb claudication, etc.) Patients with FMD do not have evidence of systemic inflammation.

- **DADA2 (deficiency of adenosine deaminase 2):** a monogenic autoinflammatory disorder where patients develop small- and medium-vessel vasculitis and/or vasculopathy that can be indistinguishable from PAN. Manifestations include transient ischemic attacks and strokes, severe skin vasculitis, inflammatory arthritis, and hematologic abnormalities including pancytopenia, pure red cell aplasia, and hypogammaglobulinemia. Most diagnoses (77%) occur before age 10 (see Chapter 69: Juvenile Systemic Connective Tissue Diseases). Diagnosis is made through *ADA2* gene sequencing or measurement of ADA2 enzyme activity. The treatment of choice is a tumor necrosis factor-alpha inhibitor.
- **VEXAS syndrome**: a disorder caused by an acquired somatic mutation in the *UBA1* gene. Patients may present with symptoms mimicking PAN, giant cell arteritis, or relapsing polychondritis, but may also have features of bone marrow involvement (macrocytic anemia, thrombocytopenia, and/or myelodysplasia). The diagnosis is made by identifying pathogenic mutations in the *UBA1* gene (see Chapter 32: Relapsing Polychondritis).

13. What causes PAN?

The cause of primary PAN is unknown. Some patients develop PAN in the setting of hepatitis B or C infection, exposure to certain medications, and hairy cell leukemia. In PAN, immune-mediated inflammation of affected blood vessels induces intimal proliferation, producing blood vessel narrowing, thrombosis, aneurysm formation, and downstream tissue ischemia.

A subset of patients felt to have PAN may have an autoinflammatory genetic disorder, such as the adult-onset VEXAS syndrome or the monogenic DADA2 syndrome (see Question 12).

14. How is PAN treated?

- The treatment for PAN depends on disease severity. Use of disease-modifying nonsteroidal agents such as methotrexate or cyclophosphamide can reduce cumulative glucocorticoid exposure and toxicity.
- Patients with **nonsevere disease** (e.g., mild systemic, joint, and/or skin symptoms, with no life- or organ-threatening manifestations), can be treated with **oral prednisone** (starting at 1 mg/kg daily, tapering over 6–12 months depending on disease status) combined with oral **methotrexate** (MTX) or **azathioprine** (AZA). Switching to cyclophosphamide (CYC) can be considered if this strategy is not effective.
- Patients with **severe disease** (e.g., mononeuritis multiplex, digital or limb ischemia, mesenteric ischemia, coronary vasculitis, or other life- or organ-threatening manifestations) can be treated with **pulse intravenous glucocorticoids**, followed by tapering doses of oral prednisone, combined with intravenous or oral **CYC**. After 3–6 months of CYC treatment, patients are transitioned to a less toxic medication such as MTX or AZA for remission maintenance.
- While not considered standard therapy for idiopathic PAN, plasmapheresis may be considered for PAN-associated with hepatitis B or C viral infection.
- Blood pressure monitoring and control is important for patients who develop renovascular hypertension from renal arteriolar involvement.

15. How does the treatment for HBV-associated PAN differ from that for idiopathic PAN?

HBV vaccination programs have reduced the incidence of HBV-associated PAN, which now accounts for less than 10% of cases. The use and timing of immunosuppression depends on the clinical severity of the vasculitis. In those with nonsevere PAN, treatment with antiviral therapy (e.g. lamivudine or entecavir) and close observation is favored. Systemic immunosuppression, similar to the regimens used for idiopathic PAN, may be considered for patients with moderate to severe PAN (e.g., mononeuritis multiplex, digital or limb ischemia, mesenteric ischemia, coronary vasculitis, or other life- or organ-threatening manifestations), or those who are intolerant of, or not responsive to, antiviral therapy. Close collaboration between the clinicians managing the immunosuppression and the viral hepatitis is needed, since immunosuppression may worsen the viral hepatitis. Plasma exchange may be considered for patients who have severe and progressive life- or organ-threatening disease or contraindications to standard treatments. Serial lab monitoring of cell counts, chemistries and liver function, HBV viral load, and HBe antigen seroconversion is advised during treatment. Typically, the PAN manifestations improve as virologic suppression is achieved.

16. What is the prognosis of PAN?

In contrast to the other vasculitis syndromes, PAN is more often **monophasic** rather than relapsing and remitting. **Relapses occur in ~30% of patients** with idiopathic PAN.

The prognosis in PAN depends on the distribution and severity of organ involvement. Major causes of death include renal failure, myocardial infarction, stroke, and intra-abdominal bleeding or intestinal perforation. Without treatment, the 5-year survival rate is 13%, which increases to 80% with appropriate treatment and monitoring.

Sources of morbidity and disability in PAN include pain or weakness from peripheral nerve infarction, symptoms resulting from visceral organ ischemia and infarction, and complications of long-term steroid therapy, including cataracts, glaucoma, opportunistic infections, osteoporosis and associated fragility fractures, and cardiovascular events.

17. Can PAN affect only one organ?

By definition, no – PAN is a systemic disease and thus cannot affect only a single organ. The 2012 Chapel Hill Consensus Conference Nomenclature of Vasculitides defined single-organ vasculitis as a discrete vasculitis category, where the name of each syndrome incorporates the singularly involved organ or vessel (e.g. cutaneous vasculitis, ciliary arteritis, testicular arteritis). A subset of patients with single-organ vasculitis may later develop vasculitis in other organs, and a new unifying diagnosis might become apparent.

Patients with single-organ vasculitis generally require a lower intensity of immunosuppression than those with systemic vasculitis. For example, effective treatment for patients with cutaneous small vessel vasculitis may consist of prednisone monotherapy tapering to low doses, or may involve colchicine, dapsone, or NSAIDs alone. Compared to those with systemic vasculitis, patients with single-organ vasculitis generally have a more favorable prognosis. In some cases, surgical resection of the affected tissue is curative.

Cutaneous medium vessel vasculitis, often historically referred to as cutaneous PAN, is another single-organ vasculitis syndrome. Patients often present with multiple, tender, nodular skin lesions (0.5–2 cm diameter) usually located on the legs and feet, but can occur on the arms and trunk as well. Diagnosis is confirmed by deep biopsy of a skin lesion, confirming the medium vessel vasculitis. Livedo is found in 60% of patients, and mild polyneuropathy can be seen in 30%. Internal organ involvement is absent, and symptoms of nerve and muscle irritability typically correlate with areas of cutaneous involvement (and hence are thought to be a secondary phenomenon). Treatment often consists of prednisone 20–40mg daily, with subsequent taper. Relapses can be common, and methotrexate, azathioprine, colchicine, and dapsone have all been described as steroid-sparing therapy.

THROMBOANGIITIS OBLITERANS (A PERIPHERAL VASCULOPATHY)

18. What is thromboangiitis obliterans (TO), and is it a true vasculitis syndrome?

TO, or Buerger disease, is an obliterative, non-atherosclerotic vascular disease of the extremities, which is strongly associated with tobacco use (and less commonly, cannabis use). It produces thrombotic occlusion of the small- and medium-sized arteries and veins. In the acute phase, an inflammatory thrombus forms in the lumen of the affected vessel which induces inflammatory changes in the vessel wall. These changes are mild compared to those seen in the vasculitis syndromes, and the internal elastic lamina is preserved. The inflammatory cellular infiltrate is concentrated in the thrombus itself rather than in the vessel wall. Therefore, TO is considered a *medium-vessel thrombotic and inflammatory vasculopathy* and not a canonical vasculitis syndrome. As the vascular lumen is compromised progressively by the thrombo-inflammatory process, downstream digital ischemia, ulceration, and gangrene occur. TO vascular disease is nearly always confined to the extremities. Visceral vascular structures are usually spared.

19. What is the etiology of TO?

Ongoing, moderate-to-heavy tobacco or cannabis use is identified in virtually every patient with TO, indicating that it is a *sine qua non* in the development of the condition. While an immunologic response to tobacco components has been hypothesized, the exact immunologic and thrombotic mechanisms underlying the pathogenesis of TO are unknown.

20. Who is affected by TO?

TO occurs worldwide, and its prevalence correlates with the regional prevalence of tobacco use. Seventy to ninety percent of affected patients are male. The mean age of onset is 40 years, though it can develop at any age. A history of active tobacco or cannabis use is believed to be required for the development and advancement of TO vascular disease.

21. What are the presenting symptoms of TO which prompt patients to seek medical attention?

The major clinical manifestations arise from thrombotic occlusion of the extremity vasculature, leading to downstream ischemia. Initially, patients may report mild pain in the calves, hands, feet, and/or digits. Migratory superficial thrombophlebitis is also an early clinical sign in TO. Patients may report cold sensitivity or arthralgias. Secondary Raynaud syndrome may develop. As thrombotic vaso-occlusion progresses, the peripheral pain symptoms intensify, claudication may occur, and digital ischemia and gangrene develop. Examination reveals cool or cyanotic hands and feet, reduced or absent peripheral pulses, sluggish capillary refill, nailbed splinter hemorrhages, and/or digital necrosis or gangrene. Rarely, TO has been reported to involve the central nervous system and gastrointestinal vasculature.

22. How is TO diagnosed?

TO is a clinical diagnosis that should be considered in any patient with active tobacco or cannabis use who develops signs or symptoms of extremity ischemia. The medium-sized vessels affected by TO are difficult to access with biopsy owing to their location deep in the dermis. As such, the diagnosis is often secured using catheter-directed angiography or pathologic review of amputation specimens. Vascular angiography reveals a characteristic pattern of vascular involvement ("corkscrew collaterals"). Disease mimickers must be excluded (see Question 25) prior to making the diagnosis. Results of laboratory testing or other imaging modalities in TO (CBC, BMP, ESR, CRP, ANA, RF, UA, C3, C4, ANCA, APLS antibodies, HBV and HCV serologies, blood cultures, TTE) are usually normal, and are generally more helpful to exclude other diagnoses. Catheter-directed arteriography is the preferred imaging technique, since CTA and MRA of the extremities have insufficient resolution to visualize the typical vascular changes of TO.

23. Describe the arteriographic findings in TO.

No single arteriographic finding is diagnostic of TO. The results must be interpreted in the context of the patient's clinical presentation. Arteriograms in patients with TO may reveal:
- thrombotic involvement of the small- and medium-sized arteries of the extremities (Fig. 27.3)
- corkscrew-shaped collaterals
- segmental disease, with alternating regions of affected and unaffected artery
- no source of thromboembolism
- no or minimal atherosclerosis.

24. Is a biopsy needed to make the diagnosis?

Biopsies are not commonly performed or required to diagnose TO, since the affected medium-sized vessels are deep in the dermis and difficult to access. When amputation specimens are reviewed, the histology reveals vascular damage with an inflammatory intramural thrombus composed of a mixed inflammatory infiltrate (giant cells, neutrophils, and lymphocytes), with relative sparing of the vessel wall and the internal elastic lamina.

25. What conditions should be included in the differential diagnosis of TO?
- Connective tissue diseases (SLE, systemic sclerosis, mixed connective tissue disease)
- Systemic vasculitis (PAN, giant cell arteritis, Takayasu arteritis, ANCA-associated vasculitis, cryoglobulinemic vasculitis, RA-associated vasculitis)
- Antiphospholipid antibody syndrome
- Hematologic disorders (hyperviscosity syndrome, polycythemia vera, essential thrombocytosis, paraproteinemia) or heritable/acquired thrombophilias
- Repetitive trauma (e.g., vibratory tools, hypothenar hammer syndrome)

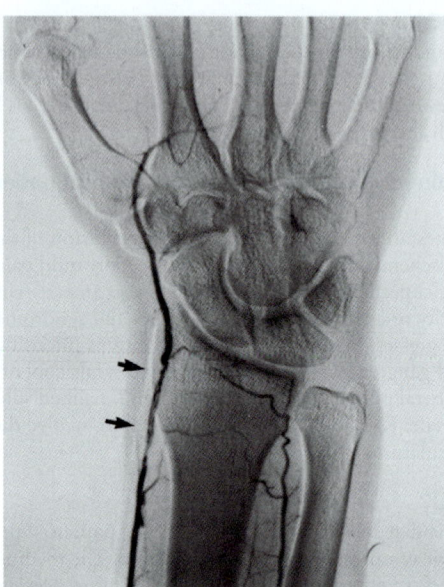

Fig. 27.3 Angiogram of hand in thromboangiitis obliterans. Note the irregularity of the radial artery (arrows) and the cut-off of the palmar arch vessels with no digital vessels.

- Embolic disease (left atrial myxoma, cholesterol emboli, atrial fibrillation, endocarditis, aneurysm, atherosclerotic plaque rupture, paradoxical embolus)
- Premature atherosclerosis
- Other: pernio, frostbite, ergotism, cocaine or methamphetamine toxicity, thoracic outlet syndrome

26. How do you treat TO?

The cornerstone of treatment for patients with TO is **total cessation of tobacco and/or cannabis use**, including the use of nicotine patches and gum. Abstinence can reduce the magnitude of ischemic limb symptoms, slow or stop the progression of vascular disease, and reduce the risk of future digital or limb amputation. Existing vascular damage and symptoms related to downstream ischemia may lessen over time, owing to the formation of collateral vessels around vascular stenoses.

Even with tobacco cessation, ischemic symptoms such as claudication, rest pain, painful ulcerations, or Raynaud phenomenon may persist. Palliative treatments for these symptoms include:

a. Regular and long-term use of intermittent pneumatic compression
b. Wound care for limb ischemic ulcerations
c. Vasodilator therapies (dihydropyridine calcium channel blockers, phosphodiesterase type 3 [e.g. cilostazol] or type 5 inhibitors [e.g. sildenafil]; intravenous prostaglandins for those with acute limb ischemia)
d. Nonsteroidal anti-inflammatory drugs for superficial thrombophlebitis

27. Are surgical or other revascularization procedures an option in the treatment of TO?

Revascularization with angioplasty or stenting is generally not possible, because the vascular lesions occur in distal limb vessels which are difficult to access endovascularly. In those with more proximal vascular disease, the feasibility of such interventions can be discussed with a vascular proceduralist. Arterial bypass surgery using an autologous vein or omental graft for limb salvage is reserved for patients with severe limb ischemia *who have intact distal target vessels.*

PRIMARY CENTRAL NERVOUS SYSTEM VASCULITIS (A SINGLE-ORGAN VASCULITIS)

28. What is primary central nervous system vasculitis (PCNSV), and who gets it?

PCNSV is a rare form of single-organ vasculitis that only affects the central nervous system (CNS) structures and spinal cord. In PCNSV, immune cells infiltrate the walls of vessels in the CNS, causing transmural inflammation. The resulting vascular thickening causes vessel narrowing and occlusion, leading to parenchymal necrosis and infarction.

The epidemiology of PCNSV is not well established. The annual incidence in a North American cohort was 2.4 cases per million. While the median age of onset is between 40 and 60 years, PCNSV also affects children. Men and women are affected equally.

29. What are the typical presenting manifestations of PCNSV?

PCNSV often has an insidious and slowly progressive presentation lasting weeks to months. Initial manifestations can be nonspecific, followed by the development of focal neurologic deficits (Table 27.3). The most common presenting features include headache and strokes. Constitutional symptoms such as fevers and weight loss are less common and may suggest an alternate diagnosis. PCNSV can present rarely (5%) with a mass-like CNS lesion with symptoms related to mass effect or potentially myelopathy and/or radiculopathy secondary to a spinal cord lesion.

30. What diagnostic evaluation should be completed if PCNSV is suspected?

The goals of the diagnostic evaluation are to (1) demonstrate that a neuro-inflammatory process is present, (2) demonstrate a vasculitic or vasculopathic process is present radiologically and/or histopathologically, and (3) rule out mimics of PCNSV (see Question 32). The diagnostic evaluation encompasses laboratory studies, imaging, and tissue biopsy.

Laboratory studies:

- **Cerebral spinal fluid (CSF) assessment** for white blood cell (WBC) count, protein, oligoclonal bands, and immunoglobulin G index, as well as testing for malignancy and infection, are the most important laboratory tests to obtain. Abnormalities in WBC count (usually a mild lymphocytic pleocytosis) and/or protein are seen in ~80–90% of patients with PCNSV. Oligoclonal bands and/or high IgG index observed in ~25%. **A normal CSF analysis suggests an alternate diagnosis.** Studies to assess for infection, autoimmune/paraneoplastic processes, and malignancy should also be obtained to evaluate for PCNSV mimics.
- CRP and ESR are typically normal, and if elevated, suggest an alternate systemic inflammatory process.

Imaging (parenchymal and vascular imaging):

- MRI of the brain is the most important parenchymal imaging test to obtain. **Over 90% of patients have abnormalities on the MRI brain.** Changes on MRI include infarcts in different vascular distributions (often of differing ages), meningeal enhancement, and hyperintense

TABLE 27.3 Clinical Manifestations in PCNSV

NONFOCAL SYMPTOMS		FOCAL SYMPTOMS	
Symptom	Frequency	Symptom	Frequency
Headaches	50–60%	Focal neurologic deficits	60%
Personality change	—	Hemiparesis	40%
Altered cognition	40–50%	Ataxia	20%
Decreased level of consciousness	30%	Aphasia	20%
Mood disorders	21%	Dysarthria	20%
		Visual disturbances	20–40%
		Strokes	40%
		Seizures	20–30%

foci on T2 FLAIR sequences. Ischemic lesions may be accompanied by subarachnoid and intraparenchymal hemorrhages. Tumor-like lesions have been reported, but are rare.

- CT angiography (CTA), MR angiography (MRA), and digital subtraction angiography (conventional catheter-based angiography, DSA) can be used to assess the vasculature.
  - CTA has higher resolution compared to MRA to assess luminal narrowing or vessel occlusion.
  - DSA has the highest resolution and is the most sensitive modality for small-medium vessels, but is invasive. Areas of narrowing and dilation ("vessel beading"), multi-locular occlusions of intracranial vessels, and/or fusiform arterial dilations can be observed. **Vessel beading is not specific for PCNSV** and can be seen in noninflammatory vasculopathies such as atherosclerosis, atrial myxomas, neurofibromatosis, infections, vasospasm, and after radiation exposure. Long segments of stenoses, microaneurysms, or complete occlusions are not common in PCNSV. DSA provides information regarding the vessel lumen but does not provide information regarding the vessel wall.
  - Importantly, a normal angiographic study does not rule out PCNSV, since the vessels involved may to too small to visualize by angiography.

Additional imaging such as echocardiography may be obtained to rule out mimics of PCNSV.

Tissue biopsy:
- A brain biopsy is often required to the confirm diagnosis of PCNSV.
- Sensitivity is ~50–75%, but the diagnostic yield can be increased by targeting an area that is abnormal on imaging studies or that is associated with the patient's deficits.
- The nondominant temporal or nondominant frontal lobe and leptomeninges can be targeted if there is no obvious area to biopsy.
- On histopathology, parenchymal or leptomeningeal vasculitis with a transmural mononuclear infiltrate and non-necrotizing granulomas is seen in 60% of patients, while a lymphocytic vasculitis or necrotizing vasculitis is seen in ~20%. A small percentage of patients will have amyloid-beta fibrils with granulomatous vasculitis, indicating amyloid-beta-related angiitis.
- The lower sensitivity of the biopsy should not preclude obtaining this critical test—brain biopsy helps rule out mimics and indicates an alternate diagnosis in > 30% of patients.

31. What is reversible cerebral vasoconstriction syndrome (RCVS), and how does it differ from PCNSV?

RCVS is the most important noninflammatory condition that mimics PCNSV, and is characterized by prolonged but reversible vasoconstriction of the cerebral vessels. It occurs in 3 per million adults and 0.2 per million hospitalized patients in the US. Triggers or risk factors for RCVS are varied and include the use of vasoactive drugs or other medications, physical exertion, Valsalva maneuvers, migraine, hypertension, orgasm, and eclampsia or being in the postpartum period. The most classic manifestation is **"thunderclap headaches"**—severe and recurrent headaches, which occur in ~90% of patients. While RCVS is generally considered a benign condition, strokes causing disability or rarely death can occur.

Laboratory studies including CSF analysis are generally unremarkable. Up to 70% of patients have normal brain imaging (CT or MRI) on initial evaluation, but up to 75% of patients can develop parenchymal lesions over time, including watershed infarcts, subarachnoid hemorrhages, and lobar intracerebral hemorrhages. Multifocal segmental cerebral artery vasoconstriction is seen on angiography, which usually resolves or substantially improves over days to weeks for more than 90% of patients. Documentation of reversal of the vasoconstriction obtained ~12 weeks after clinical onset confirms the diagnosis.

Management focuses on supportive measures, such as analgesia for headaches and avoidance of triggers. Calcium channel blockers can improve vasospasm, but their clinical impact is unclear. Use of glucocorticoids can significantly worsen outcomes. Intra-arterial vasodilator infusions can be considered in refractory cases.

PEARL: RCVS can be distinguished from PACNS by acute onset of a thunderclap headache, normal CSF exam, and reversibility of angiographic abnormalities within 1 to 3 months.

32. Outline the various conditions that can mimic PCNSV (Table 27.4)

TABLE 27.4 Disease Mimickers[a] of PCNSV & Distinguishing Characteristics

DISEASE CATEGORY	MIMICKERS & DISTINGUISHING FEATURES
Immune-Mediated CNS disease	Primary systemic vasculitis including AAV, PAN, Behcet disease, GCA, and Takayasu arteritis. *These are usually suggested by manifestations outside of the CNS.*
	ANA-related diseases including SLE, SjD, and MCTD
	Anti-phospholipid syndrome
	Autoimmune encephalopathies
	Neurosarcoidosis
	Susac syndrome: autoimmune mediated endotheliopathy with the clinical triad of BRAO, encephalopathy, and sensorineural hearing loss. Hyperintense lesions of the corpus collosum can be seen on MRI. See Chapter 74.
Cancer-Associated CNS disease	Lymphoma, leukemia, atrial myxoma, lymphomatoid granulomatosis, and other angio-centric immunoproliferative lesions. Of particular note is *intravascular lymphoma*, a subtype of extranodal diffuse large B-cell lymphoma, which is characterized by intravascular proliferation of lymphoma cells with predilection for the CNS and skin.
Infectious	Viral: VZV, HSV, HIV and West Nile virus. VZV vasculopathy can cause ischemic infarction of brain and spinal cord, cerebral aneurysm and hemorrhage, and carotid dissection.
	Bacterial: Lyme disease (B. burgdorferi), syphilis (T. pallidum), M. tuberculosis, T. whippelii, Bartonella spp., M. pneumoniae, Rickettsial diseases, S. pneumoniae, N. meningitidis
	Fungal: Aspergillus spp., Candida spp., coccidioidomycosis, Cryptococcus spp.
	Parasitic: P. falciparum and T. gondii
Genetic	CADASIL: autosomal dominant arteriopathy characterized by migraines with aura, ischemic strokes and transient ischemic attacks, and cognitive decline and dementia. Brain MRI findings include diffuse white matter hyperintensities and lacunar infarcts. Diagnosis is established by identifying a pathogenic variant in NOTCH3 in affected individuals.
	SAVI: autoinflammatory disease with vasculopathy, interstitial lung disease, & ulcerative skin lesions. Caused by dominant mutations in TMEM173
	Sneddon syndrome: mutations in CECR1 leading to ischemic strokes in young adults
	DADA2 syndrome: see Question 12.
Vascular	Subarachnoid hemorrhage causing transient cerebral vasospasm, fibromuscular dysplasia, and moya moya.

[a]The most common mimic is premature atherosclerosis and other noninflammatory cerebral vasculopathies. The list of conditions in each category is not exhaustive.

AAV, ANCA associated vasculitis; *BRAO,* branch retinal artery occlusion; *CADASIL*: cerebral autosomal-dominant arteriopathy with subcortical infarcts and leukoencephalopathy; *DADA2,* deficiency in adenosine deaminase 2; *GCA,* giant cell arteritis; *HIV,* human immunodeficiency virus; *HSV,* herpes simplex virus; *MCTD,* mixed connective tissue disease; *SAVI,* STING-associated vasculopathy with onset in infancy; *SjD,* Sjogren's disease; *VZV,* varicella zoster virus;

33. How is PCNSV treated? What is the prognosis?

No randomized controlled trials have been conducted to assess treatments for PCNSV. Treatment strategies are based on protocols for other types of organ-threatening vasculitis. The most common treatment strategy is to use glucocorticoids with another immunosuppressive agent.

Patients with severe disease frequently receive **intravenous pulse glucocorticoids** followed by high-dose oral glucocorticoids, which are tapered off over a period of months. **Cyclophosphamide** is also given orally at 2 mg/kg/day for 3–6 months, or IV 750 mg/m^2/month for up to 6 months. After completing a course of cyclophosphamide, patients are typically switched to a less toxic immunosuppressive medication such as azathioprine, methotrexate, or mycophenolate mofetil. Rituximab has been used in refractory cases but is not considered first-line therapy.

Patients with nonsevere disease are started on high-dose oral glucocorticoids (e.g., prednisone 1 mg/kg/day), which are tapered off over several months. Azathioprine, methotrexate, and mycophenolate mofetil tend to be used instead of cyclophosphamide for this group of patients.

The optimal duration of therapy has not been established. The length of treatment ranges from 12–18 months to lifelong immunosuppression, depending on clinical response.

Previous studies have shown that relapses occur in up to ~30% of patients despite adequate treatment, over a median follow-up of 19 months. Mortality ranges from 11% to 28%, and 70% of patients experience some degree of lasting functional impairment.

BIBLIOGRAPHY

Beuker C, Schmidt A, Strunk D, et al. Primary angiitis of the central nervous system: diagnosis and treatment. *Ther Adv Neurol Disord.* 2018;11.

Beuker C, Strunk D, Rawal R, et al. Primary Angiitis of the CNS: A systematic review and meta-analysis. *Neurol Neuroimmunol Neuroinflamm.* 2021;8(6):1–10.

Buerger L. Landmark publication from the American Journal of the Medical Sciences, 'Thrombo-angiitis obliterans: a study of the vascular lesions leading to presenile spontaneous gangrene'. 1908. *Am J Med Sci.* 2009;337:274.

Cacione DG, Macedo CR, do Carmo Novaes F, et al. Pharmacological treatment for Buerger's disease. *Cochrane Database Syst Rev.* 2020;5:CD011033.

Chung SA, Gorelik M, Langford CA, et al. 2021 American College of Rheumatology/Vasculitis Foundation guideline for the management of polyarteritis nodosa. *Arthritis Care Res (Hoboken).* 2021;73:1061.

Cottencin O, Karila L, Lambert M, et al. Cannabis arteritis: review of the literature. *J Addict Med.* 2010;4:191.

De Virgilio A, Greco A, Magliulo G, et al. Polyarteritis nodosa: a contemporary overview. *Autoimmun Rev.* 2016;15(6):564–570.

Fazeli B, Dadgar MM, Niroumand S. How to treat a patient with thromboangiitis obliterans: a systemic review. *Ann Vascular Surg.* 2018;49:219–228.

Forbess L, Bannykh S. Polyarteritis nodosa. *Rheum Dis Clin N Am.* 2015;41:33–46.

Grayson PC, Patel BA, Young NS. VEXAS syndrome. *Blood.* 2021;137(26):3591–3594.

Guillevin L, Mahr A, Callard P, et al. Hepatitis B virus-associated polyarteritis nodosa: clinical characteristics, outcome, and impact of treatment in 115 patients. *Medicine (Baltimore).* 2005;84:313.

Guillevin L, Mahr A, Cohen P, et al. Short-term corticosteroids then lamivudine and plasma exchanges to treat hepatitis B virus-related polyarteritis nodosa. *Arthritis Rheum.* 2004;51:482.

Gundogmus CA, Samadli V, Sorkun M, et al. The effect of smoking cessation on the technical success of endovascular treatment for thromboangiitis obliterans. *J Vasc Interv Radiol.* 2023;34:1038.

Hashem H, Kelly SJ, Ganson NJ, et al. Deficiency of Adenosine Deaminase 2 (DADA2), an inherited cause of polyarteritis nodosa and a mimic of other systemic rheumatologic disorders. *Curr Rheumatol Rep.* 2017;19(11):70.

Jennette JC, Falk RJ, Bacon PA, et al. 2012 revised International Chapel Hill consensus conference nomenclature of vasculitides. *Arthritis Rheum.* 2013;65(1).

Joviliano EE, Dellalibera-Joviliano R, Dalio M, et al. Etiopathogenesis, clinical diagnosis and treatment of thromboangiitis obliterans – current practices. *Int J Angiol.* 2009;18:119.

Junek M, Perera KS, Kiczek M, et al. Current and future advances in practice: a practical approach to the diagnosis and management of primary central nervous system vasculitis. *Rheumatol Adv Pract.* 2023;7(3):1–11.

Pagnoux C, Seror R, Henegar C, et al. Clinical features and outcomes in 348 patients with polyarteritis nodosa: a systematic retrospective study of patients diagnosed between 1963 and 2005 and entered into the French Vasculitis Study Group Database. *Arthritis Rheum.* 2010;62:616.

Schmidt WA. Use of imaging studies in the diagnosis of vasculitis. *Curr Rheumatol Rep.* 2004;6:203.

Singhal AB. Reversible cerebral vasoconstriction syndrome: a review of pathogenesis, clinical presentation, and treatment. *Int J Stroke.* 2023;18(10):1151–1160.

FURTHER READING

www.vasculitisfoundation.org.
www.nlm.nih.gov/medlineplus/vasculitis.html.

CHAPTER 28

Antineutrophil Cytoplasmic Antibody-Associated Vasculitis

Zachary S. Wallace, MD, MSc

 KEY POINTS

1. Granulomatosis with polyangiitis (GPA) predominantly affects the upper and lower respiratory tracts and kidneys and is typically associated with proteinase 3 antineutrophil cytoplasmic antibody (PR3-ANCA).
2. Microscopic polyangiitis (MPA) should be considered in all patients presenting with a pulmonary-renal syndrome and is typically associated with myeloperoxidase (MPO)-ANCA.
3. Eosinophilic granulomatosis with polyangiitis (EGPA) often presents as pulmonary infiltrates and eosinophilia in a patient with adult-onset asthma. The diagnosis is unlikely in the absence of new, severe, and/or worsening asthma and marked eosinophilia.
4. Rituximab is an effective first-line agent for induction and maintenance therapy in patients with GPA and MPA.
5. Avacopan, a complement (C5a) receptor antagonist, is a first-in-class drug that is FDA approved for use in combination with rituximab or cyclophosphamide for remission induction in patients with GPA or MPA, and can spare patients substantial glucocorticoid exposure and toxicity.
6. Mepolizumab and benralizumab, both anti-interleukin (IL)-5 therapies, are FDA approved for the treatment of EGPA, with data strongest for the treatment of eosinophilic manifestations.

1. What are the primary ANCA-associated vasculitides (AAV), and why are they classified in the current manner?

Following the discovery of ANCA in 1985, the International Chapel Hill Consensus Conference reclassified vasculitic syndromes to conform to a better understanding of their pathophysiology. Over time, this classification has been further refined as follows:

- GPA (formerly known as Wegener's granulomatosis).
- MPA.
- EGPA (formerly known as Churg–Strauss syndrome).
- Renal-limited vasculitis (RLV) with pauci-immune necrotizing/crescentic glomerulonephritis (GN), most often consistent with MPA.

Though not meant for diagnosis, the American College of Rheumatology (ACR) and European Alliance of Associations for Rheumatology (EULAR) Classification Criteria for GPA, MPA, and EGPA can provide a helpful framework for approaching the diagnosis of these conditions.

2. How are the tests to identify ANCAs performed, and how should they be interpreted?

- ANCAs are antibodies directed against specific proteins in granules of the cytoplasm of neutrophils and lysosomal proteins in monocytes. These antibodies are often detected in patients with ANCA-associated vasculitis, but can also be observed in patients with other conditions.
- ANCAs can be detected using alcohol-fixed neutrophils on a glass slide using the classic indirect immunofluorescence assay (IFA). Test serum is incubated on a slide, during which time the ANCAs bind. After washing, an antihuman IgG antibody labeled with fluorescein is incubated on the slide. After a second washing, the slide is examined using a fluorescence microscope. The highest (most dilute) titer at which fluorescence is detected, and the pattern, is noted. Two patterns are generally important in primary AAV (Fig. 28.1).
  - **Cytoplasmic (c)-ANCA pattern** is characterized by diffuse staining of the neutrophil cytoplasm. The protein recognized by c-ANCA is nearly always PR3, a serine proteinase present in primary azurophilic granules of neutrophils.
  - **Perinuclear (p)-ANCA pattern** results in perinuclear cytoplasmic staining. The protein recognized by p-ANCA is often MPO, and less commonly is elastase or other proteins (lactoferrin, cathepsin G, bactericidal/permeability-increasing protein [BPI], catalase, lysozyme, and others) within primary azurophilic or specific granules of neutrophils. Patients

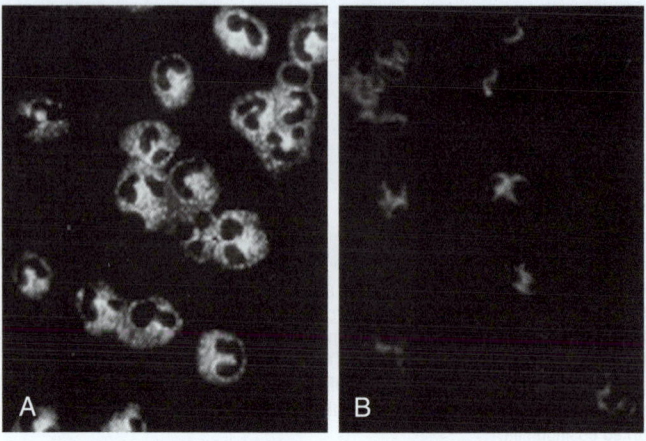

Fig. 28.1 (A) c-ANCA and (B) p-ANCA immunofluorescence patterns using alcohol-fixed neutrophils as an antigen source.

with p-ANCA with MPO specificity are those most likely to have AAV. The significance of other protein targets is uncertain, and not typically associated with AAV.
- Immunofluorescence can lack specificity and is subject to interpreter variability. As such, enzyme-linked immunosorbent assays (ELISAs) for antibodies directed against the PR3 and MPO proteins should be obtained in all patients with suspected AAV.
- Data suggest that the sensitivity of ELISA testing for PR3 and MPO antibodies (for the diagnosis of AAV) may exceed that of ANCA testing via IFA with some ELISA testing platforms. As such, ANCA testing by IFA should not be viewed as a screening test for AAV. **Owing to improved sensitivity and specificity, testing for ANCAs by IFA in addition to ELISA for PR3 and MPO should be requested when evaluating a patient for suspected AAV.**
- In patients with AAV, the presence of anti-PR3 or anti-MPO antibodies carries greater prognostic significance (disease relapse as well as clinical outcomes including response to therapy) than the clinical designation of GPA or MPA.
- In GPA, most patients are PR3+, but up to 20% may be MPO+
- ANCA-negative GPA is relatively common in patients with more limited forms of the disease, especially when manifestations are isolated to the head and neck (e.g., sinonasal disease).
- ANCA can also be detected in conditions other than AAV (including other rheumatic conditions like systemic lupus erythematosus, ulcerative colitis, infections, and following exposure to medications such as hydralazine, anti-thyroid medications, etc.; see Questions 40 and 41).

PEARL: Very high-titer MPO, dual positivity (PR3 & MPO), or discordant IFA and ELISA results (e.g. c-ANCA with MPO) should prompt one to consider a drug-induced process (e.g., hydralazine, cocaine adulterated with levamisole)

3. How do ANCAs contribute to the development of AAV? (Controversial)
It is not known how ANCAs contribute to the development of AAV, but several hypotheses have been proposed. Under certain conditions such as infections and other environmental triggers, release of cytokines (IL-1, tumor necrosis factor [TNF] α) can induce neutrophils and monocytes to transport PR3 or MPO to their cell surface. Patients with ANCA targeting PR3 or MPO can interact with the PR3 or MPO, respectively, expressed on the cell surface leading to neutrophil and monocyte activation. Cytokines (IL-1, TNFα) also upregulate adhesion molecules on endothelial cells, which the activated neutrophils can bind to and transmigrate into the vessel wall causing fibrinoid necrosis, thrombosis, and ischemia to affected areas. The circulating activated neutrophils and monocytes can degranulate and release reactive oxygen species and lysosomal enzymes, leading

to endothelial injury. Other products (e.g., PR3, MPO) released from these degranulating cells may bind to the endothelial cells and serve as target antigens for circulating ANCAs, further contributing to the cascade of events culminating in tissue injury from necrotizing vasculitis.

GRANULOMATOSIS WITH POLYANGIITIS

4. Define GPA.

GPA is a primary vasculitis characterized by:
- **Upper and lower respiratory tract** involvement with granulomatous inflammation and necrotizing vasculitis of mostly small vessels (varying levels of granulomatous inflammation, necrosis, and vasculitis may be encountered at a particular site).
- **Glomerulonephritis (GN)** that is pauci-immune, focal and segmental, necrotizing, and often crescentic.
- Strong association with **c-ANCA and anti-PR3 antibodies**.

Limited GPA tends to present as a granulomatous disorder without vasculitic features, most often involving the head and neck (e.g., sino-nasal disease). Approximately 10% of cases evolve to a more generalized form of GPA. Despite the term "limited," patients with disease limited to the head and neck may still experience substantial organ damage (e.g., saddle nose deformity, subglottic stenosis) that affects quality of life and survival.

Although GPA is considered a primary vasculitis syndrome, the inflammatory changes, including granulomatous inflammation, often occur in parenchymal sites outside vessel walls (extravascular granulomatous infiltration).

5. What is the epidemiology of GPA?

Estimates of the incidence and prevalence of GPA vary across studies depending on their design and the geographic location being studied. Regardless of this variability, it is a rare disorder and less common than other rheumatologic disorders, such as rheumatoid arthritis, systemic lupus erythematosus (SLE), polymyalgia rheumatica, and giant cell arteritis. Diagnosis usually occurs in people between 40 and 60 years of age though children, younger adults, and older adults can be affected. Males and females are equally affected. GPA is typically reported more often in White populations but can be diagnosed in patients of diverse racial and ethnic backgrounds. Limitations in the availability of ANCA testing and biopsies of affected sites may limit diagnosis in developing parts of the world, thus hindering accurate estimates of incidence and prevalence in populations outside of North America, Europe, and East Asia.

6. How does one make a diagnosis of GPA?

GPA can present in many different ways, and some manifestations mimic those observed in infectious and neoplastic etiologies. A thorough history and examination should be performed to determine the extent of organ involvement (see Questions 7–11), identify recent new medications or illicit drug exposure, and highlight clinical features that may be atypical for AAV (hard palate ulceration, single organ involvement, rapid onset without prodromal features). Laboratory and imaging studies should be conducted to assess the extent and severity of organ involvement, to determine if ANCA are present, and to rule out other etiologies. Ideally, tissue can be obtained from the lung, sinuses, skin, or kidney to identify features supportive of a diagnosis of GPA (namely vasculitis, extravascular granulomatous inflammation, and necrosis). Biopsy of these sites may ultimately fail to identify features specific to GPA, but often can be helpful nonetheless to rule out alternative diagnoses, especially in cases of limited GPA where classic organ involvement may be absent and ANCA positivity may be as low as 60%. Biopsies of the sinonasal tract are typically nonspecific. In classic presentations of more systemic forms of GPA with multi-organ involvement of usual sites (e.g., sinonasal disease, lung nodules, glomerulonephritis), the sensitivity of ANCA testing is high (90%) and the presence of concurrent c-ANCA and PR-3 antibodies is highly specific (98%); in such settings, biopsy may not be necessary and should not delay treatment if alternative diagnoses are considered unlikely or have been exonerated.

7. How is the upper respiratory tract affected clinically by GPA?

- **Paranasal sinuses**—chronic sinusitis is a common presenting manifestation (50%) that ultimately affects 80% of patients.

- **Nasal mucosa**—chronic inflammation occurs in approximately 70% of patients, resulting in chronic purulent nasal discharge, epistaxis, mucosal ulcerations, and, less commonly, perforation of the nasal septum and disruption of the supporting cartilage of the nose (leading to a **saddle-nose deformity**).
- **Oral mucosa**—oral ulcers are common and may or may not be painful.
- **Pharyngeal mucosa**—chronic inflammation may lead to obstruction of the Eustachian tube, resulting in acute suppurative otitis media or chronic serous otitis media. Hard palate lesions are atypical for GPA and should prompt the clinician to consider cocaine-induced midline destructive lesions or infiltrative malignancy (e.g., natural killer cell/T-cell lymphoma of the sinuses).
- **Laryngeal and tracheal mucosa**—chronic inflammation may lead to hoarseness and subglottic stenosis, which may result in stridor and respiratory insufficiency in severe cases.

PEARL: New-onset otitis media in an adult should make one consider GPA.

8. How does lower respiratory tract involvement manifest clinically and radiographically in GPA? What is the pathology?

Clinical evidence of pulmonary disease is common in GPA. Despite having radiographically evident pulmonary disease, some patients do not have lower respiratory tract symptoms. Patients with relatively normal chest radiographs may have abnormal computed tomography scans showing lesions not visible on the chest x-ray. Thus, consideration of cross-sectional thoracic imaging can be an important step in the evaluation of a patient with a possible GPA. The clinical manifestations of pulmonary involvement are highly variable but can be explained by the underlying pathologic process.

Chronic inflammation from GPA in the lungs typically occurs in the extravascular interstitium of the alveolar septa, but also within vessel and airway walls, where granulomatous inflammation is typically observed and necrosis may be present. This may lead to the formation of nodules and/or fixed infiltrates on chest radiographs (Fig. 28.2). The nodules may cavitate centrally. If this process is extensive, subacute or chronic respiratory insufficiency may result.

Acute inflammation results in infiltration of neutrophils and other inflammatory cells in vessel walls, extravascular interstitium, and alveolar spaces. A clinically important manifestation of acute inflammation is capillaritis, characterized by acute neutrophilic infiltration and fibrinoid necrosis within alveolar capillaries and septa, which may result in life-threatening alveolar hemorrhage.

Fibrosis may result from healing of acute or chronic inflammation. If fibrosis is diffuse, the patient may experience chronic respiratory insufficiency. Fibrosis is an uncommon manifestation of lower respiratory tract involvement of GPA, but is increasingly recognized as a manifestation of MPA, where it can be associated with interstitial lung disease (ILD). As such, ANCA testing should be considered in the evaluation of patients presenting with ILD.

9. Besides direct involvement, how else may the upper and lower respiratory tracts be affected in GPA?

- Bacterial sinusitis, most often due to *S. aureus,* commonly occurs as a result of obstruction of the paranasal sinus ostia by the inflammatory process and/or chronically damaged nasal passages. Similarly, obstruction of bronchi by nodules or intrabronchial lesions may lead to post-obstructive bacterial pneumonia.
- Infections may also result as a complication of treatment-induced immunosuppression. Patients are particularly predisposed to pulmonary infections with opportunistic organisms, including *Pneumocystis jiroveci,* mycobacteria, and fungi, as well as the common suppurative bacteria, such as *Streptococcus pneumoniae.* In the context of B cell depletion with rituximab and other immunosuppressive therapies, patients with GPA are also at risk for severe COVID-19 infection.

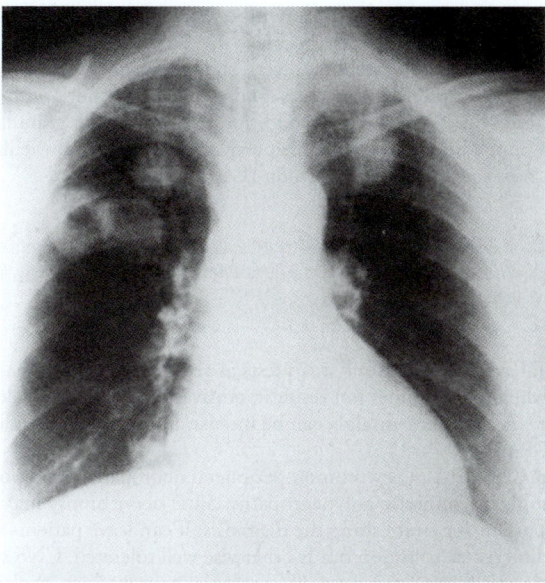

Fig. 28.2 Chest radiograph demonstrating nodules (some cavitating) in a patient with Wegener's granulomatosis. (Copyright 2014 American College of Rheumatology. Used with permission.)

- Medications may have direct toxic effects on the lungs. Cyclophosphamide, even in the relatively low doses used to treat GPA, may rarely lead to pulmonary edema or fibrosis. Methotrexate can be rarely associated with acute pneumotoxicity that typically resolves with discontinuation.

10. How does involvement of the kidney manifest clinically and pathologically in GPA?

Clinical evidence of renal disease is common in patients with GPA. It may be present at baseline or develop with a subsequent relapse. The pathologic renal lesion is a **pauci-immune, focal and segmental, necrotizing GN**. The presence of crescents is a marker of more severe disease with higher risk of progression to ESRD. Immunofluorescence studies reveal little or no deposition of immunoglobulin (Ig), immune complexes, or complement, thus the designation pauci-immune. Arteritis may be seen.

Most patients with GN have asymptomatic renal disease, manifesting as active urinary sediment (hematuria, proteinuria, and red blood cell casts) with varying degrees of kidney injury. Patients with more severe renal involvement often manifest as rapidly progressive glomerulonephritis which carries a high risk of end-stage kidney disease.

11. Besides the upper and lower respiratory tracts and kidney, what other organ systems may be affected?

All organ systems may be affected to variable degrees by GPA. Furthermore, constitutional symptoms such as anorexia, weight loss, fatigue, malaise, and fever are common.

- **Eye:** GPA may manifest as proptosis due to orbital inflammatory disease (OID). This process may result in loss of visual acuity as a result of impingement upon the optic nerve and loss of conjugate gaze due to infiltration of the extraocular muscles. The eye may also be affected by episcleritis/scleritis, peripheral ulcerative keratitis (with risk for corneal melt), uveitis, or conjunctivitis. Other manifestations include lacrimal duct obstruction, retinal vasculitis, retinal artery occlusion, and optic neuritis. Eye involvement may be the initial presentation of GPA before other manifestations occur.
- **Ear:** inner ear involvement can produce vertigo or hearing loss. Conductive hearing loss and mixed hearing loss (conductive and sensorineural) are observed. Otitis media can be

sufficiently severe to require tympanostomy tubes, which in an adult is a strong clue to the diagnosis of GPA. Mastoiditis can also occur.

- **Skin:** Lesions include palpable purpura, ulcers, subcutaneous nodules, vesicles, and livedo reticularis. Pathologic examination may reveal necrotizing vasculitis with or without granulomatous infiltration of the vessel walls, in addition to extravascular granulomatous infiltration and necrosis. A punch biopsy of a palpable purpuric lesion will show leukocytoclastic vasculitis (LCV) with non-specific Ig deposition on IFA.

> **PEARL:** IFA can be helpful in distinguishing IgA vasculitis (Henoch-Schonlein Purpura) from other forms of small vessel vasculitis such as GPA. While both conditions will have evidence of LCV on histology, IgA vasculitis will have disproportionate IgA deposition on IFA.

- **Musculoskeletal system:** commonly manifests as arthralgia and myalgia. Synovitis is less common and when present, does not result in erosive disease, articular destruction, or joint deformity. Nonetheless, the arthralgia can be intense and significantly affect quality of life in patients with GPA.
- **Peripheral and CNS:** The most common peripheral neuropathy is mononeuritis multiplex and less commonly a symmetric polyneuropathy. Sural nerve biopsy may show vasculitis and can be important for establishing the diagnosis; it can leave patients with some numbness in the sural nerve distribution but is otherwise well tolerated. CNS syndromes include pachymeningitis which can cause mass effect, cranial neuropathies, ocular palsies, cerebrovascular events, seizures, pituitary involvement, brain stem and spinal cord lesions, and brain hemorrhage (cerebral, subarachnoid, subdural). CNS manifestations are much less common than peripheral neuropathy.
- **Cardiac:** Cardiac manifestations of GPA are uncommon. Involvement of the myocardium, endocardium, and coronary vasculature is unusual but has been reported, and may result in significant morbidity and rarely, mortality.

Involvement of other organ systems, including the gastrointestinal (intestinal perforations), genitourinary tracts (bladder/urethral vasculitis, orchitis, epididymitis, prostatitis, other), salivary gland (mass), pancreas (mass), and granulomatous infiltration of liver occurs less frequently.

12. What is the natural history of GPA?

The presentation and natural history of GPA are highly variable. The spectrum of clinical presentation may range from relatively mild disease limited to the upper respiratory tract to fulminant life-threatening involvement of the upper and lower respiratory tract, kidneys, and other end-organs. Why patients can present with such variable manifestations is unknown.

The natural history of untreated GPA is rarely observed in contemporary practice because untreated, severe GPA is uniformly fatal. The standard of care is to initiate treatment quickly after the diagnosis is established, thereby reducing the risk of irreversible organ damage and death. Even in patients with limited or less severe disease, early diagnosis and initiation of treatment are important for preventing progression.

13. What is the clinical association between ANCA and GPA?

The following statements can be made about the clinical association between ANCA and GPA:

Sensitivity and specificity: ANCA positivity is seen in 90% of patients with active, non-limited GPA, whereas only 60% of patients with limited forms of GPA are ANCA-positive. Among GPA patients with positive ANCA, 80% to 90% are c-ANCA-positive with PR3 specificity, whereas 10% to 20% are p-ANCA-positive with MPO specificity.

ANCA titers and disease flares (controversial): conflicting data exist in the literature regarding the utility of ANCA titers (either increases in titer or transition from a negative to positive status) to predict subsequent flares of GPA. Some studies suggest that by limiting the target population (PR3-positive GPA patients with vasculitic manifestations), the utility of following serial ANCA measurements can be improved.

Two randomized-controlled trials compared strategies using ANCA titers and/or B cells to guide the decision of when to retreat a patient with rituximab to maintain remission. These trials, collectively, found that retreatment every 6 months was associated with numerically fewer relapses than a strategy guided by ANCA titers and/or B cell levels. Further, retreatment by ANCA titer was associated with more relapses than one guided by B cell levels. These findings support the notion that ANCA titers are imperfect markers of relapse risk. In addition, many patients with a rising ANCA titer will not go on to relapse in the near future, raising uncertainty on how to respond to these lab values. Notably, ANCA titers do not tend to rise during an acute infection, which may aid in distinguishing an exacerbation of GPA from an infectious process in patients with previously quiescent disease.

14. Besides PR3-ANCA, what other tests can be abnormal in GPA?

The systemic inflammatory nature of GPA often results in anemia of chronic inflammation, leukocytosis, thrombocytosis, and elevation of the erythrocyte sedimentation rate (ESR) and C-reactive protein (CRP). Low serum albumin and elevated globulin levels may also be present. **Importantly, leukopenia and thrombocytopenia are unusual**, often helping distinguish GPA from other autoimmune or neoplastic disorders.

Evidence of GN is suggested by the presence of hematuria, pyuria, cellular casts, and proteinuria. If renal function is compromised by the inflammatory process, elevated serum creatinine is expected. Other laboratory tests may be helpful in the investigation of specific end-organ damage, such as computed tomography of the chest to assess for nodules and other lung lesions, imaging of the sinuses to assess the extent of sinonasal disease and damage, nerve conduction velocity for mononeuritis multiplex, and magnetic resonance imaging for suspected OID.

15. The prototypic pulmonary-renal syndromes are GPA/MPA, Goodpasture disease, and SLE. Since routine hematoxylin and eosin staining of these kidney biopsies is nonspecific, what other studies performed on renal tissue may aid in distinguishing these three disorders?

Immunofluorescence studies can help in this differentiation. **Goodpasture syndrome** (anti-glomerular basement membrane [GBM] antibody disease) results from the presence of circulating antibasement membrane antibodies, which bind to epitopes (noncollagen domain 1 of α-3 chain of type IV collagen) in the basement membranes of glomeruli and alveoli. The resultant antibody–antigen interaction leads to fixation of complement and initiation of the inflammatory process, causing GN and alveolar hemorrhage. Immunofluorescence staining with antibodies against Ig detects the **linear deposition** of Ig in the GBMs.

GN due to **SLE** results from immune complex deposition in the glomerulus. Immunofluorescence studies detect **granular (lumpy) deposition** of Ig within the glomerulus, characteristic of immune complex deposition.

The pathophysiology of GN in **GPA/MPA** is unclear, but the disease does not appear to be due to immune complexes or detectable direct antibody binding to epitopes within the glomerular tissue. Thus, **immunofluorescence studies usually are negative** or reveal only scant Ig deposition, usually in areas of necrosis.

16. Compare the distinguishing features of various syndromes that may mimic GPA (Table 28.1).

17. What is appropriate induction therapy for GPA and MPA?

- GPA and MPA are typically managed using very similar approaches.
- High-dose oral or intravenous (IV) pulses of glucocorticoids are given as initial therapy, with gradual dose reduction. Glucocorticoid tapering regimens may vary considerably among clinicians, and patient-specific factors also influence the rate of taper (GPA/MPA activity/response to therapy, comorbidities such as diabetes mellitus, concurrent infection, and osteoporosis). Clinical guidelines now recommend using a reduced-dose regimen of glucocorticoids, similar to those used in recent clinical trials (see **PEXIVAS, LoVas, RITAZAREM**).
- Steroid-sparing agents (e.g., rituximab, cyclophosphamide, methotrexate) are used in combination with steroids (see below) to achieve remission.

TABLE 28.1 Distinguishing Features of Syndromes that May Mimic GPA

SYNDROME	EXAMPLE	DISTINGUISHING FEATURES
Primary vasculitis syndromes	EGPA	Atopic history with asthma (adult-onset or increasingly difficult to control)
		Marked eosinophilia
	Microscopic polyangiitis	Destructive upper airway disease unusual
		Cavitary pulmonary nodules unusual
		Absence of granuloma on pathology
Angiocentric immunoproliferative lesions	Lymphomatoid granulomatosis	Glomerulonephritis unusual
Pulmonary renal syndromes	Goodpasture disease	Anti-basement membrane antibodies
		Immunofluorescence: linear deposition
	Immune complex disease (e.g., SLE)	ANA, anti-dsDNA, and Sm antibodies
		Immunofluorescence: granular deposition
Granulomatous infections	Mycobacterium	Proper stains and cultures
	Fungi	
	Actinomycosis	
	Syphilis	
Intranasal drug abuse	Cocaine	**Antineutrophil elastase antibodies**
		Predominantly nasal septal pathology (CIMDL)
Pseudovasculitis syndromes	Atrial myxoma	Echocardiography
	Subacute bacterial endocarditis	Blood cultures
	Cholesterol emboli syndrome	Echocardiography (transesophageal)
		Angiography
		Skin biopsy
IgG4-Related Disease (IgG4-RD)		Both IgG4-RD and AAV may be associated with an elevated serum IgG4 concentration or IgG4+ plasma cell infiltrates. Granulomatous inflammation, extensive necrosis, prominent neutrophilic infiltrates, necrotizing vasculitis, and granulomas should not be seen in IgG4-RD
Neoplastic	Lethal midline granuloma	Nose/palate destruction
		NK T cell lymphoma

CIMDL, Cocaine-induced midline destructive lesion, which is usually associated with p-ANCA directed against human neutrophil elastase.

- **Cyclophosphamide** was established as truly life-saving therapy in the 1970s as daily oral treatment with 2 mg/kg daily dosing regimens. However, prolonged treatment can be complicated by myelosuppression, hemorrhagic cystitis, and bladder cancer, along with other complications. Monthly IV cyclophosphamide is associated with similar outcomes but lower cumulative exposure. Variables approaches to IV cyclophosphamide dosing have been used; doses are either based on weight or body surface area and the frequency can vary from every 2 weeks to every 4 weeks depending on the protocol being used. In general, treatment with cyclophosphamide for remission induction is limited to 3–6 months to reduce the risks of complications which include severe infection, infertility, and malignancy.

- **Rituximab** is equally as effective as cyclophosphamide for remission induction and is now the most commonly used medication in this setting. Since the publication of **RAVE**, there is now extensive real-world experience using rituximab to treat GPA/MPA across the spectrum of severity, with outcomes similar to those with cyclophosphamide. Despite this, there remains controversy over its use (without cyclophosphamide) in patients with severe renal involvement (creatinine > 4.0mg/dL) and in severe pulmonary hemorrhage requiring mechanical ventilation. In these situations, some clinicians prefer cyclophosphamide over rituximab for remission induction or use a combination of rituximab and cyclophosphamide, similar to that used in **RITUXVAS**.

- **Avacopan** is a novel, oral C5a receptor antagonist approved for use in GPA and MPA based on findings from the **ADVOCATE** trial. In this trial, patients were randomized to receive avacopan or a 20-week taper of prednisone. They also received induction with either rituximab or cyclophosphamide. Patients who received avacopan had to discontinue all prednisone within 4 weeks of randomization. At 6 months, those who received avacopan were exposed to roughly 50% less steroid than the group who received placebo, with a similar rate of remission. Thus, avacopan can now be used as part of remission induction with glucocorticoids, permitting a rapid taper of prednisone in the first 1–2 months of treatment initiation.

- **Plasmapheresis/plasma exchange (PLEX)** may be considered for extremely ill patients (diffuse alveolar hemorrhage [DAH] or advanced renal failure) and/or as salvage therapy in patients whose disease remains severe despite a combination of glucocorticoids and other immunosuppressives. The **PEXIVAS** trial is the largest trial to date in GPA/MPA and found that PLEX did not provide a significant benefit with regard to the risk of end-stage kidney disease (ESKD) or death over years of follow-up. A subsequent meta-analysis that included PEXIVAS found a short-term benefit to PLEX with regard to the risk of ESKD at 12 months, but this benefit does not appear to be maintained over time and comes at a cost of increased risk of severe infection and lack of clear mortality benefit overall. The smaller number of patients with DAH in the PEXIVAS trial may limit the interpretation of results in this subgroup. Decisions regarding the use of PLEX in the clinical setting should be tailored to the individual scenario and include a balanced risk-benefit discussion with the patient. Of importance, in patients who have an overlap with **anti-GBM disease, PLEX is still considered the standard of care**.

- Patients with subglottic stenosis can also be treated endoscopically via flexible bronchoscopy and the use of radial CO_2 laser incisions, dilation, and intralesional steroid injections with or without topical mitomycin C. Practice varies among otolaryngologists and the efficacy of these approaches have not been systematically compared to one another.

- In patients with limited GPA (absence of renal disease, pulmonary hemorrhage, orbital pseudotumor, neurologic manifestations, or CNS disease), methotrexate can be considered as a steroid-sparing therapy for induction.

- Mycophenolate mofetil has also been studied for remission induction in AAV, though data on its use remains limited.

18. What is appropriate treatment to maintain remission in GPA and MPA?

- Since it is common for GPA to relapse (especially when PR3 positive), maintenance therapy is commonly instituted once remission has been achieved. Practice varies regarding the duration of maintenance therapy, ranging from 18 months to several years or longer. There remains a risk of relapse, even after remission has been maintained for multiple years. This has been confirmed in several trials, including **MAINRITSAN 3** and **REMAIN,** which randomized patients to continue or discontinue rituximab and azathioprine, respectively.

- The most frequently used medication to maintain remission is rituximab. The **MAINRITSAN** trial demonstrated that rituximab was superior to azathioprine with regard to relapse prevention. This was confirmed in the **RITAZAREM** trial, which evaluated the efficacy of rituximab to maintain remission compared with azathioprine among patients with a history of AAV relapse.

- Other medications used to maintain remission may include azathioprine, methotrexate, leflunomide, or mycophenolate mofetil. Methotrexate and azathioprine may have similar efficacy, and are more commonly used than leflunomide or mycophenolate mofetil.
- When used to maintain remission, rituximab is typically redosed every 6 months (one 500 mg or 1,000 mg infusion). Patients at high risk for relapse, or with early B cell recovery or symptoms of relapse, may benefit from re-treatment at 4 months.
- In some circumstances, a tailored approach for rituximab maintenance therapy, guided by ANCA titers and/or B cell levels, may be considered. This approach was studied in **MAIN-RITSAN 2** as well as a single-center trial. Alternatively, some clinicians will space out the frequency of infusions (e.g., from every 6 months to every 9 months) once *sustained remission* is achieved. These approaches have been increasingly utilized since the COVID-19 pandemic, to reduce the risk of severe infection and improve vaccine effectiveness. It is less preferred in patients with a history of relapse and in those in whom a relapse could be devastating (e.g., severe kidney disease, where relapse could push the patient to end-stage renal disease).
- When cyclophosphamide without rituximab is used to achieve remission, patients are typically transitioned to a maintenance therapy with rituximab, azathioprine, or methotrexate between 3 and 6 months after cyclophosphamide initiation.
- The role of avacopan for maintenance of remission is uncertain in the context of other available therapies.
- Among patients with end-stage kidney disease from AAV and no extra-renal manifestations, the risk of subsequent relapse is thought to be low. In this scenario, the value of maintenance immunosuppression is uncertain.
- With modern therapies, the 5-year survival rate is 85% to 90%.

19. Are prophylactic antibiotics appropriate during immunosuppressive treatment?

- Oral trimethoprim/sulfamethoxazole (one double-strength tablet thrice a week or a single-strength tablet daily) provides prophylaxis against *P. jiroveci* in patients with vasculitis who are receiving high-dose (>15–20 mg/day prednisone) glucocorticoid (GC) therapy. This antibiotic therapy also limits recurrent sinus infections, which may contribute to exacerbations of GPA. Patients allergic to sulfa can receive dapsone, atovaquone, or inhaled pentamidine.
- A growing body of evidence also highlights the potential effectiveness of trimethoprim/sulfamethoxazole for preventing infections other than *P. jiroveci*, especially in the lungs.

20. What other immunosuppressive options are available in treatment-resistant cases?

- **PLEX** may be considered in life-threatening disease (rapidly progressive glomerulonephritis [RPGN] and DAH), although this is a *controversial* area (see **Question 17**). Note that PLEX removes 25% of the rituximab dose if done within 24 hours after receiving rituximab, and removes 50% of the drug if done daily for 3 days after receiving rituximab. PLEX should ideally be delayed 48–72 hours after rituximab infusions.
- **IV gammaglobulin** (2 g/kg divided over 5 days) has been described in some patients with GPA.
- A **maximal B-cell depletion strategy** (rituximab + cyclophosphamide) has been described in patients with GPA and advanced renal failure (**RITUXVAS** study; see Question 17). This is a controversial area, and head-to-head studies to determine the optimal approach (rituximab versus rituximab + cyclophosphamide) in patients with advanced renal dysfunction are lacking.
- In patients who are not responding to a specific therapy (e.g., rituximab or cyclophosphamide), the addition of the other agent may help achieve disease remission faster. For instance, in a patient treated with rituximab whose disease remains active despite appropriate therapy, a supplemental dose of cyclophosphamide may be beneficial. Similarly, a patient who received cyclophosphamide but whose disease remains difficult to control may benefit from concurrent rituximab therapy.
- Some patients with head and neck manifestations may experience the "grumblings" of disease from persistent activity in these locations. The addition of weekly oral or subcutaneous methotrexate to an existing regimen of rituximab may help achieve disease control.

- **Autologous stem cell transplant** (bone marrow transplantation) has been used rarely as salvage therapy.

21. What other treatment issues should be considered in these patients?

- Nasal irrigations to prevent sinus infections: regular use of saline rinses helps with symptoms of sinus congestion, nasal crusting, and may reduce the risk of infection. Some clinicians will recommend additives to the saline solution including:
  - 2% mupirocin (Bactroban) in 1 L of saline. This can be prepared by compounding pharmacies or patients can place a 0.5- to 1-inch strip of mupirocin into saline solution (the mupirocin does not dissolve easily, so it is recommended to mix it in warm saline and shake vigorously). Keep refrigerated after use. Irrigate sinuses with nasosinus lavage until clear return of fluid. Apply 2% mupirocin ointment with a Q-tip half-way into nasal vestibule between irrigations to diminish the carriage of *S. Aureus.*
  - Baby shampoo (acts as a surfactant): a small amount (1/2 tsp) can be added; loss of smell has been reported but is uncommon.
  - Steroids (budesonide 0.25 to 5-mg respule in rinse solution twice daily); risk of local tissue atrophy, hence should be directed by an ENT specialist.
- Therapy to prevent osteoporosis should be instituted according to guidelines.
- Cardiovascular risk factors (high blood pressure, diabetes, and lipids) should be screened for and treated as the incidence of ischemic cardiovascular disease is twofold higher in AAV.
- Malignancy screening is recommended for patients who have received cyclophosphamide. Rates of malignancy (skin and bladder cancers and acute myeloid leukemia) are increased, particularly in patients receiving a total dose of >36 g. A urinalysis should be routinely performed during follow-up for patients with prior cyclophosphamide exposure to monitor for signs of bladder cancer (e.g., hematuria).
- Patients who receive multiple courses of rituximab may be at risk of hypogammaglobulinemia. Patients with IgG levels <300 mg/dL (or <500 mg/dL with infections) may be considered for replacement doses of IV or subcutaneous immunoglobulin, as data in patients receiving rituximab for lymphoma suggest decreased risk of subsequent infections with this strategy.
- Ovarian and sperm protection should be discussed if a patient is to receive cyclophosphamide. The risk of ovarian failure is up to 50% in patients aged 20 to 30 years who receive a total dose of >20 g, among patients aged 30 to 40 years who receive a total dose of >10 g, and in those aged >40 years who receive a total dose of 5 g. Leuprolide (3.75 g monthly) has been used for ovarian protection. The risk of azoospermia occurs with a total dose of 6 to 10 g. Sperm banking and oocyte cryopreservation are the only reliable methods to assure future fertility. Some centers give testosterone 200 mg intramuscularly every 2 weeks while on cyclophosphamide therapy in an attempt to preserve testicular function.

22. Can GPA and MPA patients who go into renal failure receive a kidney transplant?

Yes. However, GPA and MPA should be under control and ideally the ANCA titer low or absent before transplant. Any patient with an estimated glomerular filtration rate of less than 20 ml/min should be referred to a transplant center for evaluation, regardless of whether they are dependent on dialysis. Kidney transplantation is associated with a survival benefit among those with AAV and end-stage kidney disease. The use of mycophenolate and cyclosporine post-transplant to prevent rejection may help prevent recurrence of GPA or MPA.

MICROSCOPIC POLYANGIITIS

23. What is MPA? How does it differ from classic polyarteritis nodosa (PAN) and GPA?

MPA is defined as a systemic necrotizing vasculitis that clinically and histologically affects small vessels (i.e., capillaries, venules, or arterioles) with few or no immune deposits. Frequently it is associated with focal segmental necrotizing GN and pulmonary capillaritis. It can be separated from classic PAN primarily because it does not cause microaneurysm formation of abdominal or renal vessels. It can be differentiated from GPA in that it does not cause granulomatous vasculitis (Table 28.2).

TABLE 28.2 Clinical Features of Polyarteritis Nodosa (PAN), MPA, and GPA

CLINICAL FEATURES	PAN	MPA	GPA
Kidney Involvement			
Renal vasculitis with infarcts and microaneurysms	Yes	No	No
Rapidly progressive glomerulonephritis with crescents	No	Yes	Yes
Lung Involvement			
Alveolar hemorrhage	No	Yes	Yes
Laboratory Data			
Hepatitis B virus infection	Yes (10%)	No	No
p-ANCA with MPO-ANCA	No	60–80%	10–20%
Abnormal angiogram with microaneurysms	Yes	No	No
Histology	Necrotizing vasculitis	Necrotizing vasculitis (no granulomatous inflammation)	Vasculitis, some granulomas possible but not typically prominent
Relapses	Rare	Common	Common

GPA, Granulomatosis with polyangiitis; *MPA*, microscopic polyangiitis; *PAN*, polyarteritis nodosa; *p-ANCA*, perinuclear antineutrophil cytoplasmic antibody.

24. Who gets MPA?

Similar to GPA, patients with MPA can be of any racial or ethnic background. In addition to being more common among people of European descent, the incidence is high (especially compared to GPA) in patients of Asian descent. In comparison, PR3+ AAV or GPA is quite less common in Asia. Men and women are affected at similar rates, with a possible female predominance in MPA. On average, people with MPA are around 10 years older than people with GPA.

25. What is the usual presentation of MPA?

Patients with MPA have variable manifestations, as with GPA. Renal involvement is very common, often presenting as rapidly progressive glomerulonephritis, although some patients can have a more indolent presentation. Patients may also have pulmonary involvement, most often with diffuse alveolar hemorrhage or fibrotic lung disease. Fibrotic lung disease is an increasingly recognized manifestation of MPA. Other manifestations can include fever, arthralgias, purpura, and peripheral neurologic disease (25–30%). Lung nodules and sinonasal disease are not typically seen in MPA. In clinical practice, differentiating MPA from GPA can be challenging in patients without a biopsy or who lack the typical granulomatous manifestation (e.g., sinonasal disease) often associated with GPA.

26. How is MPA distinguished from GPA histopathologically?

The histopathology of MPA is distinguished from GPA by the lack of granulomatous inflammation. Otherwise, features are similar, especially in the kidney where granulomatous changes are often absent in GPA.

27. How is the diagnosis of MPA made?

The diagnosis is based on a characteristic clinical presentation with a positive ANCA, often P-ANCA/MPO. The diagnosis may be supported by biopsy findings, most often of the kidney, or by characteristic findings of fibrosis or ILD on chest imaging.

28. What other pulmonary-renal syndromes must MPA be separated from?

SLE and Goodpasture syndrome can present with rapidly progressive renal dysfunction and pulmonary hemorrhage (see Question 15). The management of these conditions differs from the management of patients with MPA. When evaluating a patient with suspected MPA, an anti-GBM antibody should always be checked.

29. Describe the recommended therapy for MPA and its prognosis.

The management of MPA and GPA are essentially the same (see Questions 17 &18).

EOSINOPHILIC GRANULOMATOSIS WITH POLYANGIITIS (FORMERLY CHURG–STRAUSS SYNDROME)

30. What is EGPA ?

EGPA, previously known as Churg–Strauss, is a granulomatous inflammation of small- and medium-sized vessels, frequently involving the skin, peripheral nerves, and lungs, which is associated with peripheral eosinophilia. It occurs primarily in patients with a previous history of allergic manifestations, especially rhinitis (often with nasal polyps; 70%) and adult-onset asthma (>95%). Cytokines that affect the eosinophil (IL-5) and eosinophil granule proteins (major basic protein, cationic protein) appear to be important in the pathogenesis of this disease.

31. What are the three clinical phases of EGPA?

These phases may appear simultaneously and do not have to follow one another in the order presented here.

1. **Prodromal phase:** this phase may persist for years before presentation. It consists of allergic manifestations of rhinitis, polyposis, and most commonly asthma (80–90%). Recurrent fevers may be a characteristic feature during this stage. Asthma frequently worsens prior to entering the second phase.
2. **Peripheral blood and tissue eosinophilia** develop, frequently causing a picture resembling Löffler's syndrome (shifting pulmonary infiltrates and eosinophilia), chronic eosinophilic pneumonia, or eosinophilic gastroenteritis. Myocarditis can develop. Fevers are common during this phase. This second phase may remit or recur over years before the third phase.
3. **Life-threatening systemic vasculitis.** The onset of this phase may occur years after the onset of the prodromal phase. The asthma can abruptly abate as the patient moves into this phase. Patients can develop myocarditis, valvular insufficiency, neurologic symptoms (most commonly a vasculitic peripheral neuropathy), eosinophilic gastroenteritis, purpura, and testicular pain.

32. What are the major clinical features of EGPA (Table 28.3)?

33. What laboratory abnormalities are seen in EGPA?

The characteristic laboratory abnormality is **eosinophilia** (>1500 cells/μL). Anemia, elevated ESR/CRP, elevated IgE (70%), and a positive rheumatoid factor (70%) may be found. ANCAs are present in 50% to 65% of patients. These are directed primarily against MPO and give a p-ANCA pattern. Patients who are ANCA-positive are more likely to have or develop renal disease, alveolar hemorrhage, mononeuritis multiplex, and purpura (which are commonly considered vasculitic manifestations). There is no direct correlation between the degree of eosinophilia and disease activity.

34. How do you diagnose EGPA?

EGPA is diagnosed on the basis of its clinical and pathologic features. The diagnosis should be suspected in a patient with a previous history of allergy or asthma who presents with eosinophilia (>1500/μL), and systemic vasculitis involving two or more organs. The diagnosis is supported by biopsy of the involved tissue. The major differential diagnosis is idiopathic hypereosinophilic syndrome.

ORGAN	CLINICAL MANIFESTATIONS
Paranasal sinus	Acute or chronic paranasal sinus pain or tenderness, rhinitis (70%), polyposis, opacifications of paranasal sinus on radiographs
Lungs	Asthma (usually adult onset), patchy and shifting pulmonary infiltrates (70%), nodular infiltrates without cavitations, pleural effusions, and diffuse interstitial lung disease seen on chest radiograph. Pulmonary hemorrhage can occur.
Nervous system (60–70%)	Mononeuritis multiplex or asymmetric sensorimotor polyneuropathy; rarely central nervous system or cranial nerve involvement
Skin (50%)	Subcutaneous nodules, petechiae, purpura, skin infarction (occur mainly during the vasculitic phase)
Joints (50%)	Arthralgias and arthritis (rare)
Gastrointestinal	Eosinophilic gastroenteritis (abdominal pain, bloody diarrhea), abdominal masses
Miscellaneous	Renal failure (uncommon), congestive heart failure, conjunctivitis, OID, retinal vascular disease (AION, CRAO, CRVO), prostatitis

TABLE 28.3 Major Clinical Features of EGPA

AION: anterior ischemic optic neuropathy; CRAO: central retinal artery occlusion; CRVO: central retinal vein occlusion

35. Describe the histopathologic findings in EGPA.

The characteristic pathologic changes in EGPA include **small necrotizing granulomas** as well as **necrotizing vasculitis of small arteries and veins,** with eosinophilic infiltration. Granulomas are usually extravascular near the small arteries and veins. They are highly specific and composed of a central eosinophilic core surrounded radially by macrophages and giant cells (in contrast to a granuloma with basophilic core seen in other diseases). Inflammatory cells are also present, with eosinophils predominating with smaller numbers of polymorphonuclear leukocytes and lymphocytes.

36. What drugs have been reported to cause EGPA? (Controversial)

The cysteinyl leukotriene type I receptor antagonists, zafirlukast (Accolate), montelukast (Singulair), and pranlukast, have been associated with EGPA. Whether there is a direct cause is controversial. Some clinicians believe that EGPA is unmasked when the patient uses these drugs and subsequently tapers their GCs. Others feel that these drugs can directly contribute to the development of EGPA, as several patients have developed the disease following drug initiation even when GCs were not tapered. Consequently, leukotriene inhibitors should not be used in patients with EGPA. Similarly, dupilumab (an IL-4 and IL-13 inhibitor) has been studied for use in EGPA and while it may be effective in some patients, it can also exacerbate the disease in others. Caution should be used with these medications.

37. How is EGPA differentiated from GPA (Table 28.4)?

38. What is the five-factor score (FFS)?

The **1996 FFS** describes five classic features associated with a poor prognosis in EGPA:
- Creatinine >1.58 mg/dL.
- Proteinuria >1 g/day.
- CNS involvement.
- Gastrointestinal involvement.
- Myocardial involvement.

The original FFS was developed in 1996 to help assess prognosis in patients with EGPA (lower scores associated with higher 5-year mortality rates). In 2009, the FFS was updated and studied in GPA and MPA (in addition to EGPA).

2009 FFS (one point is given for each of the poor prognostic factors, if present):
- Creatinine >1.70 mg/dL

TABLE 28.4 Organ Involvement in Eosinophilic Granulomatosis with Polyangiitis (EGPA) and Granulomatosis with Polyangiitis (GPA)

ORGAN	EGPA	GPA
Ear/Nose/Throat	Rhinitis, polyposis	Necrotizing lesions
Allergy, bronchial asthma	Frequent	No more frequent than in general population
Renal involvement	Uncommon	Common
Cardiac involvement	Common (often subclinical, important contributor to death)	Uncommon
Eosinophilia	~10% of peripheral leukocytes	Minimally elevated
Histology	Eosinophilic necrotizing granulomatous inflammation	Necrotizing granulomatous inflammation
ANCA	MPO-ANCA+ 50–65%	PR3-ANCA ~75–80%

ANCA, Antineutrophil cytoplasmic antibodies; *c-ANCA,* cytoplasmic ANCA; *p-ANCA,* perinuclear ANCA.

- Age > 65 years old
- Gastrointestinal involvement
- Myocardial involvement
- *Absence* of ENT involvement
  When the 2009 FFS is applied to any patient with AAV, the 5-year survival is 91% for FFS of 0, 79% for FFS of 1, and 60% for FFS ≥2.

39. How do you treat EGPA? What is its prognosis?

- The management of EGPA is guided by the disease manifestations and severity of presentation.
- All patients are typically started on glucocorticoids, which are very effective. Some argue that patients with a FFS of 0 may be managed with GCs alone. However, flares are common when GCs are tapered so steroid-sparing treatments are often used, especially in those with a history of relapse. In those with non-vasculitic manifestations, mepolizumab or benralizumab, two unique anti-IL-5 therapies, are often used, especially when recurrent asthma or other eosinophilic manifestations are driving the steroid dependence. For vasculitic manifestations, cyclophosphamide, rituximab, azathioprine, mycophenolate mofetil, or methotrexate may be considered.
- Patients with poor prognostic factors (FFS ≥1) are treated with GCs (60–80 mg/day divided dose) in combination with a steroid-sparing agent. Those with severe presentations may benefit from 3 days of pulsed methylprednisolone (1 g/day). Cyclophosphamide (monthly pulse or oral) is often used in those with severe manifestations, especially vasculitis. Rituximab may also be considered, especially in those with a positive ANCA.
- Mepolizumab, an antibody to IL-5, was approved by the FDA for treatment of EGPA in 2017 and is the first medication to receive FDA approval for this condition. Approval was based on findings from the **MIRRA** trial. Of note, this trial included a patient population with low rates of renal involvement (<1%), alveolar hemorrhage (<5%), palpable purpura (13%), and ANCA positivity (20%). Mepolizumab may be particularly useful for eosinophilic manifestations and/or in those having difficulty tapering off glucocorticoids.
- Benralizumab, another anti-IL5 therapy, was approved by the FDA for the treatment of EGPA in 2024 based on findings from a large randomized controlled trial (**MANDARA**). Similar to the MIRRA trial, low rates of renal involvement (5%), palpable purpura (10%), and ANCA positivity (10%) were seen in the enrolled population.
- For maintenance therapy, rituximab, mepolizumab, benralizumab, methotrexate, azathioprine, or other steroid-sparing agents may be considered. These may reduce the risk of relapse and spare patients from glucocorticoid toxicity.

The 5-year survival rate for EGPA is 97% with FFS of 0, and 90% with FFS of ≥1. The major cause of death is cardiac involvement due to myocardial infarction and congestive heart failure.

DRUG-INDUCED ANCA-ASSOCIATED VASCULITIS

40. Does drug-induced AAV occur?

- Yes, drug-induced AAV has been reported with medications for hyperthyroidism (**propylthiouracil, methimazole,** carbimazole), **hydralazine, minocycline,** and **levamisole-cut cocaine** (in addition to other less common offending medications).
- Frequently high-titer MPO, much less commonly PR3. Dual-positivity has also been reported.
- Patients with drug-induced AAV may present with constitutional symptoms, arthralgias with occasional synovitis, and cutaneous vasculitis. Serious end-organ manifestations, including necrotizing GN and alveolar hemorrhage, occur less frequently.
- Hydralazine is the most common medication-induced AAV. Patients can develop a pauci-immune GN and DAH. Wide-ranging immunologic abnormalities can be seen: high-titer ANA and p-ANCA antibody, anti-MPO antibody, anti-histone and double-stranded DNA antibody, and hypocomplementemia. Thus, features of drug-induced lupus may be present, but renal pathology demonstrates a pauci-immune GN.
- AAV secondary to levamisole-adulterated cocaine may be associated with antibodies against PR3, MPO, and human neutrophil elastase that are simultaneously positive. Additional laboratory findings have been described including antiphospholipid antibodies and cold agglutinins that may contribute to skin necrosis. In addition, levamisole can frequently be associated with leukopenia (28%) due to bone marrow suppression. Common clinical features include retiform purpura (occasionally progressing to necrosis), arthralgias, and constitutional symptoms such as fever, night sweats, and weight loss. Necrotizing GN and alveolar hemorrhage have also been described.
- Minocycline-induced AAV frequently has elevated liver enzymes.
- Treatment involves withholding the offending drug. More serious cases require systemic GC and cytotoxic agents.

ANCA AND OTHER DISEASES

41. What other disorders are associated with ANCAs?

Commonly, c-ANCA positivity represents the presence of anti-PR3 antibodies and is associated with a small number of diseases. In contrast, p-ANCA and **"atypical ANCA"** (the term for ANCA patterns that are not clearly c-ANCA nor p-ANCA) may be due to a variety of different antibodies and can be present in a wide range of diseases. Specific antibodies that may result in positive p-ANCA or atypical ANCA patterns include antibodies directed against MPO, elastase, cathepsin G, lactoferrin, and β-glucuronidase. p-ANCA in the setting of GPA, MPA, EGPA, or RLV is usually due to anti-MPO antibodies (p-ANCA should typically be against MPO if the patient has vasculitis). p-ANCA present in other disorders is less well characterized but is usually not due to antibodies directed against MPO:

- Goodpasture (anti-GBM antibody) disease: between 10% and 40% will have positive ANCA, usually against MPO. These patients tend to have worse kidney disease prognosis.
- Most rheumatic disorders (RA, SLE, Sjögren's disease, systemic sclerosis, polymyositis, Buerger disease, relapsing polychondritis) have had positive ANCAs reported with varying but low frequency (<20%). ANCA is usually p-ANCA, directed against proteins other than MPO. The clinical significance is uncertain, but in some clinical scenarios such as lupus nephritis, ANCA presence may be associated with a worse prognosis. Several cases of p-ANCA-associated vasculitis have been reported in patients with limited and diffuse systemic sclerosis. MPO-ANCA+ tests may be present in SLE and other conditions, and while the significance is uncertain, patients should be carefully evaluated for signs of vasculitis.
- Inflammatory bowel disease: between 60% and 80% of patients with ulcerative colitis and up to 25% of patients with Crohn's disease have positive ANCAs. It is usually p-ANCA directed against a nuclear envelope or a neutrophil granule protein, but not MPO.

- Autoimmune liver disease: p-ANCA (not MPO) or atypical ANCA is seen in primary sclerosing cholangitis (70%), chronic active hepatitis, and primary biliary cholangitis.
- Cystic fibrosis: up to 80% to 90% of patients have positive p-ANCA, most commonly against BPI protein in the primary azurophilic granules of neutrophils. It is notable that patients with cystic fibrosis frequently have Gram-negative infections of their airways.
- Infections: human immunodeficiency virus, subacute bacterial endocarditis, leprosy, malaria, acute parvovirus B19, and acute infectious mononucleosis. **Note that all three ANCA patterns have been reported for patients with *Mycobacterium tuberculosis* infections**.

ACKNOWLEDGMENT

The author and editors would like to acknowledge the late Dr. Richard Brasington for his contribution to this chapter in the previous edition. Dr. Brasington has left behind a legacy in the numerous trainees he inspired to pursue a career in rheumatology.

BIBLIOGRAPHY

Charles P, Perrodeau É, Samson M, et al. Long-term rituximab use to maintain remission of antineutrophil cytoplasmic antibody-associated vasculitis: a randomized trial. *Ann Intern Med.* 2020;173(3):179–187 **MAINRITSAN 3 trial**.

Charles P, Terrier B, Perrodeau É, et al. Comparison of individually tailored versus fixed-schedule rituximab regimen to maintain ANCA-associated vasculitis remission: results of a multicentre, randomised controlled, phase III trial (MAINRITSAN2) [published correction appears in Ann Rheum Dis. 2019 Sep;78(9):e101]. *Ann Rheum Dis.* 2018;77(8):1143–1149 **MAINRITSAN 2 trial**.

Chung SA, Langford CA, Maz M, et al. 2021 American College of Rheumatology/Vasculitis Foundation guideline for the management of antineutrophil cytoplasmic antibody-associated vasculitis. *Arthritis Care Res (Hoboken).* 2021;73(8):1088–1105.

Comarmond C, Pagnoux C, Khellaf M, et al. Eosinophilic granulomatosis with polyangiitis (Churg-Strauss): clinical characteristics and long-term followup of the 383 patients enrolled in the French Vasculitis Study Group cohort. *Arthritis Rheum.* 2013;65(1):270–281.

de Groot K, Harper L, Jayne DR, et al. Pulse versus daily oral cyclophosphamide for induction of remission in antineutrophil cytoplasmic antibody-associated vasculitis: a randomized trial. *Ann Intern Med.* 2009;150(10):670–680 **CYCLOPS trial**.

Guillevin L, Pagnoux C, Karras A, et al. Rituximab versus azathioprine for maintenance in ANCA-associated vasculitis. *N Engl J Med.* 2014;371(19):1771 **MAINRITSAN trial**.

Hiemstra TF, Walsh M, Mahr A, et al. Mycophenolate mofetil vs azathioprine for remission maintenance in antineutrophil cytoplasmic antibody-associated vasculitis: a randomized controlled trial. *JAMA.* 2010;304:2381–2388 **IMPROVE trial**.

Jayne DR, Gaskin G, Rasmussen N, et al. Randomized trial of plasma exchange or high dosage methylprednisolone as adjunctive therapy for severe renal vasculitis. *J Am Soc Nephrol.* 2007;18:2180–2188 **MEPEX trial**.

Jayne DRW, Merkel PA, Schall TJ, Bekker PADVOCATE Study Group. Avacopan for the Treatment of ANCA-Associated Vasculitis [published correction appears in N Engl J Med. 2024 Jan 25;390(4):388]. *N Engl J Med.* 2021;384(7):599–609 **ADVOCATE trial**.

Jones RB, Cohen Tervaert JW, Hauser T, et al. Rituximab versus cyclophosphamide in ANCA-associated renal vasculitis. *NEJM.* 2010;363:211–220 **RITUXIVAS trial**.

Karras A, Pagnoux C, Haubitz M, et al. Randomized controlled trial of prolonged treatment in the remission phase of ANCA-associated vasculitis. *Ann Rheum Dis.* 2017;76:1662–1668 **REMAIN trial**.

Kumar B. Hydralazine-associated vasculitis: overlapping features of drug-induced lupus and vasculitis. *Semin Arthritis Rheum.* 2018;48:283–287.

Martinez V, Cohen P, Pagnoux C, et al. Intravenous immunoglobulin for relapses of systemic vasculitides associated with antineutrophil cytoplasmic autoantibodies: results of a multicenter, prospective, open-label study of twenty-two patients. *Arthritis Rheum.* 2008;58:308–317.

Pagnoux C, Mahr A, Hamidou MA, et al. Azathioprine or methotrexate maintenance for ANCA-associated vasculitis. *N Engl J Med.* 2008;359:2790–2803 **WEGENT trial**.

Stone JH, Merkel PA, Spiera R, et al. Rituximab versus cyclophosphamide for ANCA-associated vasculitis. *N Engl J Med.* 2010;363:211–232 **RAVE trial**.

Walsh M, Merkel PA, Peh CA, et al. Plasma Exchange and Glucocorticoids in Severe ANCA-Associated Vasculitis. *N Engl J Med.* 2020;382(7):622–631 **PEXIVAS trial**.

Walsh M, Collister D, Zeng L, et al. The effects of plasma exchange in patients with ANCA-associated vasculitis: an updated systematic review and meta-analysis. *BMJ.* 2022;376:e064604.

Wechsler ME, Akuthoda P, Jayne D, et al. Mepolizumab or Placebo for Eosinophilic Granulomatosis with Polyangiitis. *N Engl J Med.* 2017;376(20):1921–1932 **MIRRA trial**.

Wechsler ME, Nair P, Terrier B, et al. Benralizumab versus mepolizumab for eosinophilic granulomatosis with polyangiitis. *N Engl J Med.* 2024;390:911–921 **MANDARA trial**.

Yates M, Watts RA, Bajema IM, et al. EULAR/ERA-EDTA recommendations for the management of ANCA-associated vasculitis. *Ann Rheum Dis.* 2016;75(9):1583–1594.

FURTHER READING

www.vasculitisfoundation.org.

CHAPTER 29

Immune Complex-Mediated Small-Vessel Vasculitides

Kyle D. Maier, MD, Seth J. VanDerVeer, DO, and Ramon A. Arroyo, MD

 KEY POINTS

1. The classic cutaneous finding in small-vessel vasculitis (SVV) is palpable purpura.
2. The most common types of immune complex (IC)-mediated SVV include hypersensitivity vasculitis, IgA Vasculitis (IgAV), and cryoglobulinemic vasculitis.
3. Hypersensitivity vasculitis is most commonly idiopathic or due to a drug or infection.
4. IgAV presents with palpable purpura, arthritis, abdominal colic, and renal disease; skin biopsy shows leukocytoclastic vasculitis (LCV) with IgA deposition in vessel walls on direct immunofluorescence.
5. Urticarial lesions lasting longer than 24–48 hours and resolving with hyperpigmentation are likely vasculitic.

1. Define an immune complex (IC) and discuss its role within the immune system.

An immune complex is a molecule composed of an antigen bound to the Fab region of one or more antibodies. Normally these complexes circulate in the blood, help neutralize foreign antigens, and are cleared by the reticuloendothelial system.

2. Discuss the precipitation of immune complexes and resulting inflammation seen in small vessel vasculitis (SVV).

Under conditions of antigen excess, ICs precipitate from serum and become trapped within vascular beds. These ICs activate the classical complement pathway, leading to the release of anaphylatoxin (C5a), neutrophil recruitment, local inflammation, lysosomal enzyme release, oxygen free radical generation, and vessel wall damage. Immune complex–mediated SVV includes a variety of conditions that are often grouped together based on similar pathologic findings and common involvement of the small blood vessels of the skin, resulting in similar cutaneous findings at presentation (see Questions #5 & 6).

3. What causes this immune complex–mediated small-vessel vasculitis (IC-SVV) to occur?

Several different underlying etiologies can result in the development of cutaneous vasculitis seen in IC-SVV, and concerning findings on skin exam should prompt an evaluation for an underlying associated condition(s). All patients should be asked about **new medications or recent infections** (including risk factors for hepatitis C). Between 30% and 50% of cases have no identifiable cause. **Hypersensitivity vasculitis** is the diagnosis given to these patients when there is no identifiable cause.

4. What conditions are associated with IC-SVV? See Table 29.1.

PEARL: Malignancy is the cause of SVV in only 1% of patients. Myelodysplastic syndrome (MDS) and hairy cell leukemia are the most common.

5. Which blood vessels are affected by IC-SVV?

SVV predominately affects vessels < 50 μm in diameter, including the arterioles, capillaries, and postcapillary venules.

TABLE 29.1 Conditions Associated With Immune Complex–Mediated Small-Vessel Vasculitis

CONDITION	COMMENTS
Hypersensitivity vasculitis	Most commonly idiopathic or secondary to drug reaction
Urticarial vasculitis	If hypocomplementemic consider HUVS and SLE
IgA vasculitis	Renal and gastrointestinal involvement common in addition to skin; IgA in vessel walls
Cryoglobulinemic vasculitis	Hepatitis B and C, cancer; rheumatic disease
CTD-associated vasculitis	RA, SLE, Sjögren disease, Crohn disease
IgG4-related disease	Small vessel vasculitis with palpable purpura reported in IgG4-RD, but is not the predominant skin manifestation. Typically occurs with multi-organ disease, hypocomplementemia, ↑ serum IgG4. Pathology would reflect LCV, and not the typical lymphoplasmacytic infiltrate commonly described in IgG4-RD
Infections	SBE, *Neisseria,* influenza, mononucleosis, HIV, hepatitis B and C
Malignancy	Leukemia, lymphoma, myeloma, solid tumors, myelodysplastic syndromes, hairy cell leukemia
Anti-glomerular basement membrane disease	Pulmonary–renal syndrome (Goodpasture syndrome); *in contrast to other conditions in table, does not commonly include cutaneous manifestations*
Erythema elevatum diutinum	Occurs over the extensor surfaces of joints (hands, knees, elbows, ankles); responds to dapsone

HIV, Human immunodeficiency virus; *HUVS,* hypocomplementemic urticarial vasculitis syndrome; *RA,* rheumatoid arthritis; *SBE,* subacute bacterial endocarditis; *SLE,* systemic lupus erythematosus.

6. What is the major clinical manifestation of IC-SVV?

Palpable purpura is the most common primary lesion in IC-SVV, resulting from erythrocyte extravasation into surrounding tissue through damaged vessel walls. Therefore, purpuric lesions **do not blanch** with pressure. These lesions often begin as numerous asymptomatic, nonpalpable, purpuric macules that eventually become palpable. The presence of a **central necrotic punctum** is helpful in distinguishing vasculitic purpura from nonvasculitic etiologies. Some lesions may continue to evolve and become nodular, bullous, infarctive, or ulcerative. Purpura usually occurs in a **symmetric distribution over the dependent regions** of the body like the lower legs and feet, secondary to the increased hydrostatic pressure (Fig 29.1). The trunk, upper extremities, and other sites may also be affected.

PEARL: In contrast to IC-SVV, pauci-immune vasculitis syndromes (ANCA vasculitides) tend to involve smaller, more circumscribed areas of purpuric lesions.

7. What other cutaneous lesions can occur in IC-SVV?

- Urticaria
- Superficial ulcerations
- Splinter hemorrhages
- Erythema multiforme-like lesions
- Vesicles, pustules
- Macules, patches

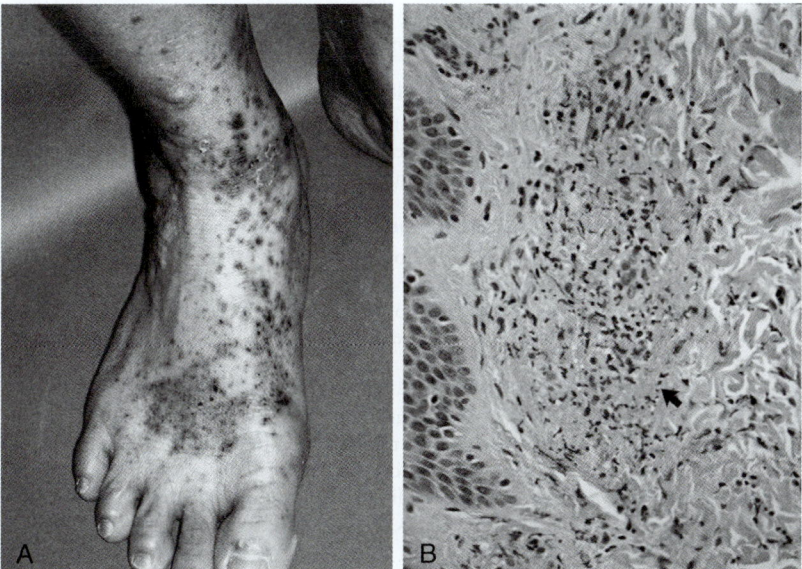

Fig. 29.1 Small-vessel vasculitis. (A) Palpable purpura. (B) Histopathology of a cutaneous blood vessel demonstrating leukocytoclastic vasculitis with nuclear dust *(arrow).*

8. What other manifestations can be seen with IC-SVV?

Constitutional – Fever, malaise
Musculoskeletal – Arthralgias, myalgias, inflammatory arthritis (less common)
Renal – Glomerulonephritis
Gastrointestinal – Abdominal pain (mesenteric vasculitis), GI bleeding
Pulmonary – Obstructive lung disease, capillaritis, alveolar hemorrhage (Goodpasture's)

9. What diseases can mimic IC-SVV?

- Pigmented purpuric dermatoses (e.g., Schamberg's disease)
- Thrombocytopenia: Immune thrombocytopenic purpura (ITP), thrombotic thrombocytopenic purpura (TTP), disseminated intravascular coagulation (DIC)
- Antiphospholipid syndrome
- Livedoid vasculopathy (atrophie blanche)
- Warfarin-induced skin necrosis
- Purpura fulminans
- Atrial myxoma
- Cholesterol emboli
- Infective endocarditis
- Meningococcemia
- Leprosy (Lucio's phenomenon)
- Amyloidosis
- Calciphylaxis
- Scurvy

10. Discuss the initial workup for a patient presenting with SVV.

These tests should be considered to help identify an etiology and assess for end-organ damage:
- CBC, CMP, UA, ESR, CRP, C3/C4, SPEP
- ANA, RF, ANCA (IFA as well as PR3 & MPO antibody by ELISA), cryoglobulins
- HIV, HBV, HCV
- Chest X-ray

This evaluation is often nonspecific but may provide reassurance regarding the extent of organ involvement and prognosis.

11. How do you diagnose IC-SVV?

Diagnosis is typically made by **skin biopsy** identifying cutaneous vasculitis.

12. Describe the defining histopathology of IC-SVV.

Leukocytoclastic vasculitis (LCV), in which small blood vessels are infiltrated with neutrophils and/or mononuclear cells. As the process evolves, **fibrinoid necrosis** of the vessel wall with leukocyte fragmentation (**leukocytoclasis**) and destruction of the vessel wall are seen.

13. Describe the optimal timing, location, and type of skin biopsy for SVV.

- Optimal timing for skin biopsy is **24–48 hours** after appearance
- If possible, biopsy a **non-ulcerated site**
- If obtaining a biopsy from an ulcerated lesion, biopsy the **ulcer's edge**
- **Punch biopsy** is sufficient (samples small vessels located within the superficial dermis

14. Describe the histopathologic assessment of a skin biopsy for SVV.

Evaluate the specimen with **light microscopy** and **direct immunofluorescence (DIF)**. Light microscopy will typically reveal LCV common to most etiologies of IC-SVV. The presence of eosinophils on biopsy may suggest a drug-induced etiology. DIF is useful for identification of IgAV or hypocomplementemic urticarial vasculitis (HUV), which will demonstrate predominant IgA deposits or intense staining for IgM, IgG, C3, C4, and C1q, respectively. Fig. 29.1

HYPERSENSITIVITY VASCULITIS

15. What is hypersensitivity vasculitis (HSV)?

HSV refers to a skin-limited IC-SVV which typically occurs **within 1–2 weeks** after an **infection or drug exposure**. In addition to purpura, arthralgias and even frank arthritis (usually large joint) can be seen.

16. What is the treatment for HSV?

Removal of the offending agent usually leads to resolution within 1–2 weeks.

Treatment with glucocorticoids is reserved for extensive disease, usually requiring a short treatment course with tapering over several weeks.

IGA VASCULITIS (FORMERLY HENOCH–SCHÖNLEIN PURPURA)

17. What is IgA Vasculitis? What are the characteristic histopathologic features?

IgA Vasculitis (IgAV) is a typically self-limited IC-SVV characterized by LCV with **predominant IgA deposition** in affected blood vessels (seen on DIF), pathologically differentiating this condition from other forms of IC-SVV. IgA can also be found in the glomerular mesangium.

> **PEARL:** Patients (especially adults) with suspected IgAV with a skin biopsy negative for IgA should be evaluated for ANCA-associated vasculitis, anti-C1q disease, or IgA paraproteinemia.

18. Describe the epidemiology of IgAV. How does the disease course differ between children and adults?

- IgAV is the prevailing form of systemic vasculitis in children, occurring primarily in those aged 2–10, but persons of any age can be affected
- IgAV is usually acute in onset and self-limited, lasting from 6 to 16 weeks except in a minority of patients (3–5%) with chronic renal disease
- Adults tend to have more severe disease with higher frequency of progressive renal disease and bullous, necrotic skin lesions

19. Discuss the pathogenesis of IgAV/HSP.

- There are two subclasses of IgA, IgA1 and IgA2. Both function in mucosal immunity, though IgA1 accounts for 80–90% of serum IgA. Importantly, IgAV and renal-limited IgA nephropathy (Berger disease) exclusively involve the deposition of **IgA1**, not IgA2. Though the reason for exclusive involvement of IgA1 is not certain, it is theorized to result from differences in **post-translational modification**. Unlike IgA2, IgA1 contains a **hinge region** with multiple O-linked glycosylation sites.
- In IgAV and Berger disease, studies have demonstrated **aberrantly glycosylated O-glycans on the hinge region of IgA1 molecules,** terminating with an *N*-acetylgalactosamine (GalNAc) or sialylated *N*-acetylgalactosamine instead of galactose. It is postulated that these galactose- deficient IgA1 molecules are recognized by **antiglycan autoantibodies** leading to IC formation, which deposit in tissues (vessel walls, renal mesangium) and activate the complement pathway.

> **PEARL:** Immunohistochemistry of IgAV and Berger disease demonstrates deposition of **galactose-deficient IgA1** in the kidney, which is *not* seen in lupus nephritis.

20. Describe the clinical manifestations of IgAV.

The classic tetrad of IgAV is palpable purpura, arthritis, abdominal pain, and renal disease (~80% of patients), and typically follows an upper respiratory infection.

Skin (100%) – Palpable purpura, urticarial papules, or plaques. The rash may begin as macular erythema and urticarial lesions but may progress rapidly to purpura. Lesions typically involve the lower extremities and buttocks. Scrotal and scalp edema can be seen, particularly in children. Bullous or necrotic lesions can be seen in adults but are rare in children.

Joints (60–84%) – Arthralgias or nonerosive arthritis. Typically oligoarticular, involving the lower extremities (knees, ankles). Upper extremity involvement (elbows, wrists) occurs less frequently. Can be migratory.

GI (60%) – Colicky abdominal pain, intussusception, hemorrhage, and, rarely, **ileal perforation** (severe presentations like intussusception are rare in adults). In cases of severe abdominal pain and concern for intussusception, ultrasound may be considered over barium enema as involvement in IgAV is typically more proximal than idiopathic cases (**ileoileal** rather than ileocecal). Abdominal symptoms result from mesenteric vasculitis causing bowel wall edema or hemorrhage.

Kidney (50%) – Usually manifests as **asymptomatic proteinuria and hematuria**. However, **nephrotic syndrome** and **acute renal failure** can occur. Most patients have complete resolution of renal manifestations with few showing persistent/progressive disease (5–10% children, 10–15% adults).

> **PEARL:** In contrast to gastrointestinal and joint involvement, which precedes skin involvement in a minority of cases (20–25%), **nephritis rarely occurs before rash** in IgA vasculitis.

21. How is IgAV treated?

Mild disease: Supportive treatment and analgesia.

- NSAIDs may help arthralgias or arthritis but may worsen gastrointestinal symptoms; should be avoided in patients with renal disease

Moderate-to-severe disease:

- **GI involvement or bleeding** - Prednisone 1 mg/kg/day × 2 weeks with tapering off over 2 weeks may be used
- **Progressive renal disease** - Difficult to treat; limited data supporting benefit of nonsteroidal immunosuppressive medications in pediatric and adult patients
- Treatment with high-dose IV glucocorticoid pulses followed by maintenance oral glucocorticoids should be considered in patients with poor prognostic factors of **proteinuria >1 g/day, nephrotic syndrome**, and/or **crescentic glomerulonephritis** (>50% crescents).

- Failure to respond after 2–3 months of corticosteroids may indicate the need for additional immunosuppression with azathioprine, cyclophosphamide, or rituximab
- Given the potential toxicity and paucity of data regarding the effectiveness of immunosuppression in this setting, some experts recommend initially treating with ACE-inhibitors or angiotensin receptor blockers for adult patients presenting with proteinuria (including nephrotic range proteinuria) prior to considering immunosuppression. However, the decision to withhold immunosuppression in this setting remains controversial.

URTICARIAL VASCULITIS

22. What is urticarial vasculitis (UV)?

Urticarial vasculitis (UV) is a rare IC-SVV that presents with urticarial lesions instead of the palpable purpura seen in other types of SVV. It can be limited to the skin or may involve other organs (kidneys, lungs, GI tract, eyes).

23. Describe the classification of urticarial vasculitis.

UV can be subcategorized into two groups based on **serum complement** levels:
1. **Normocomplementemic UV (NUV)** is a self-limited subset of hypersensitivity vasculitis. It is idiopathic and commonly benign. The clinical course can fluctuate, typically resolving within 1–4 years. In chronic cases, it must be distinguished from neutrophilic urticaria, a persistent form of urticaria not associated with vasculitis.
2. **Hypocomplementemic UV (HUV).** HUV is associated with **reduced levels of C1q, C3, and C4,** and **anti-C1q antibodies** are seen in >50% of patients. Unlike NUV, HUV is more likely to be chronic and carries a higher risk of additional organ involvement. It may have overlapping features with SLE including ANA positivity and a similar interface dermatitis with deposition of immunoglobulins and complement along the dermal-epidermal junction.
   - **Hypocomplementemic urticarial vasculitis syndrome (HUVS, McDuffie syndrome).** HUVS is the most severe subset of UV with multiorgan involvement. In addition to chronic urticaria and LCV, clinical manifestations can include:
     - **Constitutional (20%)** – Fever, malaise
     - **Allergic (40%)** – Severe angioedema, laryngeal edema
     - **Musculoskeletal (80%)** – Arthralgia, arthritis
     - **Eye (40%)** – Uveitis, scleritis, episcleritis
     - **Kidney (25%)** - Glomerulonephritis
     - **Gastrointestinal (20%)** – Recurrent abdominal pain
     - **Lung (25%)** – Obstructive lung disease (COPD)

> **PEARL:** In urticarial vasculitis, hypocomplementemia is the most sensitive marker for systemic disease, correlating with disease severity. In HUVS, **low C1q levels** (60% of patients) and **anti-C1q antibodies** (90%) can be important in helping establish the diagnosis.

24. What conditions are associated with UV?

- Autoimmune disease – SLE >> Sjögren disease > RA, JIA, MCTD
- Autoinflammatory syndromes – Cryopyrinopathies
- Infection – HBV, HCV
- Malignancy – MDS, Multiple Myeloma, NHL, various carcinomas
- IgM paraproteinemia (Schnitzler Syndrome)
- Drug reactions

25. Describe the proposed pathogenesis of HUV.

- Typically, IgG2 anti-C1q antibodies bind to the collagen-like tail of C1q, leading to IC formation (interestingly, the C1q antigenic target displays molecular mimicry with EBV-derived peptides)

- IC activation of the classical complement pathway leads to anaphylatoxin release, mast cell activation, and neutrophil recruitment. Neutrophil NETosis mediates vessel wall inflammation and vascular leakage.
- Histamine and TNF-alpha promote eosinophil influx with resultant perivascular infiltration of neutrophils, lymphocytes, and eosinophils leading to the clinical picture of UV→ wheal-like, pruritic lesions, with variable purpura and ecchymoses.
- Obstructive lung disease may result from binding of anti-C1q antibodies to pulmonary surfactant proteins.
- Accumulation of anti-C1q antibodies in glomeruli underlies the pathogenesis of renal involvement.

26. How is UV differentiated from true urticaria?

- UV lesions typically **last > 24–48 hours** and resolve with **residual hyperpigmentation**. True urticaria (hives) last < 24 hours (usually 8–12 hours) and leave no trace.
- UV lesions are characterized by **pain, burning, and tenderness** rather than pruritus, the sensory hallmark of true urticaria.
- UV lesions are typically **0.5 to 5 cm** in diameter; true urticaria may coalesce into large lesions (>10 cm).
- Signs or symptoms of systemic disease, like **fever, arthralgias, abdominal pain, lymphadenopathy, or abnormal urine sediment**, tend to occur in HUVS and rarely in true urticaria.
- The histology is **LCV** in UV, in contrast to upper dermis edema in true urticaria.
- UV tends to involve the **trunk and proximal extremities** more than the distal lower extremities, which differentiates it from other causes of LCV.

27. Discuss the treatment approach for UV.

Therapy involves supportive measures, treatment of associated/underlying disorders, and discontinuing offending medications if present. Conservative treatment is reasonable when no internal organ involvement is observed.

First line, nonsevere disease:
- **Dapsone** and **colchicine** can be used for cutaneous involvement
- NSAIDs can treat arthralgias or arthritis
- Hydroxychloroquine is generally reserved for patients with concomitant SLE
- Antihistamines address true urticaria and angioedema (occur in ~ 50%)
- Prednisone (10–60 mg daily) is often necessary for cutaneous or systemic symptom control, generally reserved for moderate-to-severe disease or after first-line treatment failure.

For severe disease and/or major organ involvement:
- Methotrexate, azathioprine, mycophenolate mofetil, or cyclosporine
- **Rituximab**; cyclophosphamide (largely fallen out of favor due to toxicity)
- **Omalizumab** (more efficacious for NUV)

For treatment-refractory disease:
- Plasmapheresis and IVIG have been proposed as potential treatment options in patients with critical organ compromise in the acute setting, particularly in patients with rapid kidney function deterioration or crescenteric glomerulonephritis.

ERYTHEMA ELEVATUM DIUTINUM

28. What is erythema elevatum diutinum (EED)?

EED is a rare form of chronic, recurrent cutaneous vasculitis typified by red-brown, violaceous, or yellowish papules and plaques. Although lesions can be asymptomatic, they are often preceded by burning or pruritus. They generally involve the extensor surfaces of joints and acral sites. EED has been associated with connective tissue diseases, infections, paraproteinemias (especially IgA), and neutrophilic dermatoses; it is not likely to represent a primary condition. Extracutaneous manifestations are less common and include arthralgias, ocular disease (panuveitis, scleritis, peripheral

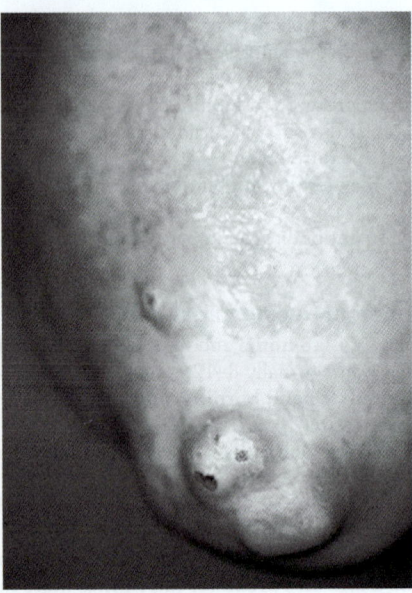

Fig. 29.2 Erythema Elevatum Diutinum. Nodules overlying the extensor elbow. (From Stone J. Immune complex-mediated small vessel vasculitis. In: *Firestein & Kelley's Textbook of Rheumatology.* 11th ed. Elsevier, Inc.; 2021:1649–1658.)

ulcerative keratitis), neuropathy, and ulcerations (oral, esophageal, penile). It is often unclear if these are symptoms of EED itself or the associated underlying condition. Fig. 29.2

29. Describe the histologic findings of EED.

Biopsy of early lesions demonstrates **LCV with fibrinoid necrosis**. As lesions progress, histiocytic inflammation predominates with formation of **granulation tissue, fibrosis, and intracellular lipoidosis**, separating it from other cutaneous vasculitides.

30. How is EED treated?

Treat the underlying condition. If none are identified, most patients respond to **dapsone** or **sulfapyridine**, but lesions often recur upon discontinuation. Other treatment options include NSAIDs, colchicine, tetracyclines, chloroquine, and plasmapheresis.

BIBLIOGRAPHY

Buck A, Christensen J, McCarty M. Hypocomplementemic urticarial vasculitis syndrome: a case report and literature review. *PubMed.* 2012. https://pubmed.ncbi.nlm.nih.gov/22328958.

Chan H, Tang YL, Lv XH, et al. Risk factors associated with renal involvement in childhood Henoch-Schonlein purpura: a meta-analysis. *PLoS One.* 2016;11(11):e0167346.

Gu SL, Jorizzo JL. Urticarial vasculitis. *Int J Women Dermatol.* 2021;7(3):290–297.

Hackl Á, Becker JU, Körner LM, et al. Mycophenolate mofetil following glucocorticoid treatment in Henoch-Schönlein purpura nephritis: the role of early initiation and therapeutic drug monitoring. *Pediatr Nephrol.* 2017;33(4):619–629.

Kolkhir P, Grakhova MA, Bonnekoh H, Krause K, Maurer M. Treatment of urticarial vasculitis: a systematic review. *J Allergy Clin Immunol.* 2019;143(2):458–466.

Marzano AV, Maronese CA, Genovese G, et al. Urticarial vasculitis: clinical and laboratory findings with a particular emphasis on differential diagnosis. *J Allergy Clin Immunol.* 2022;149(4):1137–1149.

Özen S, Marks SD, Brogan PA, et al. European consensus-based recommendations for diagnosis and treatment of immunoglobulin A vasculitis—the SHARE initiative. *Rheumatology.* 2019;58(9):1607–1616.

Sandhu JK, Albrecht J, Agnihotri G, Tsoukas MM. Erythema elevatum et diutinum as a systemic disease. *Clin Dermatol.* 2019;37(6):679–683. doi:10.1016/j.clindermatol.2019.07.028.

Selewski DT, Ambruzs JM, Appel GB, et al. Clinical characteristics and treatment patterns of children and adults with IGA nephropathy or IGA vasculitis: findings from the CUREGN study. *Kidney Int Rep.* 2018;3(6):1373–1384. doi:10.1016/j.ekir.2018.07.021.

Steffen U, Koeleman CaM, Sokolova MV, et al. IgA subclasses have different effector functions associated with distinct glycosylation profiles. *Nat Commun.* 2020;11(1):1–12.

Stone J. Immune complex-mediated small vessel vasculitis. In: Firestein G, McInnes I, Koretzky G, Mikuls T, Neogi T, O'Dell J, eds. *Firestein and Kelley's Textbook of Rheumatology.* 11th ed. Philadelphia; 1642–1652.

FURTHER READING

www.nlm.nih.gov/medlineplus/vasculitis.html.

CHAPTER 30

Cryoglobulinemia

Timothy M. Wilson, MD

No one will ever know what "In Cold Blood" took out of me.

-Truman Capote (1924–1984)

> ### KEY POINTS
>
> 1. Mixed cryoglobulinemic vasculitis is an immune complex–mediated small-vessel vasculitis most commonly associated with chronic hepatitis C virus (HCV) infection, systemic autoimmune diseases (especially Sjögren's syndrome), and lymphoproliferative disorders.
> 2. Palpable purpura, weakness, and arthralgias are the most common manifestations of mixed cryoglobulinemic vasculitis, but renal involvement is most closely associated with a poor prognosis.
> 3. Rituximab (RTX) is the recommended treatment for HCV-associated cryoglobulinemic vasculitis in the setting of progressive, organ-threatening disease, particularly when used in combination with direct-acting antiviral (DAA) agents.
> 4. Cryofibrinogenemia needs to be considered in patients presenting with lower leg ulcers or gangrene.
> 5. Cold agglutinin disease should be ruled out in patients with acrocyanosis and a complement-mediated hemolytic anemia manifested by a positive C3d direct antiglobulin test.

1. What are cryoglobulins?

Cryoglobulins are immunoglobulins (Igs) or Ig-containing complexes that spontaneously precipitate from serum and plasma at temperatures below 37°C and become soluble again with rewarming. Cryoprecipitation of human serum components was first described by Wintrobe and Buell in 1933. The term "cryoglobulin" was introduced by Lerner et al in 1947.

2. How are cryoglobulins classified?

Brouet et al. published a classification system for cryoglobulinemia in 1974, which is still in use today.

Type I: composed of a single monoclonal Ig, with IgM being the most common. Serum levels of the cryoglobulin are typically very high (5–30 mg/mL, cryocrit >5%), and precipitation occurs rapidly with cooling (usually <24 hours).

Type II: mixed cryoglobulins composed of a monoclonal IgM (typically IgM$_\kappa$) that acts as an antibody (e.g., rheumatoid factor [RF]) against polyclonal IgG. Serum levels are usually intermediate (1–10 mg/mL, cryocrit 1–5%); therefore precipitation may take a few days.

Type III: mixed cryoglobulins similar to Type II, but with polyclonal IgM with RF activity directed against polyclonal IgG. They are usually present in small quantities (0.1–1 mg/mL, cryocrit <1%) and precipitate slowly (up to 7 days); therefore they are more difficult to detect.

Type II to III: an unusual variant composed of oligoclonal IgM and faint polyclonal Igs. It is thought to represent a transition from polyclonal (type III) to monoclonal (type II) mixed cryoglobulinemia (MC) as clonal expansion of B cells progresses (see Question 11).

3. What is the overall incidence of each cryoglobulin type?

Type I: 10% to 15%, type II: 50% to 60%, type III: 25% to 30%, and type II to III: 5% to 10%. MC (type II or III) accounts for 80% to 90% of all cases.

4. Describe the requirements for collection and processing of blood specimens for cryoglobulin testing.

- Blood is collected into prewarmed tubes. The sample is then allowed to clot for 1 hour, followed by centrifugation and separation of the serum. All of these steps, including

TABLE 30.1 Classification With Typical Quantitative Amounts of the Cryoprecipitate

	MEASUREMENT AS CRYOCRIT (%)	IG CONCENTRATION (MG/ML)	IG CONCENTRATION (MG/DL)	IG CONCENTRATION (µG/ML)
Type I	>5	5–30	500–3000	5000–30,000
Type II	1–5	1–10	100–1000	1000–10,000
Type III	<1–2	0.1–1	10–100	100–1000
Normal	0	Up to 0.02	Up to 2	Up to 20

transportation of the sample after collection, must be performed at 37°C. Premature cooling may decrease the cryoglobulin concentration and result in false-negative results.

- The remaining serum is incubated at 4°C (refrigerator temperature) for 3 to 7 days. A 7-day incubation period is ideal because many mixed cryoglobulins will not be identified otherwise due to slow precipitation.
- Centrifugation at 4°C is performed. Visual inspection then allows for determination of the presence of a cryoprecipitate, which, if present, indicates a positive result (qualitative screen). The use of specialized Wintrobe tubes can allow positive results to be measured as a percentage, the cryocrit (quantitative measure). Some laboratories only report one of these two measurements, with no further testing performed.
- If a cryoprecipitate is present, further testing should be requested to phenotype the constituents of the precipitate. In this analysis, the sample is washed to remove any potential contaminates. The precipitate is then rewarmed and the contents of the cryoglobulin (specifically the Ig isotypes and assessment for clonality) and quantity can be determined by electrophoresis and immunofixation. Some laboratories may use nephelometry for Ig quantification. These tests allow for classification of the cryoprecipitate according to the Brouet system (see Question 2; Table 30.1).

5. What underlying disorders are associated with type I cryoglobulinemia?

B-cell lymphoproliferative disorders associated with monoclonal Ig production such as monoclonal gammopathy of undetermined significance (MGUS), multiple myeloma, Waldenstrom's macroglobulinemia, chronic lymphocytic leukemia, B-cell non-Hodgkin lymphoma, and lymphoplasmacytic lymphoma.

6. What conditions are associated with MC (type II or III cryoglobulinemia)?

Chronic HCV infection is the most common (70–90%), followed by autoimmune diseases (e.g., SLE and Sjogren's) (10–20%), non-HCV infections, and lymphoproliferative processes. A small fraction of cases (<5–10%) are truly "essential" cryoglobulinemia (i.e., those with no definable underlying illness).

7. Describe the relationship between HCV infection and MC.

HCV infection accounts for up to 90% of type II and up to 70% of type III cases. Overall, 30% of patients with HCV infection have detectable cryoglobulins, but <10% of these patients (or <5% of all patients with HCV infection) develop symptomatic vasculitis. The prevalence is highest in the Mediterranean area and lower in Northern Europe, the United States, and the rest of the world. Development of cryoglobulinemic vasculitis is associated with the infection duration and more often occurs after 10 years. Due to the development of DAA agents, chronic HCV infection as a cause of MC is likely to be less in the future.

8. What other infections are associated with MC?

After HCV, human immunodeficiency virus is the most common. Other infectious agents are less frequently seen and the association is not as clearly established. In many of these cases, the underlying infection is associated with the transient appearance of type III cryoglobulins, but without associated disease. Examples include hepatitis B, Epstein–Barr virus, cytomegalovirus, hepatitis A, *Coxiella burnetii* (Q fever), parvovirus B19, poststreptococcal nephritis, subacute bacterial endocarditis, tuberculosis, leprosy, brucellosis, coccidioidomycosis, parasitic infections, candidiasis, and others.

PEARL: A patient with fever, valvular heart disease, and negative cultures in the setting of MC must be evaluated for Q fever.

9. Describe the relationship between systemic autoimmune disease and MC.

Autoimmune disorders are the second most commonly associated diagnoses with MC (usually type III) after hepatitis C. Primary Sjögren's syndrome (pSS) is the most common, followed by systemic lupus erythematosus. In pSS cryoglobulins may be seen in up to 15% of patients, but associated vasculitis is seen in less than half of these patients. Levels of circulating cryoglobulins are typically lower than those seen in patients with HCV. In pSS the presence of cryoglobulins correlates with higher disease activity (elevated ESSDAI scores) and is associated with extra-glandular manifestations, development of MALT lymphoma, and mortality. Cutaneous vasculitis, peripheral neuropathy, glomerulonephritis, elevated RF, and low complement levels (specifically C4) can be associated with cryoglobulins. Less frequently, cryoglobulins can be found in multiple other rheumatologic and autoimmune disorders, such as rheumatoid arthritis, antiphospholipid antibody syndrome, Behçet's disease, antineutrophil cytoplasmic antibody (ANCA)-associated vasculitides, and inflammatory bowel disease.

10. What are the mechanisms underlying tissue injury in cryoglobulinemic vasculitis?

- Cryoglobulin aggregation and precipitation can result in vascular occlusion within small vessels leading to the hyperviscosity syndrome. This is the predominant cause of injury in type I cryoglobulinemia. This reflects the large concentration and cold-inducible characteristics of the Igs in type I disease. Cold-inducible injury is not thought to play a major role in type II and type III MC, given the fact that *in vitro* cold precipitation is much slower.
- Immune complex–mediated vasculitis is the primary cause in types II and III MC. The small vessels are most commonly affected, but medium-vessel involvement may occur. Associated complement fixation partially explains the low level of complement in this condition. The higher the thermal range that the cryoglobulin will still precipitate, the more likely it is to activate complement.

11. Describe the steps involved in mixed cryoglobulin formation and their pathogenicity.

This process has been most extensively studied in HCV-associated MC. Cryoglobulin production is the result of a persistent and progressive antigen-driven clonal selection process. HCV has a membrane protein, E2, that binds to CD81 on B and T cells leading to chronic activation of B cells with clonal expansion of atypical memory B cells. These cells produce Igs with RF activity, especially a particular variant designated the WA (VH1-69) cross-idiotype. Complexes of HCV components, Igs, RF, complement, and other particles (e.g., very low-density lipoprotein) comprise the cryoglobulin. Cryoglobulins may persist despite viral clearance following treatment (and may no longer contain viral particles), suggesting that cryoglobulin formation may initially be a virus-dependent phenomenon that eventually becomes autonomous. Tissue deposition, complement fixation, and the following inflammatory cascade result in vasculitis. The fact that a particular B-cell activating factor (BAFF) promoter polymorphism and elevated levels of BAFF are found in patients with MC suggests that it may have a pathogenic role by promoting B-cell proliferation and survival.

12. Summarize the major clinical and laboratory features of cryoglobulinemia.

The major clinical and laboratory features of cryoglobulinemia are shown in Fig. 30.1.

13. What are the common clinical manifestations of cryoglobulinemia?

Hyperviscosity syndrome (bleeding [most commonly epistaxis], vision changes, neurologic symptoms, etc.) is the most common manifestation in type I. In MC, cutaneous manifestations are the most common, with arthralgias and neuropathy being other frequent findings. The frequency of

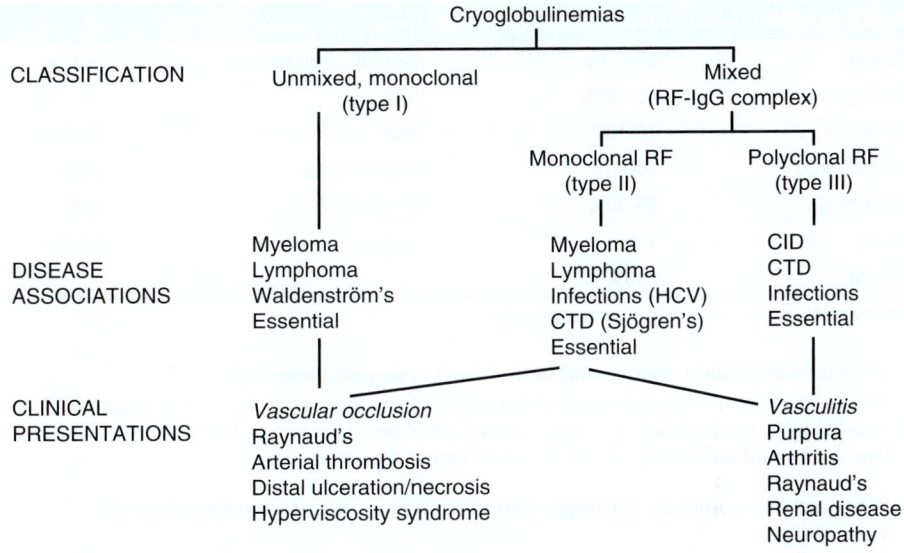

Cryoglobulinemias

CLASSIFICATION	Unmixed, monoclonal (type I)	Mixed (RF-IgG complex)

	Monoclonal RF (type II)	Polyclonal RF (type III)

| **DISEASE ASSOCIATIONS** | Myeloma Lymphoma Waldenström's Essential | Myeloma Lymphoma Infections (HCV) CTD (Sjögren's) Essential | CID CTD Infections Essential |

| **CLINICAL PRESENTATIONS** | *Vascular occlusion* Raynaud's Arterial thrombosis Distal ulceration/necrosis Hyperviscosity syndrome | | *Vasculitis* Purpura Arthritis Raynaud's Renal disease Neuropathy |

CTD = connective tissue disease; CID = chronic inflammatory disease.

Fig. 30.1 The major clinical and laboratory features of cryoglobulinemia.

manifestations in MC varies between studies, reflecting the characteristics of the patient populations (Table 30.2).

14. What are the common cutaneous manifestations in MC?

Palpable purpura is the most common manifestation, being seen in up to 100% of patients during the course of the disease. Urticarial vasculitis can also occur. Lesions typically affect the lower extremities, but can involve the trunk and upper extremities. They usually resolve spontaneously but tend to be recurrent. Because cryoglobulinemic vasculitis can involve both small and medium vessels, more severe cutaneous lesions such as large skin ulcers occurring above the malleoli are not uncommon. Digital necrosis, bullae, and livedo racemosa may also be seen.

15. What is the most common renal finding in MC?

Type 1 membranoproliferative glomerulonephritis is the most common histologic pattern (80% of cases). Frank nephrotic or nephritic syndrome can occur, but patients typically present with less substantial microscopic hematuria or proteinuria. Hypertension and elevated creatinine are common, and renal failure may be mild or severe at presentation.

16. What are the common neurologic manifestations in MC?

A painful distal sensory polyneuropathy is the most common finding. It can be symmetric or asymmetric, and insidious or abrupt in onset. Motor involvement can also occur, typically months to years after the sensory neuropathy. Mononeuritis multiplex may also be seen. Neuropathy is thought to result from vasculitis of the vasa nervorum and is always painful. Central nervous system (CNS) involvement is exceedingly rare in MC, and other causes (e.g., atherosclerotic) should be explored if CNS symptoms occur.

17. Describe the typical articular manifestations in MC.

Polyarticular arthralgias are seen in the majority of patients during the course of the disease. Patients may describe profound joint pain, but inflammatory features are lacking on examination. Nonerosive arthritis is much less commonly encountered. Immune complex deposition is thought to be the cause of joint symptoms.

TABLE 30.2 Common Clinical Manifestations in Mixed Cryoglobulinemia

Purpura	55–100%	Raynaud's phenomenon	5–35%
Arthralgias	45–100%	Renal	10–40%
Weakness	70–100%	Sicca	30–50%
Meltzer's triad[a]	40–80%	Gastrointestinal	2–6%
Neuropathy	20–80%	Pulmonary	<5%
Ulcers	10%	Malignancy	10–15%
Arthritis	<10%		

[a]**Meltzer's triad** = purpura + arthralgias + weakness/myalgias.

18. **How is malignancy associated with mixed cryoglobulinemia?**

    Symptomatic lymphoma develops in 5% to 20% of patients within 10 years of diagnosis. B-cell non-Hodgkin lymphoma (e.g., marginal zone lymphoma in spleen or liver), lymphoplasmacytic lymphoma, and diffuse large B cell lymphoma are most common.

19. **What are the common serologic abnormalities in mixed cryoglobulinemic vasculitis?**

    Elevated RF and hypocomplementemia are seen in almost all patients with MC. Notably, C4 is reduced out of proportion to C3. Polyclonal hypergammaglobulinemia or monoclonal gammopathy is also frequently seen. Autoantibodies (other than RF) are seen in more than half of patients and include antinuclear, anti-smooth muscle, ANCA, antithyroid, antimitochondrial, and antiphospholipid antibodies.

20. **How is the diagnosis of mixed cryoglobulinemic vasculitis established?**

    Detection of cryoglobulins in the right clinical setting is diagnostic. Given the fact that false-negative results are common due to sample mishandling, the absence of cryoglobulins does not exclude the diagnosis. A high level of suspicion should be maintained if characteristic clinical and laboratory features are present. Elevated RF, low complement level, and the presence of a monoclonal gammopathy (especially when found together) may serve as a surrogate marker of cryoglobulinemia. Biopsy of affected tissue (typically skin) demonstrates leukocytoclastic vasculitis, and intravascular hyaline thrombi may also be seen. Immunofluorescence typically demonstrates Ig and C3 deposition. Biopsies of liver or bone marrow may demonstrate clonal expansions of B cells.

21. **What is the prognosis of mixed cryoglobulinemic vasculitis?**

    Approximately 65% have a slow, relatively benign course, and 35% have a moderate-to-severe course. Five-year survival is 75% for MC due to HCV infection and better for other causes. Advances in antiviral therapy and use of rituximab will continue to improve survival rates. Renal involvement most strongly confers a worse prognosis. In addition, male sex, age ≥60 years, type II MC, gastrointestinal involvement, chronic HCV infection, and diffuse vasculitis are also risk factors for a poor prognosis. Complement levels, RF titers, and cryoglobulin levels have no prognostic significance. The lack of association between cryoglobulin levels and prognosis is important to note, as low cryoglobulin concentration (in the correct clinical context) can be associated with severe disease and should not be easily dismissed. Renal failure is the most common cause of death, whereas cirrhosis, widespread vasculitis, malignancy, and infection are less frequent causes.

22. **Discuss the treatment options for mixed cryoglobulinemic vasculitis.**

    Removal of the antigenic stimulus is the primary goal. In HCV-associated mixed cryoglobulinemic vasculitis, this involves use of direct-acting antiviral therapy, whereas in malignancy, other infections, and autoimmune diseases, appropriate treatment of these conditions is warranted. Immunosuppression is used to directly control the vasculitis and associated tissue damage. Most data regarding treatment are derived from studies of HCV-associated mixed cryoglobulinemic vasculitis:
    - **Glucocorticoids:** high-dose steroids should be used in patients with severe manifestations (e.g., neurologic, renal, or diffuse vasculitis), with short courses of low to intermediate doses

for minor flares. Steroids should be tapered off quickly, and there is no role for chronic therapy.
- **Plasma exchange:** although there is no controlled data supporting its use, expert opinion suggests a role in severe, life-threatening disease. It is the treatment of choice for hyperviscosity syndrome.
- **Cyclophosphamide:** it is frequently employed in combination with plasma exchange to treat severe disease. It is not recommended for use as monotherapy.
- **Other immunosuppressants:** use of azathioprine, methotrexate, cyclosporine, and other immunosuppressive agents is anecdotal, and no consensus recommendations can be made.
- **Colchicine:** it may have favorable effects on pain, weakness, purpura, and leg ulcers. The standard dose is 1 mg/day. Use for mild disease manifestations.
- **Antiviral (AV) agents and rituximab (RTX)** (see Questions 23-26).

23. Discuss the use of AV agents and RTX in the treatment of HCV-associated mixed cryoglobulinemic vasculitis.

AV agents should be used in all patients with HCV-associated and other viral-associated MC. Historically, interferon-based regimens demonstrated response rates of 30% to 80% in MC, but use was commonly limited due to contraindications, side effects (interferon-α may exacerbate vasculitis manifestations), and slow onset of action. Direct-acting antivirals (DAA), however, have transformed therapeutic outcomes in patients with HCV-associated MC. Treatment with DAA has shown an immunologic response in patients, with decreases in cryocrit in up to 80% of those treated, and clinical response in 91% of patients according to the Birmingham Vasculitis Activity Score. It is of interest to note that some patients may experience continued episodes of vasculitis despite viral clearance.

RTX has demonstrated good efficacy in treating mixed cryoglobulinemic vasculitis (clinical response in 80%) and should be considered in all patients with moderate-to-severe disease. Its use in combination with AV agents has demonstrated superiority over either agent used alone. RTX monotherapy has also been shown to be more efficacious than standard-of-care immunosuppression (high-dose steroids, azathioprine, cyclophosphamide, plasma exchange, or a combination of these). Typical response rates with combination therapy are 70% to 80%, with most patients experiencing complete clinical response. Addition of RTX to AV agents typically results in a more rapid clinical response and improved renal outcome than AVs alone. Improvement may be seen as early as 1 month, but typically occurs within 3 to 6 months. Clinical response rates are commonly higher than immunologic and virologic response, indicating that viral and immunologic responses may not be necessary for clinical efficacy.

There is no consensus regarding how RTX and AVs should be administered in patients presenting with HCV-associated MC. Patients with severe end-organ damage from vasculitis should be treated with immunomodulation first, followed by DAA after clinical stabilization (Fig. 30.2). Studies have evaluated dosing RTX 1 g every 2 weeks (2 doses) and 375 mg/m^2 weekly for 4 weeks, and both are effective.

24. Is relapse common after treatment with RTX in HCV-associated MC?

Treatment effect is usually durable and has been demonstrated for >2 years after a single treatment course. Relapse occurs in ~20% of cases and seems to be less frequent with combination therapy versus either RTX or AV monotherapy. Immunologic relapse and B-cell recovery commonly precede clinical relapse in many patients. Most patients with a clinical relapse also have viral recurrence or an initial lack of viral response. However, not all patients with an immunologic relapse (decreased C4, increased cryoglobulins, return of B cells) experience a clinical relapse; therefore, the use of lab measurements to predict relapse is limited. RTX has been proven effective in the setting of clinical relapse and should be, thus, considered in this setting.

25. Discuss the safety of RTX when used to treat mixed cryoglobulinemic vasculitis.

Overall, safety is similar when compared with other treatments. Serum sickness occurs in ~1% of cases and is usually mild. One study suggested that the administration of RTX 1 g every 2 weeks is more commonly associated with severe systemic reactions (e.g., exacerbation of vasculitis) than a weekly dosing regimen (375 mg/m^2 × 4 doses). It is hypothesized that cryoglobulins may form immune complexes with RTX by binding to it in an RF-dependent manner, resulting

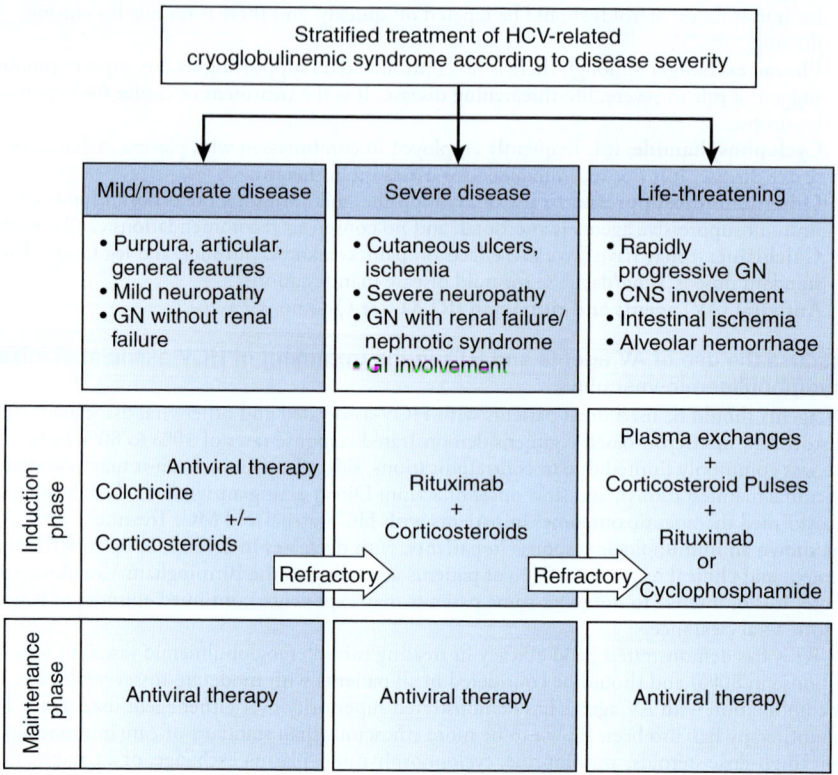

Fig. 30.2 The general treatment principles of hepatitis C virus–associated cryoglobulinemia. *CNS*, Central nervous system; *GI*, gastrointestinal; *GN*, glomerulonephritis.

in an accelerated immune complex–mediated vasculitis. This phenomenon was dependent on the level of cryoglobulins (high cryoglobulin concentration, low C4) and dose of RTX. Thus, the recommendation was to use a lower dose regimen and to consider plasma exchange prior to administration in patients with high cryoglobulin concentrations (>3%) and/or significant renal insufficiency. One approach is to carry out plasma exchange every other day for five to seven treatments while placing the patient on high-dose glucocorticoids, subsequently followed by RTX (375 mg/m^2 weekly × 4 doses). Of note, HCV viral loads may increase when RTX is used as monotherapy in the absence of AV so DAA agents should also be used. In addition, HBV may worsen or reactivate so AV therapy with oral nucleot(s)ide analogs should be instituted during RTX therapy if there is evidence of latent or active HBV infection.

26. Summarize the general treatment principles of HCV-associated MC.
The general treatment principles of HCV-associated MC are shown in Fig. 30.2.

27. Define cryofibrinogenemia and describe its diagnosis and clinical manifestations.
Cryofibrinogen (CF) is an insoluble complex of fibrin, fibrinogen, fibrin split products, fibronectin, α1-antitrypsin and α2-macroglobulin, and Igs that precipitate with cold exposure. CF does not precipitate in serum (plasma only) because the proteins consumed in the clotting process during cooling are the necessary substrates for cryofibrinogen. Cryofibrinogenemia is most commonly associated with malignancy, connective tissue diseases, and infection frequently in association with cryoglobulins. It has also been reported with oral contraceptive use, diabetes mellitus, dysfibrinogenemia, and advanced atherosclerosis. Some patients have no associated disease which is called primary or "essential" cryofibrinogenemia. Plasma levels greater than 1 g/L are more likely to cause symptoms.

Cutaneous manifestations are the most common and are the result of vascular occlusion and tissue ischemia. They tend to occur in cold-exposed areas and include purpura, livedo, ulcers, and gangrene. Eosinophilic microthrombi in small vessels and necrosis are seen in biopsy specimens, usually without vasculitis unless there are associated cryoglobulins. Thromboses in larger vessels (strokes, myocardial infarction, etc.) are seen much less frequently. Paradoxical bleeding may occur due to depletion of clotting factors. There is an association with cryoglobulins: cryofibrinogenemia is seen in 70% of patients with cryoglobulins, whereas 60% of cryofibrinogenemia occurs in isolation.

28. Discuss the appropriate collection and processing of specimens being tested for cryofibrinogenemia.

Blood is collected in nonheparinized tubes (use EDTA or citrate) that do not allow coagulation and is stored at 37°C until centrifugation. After centrifugation, the remaining plasma is stored at 4°C for 72 hours and cryofibrinogen, if present, will form during this period. Cryofibrinogen is absorbed by red blood cells (RBCs), so a delay in centrifugation or allowing the sample to cool may result in false-negative results because the RBCs are eventually discarded. Heparin tubes should not be used for collection because heparin may form a cryoprecipitate with plasma factors and lead to false-positive results. It is also recommended that a separate serum sample be obtained by collecting blood in a prewarmed tube that does allow coagulation. The serum sample should be tested for the presence of cryoglobulins as outlined in Question 4.

> **PEARL:** Cryofibrinogen will precipitate in the cold only from the plasma sample, whereas cryoglobulins precipitate in the cold from both the plasma and serum samples.

29. Discuss the treatment of cryofibrinogenemia.

Avoiding cold exposure and keeping the patient at 37°C is reasonable, as is smoking cessation if applicable. Cutaneous lesions should be treated according to standard gangrene or burn protocols. If cryofibrinogenemia is secondary to an underlying disease process such as malignancy, infection, or rheumatic disease, treatment of that condition is typically helpful. It is important to evaluate for potential conditions associated with cryofibrinogenemia. Among patients with primary (essential) cryofibrinogenemia, treatment options are derived primarily from small case series and expert opinion. Fibrinolytics such as streptokinase and stanozolol have been described as beneficial in some patients. In contrast, experience with heparin has been disappointing, with some patients actually worsening on this therapy. Experience with coumadin is similarly mixed. Some experts advocate low-dose aspirin therapy (81 mg/day) in conjunction with corticosteroids for patients with mild to moderate symptoms. Immunosuppression with corticosteroids and agents such as azathioprine, chlorambucil, and cyclophosphamide, have been described in the literature and are likely most appropriately considered in cases associated with an underlying rheumatic disease. There are limited data to support the use of plasma exchange.

30. What is cold agglutinin disease?

Cold agglutinins are typically IgM antibodies directed against I/i antigens on erythrocytes leading to hemolytic anemia due to complement-mediated RBC destruction in the reticuloendothelial system (typically the liver). Nearly all cold agglutinins causing symptoms have a titer of 1:64 or higher at 4°C and are positive for the C3d direct antiglobulin test (DAT). Occlusion of superficial vessels can occur (most commonly at exposed, cooler, acral sites) due to slowing of blood flow by agglutinated RBCs. This can lead to symptoms of acrocyanosis; Raynaud's-like symptoms; and skin ulcers on the ears, nose, and digits. Most cases with chronic manifestations are idiopathic or related to lymphoproliferative diseases. Treatment includes warmth, RTX (± fludarabine), and rarely plasmapheresis. Anti-complement agents (e.g., eculizumab, sutimlimab) are in clinical trials and show promise. Corticosteroids are not effective. Alkylating agents are mainly used for those patients requiring them for treatment of their lymphoma. Cold agglutinin disease due to infections (mycoplasma pneumoniae, infectious mononucleosis, other viruses) typically are asymptomatic or cause transient clinical manifestations that usually do not require therapy other than warmth. Cold agglutinin disease has also been described in patients with ANCA vasculitis related to levamisole-tainted cocaine.

ACKNOWLEDGMENT

The author would like to thank Dr. Duane Pearson for their contributions to this chapter in the previous edition.

BIBLIOGRAPHY

Berentsen S. New insights in the pathogenesis and therapy of cold agglutinin-mediated autoimmune hemolytic anemia. *Front Immunol.* 2020;11:590.

Blain H, Cacoub P, Musset L, et al. Cryofibrinogenaemia: a study of 49 patients. *Clin Exp Immunol.* 2000;120:253–260.

Bonacci M, Lens S, Mariño Z, et al. Long-term outcomes of patients with HCV-associated cryoglobulinemic vasculitis after virologic cure. *Gastroenterology.* 2018;155:311–315.

Brito-Zerón P, Acar-Denizli N, Ng WF, et al. How immunological profile drives clinical phenotype of primary Sjogren's syndrome at diagnosis (Sjogren's big data project). *Clin Exp Rheumatol.* 2018;S112:102–112.

Dammacco F, Lauletta G, Vacca A. The wide spectrum of cryoglobulinemic vasculitis and an overview of therapeutic advancements. *Clin Exp Med.* 2023;23:255–272.

De Vita S, Quartuccio L, al. Isola Met, et al. A randomized controlled trial of rituximab for the treatment of severe cryoglobulinemic vasculitis. *Arthritis Rheum.* 2012;64:843.

Gabbard AP, Booth GS. Cold agglutinin disease. *Clin Hematol Int.* 2020;2:95–100.

Kolopp-Sarda M, Miossec P. Cryoglobulins: an update on detections, mechanisms, and clinical contribution. *Autoimmun Rev.* 2018;17:457–464.

Kolopp-Sarda M-N, Miossec P. Practical details for the detection and interpretation of cryoglobulins. *Clin Chem.* 2022;68(2):282–290.

Moretti M, Ferro F, Baldini C, Mosca M, Talarico R. Cryoglobulinemic vasculitis: a 2023 update. *Curr Opin Rheumatol.* 2024;36:27–34.

Passerini M, Schiavini M, Magni C, et al. Are direct-acting antivirals safe and effective in hepatitis C virus-cryoglobulinemia? Virological, immunological, and clinical data from a real-life experience. *Eur J Gastro Hepatol.* 2018;30:1206–1215.

Quartuccio L, Bortoluzzi A, Scirè CA, et al. Management of mixed cryoglobulinemia with rituximab: evidence and consensus-based recommendations from the Italian Study Group of Cryoglobulinemia (GISC). *Clin Rheumatol.* 2023;42:359–370.

Ramos-Casals M, Stone JH, Cid MC, et al. The cryoglobulinemias. *Lancet.* 2012;379:348–360.

Retamozo S, Quartuccio L, Ramos-Casals M. Cryoglobulinemia. *Med Clin (Barc).* 2022;158:478–487.

Santiago MB, Melo BS. Cryofibrinogenemia: what rheumatologists should know. *Curr Rheumatol Rev.* 2022;18:186–194.

Sneller M, Hu Z, Langford C. A randomized controlled trial of rituximab following failure of antiviral therapy for hepatitis C virus-associated cryoglobulinemic vasculitis. *Arthritis Rheum.* 2012;64:835–842.

Behçet Syndrome

Yusuf Yazici, MD

1. What are the variable vessel vasculitides?

The International Chapel Hill Consensus Conference recognized two vasculitides that can affect any size and type (arteries, veins, and capillaries) of blood vessels: Behçet syndrome and Cogan's syndrome. Note that many but not all of the clinical manifestations of Behçet syndrome are due to vasculitis. Many Behçet syndrome lesions such as oral/genital ulcers and CNS lesions are associated with perivascular inflammation without vascular wall destruction.

2. What is the most commonly used criteria for Behçet syndrome?

Behçet syndrome is diagnosed clinically. There are no specific laboratory, imaging, or histologic features that can help in the diagnosis of a patient with suggestive symptoms. The diagnosis is based on a combination of clinical features in the setting of ruling out other potential causes. The most commonly used and best-performing diagnostic/classification criteria are the International Study Group (ISG) criteria (sensitivity ~92%, specificity ~96%). These criteria state that patients need to have recurrent oral ulcers plus two of the following four clinical manifestations: recurrent genital ulcers, skin lesions, eye lesions, or a positive pathergy test (Table 31.1). Another set of criteria developed by the International Criteria for Behcet's Disease (ICBD) adds vascular manifestations and neurologic manifestations and uses a point system.

PEARL: Genital ulcers that scar, pathergy, hypopyon, bilateral panuveitis, major venous thrombosis, brainstem inflammation, or pulmonary aneurysms are highly characteristic of Behcet syndrome in a patient presenting with recurrent oral ulcers. Histopathologic analysis of involved tissues ranges from a neutrophilic vascular reaction to leukocytoclastic vasculitis.

3. Behçet syndrome is a clinical diagnosis. What other diseases must be considered and ruled out in a patient presenting with possible Behçet syndrome?

Virtually all the features of Behçet syndrome can be seen in Crohn's colitis, and it may be very hard to differentiate between the two, especially in up to 20–30% of patients with Behçet syndrome who have gastrointestinal involvement. Inflammatory bowel disease must be considered particularly in patients with iron deficiency, markedly elevated erythrocyte sedimentation rate (ESR; >100 mm/hour), or even minor bowel complaints. Other diseases with oral ulcers, ocular disease, and arthritis that need to be considered include systemic lupus erythematosus, reactive arthritis, herpetic infection, systemic vasculitis, Sweet's syndrome, and periodic fever syndromes (periodic fever, aphthous stomatitis, pharyngitis, adenitis—PFAPA, hyperimmunoglobulin D syndrome [HIDS]).

TABLE 31.1 International Study Group Criteria for the Diagnosis of Behçet Syndrome

CRITERIA	FREQUENCY	COMMENTS
Oral ulcers	~97%	At least three times in a 12-month period
Plus Two Out of Four From Below:		
Recurrent genital ulcers	~80%	Usually scarring
Skin lesions	~75–80%	Erythema nodosum, pseudofolliculitis, papulopastular or acneiform lesions
Eye lesions	~50%	Anterior or posterior uveitis, retinal vasculitis
Pathergy	~50%	Evaluated for red bump in 24–48 h, after dermal insertion of a 20-gauge needle

4. Describe "pathergy".

Pathergy is the hyperreactivity occurring most commonly in the skin to any intracutaneous injection or needle stick (pathergy test), however, it can also be seen in other tissues. It frequently occurs at the sites of a blood draw. Originally described in 1937, this reaction is highly suggestive of Behçet syndrome but can also be seen in Sweet syndrome and pyoderma gangrenosum. The mechanism of pathergy in Behçet syndrome is unknown, but it is thought to be related to increased neutrophil chemotaxis. The rate of a positive reaction varies in different populations, being more common in Japan and Turkey (50–75%) and less common in England and the United States (10–20%). The **pathergy test** is done by sticking a 20-gauge needle into the alcohol-prepped skin of the volar forearm at three sites. A positive test is the appearance of a papular reaction (≥ 2 mm diameter) surrounded by erythema or the development of a pustule at a needle-stick site within 24–48 hours.

5. Who gets Behçet syndrome?

The disease occurs in both men and women equally, with the mean age of patients being approximately 25–30 years (range, 15–45 years). It is rare to occur in childhood and after the age of 50 years. The highest prevalence is in Turkey and Japan. Overall men get more severe diseases.

6. What is the relationship between this disease and the old Silk Route of Marco Polo?

Although Behçet syndrome occurs worldwide, it is much more prevalent in individuals living along the old Silk Route (trade trail of Marco Polo), extending from Japan and Korea through Turkey and into the Mediterranean basin. Japanese and Eastern Mediterranean individuals have a three to six times increased incidence of HLA-B51 in patients with Behçet syndrome compared with controls. The presence of HLA-B51 appears to be associated with a more complete expression of manifestations and a more severe clinical course of disease. HLA-B51 is not increased in frequency in patients with Behçet syndrome in the United States. Genome-wide scans have identified multiple additional loci that may contribute to the risk of developing Behçet syndrome.

7. Describe the aphthous ulcers associated with Behçet syndrome.

Aphthous-like stomatitis is commonly the initial manifestation in Behçet syndrome and is seen eventually in ~97% of patients. Preferential sites of ulceration are the mucous membranes of the cheeks (buccal mucosa), soft palate, and sides of tongue and less commonly the gingiva, inner lip, and dorsum of tongue. The hard palate, tonsils, and pharynx are rarely involved (unlike reactive arthritis or Stevens–Johnson syndrome), and the outer portions of the lips are not involved (unlike herpetic lesions). Most oral ulcers are painful, occur in crops (3 to >10 lesions), are <1 cm in diameter, heal without scarring within 1 to 3 weeks, and are recurrent. Major ulcers (>1 cm) may scar. Histamine-releasing foods (e.g., citrus fruits, nuts, and cheese) and poor oral hygiene may be triggers for oral ulcers.

8. List a differential diagnosis of aphthous stomatitis.

Underlying conditions may be identified in as many as 30% of patients with severe aphthous stomatitis. However, most cases remain idiopathic (Table 31.2).

TABLE 31.2 Differential Diagnosis of Recurrent Oral Ulcerations

CONDITION	CONDITION
Idiopathic (70% of cases)	Dermatologic Dz: pemphigoid, pemphigus, lichen planus, others
B vitamins/folate/iron/zinc deficiency	Autoinflammatory Dz: PFAPA, Hyperimmunoglobulin D
Cyclic neutropenia	Drugs (e.g., methotrexate)
Menstrual-related	Infections: herpes simplex, HIV
Recurrent (complex) aphthosis	Stevens-Johnson syndrome
Inflammatory bowel disease	Gluten-sensitive enteropathy (Celiac Dz)
Behçet's disease	Rheumatologic Dz: SLE, reactive arthritis, MAGIC syndrome

9. What is recurrent complex aphthosis?

This entity describes patients without systemic manifestations of Behçet syndrome who have recurrent oral and genital aphthous ulcers or almost constant multiple (more than three) oral aphthae. Differentiation from complex aphthosis may be difficult because the initial clinical presentation of Behçet syndrome is often confined to oral and genital ulceration. It is best to follow these patients with the possibility that they may develop further manifestations of Behçet syndrome.

10. How frequently do the various clinical symptoms of Behçet syndrome occur?

Oral aphthous ulcers	97% to 100%
Genital ulcers	75% to 90%
Ocular symptoms	30% to 80%
Arthritis	40% to 50%
Skin lesions	35% to 85%
Central nervous system disease	5% to 10%
Major vessel occlusion/aneurysm	5% to 10%
Gastrointestinal involvement	0% to 30%

11. Describe the genital ulcers in Behçet syndrome.

Aphthous ulcers similar to those in the mouth also occur on the genitalia, most frequently the scrotum and labia. They tend to heal in 1–3 weeks and are recurrent. The penis and the perianal and vaginal mucosa are less often involved. Lesions in men tend to be more painful and scar more than those in women. Scarring scrotal ulcers are considered specific for Behçet syndrome. Genital ulcers are usually deeper than oral lesions.

12. Are nonvenereal genital ulcers commonly due to Behçet syndrome?

No. Although genital ulcers are common, Behçet syndrome is a rare cause of genital ulceration overall. Venereal ulcers are the most common type of genital ulceration and include herpes simplex, syphilis, chancroid, lymphogranuloma venereum, and granuloma inguinale (donovanosis). These infections need to be ruled out in patients with suspected Behçet syndrome. Nonvenereal causes of genital ulceration include trauma (mechanical, chemical), adverse drug reactions, nonvenereal infections (nonsyphilitic spirochetes, pyogenic, yeast), vesiculobullous skin diseases, and various neoplasms such as precarcinoma (Bowen's disease) and carcinoma (basal cell carcinoma and squamous cell carcinoma). More common rheumatic causes of genital ulceration include reactive arthritis and Crohn's disease. Less common causes are A20 haploinsufficiency, MAGIC syndrome, and HIDS.

13. What are the ophthalmologic manifestations of Behçet syndrome?

Ocular lesions occur in about 50% of all patients and up to 70% of males. Intraocular inflammation and uveitis are the most common presentation and typically it is a bilateral, episodic panuveitis. Blindness is limited mostly to patients with posterior involvement (posterior uveitis, retinal vasculitis, optic neuritis) and occurs on average within the first 5 years after the onset of Behçet syndrome. Conjunctivitis, keratitis, corneal ulceration, episcleritis, and scleritis can be seen but these involve the external structures of the eye and are not typical for Behçet syndrome. Men get more severe ocular disease. All patients with Behçet syndrome need ophthalmologic screening and regular follow-up even if they do not have eye disease at onset, at least for the first 5 years after diagnosis, the time period where the likelihood of new eye disease is the highest.

14. What is a hypopyon?

It is the presence of inflammatory cells in the anterior chamber of the eye. It occurs in up to 20% of patients with Behçet syndrome-related eye disease and is a poor prognostic sign because it is frequently associated with retinal involvement. Although initially believed to be pathognomonic of ocular Behçet syndrome, hypopyon can be seen with severe B27-associated uveitis (see Chapter 74: Autoimmune Eye and Ear Disorders).

15. Describe the arthritis associated with Behçet syndrome.

Approximately 50% of patients will develop signs or symptoms of joint involvement. Arthritis is usually migratory, monoarticular or oligoarticular, and asymmetric, principally affecting the knees, ankles, elbows, and wrists. Arthritic flares typically last for 1 to 3 weeks but can last longer. Enthesopathy is common, especially in patients with acneiform lesions. Shoulders, spine, sacroiliac joints, hips, and small joints of the hands and feet are infrequently involved and should suggest another disease (e.g., HLA-B27-associated arthropathy). Arthritis may be polyarticular and occasionally resembles rheumatoid arthritis. Erosive changes are rare. Synovial fluid cell counts average 5000 to 10,000/mm³, and neutrophils predominate. Note that arthralgia is more common than arthritis in Behçet syndrome but lacks diagnostic value.

16. What are the cutaneous manifestations of Behçet syndrome?

Cutaneous lesions occur in over 75% of patients with Behçet syndrome and include the following:
- Acne or folliculitis (65%). These are histologically similar to acne vulgaris and usually not due to vasculitis; however, most patients are not teenagers, and lesions tend to occur in unusual places such as the trunk and lower extremities.
- Erythema nodosum (50%). Lobular/septal panniculitis. May have neutrophilic vasculitis.
- Superficial thrombophlebitis (25%). Any thrombotic event is a risk factor for aneurysm development so patients need to be screened for pulmonary artery aneurysms if they have thrombotic events.
- Sweet syndrome-like lesions.
- Cutaneous small-vessel vasculitis and pustular vasculitic lesions.
- Hyperirritability of skin (pathergy): common in Turkey/Japan. Rare in the United States.

17. Describe the vascular involvement in Behçet syndrome.

Behçet syndrome can involve all sizes of arteries and veins. Vascular disease is more common in men. Thrombosis of the large veins and arteries may occur, as can aortic and peripheral arterial aneurysms. Vascular thrombosis may be seen in a quarter of all patients and includes thrombosis of the superior or inferior vena cava, portal or hepatic veins (Budd-Chiari syndrome), cerebral sinuses, and pulmonary arteries. Emboli from the thromboses are rare as the thrombus is a reaction to the inflamed blood vessel walls and tends to be sticky and not form floating tails that can break off and embolize. Behçet syndrome is virtually alone among the vasculitides as a frequent cause of fatal aneurysms of the pulmonary arterial tree. **Hughes–Stovin syndrome** is a forme fruste of Behçet syndrome, characterized by deep venous thrombosis and pulmonary artery aneurysms with hemoptysis being a common presenting manifestation. In addition to large-vessel involvement, superficial thrombophlebitis and small-artery vasculitis can be seen.

18. How often do neurologic manifestations occur in Behçet syndrome?

Neurologic symptoms occur in 5% to 10% of patients, are more common in men, and tend to recur during flares of oral, genital, and joint lesions. Central nervous system (CNS) involvement, which may be life-threatening, is usually a late manifestation occurring from 1 to 7 years after the initial onset of disease. The most commonly involved region is the brainstem, particularly the mesodiencephalic junction, but any area of the brain and spinal cord can be involved and usually manifests itself as parenchymal inflammation. Parenchymal manifestations may occur in parallel with posterior uveitis. Intracranial hypertension, mostly resulting from dural sinus thrombosis, is seen in up to 20% of patients with neurologic disease and should be considered in patients with headache and ocular pain. Acute aseptic meningitis has been reported. Mortality of CNS Behçet syndrome is high (up to 40%). Unlike other vasculitic conditions, peripheral nervous system disease is rare.

19. What other organ involvement can be seen in Behçet syndrome?

- Gastrointestinal involvement is more common in Japan and the US (25–30%) and is characterized by mucosal ulcerations most commonly in the ileum and the right side of the colon. Ileocecal lesions may perforate. Stool calprotectin is elevated. Perianal involvement is rare.
- Apart from sporadic reports of valvular lesions, myocarditis, pericarditis, and coronary arteritis/aneurysms, cardiac involvement in Behçet syndrome is uncommon (5%). Usually associated with other manifestations of vascular involvement when present.
- Epididymitis occurs in 10% of men; salpingitis can occur in women.
- Renal manifestations including glomerulonephritis are uncommon (<10%).
- Amyloidosis can cause nephrotic syndrome.

20. What are the common laboratory findings in Behçet syndrome?

Laboratory parameters are nonspecific in Behçet syndrome. Inflammation markers ESR and CRP are elevated but rarely above twice the upper limit of normal. Some of the other common findings include leukocytosis, increased serum levels of immunoglobulin G (IgG), IgA, and IgM; increased α_2-globulin; elevated cerebrospinal fluid protein and cell count (in patients with neurologic involvement). These findings most often occur during disease exacerbations and can return to normal during remission.

21. What are the major causes of mortality in Behçet's disease?

- Vascular disease (ruptured pulmonary and peripheral aneurysms).
- CNS involvement
- Bowel disease (perforation).

Men, younger age at onset, and patients of Middle Eastern or Far Eastern descent usually have the worst prognosis. Mortality may be up to 15% in the first 5 years. However, disease exacerbations and mortality decrease over time. Ocular lesions causing blindness and neurologic involvement cause the most morbidity.

22. Which drugs are reported to be successful in treating the mucocutaneous lesions of Behçet's syndrome?

- Topical triamcinolone acetonide cream (0.1% in Orabase) or dexamethasone elixir (0.5 mg/5 mL) swish for 5 to 10 minutes and spit (but do not rinse) three times daily.
- Topical pimecrolimus in combination with topical corticosteroids.
- Topical sucralfate (1 g/5 mL four times a day) with or without topical corticosteroids.
- Oral colchicine, 0.6 mg two to three times daily. Especially useful for erythema nodosum and genital ulcers. Even though clinical trials have not shown major benefits in oral ulcers, colchicine is still the first choice for treatment.
- Low-dose prednisone, 5–10 mg daily as needed during flares.
- Patients who fail topicals and colchicine and cannot taper prednisone:
  - Apremilast, 30 mg twice a day. This is likely the drug of choice and also FDA approved for the oral ulcers of Behçet syndrome. It also seems to have beneficial effects on genital ulcers, skin lesions, and arthritis.
- Azathioprine, up to 2.5 mg/kg per day. Mycophenolate mofetil does not work as well as azathioprine.
- Tumor necrosis factor (TNF) α antagonists. Use with azathioprine.
- Others: dapsone, cyclosporine, thalidomide, interleukin (IL)-1 inhibitors.

23. Which immunosuppressive agents are reported to be successful in treating severe ocular Behçet syndrome?

- Topical (anterior uveitis), intraocular, and systemic corticosteroids (posterior involvement).
- Azathioprine, 2.5 mg/kg per day should be combined with corticosteroids for posterior involvement (uveitis, retina, optic nerve).
- Anti-TNFα therapy: Infliximab (5 mg/kg IV) is most commonly used. Adalimumab can also be used. Use in combination with azathioprine or other disease-modifying antirheumatic drugs.
- Cyclosporine, 2 to 5 mg/kg per day, can be added to azathioprine and anti-TNFα therapy. Cyclosporine should be used with caution in patients with CNS Behçet syndrome because it can worsen CNS symptoms. Tacrolimus, 0.1 mg/kg per day, can be used as an alternative to cyclosporine.
- Interferon-α2a is a good alternative but should be used with caution or not at all if given with azathioprine due to additive myelotoxicity (bone marrow suppression).
- Cyclophosphamide can be used in serious vascular involvement as the initial option or for other serious manifestations when other options have been tried without success.
- Others: methotrexate, mycophenolate mofetil, anakinra, tocilizumab, tofacitinib, and rituximab have been used successfully in small numbers of patients.

24. What other therapies can be useful in Behçet syndrome?

- Arthritis: colchicine. If refractory, use corticosteroids, azathioprine, methotrexate, TNF-α antagonists.
- CNS: corticosteroids, azathioprine, TNF-α antagonists, and cyclophosphamide are most commonly used. Do not use cyclosporine unless necessary to treat coexisting ocular disease.
- Gastrointestinal: corticosteroids, azathioprine, TNF-α antagonists.
- Vascular thromboses: corticosteroids and other immunosuppressives. Anticoagulation is not used commonly as the underlying cause is inflammation of the blood vessel walls. Also, patients with thrombosis are more likely to have pulmonary and other aneurysms that may rupture causing a life-threatening hemorrhage.
- Aneurysms/vasculitis: corticosteroids and azathioprine, TNF-α antagonists, cyclophosphamide. Endovascular embolization or surgery for hemorrhage.

25. Who was Behçet?

Hulusi Behçet, a Turkish dermatologist, in 1937 described a chronic relapsing syndrome of oral ulceration, genital ulceration, and uveitis that now bears his name.

26. Describe the MAGIC syndrome.

Although chondritis has been noted in association with many other rheumatic diseases, the relationship between idiopathic relapsing polychondritis and Behçet syndrome is particularly close. In 1985, Firestein and colleagues proposed the name "**M**outh **a**nd **G**enital ulceration with **I**nflamed **C**artilage" (**MAGIC**) **syndrome** in an attempt to encompass both clinical entities.

27. Describe the pathogenesis of Behçet syndrome.

The pathogenesis of Behçet syndrome remains unclear. It might not have a primary autoimmune basis. No specific antibodies or clear-cut abnormalities in B cells have been demonstrated. Infectious and other environmental triggers as well as a gut/salivary microbiota imbalance in a genetically predisposed host are postulated. Heat shock protein release interacting with Toll-like receptors can cause a release of inflammatory cytokines (e.g., IL-1) and chemokines. Genetic polymorphisms (e.g., *ERAP1*) may interfere with antigen processing and presentation leading to cytokine release (e.g., IL-12, IL-23) that promotes Th1 and Th17 cell polarization, NK cell activation, and decreased Treg cell activity. The Th1 response results in the production of proinflammatory cytokines (e.g., TNFα, IFN-ϒ) and cytotoxicity (CD8+ T cells, NK cells). The Th17 response results in production of IL-17 which promotes neutrophil chemotaxis and activation leading to NETosis. Neutrophils are a major infiltrating cell in Behcet syndrome lesions. Finally, some investigators think Behçet may be an autoinflammatory disorder; however, the rarity of fever during flares, the lack of a defined genetic locus, and the older age of onset makes this less likely.

ACKNOWLEDGMENT

The author would like to thank Dr. Sterling West for his contributions to this chapter in the previous edition.

BIBLIOGRAPHY

Bennji SM, du Preez L, Griffith-Richards S, et al. Recurrent pulmonary aneurysms: Hughes-Stovin Syndrome on the spectrum of Behçet disease. *Chest.* 2017;152:e99–e103.
Calamia KT, Schirmer M, Melikoglu M. Major vessel involvement in Behçet's disease: an update. *Curr Opin Rheumatol.* 2011;23:24–31.
Cheon JH, Kim WH. An update on the diagnosis, treatment, and prognosis of intestinal Behçet's disease. *Curr Opin Rheumatol.* 2015;27:24–31.
Esatoglu SN, Ozguler Y, Hatemi G. Disease and treatment-specific complications of Behçet syndrome. *Curr Rheumatol Rep.* 2024;26:1–11.
Hatemi G, Christensen R, Bang D, et al. 2018 update of the EULAR recommendations for the management of Behçet's syndrome. *Ann Rheum Dis.* 2018;77:808–816.
Hatemi G, Mahr A, Ishigatsubo Y, et al. Trial of apremilast for oral ulcers in Behçet's syndrome. *N Engl J Med.* 2019;381:1918–1928.
International Study Group for Behcet's Disease. Criteria for diagnosis of Behcet's disease. *Lancet.* 1990;335:1078–1080.
Imai H, Motegi M, Mizuki N, et al. Mouth and genital ulcers with inflamed cartilage (MAGIC syndrome): a case report and literature review. *Am J Med Sci.* 1997;314:330.
International Team for the Revision of the International Criteria for Behçet's Disease (ITR-ICBD). The International Criteria for Behçet's Disease (ICBD): a collaborative study of 27 countries on the sensitivity and specificity of the new criteria. *J Eur Acad Dermatol Venereol.* 2014;28:338–347.
Kalra S, Silman A, Akman-Demir G, et al. Diagnosis and management of Neuro-Behçet's disease: an international consensus recommendations. *J Neurol.* 2014;261:1662–1676.
Kidd DP. Neurological complications of Behçet's syndrome. *J Neurol.* 2017;264:2178–2183.
Kural-Seyahi E, Fresko I, Seyahi N, et al. The long-term mortality and morbidity of Behçet syndrome: a 2-decade outcome survey of 387 patients followed at a dedicated center. *Medicine.* Baltimore. 2003;82:60–76.
Saadoun D, Bodaghi B, Cacoub P. Behçet's syndrome. *N Engl J Med.* 2024;390:640–651.
Sfikakis PP, Markomichelakis N, Alpsoy E, et al. Anti-TNF therapy in the management of Behçet's disease—review and basis for recommendations. *Rheumatology.* 2007;46:736–741.
Takeuchi M, Kastner DL, Remmers EF. The immunogenetics of Behçet's disease: a comprehensive review. *J Autoimmun.* 2015;64:137–148.
Taylor J, Glenny AM, Walsh T, et al. Interventions for the management of oral ulcers in Behçet's disease. *Cochrane Database Syst Rev.* 2014;9:CD011018.
Uzun O, Erkan L, Akpolat J, et al. Pulmonary involvement in Behçet's disease. *Respiration.* 2008;75:310–321.
Vallet H, Riviere S, Sanna A, et al. Efficacy of anti-TNF alpha in severe and/or refractory Behçet's disease: multicenter study of 124 patients. *J Autoimmun.* 2015;62:67–74.
Yazici H, Seyahi E, Hatemi G, et al. Behçet syndrome: a contemporary view. *Nat Rev Rheumatol.* 2018;14:107–119.
Yazici Y, Hatemi G, Bodaghi B, et al. Behçet syndrome. *Nat Rev Dis Primers.* 2021;7:67.

FURTHER READING

http://www.niams.nih.gov/Health_Info/Behcets_Disease/.

CHAPTER 32

Relapsing Polychondritis

Meghan J. Anderson, DO and David B. Beck, MD, PhD

> ## KEY POINTS
>
> 1. Auricular chondritis can be separated from cellulitis because it does not affect the earlobe.
> 2. One-third of patients with relapsing polychondritis (RPC) will have an associated autoimmune disease (especially vasculitis) and/or hematologic disorder (myelodysplastic syndrome [MDS] most commonly).
> 3. Nasal chondritis is frequently associated with upper and lower airway involvement.
> 4. Compared to idiopathic RPC, VEXAS (vacuoles, E1, X-linked, autoinflammatory, somatic) syndrome is associated with higher mortality, greater prevalence of fevers, cutaneous disease, pulmonary infiltrates, and MDS.

1. Define RPC.

RPC is an uncommon episodic systemic disease characterized by recurrent inflammation and destruction of cartilaginous tissues. A large cohort study from the Mayo Clinic has demonstrated that 85% of patients experience episodic attacks of inflammation approximately once annually; the remaining 15% experience continuous disease activity.

2. Who gets RPC?

Patients are predominantly Caucasian, with a slight female predominance. Persons of all ages can develop RPC with a peak in the fifth decade (40–60 years). The estimated prevalence is nine cases per million. There is an association with HLA-DR4, which some studies have shown is involved in the presentation of type II collagen epitopes. A subgroup of RPC has also been linked to genetic variants in *UBA1* and *CDC42*. VEXAS syndrome is the diagnosis given to those with a pathogenic *UBA1* variant (see Question 7)

3. Briefly discuss the proposed etiopathogenesis of RPC.

The etiology of RPC is unknown but is thought to be an autoimmune process. Patients with RPC and animal models of the disease have demonstrated cellular and humoral immunity against a variety of cartilage components including collagen (types II, IX, XI), matrilin-1 (found exclusively in cartilage found in the respiratory tract and ears), and proteoglycans. In patients with RPC, the degree of immune response correlates with clinical disease activity.

An inciting agent (infectious, toxic, immunologic) has not yet been identified. However, once stimulated, activated lymphocytes and macrophages are thought to secrete mediators that induce the release of lysosomal enzymes, especially proteases. The resulting inflammatory destruction of cartilage eventually generates an attempt at repair by local fibroblasts and chondrocytes, leading to the formation of granulation tissue and fibrosis.

4. Describe the histopathology of RPC.

The histopathology of involved cartilage, regardless of location, is similar and highly characteristic. The cartilage matrix, which is normally basophilic (blue), becomes acidophilic (pink) when examined by routine hematoxylin and eosin staining. Inflammatory cell infiltrates (initially polymorphonuclear cells and later lymphocytes and plasma cells) invade the cartilage from the periphery inward. Granulation tissue and fibrosis develop adjacent to inflammatory infiltrates, occasionally resulting in sequestration of cartilage segments. Increased lipids and lysosomes in chondrocytes are demonstrated by electron microscopy. Immunofluorescence may demonstrate immunoglobulin and complement components in the tissue.

5. Is biopsy of an affected area necessary for diagnosis?

Current criteria do not require a biopsy for the confirmation of diagnosis and the procedure may precipitate severe symptoms. In addition, characteristic findings may be found in only 60% of obtained specimens. A biopsy is useful in situations where the clinical diagnosis is uncertain: lack of multiple sites of targeted cartilage involvement (bilateral ear disease is commonly considered a second site of involvement), failure to respond to prednisone and/or dapsone, or features concerning for an alternative diagnosis or associated condition. The tissue should be sent for routine histology as well as stains and cultures for mycobacteria and fungal organisms.

6. Define the McAdam and Michet diagnostic criteria for RPC (Table 32.1).

TABLE 32.1 Criteria for the Diagnosis of RPC	
(REVISED) MCADAM ET AL.[1,2]	**MICHET ET AL.[3]**
Bilateral auricular chondritis Nonerosive seronegative inflammatory polyarthritis Nasal chondritis Ocular inflammation Respiratory tract chondritis Audiovestibular damage	**Major Criteria:** • Proven inflammatory episodes involving auricular cartilage • Proven inflammatory episodes involving nasal cartilage • Proven inflammatory episodes involving laryngotracheal cartilage
The presence of 3 of 6 criteria is diagnostic of RPC. **One criterion + histologic confirmation is diagnostic.** **Two criteria + response to steroids or dapsone is diagnostic.**	**Minor Criteria:** • Ocular inflammation (conjunctivitis, keratitis, episcleritis, uveitis) • Hearing loss • Vestibular dysfunction • Seronegative inflammatory arthritis **The presence of 2 major or 1 major + 2 minor criteria is diagnostic.**

[1]McAdam LP. Relapsing polychondritis: prospective study of 23 patients and a review of the literature. *Medicine*. Baltimore. 1976;55(3):193–215.
[2]Damiani JM. Relapsing polychondritis--report of ten cases. *Laryngoscope*. 1979;89(6):929–946.
[3]Michet CJ. Relapsing polychondritis. Survival and predictive role of early disease manifestations. *Ann Intern Med*. 1986;104(1):74–78.

7. What is VEXAS Syndrome?

VEXAS is a severe, progressive, adult-onset systemic inflammatory disease due to somatic mutations in the gene *UBA1*. The acronym VEXAS stands for vacuoles, E1 enzyme, X-linked, autoinflammation and somatic, which is based on key features of the syndrome: cytoplasmic vacuoles in myeloid and erythroid progenitor cells from bone marrow aspirates, E1 refers to the ubiquitin activation enzyme that is coded by *UBA1* which is X-linked, and adult-onset autoinflammation as a result of a somatic mutation.

8. What is the pathophysiology of VEXAS syndrome?

In unaffected individuals *UBA1* expresses two protein isoforms of the E1 enzyme, the nuclear (UBA1a) and cytoplasmic (UBA1b) forms. Missense mutations affecting codon 41 (methionine) lead to a loss of the start codon of UBA1b and a shift toward an increased expression of a catalytically inactive cytoplasmic isoform (UBA1c). It remains unclear why, but the *UBA1* mutation accumulates in hematopoietic progenitor cells of the bone marrow but is restricted to myeloid cells in circulation. The exact mechanism of the disease is still unknown, but studies suggest the loss of cytoplasmic ubiquitylation results in increased cellular stress and an increase in the unfolded protein response, with subsequent elevation in multiple inflammatory cytokines.

9. What are the clinical manifestations of VEXAS syndrome?

VEXAS is a heterogenous disease, but the nearly universally shared features are late-onset disease (>50 years of age), systemic inflammation, thrombocytopenia, and macrocytic anemia in the absence of vitamin deficiency. *UBA1* variants were first identified in patients with systemic autoinflammation. However, since its discovery pathologic *UBA1* variants have increasingly been reported in Sweets Syndrome, RPC, lupus, and various vasculitides such as ANCA vasculitis, giant cell arteritis, and polyarteritis nodosa. Table 32.2 lists the clinical manifestations of VEXAS.

TABLE 32.2 Clinical Manifestations of VEXAS Syndrome

ORGAN SYSTEM	CLINICAL MANIFESTATIONS
Constitutional	Recurrent fever, elevated APR
Cutaneous	Neutrophilic dermatosis, livedo, EN, panniculitis, urticaria, ulcers
ENT	Chondritis, SNHL
Pulmonary	GGO, NSIP, bronchiolitis obliterans, nodular infiltrates
Hematologic	Thrombosis, thrombocytopenia, macrocytic anemia
Vascular	Vasculitis of any size, most commonly leukocytoclastic
Ocular	Episcleritis, uveitis, iritis, scleritis
Cardiac	<5% pericarditis or myocarditis
Neurologic	Peripheral neuropathy or mononeuritis

APR, acute phase reactant; EN, erythema nodosum; GGO, ground glass opacities; NSIP, nonspecific interstitial pneumonitis; SNHL, sensorineural hearing loss.

10. How do you diagnose VEXAS Syndrome?

Genetic testing for a somatic pathogenic variant of *UBA1* is the gold standard for diagnosis. Non-targeted testing has a low likelihood of confirming the diagnosis. However, all older males with a combination of systemic inflammation and bone marrow failure, or a bone marrow biopsy showing cytoplasmic vacuoles in myeloid and erythroid precursors, should be considered for genetic testing. Cytoplasmic vacuoles can also be seen in copper deficiency, zinc toxicity, and alcohol abuse but typically these are not associated with systemic inflammation.

PEARL: In males with relapsing polychondritis, macrocytosis, and thrombocytopenia, *UBA1* genetic testing has a 100% sensitivity and 96% specificity for the diagnosis of VEXAS syndrome.

11. Distinguish the clinical characteristics between idiopathic RPC and VEXAS-RPC.

VEXAS-RPC is more common in older men, with less airway involvement but a greater prevalence of fever, skin lesions, pulmonary infiltrates, MDS, and a higher mortality rate. See Table 32.3 for additional details.

12. Discuss the clinical features and potential complications of the auricular and nasal chondritis of RPC.

Auricular chondritis is the most frequent and characteristic clinical feature of RPC, eventually appearing in ~80% of patients. It typically presents as the sudden onset of burning pain, warmth, swelling, and purplish-red discoloration of the helix, antihelix, and sometimes tragus of one or both ears (Fig. 32.1A). Because only the cartilaginous portion is affected, the inferior soft lobules are always spared, separating it from cellulitis. Attacks may last from a few days to several weeks. Repeated inflammation may lead to cartilaginous calcification of the pinnas, which may be seen in other conditions such as frostbite as well. After one or more attacks, the external ear may lose its structural integrity owing to inflammatory dissolution of cartilage. This results in a drooping, floppy ear sometimes called "cauliflower ear" (Fig. 32.1B).

Nasal chondritis develops suddenly as a painful fullness of the nasal bridge. It is less recurrent than auricular chondritis; however, even in the absence of clinical inflammation, cartilage collapse may occur resulting in a "saddle nose" deformity (Fig. 32.2). Nasal chondritis is associated with airway involvement; its presence should prompt a computed tomography (CT) evaluation of the lungs.

TABLE 32.3 Clinical Features of RPC and VEXAS-RPC[a,b]

CLINICAL FEATURE	IDIOPATHIC RPC (%)	VEXAS-RPC (%)
Male	20	97
Fever	19	68
Auricular chondritis	67	93
Nasal chondritis	79	54
Arthritis	83	62
Ocular inflammation	28	57
Laryngotracheal symptoms	44	19
Reduced hearing	25	13
Vestibular dysfunction	52	7
Cutaneous	24	81
MDS or plasma cell dyscrasia	0	68
Pulmonary infiltrates	5	34
Cardiac	0	16
Aortitis	5	6
Death	2	13

MDS, myelodysplastic syndrome.
[a]Data from Khitri MY, Guedon AF, Georgin-Lavialle S, et al. Comparison between idiopathic and VEXAS-relapsing polychondritis: analysis of a French case series of 95 patients. *RMD Open.* 2022;8:e002255 and
[b]Ferrada MA, Sikora KA, Luo Y, et al. Somatic mutations in UBA1 define a distinct subset of relapsing polychondritis patients with VEXAS. *Arthritis Rheum.* 2021;73(10):1886–1895.

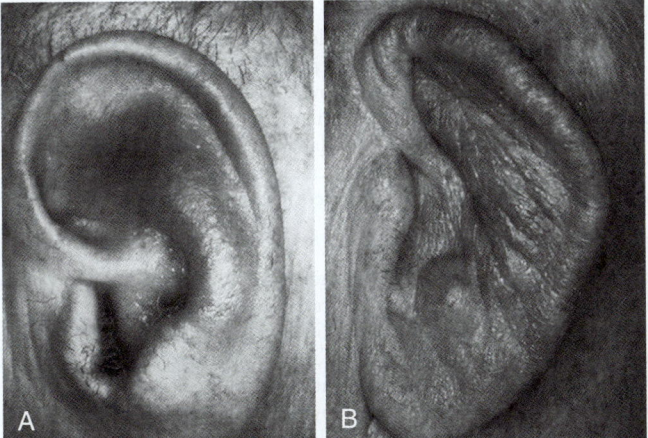

Fig. 32.1 (A) The ear in early inflammatory relapsing polychondritis. (B) Chronic collapse of the cartilaginous pinna in a patient with relapsing polychondritis (Copyright 2014 American College of Rheumatology. Used with permission.)

13. Discuss the distribution of disease, clinical symptoms, and potential complications of respiratory tract involvement in RPC.

Cartilage inflammation may occur early in the larynx and trachea, and later in the first- and second-order bronchi. In mild cases, symptoms might consist of throat tenderness, hoarseness, and a nonproductive cough. In severe cases, laryngeal and epiglottal edema may cause choking, stridor, dyspnea, or respiratory failure requiring emergency tracheostomy. Repeated or persistent

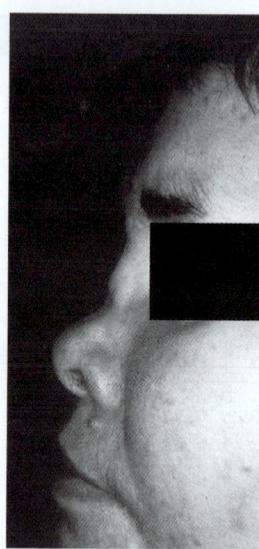

Fig. 32.2 Saddle-nose deformity due to nasal septal collapse. (Copyright 2014 American College of Rheumatology. Used with permission.)

inflammation of the airways can lead to either tracheal stenosis or dynamic airway collapse caused by dissolution of the tracheal and bronchial cartilaginous rings. Costochondritis can cause respiratory splinting and, when severe, depression of the anterior chest wall. Respiratory tract infections frequently complicate the clinical course of these patients.

14. Describe the arthritis of RPC.

The arthritis of RPC is usually an oligoarticular or polyarticular, asymmetric, nonerosive inflammatory arthritis with a predilection for the ankles, wrists, hands, and feet as well as the sternoclavicular, costochondral, and sternomanubrial joints. Tenosynovitis is common. The arthritis is typically acute, migratory, and episodic, resolving spontaneously over days to weeks. Rarely, it can become chronic. When the small joints of the hands and feet are affected, the disease may mimic seronegative rheumatoid arthritis. A report of flail chest has been described secondary to inflammatory lysis of the costosternal cartilage. Cervical, lumbar, and sacroiliac inflammation has been reported as well. The arthritis activity does not correlate with other disease manifestations of RPC.

15. Describe the ocular involvement of RPC.

Virtually every structure of the eye and surrounding tissues can be affected. Episcleritis and scleritis (including necrotizing scleritis, which can herald a systemic vasculitis) are the most common ocular manifestations occurring in about 60% of patients and potentially preceding onset of chondritis by several years. Additional manifestations include lid edema, orbital inflammatory disease, conjunctivitis, uveitis, peripheral ulcerative keratitis, retinal vasculitis, and optic neuritis. Complications due to the disease and/or therapy may include cataracts, proptosis, corneal ulcerations and thinning, and extraocular muscle palsies.

16. Discuss the audiovestibular damage in RPC.

Audiovestibular involvement presents as hearing loss, tinnitus, vertigo, and fullness in the ear (due to serous otitis media), and may occur in up to one-third of patients. Conductive hearing loss may result from inflammatory edema or cartilage collapse of the auricle, external auditory canal, and/or eustachian tubes. Sensorineural hearing loss secondary to inflammation of the internal auditory artery can also occur.

TABLE 32.4 Aortic Insufficiency: Patterns of Disease Association

PATHOLOGY	UNDERLYING CONDITION
Valvulitis	Rheumatic fever
	Rheumatoid arthritis
	Ankylosing spondylitis (AS)[a]
	Endocarditis
	Reactive arthritis (ReA)[a]
	Behçet syndrome[a]
Congenital	Bicuspid aortic valve
Dilatation of valve ring	Marfan's syndrome
	Syphilis
	Relapsing polychondritis
	Dissecting aneurysm
	Idiopathic
	Takayasu arteritis
	Giant cell arteritis
	Cogan syndrome

[a]AS, ReA, and Behçet syndrome can also cause dilatation of the valve ring.

17. Describe the cardiac manifestations of RPC.

Cardiac involvement is less common, occurring in approximately 7–20% of patients depending on the cohort examined, predominantly in male patients. Valve disease is reported in 10% of patients and typically results in aortic insufficiency. After respiratory involvement, it is the most serious complication of RPC. It is usually due to progressive dilatation of the aortic root, which may help in distinguishing it from the aortic insufficiency seen in other conditions (Table 32.4). Less frequent cardiac complications include pericarditis, myocarditis, arrhythmias, coronary aneurysms, valvulitis, and conduction defects.

18. Discuss the cutaneous manifestations of RPC.

Skin involvement occurs in about one-third of individuals and has a wide range of presentations. Oral aphthous ulcers, purpura, superficial phlebitis, livedo reticularis, ulcerations, necrosis, urticaria, and angioedema have all been described. The aphthosis may resemble Behçet disease and have the acronym **MAGIC syndrome** (mouth and genital ulcers with inflamed cartilage), an overlap of RPC and Behçet.

PEARL: Skin involvement is even more common in **VEXAS-RPC**, especially **neutrophilic dermatosis**, therefore skin involvement in the presence of chondritis should prompt systematic investigation for underlying myelodysplasia, especially in older patients.

19. How may vasculitis present in RPC?

Vasculitis may occur in up to 5% to 25% of cases and indicates a poor prognosis. Involved vessels range in size from capillaries (leukocytoclastic vasculitis) to large arteries (aortitis). Ascending thoracic aortic aneurysms may be a late manifestation. Involvement at this site may require eventual aortic grafting (see Question 30).

20. What other clinical manifestations occur in RPC?

Neurologic manifestations are rare and mainly involve the central nervous system in the form of cranial nerve damage. Other manifestations described are seizures, aseptic meningitis, encephalopathy, hemiplegia, and ataxia.

Renal disease is extremely rare (<2%) and should prompt consideration of an alternative diagnosis like ANCA-associated vasculitis.

21. What laboratory data support the diagnosis of RPC?

Laboratory abnormalities are nonspecific and generally reflective of an inflammatory state: elevated erythrocyte sedimentation rate (ESR)/C-reactive protein (CRP), leukocytosis, thrombocytosis, chronic anemia, and increased alpha and gamma globulins. Low titers of rheumatoid factor, antinuclear antibody, and ANCA may be seen. Antibodies to type II collagen have been found in approximately 30% to 40% of patients at the time of diagnosis (low sensitivity); these antibodies have also been reported in patients with rheumatoid arthritis, ankylosing spondylitis, systemic lupus erythematosus, and psoriatic arthritis among others.

22. Describe the radiographic abnormalities of RPC.

Soft-tissue radiographs of the neck may demonstrate narrowing of the tracheal air column, suggestive of tracheal stenosis. A CT and/or magnetic resonance imaging (MRI) of the lungs can more accurately define the degree of tracheal narrowing and inflammation as well as characterize the remainder of the respiratory tree. Patients with RPC and respiratory tree involvement may suffer from dynamic airway collapse; as such, CT scans should ideally include an "airway protocol" that captures dynamic images in expiration to improve sensitivity for detection of abnormalities (standard CT images are typically obtained on inspiration only).

23. What is the differential diagnosis of RPC?

Auricular chondritis due to RPC must be separated from cellulitis (*Pseudomonas, Staphylococcus*), infectious perichondritis, frostbite, recurrent trauma (wrestlers), and cocaine-induced vasculitis. Like RPC, granulomatosis with polyangiitis, syphilis, cocaine use, and lethal midline granuloma (natural killer/T cell lymphoma) can also cause saddle-nose deformities. In children, rare genetic defects can cause nasal chondritis and subsequent saddle-nose deformity, and/or myxoid degeneration of the thyroid and cricoid cartilage with laryngeal stenosis. Syphilitic aortitis, Marfan's syndrome, and several rheumatic conditions associated with ascending thoracic aortitis can cause dilatation of the aortic root (see Table 32.4). Cogan's syndrome can cause keratitis and vestibulo-auditory dysfunction.

24. Which diseases commonly coexist in patients with RPC?

Roughly one in three patients with RPC have (at the time of their diagnosis) or will develop an associated disease, with **vasculitis** and **MDS** most commonly identified. MDS with RPC is almost always due to VEXAS syndrome and should prompt genetic testing for a *UBA1* somatic mutation (see Question 11). See Table 32.5 for additional conditions associated with RPC.

25. Why is separating out ANCA-associated vasculitis from RPC important?

Several clinical features overlap between ANCA-associated vasculitis and RPC including ocular involvement (episcleritis, scleritis, orbital inflammatory disease), airway disease, and articular or auricular involvement. Low-titer ANCA antibodies can be seen in approximately 10% of true RPC as well, further contributing to difficulty in distinguishing these two conditions. Low-titer ANCA positivity in patients with RPC most often lack myeloperoxidase (MPO) and proteinase 3 (PR3) specificity, and more specific clinical features of ANCA-associated vasculitis such as cavitary lung lesions and characteristic biopsy findings (granulomatous inflammation, tissue necrosis, and vasculitis) should be absent. Distinguishing between these two conditions is important not only

TABLE 32.5 Medical Conditions Associated With RPC	
Systemic vasculitis	Behçet (MAGIC syndrome), GPA, PAN, EGPA
Rheumatologic conditions	SLE, RA, Sjogrens, spondyloarthritis, SSc
Organ-specific autoimmune conditions	Autoimmune thyroiditis, Type I diabetes, IBD, myasthenia gravis, PBC
Hematologic disorders	MDS, lymphomas, ALL, VEXAS syndrome and other myeloproliferative disorders

ALL, acute lymphoblastic leukemia; *EGPA*, eosinophilic granulomatosus with polyarteritis; *GPA*, granulomatosus with polyarteritis; *IBD*, inflammatory bowel disease; *MDS*, myelodysplastic syndrome; *PAN*, polyarteritis nodosa; *PBC*, primary biliary cholangitis; *RA*, rheumatoid arthritis; *SLE*, systemic lupus erythematosus; *SSc*, systemic sclerosis.

for prognosis but also for treatment as retrospective studies suggest a poor response to rituximab therapy in RPC unlike in ANCA vasculitis (see Question 28).

26. What clinical features help delineate prognosis in RPC?

- Nasal chondritis is associated with airway involvement and should prompt additional evaluation of the respiratory tree with CT or MRI scan imaging regardless of pulmonary symptoms.
- Airway involvement is associated with higher rates of infection as well as ICU admissions.
- Cardiac involvement is associated with a higher mortality.
- Vasculitis, male sex, and MDS (and other hematologic malignancies) are associated with a higher mortality, likely due to the high prevalence of VEXAS in these individuals.
- Neutrophilic dermatoses, including Sweet syndrome, may be especially common in patients with VEXAS-RPC and myelodysplasia.

27. Which diagnostic modalities are useful in detecting and following disease activity and cartilage damage in patients with RPC?

At baseline, all patients should undergo an evaluation by an otolaryngologist and obtain baseline pulmonary function studies (with inspiratory/expiratory flow loops), chest radiography, complete blood count (to identify anemia or other abnormalities suggestive of potential hematologic disorder), comprehensive metabolic panel, urinalysis, and ANCA, PR3, and MPO antibody testing. An ESR and CRP can be useful as well.

If patients have pulmonary symptoms, nasal chondritis (elevated risk of airway disease), or abnormal spirometry, CT or MRI of the tracheobronchial tree should be performed. Echocardiography is useful in the diagnosis and follow-up of valvular heart disease and aortic root dilatation. MR angiograms should be followed in patients with large artery involvement. Positron emission tomography has been evaluated in small research studies and may provide more accurate staging of disease as well as monitoring response to therapy, but it has not been compared with less costly imaging modalities; therefore, it is not routinely used in clinical practice. Consider a referral to ophthalmology for baseline evaluation.

28. What medications are used in the treatment of RPC?

Nonsteroidal antiinflammatory drugs, dapsone, and low-dose prednisone may be used to control minor inflammatory episodes. However, with more active disease, prednisone doses of 20 to 60 mg/day may be required until control is attained. Methylprednisolone pulses (250–1000 mg/day × 3 days) may be considered for severe disease manifestations such as acute respiratory compromise, central nervous system involvement, necrotizing scleritis, and systemic vasculitis.

Continued inflammation or an inability to taper glucocorticoids to safe maintenance doses warrants the addition of a steroid-sparing agent. Dapsone (50–200 mg/day) has been useful in patients without major organ involvement. In patients with ocular, pulmonary, or cardiovascular involvement, or with systemic vasculitis, other immunosuppressive therapies should be used. A systematic review showed that infliximab, adalimumab, tocilizumab, and methotrexate were the most effective therapies, as well as those with the most supporting data. In those with life-threatening disease, cyclophosphamide may be preferred for induction therapy along with corticosteroids, followed by maintenance therapy with a less toxic medication. Abatacept has been shown to be effective for nasal or auricular chondritis but should be avoided in cases of respiratory or neurologic disease, given reports of worsening with these specific manifestations. Results with rituximab in RPC have been largely disappointing. Plasmapheresis and intravenous immunoglobulin (2 g/kg per month) have been used as salvage therapies.

29. How do you treat VEXAS syndrome?

Patients with VEXAS syndrome are usually responsive to moderate-high dose corticosteroids (20–40 mg prednisone daily), but symptom relapse with taper below 20 mg daily is very common. There are no randomized controlled trials in VEXAS, so data is limited to case series and systematic reviews. Therapy selection is typically dictated by clinical manifestations, with most patients receiving azacytidine or bone marrow transplant in the setting of MDS. In general, conventional DMARDS, colchicine, and dapsone are ineffective. Biologic DMARDs have mixed results, with a possible trend towards greater success with inhibition of the IL-6 pathway. There have been reports of severe skin reactions in VEXAS patients receiving anakinra, so this medication is often avoided. The JAK inhibitor ruxolitinib has had promising results when used in patients with MDS. Allogeneic stem cell transplant and azacytidine are the only therapies with potential for cure. These therapies have been used with positive results in select cases, but there is a high rate of graft-versus-host disease (GVHD).

30. When does surgery play a role in the management of RPC?

Tracheostomy may be required in patients with airway collapse unresponsive to nighttime positive pressure ventilation. In such patients, extensive imaging of the entire respiratory tree is critical as severe distal involvement may be contributing primarily to symptoms and hence, tracheostomy would not be expected to aid symptoms. Caution should be taken prior to any surgical intervention as tissue disruption holds the potential for disease activation; adequate control of the inflammatory disease should occur prior to surgery if possible.

Airway obstruction caused by tracheal stenosis or tracheomalacia may require surgical resection. Endoscopic laser ablation has been described in the treatment of focal lesions. Intrabronchial stent placement has been reported as a potential remedy for dynamic airway collapse, although reports of stent-related complications are not uncommon. Aortic insufficiency may require valve replacement. In many cases, aortic insufficiency is associated with ascending aortic dilation, and improved outcomes are obtained with combined aortic valve plus aortic root/ascending aorta graft replacement (modified Bentall procedure), similar to patients with Takayasu arteritis and Behçet. Postgraft dehiscence has been described in roughly 10% of cases, unfortunately.

Surgical reconstruction of nasal septal collapse using a bone graft has been successfully described in a patient with quiescent disease, but experience in this area is limited. Cochlear implants can be used for patients with sensorineural hearing loss.

ACKNOWLEDGMENT

The authors would like to thank Dr. Marc Cohen and Dr. Jason Kolfenbach for their contributions to this chapter in prior editions.

BIBLIOGRAPHY

Cunnane G. *Relapsing Polychondritis. Kelley & Firestein's Textbook of Rheumatology.* 10th ed. Philadelphia: Elsevier; 2017:1788–1796.

Ferrada MA, Sikora KA, Luo Y, et al. Somatic mutations in UBA1 define a distinct subset of relapsing polychondritis patients with VEXAS. *Arthritis Rheumatol.* 2021;73(10):1886–1895.

Gallagher K, Al-Janabi A, Wang A. The ocular manifestations of relapsing polychondritis. *Int Ophthalmol.* 2023;43(8):2633–2641.

Imai H, Motegi M, Mizuki N, et al. Mouth and genital ulcers with inflamed cartilage (MAGIC syndrome): a case report and literature review. *Am J Med Sci.* 1997;314:330–332.

Khitri MY, Guedon AF, Georgin-Lavialle S, et al. Comparison between idiopathic and VEXAS-relapsing polychondritis: analysis of a French case series of 95 patients. *RMD Open.* 2022;8(2):1–8.

Mertz P, Sparks J, Kobrin D, et al. Relapsing polychondritis: Best Practice & Clinical Rheumatology. *Best Pract Res Clin Rheumatol.* 2023;37(1):101867.

Padoan R, Campaniello D, Iorio L, et al. Biologic therapy in relapsing polychondritis: navigating between options. *Expert Opin Biol Ther.* 2022;22(5):661–671.

Petitdemange A, Sztejkowski C, Damian L, et al. Treatment of relapsing polychondritis: a systematic review. *Clin Exp Rheumatol.* 2022;40(Suppl 134(5)):81–85.

Van Wijck RTA, Swagemakers SMA, van der Spek PJ, et al. A CDC42 Stop-loss mutation in a patient with relapsing polychondritis and autoinflammation. *J Clin Immunol.* 2023;43(1):69–71.

Axial Spondyloarthritis

Liron Caplan, MD, PhD and Rouhin Sen, MD, MS

CHAPTER 33

 KEY POINTS

1. Sacroiliitis and enthesitis are the hallmarks of the disease.
2. Non-contrast MRI of the pelvis (T1, STIR, and possibly erosion-sensitive sequences) is the preferred imaging modality for identifying the changes of axSpA.
3. HLA-B27, when negative in white patients, is good for ruling out disease.
4. Only 2–6% of HLA-B27 positive individuals develop axial spondyloarthritis during their lifetime.
5. Nonradiographic axial spondyloarthritis may be more common than radiographic axSpA.
6. TNFi, IL17i, and JAKi are very effective in axSpA for both spinal and peripheral joints.

1. What is axial spondyloarthritis? What is its relationship to ankylosing spondylitis?

Axial spondyloarthritis (axSpA) is a chronic systemic inflammatory disease affecting the sacroiliac joints, spine, and, not infrequently, peripheral joints.

Sacroiliitis evident on plain radiographs is characteristic of **ankylosing spondylitis** (AS)—the more advanced presentation of the disease. However, it typically takes 4–10 years from onset of inflammatory back pain until the development of definite radiographic sacroiliitis. Patients with axial spondyloarthritis without clear sacroiliitis on plain radiographs usually have inflammation detected on magnetic resonance imaging (MRI). These patients are said to have a **"nonradiographic" axial spondyloarthritis**, which may or may not progress over time to definite radiographic sacroiliitis. The Assessment of SpondyloArthritis International Society (ASAS) classification criteria were developed for patients with back pain greater than 3 months and age of onset less than 45 years in order to identify early disease (i.e., no clear sacroiliitis on radiographs). These criteria have a sensitivity of 83% and specificity of 84% for a patient having axSpA.

Sacroiliitis on imaging		HLA-B27
Plus	OR	plus
≥1 SpA feature		≥2 other SpA features

- **SpA features:** Inflammatory back pain, arthritis, enthesitis (heel), uveitis, dactylitis, psoriasis, Crohn's disease/ulcerative colitis, good response to NSAIDs, family history for SpA, HLA-B27 positivity, elevated C-reactive protein (CRP)
- **Sacroiliitis on imaging:** Active (acute) inflammation on MRI showing sacroiliitis; or Definite radiographic sacroiliitis

2. Describe the clinical characteristics of axSpA. How do men and women differ in their presentations?

The clinical manifestations of axSpA usually begin in late adolescence or early adulthood, with onset after age 45 being highly uncommon. It occurs slightly more commonly in males than females (2:1), though recent cohorts demonstrate a more even sex balance. AxSpA patients most commonly present with low back pain and prolonged morning (and often nocturnal) stiffness, which improves with movement and exercise. Buttock pain may initially alternate from side to side before becoming persistent. Physical examination reveals decreased spinal mobility and sometimes enthesitis, scleral injection/photophobia (uveitis/iritis), and, in advanced disease, loss of lordosis, exaggerated kyphosis, and reduced chest expansion due to costovertebral joint involvement. AxSpA is often more difficult to diagnose early in females due to less pronounced clinical features, atypical presentations (peripheral arthritis, cervical spine disease), and possibly slower development of radiographic changes.

3. **What features in the history and physical examination are helpful in differentiating inflammatory low back pain (LBP) in axSpA from mechanical low back pain?**

	Inflammatory LBP	*Mechanical LBP*
Age of onset	<40 years of age	Any age
Type of onset	Insidious	Acute (typically after injury)
Symptom duration	>3 months	<4 weeks
Morning stiffness	>60 minutes	<30 minutes
Nocturnal pain	Frequent	Absent
Effect of exercise	Improvement	Exacerbation
Effect of rest	Exacerbation	Improvement
Back mobility	Loss in all planes	Abnormal flexion
Alternating buttock pain	Present in early disease	Not present

4. **Describe three physical examination tests used to assess severity of sacroiliac joints (SIJ) and spinal joint involvement in axial spondyloarthritis. List three <u>less</u> reliable physical examination tests.**
   - **Occiput-to-wall test.** Assesses the exaggerated kyphosis in more advanced disease. Normally, with the heels and scapulae touching the wall, the occiput should also touch the wall. The distance from the occiput to the wall represents the magnitude of thoracic/cervical involvement. The tragus-to-wall test could also be used. The results of these examinations typically do not change drastically, assuming the individual is on immunosuppressive therapy.
   - **Chest expansion.** Detects limited chest mobility. Measured at the xiphisternum. Normal chest expansion varies by age and possibly sex, though usually abnormal if less than 2.5 cm and normal if 5 cm or greater.
   - **Schober test (modified).** Detects limitation of forward flexion of the lumbar spine. Place a mark at the level of the posterior superior iliac spine (dimples of Venus) and another 10 cm above in the midline (Fig. 33.1 A). With the patient in maximal forward spinal flexion with straight knees, the distance measured between the marks should increase from 10 cm to at least 14.5 cm (Fig. 33.1 B) in a young adult male. Other spinal mobility tests will show diminution in lateral flexion and spinal rotation, illustrating that the patient has a global loss of spinal mobility. Lateral flexion is measured by having the patient stand with heels and back against the wall and hands flat on the lateral thighs (neutral position, Fig. 33.1 C). The patient bends sideways toward the floor (Fig. 33.1 D) without bending knees or lifting heels. The difference in the distance of the middle finger between a neutral position and maximal lateral flexion (double-headed arrow) is recorded and averaged for left and right sides.
   - Controversial physical exam maneuvers of unclear or poor reliability: **pelvic compression**, **Gaenslen's test, Patrick's test** (knee *f*lexion, *ab*duction, and *e*xternal *r*otation (FABER) test). They also do not produce a quantifiable response. These maneuvers are <u>not</u> recommended.

5. **What is an enthesis? How does it relate to the disease process in axSpA?**
   An **enthesis** is a site of insertion of a ligament, tendon, or articular capsule into bone. In axSpA, the initial inflammatory process involves the enthesis, followed by a process that results in new

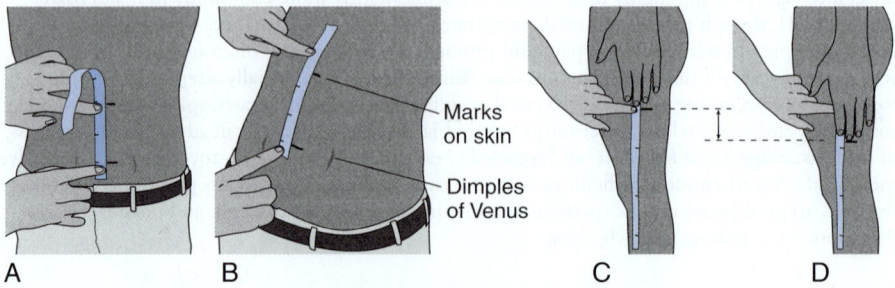

Marks on skin

Dimples of Venus

A B C D

Fig. 33.1 Schober test (modified) and lateral bending test.

bone formation or fibrosis and occasionally erosion. Sites of enthesopathy in axSpA include the sacroiliac joints (SIJ); ligamentous structures of the intervertebral discs, manubriosternal joints, symphysis pubis, attachments in the spinous processes, iliac crests (whiskering), trochanters, patellae, clavicles, and calcanei (Achilles enthesitis or plantar fasciitis).

6. Which peripheral joints are most commonly involved in axSpA?

Approximately 30% of axSpA patients develop peripheral arthritis. The hips and shoulders (girdle joints) are involved most commonly. Notably, hip involvement in axSpA is associated with a poor prognosis. Rarely, arthritis of the sternoclavicular, temporomandibular, cricoarytenoid, or symphysis pubis occurs. Involvement of the thoracic, costovertebral, sternocostal, and manubriosternal joints may cause chest pain worsened by coughing or sneezing.

7. What are the extraarticular/extraskeletal manifestations of axSpA/AS?

Remembering the first few letters of the disease's name ("Ank Spond") will help in recalling these manifestations.

A Aortic insufficiency (2–6%), ascending aortitis, and other cardiac manifestations, such as conduction abnormalities (3–5%), diastolic dysfunction, pericarditis, and ischemic heart disease (30%).

N Neurologic: atlantoaxial (C1-2) subluxation (2%), cauda equina syndrome from spinal arachnoiditis, traumatic spinal fractures with myelopathy (C5-6, C6-7 most commonly), ossification of the posterior longitudinal ligament with spinal stenosis

K Kidney: secondary amyloidosis, IgA nephropathy (5%), chronic prostatitis

S Skin: psoriasis (10%) and to a lesser extent, erythema nodosum, keratoderma blennorrhagicum, pyoderma gangrenosum

P Pulmonary: upper lobe fibrosis, restrictive changes

O Ocular: acute anterior uveitis (20–30% of patients)

N Nephropathy (IgA, 5%)

D Discitis or spondylodiscitis (Andersson lesions)

In addition, 30–60% of patients have asymptomatic microscopic colitis or Crohn's-like lesions in their terminal ileum and colon, though overt inflammatory bowel disease presents in only 7% of axSpA patients. Patients with peripheral arthritis are more likely to have colitis lesions.

8. Which human leukocyte antigen (HLA) shows a strong association with AS? Does this association vary among different racial groups?

HLA-B27 is present in 90% of white AS patients and 50–80% of non-white AS patients. The prevalence of the HLA-B27 allele is 6–9% in healthy whites and 3% in healthy North American blacks. As a result, an HLA-B27 positive individual has a 50 to 75 times increased relative risk of developing AS compared to HLA-B27 negative individuals. For white patients, this translates into a sensitivity of 90%, a positive predictive value of only 5.6%, and a negative predictive value of 99.9%. This means that a positive test is of fairly modest benefit and a negative test is good for ruling out disease, though test characteristics are generally poorer for most non-white patients.

Twin studies show a 60–75% disease concordance for AS in monozygotic twins and a 12–27% disease concordance in HLA-B27 dizygotic twins. By this analysis, genetics contributes 90% to the total risk for developing AS. HLA-B27 contributes 25–40% to the heritability of the disease. Thus, other genetic factors must contribute to the risk of developing AS (with known loci accounting for an additional 10% to the heritability), in addition to environmental factors. Over 113 non-HLA-B genetic loci have been identified, including ERAP-1 & 2, TNFα, TNFRSF1A, and IL-23R. None of these are remotely as important as HLA-B27. Genetic associations with axSpA are considerably weaker than for AS in particular. Polygenic risk scores have been published for individuals of European and East Asian descent; however, these are not available commercially or in the public domain.

9. How prevalent is AS among individuals who are HLA-B27 positive? Among individuals who are HLA-B27 positive with a relative with AS? Among different ethnic groups?

The overall prevalence of AS in the general US population is 0.3–0.5%. Only 2–6% of HLA-B27-positive persons develop AS or nr-axSpA during their lifetime. However, among those HLA-B27-positive persons with an affected first-degree relative, the rate rises to 10–20%. AS is associated with HLA-B27 in all ethnic groups, which explains why the prevalence of AS corresponds to the prevalence of HLA-B27 in a particular ethnic group. Since the prevalence of HLA-B27 in northern latitudes is high (up to 15% of Scandinavians) and low (<1% of African blacks and Asians) in ethnic populations near the equator, there is an apparent decrease in the prevalence of AS going from the north pole to the equator.

10. Describe the diagnostic algorithm for axSpA/AS. When should an HLA-B27 and other tests be ordered?

Most patients with AS can be diagnosed on the basis of history, physical examination, and the finding of sacroiliitis on radiographs, obviating the need for HLA testing. A negative HLA-B27 dramatically reduces the likelihood of AS in white patients. Up to 75% of AS patients will have an elevated ESR or CRP, which modestly predicts response to tumor necrosis factor inhibitors. However, many patients with AS will have a normal ESR and CRP. Rheumatoid factor and ANA are typically negative. IgA levels are frequently elevated in AS patients especially those who develop IgA nephropathy. See Fig 33.2.

11. What is the appropriate MRI request for evaluation of LBP in axSpA/AS?

Non-contrast MRI of the pelvis with T1 and short-tau inversion recovery (STIR) sequences. Include semi-coronal views (to visualize the SIJ along its full length). Pelvis MRI captures 95% of axSpA/AS patients—only 5% of patients require lumbar spine imaging due to a normal pelvis MRI. Emerging imaging techniques to visualize structural changes include 3D MRI sequences such as volume-interpolated breath-holding examination (VIBE) or liver acquisition with volume acceleration MRI (LAVA). These are preferred techniques for detecting SIJ erosions with higher sensitivity and reliability compared to T1-weighted sequences.

12. How is HLA-B27 hypothesized to play a role in the pathogenesis of axSpA/AS?

Infection with an unknown organism or exposure to an unknown antigen in a genetically susceptible individual (HLA-B27+) is hypothesized to result in the clinical expression of axSpA/AS. This is supported by the HLA-B27 transgenic rat model, which will spontaneously develop axial spondylarthritis in a normal habitat but will not when raised in a germ-free environment. Dysbiosis of normal bacterial flora (i.e., the microbiome) may contribute to the development of axSpA. Dysbiosis is defined as disruptions in the distribution/diversity of bacteria or perturbations in the metabolic function of these bacteria. There are four molecular hypotheses to explain the pathogenesis of axSpA:

- **Arthritogenic peptide hypothesis:** The arthritogenic response might involve specific microbial peptides that bind to HLA-B27 and then are presented in a unique manner to CD8+ (cytotoxic) T cells resulting in disease.
- **Molecular mimicry:** The induction of autoreactivity to self-antigens might develop due to similar structural elements shared by sequences or epitopes on the infecting organism or antigen and a portion of the HLA-B27 molecule or other self-peptides.
- **Free heavy chain hypothesis:** HLA-B27 heavy chains can form stable homodimers with no associated β-2 microglobulin on the cell surface. These homodimers can trigger direct activation of natural killer (NK) cells through recognition via immunoglobulin receptor (KIR)-like receptors.
- **Unfolded protein hypothesis:** HLA-B27 has a propensity to misfold in the endoplasmic reticulum causing an unfolded protein stress response. This results in the release of

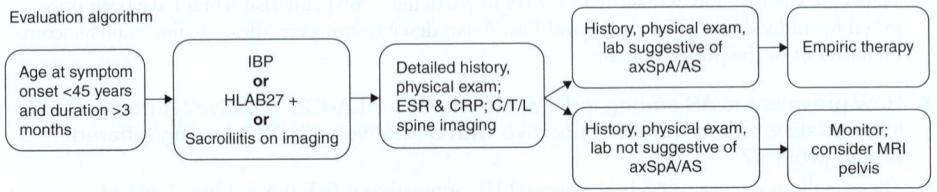

Fig. 33.2 Evaluation algorithm for axSpA/AS.

inflammatory cytokines such as IL-23 which can activate proinflammatory Th-17 cells. Notably, ERAP-1 is involved in the trimming of peptides for loading in MHC molecules (i.e. HLA-B27) in the endoplasmic reticulum. Abnormal loading may enhance misfolding of HLA-B27. As noted above, ERAP-1, ERAP-2, and IL-23R polymorphisms contribute to the genetic risk of developing AS.

13. Describe the typical features of axSpA on plain radiographs.

The radiographic changes of axSpA are predominantly seen in the axial skeleton (sacroiliac, apophyseal, discovertebral, and costovertebral) as well as at sites of enthesopathy ("whiskering" of the iliac crest, humeral greater tuberosities, ischial tuberosities, femoral trochanters, calcanei, and vertebral spinous processes). Sacroiliitis is usually bilateral and symmetric. Initially, it involves the synovial-lined lower two-thirds of the SIJ (Fig 33.3A). The earliest radiographic change is minimal erosion of the iliac side of the SIJ or sclerosis (Grade 2). Progression of the erosive process may result in moderate to significant erosions, sclerosis, widening, narrowing, or partial ankylosis of the SIJ (Grade 3), eventually followed by complete bony ankylosis or fusion of the joint (Grade 4). In cases of early sacroiliitis where plain radiographs may be normal or equivocal, a non-contrast MRI may be ordered (Fig 33.3B).

Inflammatory disease of the spine involves the insertion of the annulus fibrosis to the corners of the vertebral bodies, resulting in initial "shiny corners" (Romanus lesion) followed by "squaring" of the vertebral bodies (Fig 33.4A). Gradual ossification of the outer layers of the annulus fibrosis (Sharpey's fibers) forms intervertebral bony bridges called **syndesmophytes**. Fusion of the apophyseal joints and calcification of the spinal ligaments along with bilateral syndesmophyte formation can result in complete fusion of the vertebral column, giving the appearance of a "bamboo" spine (Fig 33.4B). Calcification of the supraspinous ligament can end caudally in a tapering point (dagger sign). Some patients develop an inflammatory destructive spondylodiscitis (Andersson lesion) that can mimic infection.

14. Name the radiographic view used to specifically visualize the sacroiliac joints.

An **anteroposterior** projection of the pelvis (AP pelvis) is often sufficient to evaluate the inferior aspects of the SIJs. The **Ferguson** view (AP with the tube angled 25°–40° cephalad) counteracts the overlap of the sacrum with the ilium, enabling a full view of the SIJ. This view is recognized because the symphysis pubis overlaps the sacrum.

15. What is the pathophysiology behind the radiographic features seen in axSpA?

Unknown. Experimental data from mouse models and cell lines support that inflammation and bone remodeling are two independent processes. These models show:
- Bone morphogenic proteins (BMP) and the WNT family of proteins may contribute to the development of calcification at sites of entheses and the SI joints. TNFα has a ying-yang effect

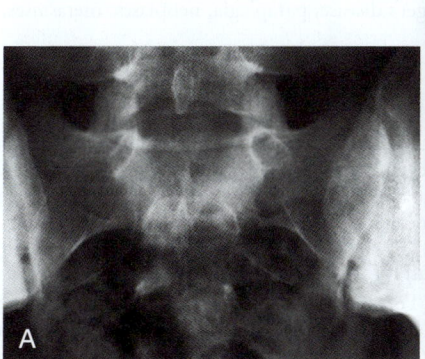
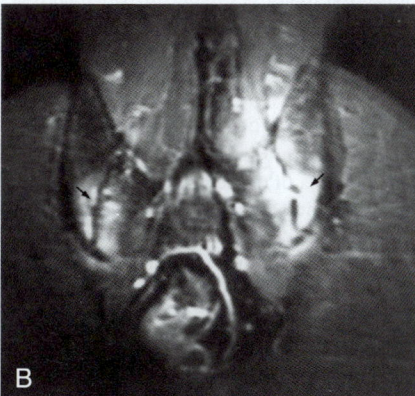

Fig. 33.3 (A) Radiograph of the pelvis demonstrating bilateral sacroiliitis. (B) Magnetic resonance image of the sacroiliac joints demonstrating edema *(arrows)* due to inflammation of these joints.

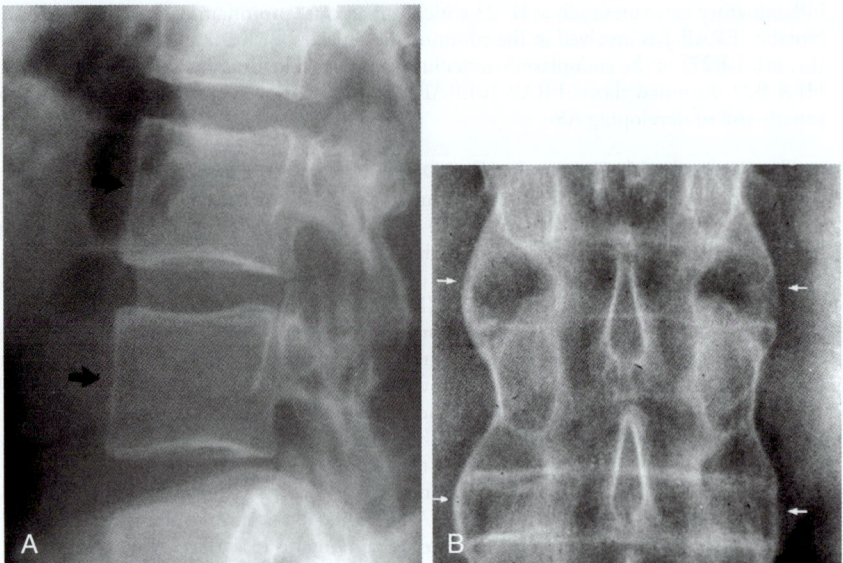

Fig. 33.4 (A) Lateral radiograph of the lumbar spine demonstrating anterior squaring of vertebrae *(arrows)*. (B) Anteroposterior radiograph of the spine demonstrating bilateral, thin, marginal syndesmophytes *(arrows)*.

on this process. It stimulates BMP production but downregulates WNT signaling through upregulation of DKK1. As of yet, genome-wide association studies have yet to implicate the WNT family of proteins in spondylarthritis.

- The presence of enthesis-resident T cells (CD3+CD4-CD8-IL-23R+) that respond to IL-23 with resultant release of IL-17 (causing local inflammation) and IL-22 (inducing osteoblast-mediated bone formation). T_H17 cells may also have direct anabolic effects on osteoblasts through the release of IL-17.
- The blood and joints of patients with SpA contain increased numbers of CD4+, CD8+, and γδ T cells as well as NK cells that elaborate granulocyte–macrophage colony-stimulating factor (GM-CSF). GM-CSF, in turn, may be partially responsible for the bone lesions in SpA.

16. What are other causes of radiographic sacroiliac joint abnormalities or the osteitis of the sacroiliac joint on MRI?

Inflammatory: spondyloarthropathies, infection (bacterial, fungal, mycobacterial septic arthritis)

Traumatic: fracture, osteoarthritis (small foci of bone marrow edema with minimal erosions), osteitis condensans ilii

Other diseases: gout, hyperparathyroidism, Paget's disease, paraplegia, neoplastic metastases, Behçet's disease

17. What is osteitis condensans ilii (OCI)?

A disorder of multiparous young women, OCI is characterized by radiographic findings of a triangular area of dense sclerotic bone only on the iliac side and adjacent to the lower half of the sacroiliac joints. Signaling on MRI T1 sequences proximal to the sacroiliac joint is hypointense with a faint rind of STIR signal surrounding the hyperintensity. This benign and typically painless condition is not a form of axSpA and is not associated with HLA-B27 status (Fig. 33.5).

18. How are AS and diffuse idiopathic skeletal hyperostosis different?

Diffuse idiopathic skeletal hyperostosis (DISH, Forestier's disease) is a noninflammatory disease occurring most commonly in obese, diabetic males aged > 50 years. It is characterized by flowing hyperostosis (bone formation), calcification of the anterior longitudinal ligament of at least four contiguous vertebral bodies, and nonerosive enthesopathies (whiskerings). The disease is not associated with sacroiliitis, apophyseal joint ankylosis, or HLA-B27. The flowing osteophytes in

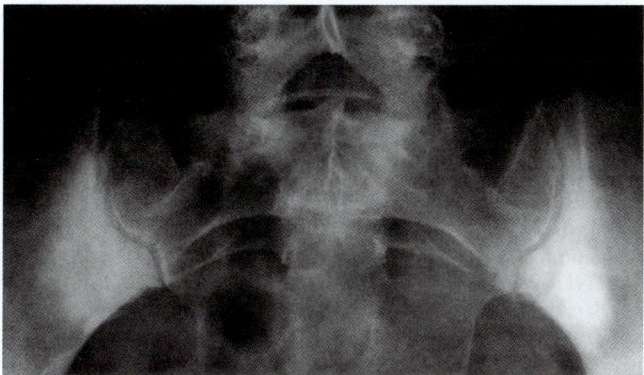

Fig. 33.5 Radiograph of the pelvis demonstrating osteitis condensans ilii.

DISH typically occur on the right side of the spine, contralateral to the heart and aorta. On a lateral spine radiograph, a linear area of radiolucency typically exists between the calcified anterior longitudinal ligament and the anterior surface of the vertebra. (See Chapter 80.)

19. Describe the typical features of axSpA on MRI.

Approximately 90% of individuals with MRI lesions typical of axSpA have a combination of both inflammatory and structural lesions and these should be evaluated contemporaneously. Active inflammatory changes on MRI include subchondral bone marrow edema on fluid-sensitive MR sequences such as STIR. Osteitis, or bone marrow edema, is especially important when proximate to the SIJ, of greater than 1 cm depth, and when associated with structural changes seen in T1 sequences. Structural changes include erosions, subchondral fat metaplasia, "backfill" (fat metaplasia in an erosion cavity), and joint space alterations (widening, narrowing, ankylosis). Sclerosis is a fairly nonspecific finding on MRI. The number of involved consecutive slices required to fulfill the definition of each feature is not universally accepted. Some have proposed for erosions in ≥2 consecutive slices or ≥3 SIJ quadrants, for bone marrow edema ≥3 consecutive slices or ≥4 SIJ quadrants, and for fat metaplasia, ≥3 consecutive slices or ≥5 SIJ quadrants.

20. Describe the natural course of axSpA.

Although the course is variable, the first 10 years predict the subsequent course of the disease. The BASDAI or ASDAS (disease activity), BASMI (spinal mobility score), and BASFI (functional index) are standardized instruments used by some clinicians to measure disease progression and response to therapy. Early factors that predict a poor prognosis include early hip joint involvement, ESR > 30 mm/hr or persistently high CRP, poor response to NSAID therapy, and early development of syndesmophytes. Extraarticular manifestations such as uveitis, cardiovascular involvement, and pulmonary fibrosis portend a poor outcome. Patients with mild axSpA have a normal life expectancy and will maintain their ability to work. However, patients with poor prognostic signs have a 3x increased risk of withdrawing from the workforce and a 1.5x increased risk of dying. Causes of death include cardiovascular disease, infections, malignancy, and (rarely) spinal fractures.

21. Which medications are helpful in the management of axSpA?

Although there is no cure for axSpA, most patients can be managed by controlling inflammatory symptoms and participating in an exercise program to minimize deformity and disability. The following modalities are helpful:

NSAIDs. These may improve symptoms to a much greater degree in axSpA compared to non-inflammatory back pain. Use of continuous celecoxib has been associated with a decrease in radiographic progression in a randomized controlled trial and observational studies. The data for other NSAIDs is less compelling. Simple analgesics can be added for additional pain relief but should not be used as primary therapy. High-dose NSAIDS for 2 weeks is considered an adequate trial, and trials with 2 NSAIDs (1 month total exposure) are recommended prior to more aggressive therapy.

TNFi therapy. These agents are highly effective in reducing the inflammatory component of axSpA including spinal mobility, function, peripheral synovitis, enthesitis, and uveitis while improving quality of life. The highest response rates (ASAS40 in 50% of patients) have been observed in younger patients with shorter disease duration and elevated CRP, but patients with advanced disease may also benefit. Concomitant therapy with methotrexate is not recommended, though some studies suggest longer drug persistence only for infliximab with methotrexate. TNFi agents should be employed for active (BASDAI ≥4) axSpA patients with predominant axial manifestations despite an adequate trial of NSAIDs. The effect of TNFi on radiographic progression is controversial. Observational data suggest that early (within 10 years of symptoms) and prolonged (>3.9 years) use decreases syndesmophyte formation. Monoclonal TNFi agents are favored in patients with uveitis or inflammatory bowel disease. Very limited data do support the use of biosimilars.

IL17Ai therapy. Secukinumab, ixekizumab, and bimekizumab have demonstrated favorable efficacy and safety profile in the axial, peripheral, and cutaneous domains of axSpA. IL17i has demonstrated a meaningful reduction in NSAID use, entheses scores, and even fatigue. Greatest effect is seen in males with elevated CRP; women with nr-axSpA had a lesser response with IL17i. IL17i does not appear to have efficacy against uveitis.

IL17A receptor therapy. In a phase III trial, brodalumab demonstrated improvements in ASAS40 response over 16 weeks. A 52-week open-label extension study is ongoing. Of note, brodalumab has been issued a black box warning for suicidal ideation that occurred in patients enrolled in RCTs.

JAKi therapy. Tofacitinib and upadacitinib appear to be effective in patients with axSpA, with improvement in disease activity, MRI scores, and physical functioning. The optimal preferred agents among TNFi, IL17i, and JAKi remains unclear.

Peripheral joint disease. Sulfasalazine (1500 mg bid)—and, to a lesser extent, methotrexate—may be beneficial in patients with NSAID-resistant peripheral arthritis but have no role in treating sacroiliitis, spondylitis, or enthesitis, according to most studies. Other conventional synthetic antirheumatic medications (leflunomide, apremilast) are not recommended.

Other biologics. Ustekinumab, abatacept, tocilizumab, and rituximab are not effective for axSpA. Although debated, **IL23i** (e.g., guselkumab) appears less effective or ineffective for axSpA, although a post hoc analysis shows a possible benefit for sacroiliitis in psoriatic arthritis patients.

Corticosteroids. Oral corticosteroids have *no* value in the treatment of the typical musculoskeletal aspects of axSpA. Local corticosteroid injections are useful in the treatment of enthesitis, peripheral synovitis (≤ 2 joints), and recalcitrant sacroiliitis.

Other treatments. Bisphosphonates and calcium/vitamin D replacement should be considered in axSpA patients with osteoporosis. Anterior uveitis can usually be managed with dilation of the pupil and corticosteroid eye drops. AxSpA patients should undergo fall evaluations and counseling.

22. How is physiotherapy used in axSpA?

Daily home exercises need to be performed to maintain good posture and chest expansion and to minimize deformities in both active and stable axSpA patients. Hydrotherapy (swimming) provides the best environment to maximize the exercise program. Patients should sleep on a firm mattress fully supine with a small neck support pillow to prevent progressive deformity. Lying prone for 15–30 minutes daily or sleeping prone at night may help prevent kyphosis. Cigarette smoking should be avoided in light of potential diminished chest expansion, apical lobe fibrosis, and its untoward cardiovascular effects.

23. When is surgery indicated in AS?

Total hip replacement is indicated in the setting of severe pain and limitation of motion. Bisphosphonates and NSAIDs may be used for 3 months after surgery to prevent postoperative calcifications around the prosthesis. Vertebral wedge osteotomy to correct severe kyphotic deformities in some patients may be considered, but it carries the risk of operative neurologic damage and should only be performed at experienced centers.

24. What is nonradiographic axial spondyloarthropathy (nr-axSpA)?

Nonradiographic axial spondyloarthritis is the diagnosis given to a patient who meets clinical criteria for axSpA but lacks evidence of sacroiliitis on plain radiographs. It may be more common than radiographic axSpA. Males and females are affected equally. Patients can have inflammatory back pain and disability that is severe. Their diagnosis is often delayed because they lack radiographic changes. MRI will show sacroiliac joint inflammation. Between 10% and 40% will progress to radiographic axSpA over 2 to 10 years. The TNFi (adalimumab, certolizumab), the IL-17i (bimekizumab, ixekizumab, and secukinumab), and JAKi (upadacitinib) are FDA approved to treat nr-axSpA.

ACKNOWLEDGMENT

The authors would like to thank Dr. Robert Janson for his contributions to this chapter in prior editions.

BIBLIOGRAPHY

Amrami KK. Imaging of the seronegative spondyloarthropathies. *Radiol Clin N Am.* 2012;50:841–854.

Lee W, Reveille JD, Weisman MH. Women with ankylosing spondylitis: a review. *Arthritis Rheum.* 2008;59:449–454.

Lories RJ, Schett G. Pathophysiology of new bone formation and ankylosis in spondyloarthropathies. *Rheum Dis Clin N Am.* 2012;38:555–567.

Magrey M, Schwartzman S, de Peyrecave N, Sloan VS, Stark JL. Nonradiographic axial spondyloarthritis: expanding the spectrum of an old disease: a narrative review. *Medicine.* Baltimore. 2022;101:e29063.

Ortolan A, Webers C, Sepriano A, et al. Efficacy and safety of non-pharmacological and non-biological interventions: a systematic literature review informing the 2022 update of the ASAS/EULAR recommendations for the management of axial spondyloarthritis. *Ann Rheum Dis.* 2023;82:142–152.

Reveille JD. Genetics of spondyloarthritis-beyond the MHC. *Nat Rev Rheumatol.* 2012;8:296–304.

Ritchlin C, Adamopoulos IE. Axial spondyloarthritis: new advances in diagnosis and management. *BMJ.* 2021;372:m4447.

Robinson PC, Brown MA. The genetics of ankylosing spondylitis and axial spondyloarthritis. *Rheum Dis Clin N Am.* 2012;38:539–553.

Sieper J, Rudwaleit M, Baraliakos X, et al. The Assessment of SpondyloArthritis International Society (ASAS) handbook: a guide to assess spondyloarthritis. *Ann Rheum Dis.* 2009;68:ii1–ii44.

Sikora KA, Colbert RA. Etiology and pathogenesis of spondyloarthritis. In: Firestein GS, Budd RC, Gabriel SE, Koretsky GA, McInnes IB, O'Dell JR, eds. *Kelley's Textbook of Rheumatology.* 11th ed. Philadelphia, PA: Elsevier; 2021:1307–1318.

van der Linden SM, Brown M, Gensler LS, et al. Ankylosing spondylitis and other forms of axial spondyloarthritis. In: Firestein GS, Budd RC, Gabriel SE, Koretsky GA, McInnes IB, O'Dell JR, eds. *Kelley's Textbook of Rheumatology.* 11th ed. Philadelphia, PA: Elsevier; 2021:1319–1343.

Voruganti A, Bowness P. New developments in our understanding of ankylosing spondylitis pathogenesis. *Immunology.* 2020;161:94–102.

Wang R, Ward MM. Epidemiology of axial spondyloarthritis: an update. *Curr Opin Rheumatol.* 2018;30:137–143.

Weber U, Lambert RGW, Ostergaard M, et al. The diagnostic utility of magnetic resonance imaging in spondylarthritis: an international multicenter evaluation of one hundred eighty-seven subjects. *Arthritis Rheum.* 2010;62:3048–3058.

Webers C, Ortolan A, Sepriano A, et al. Efficacy and safety of biological DMARDs: a systematic literature review informing the 2022 update of the ASAS-EULAR recommendations for the management of axial spondyloarthritis. *Ann Rheum Dis.* 2023;82:130–141.

FURTHER READING

www.spondylitis.org.
www.asas-group.org.

CHAPTER 34

Rheumatic Manifestations of Gastrointestinal and Hepatobiliary Diseases

Kristine A. Kuhn, MD, PhD

> **KEY POINTS**

1. Spondyloarthritis occurs in 25% of patients with IBD.
2. Episodes of SpA, axial or peripheral, often occur independent of bowel disease activity and severity.
3. Consider also celiac disease in a patient with vitamin D deficiency, GI symptoms, and an oligoarticular seronegative arthritis.
4. Autoimmune hepatitis presenting with polyarthritis and a positive ANA can mimic systemic lupus erythematosus.
5. Pancreatic cancer can release enzymes, which cause fat necrosis resulting in a triad of lower extremity arthritis, tender skin nodules, and eosinophilia (Schmidt's triad).

ENTEROPATHIC ARTHRITIDES

1. What bowel diseases are associated with inflammatory arthritis?

- Inflammatory bowel disease (IBD, Crohn's disease and ulcerative colitis) – IBD-associaited spondyloarthritis (SpA)
- Microscopic colitis (lymphocytic colitis and collagenous colitis)
- Infectious gastroenteritis
- Whipple's disease
- Celiac disease
- Bowel-associated dermatosis-arthritis syndrome (BADAS)

2. How often does a peripheral and/or axial SpA occur in patients with IBD?

Table 34.1 summarizes the prevalance of peripheral and axial SpA in IBD. Overall, the prevalance of IBD-associated SpA is ~50%. Males and females are affected equally.

TABLE 34.1 Prevalance of Arthritis in IBD (95% Confidence Interval)

ARTHRITIS PATTERN	CROHN'S DISEASE	ULCERATIVE COLITIS	ALL IBD
Peripheral	15% (12–18%)	12% (9–15%)	13% (12–15%)
Sacroiliitis*	13% (1–17%)	7% (4–11%)	10% (8–12%)
Ankylosing Spondylitis	4% (3–5%)	2% (1–3%)	3% (2–4%)

*Some of these patients have asymptomatic radiographic sacroiliitis.

3. What are the most common peripheral joints involved in ulcerative colitis (UC) and Crohn's disease?

The knees and ankles are affected most commonly, but any peripheral joint can be involved (Fig. 34.1).

4. Describe the clinical and imaging characteristics of the peripheral SpA associated with IBD.

- **Type 1:** Acute, pauciarticular, parallels IBD activity: in ~5% of IBD patients, sometimes prior to (30% of cases) or early in the course of the bowel disease and is strongly associated (80%) with flares of IBD and other extra-articular manifestations (E. nodosum, uveitis). Synovial fluid analysis reveals an inflammatory fluid [normally 5000–12,000 but can be up to 50,000

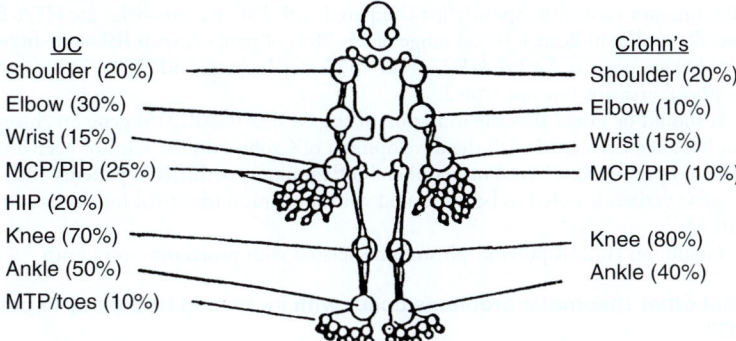

Fig 34.1. Frequency of peripheral joint involvement in ulcerative colitis and Crohn's disease.

white blood cells/mm^3 (predominantly neutrophils)] and negative crystal examination and cultures. Most arthritic episodes are self-limited with 90% resolving within 3–6 months. This type of arthritis does not result in radiographic changes or deformities. Associated with HLA-B27, B35, and DRβ1*0103.

- **Type 2:** Chronic, polyarticular, independent of IBD activity: is less common occurring in 3-4% of IBD patients. Arthritis tends to be symmetric (80%), polyarticular (MCPs> knees and ankles > other joints), runs a course independent of the activity of the IBD, and does not correlate with extraarticular manifestations (except uveitis). Active arthritis is chronic (90%) and episodes of exacerbations and remissions may continue for years. Due to its chronicity, this type of arthritis can cause erosions and deformities. Associated with HLA-B44.

5. What other extraintestinal manifestations commonly occur with IBD and peripheral SpA?

About 30 years after diagnosis, approximately 50% of patients with IBD will have developed an extra-intestinal manifestation (about 25% before diagnosis of IBD and 75% within the first 5 years of disease). Development of one extra-intestinal manifestation increases the likelihood of having a second. The most common nonarticular extra-intestinal manifestations can be remembered with the following mnemonic:

P Pyoderma gangrenosum (<2%)
A Aphthous stomatitis (<10%)
I Inflammatory eye disease (acute anterior uveitis) (2–5%): more common in Crohn's
N Nodosum (erythema) (~15%)

6. What are the clinical and imaging characteristics of axial SpA occurring in IBD?

The clinical and radiographic characteristics and course of axial arthritis in IBD are similar to those for axial SpA (see Chapter 33):

- Symptoms of inflammatory back pain are present: back pain and prolonged stiffness, particularly at night and upon awakening, that improves with exercise and movement.
- Physical examination reveals sacroiliac joint tenderness, loss of spinal motion, and sometimes reduced chest expansion (advanced cases).
- X-ray and MRI findings are compatible with axial SpA.

7. Does the activity of axial SpA correlate with the activity of the IBD?

No. The onset of sacroiliitis/spondylitis can precede by years, occur concurrently, or follow by years the onset of IBD. Furthermore, the course of the spinal arthritis is completely independent of the course of the IBD.

8. Which genes or genetic polymorphisms are linked with IBD-associated SpA?

Eight percent of normal healthy Caucasian population has the HLA-B27 gene, but a patient with IBD who possesses the HLA-B27 gene has a 7–10 times increased risk of developing an inflammatory sacroiliitis/spondylitis compared with IBD patients who are HLA-B27 negative. Overall, studies indicate a broad range of 25–78% of patients with IBD and ankylosing spondylitis (AS) are positive for HLA-B27. HLA-B27 may be increased (26%) in patients with type 1 peripheral arthritis but not type 2.

It should be noted that the mutation of the NOD2 (CARD15) gene on chromosome 16 that has been associated with the development of Crohn's disease has not been associated with an increased prevalence of axial or peripheral inflammatory arthritis in patients with IBD. However, the gene variant is noted to be associated with subclinical intestinal inflammation in patients with AS.

Finally, an IL-23R polymorphism is associated with protection from both AS and IBD.

9. What other rheumatic problems occur with increased frequency in patients with IBD?

- Achilles enthesitis/plantar fasciitis (enthesopathy)
- Granulomatous lesions of bones and joints
- Hypertrophic osteoarthropathy (periostitis) with clubbing (5%) – more common in Crohn's
- Psoas abscess or septic hip from fistula formation (Crohn's disease)
- Osteoporosis and avascular necrosis secondary to medications (i.e., prednisone)
- Vasculitis
- Amyloidosis

10. What serologic abnormalities are seen in patients with inflammatory bowel disease?

- **Inflammatory markers**: Erythrocyte sedimentation rate (ESR), C-reactive protein (CRP), serum amyloid A (SAA), and calprotectin may be elevated.
- **Autoantibodies**: Antineutrophil cytoplasmic antibody (ANCA), specifically perinuclear ANCA (pANCA), is seen in 55–70% of UC patients and < 20% of colon-predominant Crohn's patients. It is directed against lactoferrin and less commonly bactericidal permeability-increasing protein (BPI), cathepsin G, lysozyme, or elastase. It is never directed against myeloperoxidase (MPO). Rheumatoid factor and ANA are negative.
- **Antibodies to micro-organisms**: Anti-*Saccharomyces cerevisiae* (ASCA) are present in 40–70% of Crohn's disease patients and rarely (<15%) in UC patients. Antibodies to *E. coli* outer membrane protein C (OmpC) and flagellin (CBir1, Af-Fla2, Fla-X) are found in 50–60% of Crohn's and 5–10% of UC patients.

11. Which treatments are effective for IBD-associated SpA?

Table 34.2 summarizes treatments for peripheral and axial manifestations of IBD-associated SpA.

12. Why are patients with IBD prone to developing inflammatory arthritis?

The precise pathogenesis of IBD-associated SpA is unknown. There are common findings between the pathophysiology of IBD and SpA that suggest an overlap in the two disease entities. Shared genetic polymorphisms are associated with IBD and AS such as IL-23R as is microbial dysbiosis (i.e., a substantial alteration of the individual bacterial species compared to controls). In both diseases, there is a Th17-mediated inflammation characterized by increased IL-6, IL-17A, IL-17F, and IL-23. Finally, gut-derived lymphocytes and macrophages have been identified in circulation and synovial fluid of individuals with SpA; these cells express intestinal markers such as invariant T cell receptors (MAIT cells), IL-23R, IL-17a, αEβ7, α4β7, and CD163. What triggers circulation of the gut-derived cells, though, remains unknown but possibly due to microbial signals in the gut and/or increased intestinal permeability due to local inflammation.

13. What proportion of patients with AS will develop IBD?

Over half of patients with AS have microscopic inflammation of the intestine on biopsy while ~7% will have classifiable IBD. The development of worsening IBD in the setting of IL-17 inhibitors raised concern for the development of IBD in patients with AS. However, a retrospective analysis of clinical trials with secukinumab demonstrated an incidence of 0.1–0.4 cases of IBD per 100 patient-years, which is similar to the incidence of developing IBD while taking adalimumab.

TABLE 34.2 Treatment of IBD-Associated SPA

DRUG	PERIPHERAL SPA	AXIAL SPA
NSAIDs*	Yes	Yes
Corticosteroids		
Systemic	Yes	No
Intra-articular	Yes	Only for sacroiliitis
Sulfasalazine	Yes	No
Mesalamine	No	No
Methotrexate	Yes	No
Azathioprine/6MP	No	No
TNF inhibitors**	Yes	Yes
IL-23 inhibitors***	See notes	No
Other Biologics		
Vedolizumab	No	No
Ustekinumab***	See notes	No
JAK inhibitors****	Yes	Yes
Bowel Resection		
Crohn's	No	No
UC	Only for Type 1	No

*Nonsteroidal anti-inflammatory drugs (NSAIDs) may exacerbate IBD. Cox-2 selective NSAIDs may be safer.
**Anti-TNFα approved and effective include infliximab, adalimumab, golimumab, and certolizumab pegol. Etanercept is ineffective for IBD.
***Ustekinumab, risankizumab, and guselkumab are approved for use and effective in CD/UC and psoriatic arthritis.
****Tofacitinib is approved for use and effective in UC, psoriatic arthritis, RA, and AS; upadacitinib for CD, UC, psoriatic arthritis, RA, AS, GCA, and nrAxSpA.

14. Which rheumatic disorders have been associated with pouchitis, lymphocytic colitis (LC), and collagenous colitis (CC)?

Pouchitis is inflammation of the ileal pouch created following colectomy for ulcerative colitis. It occurs in up to 60% of patients having this surgery. Patients present with watery or bloody diarrhea. Treatment includes metronidazole or ciprofloxacin for 2 weeks, but some patients will develop antibiotic-refractory disease requiring immunosuppression. Surgical revision may be necessary in treatment-resistant cases. Both peripheral and axial SpA can occur.

Microscopic colitis includes both lymphocytic colitis (LC) and collagenous colitis (CC). Patients present with watery diarrhea and may develop arthritic manifestations (10–20% develop RA although peripheral and axial SpA have been reported) or autoimmune thyroiditis (>10% of patients). Patients over 65 years old (80%) and females (60%) are most commonly affected. The diagnosis is made by tissue histology obtained by colonoscopy. Budesonide is effective for inducing and maintaining clinical and histologic remission for CC and LC and loperamide may ameliorate diarrhea.

15. What rheumatic manifestations have been described in patients with celiac disease (gluten-sensitive enteropathy)?

- Arthritis (~25%)—often a seronegative, oligoarticular pattern involving predominantly large joints (knees and ankles > hips and shoulders) that may precede enteropathic symptoms in 50% of cases. There is some evidence of patients having symptoms of enthesitis or imaging evidence of sacroiliits. The arthritis responds to a **gluten-free diet** in 40–60% of cases.
- Metabolic bone disease occurs in most and can be complicated by secondary hyperparathyroidism and even osteomalacia due to steatorrhea from severe enteropathy causing vitamin D deficiency. Some of these patients are mistakenly diagnosed as fibromyalgia with irritable bowel syndrome.
- Dermatitis herpetiformis is present in 15–25% of individuals with celiac disease and usually responds to a gluten-free diet. Dapsone can also be used.
- In adults, rheumatoid arthritis is more likely (2x) to occur in patients with celiac disease while in children, juvenile idiopathic arthritis is 3x more likely to occur.

16. What human leukocyte antigen (HLA) is found in patients with celiac disease and how does it contribute to the development of the disease?

Celiac disease occurs as an autoimmune reaction to wheat gluten/gliadin by T and B lymphocytes in the gut of genetically predisposed individuals. It is a relatively common disease affecting 1:70 to 1:300, most often in individuals of Northern European ancestry. *HLA-DQ2* and/or *-DQ8* (usually in linkage with *HLA-DR3*) is seen in 99% of celiac disease patients compared with 40% of the normal population. Dietary gluten is partly digested by gastric enzymes to form a 33-amino acid peptide that is deaminated by tissue transglutaminase increasing its immunogenicity. The immunogenic gliadin peptide is then presented in the context of *HLA-DQ2* or *DQ8* to CD4+ T cells, resulting in interferon-γ release and inflammation, altered gut permeability, and villous atrophy. Only 66% have characteristic bowel symptoms whereas others will present with arthritis, vitamin D or B_{12} deficiency, iron deficiency anemia, cerebellar disease, infertility, or peripheral neuropathy. It is more likely to occur in patients with other *HLA-DR3*-associated autoimmune diseases such as Sjogren's, type I diabetes mellitus, autoimmune thyroid disease, or autoimmune liver disease.

17. How is the diagnosis of celiac disease made?

The gold standard is jejunal biopsy showing villous atrophy. However, autoantibody testing is very helpful in screening individuals prior to biopsy. On a gluten-rich diet in people who are not IgA deficient, IgA antibodies against **tissue transglutaminase** have a high sensitivity (95%) and specificity (90%) for celiac disease. Due to poor specificity, anti-gliadin antibodies are no longer used to screen for celiac disease.

18. What is bowel-associated dermatosis-arthritis syndrome (BADAS)?

BADAS is a neutrophilic dermatosis and arthritis that occurs in patients with gastrointestinal disorders. Historically it occurred in ~20% of patients who underwent intestinal bypass surgery for morbid obesity, but it can also occur in patients with IBD, diverticular disease, other bowel surgeries, and as a rare consequence of bacterial overgrowth in patients with poor intestinal peristalsis (systemic sclerosis, colorectal surgery). Affected patients develop a flu-like syndrome consisting of fevers, malaise, arthritis, myalgia, and rashes. The arthritis is nonerosive, inflammatory, oligoarticular, and frequently migratory, affecting both the upper and lower extremities, including small and large joints. The rash is maculopapular or vesiculopustular usually on the upper extremities and trunk. The pathogenesis involves bacterial overgrowth in a blind loop of bowel resulting in antigenic stimulation causing immune complex formation (frequently cryoprecipitates containing bacterial antigens, secretory IgA, and complement) in the serum that deposits in the joints and skin. Treatment includes NSAIDs, corticosteroids, and oral antibiotics, which usually improve symptoms. Only surgical reanastomosis of the blind loop can result in complete elimination of symptoms.

RHEUMATIC SYNDROMES AND PANCREATIC DISEASE

19. What pancreatic diseases have been associated with rheumatic syndromes?

Pancreatitis, pancreatic carcinoma, and pancreatic insufficiency.

20. What are the clinical features of the pancreatic, panniculitis, and polyarthritis (PPP) syndrome?

PPP is a systemic syndrome occurring in some patients (1–3%) with pancreatitis or pancreatic acinar cell carcinoma due to release of trypsin, lipase, and amylase from the diseased pancreas causing fat necrosis. It can occur at any age although most patients are older adults. A good way to remember the clinical manifestations is the mnemonic PANCREAS:

P= Pancreatitis

A= Arthritis (60%) and arthralgias, usually of the ankles and knees. Synovial fluid is typically mildly inflammatory and may be creamy in color due to lipid droplets that stain with Sudan black or oil red O. Lipid crystals may be present and are positively birefringent.

N= Nodules that are tender, red and usually on the extremities. These are frequently misdiagnosed as erythema nodosum but are areas of lobular (not septal) panniculitis with fat necrosis. Fasciitis due to subcutaneous fat necrosis can also be seen.

C= Cancer of the pancreas more commonly causes this syndrome than does pancreatitis.

R= Radiographic abnormalities due to osteolytic bone lesions from bone marrow necrosis (10%)

E= Eosinophilia. The triad of arthritis, nodules, and eosinophilia is called **Schmidt's triad**.

A= Amylase, lipase, and trypsin are elevated due to release by a diseased pancreas and cause fat necrosis in skin, synovium, and bone marrow.

S= Serositis, including pleuropericarditis frequently with fever

21. What other musculoskeletal problems can occur with pancreatic insufficiency?

Osteomalacia due to fat-soluble vitamin D malabsorption.

RHEUMATIC SYNDROMES AND HEPATOBILIARY DISEASE

22. What is autoimmune hepatitis (AIH)?

Autoimmune hepatitis (previously referred to as chronic active hepatitis) is an inflammatory disease of the liver characterized by acute hepatitis, cirrhosis, or liver failure as well as circulating autoantibodies. AIH affects all ages and races and is subdivided into type 1 (AIH-1) and type 2 (AIH-2). **Type 1 (AIH-1)** can occur in all age groups (bimodal peak 10–20, 45–70 years old), but most patients are young and predominantly female (70%). It was previously referred to as lupoid hepatitis. Many patients have clinical (e.g., arthralgias, rashes) and laboratory (e.g., ANA) manifestations that resemble systemic lupus erythematosus (SLE). Patients commonly have positive antinuclear antibodies (ANA, 70%), antibodies against smooth muscle antigen (SMA)/anti-F-actin antibodies (FA) (up to 85%), anti-soluble liver antigen/liver pancreas antibodies (SLA/LP, 10–30%), anti-dsDNA antibodies (25–35%), and anti-neutrophil cytoplasmic antibodies (atypical p-ANCA, 20–65%). Hypergammaglobulinemia is usually present. AIH-1 can overlap with other autoimmune diseases such as autoimmune thyroiditis, type 1 diabetes, IBD, celiac disease, psoriasis, and, more rarely, rheumatoid arthritis, Sjogren's syndrome, SLE, MCTD, and limited systemic sclerosis.

Type 2 (AIH-2) is predominantly a pediatric disease and presents with manifestations of liver disease/failure. These patients typically have anti-liver-kidney microsomal-1 antibodies (LKM1, 70%) and anti-liver cytosol antibodies (LC1, 30%).

23. To what degree is type 1 autoimmune hepatitis similar to SLE?

TABLE 34.3 Comparison Between Type 1 Autoimmune Hepatitis and SLE

	TYPE 1 AIH	SLE
Young women	+	+
Fever, fatigue, weight loss	+	+
Rash	+	+
Photosensitivity	–	+
Polyarthritis	+	+
Oral ulcers	–	+
Nephritis	–	+
Central nervous system disease	–	+
Polyclonal gammopathy	+	+
ANA	70%	99%
Anti-Smith (Sm) antibodies	–	25%
Anti-dsDNA antibodies	25%–35%	70%
Anti-smooth muscle antibody (ASMA)	Up to 85%	–
Anti-SLA/LP	10%–30%	–

24. List the common autoimmune diseases associated with primary biliary cirrhosis (PBC).

PBC is an autoimmune disease of the liver marked by slow progressive destruction of the small bile ducts. Bile cholestasis leads to tissue damage with fibrosis and cirrhosis. It is more common in females (9:1). Up to 80% have antimitochondrial antibodies (AMA). The most specific anti-mitochondrial antibody is the M2 antibody directed against the E2 subunit of the pyruvate dehydrogenase complex on the inner mitochondrial membrane. Many patients with PBC have one or more additional autoimmune disorders:

- Keratoconjunctivitis sicca (secondary Sjögren's syndrome)—40–60%
- Autoimmune thyroiditis (Hashimoto's disease)—10–15%
- Arthritis—5–10% with classic seropositive RA while another 10% may have a seronegative, non-RA arthritis characterized by a self-limited, symmetric, polyarticular synovitis
- Limited scleroderma occurs in 5–15% of PBC patients and antedates PBC by 14 years. Most have anticentromere antibodies.
- Others: Raynaud's phenomenon, pernicious anemia, celiac disease, IBD, SLE, polymyositis

25. What other musculoskeletal manifestations may occur in patients with PBC?

- Osteomalacia due to fat-soluble vitamin D malabsorption
- Osteoporosis due to renal tubular acidosis
- Hypertrophic osteoarthropathy

26. What dose adjustments need to be made for antirheumatic medications in patients with severe hepatobiliary disease?

Severe liver disease can be defined as a combination of one or more of the following factors: elevated bilirubin > 3 mg/dl, albumin < 3 gm/dl with ascites, elevated protime (PT/INR) not fully corrected by vitamin K, and/or cirrhosis on liver biopsy. Elevated transaminases greater than 3 times upper limit of normal should also be a concern. Also note that since creatine is synthesized in the liver, serum creatinine may be an overestimate of renal function.

Hepatobiliary disease may substantially impair the elimination or activation of drugs that the liver metabolizes or excretes. Although glucuronidation is spared, oxidation and acetylation are slowed. In addition, decreased synthesis of albumin may lead to increased free fraction of the active drug. Decreased synthesis of vitamin K–dependent clotting factors may lead to increased risk of bleeding if a medication affects platelet function or number.

The following are guidelines for antirheumatic drug therapy in severe liver disease:

- **Pro-drug metabolism**—azathioprine, leflunomide, cyclophosphamide, prednisone, and sulindac need to be converted to the active moiety by the liver. This is impaired in patients with severe hepatic insufficiency. Consequently, these drugs should be avoided or replaced with active form (i.e., 6-mercaptopurine, prednisolone).
- **Biliary excretion**—methotrexate, cyclosporine, colchicine, leflunomide, indomethacin, and sulindac are excreted in the bile and undergo enterohepatic circulation. These should be avoided in patients with impaired biliary function.
- **Change in drug dosage for severe liver disease**
  - Acetaminophen: Use up to a max dose of 2 g/day.
  - Antimalarials: Use with caution and at lower doses. ACR guidelines recommend avoidance in patients with Child-Pugh class C liver disease.
  - Anti-TNFα: Probably safe. Avoid in setting of untreated hepatitis B, but may be safe during treatment. Safe in hepatitis C. Frequent liver enzyme monitoring is advised.
  - Allopurinol: Little data. Use with caution. Can cause severe hepatitis.
  - Anifrolumab: Not metabolized by liver. Probably safe but little data.
  - Apremilast: No adjustment necessary.
  - Avacopan: Can cause liver toxicity. Avoid or use with caution. Do not use in Child-Pugh class C.
  - Azathioprine: Use 6-mercaptopurine instead but use at low dose with caution since toxicity can occur quickly.
  - Bisphosphonates: Probably safe.

- Biologics (other): Little data. Would avoid or use tocilizumab with caution since it can have liver toxicity. Avoid all in setting of viral hepatitis.
- Colchicine: Avoid.
- Cyclophosphamide: May not be converted to active form.
- Cyclosporine and tacrolimus: Eliminated by liver, so avoid.
- Febuxostat: Metabolized by the liver. Can cause liver toxicity. Avoid or use with caution at lower doses.
- JAK inhibitors: Litte data, but pharmacokinetic studies of tofacitinib indicate 70% hepatic metabolism and 30% renal excretion for clearance of the drug. Thus, a dose adjustment is likely needed for Child-Pugh class B and recommend avoidance in class C. No information on viral hepatitis. Similar recommendations for adalimumab. JAKi can cause liver enzyme elevations.
- Leflunomide: Avoid.
- Methotrexate: Avoid.
- Mycophenylate mofetil: No dosage change, but don't exceed 2 g/day.
- Narcotics: Most metabolized by liver. Fentanyl and hydromorphone safest. Need to lower dose or extend interval. Avoid meperidine.
- NSAIDs: Lower dose 50%. Avoid diclofenac, sulindac, and indomethacin. Note that NSAIDs even at low doses increase risk of bleeding and renal failure.
- Prednisone: Use prednisolone or methylprednisolone instead.
- Sulfasalazine: Use with caution and at lower doses. Can cause hepatic failure rarely. ACR guidelines recommend avoiding Child-Pugh C liver disease
- Tramadol: Double dosing interval from 6 to 12 hours. Start at dose of 25 mg.

BIBLIOGRAPHY

Altaffer AL, Weiss P. Clinical features, treatment, and outcomes of celiac-associated arthritis: a retrospective cohort study. *Pediatr Rheumatol Online J.* 2023;21(1):43. doi:10.1186/s12969-023-00822-x.

Aromolo IF, Simeoli D, Maronese CA, et al. The Bowel-Associated Arthritis-Dermatosis Syndrome (BADAS): a systematic review. *Metabolites.* 2023;13(7):790. doi:10.3390/metabo13070790.

Delco F, Tchambaz L, Schlienger R, et al. Dose adjustment in patients with liver disease. *Drug Safety.* 2005;28:529–545.

Doyle JB, Lebwohl B, Askling, et al. Risk of juvenile idiopathic arthritis and rheumatoid arthritis in patients with celiac disease: a population-based cohort study. *Am J Gastroenterol.* 2022;117(12):1971–1981.

Ellinghaus D, Jostins L, Spain SL, et al. Analysis of five chronic inflammatory diseases identifies 27 new associations and highlights disease-specific patterns at shared loci. *Nat Genet.* 2016;48(5):510–518.

Ely Garnetta M, Perruquet James L, Newman Eric D. The arthritis of primary biliary cirrhosis: clinical features and associated immune processes. *J Clin Rheumatol.* 1996;2(4):191–196.

Gatselis NK, Zachou K, Koukoulis GK, Dalekos GN. Autoimmune hepatitis, one disease with many faces: etiopathogenetic, clinico-laboratory and histological characteristics. *World J Gastroenterol.* 2015;21(1):60–83.

Karreman MC, Luime JJ, Hazes JMW, Weel A. The prevalence and incidence of axial and peripheral spondyloarthritis in inflammatory bowel disease: a systematic review and meta-analysis. *J Crohns Colitis.* 2017;11(5):631–642.

Le C, Zeffren N, Kramer N, Rosenstein ED. Rheumatologic associations of microscopic colitis: a narrative review. *Mod Rheumatol.* 2023;33(3):441–447.

Marx WJ, O'Connell DJ. Arthritis of primary biliary cirrhosis. *Arch Intern Med.* 1979;139:213–216.

Narvaez J, Bianchi MM, Santo P, et al. Pancreatitis, panniculitis, and polyarthritis. *Semin Arthritis Rheum.* 2010;39: 417–423.

Ondrejcakova L, Gregova M, Bubova K, Senolt L, Pavelka K. Serum biomarkers and their relationship to axial spondyloarthritis associated with inflammatory bowel diseases. *Autoimmun Rev.* 2024;23(3):103512. doi:10.1016/j. autrev.2023.103512.

Raiteri A, Granito A, Giamperoli A, Catenaro T, Negrini G, Tovoli F. Current guidelines for the management of celiac disease: a systematic review with comparative analysis. *World J Gastroenterol.* 2022;28(1):154–175.

Rogler G, Singh A, Kavanaugh A, et al. Extraintestinal manifestations of inflammatory bowel disease: current concepts, treatment, and implications for disease management. *Gastroenterology.* 2021;161:1118–1132.

Schreiber S, Colombel JF, Feagan BG, et al. Incidence rates of inflammatory bowel disease in patients with psoriasis, psoriatic arthritis and ankylosing spondylitis treated with secukinumab: a retrospective analysis of pooled data from 21 clinical trials. *Ann Rheum Dis.* 2019;78(4):473–479.

Selmi C, Generali E, Gershwin ME. Rheumatic manifestations in autoimmune liver disease. *Rheum Dis Clin North Am.* 2018;44:65–87.

Watt FE, James OFW, Jones DEJ. Patterns of autoimmunity in primary biliary cirrhosis patients and their families: a population-based cohort study. *Q J Med.* 2004;97:397–406.

FURTHER READING
HTTP://WWW.CELIAC.ORG.
HTTP://WWW.CCFA.ORG.
HTTP://WWW.NIDDK.NIH.GOV.
HTTP://WWW.AASLD.ORG.

CHAPTER 35

Reactive Arthritis

Itziar Quinzaños Alonso, MD

Can't see, can't pee, can't climb a tree.

—Author unknown

 KEY POINTS

1. Reactive arthritis (ReA) is a sterile inflammatory arthritis, typically preceded by a gastrointestinal or genitourinary infection occurring 1 to 4 weeks prior.
2. ReA is largely a clinical diagnosis, based on clinical findings, medical history, and direct and/or indirect detection of the pathogen.
3. Similar to other spondyloarthropathies, patients with ReA are more likely to be HLA-B27 positive, which portends a worse prognosis and more joint and extraarticular manifestations.
4. Long-term antibiotics may help chronic *Chlamydia*-induced ReA but do not affect the course of ReA associated with enteric pathogens.
5. Over 50% of patients have a self-limited course lasting 3 to 5 months, 30% have recurrent episodes, and 15% to 20% have a chronic course requiring immunosuppressive therapy.

1. Define ReA.

ReA is a sterile inflammatory synovitis occurring within 4 weeks of an infection elsewhere in the body, primarily urogenital or enteric infections. The arthritis is typically an asymmetric oligoarthritis that predominantly involves large lower extremity joints. The causative organism cannot be cultured from fluid in the joint cavity; however, in recent years it has been shown that bacterial products of the triggering microbe can be detected in the synovial fluid or synovial tissue of the affected joints. ReA patients are frequently HLA-B27 positive and commonly exhibit systemic symptoms with unique extraarticular manifestations including skin, eye, and enteropathic features.

2. What is Reiter's syndrome?

As originally described in 1916, Reiter's syndrome is the clinical triad of conjunctivitis, nongonococcal urethritis, and arthritis following infectious dysentery. For many years, ReA and Reiter's syndrome were used as synonyms. This term is no longer used due to Hans Reiter's participation in Nazi medical experimentation during World War II. The triad is now considered to be a subset of ReA because two-thirds of patients do not have all three features.

3. How is ReA acquired? What is the influence of HLA-B27?

Susceptibility to ReA may be conferred by the specific class I major histocompatibility antigen, HLA-B27. However, the development of ReA is strictly dependent on infection with certain organisms predominantly acquired through mucosal surfaces, enterogenic or urogenital (see Question 6). In hospital-based reports, HLA-B27 is present in 60% to 80% of patients with ReA. These patients tend to have more severe arthritis, extraarticular manifestations, higher prevalence of sacroiliitis, and a protracted course. Notably in population-based studies, patients with ReA are less likely to be HLA-B27-positive (30% or less in some ethnic groups). These cases have a milder oligoarthritis with fewer systemic symptoms or extraarticular manifestations.

4. What is the role of HLA-B27 in ReA pathogenesis?

There are several hypotheses to date. (1) **Misfolding hypothesis:** HLA-B27 folds more slowly than other HLA types when assembled in the endoplasmic reticulum. This may cause inadequate folding and instability of HLA-B27 leading to accumulation of such molecules with activation of inflammatory processes. (2) **Arthritogenic peptide hypothesis:** postulates that HLA-B27 on antigen-presenting cells present microbial peptides that may mimic certain self-peptides (molecular mimicry) to CD8 cytotoxic T lymphocytes, leading to autoimmunity. Alternatively, the similarity between the microbial and self-peptides may allow microbial fragments to persist due to an inadequate immune response. (3) **Heavy-chain homodimer hypothesis:** HLA-B27 can be expressed on the cell surface as a homodimer of heavy chains without ß-2 microglobulin. These abnormal chains can activate natural killer, T, and B cells.

5. What are other potential factors involved in the pathogenesis of ReA?

Since patients who are HLA-B27-negative also develop ReA, other focus of investigations favors the role of microbial factors. Some examples of these theories are (1) the ability of certain outer membrane proteins of some of the involved organisms (*Salmonella*) to stimulate specific interleukin (IL) responses (IL-17 and IL-23) in synovial cells; (2) finding metabolically active particles (*Chlamydia*) in the synovial tissue of patients with chronic ReA; and (3) alteration of the gut microbiota leading to an abnormal immune response.

6. What infectious agents trigger ("cause") ReA?

Urogenital	***Chlamydia*** *trachomatis*[a,f], *Ureaplasma urealyticum*[b,f], *Mycoplasma genitalium*[b,f]
Enterogenic	***Salmonella***[a,f] *typhimurium, S. enteritidis, S. heidelberg, S. cholerae-suis, Paratyphi B and C*
	Shigella[a,f] *flexneri, S. dysenteriae, S. sonnei*
	Yersinia[a,f] *(especially O:3, O:8 and O:9), Y. pseudotuberculosis*
	Campylobacter[a,f] *jejuni, C. Coli*
	Clostridium difficile[b]
	Escherichia coli[b], *Diarrhogenic strains*
	Giardia lamblia[b]
Respiratory	*Chlamydia pneumoniae*[b,f]
	Group A beta-hemolytic Streptococcus[b,c]
Viral	*Human immunodeficiency virus*[b,d]
	SARS-CoV2[a]
Multiple sources, case reports only[e]	*Helicobacter pylori*
	Vibrio parahaemolyticus
	Mycobacterium bovis
	Calmette-Guerin Bacillus
	Klebsiella pneumonia
	Strongyloides stercoralis[d]

Note: In up to 40% of ReA patients, an infectious agent cannot be identified. Serologic tests especially for *Chlamydia* may identify a previous infection if cultures/PCR are negative.
[a]Common infections associated with ReA. Also, most common infections are associated with HLA-B27-patients.
[b]Uncommon infections associated with ReA.
[c]Typically causes acute rheumatic fever, but has been described to cause ReA.
[d]ReA has occurred in the setting of HIV, but usually the virus is not directly associated and other pathogens may be implicated.
[e]Not full list but prominent case reports. For a more comprehensive list please consult the article by Zeidler H et al in bibliography.
[f]Documented reports of identification of bacterial products in the joint by various methods.
[g]Controversial, case series/reports from worldwide compilations present 50 + patients with a ReA pattern arthritis (a lower limb predominant, oligoarticular, asymmetric pattern with axial and enthesitis symptoms often coexistent) after documented COVID-19 infection.

7. Who gets ReA?

Primarily young adults aged 20 to 40 years. Because the prevalence of bacterial triggers can vary widely in populations and over time, the incidence and prevalence also vary accordingly. Patients with enterogenic ReA exhibit higher relative risk for women than for men (1.5:1), whereas those with the urogenital form are predominantly men. ReA is rare in children and less common in African Americans. ReA is one of the most common types of inflammatory arthritis affecting young adult men. Approximately 1% to 3% of patients with nonspecific urethritis develop a ReA.

8. After the initial infection, when do symptoms of ReA first appear?

Although the initial infection may be mild or inapparent (10–30%), most patients will develop systemic symptoms within 1 to 4 weeks.

9. **List the extraarticular manifestations associated with ReA.**

Constitutional	Genitourinary
Low-grade fever	Infectious urethritis
Weight loss (rare)	Sterile dysuria
	Prostatitis
Ocular	Hemorrhagic cystitis
Sterile conjunctivitis (35%, typically during acute stages only)	Salpingitis, vulvovaginitis
Anterior uveitis (20%) (acute unilateral, HLA-B27-positive)	**Mucocutaneous** Circinate balanitis (30%, most frequently associated with *Chlamydia*)
Scleritis, pars planitis, iridocyclitis (rare)	Keratoderma blennorrhagicum (15%)
Gastrointestinal	Hyperkeratotic nails (10%)
Infectious ileitis/colitis	Painless oral ulcers (25%)
Sterile ileitis/colitis (60%)	Erythema nodosum (*Yersinia*)
	Renal (case reports only)
Cardiac (rare in acute disease)	IgA nephropathy
Heart block (1%)	Renal amyloidosis
Aortic regurgitation	**Other** (case reports only)
Aortitis (1%)	Thrombophlebitis, livedo reticularis
Pericarditis (rare)	Neuropathy (cranial or peripheral nerve)

Note: The frequency of the various extraarticular manifestations depends on both the inciting infectious agent and if the patient is HLA-B27-positive.

10. **What two cutaneous lesions are characteristic of ReA?**

Circinate balanitis and **keratoderma blennorrhagicum** are relatively specific for ReA. Circinate balanitis is a painless, serpiginous ulceration of the glans penis. Similarly, keratoderma blennorrhagicum refers to psoriasiform lesions occurring primarily on the plantar surface of the heel and metatarsal heads. Both lesions are predominantly associated with urogenital ReA (*Chlamydia*) and resolve spontaneously.

11. **Describe the musculoskeletal manifestations of ReA.**

Arthritis: In ReA, the joints tend to be moderately inflamed and characterized by prolonged stiffness. Joint involvement is typically asymmetric, oligoarticular (less than five joints), and confined to the knees, ankles, and/or feet. Large joint effusions, especially in the knees, are not unusual. Hip involvement is rare. Upper limb arthritis (e.g., wrist and digits) may also occur (50%) but is never more prominent than the lower extremity arthritis. Uncommonly it can be a polyarthritis. Arthritis always lasts over 1 month, though usually longer. Joint erosions may result from chronic disease.

Enthesitis: An inflammation of the ligament, tendon, joint capsule, or fascia insertion site into bone (enthesis). In ReA, enthesitis commonly causes heel pain (Achilles tendon and plantar fascia), metatarsalgia (plantar fascia), and iliac spine/crest pain. Enthesitis is common in ReA and may help distinguish it from other differential diagnoses.

Dactylitis: "Sausage" digits of fingers and toes are due to a combination of arthritis, enthesitis, and tendinitis.

Sacroiliitis/spondylitis: Up to 40% of patients with ReA may have axial skeleton symptoms, and 25% develop radiographic changes. The risk of developing sacroiliitis and/or spondylitis is related to disease chronicity and HLA-B27.

12. **What is the differential diagnosis for ReA?**

Most Likely	Less Likely
Gonococcal arthritis	Ankylosing spondylitis
Acute septic arthritis	Rheumatic fever
Psoriatic arthritis	Gout/pseudogout
Inflammatory bowel disease arthritis	Lyme disease
Rheumatoid arthritis	Behçet's syndrome
	Secondary syphilis

13. Compare the clinical features of ReA with gonococcal arthritis.

A comparison of the clinical features of ReA with gonococcal arthritis is given in Table 35.1.

14. Compare the clinical features of ReA with rheumatoid arthritis.

A comparison of the clinical features of ReA with rheumatoid arthritis is given in Table 35.2.

TABLE 35.1 A Comparison of the Clinical Features of Reactive Arthritis With Gonococcal Arthritis

FEATURE	REACTIVE	GONOCOCCAL
Sex ratio	Male > female	Female > male
Age	20–40 years	All ages, most 20–40 years
Migratory arthralgias	No	Yes
Arthritis	Lower limbs	Upper limbs, knees
Enthesitis	Yes	No
Spondylitis	Yes	No
Tenosynovitis	Yes	Yes
Dactylitis	Yes	No
Urethritis	Yes	Yes
Uveitis	Yes	No
Oral ulcers	Yes	No
Cutaneous lesions	Keratoderma, balanitis	Pustules
Culture-positive	No	Yes (<50%)
HLA-B27-positive	Yes (up to 80%)	Same as general population
Cephalosporin responsive	No	Yes

TABLE 35.2 A Comparison of the Clinical Features of Reactive Arthritis With Rheumatoid Arthritis

FEATURE	REACTIVE ARTHRITIS	RHEUMATOID ARTHRITIS
Sex ratio	Male > female	Female > male
Age	20–40 years	All ages (most frequently: women aged 40–60 years, men older)
Arthritis	Oligoarticular	Polyarticular
	Large joints (asymmetric)	MCP, PIP, wrist, MTP (symmetric)
Enthesitis	Yes	No
Spondylitis	Yes	No
Ocular disease	Conjunctivitis, uveitis	Keratitis, scleromalacia, sicca, scleritis
Lung disease	No	Yes
Urethritis	Yes	No
Cutaneous lesions	Keratoderma, balanitis	Subcutaneous nodules, vasculitis
Rheumatoid factor positive	No	Yes (85%)
HLA association	HLA-B27 (80% of white males)	HLA-DR4 (70%)

HLA, human leukocyte antigen; *MCP*, metacarpophalangeal; *MTP*, metatarsophalangeal; *PIP*, proximal interphalangeal.

15. Which laboratory investigations are useful in confirming the diagnosis of ReA?

The diagnosis of ReA is clinical, and no laboratory investigation can substitute for a proper history and physical examination. However, they can be used in confirming the clinical diagnosis. Arthrocentesis is the most valuable test because it excludes septic and crystalline arthritis (Table 35.3).

16. What are the usual synovial fluid findings from a patient with ReA?

The synovial fluid typically reveals a predominance of leukocytes, ranging from 2000 to 50,000 cells/mm^3. In acute ReA, most of these cells are neutrophils, but in chronic disease, either lymphocytes or monocytes may be prevalent.

Other synovial fluid characteristics include decreased viscosity, normal glucose level, and increased protein. Large vacuolar macrophages (Reiter's cells) containing intact lymphocytes or fragmented nuclei are occasionally seen but are not specific for ReA. Synovial fluid polymerase chain reaction (PCR) for *Chlamydia* can be done but has not been validated.

TABLE 35.3 Laboratory Investigations Useful in Confirming the Diagnosis of Reactive Arthritis

	EXPECTED RESULT
Primary (essential)	
ESR and/or CRP	Elevation
Complete blood count and differential	Polymorphonuclear leukocytosis
	Thrombocytosis and anemia of chronic disease
Rheumatoid factor	Negative
Urinalysis	Pyuria, microhematuria +/− bacteria
Synovial fluid analysis	Moderate leukocytosis
	Negative Gram stain and no crystals
Cultures and/or PCR	
—Throat	(+/−) (*Chlamydia*)
—Urine	(+/−) (*Chlamydia*)
—Stool	(+/−) (*Yersinia* and *Salmonella* can persist for weeks)
—Synovial fluid	Negative cultures
—Urethra/cervix	(+/−) (*Chlamydia*)
—Sputum	(+/−) (*Chlamydia pneumonia*)
Secondary (optional)	
Antinuclear antibody	Negative
Antibody serology	Positive (e.g., *Yersinia*, *Shigella*, and *Chlamydia*)
Blood cultures	Negative, unless septic
Radiographs	
• Peripheral joints	Arthritis, enthesitis
• Axial joints	Spondylitis, enthesitis
• Anteroposterior pelvis	Sacroiliitis
Electrocardiogram	Heart block
Colonoscopy	Ileitis/colitis

Note: In 40% of reactive arthritis patients an infectious agent cannot be identified. Urine polymerase chain reaction for *Chlamydia* and stool cultures may be helpful in patients with urethritis or diarrhea, respectively. Serologic tests for *Chlamydia*, *Salmonella*, and *Yersinia* can be done depending on the suspected inciting agent.
CRP, C-Reactive protein; *ESR*, erythrocyte sedimentation rate; *PCR*, polymerase chain reaction.

17. Describe the radiographic features seen in patients with ReA.

Remember your **ABCDE'S.** These radiographic features are typical of all seronegative spondyloarthropathies.

A—**A**nkylosis of the spine occurs in up to 20% to 25% of patients. There are large nonmarginal syndesmophytes called "jug-handle" syndesmophytes, which usually occur in an asymmetric distribution. These syndesmophytes can also occur in psoriatic spondylitis but differ from the thin, marginal, bilateral syndesmophytes seen in ankylosing spondylitis (Fig. 35.1).

B—**B**ony reactivity and proliferation at enthesis sites (Achilles tendon and plantar fascia insertions) and periostitis are common. Ossification of tendons may occur. **Bone demineralization** (periarticular osteopenia) may be observed.

C—**C**artilage space narrowing occurs uniformly across the joint space of weight-bearing joints compatible with inflammatory arthritis. No soft tissue **calcifications** are seen.

D—**D**istribution of arthritis is primarily in the lower extremity, whereas psoriatic arthritis usually affects the upper extremity. The sentinel joint involved may be the interphalangeal joint of the great toe (Fig. 35.2).

E—**E**rosions are common in the metatarsophalangeal joints (Fig. 35.2). Sacroiliac joint erosions tend to involve one joint more than the other (asymmetric), which contrasts to the symmetric involvement of ankylosing spondylitis (Fig. 35.3).

S—**S**oft tissue swelling and dactylitis (diffuse swelling of toes).

18. How do the radiographic features of sacroiliac and spine involvement in ReA compare with those in ankylosing spondylitis?

Note that 100% of patients with ankylosing spondylitis develop radiographic changes in the sacroiliac joints compared with only 20% to 25% of ReA patients (Table 35.4). Patients with inflammatory bowel disease also develop radiographic changes of their spine similar in appearance to those of ankylosing spondylitis, whereas psoriatic arthritis produces changes similar to ReA.

Note: Unilateral sacroiliitis without peripheral arthritis does not occur in ReA and should suggest another diagnosis (e.g., infection).

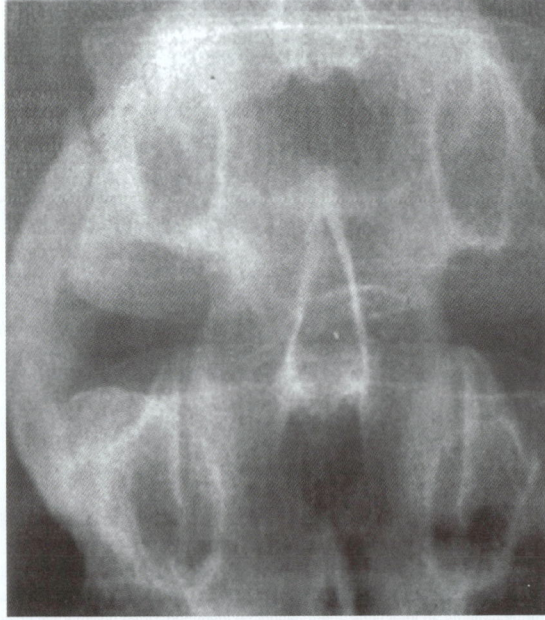

Fig. 35.1 Radiograph of the spine showing a large "jug-handle" syndesmophyte.

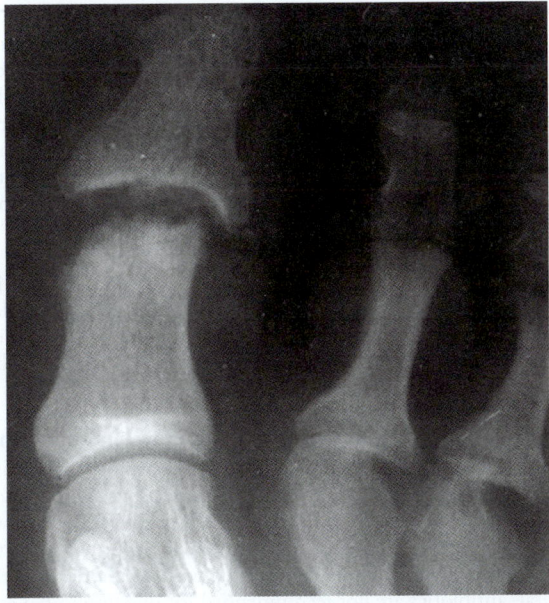

Fig. 35.2 Radiograph of the foot in a patient with reactive arthritis showing erosions of the interphalangeal joint of the great toe and second and third metatarsophalangeal joints.

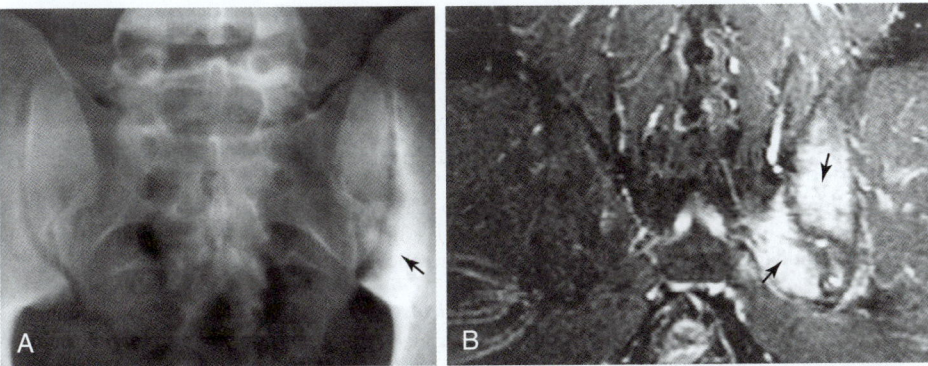

Fig. 35.3 (A) Radiograph of pelvis showing left sacroiliitis *(arrows)*. (B) Magnetic resonance image of pelvis showing left sacroiliitis *(arrows)*.

TABLE 35.4 Radiographic Features of Sacroiliac and Spine Involvement in Reactive Arthritis in Comparison With Those in Ankylosing Spondylitis

	ANKYLOSING SPONDYLITIS	REACTIVE ARTHRITIS
Sacroiliitis	Bilateral, symmetric	Unilateral or asymmetric
Spondylitis	Bilateral, thin, marginal syndesmophytes	Asymmetric, nonmarginal, "jug-handle" syndesmophytes

19. Is HLA-B27 determination useful?

A sufficient number of patients with ReA will not be HLA-B27-positive, thus rendering HLA-B27 determination a poor diagnostic test in screening patients for ReA, especially because 7% of the normal white population will be positive. Patients with ReA can usually be successfully diagnosed and managed without HLA-B27 determination. However, many rheumatologists find it useful to classify patients as having either "HLA-B27-associated" or "non-associated" forms of ReA since HLA-B27 positivity correlates with an increase in disease severity, chronicity, and frequency of exacerbations as well as development of aortitis, uveitis, and spondylitis.

20. Describe the nonpharmacologic management of ReA.

Initial management begins with rest of the affected joints. Transient relief of joint inflammation may be obtained by use of ice packs and/or warm compresses. Once inflammation subsides (1–2 weeks), **passive** strengthening and range of motion exercises should be initiated. Progression to **active** exercises reduces the likelihood of muscle atrophy. Avoidance of behavior promoting reinfection is critical.

21. Describe the pharmacologic management of the initial infection in ReA.

Elimination of the "triggering" infection with appropriate antibiotics is the first therapeutic goal in ReA. This is especially true for acute *Chlamydia* infections (azithromycin 1 g single dose or doxycycline 100 mg twice daily for 7 days, patient and partner). Patients with a history of *Chlamydia*-related ReA should be evaluated for recurrent genitourinary infection if arthritis or genitourinary symptoms recur and should be retreated with antibiotics if testing for *Chlamydia* is positive. In general, antibiotics are not recommended for uncomplicated enteric infections. However, some patients with enteric infections may require treatment depending on their comorbidities (e.g., age, immunocompromised) and/or severity of disease and type of organism (e.g., *C. difficile*).

22. Describe the pharmacologic management of the extraarticular manifestations in ReA.

The mucocutaneous features of ReA are usually self-limited and may require no specific therapy. Topical corticosteroids and keratolytic agents may help keratoderma blennorrhagicum. Symptoms of uveitis should be referred for urgent ophthalmologic evaluation.

23. Describe the pharmacologic management of the arthritis in ReA.

The following algorithm is a stepwise approach to the treatment of acute and chronic ReA (Fig. 35.4). Chronic ReA is defined as symptoms lasting >6 months not controlled with nonsteroidal antiinflammatory drugs (NSAIDs) and intraarticular glucocorticoids.

24. Should long-term antibiotics be used in *Chlamydia*-related ReA?

In chronic *Chlamydia*-related ReA, chlamydial organisms have been demonstrated in a metabolically active state in the synovial tissue; therefore, antibiotic therapy has been trialed. Results are mixed in randomized trials of long-term therapy with single antibiotics, and most do not show benefit. By contrast, there is one prospective, double-blind, triple-placebo trial of the combination of either doxycycline (100 mg twice a day) plus rifampin (300 mg daily) or azithromycin (500 mg daily for 5 days, then twice a week) plus rifampin for 6 months that showed antibiotics to be effective therapy in patients with chronic *Chlamydia*-induced ReA. Improvement of joint symptoms (63% versus 20%) and increased rate of remission (22% versus 0) was seen. Further studies with larger numbers of patients are required to confirm these findings, but a trial of antibiotics in patients with chronic *Chlamydia*-related ReA could be trialed.

25. Should long-term antibiotics be used in enteric-ReA?

No. Antibiotic therapy for common postenteric-associated ReA has not been demonstrated in trials to reduce the severity of arthritis. The demonstration of bacterial cell wall antigens but not nucleic acid in the synovial tissue suggests that bacterial antigens alone (not viable microorganisms) may perpetuate this type of ReA and therefore antibiotics are not effective.

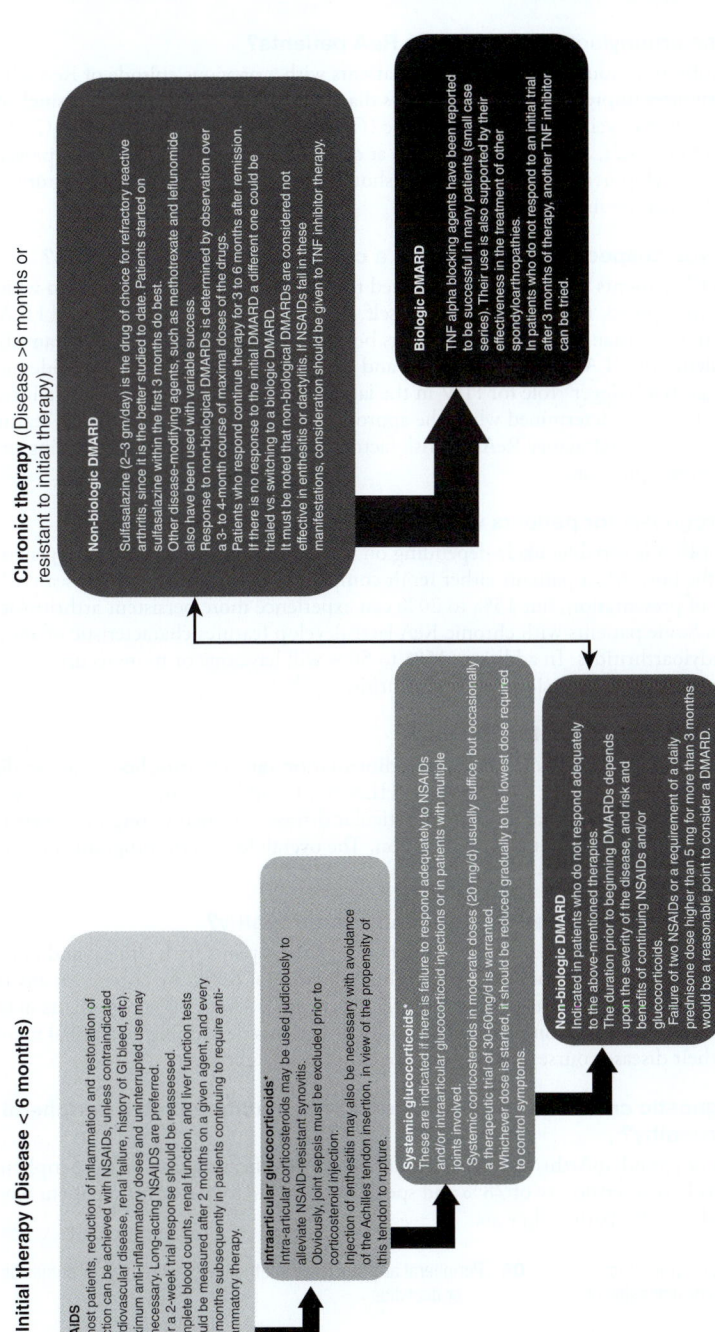

Initial therapy (Disease < 6 months)

NSAIDS

In most patients, reduction of inflammation and restoration of function can be achieved with NSAIDs, unless contraindicated (cardiovascular disease, renal failure, history of GI bleed, etc). Maximum anti-inflammatory doses and uninterrupted use may be necessary. Long-acting NSAIDS are preferred.
After a 2-week trial response should be reassessed.
Complete blood counts, renal function, and liver function tests should be measured after 2 months on a given agent, and every 3-6 months subsequently in patients continuing to require anti-inflammatory therapy.

Intraarticular glucocorticoids*

Intra-articular corticosteroids may be used judiciously to alleviate NSAID-resistant synovitis.
Obviously, joint sepsis must be excluded prior to corticosteroid injection.
Injection of enthesitis may also be necessary with avoidance of the Achilles tendon insertion, in view of the propensity of this tendon to rupture.

Systemic glucocorticoids*

These are indicated if there is failure to respond adequately to NSAIDs and/or intraarticular glucocorticoid injections or in patients with multiple joints involved.
Systemic corticosteroids in moderate doses (20 mg/d) usually suffice, but occasionally a therapeutic trial of 30-60mg/d is warranted.
Whichever dose is started, it should be reduced gradually to the lowest dose required to control symptoms.

Non-biologic DMARD

Indicated in patients who do not respond adequately to the above-mentioned therapies.
The duration prior to beginning DMARDs depends upon the severity of the disease, and risk and benefits of continuing NSAIDs and/or glucocorticoids.
Failure of two NSAIDs or a requirement of a daily prednisone dose higher than 5 mg for more than 3 months would be a reasonable point to consider a DMARD.

Chronic therapy (Disease >6 months or resistant to initial therapy)

Non-biologic DMARD

Sulfasalazine (2–3 gm/day) is the drug of choice for refractory reactive arthritis, since it is the better studied to date. Patients started on sulfasalazine within the first 3 months do best.
Other disease-modifying agents, such as methotrexate and leflunomide also have been used with variable success.
Response to non-biological DMARDs is determined by observation over a 3- to 4-month course of maximal doses of the drugs.
Patients who respond continue therapy for 3 to 6 months after remission.
If there is no response to the initial DMARD a different one could be trialed vs. switching to a biologic DMARD.
It must be noted that non-biological DMARDs are considered not effective in enthesitis or dactylitis. If NSAIDs fail in these manifestations, consideration should be given to TNF inhibitor therapy.

Biologic DMARD

TNF alpha blocking agents have been reported to be successful in many patients (small case series). Their use is also supported by their effectiveness in the treatment of other spondyloarthropathies.
In patients who do not respond to an initial trial after 3 months of therapy, another TNF inhibitor can be tried.

*There is no evidence (anecdotal or published) of the disease worsening with the use o f intraarticular or systemic glucocorticoids, despite the infectious trigger of ReA.

NSAID- Nonsteroidal anti-inflammatory drugs
DMARD- Disease-modifying antirheumatic drugs

Fig. 35.4 Algorithm for initial and chronic therapy for reactive arthritis.

26. Should you use prophylactic antibiotics in ReA patients?

Prophylactic antibiotics should be considered in patients with a previous episode of ReA who later develop urethritis after unprotected sex or traveler's diarrhea. Azithromycin (1 g) as a single dose for urethritis, or azithromycin (1 g) as a single dose (*Campylobacter*) plus ciprofloxacin (750 mg) as a single dose (*Salmonella*, *Shigella*, and *Yersinia*) at onset of diarrhea has anecdotally prevented the subsequent redevelopment of ReA. Probiotics should be used in patients with a history of ReA due to *C. difficile* when antibiotics must be used.

27. When should you suspect that ReA may be a complication of HIV infection?

ReA is seen in HIV patients but is generally believed to be related to other infections to which patients have been exposed, rather than to HIV itself. An association between ReA and HLA-B27 has been noted in Caucasian HIV-infected patients but not in patients from sub-Saharan Africa where the prevalence of HLA-B27 is much lower and ReA was rare before the HIV epidemic. This finding suggests a "trigger" role for HIV in the latter population. Given the uncertainty, HIV antibody status should be determined when the appropriate risk factors and/or clinical features are present. Patients with refractory ReA and risk factors for HIV should also have testing prior to the use of immunosuppression.

28. What is the prognosis for patients with ReA?

The prognosis of ReA is variable, likely depending on the triggering pathogen and the genetic background of the host. Most patients either remit completely or have little active disease within 6 to 18 months of presentation, but 15% to 20% can experience more persistent arthritis/or axial skeleton disease. Some patients with chronic ReA later develop features characteristic of another one of the spondyloarthritides. In addition, 15% to 50% will have one or more recurrences of ocular disease, mucocutaneous lesions, and/or arthritis.

29. What are poor prognostic factors in ReA?

Reinfection, male sex, hip arthritis, erythrocyte sedimentation rate >30 mm/hour, sausage digits, poor response to NSAIDs, genetic susceptibility (HLA-B27), and heel pain are associated with a poorer prognosis. In general, disability due to articular disease is related to responsiveness to medication in the absence of spontaneous remission. The overall long-term prognosis for post-dysenteric ReA is better than post-*Chlamydia* ReA.

30. What is an undifferentiated peripheral spondyloarthropathy?

The term *undifferentiated spondyloarthritis* is used to designate patients with clinical and radio-graphic features consistent with spondyloarthritis but who do not fulfill the criteria for any of the established disease categories (e.g, ReA or psoriatic arthritis). About 40% of patients may be undifferentiated upon presentation, with the majority of patients developing additional manifestations later in their disease course enabling a more definitive diagnosis.

31. Are there diagnostic criteria to identify patients with undifferentiated peripheral spondyloarthropathy?

The Assessment of SpondyloArthritis International Society classification criteria for peripheral spondyloarthritis have a sensitivity of 78% and specificity of 83% for detecting a patient who has peripheral spondyloarthropathy. They are:

Peripheral arthritis (asymmetric lower extremity) or enthesitis or dactylitis	**OR** Peripheral arthritis (asymmetric lower extremity) or enthesitis or dactylitis
Plus, one of the following: HLA-B27; genitourinary/gastrointestinal infection; psoriasis; inflammatory bowel disease; or magnetic resonance imaging showing sacroiliitis.	Plus, two of the following: arthritis; enthesitis; dactylitis; inflammatory back pain; family history of spondyloarthropathy.

ACKNOWLEDGMENT

The author would like to thank Dr. Richard Meehan for his contributions to this chapter in the previous editions.

BIBLIOGRAPHY

Adizie T, Moots RJ, Hodkinson B, et al. Inflammatory arthritis in HIV positive patients: a practical guide. *BMC Infect Dis.* 2016;16:100.

Barber CE, Kim J, Inman RD, et al. Antibiotics for treatment of reactive arthritis: a systematic review and metaanalysis. *J Rheumatol.* 2013;40:916–928.

Carter JD, Hudson AP. Recent advances and future directions in understanding and treating chlamydia-induced reactive arthritis. *Expert Rev Clin Immunol.* 2017;13:197–206.

Carter JD, Hudson AP. Reactive arthritis. In: Firestein GS, Koretsky GA, Budd RC et al, eds. *Firestein & Kelley's Textbook of Rheumatology.* 11th ed. Philadelphia, PA: Elsevier; 2021:1344–1358.

Colmegna I, Cuchacovich R, Espinoza LR. HLA-B27-associated reactive arthritis: pathogenetic and clinical considerations. *Clin Microbiol Rev.* 2004;17:348–369.

Courcoul A, Brinster A, Decullier E, et al. A bicentre retrospective study of features and outcomes of patients with reactive arthritis. *Joint Bone Spin.* 2018;85:201–205.

Hannu T. Reactive arthritis. *Best Pract Res Clin Rheumatol.* 2011;25(3):347–357.

Manasson J, Shen J, Helga R, et al. Gut microbiota perturbations in reactive arthritis and post-infectious spondyloarthritis. *Arthritis Rheumatol.* 2018;70:242–254.

Meyer A, Chatelus E, Wendling D, et al. Safety and efficacy of anti-tumor necrosis factor α therapy in ten patients with recent-onset refractory reactive arthritis. *Arthritis Rheum.* 2011;63:1274–1280.

Migliorini F, Bell A, Vaishya R, Eschweiler J, Hildebrand F, Maffulli N. Reactive arthritis following COVID-19 current evidence, diagnosis, and management strategies. *J Orthop Surg Res.* 2023;18:205.

Schmitt SK. Reactive arthritis. *Infect Dis Clin North Am.* 2017;31:265–277.

Zeidler H, Hudson AP. Reactive arthritis update: spotlight on new and rare infectious agents implicated as pathogens. *Curr Rheumatol Rep.* 2021;23:53.

FURTHER READING

https://www.spondylitis.org.

CHAPTER 36

Arthritis Associated With Psoriasis and Other Skin Diseases

Elena Weinstein, MD

> ### KEY POINTS
>
> 1. Inflammatory joint disease occurs on average in 20% to 25% of patients with psoriasis.
> 2. Psoriatic arthritis (PsA), like other forms of spondyloarthritis, can be associated with uveitis, bowel inflammation, and mucosal ulcerations.
> 3. Dactylitis, enthesitis, and tenosynovitis are common musculoskeletal features accompanying PsA.
> 4. Agents that inhibit tumor necrosis factor α (anti-TNFα), interleukin (IL)-12/23, IL-17, and IL-23 are effective for peripheral arthritis as well as skin disease.
> 5. Psoriatic patients have a higher mortality rate due to an increased incidence of metabolic syndrome and premature atherosclerosis.

1. How prevalent is psoriasis and PsA in the general population?

Epidemiologic studies suggest that the prevalence of psoriasis is approximately 2% to 3%. Whites are affected (two times) more often than other ethnic groups. Men and women are equally affected. Peak incidence is in the fourth decade of life. A meta-analysis in 2019 demonstrated that while there is variability among ethnic groups and severity of psoriasis, 20–25% of patients with psoriasis develop psoriatic arthritis.

2. Do genetic and environmental factors play a role in PsA?

Yes. Twin studies, family studies, and genome-wide association studies (GWAS) suggest a genetic predisposition to PsA. Concordance among monozygotic twins ranges from 35% to 70%, versus 12% to 20% for dizygotic twins. Epidemiologic studies have found that first-degree relatives of PsA patients are 40 times more likely to develop arthritis. Up to 40% of patients with PsA have a family history of psoriasis.

PsA is a polygenic disorder. GWAS have identified numerous possible associated genes. HLA-C*06:02 is associated with severe, early-onset skin psoriasis but less clearly with PsA. HLA-B*08 is associated with asymmetric sacroiliitis while HLA-B*27 is associated with symmetric sacroiliitis and spondylitis. Major histocompatibility complex class I genes (HLA-B*08:01, B*27:05, B*38:01, B*39:01) with a glutamate at position 45 as well as 30 non-HLA susceptibility loci (e.g. IL-23R) have been found to be associated with peripheral and/or axial PsA.

Evidence suggests that trauma and infection may play a role in PsA. Trauma to a joint (deep Koebner phenomenon) is reported in 25% of patients before the onset of a patient's PsA. Subclinical trauma may explain distal interphalangeal (DIP) involvement. Bacterial agents such as streptococcal pharyngitis have been reported before the onset of guttate psoriasis. Obesity increases the risk of PsA in psoriasis patients.

Gut dysbiosis and gut inflammation are associated with SpA including PsA but clarity as to whether this is a cause-effect relationship, or a correlation, is still needed from ongoing and future studies.

3. How does juvenile PsA typically present?

Notably, only 2% of children with psoriasis develop PsA. Unlike adults in whom skin psoriasis precedes the development of PsA, patients with juvenile PsA typically develop their skin psoriasis years after they present with their musculoskeletal manifestations. Therefore, a family history of psoriasis or PsA may be an important clue to diagnosing juvenile PsA. Juvenile PsA accounts for only 5% of all children with juvenile idiopathic arthritis (JIA) and may be difficult to separate from other JIA subsets. There are two main ways that juvenile PsA presents:

- *Polyarticular or oligoarticular-extended subset*: typically occurs between the ages of 6 and 12 years (usually adolescents) and affects boys and girls equally. There is a high association with HLA-B27. Enthesitis, dactylitis, nail pitting, and axial involvement are common.

- *Oligoarticular subset*: typically presents around 2 years of age, is more common in females, and is associated with positive antinuclear antibody, dactylitis, and painless chronic uveitis.

4. Is there a relationship between the onset of psoriasis and the onset of arthritis?
- Psoriasis precedes arthritis by an average of 8 to 10 years in ~70% of patients.
- Arthritis precedes psoriasis in ~10% to 15% of patients (particularly in juvenile PsA).
- Simultaneous onset of PsA and psoriasis occurs in ~15% patients (this subgroup tends to flare skin and arthritis simultaneously during their disease course).
- Patients with psoriasis who have nail involvement or a family history of PsA are more likely to develop PsA.

5. If psoriasis is not obvious, what areas should be closely examined?
Always check the umbilicus, scalp, perineum, and behind the ears.

6. Is there a relationship between the extent or location of skin involvement and arthritis?
No particular pattern (plaque, pustular, or guttate) or extent of psoriasis is associated with arthritis. However, some suggest that arthritis is more deforming and widespread with extensive skin involvement as indicated by a Psoriasis Assessment Severity Index (PASI) >10 (range of PASI score: 0–72). Up to 35% report that flares of their skin and joint disease occur simultaneously. Some population-based studies have suggested that in addition to nail dystrophy, scalp lesions and intergluteal or perianal psoriasis are associated with an increased frequency of developing PsA.

7. What are the current classification criteria for PsA?
Always keep in mind that the purpose of classification criteria is to standardize patients for clinical trials. Nonetheless, they can be useful in making the diagnosis of PsA. The most widely used criteria are the Classification of Psoriatic Arthritis (CASPAR) criteria. The Moll and Wright criteria and European Spondyloarthropathy Study Group criteria are also used, but CASPAR has the highest sensitivity. CASPAR presumes a clinical assessment of inflammatory arthritis.
The **CASPAR** criteria are:
1. Evidence of psoriasis (current, past, family): two points if current history of psoriasis; one point for others.
2. Psoriatic nail dystrophy (onycholysis, pitting): one point
3. Negative rheumatoid factor: one point.
4. Dactylitis (current, past history): one point.
5. Radiographic evidence of juxtaarticular new bone formation: one point.
   Three or more points have 99% specificity and 92% sensitivity for diagnosis of PsA.

8. What are the characteristic patterns of joint involvement in PsA?
Approximately 95% of patients with PsA have peripheral joint disease (synovitis, tenosynovitis [dactylitis], enthesitis) with or without axial disease. Another 5% have axial spine involvement exclusively. In 1973, Moll and Wright divided PsA into five broad categories. These categories overlap, creating a heterogeneous combination of joint diseases. For instance, only 2% to 5% of PsA patients have predominantly DIP involvement, whereas over 50% of patients have DIP involvement in association with another pattern. As mentioned earlier, 5% of patients have only axial spine involvement, but up to 40% of patients with one of the other patterns of PsA will also have coexistent axial involvement (Table 36.1). Importantly, these patterns are not mutually exclusive. Treatment recommendations generally take into consideration severity of skin involvement, number of peripheral joints affected, and whether or not there is axial disease.

9. What other features are associated with certain subtypes?
- Asymmetric oligoarthritis—dactylitis.
- Predominant DIP involvement—nail changes.
- Arthritis mutilans—osteolysis of involved joints, "telescoping" of digits.
- "Rheumatoid-like" disease—fusion of wrists.
- Axial involvement—asymmetric sacroiliitis and "jug handle"-like syndesmophytes.
- Dactylitis—increased risk of radiographic damage

TABLE 36.1 Classification of Joint Involvement in Psoriatic Arthritis

SUBTYPE	%	TYPICAL JOINTS
1. Asymmetric oligoarticular disease	15–20	DIP and PIP joints of hands and feet. MCP joints, MTP joints, knees, hips, and ankles
2. Predominant DIP involvement	2–5	DIP joints
3. Arthritis mutilans	5	DIP joints, PIP joints
4. Polyarthritis "rheumatoid-like"	50–60	MCP joints, PIP joints, and wrists
5. Axial involvement (isolated)	2–5	Sacroiliac, vertebral

DIP, Distal interphalangeal; *MCP*, metacarpophalangeal; *MTP*, metatarsophalangeal; *PIP*, proximal interphalangeal.

10. Which is the most "classic" pattern of PsA?

Predominant DIP involvement. Note that this is one of the least common patterns. However, very few inflammatory arthritides involve the DIP joints. When a patient has DIP inflammatory arthritis, PsA should be high on the differential.

11. How does the axial involvement in PsA differ from that in other seronegative spondyloarthropathies?

Asymmetric sacroiliac involvement is typical of PsA. However, some patients can have symmetric sacroiliitis. Notably, patients with asymmetric sacroiliitis tend to be HLA-B*08 positive (63%) while those with symmetric sacroiliitis are more likely to be HLA-B27 positive (61%). Additionally, syndesmophytes are characteristically large, nonmarginal ("*jug handle*"-*like*), as opposed to the thin, marginal, symmetric syndesmophytes that occur in ankylosing spondylitis (see Chapter 33: Axial Spondyloarthritis) and may skip vertebral levels. Age of onset for PsA is typically older than other spondyloarthropathies, and the ratio of female to male patients is 1:1, whereas other spondyloarthropathies have a male predominance.

12. What clinical features suggest PsA rather than other polyarticular arthritic diseases such as rheumatoid arthritis?

- Asymmetric, often oligoarticular joint involvement.
- Absence of rheumatoid factor.
- Significant nail pitting or nail dystrophy.
- Involvement of DIP joints in the absence of osteoarthritis.
- "Sausage digits" (dactylitis): seen in 30% to 50%, due to synovitis and flexor tenosynovitis.
- Enthesitis: seen in 35% to 40%. Most common sites: Achilles and plantar fascia insertion.
- Family history of psoriasis or PsA.
- Axial radiographic evidence of sacroiliitis, paravertebral ossification, and syndesmophytes.
- Peripheral radiographic evidence of erosive arthritis with relative lack of periarticular osteopenia.
- Synovial biopsies show increased vascularity and the presence of macrophages (CD163+), lymphocytes (many CD8+ T cells), and neutrophils.

13. Are there any extraarticular features associated with PsA?

Nail changes are seen in 80% of patients with arthritis, as opposed to 30% with psoriasis only. These changes include pitting, onycholysis, oil spot sign, hyperkeratosis, and nail crumbling. **Eye disease** includes conjunctivitis in 20% and iritis/uveitis in 7–20% of cases. Iritis/uveitis tends to be chronic and bilateral. It can be an anterior, posterior, or panuveitis. Acute anterior uveitis can occur and is more common in PsA patients who are HLA-B*27 positive and have axial involvement. Other, less common features include oral ulcers, urethritis, nonspecific colitis, and, rarely, dilatation of base of aortic arch causing aortic insufficiency.

14. What other comorbidities are commonly associated with PsA?

Some important comorbidities that are linked with PsA include cardiovascular disease risk, obesity, fatty liver disease, fibromyalgia, and mood disorders. Due to obesity, the metabolic syndrome and obstructive sleep apnea are more common in patients with psoriasis. When choosing therapy for a particular patient, it is essential to take into account how comorbidities may impact treatment (e.g., avoiding methotrexate and leflunomide in fatty liver disease). Treatment of patients with PsA often involves a multidisciplinary approach and should always include communication with the patient's primary care provider.

15. Is there an association between flares of skin and nail disease and flares of PsA?

The relationship between skin and joint disease activity is variable. Patients with simultaneous onset of psoriasis and PsA have reported that when one manifestation flares, the other is likely to flare. However, for most patients the skin and arthritis run separate courses. Patients with DIP involvement are more likely to have worse nail involvement. This is partly because the extensor tendon enthesis inserts in an area adjacent to the nail root. When the enthesis becomes inflamed, nail growth is adversely affected.

16. Are there specific comorbid diagnoses to consider when someone presents acutely with severe psoriasis or PsA?

In this scenario, one needs to consider concurrent human immunodeficiency virus (HIV) infection. Clinically, psoriasis or PsA associated with HIV infection is more aggressive and difficult to control with traditional medical therapy. In the modern era of highly active antiretroviral therapy (HAART) for HIV, this is seen less frequently, as psoriasis is often associated with T-cell counts of <100 cells/μL. Treatment for psoriasis and PsA associated with HIV involves treating HIV with antiretroviral drugs in addition to treating the skin and joint disease. Case reports suggest that anti-TNF agents may be relatively safe in this population when used in conjunction with HAART (for additional details on HIV, see Chapter 41: HIV-Associated Rheumatic Syndromes).

17. Can laboratory tests help in diagnosing PsA?

PsA is classified as a "seronegative" arthritis, meaning that the rheumatoid factor is typically negative. However, low-titer rheumatoid factor can be detected in 2% to 10% and anticitrullinated peptide antibodies in 8% to 16% of PsA patients, particularly those with polyarthritis. This can make it difficult to separate from rheumatoid arthritis. However, the presence of DIP involvement, enthesitis, and dactylitis supports a diagnosis of PsA regardless of serologies. Antinuclear antibodies at titers of ≥1:80 are reported in 10% to 15%. As in other inflammatory diseases, erythrocyte sedimentation rates (ESR), C-reactive protein (CRP), and anemia may vary with disease activity. Patients with an elevated ESR and CRP are more likely to have polyarticular disease and a worse prognosis. It is important to note that only 40% of patients with PsA have elevated ESR and/or CRP. Hyperuricemia is seen in 20% and is not due to the extent of skin involvement but related to the increased incidence of the metabolic syndrome seen in patients with psoriatic disease (this is important to keep in mind when distinguishing between PsA and gout; hence, synovial fluid analysis is paramount). Analysis of synovial fluid typically reveals inflammatory fluid with a neutrophilic predominance. HLA-B27 is positive in 19–40% of all cases.

18. What is known about the pathogenesis of PsA?

It is thought that psoriasis and PsA result from a complex interaction between genetic and environmental factors. The mechanism that triggers the skin disease is unclear, but notably psoriasis can be induced or exacerbated by nonspecific triggers (e.g., Streptococcus infection, physical injury, or antimalarials) and/or by the release of the antimicrobial peptide LL-37 from keratinocytes. LL-37 promotes the release of interferon-alpha from plasmacytoid dendritic cells. This activates dermal dendritic cells and T cells that circulate to the lymph node and return to the dermis where they differentiate into Th1 and type 17 cells in response to IL-12/interferon-gamma and IL-23, respectively. The Th1 cells release interferon-gamma and TNFα contributing to hyperkeratosis. The type 17 cells [CD4+ helper T cells (Th17) and CD8+ cytotoxic T cells (Tc17)] secrete IL-17 and other cytokines contributing to inflammation. Innate immune cells (e.g. NK cells, γδ T cells, neutrophils) are also present. All these cells stimulate the secretion of cytokines, chemokines, and antimicrobial peptides (from keratinocytes) amplifying the inflammatory responses in the dermis and epidermis.

In addition to the inflamed skin, there is now evidence that the gastrointestinal tract may contribute to the development of PsA. Intestinal dysbiosis may enhance the release of bacterial products causing the local production of proinflammatory cytokines leading to mucosal inflammation and disruption of the epithelial barrier. Macrophages and dendritic cells in the gut mucosa present peptide fragments mainly to CD8+ T cells. These antigen presenting cells also produce IL-23 and TNFα. IL-23 stimulates resident Th17 and Tc17 cells. Other microbial antigens directly stimulate innate-like T cells (γδ T cells, mucosal-associated invariant (MAIT) cells, and invariant NK T cells), which also produce IL-17 among other cytokines. Due to the "leaky gut," microbial products/antigens and activated gut mucosal immune cells can enter the bloodstream and circulate to the joints and entheses where they promote inflammation. Most importantly, the production of IL-17 by all these cells causes activation of synovial fibroblasts, chondrocytes, and osteoclasts inducing synovial proliferation and bone reabsorption. Surface markers on CD8+ T cells in the synovium indicate their potential to migrate between joint, skin, and intestine. IL-17, IL-23, and TNFα are pivotal cytokines in the pathogenesis of psoriasis and psoriatic arthritis.

19. What radiographic features help differentiate PsA from other inflammatory diseases?

Historically, 45% to 50% of patients will develop erosions within the first 2 years of their disease, and 67% will eventually develop radiographic changes. Some relatively unique findings in PsA include:
- Asymmetric distribution; involvement of DIP joints
- Eccentric erosions, periostitis, and bony ankylosis
- Relative absence of periarticular osteopenia
- Whittling of the phalanges, pencil-in-cup deformity, osteolysis of bones (arthritis mutilans), and erosion of the terminal tufts (acroosteolysis)
- Polyarticular unidigit—metacarpophalangeal, proximal interphalangeal (PIP), and DIP of same finger involved.
- Erosions at entheseal sites
- Musculoskeletal ultrasound and/or magnetic resonance imaging showing signs of enthesitis and dactylitis.
- Sacroiliac and spondylitic changes (usually asymmetric).

A radiograph from a patient with PsA showing erosions and ankylosis of DIP and PIP joints is shown in Fig. 36.1.

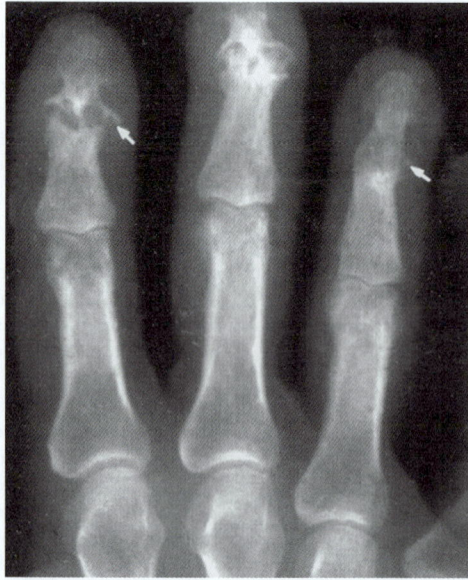

Fig. 36.1 Psoriatic arthritis, showing erosions and ankylosis of distal interphalangeal (arrows) and proximal interphalangeal joints. *DIP,* distal interphalangeal; *PIP,* proximal interphalangeal. (From Perlman SG, Barth WF. Psoriatic arthritis: diagnosis and management. *Compr Ther.* 1979;5:60–66 with permission.)

20. What principles guide treatment of PsA? What classes of medications can be used to treat PsA?

Patients should be treated with similar goal-directed therapy as in other inflammatory arthritides. Remission or sustained low disease activity should be the goal for most patients. The **Disease Activity index for Psoriatic Arthritis (DAPSA)**, which measures tender/swollen joint counts, CRP, and patient's assessment of disease activity/pain, can be used to document remission (score ≤ 4) or low disease activity (5–14). The **Psoriatic Area and Severity Index (PASI)** measures the extent and severity of skin disease (>10 severe, range 0-72). **Minimal Disease Activity (MDA)** has been derived from components of the DAPSA, PASI, and HAQ-DI.

Polyarticular disease, dactylitis, joint erosions, an elevated ESR/CRP, and DAPSA > 28 indicate a worse prognosis. Patients with mild oligoarticular disease can sometimes be managed with nonsteroidal anti-inflammatory drugs (NSAIDs) and intraarticular steroid injections, but in general clinicians should have a low threshold to initiate disease-modifying antirheumatic drugs (csDMARDs, JAKi, or bDMARDs). The choice of DMARD should be undertaken with the guiding principle of treating as many manifestations of a particular patient's disease as possible. Even when a DMARD is initiated, NSAIDs, physiotherapy, and glucocorticoid injections remain useful adjuncts for psoriatic arthritis.

- **Methotrexate and leflunomide** are csDMARDs that have been reported to have a small effect on skin involvement, peripheral arthritis, enthesitis, and dactylitis. There is less evidence for leflunomide than for methotrexate for treatment of skin disease. These medications have been shown to neither halt radiographic progression nor effectively treat axial disease or nail disease. Recent data strongly support the superiority of some biologics over these csDMARDs in early disease. If shared decision-making leads to initiation of a csDMARD as first-line therapy, regular assessment of response is essential to determine if escalation of therapy to apremilast, JAKi, or a bDMARD (TNFi, IL-17i, IL-12/23i, IL-23i, abatacept) is required.
- **Anti-TNFα agents** with or without methotrexate have been shown to be effective therapy for arthritis, dactylitis, enthesitis, spondylitis, and skin disease. It is important to note that if a patient with PsA has related conditions of inflammatory eye disease or inflammatory bowel disease, etanercept should not be used. Of note, obesity and smoking appear to reduce the effectiveness of anti-TNF agents.
- **Ustekinumab** is a monoclonal antibody that binds to the p40 subunit common to both IL-12 and IL-23, which prevents cytokine binding to their respective receptors. Ustekinumab is not effective in treating axial PsA.
- **Guselkumab and Risankizumab** are fully human and humanized (respectively) monoclonal antibodies that block IL-23 by inhibiting the p19 subunit of IL-23. Importantly, it is not clear whether these agents have adequate effectiveness in treating axial PsA. This may be due to MAIT cells' predilection to home to the axial skeleton. MAIT cells can produce IL-17 without the need for IL-23 stimulation.
- **Secukinumab, Bimekizumab, and Ixekizumab** block IL-17 and are effective for treating both skin and musculoskeletal manifestations of PsA. They are not effective for treating uveitis. These agents also may exacerbate IBD and should not be used in patients with this condition.
- **Apremilast,** an inhibitor of phosphodiesterase 4, also treats both psoriasis and PsA, but the magnitude of response is typically less than that of biologic agents. It is best used for mild skin and oligoarthritic manifestations.
- **Abatacept (CTLA4-Ig),** is an agent that blocks the CD80 and CD86 pathways of T-cell costimulation. Its efficacy is demonstrated more clearly in peripheral PsA, and it lacks clear efficacy in treating psoriasis.
- **Tofacitinib and Upadacitinib** are oral Janus kinase (JAK) inhibitors approved for the treatment of PsA and have demonstrated efficacy in axial and peripheral disease, with similar safety profile as in rheumatoid arthritis. These agents need to be used with caution or not at all in patients over age 65 and in those with cardiovascular, malignancy, or venous thromboembolism risk factors.

Exacerbation of psoriasis and erythroderma can occur with antimalarials (e.g., hydroxychloroquine), and consequently many consider them to be contraindicated. Systemic glucocorticoids should also be used cautiously or not at all because of the risk of inducing a flare of skin disease if tapered too rapidly. The ACR, EULAR, and GRAPPA have all issued treatment guidelines for PsA.

21. What is the best DMARD to use for PsA? Can DMARDs ever be stopped in a patient with PsA who is in remission?

Methotrexate (MTX), leflunomide, and apremilast should only be used as first-line agents in PsA patients with mild skin and/or oligoarticular disease without poor prognostic factors. Unlike rheumatoid arthritis, MTX does not need to be used with bDMARDs to prevent anti-drug antibodies. MTX and leflunomide should be avoided in patients with fatty liver disease. Intraarticular glucocorticoids can be an effective adjunctive therapy.

For patients with peripheral arthritis who have poor prognostic factors (polyarticular disease, erosions/deformities, high CRP), there is no specific order of preference for use of bDMARDs or JAKi. Therefore, choice of therapy depends on the presence of axial disease, extraarticular manifestations, and comorbidities.

- **Axial disease:** all bDMARDs and JAKi can be used. Ustekinumab and IL-23 inhibitors may be less effective than other bDMARDs.
- **Uveitis:** Anti-TNFα agents (except etanercept) should be used, since they treat uveitis.
- **Severe skin disease:** IL-17, IL-23, and IL-12/23 inhibitors work best for severe skin disease.
- **Inflammatory bowel disease:** IL-17 inhibitors and etanercept should not be used.
- **Coexistent cardiovascular/thrombotic risk factors:** If used, JAKi should be used with caution.

Patients with PsA who achieve remission (DAPSA ≤4, MDA) can be considered for tapering of medications. Patients on csDMARDs (e.g, methotrexate) or corticosteroids should be tapered off these medications first. Patients should not have bDMARDs or JAKi stopped due to risk of disease recurrence. Some physicians may try to taper but not stop the DMARDs.

22. How does the prognosis of PsA compare with that of rheumatoid arthritis?

PsA and rheumatoid arthritis have a similar prognosis and effect on quality of life. Historically, 60% of patients have erosive arthritis in five or more joints and 40% have joint deformities and/or spine involvement. Up to 20% will develop ACR class III or IV functional impairment with disability. Polyarticular disease, dactylitis, early development of erosions, and elevated ESR/CRP all predict a poor prognosis. In addition, mortality is increased, with a standardized mortality ratio of 1.36. Studies have established a link among psoriasis, obesity, metabolic syndrome, hyperuricemia, and premature atherosclerosis. Obstructive sleep apnea may occur in obese patients, causing fibromyalgia.

23. Can combination immunomodulatory therapy be used in PsA?

Unfortunately, only about 50% of patients with PsA achieve MDA regardless of the JAKi or bDMARD used. Combining MTX with a bDMARD improves this minimally. Due to insurance restrictions, combining apremilast with a JAKi or bDMARD or combining bDMARDs cannot be done. Notably, anecdotal reports combining an anti-TNFα agent with ustekinumab or an IL-23i have shown marked improvement in PsA and skin disease without increased safety issues. More studies with other combinations of immunomodulatory medications in PsA are warranted.

24. Are there any other medications that may be available now or in the future to treat PsA?

Additional biologic therapies for PsA are in phase III trials. Brodalumab is a monoclonal antibody against subunit A of the IL-17 receptor and therefore able to inhibit all members of the IL-17 cytokine family. It is FDA approved for treatment of skin psoriasis, and phase III trials for PsA are pending. It has a blackbox warning for suicidality. Izokibep is an IL-17A trap that is comprised of two IL-17A-specific binding Affibody domains and one albumin-binding domain. It may be more effective than a monoclonal antibody against IL-17 due to its small size and superior tissue penetration. Deucravacitinib is a selective TYK2 inhibitor that in trials has shown effectiveness in both psoriasis and psoriatic arthritis. There are an additional six tsDMARDs and five bDMARDs in development for treating PsA.

25. What other dermatologic conditions have been associated with arthritis? What musculoskeletal manifestations are typically associated with these?

Palmoplantar pustulosis, acne conglobata, acne fulminans, psoriatic onychopachydermoperiostitis, interstitial granulomatous dermatitis, and hidradenitis suppurativa. Note that acne vulgaris is not included. These typically are associated with anterior chest wall pain and swelling, involving the sternoclavicular, manubriosternal, and sternocostal joints. Chronic cervical and lumbar pain as well as pain at the symphysis pubis are common. Less often, oligoarticular or monoarticular peripheral arthritis can occur. Wrists, PIPs, elbows, acromioclavicular joints, and metatarsophalangeal joints are the most commonly involved.

26. What is SAPHO syndrome? How is it treated?

S—Synovitis (90% of patients): oligo-asymmetric (large > small joints), axial (sternal), and sacroiliac joints (unilateral).

A—Acne (18%): cystic acne conglobata, acne fulminans.

P—Pustulosis (66%): pustular psoriasis, palmoplantar pustulosis, or hidradenitis suppurativa.

H—Hyperostosis: especially of anterior chest wall with sternocostoclavicular hyperostosis.

O—Osteitis: symphysis pubis, sacroiliitis (33%), spondylodiscitis, anterior chest wall and vertebral sclerosis, more so than long bones.

The name was proposed in 1987 by Chamot et al. because they were impressed by the association of sterile arthritis (frequently involving the anterior chest) and various skin conditions. Etiology is unclear; however, Cutibacterium acnes (formerly Propionibacterium acnes) as a causative agent has been implicated. HLA-B27 is positive in 13% of cases. Inflammatory cytokines IL-8, IL-18, IL-17, and TNFα are often elevated. It is thought to be an innate immunity-linked autoinflammatory disease. NSAIDs and antibiotics (especially doxycycline) are typically used as first-line therapy. Conventional synthetic DMARDs, such as methotrexate, sulfasalazine, leflunomide, and cyclosporine, have variable results reported in the literature. Intravenous bisphosphonates, pamidronate in particular, may be an effective treatment for bone and osteoarticular manifestations. Anti-TNF agents, particularly infliximab, have been consistently effective in treating bone and joint symptoms but not necessarily skin lesions (reports of exacerbation of pustular psoriasis). Ustekinumab, IL-17 inhibitors, IL-1 inhibitors, and JAKi have been effective in case reports.

27. What is chronic recurrent multifocal osteitis (CRMO) and how does it relate to SAPHO?

CRMO is a chronic, sterile, inflammatory, and multifocal disease of bone that preferentially affects children. Bone sites involved differ according to the patient's age. **The metaphysis of the long bones is preferentially affected in children and adolescents** (which is different than common sites of involvement in SAPHO syndrome), whereas **anterior thoracic, vertebral, and/or unilateral sacroiliac lesions predominate in adults** (similar to SAPHO). Bone biopsies are necessary to rule out bacterial osteomyelitis, tumor, and eosinophilic granuloma. Adult patients with suspected CRMO should be closely assessed for underlying Crohn's disease, psoriasis, or another spondyloarthropathy. In addition, clinicians should monitor for the development of characteristic skin lesions that would otherwise classify the patient as having SAPHO syndrome. The treatments used have been similar to those used in SAPHO.

BIBLIOGRAPHY

Adizie T, Moots RJ, Hodkinson B, et al. Inflammatory arthritis in HIV positive patients: a practical guide. *BMC Infect Dis.* 2016;16:100.

Alinaghi F, Calov M, Kristensen LE, et al. Prevalence of psoriatic arthritis in patients with psoriasis: a systematic review and meta-analysis of observational and clinical studies. *J Am Acad Dermatol.* 2019;80:251–265.

Azuaga AB, Ramírez J, Cañete JD. Psoriatic arthritis: pathogenesis and targeted therapies. *Int J Mol Sci.* 2023;24:4901.

Bogliolo L, Alpini C, Caporali R, et al. Antibodies to cyclic citrullinated peptides in psoriatic arthritis. *J Rheumatol.* 2005;32:511.

Brunello F, Tirelli F, Pegoraro L, et al. New insights on juvenile psoriatic arthritis. *Front Pediatr.* 2022;10:884727.

Chandran V, Schentag CT, Gladman DD. Reappraisal of the effectiveness of methotrexate in psoriatic arthritis: results from a longitudinal observational cohort. *J Rheumatol.* 2008;35:469.

Cheng W, Li F, Tian J, et al. New insights in the treatment of SAPHO syndrome and medication recommendations. *J Inflamm Res.* 2022;15:2365–2380.

Cianci F, Zoli A, Gremese E, Ferraccioli G. Clinical heterogeneity of SAPHO syndrome: challenging diagnosis and treatment. *Clin Rheumatol.* 2017;36:2151–2158.

Coates LC, Fransen J, Helliwell PS. Defining minimal disease activity in psoriatic arthritis: a proposed objective target for treatment. *Ann Rheum Dis.* 2010;69:48–53.

Coates LC, Soriano ER, Corp N, et al. Group for Research and Assessment of Psoriasis and Psoriatic Arthritis (GRAPPA): updated treatment recommendations for psoriatic arthritis 2021. *Nat Rev Rheumatol.* 2022;18:465–479.

Fotiadou C, Lazaridou E. Psoriasis and uveitis: links and risks. *Psoriasis (Auckl).* 2019;9:91–96.

Furst DE, Belasco J, Louie JS. Genetic and inflammatory factors associated with psoriatic arthritis: relevance to diagnosis and management. *Clin Immunol.* 2019;202:59–75.

Gracey E, Vereecke L, McGovern D, et al. Revisiting the gut-joint axis: links between gut inflammation and spondyloarthritis. *Nat Rev Rheumatol.* 2020;16:415–433.

Gupta S, Syrimi Z, Hughes DM, Zhao SS. Comorbidities in psoriatic arthritis: a systematic review and meta-analysis. *Rheumatol Int.* 2021;41:275–284.

Haberman RH, Castillo R, Scher JU. Induction of remission in biologic-naive, severe psoriasis and PsA with dual anti-cytokine combination. *Rheumatology (Oxford).* 2021;60:e225–e226.

Hassan M, Assi H, Hassan M, et al. Chronic recurrent multifocal osteomyelitis: a comprehensive literature review. *Cureus.* 2023;15:e43118.

Karmacharya P, Chakradhar R, Ogdie A. The epidemiology of psoriatic arthritis: a literature review. *Best Pract Res Clin Rheumatol.* 2021;35:101692.

Laborde CM, Larzabal L, González-Cantero Á, Castro-Santos P, Díaz-Peña R. Advances of genomic medicine in psoriatic arthritis. *J Pers Med.* 2022;12:35.

Lindsey SF, Weiss J, Lee ES, Romanelli P. Treatment of severe psoriasis and psoriatic arthritis with adalimumab in an HIV-positive patient. *J Drugs Dermatol.* 2014;13:869–871.

McDonagle D, Lories RJ, Tan AL, et al. The concept of a "synovio-entheseal complex" and its implications for understanding joint inflammation and damage in psoriatic arthritis and beyond. *Arthritis Rheum.* 2007;56:2482.

Moll JM, Wright V. Psoriatic arthritis. *Semin Arthritis Rheum.* 1973;3:55–78.

Ogdie A, Coates LC, Gladman DD. Treatment guidelines in psoriatic arthritis. *Rheumatology (Oxford).* 2020;59(suppl 1):i37–i46.

Ritchlin CT, Colbert RA, Gladman DD. Psoriatic arthritis. *N Engl J Med.* 2017;376:957–970.

Saad AA, Symmons DP, Noyce PR, et al. Risks and benefits of tumor necrosis factor-alpha inhibitors in the management of psoriatic arthritis: systemic review and metaanalysis of randomized controlled trials. *J Rheumatol.* 2008;35:883.

Siannis F, Farewell VT, Cook RJ, et al. Clinical and radiological damage in psoriatic arthritis. *Ann Rheum Dis.* 2006;65:478.

Singh JA, Guyatt G, Ogdie A, et al. Special article: 2018 American College of Rheumatology/National Psoriasis Foundation guideline for the treatment of psoriatic arthritis. *Arthritis Rheumatol.* 2019;71:5–32.

Taylor W, Gladman D, Helliwell P, et al. Classification criteria for psoriatic arthritis: development of new criteria from a large international study. *Arthritis Rheum.* 2006;54:2665.

Wilson FC, Icen M, Crowson CS, McEvoy MT, Gabriel SE, Kremers HM. Incidence and clinical predictors of psoriatic arthritis in patients with psoriasis: a population-based study. *Arthritis Rheum.* 2009;61:233–239.

FURTHER READING

http://www.psoriasis.org.

https://rarediseases.info.nih.gov/diseases/7606/sapho-syn.

Bacterial Septic Arthritis, Bursitis, and Osteomyelitis

Laura Damioli, MD and Michael Haden, MD

CHAPTER 37

 KEY POINTS

1. *Staphylococcus aureus* is the most common causative agent of septic arthritis and osteomyelitis.
2. Large weight-bearing joints, particularly the knee, are most prone to developing septic arthritis.
3. In a hemodynamically stable patient, joint aspirate or bone biopsy for culture should be obtained prior to initiation of antibiotics.
4. Initial choice of antibiotic therapy is based on the Gram stain and clinical situation.
5. More than 50% of women who develop disseminated gonococcal infections (DGIs) do so within 1 week of onset of menses.
6. Any patient with fever, arthralgias, and tenosynovitis should be evaluated for DGI.

---

1. How do gonococcal and nongonococcal septic arthritis differ?

	Gonococcal	*Nongonococcal*
Host	Young, healthy adults	Small children, elderly, Immunocompromised
Pattern	Migratory polyarthralgias/arthritis	Monoarthritis
Tenosynovitis	Common	Rare
Skin rash	Common	Rare
Positive joint cultures	<25%	~70–95%
Positive blood cultures	Rare	40–50%
Outcome	Good in >95%	Poor in 30–50%

2. What clinical manifestations are typical of nongonococcal septic arthritis?

Classic presentation includes abrupt onset of swelling, warmth, and pain involving the affected joint. Presentation in those with prosthetic joints may be more indolent (delayed onset type). Many patients have serious underlying illnesses and 40% to 60% may be febrile or have chills. Large joints (knee, hip) are most commonly involved. Patients keep the knee or hip flexed, abducted, and externally rotated to maximize intracapsular volume. Both passive and active ranges of motion are very painful. Children and most adults refuse to use the involved extremity.

3. How do organisms reach the synovium to cause septic arthritis?

- Hematogenous spread (most common)
- Contiguous spread from adjacent osteomyelitis (especially in children) or soft tissue infection.
- Iatrogenic infections from arthrocentesis or arthroscopy (rare)
- Penetrating trauma from plant thorns or other contaminated objects.

4. What factors predispose an individual to develop septic arthritis?

- Preexisting joint disease including rheumatoid arthritis (RA), osteoarthritis (OA), hemarthrosis, and in those with prosthetic joint replacements
- Chronic, severe illness, including alcohol use disorder, diabetes, cirrhosis, end-stage renal disease, human immunodeficiency virus (HIV)
- Intravenous drug use
- Impaired host defense such as those on immunosuppressive agents, SLE and sickle cell disease (functional asplenia), hypogammaglobulinemia, or with late complement deficiencies (susceptible to *Neisseria*)
- Elderly (>80 years old) or children (<5 years old)

- Cutaneous ulcers and skin infections
- Direct penetration, such as penetrating trauma or rarely invasive procedures (arthroscopy, arthrocentesis, or intra-articular corticosteroid injections)

5. Which joints are most commonly involved in nongonococcal septic arthritis in adults?

Knee	45%
Hip	15%
Ankle	9%
Elbow	8%
Wrist	6%
Shoulder	5%
Polyarticular	10–20% (usually only two or three joints)

6. Which bacteria are usually responsible for nongonococcal septic arthritis in adults?

Overall causative pathogens are documented by culture in approximately 70% to 90% of septic arthritis patients and include:

S. aureus	52% (increasing rates of methicillin resistance)
Streptococci	16% (group B more common in elderly and diabetics)
Gram-negative bacilli	10–15%
Polymicrobial	5%
Coagulase-negative Staphylococci	3%
Culture-negative	~20%

7. Why does *S. aureus* cause most cases of septic arthritis?

S. aureus produces many virulence factors including extracellular toxins, enzymes, as well as several surface adhesins that bind to connective tissue and extracellular matrix proteins. Clumping factors (A and B) bind to fibrinogen, and fibronectin-binding protein (A and B) binds to fibronectin. Exotoxins produced by the bacteria contribute to the inflammatory response and bacterial survival. Some strains of *S. aureus* contain the virulence factor Panton-Valentine leucocidin (PVL), which allows survival within neutrophils, with these strains being associated with more fulminant infections, including those in healthy patients.

8. Which organisms are commonly involved in septic arthritis in children?

Considerable institutional variation exists, but the most common organisms in various age groups are as follows:

Neonates (<3 Months Old)	Age 3 Months to 5 Years Old	Age 5–15 Years Old
S. aureus	S. aureus	S. aureus
Group B Streptococci	Kingella kingae	Streptococcus pyogenes
E.coli and other Gram-negative bacteria	Streptococcus pyogenes	Neisseria gonorrhoeae (sexually active adolescents)
Neisseria gonorrhoeae (newborns)	Streptococcus pneumoniae	
	Hemophilus influenza (less common due to vaccination)	

9. Name the organisms that are associated with underlying disorders in septic arthritis.

RA	S. aureus (frequently polyarticular)
Immunocompromised/alcoholics	S. aureus, Streptococci, Gram-negatives, Listeria
Malignancies/Diabetics	S. aureus, group B Streptococci
Intravenous drug use	S. aureus
	Gram-negative (Pseudomonas among others)
Dog/cat bites	Pasteurella multocida, Capnocytophaga, anaerobes
Human bites	Streptococci, Eikenella, oral anaerobes including Prevotella, Fusobacterium, and Peptostreptococcus
Terminal complement-deficiency	Neisseria species

Sickle cell disease (functional asplenia)	*Streptococcus pneumoniae*
	Salmonella spp. (osteomyelitis)
Hemochromatosis	*Vibrio vulnificus* (oyster-eating)
	Yersinia species (esp prosthetic joints)
Hypogammaglobulinemia	*Mycoplasma* and Ureaplasma
Raw milk/dairy products	*Brucella* spp.—often involves sacroiliac joints
Systemic lupus erythematosus (SLE) (functional asplenia)	Encapsulated organisms (*Neisseria, Salmonella*)

10. How helpful is synovial fluid analysis and culture in nongonococcal septic arthritis?

Arthrocentesis with demonstration of the bacteria on Gram stain or culture establishes the diagnosis of septic arthritis. Of the tests that can be done on the synovial fluid, culture, Gram stain, and leukocyte (white blood cell [WBC]) counts are the most helpful. Both universal polymerase chain reaction (PCR) and organism-specific PCR (higher sensitivity) can help identify organisms in the setting of prior antibiotic use or in cases of culture-negative infection.

Laboratory Tests of Synovial Fluid in Nongonococcal Septic Arthritis:

Procedure	*Technical Aspects*	*Diagnostic Yield*
Culture	Plate or inoculate culture bottles immediately	70–95% positive in nongonococcal arthritis
Gram stain	May increase yield by centrifuging synovial fluid	Sensitivity 30–50%
WBC count	Usually >50,000 cells/mm³ with neutrophilic predominance	Counts often overlap other inflammatory disease (gout, RA, ReA)
Glucose	<50% of serum glucose	Helpful if present
Miscellaneous tests	Alpha defensin very sensitive for prosthetic joint infections	NAAT if concerned for *Mycoplasma, Ureaplasma, Brucella, Yersinia*

NAAT, nucleic acid amplification test; *ReA,* reactive arthritis.

PEARL: Only 40% to 50% of all patients with septic arthritis have synovial fluid WBC counts over 100,000 cells/mm³. So even if the synovial fluid WBC is not "classic" for septic arthritis, there can still be an infection even with WBC counts less than 50,000 cells/mm³, especially in immunocompromised and neutropenic patients. Notably, crystal-induced arthritis (gout, pseudogout) can coexist with septic arthritis.

11. Are any blood tests useful in septic arthritis?

Blood cultures in nongonococcal arthritis can be positive in 40–50% of adult cases but much less likely in children. Whenever blood cultures are positive for *S. aureus*, a transthoracic echo should be performed to assess for endocarditis. Also consider endocarditis in patients with enterococcal or streptococcal septic arthritis who do not have an obvious source for septic arthritis. Blood cultures may be positive while synovial fluid cultures are negative in up to 14% of cases. **Leukocytosis, elevated erythrocyte sedimentation rate** (ESR), and **elevated C-reactive protein** (CRP) are seen in most individuals (60–90%) but are not discriminative due to overlap with other inflammatory arthritic diseases. Over 90% of patients with septic arthritis have an elevated CRP >2 mg/dL (20 mg/L), so values lower than this are helpful in excluding septic arthritis. It is important to remember that that some patients are unable to mount an adequate immune response and can have a low CRP value. It can be helpful to review prior laboratory results to see if the patient has had an elevated CRP in the past. An elevated serum **procalcitonin** level may be supportive of the diagnosis but nondiagnostic by itself. Serial measurements of ESR and CRP are helpful in monitoring response to therapy.

12. Do plain radiographs play a role in diagnosing septic arthritis?

Initial radiographs can be used to assess baseline joint damage. Radiographs are likely to show a joint effusion demonstrated by widening of the joint space and soft tissue swelling. Periarticular osteopenia occurs within a few days. As the disease progresses over the following 2–3 weeks there may be development of adjacent osteomyelitis demonstrated by periosteal reaction, bony destruction, erosions, and osteonecrosis. Joint space loss indicates cartilage destruction.

13. Can any other radiographic studies be helpful in septic arthritis?

CT or MRI can be helpful to confirm presence of effusions and inflammation in joints that are difficult to assess clinically (e.g., hip, sacroiliac, and sternoclavicular joints). Both CT and MRI are more sensitive at diagnosing adjacent osteomyelitis than plain radiographs are. Intravenous contrast is useful for evaluating soft tissue abscesses and synovial thickening.

14. How do you treat nongonococcal septic arthritis?

- Choose effective antibiotic based on patient age, clinical situation, Gram stain, and culture results.
- Prompt and adequate drainage of the joint by either surgical drainage (arthroscopically or open arthrotomy) or serial closed needle arthrocentesis (often more than once a day). There is debate on which modality is best, though serial closed needle arthrocentesis has the advantage of measurement of clinical response through leukocyte counts and culture of the synovial fluid. Surgical drainage tends to be preferred in those who are optimal surgical candidates, with closed needle aspiration reserved for those not fit for surgery. Surgical drainage should be considered in those who do not improve with closed needle arthrocentesis, as well as for complicated cases such as prosthetic joints, extensive soft tissue or bone involvement, or joints poorly accessible to needle aspiration such as the hip (see Question 16).
- Early physical therapy is important.

15. Which antibiotic should you choose? How long do you treat nongonococcal septic arthritis?

Antibiotics should be started after cultures are obtained, with the choice of antibiotics determined by the suspected organism based on initial Gram stain and clinical situation.

- **Gram-positive cocci on Gram stain:**
  - High prevalence for MRSA: vancomycin
  - Low prevalence for MRSA: cefazolin
- **Gram-positive rod:** often *C. acnes,* start ceftriaxone 2 g IV every 24 hours; if allergic to beta-lactams, could use vancomycin.
- **Gram-negative cocci:** suspect disseminated gonococcal infection or usually *Neisseria meningitidis.* Treat with a third-generation cephalosporin, such as ceftriaxone.
- **Gram-negative rod:** start a third-generation or fourth-generation cephalosporin such as ceftriaxone or cefepime, or piperacillin-tazobactam.
- **Negative Gram stain:** start vancomycin plus ceftriaxone or antipseudomonal beta-lactam, such as cefepime or piperacillin-tazobactam.
- **Human, dog, or cat bites:** ampicillin-sulbactam.

  Once the organism has been identified, the antibiotic regimen should be narrowed based on sensitivity data.

  Total duration of therapy is variable, ranging from 2 to 6 weeks depending on the patient's clinical response and improvement in inflammatory markers.

PEARL: If the patient was on antibiotics prior to synovial fluid aspiration, then need to consider treating organisms that may have been present but have had their growth inhibited. *S. aureus* and *Pseudomonas* if present will almost always grow.

16. When is surgical drainage absolutely indicated for a septic joint?

- Infected hip and shoulder joints.
- Vertebral osteomyelitis with cord compression.
- Anatomically difficult-to-drain joints (i.e., sternoclavicular joint).
- Inability to remove purulent fluid by needle drainage because fluid is too thick or loculated.

- Joints failing to respond to needle drainage (i.e., persistent positive cultures of synovial fluid or failure of synovial WBC to decrease).
- Prosthetic joints.
- Associated osteomyelitis requiring surgical drainage.
- Arthritis associated with foreign body.
- Delayed onset of therapy (>7 days)—irreversible cartilage damage starts within 1 week.

17. What is the prognosis in patients with nongonococcal septic arthritis?

Despite better drainage and antibiotics, this remains a serious disease with a mortality rate of 5% to 15%. Most of these patients have a chronic debilitating underlying disease contributing to the mortality. Of the surviving patients, up to 50% have residual abnormalities (pain or limited motion of the joint).

18. What factors suggest a poor outcome in nongonococcal septic arthritis?

- Rheumatoid arthritis
- Immunosuppressive therapy
- Age > 65 years old
- Polyarticular involvement
- Delayed diagnosis
- End stage renal disease or cirrhosis

19. How does septic arthritis differ in children?

- Age of patient is very helpful in determining the likely organism (see Question 8).
- Children have a higher incidence of hip involvement than adults.
- Blood cultures are less likely to be positive compared to adults.

20. Discuss the important aspects in the association of RA and septic joints.

The combination of existing joint damage and immunosuppressive medication use in RA patients place them at high risk for bacterial arthritis. Polyarticular involvement is common. Functional outcomes are worse and mortality is high, in part due to delays in diagnosis because septic arthritis is often mistaken for an RA flare.

21. Are there any peculiarities about septic arthritis in IV drug users?

Higher incidence of Gram-negative organisms, but *S. aureus* remains the most common organism. There is also an increased propensity to affect the axial skeleton (especially the lumbar vertebrae, as well as cartilaginous joints such as the sacroiliac, sternoclavicular, and pubic symphysis).

22. What is the incidence of prosthetic joint infections? What are the risk factors?

The overall infection rate in primary total joint replacement is approximately 1% to 2%, with knee prostheses having the highest risk of infection. Risk factors include smoking, obesity, diabetes, RA, immunosuppressive therapy, malignancy, distant site of infection, and those who undergo revision arthroplasty (likely due to increased operative time for revisions).

23. What are the most common organisms causing prosthetic joint infection?

Early infections (<3 months post–total joint arthroplasty) are caused by *S. aureus, Streptococcus,* or Gram-negative bacilli. Usually due to surgical contamination. These patients present with fever and local signs of wound infection typical of septic arthritis.

Delayed infections (3–24 months) are usually caused by indolent organisms such as coagulase-negative *Staphylococci, Enterococci,* or *C. acnes*. Patients present with progressive joint pain but frequently do not have other symptoms typical of septic arthritis. Fever occurs in <50% and leukocytosis in 10%. Elevated ESR and CRP are common.

Late infections (>24 months) are due to hematogenous seeding from a distant site of infection. *S. aureus* is the most common in this setting. Patients have acute onset of joint pain, swelling, and fever typical of septic arthritis.

> **PEARL:** *C. acnes* often takes 7–10 days to grow (ask the microbiology lab to hold the plates).

24. How can a prosthetic joint infection (PJI) be separated from aseptic loosening?

Infection should be suspected in any patient with progressive pain in a prosthetic joint.

Unfortunately, there is no single test that is 100% accurate for PJI diagnosis, but instead it is achieved through a combination of clinical findings, laboratory results from peripheral blood and synovial fluid, microbiological data, histological evaluation of tissue, intraoperative inspection, and radiographic results. Fever may or may not be present, but ESR and CRP are frequently elevated. Synovial fluid has a high sensitivity and specificity for PJI. The fluid will be inflammatory, though it should be noted neutrophil counts are much lower than in native joint disease, with thresholds indicating infection as low as 1100 nucleated cells per microliter. Plain radiographs may show periprosthetic lucency, effusion, adjacent soft tissue gas or fluid collection, or periosteal new bone formation; however, none of these are sensitive or specific. MRI, CT scan, and positron emission tomography-fluorodeoxyglucose scans do have the advantage of high spatial resolution to evaluate for infection in periprosthetic tissues, though added benefit of these tests beyond history and physical exam findings are unclear. Three-phase bone scintigraphy has high sensitivity but poor specificity for PJI, as any cause of increased bone formation (such as physiologic bone remodeling or aseptic prosthetic loosening) can cause activity on the scan. In the setting of a positive three-phase bone scan, the addition of white blood cell scintigraphy leads to higher diagnostic accuracy for PJI.

25. How are prosthetic joint infections treated? What measures can be done to prevent them?

1. Prior to total joint arthroplasty (TJA), patients should be encouraged to have dental work to ensure healthy teeth at time of TJA. Dental work should be postponed 3–6 months after TJA. There is no need for routine antimicrobial prophylaxis prior to dental work following TJA; patients at particularly high risk may be an exception (i.e., history of transplant or history of PJI). Patients should also be encouraged with smoking cessation, weight loss, optimization of diabetes, and appropriate timing of immunosuppressive agents around time of TJA.
2. Debridement, antibiotics, and implant retention (DAIR): considered for patients with a well-fixed prosthesis without a sinus tract who develop an acute infection. Treated for 6 weeks with IV antibiotics followed by oral antibiotics to complete a total of 3 months of antimicrobial therapy for total hip arthroplasty or a total of 6 months of antimicrobial therapy for all other joints. Consideration for lifelong oral suppression to be based on patient and microbial factors. Success rates varies from 31% to 82%.
3. One-stage replacement: removal of prosthesis, washout, and immediate placement of new prosthesis. Performed more frequently in Europe than in the United States. Can be considered when a good soft tissue envelope is present and the infecting pathogen is known preoperatively. Antimicrobial therapy is the same as for DAIR. Success rate 70% to 90%.
4. Two-stage replacement: (1) prosthesis and cement removal with stabilization of joint using an antibiotic-impregnated spacer, followed by 6 weeks of systemic antibiotics, followed by (2) reimplantation after completion of antimicrobial therapy. Success rate 87% to 100%.

> **PEARL:** Rifampin is often added to the antibiotic regimen to penetrate biofilm for infections caused by susceptible *Staphylococci*.

26. What is "pseudoseptic" arthritis?

Pseudoseptic arthritis is seen in the setting of poorly controlled RA in which the patient presents with one or more inflamed joints with very high synovial fluid WBC counts (>100,000 cells/mm^3). The cultures are negative, and patients respond to increased corticosteroids rather than antibiotics. However, infection always needs to be ruled out first! This presentation may also be seen in crystal-induced arthritides, seronegative spondyloarthropathies, and viscosupplementation for osteoarthritis, especially in a patient with calcium pyrophosphate dihydrate deposition disease who gets Synvisc.

27. Who is at risk for DGI?

Unlike nongonococcal septic arthritis, the typical patient who develops gonococcal arthritis is a young, healthy person. Women are more commonly affected than men and are more prone to develop DGI around menstruation and pregnancy. Other risk factors include HIV, high-risk sexual activity, low socioeconomic status, and terminal complement deficiency. Septic arthritis due to DGI used to be the most common cause of septic arthritis in adults aged <30 years. At the time of writing, the incidence has declined to about 1% of all septic arthritis due to effective sexually transmitted infection control programs.

28. How soon after infection do arthritic symptoms develop in DGI?

Arthritis complicates 1% to 3% of patients with gonorrhea. Typically, symptoms develop 1 day to several weeks after the sexual encounter and commonly (50% of female patients) occur during the week of the menstrual period in women.

29. What host factors enhance susceptibility to DGI?

1. High-risk sexual practices (i.e., multiple sexual partners, prostitutes).
2. Local environment of the cervix (i.e., changes in pH that occur during menstruation).
3. Congenital or acquired complement deficiencies, especially of C5–C8, predispose to recurrent *Neisseria* infections. The interaction between the Neisseria organisms and the complement system is critical to eradicating them from the bloodstream.

> **PEARL:** Always get a serum CH50 level in a patient with recurrent Neisseria infections. If it is 0, evaluate the patient for complement deficiency.

4. Asplenia or reticuloendothelial dysfunction such as may occur in SLE and sickle cell anemia patients.

30. What patterns of arthritis are associated with gonorrhea?

Migratory polyarthralgia	70%
Tenosynovitis	67%
Purulent arthritis	42%
Monoarthritis	32%
Polyarthritis	10%

When the arthritis is monoarticular, the knee is most commonly involved, followed by the wrist, ankle, and elbow. Unlike other causes of septic arthritis, the small joints of the hand are frequently involved. Less than 50% patients develop purulent arthritis. An important diagnostic clue is **tenosynovitis.** It most commonly affects the dorsum of wrists, fingers, toes, and ankles. The pain is often out of proportion to what is seen on physical examination. Patients should also be examined for meningitis and endocarditis.

31. Besides the articular complaints, what other symptoms are associated with DGI?

- **Skin rash** (66% of patients): typically 2 to 10 small painless macules, papules, or pustules on the distal extremities; patients are often unaware of these lesions and they may be easily overlooked on physical examination (Fig. 37.1).
- **Tenosynovitis** (66% of patients): usually involves wrists (extensors), fingers (flexors), ankles, and toes. Can involve multiple sites. Patients may present with only migratory polyarthralgias, tenosynovitis, and skin lesions.
- It is important to note that only 25% of patients with DGI have **genitourinary symptoms** (i.e., pelvic inflammatory disease [PID]) consistent with a localized gonorrhea infection. Therefore, lack of symptoms of PID either in the past or present does not rule out DGI.

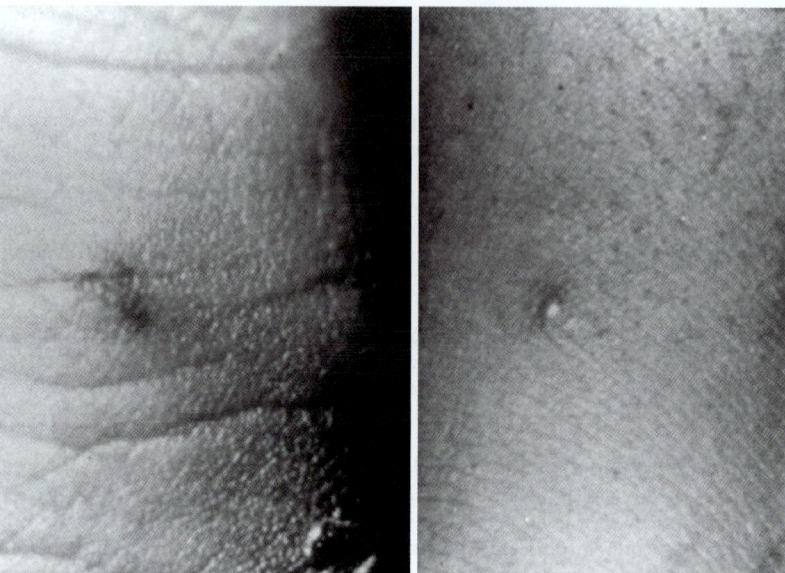

Fig. 37.1   The vesicle and pustular rash of disseminated gonococcal infection. (Copyright 2014 American College of Rheumatology. Used with permission.)

32. How useful are cultures and Gram stains in diagnosing gonococcal septic arthritis?

Unlike nongonococcal arthritis, the Gram stains of synovial fluid are positive in <25% in gonococcal arthritis. Cultures improve the diagnostic yield, but gonococci are recovered in less than 50% of cases. Because urethritis is often asymptomatic, all patients should have a urine specimen as well as urethral/rectal/pharyngeal swabs sent for Gram stain, culture, and NAAT testing. Urethral smears and cultures are more useful in men (>90% sensitivity) than in women.

Culture Positivity in DGI

Site	Isolation Rate
Genitourinary	80%
Synovial fluid	50%
Rectum	20%
Pharynx	10%
Blood	<30%
Skin	Rare

33. Are other laboratory tests helpful in DGI?

Much like nongonococcal septic arthritis, in DGI, leukocytosis and elevated ESR/CRP are common but nonspecific. Synovial fluid WBC counts range from 34,000 to 68,000 cells/mm^3 with a mean of 50,000/mm^3. While a NAAT for the synovial fluid is not commercially available, patients should have NAAT sent from specimens where insertive intercourse occurs (urine, pharyngeal swab, and rectal swab).

34. How is DGI treated?

Local (cervicitis, urethritis, proctitis)	**Ceftriaxone**, 500 mg intramuscularly × 1 dose -Treat for Chlamydia if this has not been excluded.
DGI	**Ceftriaxone** 1g IV every 24 hours until clinical improvement (often > 7 days)

If patient has a cephalosporin allergy, then infectious disease should be consulted.
All patients should also be tested for syphilis and HIV.

35. Can *N. meningitides* cause septic arthritis?

Infectious arthritis can be seen in as many as 14% of those with invasive meningococcal disease, though rarely patients can have isolated meningococcal arthritis. It typically affects the knee or other large joints. Joint fluid is often sterile. Joint outcomes are typically good with preservation of function.

36. Can syphilis cause arthritis?

Infection with *Treponema pallidum*, otherwise known as syphilis, can cause a polyarthritis that can be confused with other connective tissue diseases. This can occur during any stage of syphilis, though most musculoskeletal manifestations occur during the secondary stage. Knee involvement has been reported most, but shoulders, elbows, wrists, ankles, and sacroiliac joints are common as well. Syphilitic arthritis should be suspected in patients with polyarthritis, along with other symptoms suggestive of syphilis infection, such as genital chancre with localized lymphadenopathy, maculopapular rash on the palms and soles, fever, and malaise. Tenosynovitis may be present. Synovial fluid cell counts range from 4000 to 13,000/mm^3. Diagnosis is made by either treponemal antibody testing or nontreponemal testing (rapid plasma reagin test). Treatment for secondary syphilis is benzathine penicillin 2.4 million units intramuscularly (IM) once or doxycycline 100 mg twice daily for 14 days. Treatment for late latent or tertiary syphilis with associated arthritis is benzathine penicillin 2.4 million units IM weekly for 3 weeks or doxycycline 100 mg twice daily for 28 days. Concomitant HIV infection should always be ruled out.

37. Can bursae become infected?

The olecranon (adults) and prepatellar (children) bursae are the most common sites of septic bursitis. Most septic bursitis occurs in patients who repeatedly traumatize the skin in these areas via manual labor or recreational activities. Alcoholism, diabetes, glucocorticoid therapy, and rheumatoid arthritis are also risk factors. Over 80% of septic bursitis is due to *S. aureus*. Blood cultures are rarely positive because the organisms get into the bursa by transcutaneous spread through skin abrasions. Patients usually have abrupt onset of pain, swelling, and erythema. Diagnosis is made by aspiration, Gram stain, and culture of bursal fluid. Bursal fluid cell counts are elevated but not as much as in septic joints. Antibiotics should be administered based on Gram stain results. Role for surgical incision and drainage is not standardized but should be considered in those with severe infection or infections that do not respond to antibiotic therapy alone.

38. What are the different etiologies and classifications of osteomyelitis?

Etiology:
- **Hematogenous:** Seen mostly in children and elderly adults, usually monomicrobial, more common in children; typical route for vertebral osteomyelitis/discitis in adults.
- **Contiguous spread** from adjacent foci of infection (such as diabetic foot infections), usually polymicrobial.
- **Direct inoculation from trauma**
  Classification:
- **Acute:** osteomyelitis prior to the development of osteonecrosis; can be treated with antibiotics +/– surgery.
- **Chronic:** osteomyelitis with development of osteonecrosis. Defined by the presence of sequestra—separated fragments of necrotic bone devoid of blood supply that can harbor bacteria despite antibiotic treatment. Other indications of chronic osteomyelitis are involucrum (new bone growth around areas of sequestra), sinus tracts, and bone loss. Treatment requires surgical resection of sequestra followed by antibiotics.

39. How is osteomyelitis diagnosed?

- Gold standard: culture and histopathology of infected bone.
- Probe-to-bone: exposed bone or ability to probe to bone has sensitivity of 60% and specificity of 91% in diabetic foot ulcers.
- Plain radiographs: can detect osteomyelitis after ~2 weeks of symptoms (may miss early osteomyelitis).
- MRI: highest sensitivity with detection within 3 to 5 days of symptom onset.
- CT: more sensitive than plain radiographs, less sensitive than MRI. Useful for evaluating for the presence of sequestra and involucrum.

- Laboratory tests will usually reveal leukocytosis and elevations in ESR/CRP. Blood cultures are positive in ~50% of acute hematogenous osteomyelitis cases.

PEARL: Cultures of sinus tracts are not predictive of the organisms found in bone with the exception of *S. aureus*.

40. What is the difference between sequestrum and Brodie's abscess?

- <u>Sequestra</u>: Segments of necrotic bone separated from living bone by granulation tissue. Must be removed by debridement owing to inability of antibiotics to sterilize it.
- <u>Brodie's abscess</u>: Subacute form of osteomyelitis presenting as purulent collection within bone, often with insidious onset and can be mistaken for bone tumor, leading to delay in diagnosis.

ACKNOWLEDGMENT

The authors would like to acknowledge the contributions of Dr. Steven C. Johnson to this chapter in the previous edition.

BIBLIOGRAPHY

Chihara S, Segreti J. Osteomyelitis. *Disease-a-Month*. 2010;56:6–31.

Hariharan P, Kabrhel C. Sensitivity of erythrocyte sedimentation rate and C-reactive protein for the exclusion of septic arthritis in emergency department patients. *J Emerg Med*. 2011;40:428.

Johnson AJ, Zywiel MG, Stroh A, Marker DR, Mont MA. Serological markers can lead to false negative diagnoses of periprosthetic infections following total knee arthroplasty. *Int Orthop (SICOT)*. 2011;35:1621–1626.

Lormeau C, Cormier G, Sigaux J, Arvieux C, Semerano L. Management of septic bursitis. *Joint Bone Spine*. 2019;86:583–588.

Manadan AM, Block JA. Daily needle aspiration versus surgical lavage for the treatment of bacterial septic arthritis in adults. *Am J Ther*. 2004;11:412–415.

Margaretten ME, Knowles J, Moore D, Brent S. Does this adult patient have septic arthritis? *JAMA*. 2007;297:1478–1488.

Mathews CJ, Kingsley G, Field M, et al. Management of septic arthritis: a systematic review. *Ann Rheum Dis*. 2007;66:440–445.

Mathews CJ, Weston VC, Jones A, et al. Bacterial septic arthritis in adults. *Lancet*. 2010;375:846–855.

Osmon DR, Berbari EF, Berendt AR, et al. Diagnosis and management of prosthetic joint infection: clinical practice guidelines by the Infectious Diseases Society of America. *Clin Infect Dis*. 2013;56:e1–e25.

Palestro CJ, Love C, Miller TT. Diagnostic imaging tests and microbial infections. *Cell Microbiol*. 2007;9:2323–2333.

Quinn RH, Murray JN, Pezold R, Sevarino KS. Members of the Writing and Voting Panels of the AUC for the Management of Patients with Orthopaedic Implants Undergoing Dental Procedures. The American Academy of Orthopaedic Surgeons appropriate use criteria for the management of patients with orthopaedic implants undergoing dental procedures. *J Bone Joint Surg Am*. 2017;99:161–163.

Ravindran V, Logan I, Bourke BE. Medical vs surgical treatment for native joint in septic arthritis: a 6-year, single UK academic centre experience. *Rheumatology*. 2009;48:1320–1322.

Rice PA. Gonococcal arthritis. *Infect Dis Clin North Am*. 2005;19:853–861.

Ross JJ. Septic arthritis of native joints. *Infect Dis Clin North Am*. 2017;31:203–218.

Rupasov A, Cain U, Montoya S, Blickman JG. Imaging of posttraumatic arthritis, avascular necrosis, septic arthritis, complex regional pain syndrome, and cancer mimicking arthritis. *Rad Clin North Am*. 2017;55:1111–1130.

Saavedra-Lozano J, Falup-Pecurariu O, Faust SN, et al. Bone and joint infections. *Ped Infect Dis J*. 2017;36:788–799.

Signore A, Sconfienza LM, Borens O, et al. Consensus document for the diagnosis of prosthetic joint infections: a joint paper by the EANM, EBJIS, and ESR (with ESCMID endorsement). *Eur J Nucl Med Mol Imaging*. 2019;46:971–988.

Singleton JD, West SG, Nordstrom DM. "Pseudoseptic" arthritis complicating rheumatoid arthritis: a report of 6 cases. *J Rheumatol*. 1991;18:1319.

Tande AJ, Patel R. Prosthetic Joint Infection. *Clin Microbiol Rev*. 2014;27:302–345.

Traczuk A, Chetrit DA, Balasubramanya R, et al. Musculoskeletal manifestations of syphilis in adults: secondary syphilis presenting with ankle inflammatory arthritis and bone involvement with calvarial and sternal lesions. What the rheumatologist needs to know? *Clin Rheumatol*. 2023;42:1195–1203.

Van Der Naald N, Smeeing DPJ, et al. Brodie's abscess: a systematic review of reported cases. *J Bone Joint Infect*. 2019;4:33–39.

Zhou MX, Berbari EF, Couch CG, Gruwell SF, Carr AB. Viewpoint: periprosthetic joint infection and dental antibiotic prophylaxis guidelines. *J Bone Jt Infect*. 2021;6:363–366.

CHAPTER 38

Lyme Disease

Trevor McKown, MD and Tiffany Lin, MD

> **KEY POINTS**
>
> 1. Lyme disease is the most common vector-borne disease in the United States, with peak onset in spring and summer months.
> 2. Erythema migrans (EM) is the diagnostic skin lesion occurring at the site of the tick bite.
> 3. Disseminated infection can affect the nervous system, heart, and joints.
> 4. Diagnosis of disseminated infection is confirmed by a positive screening immunoassay and immunoblot or alternate assay for *Borrelia burgdorferi* in the serum of a patient with appropriate clinical findings.
> 5. Oral antibiotics are effective for prevention of late disease manifestations and early disease (EM), but intravenous antibiotics may be necessary for disseminated disease.
> 6. Coinfection with *Babesia* or *Anaplasma* should be considered in any patient with hemolysis, neutropenia, and/or thrombocytopenia.

1. How was Lyme disease recognized as a distinct clinical entity?

Lyme disease was first recognized as a distinct entity in Lyme, Connecticut, in 1975. Neighborhood outbreak of juvenile rheumatoid (idiopathic) arthritis was reported to the state public health department by the mothers of the affected children because they believed the neighborhood clustering to be more than coincidence. The outbreak in this rural community was consistent with an infectious etiology transmitted by an arthropod vector.

2. What is the etiology of Lyme disease?

Lyme disease in the United States is caused by an infection with the tick-borne spirochete, *B. burgdorferi*, which was discovered in 1982. A cluster of closely related spirochete species is classified as *B. burgdorferi* sensu lato; this cluster includes over 20 species, of which 9 have been shown to cause disease in humans. *B. burdorferi* sensu stricto causes the vast majority of infections in the United States, while three species (*B. afzelii, B. garinii,* and *B. bavariensis*) cause most infections in Europe. There are many similarities to syphilis; it is a multisystem disease occurring in stages that can mimic other diseases. *Borrelia* can only rarely be cultured from the blood or other infected tissues. The incubation period is 3 to 32 days.

3. What is the geographic distribution and seasonal occurrence of Lyme disease in the United States? In what other countries has it been reported?

Lyme disease is most prevalent from April or May to November in the endemic areas. The peak incidence is in the late spring and early summer months of June and July. In the United States, there are an estimated 476,000 people who contract Lyme disease every year. Lyme disease has been reported in many of the 48 contiguous states, but most cases occur in two high-incidence regions:

- Northeast and Atlantic Coast (Maine, Vermont, New Hampshire, New York, Pennsylvania, Connecticut, Massachusetts, Rhode Island, Delaware, Maryland, Virginia)
- Upper Midwest (Wisconsin and Minnesota)

Lyme disease is also present in the Pacific Northwest (Northern California and Oregon), but rates of disease are much lower (likely due to lower rates of Borrelia infection in tick vectors in this region, as discussed below).

Lyme disease also occurs in Europe (highest in the Netherlands, Belgium, Slovenia, Austria, Lithuania, and Estonia) and cases have been reported in Asia (China and Mongolia). Lyme disease is the most common vector-borne disease in the United States and Europe and the second most common in the world (malaria being the most common).

4. Name the arthropod vector of *B. burgdorferi*, its animal hosts, and describe how Lyme disease is transmitted?

Ixodes scapularis is the tick that represents the major vector in the Northeastern and Midwest United States. *I. scapularis* egg mass is typically laid in the leaf clutter at the bottom of a forest; consequently, this tick does not thrive in dry climates. Larvae (the first stage of tick development) emerge in the summer and fall. They require a blood meal that they obtain from rodents, an asymptomatic reservoir for *Borrelia*. After the tick larvae acquire *Borrelia* with their blood meal, they fall off the mouse and molt to nymphs (the second stage of tick development) that lay dormant until late spring and summer of the following year. Infected nymphs can then pass *Borrelia* on to other mice and humans (transmission of infection) when they take a blood meal. Subsequently, the nymphs become adults (final stage of tick development), and the females feed on white-tailed deer to get blood nutrients to make eggs. The eggs are laid in leaf clutter, completing the 2-year life cycle. Of note, the eggs are not infected with *Borrelia* even if the female tick is (the tick subsequently acquires the spirochete during the larvae stage from the rodent host population). Up to 50% of adult ticks are infected in endemic areas.

I. pacificus is the vector on the West Coast of the United States; its preferred host is lizards, which are resistant to infection with *Borrelia,* resulting in lower rates of *Borrelia* carriage among *I. pacificus.* Other ixodid species are the vectors in other parts of the world. *Ixodes* species in Europe feed on mammals, birds, and reptiles; birds are an important reservoir for *B. garinii*, and rodents are an important reservoir for *B. afzelii*.

The bite of an ixodid tick is remembered by only half of the patients with Lyme disease—a key point to remember when taking a history. The tick is very small (size of a freckle) and often simply overlooked. The intestinal tract of the tick is the reservoir for *Borrelia*. The blood meal ingested by the tick stimulates local spirochetes to enter a state that allows them to invade the salivary glands of the tick and subsequently be transmitted to the human (or rodent) on which it is feeding, typically hours after initial attachment.

5. What organ systems are involved in Lyme disease?

The disease is often thought of as a "rash-arthritis" complex, but not all patients have rash or arthritis. In the United States, 80% of patients infected with *B. burgdorferi* develop the typical skin rash, EM. Joint involvement is common, with polyarthralgia an early finding, and inflammatory oligoarthritis a later manifestation. In addition, the nervous system (both central and peripheral) and the cardiac system are frequently involved. In Europe, arthritis is less common but skin and neurologic involvement are more common.

6. What are the three stages of Lyme disease, and which organ systems are involved in each stage?

The manifestations of Lyme disease can be organized into three stages, although not all patients experience a linear progression through these stages.
- Early localized: skin (EM), regional lymphadenopathy, flu-like symptoms.
- Disseminated infection: nervous, cardiac, skin, and musculoskeletal systems.
- Persistent infection (late disease): musculoskeletal and nervous systems.

The first stage of Lyme disease occurs days to weeks after inoculation. "Flu-like" symptoms such as headache, fatigue, arthralgias often occur, as can fever (15%) and regional lymphadenopathy (25%). EM usually resolves in several days to a few weeks. The second stage, or disseminated infection, occurs weeks to months after EM occurs and is due to hematogenous spread. The third stage occurs at a mean of 6 months after disease onset (but may occur as soon as days to as late as 2 years after disease onset).

7. Describe the typical rash of Lyme disease.

In 80% to 90% of patients with Lyme borreliosis in the United States, the disease begins with EM, which usually occurs at the site of the tick bite. EM is most frequently found in the groin, axilla, waist, back, and legs. In children, the head is also a common site. EM begins as a red macule or papule that expands to form a **large annular lesion** measuring ≥20 cm in diameter. Classically, it has an area of **central clearing** and a bright red outer border (Fig. 38.1), but more commonly lesions are uniform in color or have enhanced central erythema. **An EM-like lesion can also be a sign of Southern tick-associated rash illness** (STARI), which is associated with

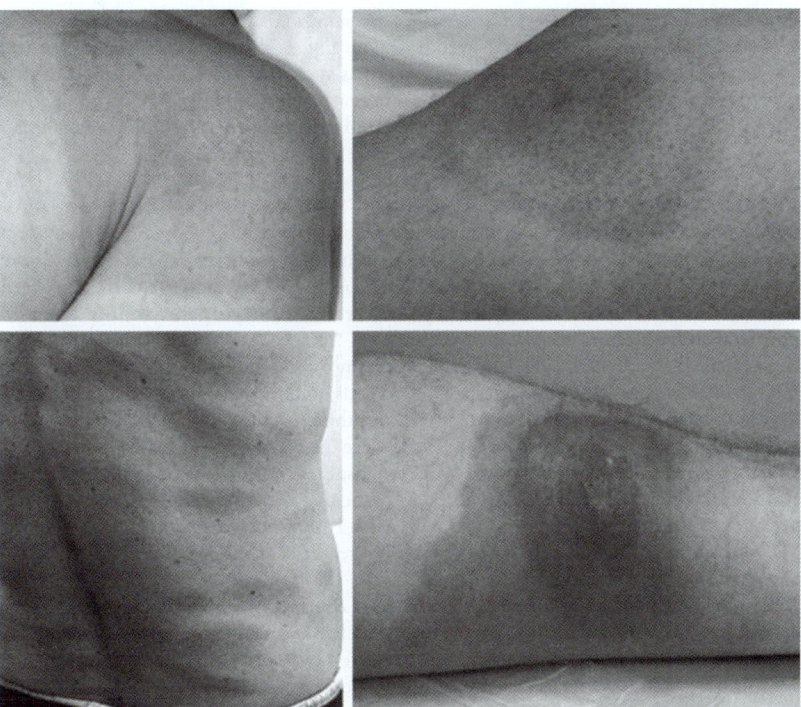

Fig. 38.1 The lesions of erythema chronicum migrans. (Courtesy Juan Salazar, MD, University of Connecticut Health Center.)

bites from the lone star tick, *Amblyomma americanum,* present in the southeastern and south-central United States. The causative agent of STARI is unknown, as is whether antibiotic treatment is helpful for treatment of STARI.

8. What clinical manifestations occur in the second stage (disseminated infection) of Lyme disease?

The nervous, cardiac, skin, and musculoskeletal systems are classically involved in the second stage of Lyme disease. Approximately 10% of patients develop neurologic symptoms 1 to 2 weeks into the disease. The most common neurologic manifestations are cranial nerve palsy (especially unilateral or bilateral Bell's palsy), lymphocytic meningitis, or a motor or sensory radiculoneuritis. Cardiac manifestations occur in <3% of untreated patients during this stage and include varying degrees of atrioventricular block (usually temporary) and myo- or pancarditis. The heart valves are not involved, distinguishing it from acute rheumatic fever. Secondary (satellite) skin lesions are common (50%) and indicate spirochetal dissemination. Migratory arthralgias are common, but frank arthritis is usually not prevalent until the third stage. Lymphadenopathy, splenomegaly, mild hepatitis, sensorineural hearing loss, iritis/keratitis, and severe fatigue can also occur.

9. Describe the clinical manifestations of the third stage (late disease) of Lyme disease.

The third stage of Lyme disease occurs in 10% of untreated patients and represents persistent infection due to *B. burgdorferi,* which has mechanisms that enable it to evade the immune system. This stage usually involves episodic attacks of an **asymmetric oligoarticular arthritis** affecting the large joints (knee in 80% of cases). Epidemiologic surveillance data suggest about 30% of patients with Lyme disease present with arthritis. Over time, the arthritic attacks typically resolve. In <10% of patients, the arthritis becomes more persistent and chronic, again usually affecting the knee. Fatigue frequently accompanies the arthritis episodes, but in general fever and other systemic symptoms do not. Synovial fluid is typically inflammatory (white blood cell count averaging around 15,000 mm^3 in adults; WBC counts are frequently higher in children). In Europe a progressive skin lesion, *acrodermatitis chronica atrophicans,* is the most common late manifestation. The lesions are red or bluish-red swellings, typically on the extensor surfaces of extremities, which eventually become atrophic. **Chronic nervous system involvement** may occur in the third stage but is rare. Manifestations include a chronic severe encephalomyelitis, primarily described in Europe. Stroke-like presentations, a mild sensory polyneuropathy, and mild encephalopathy have also been described.

10. What other tickborne diseases can co-occur with Lyme disease?

I. scapularis can transmit other pathogens at the time it transmits *B. burgdorferi.* The two most common in the United States are *Babesia microti* (which causes babesiosis) and *Anaplasma phagocytophilum* (which causes human granulocytic anaplasmosis). **Any patient with suspected Lyme disease who has hemolytic anemia, leukopenia, or thrombocytopenia should be investigated for coinfection with one of these pathogens.**

Babesiosis causes fever, headaches, myalgias, hemolytic anemia, thrombocytopenia, and elevated liver enzymes. *Babesia* invades red blood cells, and intraerythrocytic organisms may be seen on peripheral blood smear. Treatment requires therapy with azithromycin plus atovaquone, or clindamycin plus quinine, for 7 to 10 days. Severe disease may require hospitalization and IV treatment. **Human granulocytic anaplasmosis** causes fever, headache, arthralgias, leukopenia, and thrombocytopenia. If it is misdiagnosed as Lyme disease, it still responds to doxycycline but not to amoxicillin therapy. Treatment is doxycycline 100 mg twice daily for 10 days. Patients allergic to or unable to take doxycycline should be treated with rifampin 300 mg twice daily (or 10 mg/kg twice daily for children) for 7 to 10 days.

I. scapularis can rarely transmit other pathogens. *Borrelia miyamotoi* causes relapsing fever, headache, myalgia, arthralgia, and fatigue; unlike in Lyme disease, these individuals will not have a rash. Powassan virus is a flavivirus that is transmitted by *I. scapularis* bites in the Northeast and Upper Midwest. Powassan virus infection causes an encephalitis, which is fatal in about 10% of patients and often leads to long-term morbidity in survivors. Treatment is supportive.

11. How is EM treated?

Doxycycline is the drug of choice. Doxycycline has good penetration into the central nervous system (CNS) and is also effective against coinfection with *Anaplasma.* In younger children (<8 years old), pregnant and breastfeeding women, doxycycline has been traditionally avoided due to concern for staining of permanent teeth; however, more recent data suggest short courses of doxycycline are safe in children, although there is still lack of data in pregnant and breastfeeding women. Amoxicillin or cefuroxime axetil is recommended if doxycycline cannot be used. Azithromycin has lower efficacy so it is used only if beta-lactams are contraindicated. Treatment shortens the duration of EM and greatly reduces the occurrence of later manifestations of Lyme disease.

2020 IDSA/AAN/ACR TREATMENT GUIDELINES FOR ERYTHEMA MIGRANS

Age Category	Drug	Dosage	Maximum Dose	Duration (Days)
Adults	Doxycycline	100 mg twice daily or 200 mg once daily, orally	N/A	10
	Cefuroxime axetil	500 mg twice daily orally	N/A	14
	Amoxicillin	500 mg three times daily orally	N/A	14
	Azithromycin[a]	500 mg once daily orally	N/A	7
Children	Doxycycline	4.4 mg/kg per day orally, divided into two doses	200 mg daily	10
	Amoxicillin	50 mg/kg per day orally, divided into three doses	500 mg per dose	14
	Cefuroxime axetil	30 mg/kg per day orally, divided into two doses	500 mg per dose	14
	Azithromycin[a]	10/mg kg per day orally	500 mg per dose	7

[a]Reserved for patients for whom beta-lactam antibiotics are contraindicated.

12. What diagnostic tests are available for Lyme disease?

In addition to the clinical diagnosis (tick bite in an endemic area followed by EM), serologic antibody testing is commonly used. Detection of antibodies to *B. burgdorferi* may be performed by one of two approaches for two-tiered testing: standard two-tiered testing (STTT) and modified

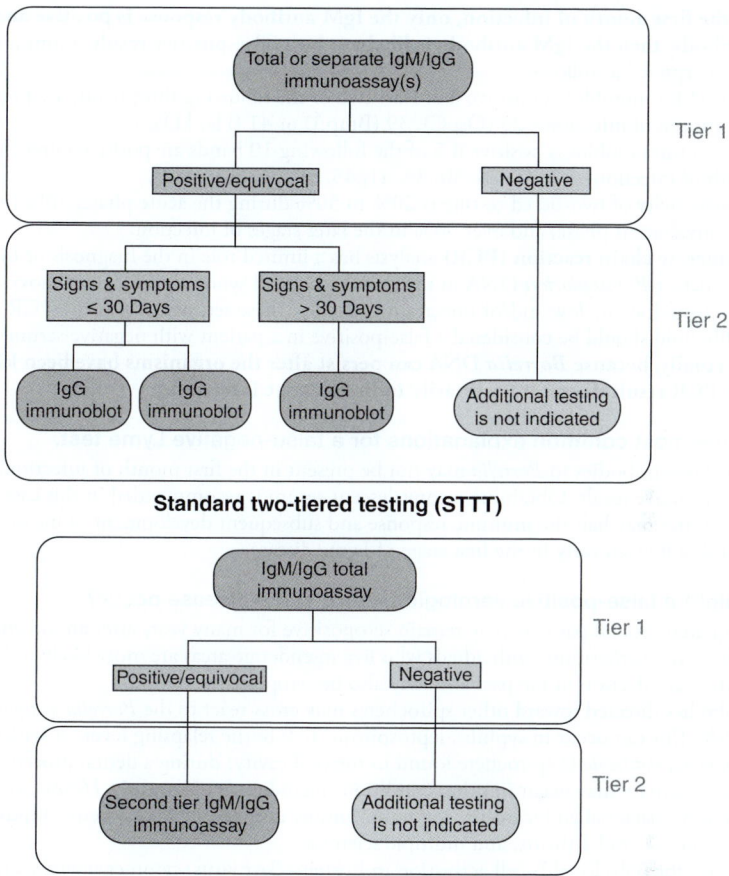

Standard two-tiered testing (STTT)

Modified two-tiered testing (MTTT)

Fig. 38.2 Standard two-tiered testing (STTT) and Modified two-tiered testing (MTTT) for Lyme Disease Standard two-tiered testing (STTT) Modified two-tiered testing (MTTT).

two-tiered testing (MTTT). STTT utilizes an immunoassay for screening, followed by immunoblot testing for confirmation. MTTT uses two separate immunoassays (one for screening, the other for confirmation) that together have been cleared by the FDA for diagnosis. These tests should be performed and interpreted according to Centers for Disease Control criteria to ensure accuracy (Fig. 38.2).

For screening tests, 70% to 80% of patients will be IgM-positive within 2 to 4 weeks following infection. IgM antibodies peak at 6 to 8 weeks. IgG antibodies are positive after 4 weeks and peak at 4 to 6 months after infection. **It is important to note that screening tests may lead to false negative results within the 1st month of disease onset.** Therefore, in a patient with acute disease, IgM and IgG antibody responses should be measured in both acute and convalescent sera, and patients with EM should be treated empirically at onset regardless of the results from the initial sample. Both IgM and especially IgG antibodies can remain positive for years after successful therapy with antibiotics. Therefore, persistent IgM antibodies following adequate antibiotic therapy do not indicate active or inadequately treated infection.

For confirmatory testing in the STTT, immunoblot is more specific but less sensitive than the immunoassay for diagnosing Lyme disease. In the MTTT, the second tier (confirmatory) immunoassay will have comparable test characteristics to immunoblot. After the first month of infection, only the IgG antibody response should be used to support the diagnosis (Fig. 38.2).

If after the first month of infection, only the IgM antibody response is positive and not the IgG antibody, then the IgM antibody is likely to be a false-positive result. Immunoblot positivity is interpreted as follows:

- The IgM immunoblot is positive if at least two of the following three bands are present (first month of infection): 23 (OspC), 39 (BmpA) or 41 (Fla) kDa
- The IgG immunoblot is positive if 5 of the following 10 bands are positive (after the first month of infection): 18, 21, 28, 30, 39, 41, 45, 58, 66, or 93 kDa.

The sensitivity of two-tiered testing is 20% to 50% during the acute phase, 70% to 80% during the convalescent phase, and over 90% in the later stages of infection.

Polymerase chain reaction (PCR) analysis has a limited role in the diagnosis of Lyme disease. PCR can detect *B. burgdorferi* DNA in the skin, spinal and synovial fluid, and synovial tissue, but the sensitivities are low and/or uncertain in each of these settings. A positive PCR result from any bodily fluid should be considered a false-positive in a patient with negative serum two-tiered testing. **Finally, because *Borrelia* DNA can persist after the organisms have been killed, a positive PCR result does not necessarily indicate active infection.**

13. Name the most common explanations for a false-negative Lyme test.

IgM and IgG antibodies to *Borrelia* may not be present in the first month of infection, leading to a false-negative result. Obtaining a convalescent serum is recommended in this case. Additionally, antibiotics may halt the immune response and subsequent development of measurable levels of antibodies if given early in the first stage of Lyme disease.

14. Why might a false-positive serologic test for Lyme disease occur?

- Adequately treated patients may remain seropositive for many years after an infection is eradicated. Furthermore, individuals who live in endemic areas are more likely to have had a subclinical infection in the past and may also be seropositive.
- Antibodies directed toward other spirochetes may cross-react to the *Borrelia* antigen(s) used in ELISA. This can occur in syphilis, leptospirosis, tick-borne relapsing fever, or with exposure to *Treponema denticola* (a spirochete found in the oral cavity) during a dental procedure.
- Cross-reactivity may occur in other conditions including anaplasmosis, *Helicobacter pylori* infections, bacterial endocarditis, and autoimmune diseases, such as systemic lupus erythematosus, rheumatoid arthritis, and multiple sclerosis.
- Nonspecific polyclonal B-cell activation in Epstein–Barr virus, cytomegalovirus, and malaria may also produce cross-reactive antibodies.
- The use of unvalidated methods for interpretation of immunoblots may lead to false-positive results.

Due to these limitations, Lyme testing should only be used to confirm the diagnosis in patients with a compatible clinical presentation and should be avoided as a screening method in patients who have multiple vague complaints.

15. Describe additional laboratory abnormalities that may be seen in Lyme disease.

In patients with neuroborreliosis, cerebrospinal fluid (CSF) analysis typically shows a lymphocytic pleocytosis, mildly elevated protein concentration (100–200 mg/dL), and normal glucose concentration. Additionally, a high IgG index and oligoclonal bands may be present. Specific testing includes intrathecal antibodies against *Borrelia*. The most sensitive and specific application of this test is through the calculation of an antibody index (the ratio of *Borrelia*/total antibody in the CSF versus the same ratio in the serum). PCR testing of CSF may also be performed, but the sensitivity is very low (<20%). While CSF testing lacks the sensitivity of serum testing, it is a useful and often necessary undertaking required to rule out other causes of meningitis and encephalomyelitis.

During episodes of arthritis, synovial fluid white cell counts range from 500 to 110,000/mm^3 (mean 15,000/mm^3) with a polymorphonuclear predominance. PCR can detect *B. burgdorferi* DNA in synovial fluid and synovial tissue; however, PCR is less sensitive than two-step serologic testing so is not used in routine diagnosis of Lyme arthritis. PCR from synovial fluid or tissue may also remain positive for weeks or months after antimicrobial therapy, complicating interpretation of results. Synovial PCR may assist a diagnosis of Lyme arthritis in patients presenting with arthritis and known prior Lyme infection, since serologic testing may remain positive for years in these patients and will be unable to differentiate current infection from prior infection.

Significant hematologic or liver function abnormalities are not characteristic of Lyme disease and, if present, should raise concern for co-infection with other tickborne diseases (see Question #10.)

16. How should the second (disseminated disease) and third (late disease) stages of Lyme disease be treated?

Disease Manifestation	Antibiotic	Treatment Duration in Days (Range)
Second Stage (Disseminated Disease)		
Meningitis, radiculopathy or peripheral neuropathy	Ceftriaxone 2 g intravenous (IV) daily (pediatric dosage 50–75 mg/kg IV daily)	14–21
	Doxycycline 100 mg orally twice daily (pediatric dosage for children aged ≥8 years 4–8 mg/kg daily divided in two doses)	14–21
Isolated facial nerve palsy	Same oral antibiotics as used in the treatment of erythema migrans	14–21
Carditis[a,b]	Ceftriaxone 2 g IV daily (pediatric dosage 50–75 mg/kg IV daily) initially for hospitalized patients	14–21
	Same oral antibiotics as used in the treatment of erythema migrans (outpatients or for the remainder of treatment in hospitalized patients)	14–21
Third Stage (Late Disease)		
Arthritis	Same oral antibiotics as used in the treatment of erythema migrans	28
	If partial improvement with initial oral antibiotic, observe vs. re-treat with oral antibiotics	28 with oral antibiotics
	If no response to initial oral antibiotics, treat with IV ceftriaxone versus another course of oral antibiotics	14–28 with IV ceftriaxone 28 with oral antibiotics
Encephalomyelitis	Ceftriaxone 2 g IV daily (pediatric dosage 50–75 mg/kg IV daily)	14–28

[a]Hospitalization and continuous cardiac monitoring in patients with chest pain, dyspnea, syncope, first-degree heart block with PR interval ≥300 ms, second- or third-degree heart block.
[b]Advanced heart block may require a temporary pacemaker.

17. What is post-antibiotic Lyme arthritis and how is it treated?

Up to 10% of patients with Lyme arthritis continue to experience synovitis despite completion of two courses of antibiotics, which is referred to as **post-antibiotic Lyme arthritis** (previously termed *antibiotic-refractory*). PCR testing of synovial fluid and/or tissue specimens usually yields negative results in these patients. It has been hypothesized that these patients carry particular class II major histocompatibility genes (HLA-DR4 and DRB1*1501 alleles) which can bind an epitope of *B. burgdorferi* outer surface protein A (OspA) that cross-reacts with a self-protein, leading to autoimmune joint inflammation. Additional courses of antibiotic therapy are not recommended given the absence of persistent infection. Initial treatment includes nonsteroidal anti-inflammatory drugs and intraarticular corticosteroid injections; if persistent, disease-modifying antirheumatic drugs including hydroxychloroquine, methotrexate, or TNF inhibitors are used. If synovitis persists despite these treatments, arthroscopic synovectomy is advised.

18. How can Lyme disease be prevented?

It is optimal to avoid tick-prone habitats (tall grasses, brush) while in an endemic area. Individuals should wear long-sleeved shirts tucked into pants, and the pant legs should be tucked into socks. Light-colored clothing allows detection and removal of ticks. Tick repellents including DEET, picaridin, and IR3535 can be applied to skin and clothing. Permethrin can only be applied to clothing but is highly effective at repelling ticks. Clothing that has been commercially impregnated with permethrin may also be purchased. Body checks should be performed on a daily basis, and attached ticks should immediately be removed with forceps. If there are any mouth-parts left in the skin, they should be left alone and be allowed to naturally fall out over time. In the case of a confirmed *Ixodes* tick attached for over 36 hours, postexposure antibiotic prophylaxis can be given (see question #19).

A human vaccine using a recombinant OspA antigen, LYMErix, was marketed in the United States in 1998 but was withdrawn in 2002 due to modest efficacy, safety concerns, and poor sales. There are currently several ongoing clinical trials for vaccine candidates including a multivalent recombinant protein and mRNA vaccines.

19. When is antibiotic prophylaxis indicated after a tick bite?

Only tick bites that are at high risk of transmitting Lyme infection require prophylaxis. A high-risk bite is one from a tick that has been identified as an *Ixodes* vector, in a region of high Lyme disease endemicity, and with a prolonged attachment (>36 hours) leading to visible engorgement. If all these criteria are met, a single dose of doxycycline (200 mg PO for adults, 4.4 mg/kg up to 200 mg for children) should be given within 72 hours of tick removal. This regimen has been shown to significantly reduce the risk of subsequent Lyme disease. For tick bites not meeting these criteria, patients should be advised to seek medical attention if they develop symptoms (particularly an erythematous lesion at the bite site).

DIFFICULT CLINICAL SITUATIONS

20. A patient reports she has had diffuse arthralgias/myalgias for many months and has a diagnosis of fibromyalgia. She reports she used to visit New York, although never went camping or hiking. Her physician ordered a Lyme test, and the IgM immunoassay returned positive. Should she get antibiotics?

No. The immunoassay test leads to many false-positive results. The IgM immunoblots can also lead to false-positive results and are useful only in the first few weeks of an infection. Patients with symptoms for >1 to 2 months who have a negative IgG immunoassay and/or IgG immunoblot do not have Lyme disease. In other words, IgG seropositivity is virtually universal in the later stages of Lyme disease.

21. A patient with a history of definite Lyme disease in the past has been treated with two courses of appropriate IV antibiotics for 1 month each time. She continues to experience myalgias and has been diagnosed with fibromyalgia. Should she receive another course of therapy with a different antibiotic?

No. This patient has post treatment Lyme disease syndrome (PTLDS), a condition that occurs in <10% of patients with Lyme disease. Symptoms last for over 6 months and resemble fibromyalgia with subjective cognitive and memory difficulty, widespread pain, sleep disturbance, and fatigue. This condition has been referred to by laypeople as "chronic Lyme disease"; however, there is no clinical evidence of ongoing infection in these individuals. (The term chronic Lyme disease was also used in the medical literature to refer to active disease in second or third stage Lyme disease, but the preferred nomenclature is now late Lyme disease.)

The pathophysiology of PTLDS is unclear, but some theories have suggested that the inflammatory state may last after the infection has been eradicated. Three National Institute of Health–funded placebo-controlled clinical trials in patients with PTLDS have shown a lack of benefit with antibiotic therapy when compared with placebo. In addition, there was an adverse event rate with parenteral antibiotics in these studies. Therefore, this population of patients should not be treated with antibiotics. Instead, symptomatic treatment and exclusion of other medical conditions are recommended.

22. An adult is referred to you for a positive IgG EIA and immunoblot test for exposure to *B. burgdorferi*. The test was obtained by his primary care physician as part of an annual physical exam, since the patient frequently hikes and camps in an area with known Lyme disease. He has never had symptoms of Lyme disease and is asymptomatic. Do you treat him with antibiotics?

There are no formal guidelines for this scenario, since routine screening for Lyme disease is not recommended in asymptomatic patients who may have a greater exposure to *Ixodes* ticks. Some argue that a 1-month course of oral antibiotics is indicated to assure eradication of the spirochete, similar to the treatment of an asymptomatic patient found to have a positive fluorescent treponemal antibody absorption test for syphilis. Others argue that the patient had a subclinical infection and the patient's immune system has already eradicated the *Borrelia*.

ACKNOWLEDGMENT

The authors would like to acknowledge the contributions of Dr. Kevin McKown to this chapter in the previous edition.

BIBLIOGRAPHY

Association of Public Health Laboratories. *Suggested Reporting Language, Interpretation and Guidance Regarding Lyme Disease Serologic Test Results.* 2024. https://www.aphl.org/aboutAPHL/publications/Documents/ID-2024-Lyme-Disease-Serologic-Testing-Reporting.pdf.

Koedel U, Fingerle V, Pfister HW. Lyme neuroborreliosis-epidemiology, diagnosis and management. *Nat Rev Neurol.* 2015;11:446–456.

Kugeler KJ, Schwartz AM, Delorey MJ, Mead PS, Hinckley AF. Estimating the frequency of Lyme disease diagnoses, United States, 2010–2018. *Emerg Infect Dis.* 2021;27:616–619.

Lantos PM, Rumbaugh J, Bockenstedt LK, et al. Clinical practice guidelines by the Infectious Diseases Society of America (IDSA), American Academy of Neurology (AAN), and American College of Rheumatology (ACR): 2020 guidelines for the prevention, diagnosis, and treatment of Lyme disease. *Arthritis Rheumatol.* 2021;73:12–20.

Lochhead RB, Strle K, Arvikar SL, Weis JJ, Steere AC. Lyme arthritis: linking infection, inflammation and autoimmunity. *Nat Rev Rheumatol.* 2021;17:449–461.

Radolf JD, Strle K, Lemieux JE, Strle F. Lyme disease in humans. *Curr Issues Mol Biol.* 2021;42:333–384.

Schwartz AM, Hinckley AF, Mead PS, Hook SA, Kugeler KJ. Surveillance for Lyme Disease—United States, 2008–2015. *MMWR Surveill Summ.* 2017;66:1–12.

Steere AC, Malawista SE, Snydman DR, et al. Lyme arthritis: an epidemic of oligoarticular arthritis in children and adults in three Connecticut communities. *Arthritis Rheum.* 1977;20:7–17.

Swanson SJ, Neitzel D, Reed KD, Belongia EA. Coinfections acquired from *ixodes* ticks. *Clin Microbiol Rev.* 2006;19:708–727.

FURTHER READING

www.cdc.gov/Lyme.
www.idsociety.org/Lyme.

CHAPTER 39

Mycobacterial and Fungal Joint and Bone Diseases

Jared J. Eddy, MD, MSc and Michael Haden, MD

There is a fungus among us.
    —Terry Nolan, 1958

> **KEY POINTS**
>
> 1. Osteoarticular tuberculosis (TB) accounts for about 10% of all cases of extrapulmonary TB disease.
> 2. Many patients with osteoarticular TB will have a normal chest radiograph.
> 3. Nontuberculous mycobacterial (NTM) musculoskeletal infections most commonly present as hand tenosynovitis but may also cause vertebral osteomyelitis.
> 4. Treatment of NTM infections often requires surgical debridement given the extensive drug resistance and limited effectiveness of active antibiotics.
> 5. Fungal osteoarticular infections are often indolent with symptom onset over several weeks to months.

1. What percentage of patients with TB have bone or joint involvement?

About one-fourth of the world's population is estimated to be infected with *Mycobacterium tuberculosis* (MTB) leading to about 10 million annual cases of TB including some 1.5 million annual deaths. Extrapulmonary disease accounts for 20% of all cases of TB, of which about 10% have osteoarticular involvement. Of all TB cases, 1–3% have skeletal system involvement. In the United States, up to 13 million people are living with latent TB infection and 8331 cases of active TB were reported in 2022. A review of extrapulmonary TB in the United States (1993–2006) found that 18.7% of cases were extrapulmonary, of which 11.3% involved bone and/or joint. Osteoarticular TB is more prevalent in economically developing countries.

2. How does TB disseminate to the bone and joint?

- Hematogenous spread during primary infection through the arterial circulation or Batson's paravertebral plexus of veins.
- Lymphatic spread from a distant focus.
- Contiguous spread from infected areas.

    In immunocompetent patients, the disease generally starts in the synovium with granulation tissue extending to involve the surrounding bone. Therefore, both bone and joint are usually affected, though each may occur without the other. Osteoarticular TB generally develops 2–3 years after the primary focus.

3. Who is at risk for osteoarticular TB?

- Female sex
- Children in the first decade of life
- Young adults 20–30 years of age
- Age >65 years
- **Immigrants from endemic countries**
- Alcoholics and drug abusers
- Malnutrition
- **HIV-positive patients**
- Immunosuppressed patients
- Patients treated with iatrogenic immunosuppressive therapy including biologics (tumor necrosis factor [TNF] antagonists > others) or corticosteroids at prednisone ≥ 10 mg/day equivalent.

A considerable percentage of cases in the literature are lacking any significant risk factor for dissemination. *M. bovis,* when administered as intravesicular BCG for bladder cancer, may disseminate and cause vertebral osteomyelitis.

4. Which bones and joints are commonly affected with osteoarticular TB?

Spine involvement (Pott's disease) accounts for >50% of cases with the lower thoracic and upper lumbar spine most frequently involved. It usually involves the anterior vertebral border and disc, ultimately progressing to disc narrowing, vertebral collapse, and kyphosis (gibbus deformity). Although TB may affect only the vertebral body, it usually will cross the disc and involve the adjacent vertebrae. Complications may include paravertebral cold abscess, spread beneath anterior longitudinal ligament causing scalloping of anterior vertebral bodies, psoas abscess, sinus tract formation, and neurologic compromise. Sacroiliac joint involvement accounts for 10% of osteoarticular TB, is usually unilateral when it occurs, and may be misdiagnosed as a spondyloarthropathy.

Peripheral joint involvement typically involves weight-bearing joints: usually the hip, knee, and ankle, and is monoarticular. Subchondral bone involvement may precede cartilage destruction, so that joint space narrowing is often a late finding. Adjacent osteomyelitis is very common. It accounts for approximately 30% of all cases of osteoarticular TB.

Multifocal osteomyelitis and **dactylitis** account for 2% to 3% of all osteoarticular TB. It may only involve the appendicular skeleton; peripheral involvement is dependent on the age of the patient. In adults, metaphyseal regions of the long bones with femur and tibia are most commonly affected. Ribs as well as other bones may be involved. In children, metacarpals and phalanges are more likely to be affected and resemble dactylitis.

Tenosynovitis and **bursitis** occur more commonly in NTM infections.

5. What are the typical signs and symptoms of osteoarticular TB?

Constitutional Symptoms (Fever, Weight Loss, Malaise) Occur Infrequently (<30%)

Spinal TB	Back pain (especially with movement), spasm, local tenderness, kyphosis, cord compression, weakness, tingling, paraplegia, mycotic aneurysm of aorta
Peripheral joints	Slow onset, chronic monoarthritis Hip—pain in thigh and groin with limited range of motion Knee—insidious pain, swelling, limp (especially children) Hand/wrist—carpal tunnel syndrome, swelling, pain
Multifocal Osteomyelitis	Pain, lytic lesions on radiographs without periosteal reaction Dactylitis (85% of cases occur in children aged <6 years)

If the disease damages the growth centers in childhood, then shortening of bones and angulation of the region may result. Note that patients with active pulmonary TB can be rheumatoid factor and/or anti-CCP positive, which may cause confusion when diagnosing a patient presenting with peripheral arthritis due to tuberculosis.

6. What is Poncet's disease?

Active TB (pulmonary, extrapulmonary, or miliary) may rarely cause acute symmetric polyarthritis (presumably reactive and immune mediated), accompanied by fever. Tuberculous organisms are not cultured from the involved joints, as there is no evidence of active TB in these joints. While any joint may be involved (large or small), knees, ankles, and elbows are most common. Arthritis generally resolves a few weeks after initiation of anti-TB therapy without lasting joint damage. HIV infection appears to be a risk factor.

7. How do you diagnose osteoarticular TB?

Diagnosis should include microscopy and culture of infected tissue. Culture of draining sinuses may yield a pathogen but risks isolating colonizing organisms. Isolating MTB from other sites (e.g., urine) can be helpful. Diagnosis may be difficult and is often delayed up to 12 to 18 months due to the insidious onset of nonspecific symptoms. Additionally, the chest radiograph may be normal in 50% of patients with osteoarticular TB. Purified protein derivative (PPD) skin test is useful for demonstrating an immune response presumed to represent infection with TB (latent or active), but this method has a few drawbacks. Some patients will have anergy and a false-negative test may result, the test requires patients to return for it to be interpreted at 48–72 hours, and it can be falsely positive in patients who have received the Bacillus Calmette–Guérin (BCG) vaccination. Interferon-γ release assays (QuantiFERON-TB Gold and T-SPOT.TB) (IGRAs) are more sensitive than the PPD test and not affected by previous BCG vaccination.

PEARL: PPD and IGRA may be falsely negative in immunocompromised patients. T-spot has higher sensitivity than quantiferon gold in immunocompromised patients.

A definitive diagnosis is established by demonstrating MTB in the tissue or synovial fluid. Sensitivity increases with increasing MTB bacillary load. The general sensitivity of common procedures is as follows:

Synovial fluid smear for TB	20%
Synovial fluid adenosine deaminase (>31 U/L)	80%
Synovial fluid culture for TB	80%
Synovial biopsy and culture	>90%
Nucleic acid amplification tests (NAATs)	70%
	ca. 80% (Xpert MTB/RIF)
	ca. 90% (Xpert MTB/RIF Ultra)

The advantage of **NAAT** is related to the rapid result time of a few hours to days instead of 3 to 6 weeks with conventional culture. The GeneXpert assay has been studied in osteoarticular disease and has the additional ability to detect rifampin resistance. It may also detect nonviable MTB bacilli in patients who have already started anti-TB treatment prior to specimen collection. However, culture and phenotypic drug susceptibility remains the gold standard for diagnosis. Histological examination of tissue sampling can aid the diagnosis, but both false-positive and false-negative results may be seen.

8. What are the characteristics of the synovial fluid and tissue biopsies in osteoarticular TB?

Synovial fluid analysis reveals elevated protein in virtually all patients with arthritis, whereas low glucose level is seen in 60%. Cell counts are highly variable and range from 1000 to 100,000 cells/mm^3, but most fall in the 10,000 to 20,000 cells/mm^3 range. Polymorphonuclear cells usually predominate, but fluid may also be primarily lymphocytic. The specificity of synovial fluid alone is poor but increases in the clinical context and with radiology and further laboratory results. Synovial membrane biopsies typically show caseating granulomas in 80% of cases. Osteomyelitis is diagnosed by needle or surgical biopsy, which usually reveals granulomata that may or may not be associated with caseating necrosis.

9. What are the characteristic radiographic features of osteoarticular TB?

No pathognomonic radiographic signs of TB exist. However, several signs may be helpful:
Spine
  Narrowing of joint space with vertebral collapse (vertebra plana)
  Anterior > posterior vertebral damage, leading to wedge-shaped collapse and angulation/hunchback (gibbus)
  Anterior vertebral scalloping and soft tissue swelling (paravertebral or psoas abscess)
  Extensive vertebral destruction with relative preservation of disc space (Fig. 39.1)
Peripheral joint
  Soft tissue swelling with effusion
Phemister triad
  Juxta-articular osteopenia/osteoporosis
  Peripheral subchondral osseous erosions
  Joint space narrowing occurs as a late finding
Osteomyelitis
  Lytic lesion with lack of periosteal reaction
Dactylitis (mainly children)
  Ballooned-out lytic appearance of a short bone of the hand with lack of periosteal reaction (spina ventosa)

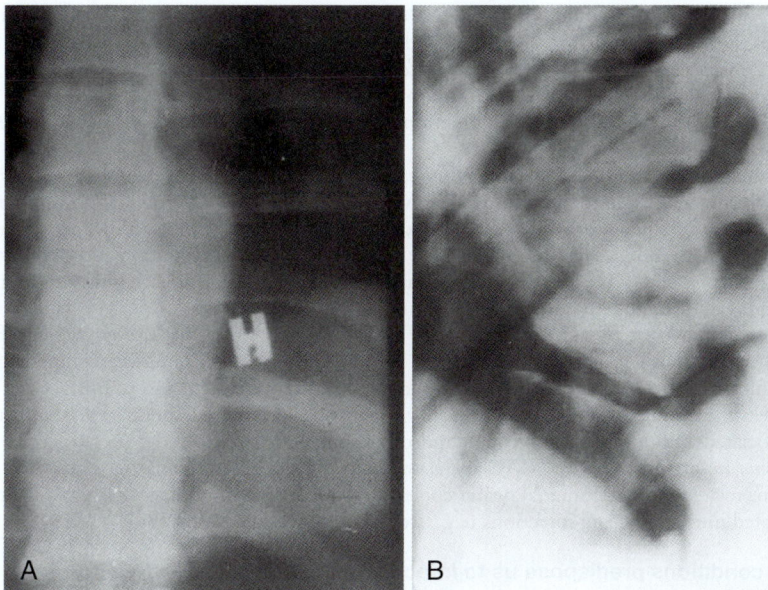

Fig. 39.1 (A) Abscess formation on an anterior view of the thoracic spine. (B) Vertebral collapse with angulation (Pott's disease) on a lateral view. (Copyright 2014 American College of Rheumatology. Used with permission.)

10. How do you treat osteoarticular TB?

Current guidelines from the Centers for Disease Control and Prevention, the American Thoracic Society, and the Infectious Disease Society of America recommend 6–9 months of therapy with first-line agents identical to those used for pulmonary tuberculosis. Standard treatment includes four drugs initially: **isoniazid** (5 mg/kg, up to 300 mg daily), **rifampin** (10 mg/kg, up to 600 mg daily), **ethambutol** (15 mg/kg daily, up to 1600 mg daily), and **pyrazinamide** (15–30 mg/kg, up to 2 g daily). Once the MTB is confirmed to be sensitive to isoniazid, ethambutol can be discontinued. Pyrazinamide is administered only in the intensive phase (first 2 months). Patients with drug-susceptible TB are treated with isoniazid and rifampin daily in the continuation phase of therapy. The CDC does not recommend the newer 4-month treatment of rifapentin and moxifloxacin for most types of extrapulmonary TB.

Patients with rifampin-resistant or multidrug-resistant TB (1% of all cases in the United States) should be treated with other drug regimens prescribed by an expert in TB therapy. Such regimens have traditionally been continued for 18 to 24 months or longer. The WHO now endorses shorter 9-month and 6-month regimens incorporating bedaquiline for drug-resistant pulmonary TB, but trials for these regimens excluded patients with osteoarticular TB.

For those with arthritis or minimal osteomyelitis, antituberculous therapy is often the only therapy needed. However, if bone involvement is extensive, there is poor response to chemotherapy with ongoing infection/deterioration, spinal kyphosis is greater than 40 degrees, multidrug-resistant TB is present, or there is neurologic compromise, surgery is often necessary to debride the abscess and hasten recovery.

11. What musculoskeletal problems can be caused by nontuberculous mycobacteria (NTM)?

Unlike MTB, NTM do not spread human to human. Known also as "atypical" or "environmental" mycobacteria, they are natural inhabitants of our environment. NTM are primarily pulmonary pathogens but may involve bone and joint either through direct inoculation (typically via injury or surgery) or through hematogenous spread, the latter especially in immunocompromised hosts. HIV is the most well-established risk factor for disseminated infection, especially with CD4 count <100 cells/mm^3. NTM have a propensity to involve the tendons and joints of the hands.

In fact, 50% affect the hands, while only 20% affect the knees. Polyarticular disease and involvement of the spine are much less common and usually associated with dissemination.

Rapid growers: *M. abscessus* complex, *M. chelonae*, *M. fortuitum* complex

Infection usually follows trauma or surgical procedures, leading to direct inoculation.

Due to inherent drug resistance, combination antimycobacterial therapy and surgical resection is key to treatment.

Most often HIV associated: *M. haemophilum*, *M. avium* complex (MAC), and *M. kansasii*

Most likely to cause vertebral osteomyelitis: MAC, *M. xenopi*, *M. fortuitum*, and *M. abscessus*.

M. marinum: an aquatic organism that is an occupational hazard of oyster shuckers and aquarium enthusiasts. Tenosynovitis of the hands or wrist is the classic presentation, although synovitis and osteomyelitis have been reported. May also present as a chronic draining wound to the hand, i.e. "fish tank granuloma" or "swimming pool granuloma."

M. ulcerans: the agent of Buruli ulcer, mainly found in West Africa, but also rarely identified in South America, Mexico, Australia, Papua New Guinea. Occurs in immunocompetent hosts in tropical rainforests. Starts as a painless nodule, most frequently on an extremity. Over days to weeks the nodule breaks down to a slowly progressive ulceration. About 13% of infections are associated with tendon involvement and/or osteomyelitis.

M. chimaera: organism within MAC associated with the global outbreak of postoperative infections related to contaminated heater cooler units used in cardiothoracic surgery, leading to related musculoskeletal infections (e.g., sternal or vertebral osteomyelitis).

12. What conditions predispose us to infection with NTM?

- Prior surgery
- Direct inoculation and/or environmental exposure (soil, water), typically after trauma
- Intraarticular steroid injections and preexisting joint disease
- Open wounds in the hands or fingers
- Intravenous drug use (IVDU)
- Diabetes mellitus
- Immunosuppression and biologic therapy

13. How are NTM osteoarticular infections treated? What is the prognosis?

Require multidrug regimens, with antibiotic selection specific to the causative organism (consult an infectious disease specialist, preferably with specialty in NTM infections).

Antibiotics should be guided by susceptibility results but not all susceptibilities are reliable (consult an NTM specialist).

Surgical debridement plays an important role to debulk the infection.

Unless the infection is severe or rapidly progressive, antibiotics may be held until surgery can be undertaken for three reasons: (1) antibiotic effectiveness will be limited until source control is achieved, (2) to limit prolonged (unnecessary) antibiotic side effects, and (3) to confirm the causative organism and susceptibility pattern (i.e., decreased ability to isolate an organism while on antibiotics).

Prolonged therapy is necessary, commonly 6 to 12 months. In general, the more thorough the debridement, the shorter the treatment course.

Relapses are common even with optimal therapy, emphasizing the need for adequate debridement sooner in the infection.

14. What are the consequences of the administration of corticosteroids for patients with NTM osteoarticular infection?

Extrapulmonary osteoarticular infections are frequently mistaken for immunologic conditions (e.g., erythema nodosum, autoimmune inflammatory arthritis) that are treated with corticosteroids. Administration of injections or systemic corticosteroids leads to a worsening of the infection with contiguous expansion, and potentially also dissemination to more distant sites.

15. List guidelines for mycobacterial infection prevention in patients who are to receive biologic agents?

- All patients who are to receive biologic agents should undergo screening for MTB infection (latent and active) and NTM screening.

- All patients should have risk factor assessment, physical examination, and a chest radiograph.

NTM:
- If there is clinical suspicion for NTM, no guidelines exist, but chest CT and at least one sputum for AFB smear/culture are prudent for pulmonary disease; imaging (MRI/CT) plus tissue sampling should be performed for extrapulmonary disease.
- In the United States, NTM (especially MAC) is much more common than MTB. There are no skin tests or blood tests to detect NTM infection.
- In general, immune suppression is avoided or minimized/weaned (as able) in NTM disease.
- The 2007 NTM guidelines suggest starting adequate multidrug treatment for NTM if NTM are present and an anti-TNFα agent is given, while other societies consider NTM infection a contraindication to initiation of TNFα inhibition.
- Patients with prior history of treated NTM infection should be evaluated by a specialist before a biologic is used. Some NTM are difficult to cure, and anti-TNFα agents should be avoided. Rituximab or abatacept may be safer agents.

MTB:
- Tuberculin skin test only has a sensitivity and specificity of 70%. PPD induration >5 mm at 48–72 hours should be considered positive regardless of prior history of BCG vaccination.
- Many patients with immune-mediated inflammatory diseases are on prednisone and other immunosuppressants, which can make PPD unreliable. Therefore, IGRA screening is also recommended. Notably, up to 10% of IGRA tests can be indeterminate in patients on immunosuppressants. Consequently, a dual testing strategy (perform one test and, if negative, perform the other) may be used, in which a positive result from either test would be considered positive.
- Screening procedures decrease reactivation of MTB by 80%.
- Biologic therapy: Monoclonal antibodies (especially infliximab) against TNFα have the highest risk. Janus kinase (JAK) and IL-6 inhibitors are also thought to confer a higher risk than other biologics (e.g., abatacept and rituximab as well as IL-17 and IL-23 blockade). Reactivation of MTB tends to occur within 6 months of starting anti-TNFα therapy and usually presents as extrapulmonary disease, especially lymphadenitis.
- Patients with latent MTB and normal chest radiograph should delay biologic initiation (especially anti-TNFα agents) until 1 month of latent TB therapy has been administered. Patients should receive a complete course for latent MTB (typically 9 months of isoniazid or 4 months of rifampin).
- Patients should have an assessment for active TB before initiating any treatment for latent TB, including sputa x3 for AFB smear/culture and MTB NAAT x2 if symptoms and/or imaging findings warrant this. Never treat a patient for latent TB who has active TB.
- Patients with active MTB should have a complete course of anti-tuberculous therapy before starting a biologic (especially anti-TNFα agent).
- The decision whether or not to restart an anti-TNFα agent in a patient who has developed active TB should be individualized and in general may be considered after at least 2 months of effective antituberculosis treatment.

16. **Are any musculoskeletal conditions associated with *M. leprae* (leprosy)?**
The prevalence of leprosy-related arthritis ranges from 1–78% in various studies and is the third most common disease manifestation (following dermatologic and neurologic). Arthritis takes many forms from arthralgias to inflammatory or septic arthritis:
Erythema nodosum leprosum—It is seen in immunologic reactions to lepromatous leprosy and probably represents a "reactive" arthritis. Clinical manifestations include fever, subcutaneous nodules, arthralgias, and acute or subacute onset of frank arthritis that is symmetric and polyarticular, compromising small and large joints and generally self-limited.
Insidious chronic polyarthritis (with rheumatoid arthritis-like picture)—It usually involves the wrist, small joints of the hands and feet, and knees. Onset is insidious and months to years after initial infection. It is most often seen in tuberculoid or borderline leprosy. Patients may be rheumatoid factor positive.
Bony abnormalities secondary to neuropathy—These include resorption of the distal metatarsals, aseptic necrosis, "claw" hands, and Charcot joints.

Direct infection of the bone—This typically affects the distal phalanges including resorption, fragmentation, and malaligned fractures.

Lucio's phenomenon (erythema necroticans)—Necrotizing vasculitis of skin due to lepromatous leprosy.

Other rheumatologic manifestations include enthesitis, sacroiliitis (can be bilateral), isolated tenosynovitis, swollen hands and feet, and systemic lupus erythematosus-like and dermatomyositis-like presentations.

17. How do fungal infections of the bones and joints present clinically? What are the risk factors?

Typical presentation of fungal osteoarticular infections include localized pain, tenderness, and decreased range of motion at the site of infection; fever is infrequent. Osteomyelitis is more common than septic arthritis. Onset is often insidious over several weeks to months. Acute arthritis is unusual except in *Candida* and *Blastomyces* infections. The three mechanisms for fungal osteoarticular infections include: hematogenous dissemination, direct inoculation, and contiguous spread from an adjacent site. Risk factors include: environmental exposure, immunocompromised status (especially those on TNF inhibitors), and nosocomial exposure.

18. How helpful are synovial fluid analyses and cultures in fungal septic arthritis?

Similar to TB, synovial fluid white blood cell counts are highly variable, ranging from 10,000 to 60,000/mm^3 with either polymorphonuclear or mononuclear cells predominating.

Culture of synovial fluid is critically important in establishing the diagnosis, but colony counts are often low. Laboratory personnel must be alerted to the possibility of fungal disease, so they take proper precautions and do not use inhibitory media.

Recently, polymerase chain reaction–based amplification techniques have been developed for many species of fungi that may be useful diagnostic techniques in the future.

19. Describe the epidemiology of some of the fungi causing bone and joint infections.

Organism	Geographic Area	Mode of Infection
Candida species	Worldwide, endogenous	Often hematogenous spread from Candidemia secondary to intravenous catheters, immunosuppression, antibiotic use, intravenous drug use
Aspergillus species	Worldwide, found in soil and decaying vegetative material	Inhalation of spores, followed by pulmonary infection and hematogenous dissemination or contiguous spread. Also, direct inoculation via trauma or surgery.
Coccidioides immitis	Southwestern United States, Central and South America (especially in arid and semiarid regions)	Inhalation and pulmonary infection, followed by hematogenous or lymphangitic dissemination
Blastomyces dermatitidis	Mississippi and Ohio River basins, Middle Atlantic states, Canada, Europe, Africa, and northern South America	Inhalation of spores, followed by pulmonary infection and dissemination. Less commonly from direct cutaneous inoculation.
Histoplasma capsulatum	Worldwide, but highest in Ohio and Mississippi River valleys in damp soil containing bird excreta or bat guano	Inhalation, followed by pulmonary infection and dissemination. Very rarely via direct inoculation.
Cryptococcus neoformans	Worldwide, associated with bird excreta	Inhalation and pulmonary infection, followed by hematogenous spread
Sporothrix schenckii	Worldwide	Direct inoculation following skin injury from scratch or thorn prick, or through hematogenous dissemination.

20. How frequently is bone or articular involvement seen with these fungi and at what locations?

- *Candida* species: Most common fungal organism causing osteoarticular infections, often preceded by Candidemia. Knees are the most common site for septic arthritis; adjacent osteomyelitis is common. Osteomyelitis most commonly affects the vertebrae in adults and long bones in the pediatric population. Prior abdominal surgery, recent antibiotic use, intravenous access including central venous catheters and illicit intravenous drug use, and immunosuppressed status are major risk factors. High index of suspicion is necessary due to wide range from time of presentation to diagnosis.

- *Aspergillus* species: Second most common organism causing fungal osteoarticular infections, typically in immunocompromised patients. Occurs via hematogenous or contiguous spread often from a pulmonary source. Ribs and vertebrae are most common sites of osteomyelitis due to adjacent pulmonary aspergillosis. Knee is the most affected joint. Tissue biopsy or synovial fluid preferred to establish diagnosis; serum galactomannan is elevated in only a minority of cases.

- *C. immitis*: Osteoarticular infection is common in disseminated disease in immunocompromised patients or pregnant women, and generally manifests as vertebral osteomyelitis, or septic arthritis of the knee, wrist, or ankle. Serologic testing and tissue biopsies with stains and cultures are necessary to confirm the diagnosis. Synovial fluid cultures are rarely positive.

- *B. dermatitidis*: Osteoarticular involvement present in 5–20% of those with disseminated blastomycosis. Typically affects long bones, vertebrae, and ribs. Septic arthritis occurs via contiguous spread. Diagnosed by tissue culture, blood or urine antigen testing, though antigen testing has cross-reactivity with Histoplasma.

- *H. capsulatum*: Osteoarticular infections are rare, occurring in disseminated disease mostly in immunocompromised patients. Osteomyelitis is most common in long bones and vertebrae, septic arthritis most common in the knee. Can be clinically and histologically indistinguishable from tuberculosis arthritis. Serum and urine antigen testing preferred, along with tissue/body fluid for histopathology and culture.

- *C. neoformans*: Osteoarticular infection is a rare consequence of disseminated infection typically in the immunocompromised population. Osteomyelitis occurs in less than 10% of infections affecting the vertebrae most commonly. Septic arthritis is very rare and almost always involves the knee. Tissue biopsy for histopathology and culture can confirm the diagnosis.

- *S. schenckii*: Osteoarticular infection is a rare consequence of either contiguous spread or hematogenous dissemination. Long bones and knees are most common. Hand and wrist involvement is more common compared to other fungal infections. Tissue for histopathology and culture can confirm the diagnosis.

- *Madurella* species: Bone and joint involvement is common with spread of the soft tissue infection to the bone, fascia, and joint.

- *Scedosporiosis* species: Have a predilection for bone and cartilage after cutaneous inoculation and dissemination.

21. What is mucormycosis and how is the treatment of this fungus unique?

Mucormycosis is a rapidly progressive angioinvasive disease caused by fungi in the class zygomycetes (Rhizopus, Mucor, and Rhizomucor), which are ubiquitous in the environment. It is associated with high mortality and requires emergent aggressive surgical debridement followed by antifungal therapy (liposomal amphotericin B +/− an echinocandin or triazole). Risk factors for disease include prolonged neutropenia, iron overload, uncontrolled diabetes with hyperglycemia and acidosis, and treatment with glucocorticoids. The fungus has a predilection for sinus cavities but may involve any bone or joint.

22. How do you treat fungal septic arthritis?

Treatment approach should include surgical debridement of infected tissues, removal of infected hardware when possible, as well as prolonged courses of antifungal therapy. In patients with ongoing immune suppression sometimes chronic prophylaxis or suppression is used to prevent relapse or recurrence of infection. Consultation with an infectious disease specialist is recommended.

23. List some other organisms that may cause osteoarticular problems in other areas of the world, although rarely within the United States.

- **Brucellosis:** Acquired by contaminated animal products, typically unpasteurized dairy products. Presents as nonspecific flu-like illness and osteoarticular involvement is common, predominantly causing sacroiliitis (50%), peripheral arthritis (monoarticular or polyarticular) (35%), spondylitis (25%), and osteomyelitis of the lumbar spine (5%).
- **Parasitic infection:** Parasitic rheumatism should be considered in patients from endemic areas who do not respond to antirheumatic treatment. Eosinophilia should also prompt consideration for a parasitic infection. Anti-IL-17 therapy can potentially increase susceptibility to parasitic infections.

ACKNOWLEDGMENT

The authors would like to thank Dr. Laura Damioli and Dr. Shannon Kasperbauer for their contributions to this chapter in the previous edition.

BIBLIOGRAPHY

Adetunji SA, Ramirez G, Foster MJ. Arenas-Gamboa AM. A systematic review and meta-analysis of the prevalence of osteoarticular brucellosis. *PLoS Negl Trop Dis*. 2019;13:e0007112.

De Vuyst D, Vanhoenacker F, Gielen J, et al. Imaging features of musculoskeletal tuberculosis. *Eur Radiol*. 2003;13(8):1809–1819.

El-Gendy H, El-Gohary RM, Shohdy KS, et al. Leprosy masquerading as systemic rheumatic diseases. *J Clin Rheumatol*. 2016;22:264–271.

Gamaletsou MN, Rammaert B, Brause B, et al. Osteoarticular mycoses. *Clin Microbiol Rev*. 2022;35:e00086–e00119.

Griffith DE, Aksamit T, Brown-Elliot BA, et al. An official ATS/IDSA statement: diagnosis, treatment, and prevention of non-tuberculous mycobacterial diseases. *Am J Resp Crit Care Med*. 2007;175:367–416.

Held MFG, Hoppe S, Laubscher M, et al. Epidemiology of musculoskeletal tuberculosis in an area with high disease prevalence. *Asian Spine J*. 2017;11:405–411.

Henry MW, Miller AO, Walsh TJ, Brause BD. Fungal Musculoskeletal Infections. *Infect Dis Clin North Am*. 2017;31:353–368.

Johansen IS, Nielsen SL, Hove M, et al. Characteristics and clinical outcome of bone and joint tuberculosis from 1994 to 2011: a retrospective register-based study in Denmark. *Clin Infect Dis*. 2015;61:554–562.

Kroot EJ, Hazes JM, Colin EM, et al. Poncet's disease: reactive arthritis accompanying tuberculosis. Two case reports and a review of the literature. *Rheumatology (Oxford)*. 2007;46:484–489.

Lewinsohn DM, Leonard MK, LoBue PA, et al. Official American Thoracic Society/Infectious Diseases Society of America/Centers for Disease Control and Prevention Clinical Practice Guidelines: Diagnosis of tuberculosis in adults and children. *Clin Infect Dis*. 2017;64:111–115.

Mazi PB, Rauseo AM, Spec A. Blastomycosis. *Infect Dis Clin North Am*. 2021;35:515–530.

Maziarz EK, Perfect JR. Cryptococcosis. *Infect Dis Clin North Am*. 2016;30:179–206.

Moni BM, Wise BL, Loots GG, Weilhammer DR. Coccidioidomycosis osteoarticular dissemination. *J Fungi*. 2023;9:1002.

Nahid P, Dorman SE, Alipanah N, et al. American Thoracic Society/Centers for Disease Control and Prevention/Infectious Diseases Society of America guidelines for treatment of drug-susceptible tuberculosis. *Clin Infect Dis*. 2016;63:e147–e195.

Peto HM, Pratt RH, Harrington TA, et al. Epidemiology of extrapulmonary tuberculosis in the United States, 1993–2006. *Clin Infect Dis*. 2009;49:1350–1357.

Ranches GP, Winthrop KL. Nontuberculous mycobacteria infections in patients receiving immunosuppressive agents. Bronchiectasis. In: Chalmers JD, Polverino E, Aliberti S, eds. *ERS Monograph*. Sheffield, UK: ERS Publications; 2018:238–253 (9781849840989).

Sun Q, Wang S, Dong W, et al. Diagnostic value of Xpert MTB/RIF Ultra for osteoarticular tuberculosis. *J Infect*. 2019;79:153–158.

Tsantes AG, Papadopoulos DV, Markou E, et al. *Aspergillus* spp. osteoarticular infections: an updated systematic review on the diagnosis, treatment and outcomes of 186 confirmed cases. *Med Mycol*. 2022;60:myac052.

Tuli SM. Tuberculosis of the Skeletal System (Bones, Joints, Spine and Bursal Sheaths). 5th ed. New Delhi, India: Jaypee Brothers Medical Publishers (P) Ltd.; 2016.

Wheat LJ, Azar MM, Bahr NC, Spec A, Relich RF, Hage C. Histoplasmosis. *Infect Dis Clin North Am*. 2016;30:207–227.

Zeidler H, Hudson AP. Reactive arthritis update: spotlight on new and rare infectious agents implicated as pathogens. *Curr Rheumatol Rep*. 2021;23:53.

Viral Arthritides

Meredith Morcos, MD

1. What are the general characteristics of viral arthritis?

Viral arthritis constitutes approximately 1% of acute arthritis. While virtually all viruses can cause arthralgia and arthritis, parvovirus B19, hepatitis B and C, and alphaviruses are the most common causative agents. Viral arthritis typically presents as an acute self-limited, nonerosive, inflammatory arthritis (in a pattern that may mimic rheumatoid arthritis [RA]). When a viral arthritis is suspected, an accurate history (with exposures and travel) and a careful physical examination are essential to diagnosis. While antiviral antibody titers may be helpful diagnostically, many causative viruses have not yet been described or serologic tests have not been developed for clinical use. Therefore, the diagnosis of viral arthritis is usually presumptive and retrospective based on the history and physical examination as well as resolution of arthritis within weeks to months after minimal therapy.

2. What autoantibodies can be seen in the course of viral infection and what are their implications?

Low-titer autoantibodies such as rheumatoid factor (RF) and antinuclear antibody (ANA) can be detected in patients with many viral infections. Because these patients can develop symptoms and signs that mimic rheumatic diseases, such as RA, systemic lupus erythematosus (SLE) or Sjögren disease (SjD), the clinician must be careful to avoid inappropriate laboratory testing, diagnosis, and treatment.

HEPATITIS B

3. Describe the general characteristics of hepatitis B virus (HBV).

HBV is a hepatotropic, enveloped, double-stranded DNA virus of Hepadnaviridae family consisting of a nucleocapsid core with two antigenically distinct constituents, hepatitis B core antigen (HBcAg) and hepatitis B envelope antigen (HBeAg). The core is surrounded by a nucleocapsid coat, known as the hepatitis B surface antigen (HBsAg).

4. What is the prevalence, transmission, and clinical course of HBV infection?

HBV is estimated to affect approximately 350 million people worldwide and is transmitted parenterally, through sexual contact, or vertically (during childbirth). Most adults exposed to this virus experience a clinically silent, self-limited infection resulting in an antibody response to HBsAg. If the patient is immunocompetent, IgM antibodies against HBcAg indicate an acute HBV infection. The acute infection resolves in 90% to 95% of adult cases and is serologically indicated by absence of HBsAg, HBeAg, and viral DNA and the development of hepatitis B surface antibody (HBsAb) and hepatitis B core antibody (HBcAb). In approximately 5% to 10% of cases of adult infection, HBV infection proceeds to a chronic illness.

5. Briefly describe the chronic HBV infection.

Chronic HBV infection is characterized serologically by the presence of HBsAg and HBcAb (IgG). Patients (30%) with chronic HBV infection proceed to chronic active hepatitis, during which the virus is actively replicating (typically with +HBeAg and detectable viral load) and patients develop transaminitis. Risk factors for chronicity include male sex and immunocompromised state.

6. Describe the rheumatologic manifestations of HBV.

A variety of extrahepatic rheumatic manifestations may occur during HBV infection including arthralgias, arthritis, arthritis–dermatitis syndrome, membranous nephropathy, cryoglobulinemia, and systemic necrotizing vasculitis (HBV-associated polyarteritis nodosa [PAN]).

7. How does HBV infection produce articular symptoms and signs?

HBV-related rheumatic manifestations are usually attributed to the deposition of immune complexes (HBsAg-HBsAb, HBeAg-HBeAb) in the tissues (e.g., synovium or vessel wall) leading to a secondary inflammatory response. Arthritis is more common in acute HBV infection than in chronic infection.

8. Describe the articular symptoms and signs associated with HBV infection.

As in all viral illnesses, arthralgia is much more common than arthritis in HBV infection (20% with arthralgia, <10% with arthritis). This immune complex–mediated arthritis can occur in both the prodromal phase of acute infection and during a chronic infection, although the prodromal phase is more common. During this phase of acute infection, patients develop either a migratory or additive arthritis resulting in a symmetric polyarthritis involving the proximal interphalangeal (PIP), knees, and ankle joints mimicking RA. The arthritis typically precedes jaundice and transaminitis; it may last for days or months and resolves with the onset of jaundice. Accompanying symptoms include fever, malaise, myalgia, and rash (maculopapular, urticarial, petechial; the so-called **arthritis–dermatitis syndrome**).

9. Describe the clinical course of articular manifestations in HBV infection and their treatment.

In patients with acute HBV infection, arthritis is typically self-limited and does not cause permanent joint damage. In patients with chronic active hepatitis, arthralgia is reported in up to 25% of patients. Treatment is generally supportive and includes joint rest and NSAIDs.

10. What serum antibodies and other laboratory findings are commonly seen with HBV infection and arthritis?

In acute hepatitis B, aspartate transaminase (AST) and alanine transaminase (ALT) are significantly elevated (1000s IU/mL) and HBsAg and HBeAg are present. With the onset of jaundice and resolution of arthritic symptoms, the HbsAg titer decreases and IgG HbsAb and IgM HbcAb titers increase. As the remainder of the virus is cleared, IgG HbcAb appears. Other abnormal laboratory findings include a positive RF (25% of patients) and depressed C3 and C4 levels (as much as 40% of patients). Synovial fluid is typically inflammatory.

11. What vasculitis is associated with HBV infection and when should it be suspected?

Secondary PAN can be seen in patients infected with HBV, although this is becoming less common in developed countries with established vaccination programs and systemic screening of blood transfusions. Patients with HBV-associated PAN have active viral replication, persistent antigenemia, and circulating immune complexes.

12. What are the typical features, treatment, and prognosis of HBV-associated PAN?

HBV-associated PAN has a more severe course with more frequent nerve, gastrointestinal, and cardiac involvement and less skin involvement compared with non-HBV-associated PAN. Treatment includes combination of plasmapheresis and antiviral agents. Immunosuppressive medications are used in patients with severe manifestations or those not responding adequately to antiviral treatment. HBV-associated PAN has a higher (34%) mortality than non-HBV-associated PAN (see Chapter 27: Medium-Vessel Vasculitides).

13. Can HBV cause cryoglobulinemic vasculitis?

Yes. HBV can also cause cryoglobulinemic vasculitis, although it is much less common than seen in hepatitis C virus (HCV) infection.

14. Which immunosuppressive drugs can contribute to the reactivation of HBV?

Certain biologic disease-modifying antirheumatic drugs (bDMARDs) have been associated with HBV reactivation. Rituximab appears to pose the highest risk among available immunosuppressive agents. Before prescribing bDMARDs, testing HbsAb, HbcAb, and HbsAg is recommended. Non-bDMARDs are considered low risk for reactivation, but screening patients on these medications to risk stratify is reasonable. Chronic low-dose prednisone (<10 mg per day) is also considered low risk for reactivation except for individuals who are chronic carriers (HBsAg+). Prophylactic antiviral therapy is typically recommended if there is a moderate (1–10%) or high (>10%) risk of hepatitis B reactivation (Table 40.1). Avoiding medication classes that pose a high risk of hepatitis B reactivation is preferable if reasonable alternative treatment options exist. Seeking guidance from hepatology or infectious disease is sensible if planning use of a medication that poses a high risk of hepatitis B reactivation or in individuals with chronic active infection (positive HBV viral load).

HEPATITIS C

15. Discuss the epidemiology and transmissibility of HCV infection.

HCV is a linear, single-stranded RNA virus. Chronic HCV infection affects more than 180 million people worldwide. HCV is transmitted through blood transfusion, needle stick, sharing drug delivery paraphernalia, and sexual intercourse.

TABLE 40.1 Hepatitis B Prophylaxis Recommendations for Immunosuppression

	RESOLVED INFECTION (HBSAG−, HBCAB+, HBSAB+/−, UNDETECTABLE VIRAL LOAD [VL])	CHRONIC CARRIER (HBSAG+, HBCAB+, HBSAB−, UNDETECTABLE VL)	CHRONIC ACTIVE (HBSAG+, HBCAB+, HBSAB−, POSITIVE VL)
TNFi	No routine prophylactic antiviral therapy recommended. Monitor LFTs and VL periodically.	Prophylactic antiviral therapy recommended*	Avoid
Other non-TNFi bDMARDs	No routine prophylactic antiviral therapy recommended. Monitor LFTs and VL periodically.	Prophylactic antiviral therapy recommended*	Avoid
Rituximab	Prophylactic antiviral therapy recommended+	Prophylactic antiviral therapy recommended+	Avoid
Low-dose prednisone (<10 mg daily for ≥ 4 weeks)	No routine prophylactic antiviral therapy recommended. Monitor LFTs and VL periodically.	Prophylactic antiviral therapy recommended*	Avoid
Moderate/high-dose prednisone (>10 mg daily for ≥ 4 weeks)	Prophylactic antiviral therapy recommended*	Prophylactic antiviral therapy recommended+	Avoid

*Moderate risk of hepatitis B reactivation.
+High risk of hepatitis B reactivation; avoid, if possible, use with guidance from infectious disease or hepatology.

16. Describe the clinical course of hepatitis in HCV.

Most acute HCV infections are asymptomatic. More than 60% of acute infections, however, lead to chronic hepatitis, and this latter group will progress to cirrhosis in roughly 30% of cases (with a subset that may progress to hepatocellular carcinoma). It is estimated that 60% to 80% of untreated patients with HCV-associated cirrhosis will die of liver-related causes.

17. What are the autoantibodies that may be present in HCV infection?

Patients with HCV may produce autoantibodies including ANA (10–40%), anticardiolipin antibodies (15–20%), antithyroid antibodies, anti–smooth muscle antibodies, anti–liver-kidney microsomal antibody 1, RF (45–70%), and celiac disease autoantibodies as a consequence of non-specific B-cell activation. In HCV-related arthritis, the frequency of RF that can be high titer is as high as 80%, whereas anticyclic citrullinated peptide (anti-CCP) antibodies are uncommon and, if present, should prompt consideration of a diagnosis of concurrent RA.

18. What are the main rheumatic manifestations related to HCV?

- HCV-associated arthritis
- Cryoglobulin-related arthritis and vasculitis

19. Describe the pattern of arthritis associated with HCV.

Up to 20% of patients with HCV may develop an immune complex–mediated arthritis. Two-thirds of the patients experience a symmetric, nonerosive arthritis affecting the hands and feet similar to RA. The remaining patients develop a monoarticular or oligoarticular medium and/or large joint (most commonly ankles) arthritis often associated with mixed cryoglobulinemic vasculitis.

20. How do we differentiate HCV-associated arthritis from RA, and how do we manage it?

When a patient with HCV infection has a positive RF and a nonerosive, non-nodular polyar-thritis in a RA distribution for >8 weeks, it can be challenging to differentiate HCV-associated arthritis from RA. However, the presence of anti-CCP antibody and/or erosions on radiograph is indicative of RA. The management of HCV-associated arthritis includes NSAIDs, analgesia, and treatment of HCV. Resistant cases can be treated with low-dose prednisone and/or hydroxy-chloroquine, but persistent arthritis despite virologic response to antiviral therapy should prompt consideration of an alternative diagnosis.

21. Describe the clinical manifestations of HCV-associated cryoglobulinemic vasculitis.

Cryoglobulins (types II and III) can be detected in 40% to 50% of patients with chronic HCV infection. However, <5% of patients develop cryoglobulinemic vasculitis. Positive RF and low complement levels (especially C4) are frequently present due to immune complex formation and activation. Details on the management of HCV-associated cryoglobulinemic vasculitis can be found in an earlier chapter (see Chapter 30: Cryoglobulinemia).

22. Describe the HCV-associated keratoconjunctivitis sicca.

Sicca symptoms are commonly reported in chronic HCV patients, which may result from impair-ment of the exocrine glands caused by mild sialadenitis. Clinically, it may be indistinguishable from SjD.

23. How can we differentiate HCV-associated sicca syndrome from SjD?

This can be difficult because patients with HCV can also produce anti-SSA and anti-SSB antibodies. However, a minor salivary gland biopsy helps to differentiate them. HCV-related sialadenitis has focal $CD8^+$ T-cell infiltrates. In contrast, SjD is characterized by the infiltration of $CD4^+$ T cells.

24. **How can coexistent HBV or HCV infection influence the treatment of rheumatic conditions?**

Certain DMARDs such as methotrexate and leflunomide are hepatotoxic. The hepatotoxicity of these medications increases in patients who have HBV or HCV infection. Thus, methotrexate and leflunomide should be used with caution in HBV- or HCV-infected patients, if at all, and alternative DMARDs such as hydroxychloroquine, sulfasalazine, and azathioprine are preferred. The use of TNF inhibitors in HCV patients appears to be safe. See Table 40.1 for information regarding indications for hepatitis B prophylaxis.

PARVOVIRUS

25. **Describe the general characteristics of parvovirus B19 (parvo B19)?**

Parvo B19 is a member of the Parvoviridae family. It is a small, single-stranded, species-specific DNA virus that replicates within dividing cells, especially human erythroid progenitor cells.

26. **What diseases are associated with human parvo B19 infection?**

It is responsible for several diseases, including erythema infectiosum ("fifth disease") in children, transient aplastic crisis in adults, fetal hydrops in infected mothers, and pseudorheumatoid inflammatory arthritis. Parvo B19 infection can mimic lupus with clinical features including fever, rash, myalgia, arthritis (adults > children), cytopenia, hypocomplementemia, a positive ANA, and transient antiphospholipid antibodies.

27. **How is parvo B19 transmitted?**

Parvo B19 is likely transmitted via respiratory secretions. Infection with parvo B19 tends to occur in late winter and early spring but can happen at any time of the year. Risk factors for infection include immunocompromised status and working among children (e.g., daycare, schoolteachers).

28. **What is the clinical course of parvo B19 infection?**

The incubation period can last up to a few weeks with symptoms typically developing 10 to 14 days after exposure. Individuals may develop flu-like symptoms, and adults may notice a morbilliform rash on their trunk and extremities. The classic presentation of parvo B19 in children is the erythema infectiosum or "fifth disease," manifesting as fever and a maculopapular or reticular rash appearing as a bright red facial rash (i.e., slapped cheeks).

29. **Describe the articular manifestations associated with parvo B19 infection.**

The articular manifestations of parvo B19 are more common in adults than in children and in women than in men. The reported frequency of arthritis in adults with parvo B19 is as high as 50% to 80%. Symptoms initially begin in a few joints and rapidly involve more joints in an additive fashion. In adults, the pattern is more RA-like, symmetrically affecting the wrists, metacarpophalangeal, and PIP joints. In children, the pattern is usually asymmetric and oligoarticular involving the large joints (e.g., knees).

30. **What is the prognosis of parvo B19 infection?**

In general, the symptoms due to parvo B19 are self-limited (resolve within several weeks to months), but a small percentage of adults may develop chronic arthritis. As with other viral arthritis, no long-term joint damage has been reported after isolated parvo B19-associated arthritis.

31. **How does parvo B19 virus cause arthritis?**

It is believed that during viremia, the deposition of immune complexes comprised of the virus and anti-parvovirus IgM antibodies leads to a nonspecific inflammatory response. This includes the recruitment of immune cells and the production of several proinflammatory cytokines. In acute arthritis, viral DNA has been documented in the synovial fluid. Patients with chronic joint symptoms may have parvo B19 DNA in their synovium and bone marrow.

32. Describe the serologic diagnosis of parvo B19 infection.

The definitive diagnosis of parvo B19 infection relies on the detection of IgM antibodies or viral B19 DNA in the correct clinical context. Anti-parvo B19 virus IgM antibodies peak around 1 month post-infection and are largely undetectable by 2 to 3 months, with appearance of anti-parvo B19 IgG antibodies. IgG antibodies may persist for many years. Thus, the finding of IgG anti-parvo B19 antibodies without IgM antibodies indicates past infection of indeterminate timing (IgG antibodies are present in 60–80% of the adult population).

33. Which autoantibodies can be seen during parvo B19 infection?

Parvo B19 infection can induce a spectrum of autoantibodies, often transiently, including RF, ANA, anti-dsDNA, anti-extractable nuclear antigen antibodies, and antiphospholipid antibodies, among others.

34. Why is it important to make a diagnosis of parvo B19 infection?

The clinical presentation of parvo B19 infection (fever and symmetric pattern of small joint involvement) in conjunction with autoantibody positivity may resemble RA, juvenile idiopathic arthritis, or SLE. If patients are misdiagnosed, this potentially self-limited disease would be unnecessarily treated with DMARDs or immunosuppressants.

35. How are patients with chronic joint symptoms arising from parvo B19 treated?

Treatment of the acute arthritis associated with parvo B19 is generally supportive, which includes NSAIDs and rest. Persistent arthritis is reported in only a small percentage of patients, and hydroxychloroquine may be successful in this setting. Some patients with chronic parvo B19 arthropathy are unable to develop IgG antibodies to the minor capsid protein VP1, which encodes neutralizing epitopes. This may account for their inability to clear viral B19 DNA. In these patients with chronic joint pain and persistent B19 IgM antibodies and/or viral B19 DNA, intravenous immunoglobulin may be an effective treatment, although it appears to be more effective in immunocompromised (hypogammaglobulinemic) patients.

CHIKUNGUNYA AND OTHER ALPHAVIRUSES

36. Describe the general characteristics, clinical course, and the management of alphavirus infections.

Alphaviruses are a genus of ssRNA viruses (Togaviridae family) that are primarily transmitted by mosquitoes. The six alphaviruses that may have musculoskeletal manifestations are listed in Table 40.2. Treatment is generally supportive and consists of analgesics and hydration. NSAIDs and aspirin are typically avoided until co-infection with Dengue is excluded.

37. What is the general clinical course and pathology of alphavirus infections?

The incubation period for most alphaviruses is approximately 3–15 days. Alphaviruses share several typical clinical features including fever, arthralgia, arthritis, and rash. Arthritis is typically symmetric and polyarticular and frequently affects the hands, wrists, elbows, knees, and ankles. In

TABLE 40.2 Geographic Distribution of Various Alphaviruses	
ALPHAVIRUS	**GEOGRAPHIC DISTRIBUTION**
Chikungunya	East Africa, India, Southeast Asia, the Philippines, Europe, the Caribbean, the United States, Central/South America
O'nyong-nyong	East Africa
Ross River	Australia, New Zealand, South Pacific Islands
Mayaro	South America (Bolivia, Brazil, Peru)
Sindbis (Karelian fever)	Sweden, Finland, Isthmus of Russia
Igbo-ora virus	Nigeria

most alphavirus infections, joint symptoms resolve after 7 to 10 days but may persist for >1 year. Researchers speculate that the inflammation associated with an alphavirus infection is due to macrophages releasing proinflammatory cytokines and matrix metalloproteinases.

38. Describe the epidemiology of chikungunya virus (CHIK).

CHIK is transmitted by Aedes aegypti or Aedes albopictus mosquitoes. Before 2013, CHIK outbreaks had been identified only in Africa, Asia, Europe, and the Indian and Pacific Oceans. In late 2013, the first local transmission of CHIK was identified in the Western hemisphere (Caribbean countries, with subsequent reports in Central and South America and in the United States in Puerto Rico, Florida, and Texas).

39. Describe the clinical course of CHIK infection.

CHIK infection may have two consecutive phases. The acute phase consists of two stages— viral (5–10 days) and subacute post-viremic phase, indicated by IgM antiviral antibody (6–21 days). The viral stage is characterized by high fever, rash, myalgia, headache, arthralgia, and conjunctivitis. Most patients develop symmetric arthralgias or less commonly arthritis involving small and large joints. The arthralgias may be severe and debilitating. Laboratory abnormalities include thrombocytopenia and leukopenia, elevated levels of AST and ALT, and elevated muscle enzymes (creatinine kinase and lactate dehydrogenase). Treatment is supportive.

40. Describe the remitting-relapsing articular symptoms/signs due to CHIK infection.

Rarely, arthralgias/arthritis can follow a chronic remitting-relapsing course, with symptoms persisting as long as six years following initial infection in some patients. Less commonly, a pattern of chronic persistent arthritis/arthralgia may develop. The proper laboratory assessment includes the detection of virus-specific antibodies (IgM and IgG). Treatment is generally supportive, but the use of hydroxychloroquine, sulfasalazine, methotrexate and even biologic DMARD therapy has been described in patients with persistent post-CHIK arthritis. In those with chronic arthritis, checking autoimmune serologies (such as RF or anti-CCP) is recommended.

OTHER VIRUSES

41. Describe the rheumatic manifestations of severe acute respiratory syndrome coronavirus 2 (SARS-CoV-2).

SARS-CoV-2 is a ssRNA virus in the Coronavirus family. Human infection is transmitted by respiratory droplets/aerosols or by touching their face after contact with an infected surface. In addition to respiratory symptoms, it can cause arthralgias and myalgias (30–60%). Much less commonly it can cause an oligoarticular reactive arthritis (20% HLA-B27+). The arthritis is treated similar to other forms of viral arthritis. Case reports have also implicated the virus as causing chilblains, cutaneous vasculitis, Kawasaki disease, autoimmune hemolytic anemia, immune thrombocytopenia, autoimmune encephalitis, and antiphospholipid syndrome. Infected patients may develop autoantibodies including ANA, anti-SS-A, and antiphospholipid antibodies. There are case reports of SARS-CoV-2 infection triggering the onset of RA, SLE, and myositis as well as causing flares in patients who already have a systemic autoimmune rheumatic disease. This is most likely to occur in unvaccinated patients who have had severe infections with the delta variant of the virus.

Long-term sequalae following an acute infection, commonly referred to as long COVID, occurs in up to 30% of patients. It can manifest as persistent or relapsing arthralgias, myalgias, sleep disorders, cognitive impairment, as well as other symptoms which can mimic a rheumatic disease. COVID-19 vaccination has been reported to cause arthritis, arthralgias, and/or myalgias requiring anti-inflammatory medications.

42. Describe the epidemiology and clinical picture of Dengue fever.

Dengue virus is a ssRNA virus that belongs to the Flaviviridae family and is transmitted by the same mosquito as CHIK. The incidence is high in Asia, the Pacific, Africa, South and Central Americas, and the Caribbean. Nearly all dengue cases reported in the continental United States were acquired elsewhere by travelers or immigrants. Clinically it has gained the title "break-bone fever" and is characterized by fever, headache, retroorbital pain, deep bone pain, arthralgia, rash, and hemorrhagic manifestations. A small percentage of patients may deteriorate and develop hemorrhagic fever and shock.

43. How can we distinguish dengue fever from CHIK infection?

Arthralgia without synovitis is more frequent in dengue fever, whereas **arthritis is more common in CHIK infection.** Certain other manifestations including abdominal pain, leukopenia, and **hemorrhagic manifestations are more common in dengue fever** than in CHIK.

44. Describe the epidemiology and clinical picture of Zika virus infection.

The Zika virus is a ss-RNA virus that belongs to the Flaviviridae family and is transmitted by the same mosquito as CHIK and dengue viruses. Historically, outbreaks of Zika virus have occurred in Africa, Southeast Asia, and the Pacific. However, since 2015, the Zika virus epidemic has spread to the Caribbean and the Americas (South America, Central America, Mexico and the United States). Zika virus is transmitted via mosquito bite, transfusion of blood products, sex, and maternal-fetal route. Clinically, most cases are asymptomatic or mild and self-limited. Symptomatic cases may manifest with fever, pruritic rash, conjunctivitis, myalgia, and arthralgia without arthritis. Zika virus infection during pregnancy causes congenital microcephaly and fetal loss.

45. Describe the diagnosis, management, and complications of Zika virus infection.

The diagnosis is established by epidemiologic exposure, serology, and reverse transcriptase polymerase chain reaction for viral RNA. Treatment is supportive and includes rest, hydration, and acetaminophen. **NSAIDs and aspirin use is controversial** because these drugs have caused bleeding in patients with other Flaviviridae infections.

46. Describe the musculoskeletal manifestations of the human T-lymphotropic virus type I (HTVL-I) infection.

Patients with HTLV-I infection may present clinically with a symmetric small joint arthritis (pseudo-RA presentation). It can also cause a chronic oligoarthritis affecting the shoulders, wrists, and knees. Infection with this virus may cause the production of RF and ANA. Additional details on the epidemiology of HTLV-1 and its rheumatic manifestations can be found in the next chapter (see Chapter 41: HIV-Associated Rheumatic Syndromes).

47. What other viruses are known to cause arthritis?

Other viruses including HIV, mumps, rubella, Epstein–Barr, coxsackievirus, echovirus, adenovirus, herpes viruses (herpes simplex, cytomegalovirus, and varicella-zoster) have been implicated as causes of self-limited arthritis.

ACKNOWLEDGMENT

The author would like to acknowledge the contributions of Dr. Afzal Wais and Dr. Seth Mark Berney who were the authors of this chapter in the previous edition.

BIBLIOGRAPHY

Ciaffi J, Meliconi R, Ruscitti P, et al. Rheumatic manifestations of COVID-19: a systematic review and meta-analysis. *BMC Rheumatol.* 2020;4:65.

Colmegna I, Alberts-Grill N. Parvovirus B19: its role in chronic arthritis. *Rheum Dis Clin North Am.* 2009;35:95–110.

Fedorchenko Y, Zimba O. Long COVID in autoimmune rheumatic diseases. *Rheumatol Int.* 2023;43:1197–1207.

Forbess L. Polyarteritis nodosa. *Rheum Dis Clin North Am.* 2015;41:33–46.

Fragoulis GE, Nikiphorou E, Dey M, et al. 2022 EULAR recommendations for screening and prophylaxis of chronic and opportunistic infections in adults with autoimmune inflammatory rheumatic diseases. *Ann Rheum Dis.* 2023;82:742–753.

Guzman MG, Harris E. Dengue. *Lancet.* 2015;385:453–465.

Halani S, Tombindo PE, O'Reilly R, et al. Clinical manifestations and health outcomes associated with Zika virus infections in adults: a systematic review. *PLoS Negl Trop Dis.* 2021;15:e0009516.

Koutsianas C, Thomas K, Vassilopoulos D. Hepatitis B reactivation in rheumatic diseases: screening and prevention. *Rheum Dis Clin North Am.* 2017;43:133–149.

Lambert N, Strebel P, Orenstein W, et al. Rubella. *Lancet.* 2015;385:2297–2307.

Loomba R, Liang TJ. Hepatitis B reactivation associated with immune suppressive and biological modifier therapies: current concepts, management strategies, and future directions. *Gastroenterology.* 2017;152:1297–1309.

Marks M, Marks JL. Viral arthritis. *Clin Med (Lond.).* 2016;16:129–134.

Moghoofei M, Mostafaei S, Ashraf-Ganjouei A, et al. HBV reactivation in rheumatic diseases patients under therapy: a meta-analysis. *Microb Pathog.* 2018;114:436–443.

Palazzi C, D'Amico E, D'Angelo S, et al. Rheumatic manifestations of hepatitis C virus chronic infection: indications for a correct diagnosis. *World J Gastroenterol.* 2016;22:1405–1410.

Priora M, Borrelli R, Parisi S, et al. Autoantibodies and rheumatologic manifestations in hepatitis C virus infection. *Biology (Basel).* 2021;10:1071.

Robinson WH, Younis S, Love ZZ, et al. Epstein–Barr virus as a potentiator of autoimmune diseases. *Nat Rev Rheumatol.* 2024;20:729–740.

Sapkota HR, Nune A. Long COVID from rheumatology perspective—a narrative review. *Clin Rheumatol.* 2022;41:337–348.

Suhrbier A. Rheumatic manifestations of chikungunya: emerging concepts and interventions. *Nat Rev Rheumatol.* 2019;15:597–611.

Terrault NA, Lok ASF, McMahon BJ, et. al. Update on Prevention, Diagnosis, and Treatment of Chronic Hepatitis B: AASLD 2018 Hepatitis B Guidance. *Hepatology.* 2018 Apr;67(4):1560–1599.

FURTHER READING

https://www.cdc.gov/chikungunya/geo/index.html.
https://www.cdc.gov/dengue/index.html.
https://www.cdc.gov/vhf/ebola/index.html.
https://www.cdc.gov/zika/index.html.

CHAPTER 41

HIV-Associated Rheumatic Syndromes

Sarah Goglin, MD

1. How common are rheumatic manifestations in PWH? Has ART affected this?

It is estimated that 38 million people are infected with HIV worldwide. The overall prevalence of rheumatic manifestations associated with HIV is approximately 9%. With the use of ART, the overall prevalence of SpAs, DILS, and painful articular syndrome has decreased significantly. In contrast, the complications of HIV and its therapy (osteopenia, avascular necrosis, and IRIS) have increased. With ART, a normal life expectancy for HIV patients can be anticipated, with an increasing prevalence of chronic musculoskeletal conditions.

2. What are the rheumatic manifestations associated with HIV?

Pre-ART Therapy	ART Therapy
Articular	**IRIS**
Arthralgias (5%)	Sarcoidosis
HIV-associated arthritis (1%)	RA
ReA	SLE
Psoriatic arthritis	ReA
Undifferentiated SpA	Sjögren's syndrome
Painful articular syndrome (10%)	Subacute cutaneous lupus
Muscular	Graves' disease
Myalgias/fibromyalgia (30%)	**Drug-induced conditions**
Polymyositis (2%)	Zidovudine myopathy
Nemaline rod myopathy	Mitochondrial myopathies from newer NRTIs
Inclusion body myositis	Rhabdomyolysis
HIV-wasting syndrome	Gout/hyperuricemia
DILS (3%)	Lipodystrophy
Vasculitis (<1%)	**Osseous conditions**
Infection	Osteopenia/osteoporosis
Septic arthritis	Osteomalacia
Pyomyositis	Osteonecrosis
Gout/Hyperuricemia	Osteomyelitis

NRTIs, nucleoside reverse transcriptase inhibitors; *RA,* rheumatoid arthritis; *SLE,* systemic lupus erythematosus.
Adapted from Patel N, Patel N, Espinoza LR. HIV infection and rheumatic diseases: the changing spectrum of clinical enigma. *Rheum Dis Clin N Am.* 2009;35:139–161.

3. Does HIV infection have a direct role in the pathogenesis of rheumatic diseases?

A wide range of rheumatic syndromes/diseases have been observed in PWH, although the direct involvement of HIV in these conditions remains uncertain. Many of these rheumatic syndromes, such as polymyositis (PM), vasculitis, HIV-associated arthritis, and DILS, tend to occur in individuals with severe immune deficiency. The prevalence of certain rheumatic syndromes/diseases appears to decrease in HIV-infected individuals who receive antiretroviral therapy (ART), which suggests an indirect role of HIV infection in their development.

Moreover, as the CD4+ T-cell count decreases, diseases characterized by CD8+ T-cell predominance, like psoriasis, ReA, and DILS, are more frequently observed. In patients with HIV infection, the depletion of T regulatory cells (a subset of CD4+ T cells responsible for maintaining self-tolerance and preventing the development of autoimmunity) is observed. This depletion, along with the production of various cytokines, is believed to contribute to the pathogenesis of HIV and may lead to the production of autoantibodies and the development of autoimmune complications.

As CD4+ T-cell numbers decline to less than 300/µL, the risk of opportunistic infections increases. Additionally, viral particles have been identified in the synovium and synovial fluid of individuals with arthritis, suggesting a direct inflammatory effect. However, further research is needed to fully understand the mechanisms underlying these rheumatic syndromes/diseases in the context of HIV infection.

4. What role do autoantibodies have in HIV-associated rheumatic syndromes?

In untreated HIV-positive patients, several laboratory abnormalities are commonly observed. These include polyclonal gammopathy in approximately 45% of patients, low-titer rheumatoid factor (RF) and antinuclear antibodies (ANAs) in up to 20% of patients, and IgG anticardiolipin antibodies in over 90% of patients. It's important to note that anticardiolipin antibodies are generally not clinically significant as they are not associated with anti-β2-glycoprotein I antibodies. Double-stranded DNA antibodies are rare in this population. Cryoglobulins can occur in HIV patients with or without coexistent hepatitis C infection. Although both cytoplasmic and perinuclear antineutrophil cytoplasmic antibodies have been described, characteristic vasculitis is not commonly associated with them.

While autoantibodies are frequently found in HIV-positive patients, there is no clear correlation between the presence of these autoantibodies and the development of a specific rheumatic syndrome. Notably, patients with arthralgias and one of these autoantibodies may initially be misdiagnosed as having a particular rheumatic disease rather than an HIV infection.

With the advent of ART, antibody titers often decrease or disappear entirely, making them less common in the current era of HIV treatment. However, it's important to mention that the erythrocyte sedimentation rate (ESR), a nonspecific marker of inflammation, can remain chronically elevated in patients with HIV, even with consistent use of ART. Therefore, caution should be exercised when interpreting ESR values in patients with HIV and concurrent rheumatic disease, as they may not correlate with rheumatic disease activity.

5. What are the unique types of HIV-associated arthritis? How does HIV-associated arthritis differ from the painful articular syndrome?

HIV infection is associated with several distinct arthritis syndromes. Additionally, seroconversion (the development of detectable antibodies against HIV) can be accompanied by nonspecific symptoms such as arthralgia (joint pain), myalgia (muscle pain), and polyarthritis (inflammation of multiple joints).

HIV-associated arthritis typically presents as oligoarticular arthritis, affecting the joints of the lower extremities, such as the knees and ankles. It is more commonly observed in men and can occur at any stage of HIV infection. The synovial fluid analysis is noninflammatory, with negative cultures, and radiographs and tests for RF, ANA, and HLA B27 genotypes are usually negative. The symptoms of HIV-associated arthritis are typically self-limited, lasting from 1 to 6 weeks, and they usually respond well to rest, physical therapy, nonsteroidal anti-inflammatory drugs (NSAIDs), and low-dose corticosteroids. Once the clinical disorder resolves, medications can be safely discontinued. In rare cases, more prolonged arthritis can develop, leading to joint-space narrowing and erosions that resemble rheumatoid arthritis (RA). Another form of arthritis called Jaccoud arthropathy, characterized by reducible deformities at the metacarpophalangeal and interphalangeal joints, has also been described in HIV-infected individuals. These patients may respond to treatment with NSAIDs, hydroxychloroquine, and/or sulfasalazine.

The **painful articular syndrome** is characterized by the acute onset of severe joint pain, commonly affecting the knees, shoulders, and elbows, and it typically resolves within 24 hours. This syndrome is observed in the late stages of HIV infection. It is speculated that this syndrome may be due to transient bone ischemia (lack of blood supply to the bone), as there is no evidence of inflammatory synovitis. Narcotics are often required to relieve the severe pain associated with this syndrome.

6. How does reactive arthritis typically present in a person living with HIV?

The incidence of reactive arthritis (ReA) associated with HIV infection ranges from 0.5% to 3%, but it has significantly decreased since the introduction of antiretroviral therapy (ART). ReA can manifest in different ways: it may precede the diagnosis of acquired immunodeficiency syndrome (AIDS) by up to 2 years, co-occur, or, more commonly, present in individuals with severe established immunodeficiency. Common symptoms include seronegative oligoarthritis of the lower extremities and urethritis, while conjunctivitis is rarely observed. Enthesitis, plantar fasciitis, dactylitis, stomatitis, and skin and nail changes are frequently seen, and balanitis may also occur. However, axial skeletal involvement and uveitis are uncommon. Synovial fluid analysis typically shows inflammation with a cell count ranging from 2000 to 10,000 cells/μL; cultures are usually negative. The clinical course of HIV-associated ReA is generally characterized by mild arthritis with periods of remission and recurrence. However, in some cases, severe erosive arthritis can develop, leading to significant disability.

The frequency of HLA-B27 in HIV-positive ReA patients is similar to that found in HIV-negative ReA patients of the same ancestry. Rates of ReA tend to be higher in areas where HIV is primarily transmitted through sexual encounters, such as Central and South America and Africa, compared to areas where intravenous drug use is the primary mode of transmission. However, in Asian cohorts, few cases of ReA have been reported despite the majority of HIV cases being transmitted sexually. The lower rates of ReA in the United States may be attributed to the early introduction of ART and changes in sexual practices. The association between HIV and ReA may primarily be due to coinfection with organisms such as Chlamydia trachomatis and Ureaplasma urealyticum, which are known to cause ReA but may be asymptomatic or not commonly tested for (in the case of U. urealyticum).

7. What is the association between psoriasis and HIV infection?

Psoriasis and psoriatic arthritis typically manifest later in the course of HIV infection. A wide range of psoriasiform skin manifestations can be observed in the same patient. Antiretroviral therapy (ART) can be highly effective in managing both psoriasis and psoriatic arthritis. However, medications such as methotrexate, biologics, and phototherapy may be necessary to control skin and joint disease and may be used with appropriate monitoring in many PWH (see Question 9). Any patient experiencing a severe and unexplainable flare-up of psoriasis, the simultaneous presence of different subtypes of psoriasis, or the onset of psoriasis that does not respond to conventional therapy should be screened for HIV infection. Additionally, in HIV-infected individuals with widespread psoriasiform lesions, cutaneous T-cell lymphoma should be considered as a possible differential diagnosis.

8. Why are many PWH with arthritis categorized as having an undifferentiated SpA?

Many patients with HIV-associated arthritis develop a pattern of oligoarthritis, enthesitis, dactylitis, onycholysis, balanitis, uveitis, or spondylitis without sufficient criteria to be classified as having ReA or psoriatic arthritis. These patients are ultimately given the diagnosis of an undifferentiated SpA.

9. What is conventional treatment for arthritis and autoimmune disease in HIV-infected patients? Can treatment with anti-tumor necrosis factor (TNF) α therapy be considered?

The choice of treatment for individuals living with HIV depends on the specific autoimmune/inflammatory disease, the severity of the disease, and the status of the HIV infection. NSAIDs, low-dose oral corticosteroids, hydroxychloroquine, sulfasalazine, and methotrexate are generally considered safe and can be used when indicated.

The use of other immunosuppressive medications, such as leflunomide, azathioprine, mycophenolate mofetil, cyclosporine, TNFα antagonists, and rituximab, has been described in the literature for patients with HIV. Many experts suggest that these medications may be used safely in patients who consistently take antiretroviral therapy (ART), who have successfully suppressed viral activity, and who have CD4+ T-cell counts above 200/μL. There is less experience in using other classes of biologics and novel small molecule inhibitors in PWH; thus, assessing the risk-benefit ratio in an individual and engaging in shared decision-making are essential.

It is recommended to screen for comorbid infections such as tuberculosis and hepatitis B/C before initiating any new immunosuppressive medication. Before starting a new immunosuppressive medication, it is essential to assess for potential drug interactions due to the complex pharmacology of ART therapy. Patients on immunosuppressive therapy should be closely monitored to ensure there is no evidence of worsening control of HIV, development of HIV-associated complications (e.g., Kaposi's sarcoma), or opportunistic infections.

10. What are the HIV-associated muscle diseases?

Muscle involvement is common in PWH and can manifest at any stage of the disease as either an inflammatory or noninflammatory condition. **HIV-associated wasting syndrome**, which is a noninflammatory necrotizing myopathy, has been reported in over 40% of people with HIV (PWH) diagnosed with myopathy. However, it is important to note that this prevalence is likely significantly lower in the modern era of HIV treatment. Muscle biopsies of individuals with HIV-associated wasting syndrome typically show muscle atrophy and necrosis without evidence of inflammation. The exact underlying mechanism is still uncertain, although there is speculation regarding immune-mediated, metabolic, or nutritional factors.

Given that the clinical presentation of HIV-associated myopathy can resemble other forms of myopathy, performing a muscle biopsy can be beneficial in distinguishing this condition from inflammatory myositis or toxic (drug-induced) myopathy. In pre-antiretroviral therapy (pre-ART) HIV-infected patients, polymyositis (PM), HIV-associated inclusion body myositis, nemaline rod myopathy (which is rare), pyomyositis, and HIV-associated wasting syndrome are more commonly observed. On the other hand, patients receiving ART tend to develop drug-induced conditions such as mitochondrial myopathy, rhabdomyolysis, and lipodystrophy. It is essential to be cautious about the concurrent use of protease inhibitors and statins, as this combination has been associated with an increased risk of rhabdomyolysis.

11. How can HIV-associated PM and zidovudine (AZT) myopathy be clinically distinguished?

HIV-associated polymyositis (PM) presents with clinical features identical to idiopathic PM, including proximal muscle weakness, elevated creatine kinase (CK) levels, myopathic electromyography (EMG) findings, abnormal muscle magnetic resonance imaging (MRI) results, and an inflammatory muscle biopsy showing CD8+ infiltrates and viral antigen. However, CK levels in HIV-associated PM patients may be lower than those in non-HIV-associated PM patients or even within the normal range. Additionally, myositis-specific autoantibodies are typically absent. It is essential to exclude other potential causes, such as infection with Toxoplasma gondii.

Most patients with HIV-associated PM respond well to corticosteroid therapy (0.5 mg/kg per day) for a period of 6 to 12 weeks, and the dosage can be adjusted based on the individual's clinical course. Combining corticosteroids with antiretroviral therapy (ART) may be beneficial. In selected patients with persistent myositis, second-line therapy with methotrexate or other immunosuppressants may be considered, but close monitoring for potential complications is necessary.

AZT-induced myopathy typically occurs after an average duration of therapy of 11 months with a daily dosage of AZT exceeding 600 mg. This syndrome presents clinically in a manner that is indistinguishable from polymyositis (PM). It is characterized by a mild elevation of muscle enzymes, myopathic EMG findings, and an inflammatory muscle biopsy. In some cases, the muscle biopsy may reveal AZT-induced toxic mitochondrial myopathy, characterized by "ragged red fibers," which indicates abnormal mitochondrial function and the presence of paracrystalline inclusions. In general, performing an EMG and muscle biopsy is not necessary in cases of suspected AZT-induced myopathy.

The recommended approach for evaluating muscle weakness in a patient receiving AZT is to temporarily discontinue the drug for four weeks and reassess the patient through clinical examination and measurement of creatine kinase (CK) levels. Symptoms and laboratory abnormalities associated with AZT-induced myopathy typically improve within four weeks, and muscle strength usually returns to normal within eight weeks after discontinuation of the drug. It is worth noting that with the introduction of antiretroviral therapy (ART), high-dose AZT is rarely used, resulting in a significant decrease in the incidence of AZT-induced myopathy. It is also essential to be aware that other nucleoside reverse transcriptase inhibitors (NRTIs), such as didanosine, may also be associated with the development of myopathy.

12. Describe DILS (diffuse infiltrative lymphocytosis syndrome) in a patient with HIV

DILS is a benign lymphoproliferative disorder in PWH. It is characterized by (1) HIV-positivity, (2) the presence of bilateral, painless salivary gland enlargement or xerostomia persisting

>6 months, and (3) histologic confirmation of salivary or lacrimal gland lymphocytic infiltration with predominantly CD8+, CD29 T cells in the absence of granulomatous or neoplastic enlargement, or confirmatory ^{67}Ga scintigraphy. There is a much higher prevalence of DILS in Africa than in the United States. It is characterized by xerophthalmia, xerostomia, parotid gland enlargement, parotid cysts, persistent circulating CD8+ T-cell lymphocytosis, and diffuse visceral lymphocytic infiltration. Lymphocytic interstitial pneumonitis is the most severe complication of DILS and has decreased significantly with ART. Cranial nerve palsies (VII due to parotid compression), aseptic meningitis, and symmetric peripheral motor neuropathy may occur. Lymphocytic hepatitis, interstitial nephritis, type IV renal tubular acidosis, PM, and lymphoma have also been observed. Low to moderate doses of corticosteroids for glandular enlargement and sicca symptoms are beneficial. Topical treatment is usually satisfactory, but pilocarpine (5–10 mg thrice a day) may be necessary for severe sicca symptoms. High-dose corticosteroids and ART are used for severe extraglandular involvement.

13. Compare DILS with Sjögren's syndrome. See Table 41.1.

TABLE 41.1 Comparison of Sjögren's Syndrome and DILS

	SJÖGREN'S	DILS
Parotid swelling	Uncommon	Common
Sicca symptoms	Common	Common
Extraglandular manifestations	Uncommon	Common
Infiltrative lymphocytic phenotype	CD4+ T cells	CD8+ T cells
Autoantibodies (RF, ANA, anti-SS-A/SS-B)	Common	Rare
HLA association	DRB1*0301	DRB1*1102, 1301, 1302
Corticosteroids for glandular symptoms	Rarely helpful	Beneficial

14. List the forms of vasculitis that have been described with HIV infection and/or following the institution of ART.

Vasculitis is a rare manifestation (<1%) of HIV infection. All vasculitis subtypes (small, medium, large, and variable vessel) have been reported. The CD4+ count is typically >200 cells/uL in PWH with primary vasculitis. Opportunistic co-infections (e.g., hepatitis B, hepatitis C, CMV, EBV, VZV, herpes, fungal, mycobacterial, and others) as the cause of the vasculitis must always be ruled out regardless of the CD4+ count.

- Polyarteritis nodosa: usually a sensorimotor neuropathy
- Large artery/aorta vasculitis: more common in Africa
- Hypersensitivity angiitis due to AZT and didanosine
- Henoch–Schönlein purpura
- Primary angiitis of the central nervous system
- Behçet's syndrome
- Cryoglobulinemia: types 2 and 3
- Kawasaki-like syndrome: in both children and adults
- Erythema elevatum diutinum
- ANCA-associated vasculitis: more commonly reported post-ART
  Importantly, PWH who have had vasculitis are at increased risk of accelerated atherosclerosis and future cardiovascular events due to the inflammation, vascular damage, and side effects of ART.

15. What is HIV-associated immune complex kidney disease, and why is it helpful for a rheumatologist to be aware of this HIV-associated condition?

Renal disease can occur in individuals with HIV due to various causes, including the viral infection itself (known as HIV-associated nephropathy or HIVAN), medication toxicity associated with antiretroviral therapy (ART), infection, and immune-mediated injury resulting from the systemic response against HIV. With the introduction of ART, renal disease secondary to HIV and opportunistic infections has become less common. Recent studies suggest that **HIV-associated**

immune complex (HIVIC) kidney disease is now the most frequently observed pathological finding in renal biopsy specimens from patients with HIV.

Patients with HIVIC typically present with renal insufficiency, proteinuria, active urinary sediment, and hypocomplementemia. HIVIC is associated with a wide range of histopathologic findings, including a lupus-like glomerulonephritis characterized by a "full-house pattern" (presence of IgG, IgM, IgA, C3, and C1q) on immunofluorescence. These features may mimic lupus nephritis, so rheumatologists need to recognize the presence of HIVIC. It is also essential to rule out coinfection with hepatitis B and C, syphilis, as well as other coexisting conditions such as cryoglobulinemia and DILS, as they can also contribute to immune complex deposition in the kidneys.

Treatment for HIVIC involves the use of ART, which is the cornerstone of management. In some instances, immunosuppressive therapy may be considered, although its use remains controversial due to limited data. Severe cases, such as those with crescentic glomerulonephritis, may require additional medications along with corticosteroids.

16. Is septic arthritis or bone infection more common in HIV-infected patients?

No, bone and joint infections from bacteria do not occur any more frequently in PWH compared with HIV-negative individuals. *Mycobacterium tuberculosis* arthritis and osteomyelitis can occur at any time in the course of HIV infection and may be multifocal (30%). Atypical mycobacterium and fungal musculoskeletal infections typically occur with severe immunosuppression (CD4+ count <100 cells/μL).

17. How does pyomyositis present clinically?

Pyomyositis, a bacterial muscle infection, is relatively rare in developed countries but remains frequently diagnosed in Africa and India. It typically affects individuals in the late stage of HIV disease with CD4+ counts below 200/μL. The characteristic symptoms of pyomyositis include fever, localized muscle pain, erythema, swelling, and leukocytosis. This infection commonly affects the quadriceps muscle, and about 75% of cases involve a single abscess. Staphylococcus aureus is the most frequently identified bacteria, although opportunistic infections may also occur.

The diagnosis of pyomyositis is made using imaging techniques such as ultrasound, computed tomography (CT) scan, magnetic resonance imaging (MRI), and cultures to identify the causative bacteria. Treatment typically involves conventional surgical drainage of the abscess and administration of appropriate antibiotics.

18. Name the rheumatic diseases that may remit or improve in association with AIDS.

Both systemic lupus erythematosus (SLE) and rheumatoid arthritis (RA) involve the interaction between major histocompatibility complex class II gene products and CD4+ T lymphocytes. As a result, SLE and RA may become less active as HIV infection progresses and CD4+ T-cell counts decline, although this is not always the case. When individuals with comorbid HIV and SLE present, they may exhibit overlapping features such as rash, arthralgia (joint pain), myalgia (muscle pain), adenopathy (enlarged lymph nodes), and cytopenia (low blood cell counts). Generally, these patients tend to have less severe disease and lower antibody titers compared to those with SLE alone or HIV alone.

However, it's important to note that in people living with HIV who have previously been diagnosed with SLE or RA and are being treated with antiretroviral therapy (ART), immune reconstitution resulting from ART can lead to a reactivation of their dormant SLE or RA, which had previously been inactive.

19. What is the immune reconstitution inflammatory syndrome (IRIS)?

After initiating antiretroviral therapy (ART) in an individual with HIV, cellular immunity improves. This improvement is characterized by increased CD4+ cells, CD4+/CD8+ ratio, and the levels of cytokines such as interleukin-6 and interferon-γ. There is also an imbalance in Th1/Th2 immune responses and changes in the expression of specific markers on immune cells, such as CCR-3 and CCR-5 on monocytes and granulocytes. As a result, some patients (up to 13%) may experience a profound inflammatory systemic response known as immune reconstitution inflammatory syndrome (IRIS) within 3 to 27 months (average = 9 months) after starting ART.

The likelihood of developing IRIS is lower if the CD4+ count is above 200 to 350/μL at ART initiation. Conversely, the risk of IRIS is higher in individuals with lower CD4+ counts and higher viral loads. A diagnosis of IRIS can be made in a patient with AIDS if they experience severe systemic inflammatory symptoms while on ART, accompanied by increasing CD4+ counts and decreasing HIV-1 viral load, and if another new infection or etiology cannot explain these symptoms.

IRIS occurs in two phases. The first phase, which occurs within 8 to 12 weeks after starting ART, is associated with an increase in memory CD4+ cells and can exacerbate preexisting conditions such as rheumatoid arthritis (RA), systemic lupus erythematosus (SLE), or sarcoidosis. The second phase occurs after six months of ART and involves naive CD4+ cells and their cytokines. This phase can be associated with developing new systemic or organ-specific autoimmune diseases, including RA, SLE, sarcoidosis, Still's disease, PM, ReA, autoimmune thyroid disease, subacute cutaneous lupus, or Guillain-Barré syndrome. Additionally, opportunistic infections that are being treated can worsen during this phase.

IRIS is typically self-limited, and ART is generally continued. However, discontinuing ART and administering corticosteroids may be necessary if the inflammatory response is severe and poses a risk of irreversible damage to the eyes or central nervous system.

20. When should screening for HIV be considered by the rheumatologist?

Traditionally, HIV screening has been recommended in the following situations encountered by the rheumatologist:
1. Diagnosis of reactive arthritis (ReA) with sexual or unknown mode of acquisition.
2. History of intravenous drug use or other potential exposures.
3. Patients with septic arthritis or pyomyositis.
4. Psoriatic arthritis with refractory or atypical rash subtypes.
5. Atypical lupus or multiple unexplained autoantibodies.
6. Sicca symptoms in the absence of SSA or SSB autoantibodies.
7. Autoimmune disease is refractory to typical therapy.

However, due to the significant benefits of early identification and initiation of antiretroviral therapy (ART), the Centers for Disease Control and Prevention (CDC) now recommends universal screening for HIV in all patients with their consent. Therefore, rheumatologists should have a very low threshold to screen for HIV in all patients.

21. What other miscellaneous rheumatic syndromes are described in patients with HIV?

Fibromyalgia is reported in 10% to 30% of HIV-infected patients. Nonspecific musculoskeletal complaints are common, affecting up to 60% of patients at some point during HIV infection and treatment. Conditions such as tendinitis, bursitis, carpal tunnel syndrome, adhesive capsulitis (frozen shoulder), and Dupuytren's contracture may occur, particularly in patients treated with protease inhibitors like indinavir. Hyperuricemia is also common in HIV patients, and gout can occur. There may be an association between ritonavir and indinavir, two protease inhibitors, and the development of gout.

22. What bone diseases occur more commonly in HIV patients?

- **Osteoporosis:** PWH have a three times higher risk of developing low bone mass than the general population. The causes of osteoporosis in PWH are multifactorial and include factors such as vitamin D deficiency, hypogonadism, low body mass index, side effects of antiretroviral therapy (ART), and chronic inflammation. As the life expectancy of PWH increases and the duration of ART use extends, the prevalence of bone disease in this population is expected to rise. Screening for bone density is essential to identify individuals who may require treatment, which may involve ensuring adequate calcium and vitamin D intake and initiating specific osteoporosis medications.

- **Osteonecrosis (avascular necrosis):** Osteonecrosis can occur in any joint, although it is most commonly observed in the hip, with a prevalence estimated at 4–5% in PWH. Bilateral disease and earlier onset are more common in this population. Risk factors for osteonecrosis in PWH include dyslipidemia associated with protease inhibitors, corticosteroid use, and HIV infection itself, particularly in individuals with very low CD4 counts (<60 cells/μL).

- **Hypertrophic osteoarthropathy:** This condition can develop in patients with Pneumocystis jiroveci pneumonia, a lung infection commonly seen in advanced stages of HIV infection. Treatment of pneumonia typically leads to improvement in hypertrophic osteoarthropathy symptoms.

23. Do any other retroviruses cause rheumatic diseases?

Human T lymphotropic virus type I (HTLV-I) is a complex type C RNA retrovirus. It is prevalent in certain regions worldwide, including the Caribbean, southern Japan, South Africa, and South America (particularly Brazil). HTLV-I is transmitted through breast milk, sexual intercourse, and blood products. The virus is associated with two types of diseases: adult T-cell leukemia/non-Hodgkin's lymphoma (lifetime risk of 5%), which often presents with hypercalcemia and skin involvement, and various chronic inflammatory syndromes (lifetime risk of 2%). These inflammatory syndromes encompass seronegative oligo- or polyarthritis with tenosynovitis and nodules featuring fibrinoid necrosis. Other syndromes associated with HTLV-I include polymyositis-like disease, dermatitis, uveitis, and transverse myelitis, also known as HTLV-1-associated myelopathy/tropical spastic paraparesis. Diagnosis typically involves detecting antibodies through enzyme-linked immunosorbent assay, confirming with Western blot, and observing "flower cells" on a peripheral smear. Unfortunately, treatment options for HTLV-I are limited. Cases of this viral infection are being observed more frequently in the United States due to immigration.

ACKNOWLEDGMENT

The author would like to thank Dr. Katrina M. Lawrence-Wolff and Dr. Daniel F. Battafarano for their contributions to this chapter in the previous edition.

BIBLIOGRAPHY

Adizie T, Moots RJ, Hodkinson B, et al. Inflammatory arthritis in HIV positive patients: a practical guide. *BMC Infect Dis.* 2016;16:100.

Akram B, Khan M, Humphrey MB. HIV-associated rheumatic diseases: a narrative review. *J Clin Rheumatol.* 2024;30:e42–e45.

Biver E. Osteoporosis and HIV Infection. *Calcif Tissue Int.* 2022;110:624–640.

Branson BM, Handsfield HH, Lampe MA, et al. Revised recommendations for HIV testing of adults, adolescents, and pregnant women in health-care settings. *MMWR.* 2006;55(RR14):1–17.

Cohen SD, Kopp JB, Kimmel PL. Kidney Diseases Associated with HIV Infection. *NEJM.* 2017;377:2363–2374.

Fox C, Walker-Bone K. Evolving spectrum of HIV-associated rheumatic syndromes. *Best Pract Res Clin Rheumatol.* 2015;29:244–258.

Medina F, Pérez-Saleme L, Moreno J. Rheumatic manifestations of human immunodeficiency virus infection. *Infect Dis Clin North Am.* 2006;20:891–912.

Maganti RM, Reveille JD, Williams FM. Therapy insight: the changing spectrum of rheumatic disease in HIV infection. *Nat Clin Pract Rheumatol.* 2008;4:428–438.

Muller M, Wandel S, Colebunders R, et al. Immune reconstitution inflammatory syndrome in patients starting antiretroviral therapy for HIV infection: a systemic review and meta-analysis. *Lancet Infect Dis.* 2010;10:251–261.

Patel N, Patel N, Espinoza LR. HIV infection and rheumatic diseases: the changing spectrum of a clinical enigma. *Rheum Dis Clin N Am.* 2009;35:139–161.

Robinson-Papp J, Simpson DM. Neuromuscular diseases associated with HIV-1 infection. *Muscle Nerve.* 2009;40:1043–1053.

Steve RJ, Alex D, Yesudhason BL, et al. Autoantibodies among HIV-1 infected individuals and the effect of anti-retroviral therapy (ART) on it. *Curr HIV Res.* 2021;19:277–285.

Vega LE, Espinoza LR. Vasculitides in HIV infection. *Curr Rheumatol Rep.* 2020;22:60.

Vega LE, Espinoza LR. Human immunodeficiency virus infection (HIV)-associated rheumatic manifestations in the pre- and post-HAART eras. *Clin Rheumatol.* 2020;39:2515–2522.

Walker NF, Scriven J, Meintjes G, Wilkinson RJ. Immune reconstitution inflammatory syndrome in HIV-infected patients. *HIV AIDS (Auckl).* 2015;7:49–64.

Walker-Bone K, Doherty E, Kaushik S, et al. Assessment and management of musculoskeletal disorders among patients living with HIV. *Rheumatology.* 2017;56:1648–1661.

FURTHER READING

htpps://www.hivguidelines.org.
htpps://www.clinicalinfo.hiv.gov.
htpps://www.cdc.gov/hiv/guidelines.

CHAPTER 42

Whipple Disease

Lisa Davis, MD, MsCS

KEY POINTS

1. Whipple disease (WD) is a rare, systemic, infectious disorder caused by the actinomycete *Tropheryma whipplei*.
2. Joint manifestations of WD often precede the gastrointestinal symptoms by approximately 6 years, and typically affect large joints in a migratory, intermittent, pattern resembling palindromic rheumatism.
3. The diagnosis is often established by demonstrating foamy macrophages on biopsy of the small bowel (or other affected organs) or by using quantitative polymerase chain reaction (qPCR) analysis.
4. Treatment consists of prolonged antibiotic therapy, and patients should be followed lifelong, as recurrences are frequent.

1. What is the spectrum of *Tropheryma whipplei* infections, and what is Whipple disease?

There are four commonly recognized manifestations of *T. whipplei* infections: (1) classic Whipple disease, (2) localized chronic infections, (3) acute infections, and (4) asymptomatic bacterial carriage. Classic Whipple disease is an uncommon, chronic, multisystem disorder. First described by Dr. George Hoyt Whipple in 1907, classic Whipple disease generally presents with arthritis/arthralgia and fevers, followed years later by diarrhea, malabsorption, abdominal pain, and weight loss; patients may subsequently develop central nervous system (CNS) or cardiovascular manifestations. Due to its nonspecific presentation, the condition is usually diagnosed at an advanced stage.

Localized chronic infections do not have signs of gastrointestinal involvement and can include joint infections, culture-negative endocarditis, uveitis, and isolated encephalitis. *T. whipplei* acute infections include pneumonia, gastroenteritis, and bacteremia. *T. whipplei* asymptomatic carriage can be found in saliva and stool samples.

2. Describe the epidemiology of T. whipplei, T. whipplei infections, and Whipple disease

T. whipplei has a high occurrence in the environment, and human exposure to *T. whipplei* is widespread. *T. whipplei* is found in wastewaters and is thought to be transmitted via feces and saliva. Varying with the population and environment, 48% to 72% of general populations have antibodies to *T. whipplei*. *T. whipplei* carriage has been found in sampling healthy individuals, including in saliva, stool, and dental plaque samples and in duodenal biopsies. *T. whipplei* has been found in 1.5–4% of fecal samples of asymptomatic individuals and in 12–25% of individuals in at-risk populations such as sewage workers and undomiciled individuals.

In a retrospective study of patients who had rheumatologic symptoms, 2.6% had chronic arthritis associated with *T. whipplei*. *T. whipplei* was responsible for 2–6% of culture-negative endocarditis in France and 6% in Germany, making *T. whipplei* the fourth most frequent pathogen found in culture-negative endocarditis.

Classic Whipple disease (WD) prevalence is estimated at 1.1 cases per 1 million people. The mean age of diagnosis is 55 years, and 85% of cases are males, although the prevalence in females has increased over the last 30 years. Over 66% of patients who develop WD have had occupational exposure to soil (farmers), sewage water, or animals.

3. Describe the biology of T. whipplei.

The bacterium that causes Whipple disease was named in 1991. Initially, it was named *Tropheryma whippelii* (from Greek *trophe-* "nourishment", *-eryma* "barrier"), which refers to the malabsorption caused by Whipple disease. In 2001, the bacterium was renamed *T. whipplei* to correct the spelling to that of its eponym, Dr. Whipple. *T. whipplei* is categorized in the phylum Actinomycetota. It is a small (1–2 × 0.2 μm) rod-shaped bacterium with a plasma membrane surrounded by a thin homogenous wall, and another plasma membrane-like structure, resulting in trilaminar appearance. It is Gram variable (often Gram-negative when grown in media but Gram-positive in clinical samples) and periodic acid–Schiff (PAS) positive. It has a single circular genome of 0.93 Mbp (approximately 800 open reading frames, GC content 46.3%). It is one of the slowest-growing human pathogenic bacteria, requiring 30 days to detect in cultures, with a generation time of 18 days. *T. whipplei* lacks genes for several amino acid pathways and for the tricarboxylic acid cycle and was initially thought to require intact eukaryotic cells for culture. In 2003, an axenic culture medium was created, which indicates that while *T. whipplei* is not a strict obligate intracellular organism, it requires a close relationship with its host. In fibroblast cell cultures, *T. whipplei* has an intracellular form within vacuoles and an extracellular form as aggregates of bacteria embedded in a polysaccharidic matrix. The intracellular form in macrophages is surrounded by an inert material, which is thought to be an intracellular biofilm. *T. whipplei* has a large collection of genes encoding surface proteins called WiSP (Wnt-1-inducible signaling pathway). It is theorized that the bacteria commandeer the mechanisms of the host macrophages to produce glycosylation of the WiSP proteins, and that these glycosylated proteins play a role in immune evasion.

4. What is the immunopathogenesis of Whipple disease?

Most exposures to *T. whipplei* result in either a self-limited infection or asymptomatic carriage, and then immunity. Due to the low number of individuals who develop Whipple disease (WD) relative to the exposure rate, it is postulated that development of WD is dependent on host predisposition. Studies have suggested a genetic heterogeneity of susceptibility to chronic infections with *T. whipplei*. A German study found potential association between classic WD and human leukocyte antigen (HLA)-B27, while a larger study found a higher frequency of HLA alleles DRB∗13 and DQB1∗06. HLA-B*51 and HLA-B*44 are correlated with cardiac and neurological forms, while HLA-DQB1*06 has been correlated with immune reconstitution inflammatory syndrome (IRIS). Whipple disease has been linked to increased expression of interleukin (IL)-4, IL-10, and Th2 cells, with decreased expression of interferon-γ and IL-12 and diminished functionality of Th1 cells, macrophages, and monocytes. It has been proposed that *T. whipplei*- and IL-16-mediated interference with the macrophage endocytic pathway allows the bacteria to be phagocytosed but disallows the macrophages to neutralize the bacteria, thereby contributing to the spread of *T. whipplei*. This manipulation of the immune system results not only in a decreased ability to clear the infection but also in a utilization of macrophages and immature dendritic cells for multiplication and dispersion throughout the body. Individuals with WD do not have associated opportunistic infections, but they do have a susceptibility to reinfections with new strains.

5. How is the diagnosis of Whipple disease made?

Before the advent of quantitative polymerase chain reaction (qPCR), a definitive diagnosis of Whipple disease (WD) was established only when microscopic examination of a small bowel mucosal biopsy by hematoxylin and eosin (H&E) and PAS staining showed infiltration of the mucosa and lamina propria by large "foamy" macrophages that contained PAS-positive inclusions. The culture of *T. whipplei*, even with the advent of a specific axenic medium, can only be performed in a few laboratories. Today, the most common means of diagnosis include pathology and qPCR. When classic WD is suspected, current recommendations include an initial screen of both stool and saliva with qPCR. When both saliva and stool samples are positive, qPCR has a 95% positive predictive value (PPV) for classic WD, and when both are negative, a 98% negative predictive value (NPV). However, the sensitivity of qPCR in patients with focal *T. whipplei* infections decreases to 36% for saliva and 64% for stool. Urine has been proposed as another noninvasive sample source; however, at this time, the PPV and NPV are not yet known.

The current gold standard for diagnosis of *T. whipplei* infection is the demonstration of the organism in one involved tissue (usually small bowel) by at least two evaluative methods or the demonstration of the organism by qPCR testing in two involved sites (e.g., synovial fluid and cerebrospinal fluid, CSF). All patients, regardless of the presence or absence of neurologic symptoms, should have a qPCR of their CSF to rule out occult CNS infection. The methods now available for tissue examination include PAS stain with supplementary Ziehl-Nelsen stain (as some bacterial species such as *Mycobacterium avium* can also be stained by PAS), qPCR, immunohistochemical staining with antisera specific for *T. whipplei* with electron microscopy, or fluorescence in situ hybridization (FISH) with laser scanning confocal microscopy to confirm the presence of *T. whipplei* bacterial rRNA. Treatment of patient samples with a glycosidase cocktail increases the detection rate by both qPCR and FISH by removing the polysaccharidic matrix surrounding *T. whipplei*. Serological antibody tests are not recommended given the high environmental exposure.

6. Describe the clinical presentation of patients with Whipple disease.

Classic Whipple disease (WD) symptoms are typically arthralgia/arthritis followed by gastrointestinal symptoms and CNS symptoms. Classic WD is often divided into early (<6 years), middle (6–8 years), and late (>8 years) phases (Table 42.1). **Early-phase** WD manifestations are dominated by intermittent arthritis or arthralgias. The delay between the first clinical manifestations and the appearance of gastrointestinal signs often exceeds six years. However, this delay may be shortened considerably if immunosuppressive therapy is given mistakenly to treat the arthritis that has been attributed to another disease. Several studies have shown a correlation between the use of immunosuppressive therapy and aggressive progression of WD. In WD patients who were treated for an unclear arthropathy with TNF-inhibitors, the incidence of endocarditis was 12.2%, while it was 1.6% in those who did not receive TNF-inhibitors.

Middle phase WD manifestations primarily include diarrhea, malabsorption, weight loss, abdominal pain, lymphadenopathy, anemia, and skin hyperpigmentation. Hyperpigmentation of the skin is found in 50% of patients and may be related to vitamin malabsorption. **Late phase** WD manifestations can include CNS symptoms and cardiovascular manifestations.

The multisystem manifestations of WD can be remembered using the following mnemonic:

Wasting/weight loss	**D**iarrhea
Hyperpigmentation of skin	**I**nterstitial nephritis
Intestinal pain	**S**kin lesions
Pancytopenia	**E**ye inflammation
Psychiatric symptoms	**A**rthritis
Lymphadenopathy	**S**upranuclear ophthalmoplegia
Encephalopathy	**E**ndocarditis
Steatorrhea	

7. Describe the arthritis, synovial fluid analysis, and microscopic results from arthrocentesis and synovial biopsies for patients with Whipple disease.

The pattern of arthritis associated with Whipple disease (WD) is a seronegative, migratory, oligo- or polyarthritis primarily involving large- and medium-joints (knees, ankles, and wrists). This arthritis is characterized by brief (a few days) episodic attacks of redness, swelling, pain, and decreased function. Less commonly affected joints are elbows, hips, and shoulders; small joints of the hands are even less frequently involved, and never in isolation. WD arthritis should evoke the

TABLE 42.1 Common Disease Course for Classic Whipple Disease

EARLY PHASE (<6 YEARS)	MIDDLE PHASE (6–8 YEARS)	LATE PHASE (>8 YEARS)
Intermittent arthralgias or arthritis (60–80%)	Diarrhea (80%)	CNS symptoms (6–63%)
Fevers (19–54%)	Weight loss (93%)	Cardiovascular
	Abdominal pain (23–60%)	
	Lymphadenopathy (35–66%)	
	Skin hyperpigmentation (50%)	
	Anemia (80%)	
Less common manifestations		
Cutaneous lesions	Pancytopenia	Ocular (4–27%)
Subcutaneous lesions		

differential diagnosis of palindromic rheumatism, spondyloarthritis, or seronegative rheumatoid arthritis. Some experts posit that a middle-aged man with a palindromic rheumatism-like presentation and a lack of response to steroids and biologic medications (TNF inhibitors, IL-6 antagonists) should prompt consideration of WD. Arthritis is the presenting symptom in 60–70% of cases and is present in 90% of all patients. The arthritis precedes the intestinal manifestations in 75% of patients by a mean interval of six years. Sacroiliitis is present in 7% and spondylitis in 4% of cases.

Arthrocentesis for patients with WD arthritis usually reveals an inflammatory fluid with white blood cell counts between 2000 and 30,000 cells/mm^3 with >50% of polymorphonuclear cells; repeat arthrocentesis after antibiotic therapy shows resolution of inflammation. Synovial fluid examination may reveal PAS-positive or qPCR-positive material, and cultures are typically negative. Synovial biopsy demonstrates focal synovial-lining hyperplasia and moderate perivascular lymphocytosis. The synovial membrane should contain PAS-positive granules in macrophages (foamy macrophages) or should test positive by qPCR, immunohistochemical staining, or FISH.

Rarely, patients with prolonged, untreated, WD may develop radiological evidence of destruction, such as joint space narrowing (thought to be due to septic arthritis). Hypertrophic osteoarthropathy is a very rare manifestation. *T. whipplei* has been implicated in some cases of discitis and joint prosthesis infection.

8. What are some of the late-phase manifestations of Whipple disease?

- **CNS manifestations:** CNS manifestations affect 6–63% of individuals with Whipple disease (WD). Symptoms can be central or peripheral, isolated or multifocal. Even in WD patients *without* neurologic symptoms, 50% can have qPCR-positive CSF. All patients should have CSF tested before therapy, regardless of symptoms. Postmortem examination of WD patients and *T. whipplei* carriers found that 90% of these individuals had brain and spinal cord lesions. The CNS lesions typically consist of necrosis with inflammatory cells and astrogliosis with perivascular macrophages containing intracellular PAS-positive rod-shaped structures. Of patients who develop neurologic symptoms, the most common manifestations include dementia (70%), psychiatric symptoms (50%), supranuclear vertical gaze palsy (50%), hypothalamic involvement (33%), and myoclonus (25%); other neurological signs include facial weakness and bilateral ptosis. The classic CNS WD triad of dementia, supranuclear ophthalmoplegia, and myoclonus is very specific and should warrant further investigation. Oculomasticatory myorhythmia (OMM) and oculofacial-skeletal myorhythmia (OFSM) are virtually pathognomonic of CNS WD. OMM is characterized by smooth, slow, convergent-divergent pendular nystagmus of the eyes at 1–3 Hz, with synchronous contractions of the masticatory muscles, supranuclear vertical gaze palsy, and occasionally rhythmic movements of the proximal and distal skeletal muscles. OFSM is similar to OMM, but with rhythmic movements of non-facial skeletal muscles. Brain biopsy and positive qPCR of CSF are diagnostic in 90% of cases. The prognosis for patients with symptomatic CNS involvement is poor; the 4-year survival rate is <75% and major sequelae are seen in 25%.
- **Cardiovascular involvement:** *T. whipplei* has been noted as the fourth most common cause of culture-negative endocarditis, depending on the region. Cardiac involvement of the pericardium, myocardium, and endocardium (including valves) is found at autopsy in almost all patients with classic WD. However, only 17–55% of cases are symptomatic.
- **Ophthalmologic manifestations:** Panuveitis is the most common ocular manifestation and diagnosis is made by PAS stain for macrophages and qPCR testing of the vitreous humor. Other manifestations include keratitis, retinitis, choroiditis, optic neuritis, and orbital inflammatory disease including orbital pseudotumor. Crystalline keratopathy has been reported as a characteristic of ocular WD.
- Other manifestations that may accompany classic WD include pulmonary involvement (30%), mesenteric more than peripheral adenopathy with noncaseating granulomas (9%), and, rarely, genitourinary involvement.

9. Describe some of the localized chronic infections that can occur with T. whipplei infections.

T. whipplei can cause localized infections that are not manifested as the classic, multisystem form of WD. Stool and saliva samples and duodenal biopsies are frequently negative.

- **Endocarditis:** In this form of endocarditis, the bacterium is an intracellular infection rather than biofilm colonization. Clinical signs are similar to those of patients with culture-negative endocarditis of other etiologies. The majority (79%) of patients with diagnosed localized endocarditis due to *T. whipplei* displayed vegetations. When compared with cardiac valves from patients with endocarditis of other etiologies, those with endocarditis due to *T. whipplei* displayed more fibrosis, lack of calcification, slightly less vegetation, reduced vascularization, and reduced inflammation.
- **Encephalitis:** In cases of localized encephalitis due to *T. whipplei* the most common symptoms reported are cognitive impairment, ataxia, and supranuclear ophthalmoplegia. Ataxia and dementia have been shown to be more severe in patients with encephalitis than in those with classic WD.

10. What is the therapy and follow up currently recommended for Whipple disease?

Before the use of antibiotics, Whipple disease was uniformly fatal. Though antibiotic treatment of *T. whipplei* often leads to a rapid improvement of symptoms (typically within 1–2 weeks), prolonged treatment is required to ensure eradication of the bacterium. Since lifetime susceptibility to *T. whipplei* has been shown, many experts recommend lifelong follow-up. This may include follow-up qPCR of feces every 3 months, or follow-up gastroscopy with the schedule of at 6 and 12 months, yearly for 3 years, then every 3 years lifelong. While histologic samples will remain PAS-positive for many years, the number of PAS-positive macrophages decreases and the appearance changes over years. Of importance, qPCR of tissue for *T. whipplei* becomes negative very quickly following treatment.

Although there are no large, randomized trials on the best antibiotic regimen for treatment of *T. whipplei*, treatment regimes relying on trimethoprim/sulfamethoxazole (TMP/sulfa) have shown high rates of relapse and are not recommended by many experts. Doxycycline is active against *T. whipplei* in vitro, and hydroxychloroquine causes increased intravacuolar pH, thereby decreasing *T. whipplei* viability (vacuole acidification is critical to the survival of *T. whipplei* in phagosomes). If a patient has CNS involvement, many experts recommend induction with an intravenous (IV) regimen that can penetrate the blood-brain barrier, followed by an oral regimen. The following are the most recent recommendations:

- **Primary regimen for classic Whipple disease *without* neurologic involvement:**
  Induction: doxycycline 100 mg twice daily + hydroxychloroquine 200 mg three times daily for 1 year.
  Maintenance: lifelong antibiotic prophylaxis with doxycycline 100 mg twice daily.
- **Alternative regimens to be considered for Whipple disease (with or without neurologic symptoms), in an asymptomatic patient with a positive CSF qPCR, or in a patient with endocarditis:**
  Induction: ceftriaxone 2 g IV once or twice daily, meropenem 1g IV every 8 hours, or penicillin G 4 MU IV every 4 hours for 14–28 days. Consider using higher doses for longer periods (i.e., 28 days) in patients with overt neurologic symptoms.
  Maintenance: doxycycline 100 mg twice daily + hydroxychloroquine 200 mg three times daily for at least a year, or one double-strength TMP/sulfa 160 mg/800 mg twice daily for 1 year
- **Localized chronic infections**
  Induction: doxycycline 100 mg twice daily + hydroxychloroquine 200 mg three times daily for 12-18 months.
  Maintenance: none

11. How frequently do patients experience clinical relapses of the disease following one year of treatment?

It is estimated that up to 35% of patients with Whipple disease who had long-term treatment relapsed after an average of 5 years. Neurologic relapses are most common and are particularly hard to treat. Recommendations for treating disease relapses include using an alternative antibiotic regimen from the initial regimen versus prolonged treatment.

Treatment regimens for relapse include:
Induction: ceftriaxone (2 g IV twice daily), meropenem 1g IV every 8 hours, or penicillin G 4 MU IV every 4 hours, for 4 weeks

Maintenance: doxycycline 100 mg twice daily + hydroxychloroquine 200 mg three times daily for at least a year or one double-strength TMP/sulfa 160 mg/800 mg twice daily for 1 year

12. Describe the immune reconstitution inflammatory syndrome (IRIS) that can occur during antibiotic therapy for Whipple disease.

Immune reconstitution inflammatory syndrome (IRIS) occurs in approximately 10–20% of patients with classic Whipple's disease, most commonly within the first few weeks of initiation of antibiotic therapy. IRIS occurs at a higher rate in those who received immunosuppressive therapies or in those who have CNS involvement. The mortality rate of Whipple disease with IRIS is approximately 10%. IRIS may manifest as a patient having had an initial response to antibiotic therapy, but they then develop recurrence of local or systemic inflammation (such as arthralgia and fever) for at least a week, but with no evidence of recurrence of infection. Corticosteroids can be beneficial in the control of these symptoms and thalidomide may be an alternative treatment for those with corticosteroid resistance.

BIBLIOGRAPHY

Bonhomme CY, Renesto P, Desnues B, et al. Tropheryma whipplei glycosylation in the pathophysiologic profile of whipple's disease. *J Infect Dis.* 2009;199:1043–1052.

Boumaza A, Ben Azzouz E, Arrindell J, Lepidi H, Mezouar S, Desnues B. Whipple's disease and Tropheryma whipplei infections: from bench to bedside. *Lancet Infect Dis.* 2022;22:e280–e291.

Cappellini A, Minerba P, Maimaris S, Biagi F. Whipple's disease: a rare disease that can be spotted by many doctors. *Eur J Intern Med.* 2024;121:25–29.

Dolmans RAV, Edwin Boel CH, Lacle MM, Kusters JG. Clinical manifestations, treatment, and diagnosis of Tropheryma whipplei infections. *Clin Microbiol Rev.* 2017;30:529–555.

El-Abassi R, Soliman MY, Williams F, England JD. Whipple's disease. *J Neurol Sci.* 2017;377:197–206.

Fenollar F, Lagier JC, Raoult D. Tropheryma whipplei and Whipple's disease. *J Infect.* 2014;69:103–112.

Feurle GE, Junga NS, Marth T. Efficacy of ceftriaxone or meropenem as initial therapies in Whipple's disease. *Gastroenterology.* 2010;138:478–486.

Lagier JC, Fenollar F, Lepidi H, Giorgi R, Million M, Raoult D. Treatment of classic Whipple's disease: from in vitro results to clinical outcome. *J Antimicrob Chemother.* 2014;69:219–227.

La Scola B, Fenollar F, Fournier P-E, Altwegg M, Mallet M-N, Raoult D. Description of *Tropheryma whipplei* gen. nov., sp. nov., the Whipple's disease bacillus. *Int J Syst Evol Microbiol.* 2001;51:1471–1479.

Martinetti M, Biagi F, Badulli C, et al. The HLA Alleles DRB1*13 and DQB1*06 are associated to Whipple's disease. *Gastroenterology.* 2009;136:2289–2294.

Acute Rheumatic Fever and Poststreptococcal Arthritis

Katherine D. Nowicki, MD and Jennifer B. Soep, MD

> **KEY POINTS**
>
> 1. Acute rheumatic fever (ARF) causes migratory polyarthritis, typically in children, and is the most common cause of acquired valvular heart disease worldwide.
> 2. The diagnosis of ARF is made with the Jones criteria, which were updated in 2015 to account for population risk and the echocardiographic diagnosis of rheumatic heart disease.
> 3. Salicylates and antibiotics (ideally with beta-lactams and penicillin in particular) are the mainstays of acute treatment of ARF, with long-term antibiotic prophylaxis regimens of varying lengths indicated thereafter.
> 4. ARF is described as the prototypical disease of molecular mimicry, although a complex range of host factors and characteristics of group A streptococcus (GAS) may contribute to pathogenesis.
> 5. Poststreptococcal reactive arthritis is characterized by nonmigratory, additive polyarthritis; when compared to the arthritis of ARF, it is less responsive to salicylates and occurs after a shorter latent period.

1. What is acute rheumatic fever (ARF)?

ARF is a **systemic inflammatory syndrome** occurring in a subset of patients (1–6%) infected with Group A *Streptococcus* (GAS), most commonly in the setting of pharyngitis. ARF typically presents **2 to 4 weeks following a GAS infection**. The most common manifestations are migratory arthritis and carditis. Other manifestations include Sydenham's chorea, subcutaneous nodules, and erythema marginatum (EM). **Rheumatic heart disease (RHD)** represents the most devastating manifestation of the illness and is the most common cause of acquired valvular disease worldwide.

2. What is the impact of ARF on public health?

In developed nations, ARF has dramatically declined in incidence over recent decades, although it is unclear to what degree this is due to changes in socioeconomic conditions and antibiotic availability versus shifts in bacterial serotypes. Unfortunately, **ARF remains a considerable public health burden worldwide,** particularly in India, south and east Africa, Aboriginal Australia, and Oceania. Recent estimates suggest a prevalence of 33.4 million RHD cases worldwide, with an annual incidence of over 200,000. RHD represents 25–40% of all cardiovascular diseases in many developing countries.

3. Why does GAS cause ARF?

ARF is thought to result (at least in part) from damaging immune responses to cross-reactive self-antigens following GAS infection (**molecular mimicry**) in **genetically predisposed individuals**. Specifically, the structural and immunologic similarities between streptococcal antigens, including M protein and surface carbohydrates, and host antigens, including cardiac myosin and laminin, may be what trigger the cellular and antibody-mediated autoimmune responses that cause ARF.

4. Does GAS cause ARF through any other mechanisms?

Yes, a direct pathogenic binding effect of GAS M-proteins to collagens may initiate a local immune reaction. Anti-Group A carbohydrates can also cross-react with the glycosides of heart valves. So-called heart-reactive antibodies are found in higher titers in 33–85% of patients with RHD than in patients without RHD. These antibodies may also target the basal ganglia and play a role in the pathogenesis of chorea.

5. Do host factors contribute to the pathogenesis of ARF?

Yes. For example, ARF is **most frequent in children (5–15 years)**. Incidence also varies according to geography and is partially explainable by socioeconomic disparities, healthcare factors (e.g., distance to healthcare access), and other environmental factors, but bacterial serotype variation and host genetic factors also contribute. Twin concordance studies suggest an overall heritability of 60%. HLA Class II association studies have resulted in conflicting data, although many were performed in relatively low-incidence (European) populations. **HLA-DR7 and HLA-D8/17** have been most frequently associated with RHD. Expression of a B lymphocyte alloantigen (recognized by the antibody D8/17) has been found in 66–100% of ethnically diverse ARF patients and 10% of controls.

6. What is the major GAS serotype classification system?

Regardless of mechanism, M protein appears to be the key virulence factor of GAS and is commonly used to classify GAS into serotypes. Associations between M-serotype and pathogenicity are described (i.e., rheumatogenic strains versus those associated with pyoderma/impetigo or other GAS manifestations), although these associations are not uniform across host population groups or geography. This fact, along with the vast diversity in M serotypes, has been a major impediment to GAS vaccine development despite extensive efforts.

7. How is the diagnosis of ARF established and how have the criteria changed?

The **Jones criteria** for guidance in the diagnosis of ARF were first published by T. Duckett Jones, MD, in 1944. The American Heart Association (AHA) modified the criteria in 1992 and again in 2015 to account for baseline population-specific risk and subclinical valvulitis (i.e. no auscultatory findings, but evidence on echocardiography). Low-risk populations (low incidence/prevalence of ARF) include patients in the United States and Europe. Moderate to high-risk populations include those from African, Asia-Pacific, indigenous Australian, and other populations in which the incidence of ARF exceeds 2 cases per 100,000 school-aged children. A summary of current criteria is listed in Table 43.1. It is important to note that evidence of a preceding GAS infection is required for the diagnosis of ARF, since other conditions such as systemic juvenile idiopathic arthritis (sJIA) may closely resemble it.

8. Is there an easy way to remember the major manifestations of the Jones criteria for ARF?

Yes. **Remember the word "Jones", with "O" as a "heart":**

J—joints
♥—carditis
N—nodules
E—erythema marginatum
S—Sydenham's chorea

9. Describe scenarios where a diagnosis of ARF might be made without strict adherence to the Jones criteria.

1. **Isolated chorea** many months after the initial streptococcal infection when serologic evidence of an antecedent infection is lacking.
2. **Indolent carditis and/or typical chronic valve lesions** (mitral, aortic) may also present as the only manifestation of ARF. The latent period between clinical infection and discovery makes proof of antecedent streptococcal infection difficult.
3. In **patients with a history of RHD**, recurrent ARF may be difficult to diagnose without development of a different heart lesion; therefore, a presumptive diagnosis based on only one major or one minor criterion may be reasonable.

10. When should a diagnosis of ARF be on the differential?

ARF should be on the differential in the setting **of persistent fever, systemic inflammation, carditis, polyarthritis, and/or chorea**. One in three patients does not recall an illness prior to developing symptoms of ARF, so it should remain on the differential even in the absence of preceding illness. Only 5% of ARF cases occur in children under age 5. Most initial episodes of ARF occur in school-aged children, and the incidence wanes during the second decade of life.

11. What specific laboratory tests are used to confirm a recent GAS infection?

Evidence for an infection may be shown through one of three ways: **(1) a positive throat culture for GAS**, **(2) a positive rapid streptococcal antigen test** in an individual whose clinical

TABLE 43.1 2015 Revised Jones Criteria

Evidence of antecedent GAS infection by at least 1 of the following:
- + throat culture
- + rapid streptococcal antigen test in a child whose clinical presentation suggests a high pretest probability of streptococcal pharyngitis
- increased or rising streptococcal antibody titer

Diagnosis of initial ARF	**Diagnosis of recurrent ARF:**
• 2 major manifestations OR • 1 major + 2 minor manifestations	• 2 major OR • 1 major + 2 minor manifestations OR • 3 minor manifestations*

Major Criteria	
Low-risk populations+	*Moderate to high-risk populations*+
Carditis (clinical or subclinical)	Carditis (clinical or subclinical)
Polyarthritis	Polyarthritis OR monoarthritis OR polyarthralgia
Chorea	Chorea
Subcutaneous nodules	Subcutaneous nodules
Erythema marginatum	Erythema marginatum
Minor Criteria	
Low-risk populations	*Moderate to high-risk populations*
Polyarthralgia	Monoarthralgia
Fever ≥38.5C	Fever ≥38C
ESR ≥60 mm/hr and/or CRP ≥3 mg/dL	ESR ≥30 mm/hr and/or CRP ≥3 mg/dL
Prolonged PR interval (in absence of carditis)	Prolonged PR interval (in absence of carditis)

ARF, acute rheumatic fever; *CRP,* C-reactive protein; *ESR,* erythrocyte sedimentation rate; *GAS,* group A streptococcus.
*When minor manifestations alone are used to make a diagnosis of recurrent ARF, it is critical to exclude other more likely causes of the clinical presentation.
+Population risk based on the incidence/prevalence of ARF in that community. For example, an incidence of ARF > 2 cases per 100,000 school-aged children is considered a moderate- to high-risk population for ARF (see Question 7).

presentation suggests a high pretest probability of streptococcal pharyngitis, or **(3) an increased or rising streptococcal antibody titer**. Antibody-based testing may be particularly useful since only 25% of ARF patients will have a positive throat culture or rapid antigen test due to the latent period (mean 18 days; range 1–4 weeks) between infection and development of ARF symptoms. Neither culture nor antigen-based testing distinguishes between a carrier state and active infection. Consequently, a rise in streptococcal antibodies may provide the best evidence for recent infection. While antistreptolysin-O (ASO) and antideoxyribonuclease-B (antiDNase-B or ADB) are the most common streptococcal antibodies used, others include antistreptokinase, anti-hyaluronidase, and anti-NADase. Using ASO antibody testing in conjunction with an additional serologic test can generate a sensitivity >90% for the diagnosis.

12. How are antistreptococcal antibodies interpreted?

"Normal" ranges for these antibody titers depend on the patient's age (higher titers are expected in school-aged children), geographical location, epidemiologic circumstances, and the time of the year. In the United States, an **ASO titer is considered elevated at 240 Todd units in adults and 320 Todd units in children. ADB titers above 85 Todd units in adults and 170 Todd units in children are typically considered elevated**. Trending serologic levels of anti-ASO and/or anti-DNAse B antibodies at 2- to 4-week intervals may be more helpful than obtaining one-time levels when suspicion is high for ARF, since rising titers are expected in ARF. Antibody levels begin to rise starting about a week after a GAS infection and then peak at 4 to 8 weeks after the pharyngeal infection (with ADB peaking latest).

13. How specific are antistreptococcal antibodies?

ASO is relatively nonspecific, whereas ADB is somewhat more specific. High ASO titers or other antistreptococcal antibodies can also be found in patients (particularly children) with other rheumatic diseases and no associated ARF. This is usually a result of past streptococcal exposure and nonspecific immune stimulation resulting in a polyclonal gammopathy. Furthermore, **in more than 50% of school-aged children, anti-GAS antibodies remain elevated for over a year** following infection, which makes estimation of the timing of a GAS infection challenging.

14. How does the arthritis of ARF typically present?

The arthritis of ARF usually involves **larger joints**, particularly the knees (75%) and ankles (50%), and less commonly elbows/wrists/hips (15%). The shoulder, spine, and smaller joints of the hands and feet are not commonly involved. Most often, several joints are involved at a time in a **migratory polyarthritis pattern**, along with an acute febrile illness. Arthritis in ARF is self-limited and even in the absence of therapy resolves by 4 weeks. ARF does not cause erosions or permanent joint damage, with the rare exception of Jaccoud deformity, which can occur following multiple recurrences of ARF. Synovial fluid is sterile and inflammatory. Since the arthritis of ARF is typically **highly responsive to salicylates** and nonsteroidal anti-inflammatory drugs (NSAIDs), use of such medications before diagnosis can complicate determination of whether a patient has polyarthralgias (a minor criteria in low-risk populations) or polyarthritis (a major criterion).

15. What is Sydenham chorea?

Sydenham's chorea (or "St Vitus" dance) is characterized by uncoordinated, involuntary, and often rapid asymmetric movements of the trunk and/or extremities. It can be associated with muscle weakness and emotional lability. Sensation is not affected. The choreiform movements disappear during sleep. The latent interval between streptococcal pharyngitis and chorea onset may be prolonged, frequently >6 to 8 weeks. Consequently, anti-streptococcal antibody titers may be normal (especially ASO titers which decrease sooner than ADB). Brain magnetic resonance imaging shows inflammation in the basal ganglia. Symptoms can last 2 to 4 months. Treatment is supportive care. Chorea may be the only manifestation of ARF, but it occurs with RHD in up to 33% of patients. Patients may also be at increased risk for developing future neuropsychiatric disorders such as obsessive-compulsive disorder (OCD).

16. What are the other major manifestations of ARF and their prevalence?

- **Carditis** (50–80% of ARF cases): Pericardium, myocardium, and valves may be involved. The mitral valve is most often affected resulting in mitral regurgitation much more often than mitral stenosis. The aortic valve is the next most affected valve. Echocardiography often shows involvement not appreciated clinically. *Echocardiographic criteria for diagnosing RHD have been defined in the 2023 World Heart Federation guidelines.* Congestive heart failure from myocarditis occurs in 5% to 10% of patients, never occurs without valve involvement, and is more likely to occur in cases of recurrent ARF as opposed to initial cases. All degrees of heart block can occur.
- **Subcutaneous nodules** (<10% of ARF cases): They are firm, painless, a few millimeters to 2 cm in size, and often resolve within days. These nodules have been reported on the occiput, spinous processes of the thoracic and lumbar vertebrae, and the extensor surfaces of the knees, elbows, and wrists.
- **Erythema marginatum** (<6% of ARF cases): EM is an irregular, serpiginous, nonpruritic pink rash that is present on the trunk and proximal extremities, but never the face.

17. What are the minor manifestations of ARF?

Fever (≥38.5C or higher in low-risk populations), **prolonged PR interval** on ECG, elevated erythrocyte sedimentation rate (**ESR**), elevated C-reactive protein (**CRP**), and **history of rheumatic fever or rheumatic heart disease** are the minor manifestations. Fever can be high, especially in the first week. However, in up to 30% of patients, the body temperature does not exceed 38°C. Fever does not last longer than 4 weeks. Normal ESR and CRP levels are not consistent with ARF except in cases of isolated chorea. The CRP should be ≥3 mg/dL (typically greater than 7.0 mg/dL) and the ESR should be ≥60 mm/hr in low-risk populations (≥30 mm/hr in high-risk populations).

18. How is ARF managed?

1. **Treatment of acute manifestations:**

    Hospitalization may be warranted to facilitate prompt access to echocardiograms, consultant providers, and treatment.

    All patients: Treatment with **antibiotics** to eradicate the pharyngeal carriage of GAS is indicated, even if the throat culture is negative. *Specific guidance on antibiotic treatment of ARF has been published by the American Heart Association (AHA), the World Health Organization, and in the Red Book published by the American Academy of Pediatrics (AAP).*

    Carditis: Aspirin is first-line therapy for carditis, frequently at doses of 80 to 100 mg/kg per day (divided into doses every 4–6 hours) and tapered down after 4 to 8 weeks of treatment. Lower doses of 50 mg/kg per day should be tried initially in children (to reduce the risk of salicylate toxicity). Severe carditis and congestive heart failure may require treatment with oral prednisone, which has been found to be more effective than IV steroids in one study. Some patients require medical management of heart failure, and some with severe valvular disease require surgical repair or replacement.

    Arthritis: Arthritis in ARF is typically responsive to salicylates. While aspirin has historically been used, NSAIDs such as naproxen and ibuprofen are also effective and have fewer side effects. Consistent NSAID use for 1–2 weeks followed by gradual tapering is often sufficient. Steroids are generally not required.

    Chorea: Supportive care including reassurance and creating a calm environment for the patient are generally sufficient. In more severe cases, carbamazepine or valproic acid may be used as some small studies have shown efficacy.

2. **Education for patients and their families.**
3. **Testing of and treatment for GAS carriage in household contacts.**
4. **Secondary prophylaxis** (see Questions 19 and 20).

19. How is ARF prevented?

Prevention of ARF in patients without a prior history of ARF (primary prevention) centers around **antimicrobial therapy for acute GAS infections.** Antibiotic treatment of pharyngitis caused by group A streptococcus started within 9 days of sore throat onset decreases the risk of subsequent ARF by 80%. However, prevention is limited by many factors, including the fact that up to two-thirds of patients do not experience sore throat before developing ARF.

Those with a prior history of ARF are at progressively increasing risk for developing recurrent ARF with each streptococcal infection, with recurrence rates as high as 50% in the first year. **Prophylaxis to prevent intercurrent streptococcal infections** (secondary prevention) is indicated to reduce this risk. In most circumstances, the preferred regimen for secondary prevention is intramuscular benzathine penicillin G every 4 weeks. Additional pharmacologic options can be found in the AAP's Red Book.

20. For how long does a patient with ARF need antibiotic prophylaxis?

According to the AHA, the **duration of prophylaxis varies depending on multiple factors** including "number of previous attacks, the time elapsed since the last attack, the risk of exposure to GAS infections, the age of the patient, and the presence or absence of cardiac involvement" (Gerber, 2009). Patients with a history of ARF without cardiac involvement should receive antibiotic prophylaxis for 5 years after the last episode or to age 21 (whichever is longer). Patients with a history of cardiac involvement and no residual damage/valvular disease should be on prophylaxis for 10 years or until age 21 (whichever is longer). Patients with a history of carditis and residual heart disease (including persistent valvular damage) should receive antibiotics for 10 years or to age 40, with consideration for lifelong prophylaxis. Even without cardiac involvement, ARF patients who have frequent exposure to children (parent of school-aged children, teacher, day-care worker, healthcare professional, etc.) or who live in crowded situations (e.g., college dormitories) should receive prophylaxis for as long as the exposure continues.

21. Can infection with GAS result in arthritis distinct from ARF?

Yes, post-streptococcal reactive arthritis (PSRA) is a distinct phenotype of arthritis following GAS infection that is not associated with carditis or other ARF manifestations. PSRA occurs after a **shorter latent period** (~10 days) than ARF, but **symptoms often last longer** than that of ARF (often months). Whereas arthritis in ARF is typically migratory, transient, and involves the large joints, **PSRA involves large joints, small joints, and the axial skeleton in a cumulative and persistent manner**. PSRA does not respond as readily to anti-inflammatory therapy compared to patients with ARF. Epidemiologically, PRSA most commonly affects young adults rather than children. PSRA in adults is more likely to be missed since symptomatic pharyngitis is less common and GAS testing may not be performed.

22. Should PRSA be treated like a "reactive" arthritis or on the continuum of ARF?

While some literature suggests PSRA is an entirely distinct clinical entity, with diagnostic criteria based on arthritis after GAS infection without other Jones criteria, others have argued that PSRA is simply an incomplete phenotype of ARF. The AHA and AAP Red Book recommend **1 to 2 years of clinical monitoring for carditis as well as consideration of secondary prophylaxis during this timeframe**, since a very small proportion of patients with PSRA have been reported to later develop valvular heart disease. If carditis develops, the patients should be diagnosed with ARF and started on secondary prophylaxis.

23. What is PANDAS?

PANDAS stands for **pediatric autoimmune neuropsychiatric disorder associated with group A streptococci** and is a subtype of Pediatric Acute-Onset Neuropsychiatric Syndrome (PANS). A diagnosis of PANDAS is established based on five clinical criteria which were proposed by Swedo et al. in 1998: (1) OCD and/or tic disorder, (2) pediatric onset between age 3 and the onset of puberty, (3) abrupt onset and episodic course of symptoms, (4) temporal relation between GAS infection and onset and/or exacerbation(s), and (5) neurologic abnormalities such as motor hyperactivity, severe separation anxiety, mood swings, and hallucinations. PANDAS is a diagnosis of exclusion and a thorough evaluation is warranted for alternative diagnoses including autoimmune encephalitis, psychiatric disorders, and Sydenham's chorea as part of ARF. The pathogenesis of this disorder and the role of GAS are not well characterized and somewhat controversial. Some hypothesize that PANDAS is an autoimmune condition wherein anti-GAS antibodies target proteins in the basal ganglia or other components of the central nervous system. Questions about whether PANDAS is sufficiently different from OCD and tic disorder to be considered a distinct entity also persist.

24. How is PANDAS treated?

Controversy also exists surrounding management, particularly the role of long-term prophylactic antibiotics and immune-modulating therapy, although intravenous immunoglobulin has been suggested as an effective treatment in some literature. Acute treatment with GAS-directed antibiotics may be reasonable in confirmed cases, although no randomized trials exist. Otherwise, **symptomatic treatment of neuropsychiatric symptoms including behavioral interventions and potentially psychiatric medications** is indicated.

ACKNOWLEDGMENT

The authors wish to thank Drs. Carolyn Coyle and Patrick R. Wood for their contributions to this chapter in the prior editions.

BIBLIOGRAPHY

Auala T, Zavale BG, Mbakwen AC, et al. Acute rheumatic fever and rheumatic heart disease: highlighting the role of group A *Streptococcus* in the global burden of cardiovascular. *Dis Pathogens*. 2022;11(5):496.

Barash J, Mashihach E, Navon-Elkan P, et al. Differentiation of post-streptococcal reactive arthritis from acute rheumatic fever. *J Pediatr*. 2008;153(5):696–699.

Câmara EJ, Braga JC, Alves-Silva LS, et al. Comparison of an intravenous pulse of methylprednisolone versus oral corticosteroid in severe acute rheumatic carditis: a randomized clinical trial. *Cardiol Young*. 2002;12(2):119–124.

Carapetis JR, McDonald M, Wilson NJ. Acute rheumatic fever. *Lancet*. 2005;366:155–168.

Gerber MA, Baltimore RS, Eaton CB, et al. Prevention of rheumatic fever and diagnosis and treatment of acute *Streptococcal pharyngitis*: a scientific statement from the American Heart Association Rheumatic Fever, Endocarditis, and Kawasaki Disease Committee of the Council on Cardiovascular Disease in the Young, the Interdisciplinary Council on Functional Genomics and Translational Biology, and the Interdisciplinary Council on Quality of Care and Outcomes Research: endorsed by the American Academy of Pediatrics. *Circulation*. 2009;119(11):1541–1551.

Gewitz MH, Baltimore RS, Tani LY, et al. Revision of the Jones Criteria for the diagnosis of acute rheumatic fever in the era of Doppler echocardiography: a scientific statement from the. *Circulation*. 2015;131:1806–1818.

Hatanu A, Reddy LN, Matthew J, et al. Pediatric autoimmune neuropsychiatric disorders associated with group A *Streptococci*: etiopathology and diagnostic challenges. *Cureus*. 2022;14(8):e27729.

Pathak H, Marshall T. Post-streptococcal reactive arthritis: where are we now. *BMJ Case Rep*. 2016 bcr2016215552.

Red Book. Report of the Committee on Infectious Diseases (32nd Edition). In: Kimberlin, D.W., Barnett, E.D., Lynfield, R., Sawyer, M.H. *American Academy of Pediatrics*. Itasca, IL, 2021. 60143.

Rwebembera J, Marangou J, Mwita JC, et al. 2023 World Heart Federation guidelines for the echocardiographic diagnosis of rheumatic heart disease. *Nat Rev Cardiol*. 2024;21:250–263.

Seckeler MD, Hoke TR. The worldwide epidemiology of acute rheumatic fever and rheumatic heart disease. *Clin Epidemiol*. 2011;3:67–84.

World Health Organization. *Antibiotic Use for the Prevention and Treatment of Rheumatic Fever and Rheumatic Heart Disease in Children: Report of the 2nd Meeting of WHO's Subcommittee of the Expert Committee of the Selection and Use of Essential Medicines*. Geneva: WHO; 2008. Accessed November 1, 2024. https://www.researchgate.net/publication/242186730_Antibiotic_use_for_the_Prevention_and_Treatment_of_Rheumatic_Fever_and_Rheumatic_Heart_Disease_in_Children.

FURTHER READING

https://www.cdc.gov/groupastrep/diseases-hcp/acute-rheumatic-fever.html.
https://www.ncbi.nlm.nih.gov/books/NBK594238/.

Gout

CHAPTER 44

Lindsay N. Helget, MD and Ted R. Mikuls, MD, MSPH

I've been shot, beaten up, stabbed, and thrown out of a helicopter, but none of that compared to gout.

–U.S. Veteran with gout, c. 2001

KEY POINTS

1. Gout is the most common cause of inflammatory arthritis.
2. Gout is rare in a premenopausal woman and in men under the age of 25 years.
3. Hyperuricemia is a necessary but insufficient risk factor in gout development.
4. Hyperuricemia and gout are strongly associated with obesity and the metabolic syndrome.
5. Dietary and lifestyle modifications are recommended as adjuvant therapies in the management of gout, although in isolation are not often sufficiently effective in lowering serum urate.
6. Always look for gout in all undiagnosed joint conditions even if the serum urate level is normal, the involved joint is atypical, and the flare is chronic and polyarticular.
7. Assess the patient's comorbid medical conditions including renal and hepatic function to guide the safest treatment options for flares and chronic symptomatic hyperuricemia with a goal serum urate <6.0 mg/Dl.

1. What is gout? How was the term derived?

Gout is a disease in which tissue deposition of monosodium urate (MSU) crystals occurs as a result of hyperuricemia, resulting in one or more of the following manifestations:

- Gouty arthritis
- Tophi (aggregated deposits of MSU occurring in articular, osseous, cartilaginous, or soft tissue areas)
- Gouty nephropathy
- Uric acid nephrolithiasis

The term *gout* is derived from the Latin word *gutta*, which translates as "a drop." In the 13th century, it was thought that gout resulted from a drop of evil humor affecting a vulnerable joint. This explains why a majority of early gout therapies were aimed at removing excess humor (e.g. the use of bloodletting and cupping).

2. How is hyperuricemia defined? What are the most common factors associated with hyperuricemia and gout?

Hyperuricemia is defined by a serum urate concentration exceeding its solubility threshold, promoting the formation and deposition of MSU. At a physiologic pH, hyperuricemia is defined as a serum concentration >6.8 mg/dl (>360 μmol/L). Serum urate concentrations increase with age and are higher in men than in women, increasing in association with the onset of puberty in young men and menopause in women (the latter owing to uricosuric properties of estrogen). Gout is rare in men under the age of 25 and in premenopausal women; when it occurs in these populations, it is often attributed to an inherited defect in purine metabolism, alcohol use, and/or renal insufficiency including familial juvenile hyperuricemic nephropathy or medullary cystic kidney disease. In addition to older age and male sex, other factors commonly associated with hyperuricemia and gout include obesity, hypertension and other elements of metabolic syndrome, high purine intake, a family history of gout, alcohol use disorder, renal insufficiency, the use of select medications such as low-dose aspirin, diuretics, and cyclosporine among others.

3. How prevalent is gout? Discuss the epidemiology of gout.

The overall prevalence of gout in the U.S. is estimated to be 3.9% (affecting 5.2% of men and 2.7% of women, for a total of 9.2 million individuals), representing by far the most common form of inflammatory arthritis. Hyperuricemia is a necessary, but insufficient, risk factor in gout onset and is seen in approximately 1 of every 5 adults in the U.S. Although only a small proportion of individuals with hyperuricemia eventually develop gout (~15%), the risk increases to 30–50% in the context of marked hyperuricemia (e.g. >9–10 mg/dl). The risk of gout increases with advancing age and parallels age-related increases in serum urate. The frequency of gout in those over the age of 80 is >30-fold higher than in individuals between the ages of 20 and 29. It has been estimated that the prevalence of gout has increased by almost 50% in recent decades, an increase that appears to be in part related to rising rates of obesity and metabolic syndrome.

4. Uric acid is a product of the metabolism of which group of nucleotides?

Uric acid is the end-product of purine degradation. Humans lack the enzyme *uricase*, which in other mammalian species converts uric acid (sparingly soluble) into highly soluble allantoin. The lack of this enzyme subjects humans to the potential risk of tissue deposition of MSU crystals. Although humans possess the uricase gene, it is inactive. It is postulated that humans have acquired the propensity to become hyperuricemic because uric acid may exert potent antioxidant properties.

5. What pathogenic processes are responsible for the development of hyperuricemia?

- Overproduction of urate (endogenous production or exogenous dietary purine precursors)
- Underexcretion of urate (abnormal renal handling of urate)
- A combination of both processes.
  Most patients with hyperuricemia and gout are underexcreters of uric acid (80–90%).

6. How do you determine if a patient with gout is an overproducer or underexcreter of uric acid?

Although not routinely required in clinical management, a 24-hour urine collection can be obtained to determine uric acid and creatinine excretion (the latter to ensure an adequate 24-hour collection). On a regular purine diet, a urate value >800 mg/24 hr suggests overproduction while a value <800 mg suggests underexcretion. Historically this distinction had clinical implications, as the use of uricosurics was recommended only for patients with documented underexcretion of uric acid. In clinical practice, however, the use of xanthine oxidase inhibitors (XOIs) has largely supplanted uricosurics, with the latter commonly prescribed in conjunction with a XOI rather than as monotherapy. In fact, the 2020 American College of Rheumatology (ACR) Guideline for the Management of Gout strongly recommends allopurinol as the preferred first-line agent for urate-lowering therapy (ULT), and conditionally recommends against routine measurement of urinary uric acid in patients in whom uricosuric therapy is considered. *Although controversial*, the rare gout patient with contraindications to XOIs (and no contraindication to uricosurics) might benefit from 24-hour urine uric acid testing to confirm they are not a hyperexcreter of uric acid (in which case pegloticase may be considered).

7. Name the two inherited enzyme abnormalities in the urate biosynthesis pathway that can cause urate overproduction.

- Overactivity of phosphoribosylpyrophosphate (PRPP) synthetase
- Partial deficiency of hypoxanthine-guanine phosphoribosyltransferase (HGPRT) (Kelley-Seegmiller syndrome)
  These enzyme abnormalities, which cause urate overproduction, are inherited as X-linked traits. Men with these abnormalities often present with early-onset gout (<25 years of age) and a high incidence of uric acid nephrolithiasis. Complete HGPRT deficiency results in **Lesch-Nyhan syndrome** (intellectual disability, spasticity, choreoathetosis, and self-mutilation). In addition, patients with **glucose-6-phosphatase deficiency** (von Gierke's disease) also exhibit urate overproduction due to an accelerated ATP breakdown during hypoglycemia-induced glycogen degradation. Inhibition of renal tubular urate secretion can also occur in this disease as a result of competitive anions from lactic acidosis. Finally, patients with hereditary fructose intolerance caused by **fructose-1-phosphate aldolase deficiency** can develop hyperuricemia in part because of accelerated ATP catabolism.

8. **What are the acquired causes of hyperuricemia?**

Urate overproduction: excess dietary purine consumption, accelerated hepatic ATP degradation in alcohol abuse or fructose ingestion, and increased nucleotide turnover in myeloproliferative and lymphoproliferative disorders.

Urate underexcretion: renal disease, lead nephropathy (saturnine gout), inhibition of tubular urate secretion (keto- and lactic acidosis), select drugs (see question #9), and miscellaneous causes such as hyperparathyroidism, hypothyroidism, and respiratory acidosis.

9. **Name the drugs that cause hyperuricemia due to decreased renal excretion of urate.**

The mnemonic **CAN'T LEAP** can be used to remember these drugs:

Cyclosporine	Lasix (furosemide) (and other loop diuretics)
Alcohol	Ethambutol
Nicotinic acid	Aspirin (low dose)
Thiazides/Tacrolimus	Pyrazinamide

Other drugs that can cause hyperuricemia include levodopa, theophylline, and didanosine (ddI). In contrast, the following commonly used drugs exert mild uricosuric effects and produce modest urate lowering: amlodipine, atorvastatin, fenofibrate, leflunomide, losartan, rosuvastatin, SGLT2 inhibitors, and high-dose salicylates.

10. **Why does excessive alcohol consumption often lead to hyperuricemia and gout?**

The quantity of alcohol consumption strongly correlates with the risk of developing gout. Consuming over 30–50 grams of alcohol a day (3–4 beers, glasses of wine, or liquor shots) increases gout risk by 2–2.5-fold compared to someone who does not drink alcohol. Alcohol consumption increases urate synthesis by accelerating the hepatic degradation of ATP. Alcohol consumption is also associated with lactate production, which further reduces renal urate excretion. In addition to alcohol content, beer contains a substantial amount of the purine guanosine and confers a more than twofold risk of gout over liquor. Moderate wine consumption does not appear to increase serum urate or gout risk. Additional data suggest that among those with established gout, episodic consumption of all alcohol types (wine, beer, and liquor) may act as a trigger for recurrent flare in a dose-dependent fashion.

11. **What is the typical natural history of hyperuricemia leading to gout?**

Among those developing gout, most will have an extended period (often 20 years or more) of asymptomatic hyperuricemia preceding symptom onset. Gout flares are typically the initial symptomatic manifestation and involve a single joint in the vast majority (85–90%) of patients experiencing their first episode. Subsequent gout flares are typically separated in time by asymptomatic intervals, periods that are termed "intercritical gout". It has been estimated that approximately half of individuals experiencing an initial flare will experience a second episode within 1–2 years. If left untreated, these intercritical periods often become progressively shorter in duration with a corresponding increase in gout flare frequency. A minority of these individuals may progress to develop chronic tophaceous (advanced) gout, characterized by the progressive development of subcutaneous, synovial, or subchondral MSU deposits. Subcutaneous tophi typically develop after 10 years or more of symptomatic gout that has been inadequately treated.

12. **Describe the characteristics of a gout flare.**

Early gout flares are typically **monoarticular** (85–90%), begin abruptly, and reach maximal intensity within hours. Flare onset often occurs during the **night** or **early morning** when the joint is most cool. The affected joint becomes exquisitely painful, warm, red, and swollen. A low-grade fever may be present. **Periarticular erythema and swelling** may progress to resemble an aseptic cellulitis that can be confused with an infectious process. Acute flares also occur in periarticular sites, such as the Achilles tendon or olecranon or prepatellar bursa. Early in the course of gout, flares are self-limited and typically resolve over 3–10 days with a return to "baseline". **Desquamation of the skin** overlying the affected joint can occur with resolution of the inflammation. Subsequent attacks of gout can occur more frequently, become polyarticular, and persist longer.

13. Which joints are most commonly involved in gout?

The joints of the lower limbs are typically involved most often, although gout has been reported to involve almost any joint. Termed **podagra**, the **first metatarsophalangeal** (MTP) is involved in >50% of initial flares and over time is affected in the vast majority of patients (*in mythology, the goddess Podagra was a 'foot-torturess' associated with gout, born of the seduction of Venus by Bacchus*). Other commonly involved sites include joints of the mid- and hind-foot, ankles, knees, wrists, fingers, and elbows. Flares involving axial sites (spine or sacroiliac joint) are rare. Gout and tophi have a predilection for cooler, acral sites, where the solubility of monosodium urate crystals (as well as circulation) may be diminished as a result of the cooler temperatures. In addition, joints that have undergone degenerative changes appear to provide a nidus that facilitates crystal formation.

14. What events may trigger an acute attack of gout?

Alcohol ingestion	Initiation of urate lowering therapy (ULT)
Dietary excess of purines	Acute medical illness including infections
Exercise	Drugs
Trauma	Radiation or chemotherapy
Fructose ingestion	Surgery (postoperative days 3–5)
Dehydration	Other physiologic stressors
Extreme temperature variations	Air pollution

15. Can symptomatic hyperuricemia (gout) be managed by diet alone?

Unfortunately, gout is difficult to manage by diet alone because the purine content of the diet typically contributes only modestly to the total serum urate concentration. Patients should limit/moderate their consumption of purine-rich foods such as red meats (particularly organ meats) and seafood (particularly shellfish, sardines, and anchovies). Excessive fructose consumption (sodas, fruit juices, energy drinks) is also associated with an increased gout risk. Fructose is metabolized in the liver to ATP that contributes to the urate production. In contrast, moderate intake of purine-rich vegetables (asparagus, cauliflower, spinach, and mushrooms), nuts, legumes (beans and peas), and vegetable protein is not associated with an increased risk of gout. Coffee intake through a non-caffeine mechanism, vitamin C (500 mg/day), reduced-fat dairy intake (low-fat milk, yogurt), and tart cherries can reduce serum urate levels and the risk of gout.

16. How is the diagnosis of gout established?

The demonstration of MSU crystals in aspirates of synovial fluid or tophi remains the gold standard for diagnosis. Intra- or extra-cellular MSU crystals are needle-shaped, approximately the size of a white blood cell, and are strongly negatively birefringent (yellow when parallel to the axis of a red compensator) on polarized microscopy (Figure 44.1; see Chapter 7: Arthrocentesis, Synovial Fluid Analysis and Biopsy). MSU crystals can be identified in joint aspirates during intercritical (asymptomatic) periods. Synovial fluids during a gout flare are inflammatory (typically 20,000–100,000 leukocytes/mm3) with a predominance of neutrophils. Septic synovial fluids may contain MSU crystals; as such, it is important to consider a Gram stain and culture to rule out concomitant septic arthritis in the appropriate setting. This is particularly important as gout flares may present with overlapping signs and/or symptoms of infection such as low-grade fever, elevated acute phase responses, and mild leukocytosis.

17. Can serum urate levels be used to diagnose gout?

Serum urate levels alone cannot be used to diagnose gout. Although serum urate levels are elevated (>6.8 mg/dl) at some time in almost all gout patients, serum concentrations are normal at the time of an acute flare in up to one-third (false-negative results). This appears to be due in part to the generation of pro-inflammatory cytokines such as IL-6, which exert a uricosuric effect. It is equally important to recognize that many individuals may have hyperuricemia in the absence of gout (false-positive results).

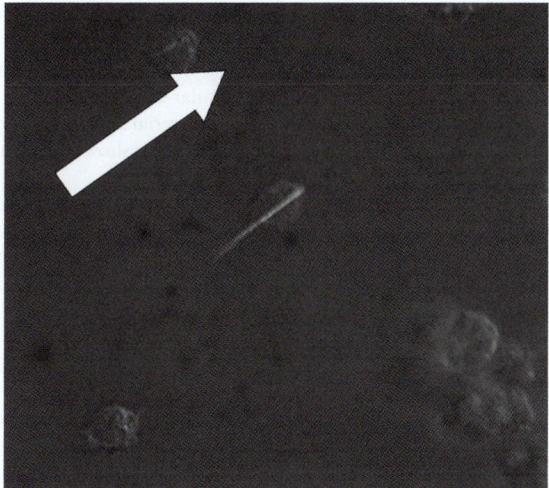

Fig. 44.1 Polarized microscopy showing needle-shaped MSU crystal within a neutrophil in synovial fluid. Arrow shows plane of red compensator. In color, the MSU crystal appears yellow when parallel to the red light, and blue when its orientation is perpendicular (negative birefringence).

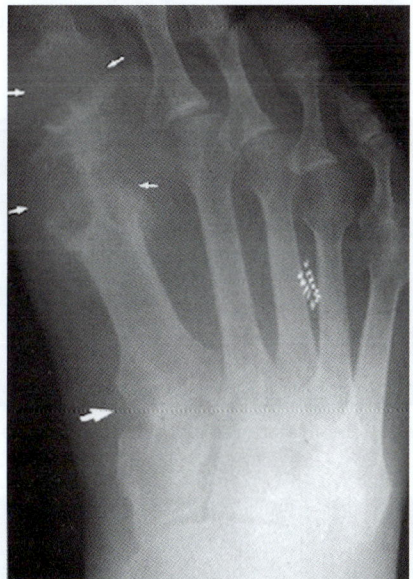

Fig. 44.2 Radiograph of the foot showing erosive changes (arrows) of chronic tophaceous gout.

18. What are the typical radiographic features of gout?

Soft tissue swelling around the affected joint can accompany gout flare. In chronic gout, **tophi** and **bony erosions** can be seen (Figure 44.2). Articular tophi produce irregular soft tissue densities that occasionally are calcified, although urate/MSU is radiolucent in isolation. Bony erosions in gout appear "punched-out" with sclerotic margins and **overhanging edges**, sometimes described as **rat bite erosions**. In stark contrast to rheumatoid arthritis, the joint space is typically preserved until late in the disease and juxta-articular osteopenia is absent.

19. **What are the roles of ultrasonography and dual energy CT (DECT) scan in gout diagnosis?**
    - **Ultrasonagraphy (US):** Musculoskeletal US can show a superficial, hyperechoic band (deposition of urate crystals) on the surface of articular cartilage ("double contour sign") in gout (Fig. 44.3). Tophi appear as nonhomogenous material surrounded by an anechoic rim. Although highly "operator" dependent, recent studies have shown the sensitivity of US for gout diagnosis to be 77% with a specificity of 84%.
    - **Dual energy CT (DECT) scan:** DECT allows identification of MSU deposits because the chemical composition of urate causes less attenuation of x-ray photons tracking through it compared to bone calcium. Thus, urate deposits can be distinguished from surrounding tissues with a high degree of sensitivity and specificity. However, false-negative findings have been reported early in the course of gout, while false positives most commonly accompany osteoarthritis of the knee.

20. **Where do subcutaneous tophi commonly occur?**
    In addition to involving the synovium and subchondral bone, tophi can develop at a multitude of subcutaneous sites including on digits of the hands and feet, olecranon bursa, extensor surface of the forearm, Achilles tendon, and, less commonly, the antihelix of the ear (Fig. 44.4). Tophi can ulcerate through the skin and extrude a white, chalky material consisting of a dense concentration of MSU crystals. Although rare, an ulcerated tophus can become infected.

21. **What medical conditions associated with hyperuricemia and gout should be assessed for as part of your evaluation of a gout patient?**
    Common medical conditions associated with hyperuricemia and gout:
    - Obesity: weight loss can improve hyperuricemia

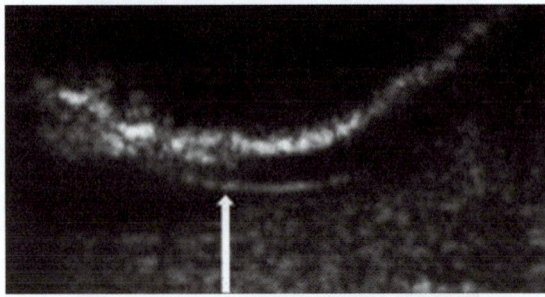

Fig. 44.3 Ultrasound of a metatarsaophalangeal joint showing the "double contour" sign.

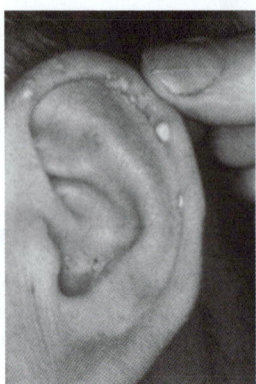 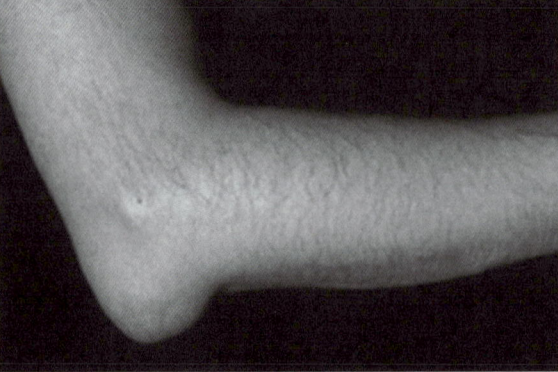

Fig. 44.4 (A) Tophi in the antihelix of the ear. (B) Tophi within the olecranon bursa. Images courtesy of ACR Image Library.

- Alcohol abuse
- Renal insufficiency
- Cardiovascular conditions
- Diabetes
  Other medical conditions associated with hyperuricemia and gout:
- Select drugs (See Question #9)
- Hypothyroidism
- Lead toxicity (look for other signs/symptoms such as renal failure, cognitive impairment, neuropathy, anemia, among others)
- Myeloproliferative disease, lymphoproliferative diseases, hemolytic anemias, polycythemia vera, sickle cell disease
- Hyperparathyroidism, diabetic ketoacidosis, diabetes insipidus, Bartter's syndrome
- Autosomal dominant medullary cystic kidney disease, lead nephropathy, familial **juvenile** hyperuricemic nephropathy
- Psoriasis

22. Does gout impact comorbidity or survival?

Patients with gout have reduced survival compared to individuals without gout, and this appears to be driven by a disproportionate burden of comorbidity. Gout patients suffer disproportionately from the effects of metabolic syndrome and more frequently have hypertension, dyslipidemia, coronary artery disease, chronic kidney disease, nephrolithiasis, and diabetes.

23. How do women with gout differ from men with regard to disease onset and clinical features?

Compared to men, women develop gout at an older age (typically after menopause) and more often suffer from polyarticular flares. Women with gout frequently have osteoarthritis, hypertension, and mild chronic renal insufficiency or are being treated with diuretics. Tophi developing in women are particularly common in previously damaged joints including Heberden's nodes, and in the finger pads (Fig. 44.5).

24. Discuss the pathophysiology of gout flares.

Gout flares are triggered by the precipitation of MSU crystals in the joint or surrounding tissues. The initial recognition of "naked" MSU crystals by toll-like receptors (TLR)-2 and -4 on chondrocytes and macrophage lineage cells appears to be critical to the expression of proinflammatory cytokines and initiation of the inflammatory response. MSU crystals stimulate the production of chemotactic factors, cytokines [IL-1β and IL-18 (through activation of the NLRP3

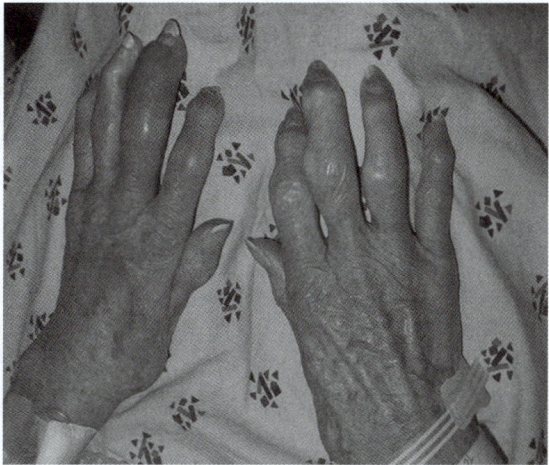

Fig. 44.5 Multiple tophi within Heberden's nodes of an elderly female patient.

inflammasome), IL-6, IL-8, and TNF], prostaglandins, leukotrienes, and oxygen radicals by neutrophils, monocytes, and synovial cells in addition to activating complement and inducing lysosomal enzyme release.

25. Why are gout flares typically self-limited?

The following mechanisms have been postulated:
- Inflammation allows for an influx of apolipoprotein-B into the joint, where it coats crystals and reduces their inflammatory potential.
- Phagocytosis and clearance by neutrophils decrease the crystal burden; neutrophil extracellular traps (NETs) are formed, and NET-related proteases digest inflammatory mediators, followed by apoptosis of inflammatory cells.
- Heat generated from inflammation enhances urate solubility.
- ACTH secretion in response to pain/stress suppresses inflammatory responses.
- Proinflammatory cytokines (IL-1 and TNF) are balanced by the production of **cytokine** inhibitors and regulatory cytokines such as transforming growth factor-β (TGF-β).

26. Name the types of renal diseases associated with hyperuricemia.

- **Urate nephropathy**. Deposition of MSU crystals in renal interstitial tissues with a surrounding giant cell reaction; may cause low-grade, intermittent proteinuria but only rarely causes significant renal dysfunction.
- **Uric acid nephropathy**. Precipitation of uric acid crystals in the collecting ducts and ureters results in acute renal failure, as occurs in acute tumor lysis syndrome; characteristically following chemotherapy for lymphoma or leukemia.
- **Uric acid nephrolithiasis**. Occurs in 10–25% of gout patients; risk parallels **increases** in serum and urinary urate concentrations as well as urine acidity. In contrast to calcium stones, uric acid stones are radiolucent; thus, DECT may be useful in detection of uric acid stones. The incidence of calcium stones is also increased in patients with gout, particularly those with hyperuricosuria as uric acid serves as a nidus for calcium stone formation.
- **Other**. Autosomal dominant medullary cystic kidney disease (one-third of patients **have** gout), lead intoxication (saturnine gout), and familial juvenile hyperuricemic nephropathy (an inherited uromodulin defect).

27. Discuss the renal transport of uric acid and how this can contribute to hyperuricemia and gout.

Renal urate transport consists of glomerular filtration followed by near-complete reabsorption, subsequent secretion back into the tubule, and reabsorption in the distal proximal tubule with a net renal excretion of ~10% of filtered urate. **URAT1** is an important renal urate-anion exchanger on the apical surface of the proximal tubular epithelial cell responsible for the reabsorption of filtered urate. Inhibition of URAT1 results in enhanced uricosuria and lower serum urate levels. Drugs that inhibit URAT1 include probenecid, sulfinpyrazone, benzbromarone, metabolites of losartan, high-dose salicylates, and lesinurad (the latter highly specific for URAT1 but no longer commercially available in the U.S.). Conversely, URAT1 is stimulated by other drugs/ compounds (lactate, nicotinate, pyrazinoate, low-dose aspirin, and possibly diuretics), resulting in decreased urate excretion and hyperuricemia. **GLUT9a** is the major transporter on the basolateral surface of the proximal tubular epithelial cell and facilitates the transport of urate from the tubular cell into the renal interstitium. Other transport proteins in the renal proximal tubular epithelial cell that regulate urate secretion include **OAT1** and **OAT3** on the basolateral surface while **ABCG2** and MRP4 are the two major proteins on the apical surface.

28. What is the role of genetics in hyperuricemia and gout?

ABCG2 gene: encodes for ATP-binding cassette G2 transporter, an important urate transporter in the kidney. Certain polymorphisms in this gene can lead to hyperuricemia, early onset gout, tophi formation, and poor response to allopurinol.

SLC2A9 gene: encodes for GLUT9a. Certain polymorphisms of the SLC2A9 gene can result in reduced urate reabsorption, lower serum urate concentrations, and lower risk of developing gout.

29. When should treatment of asymptomatic hyperuricemia be considered?

In the absence of symptomatic flares or tophi, there are currently no widely accepted indications for the treatment of asymptomatic hyperuricemia. An exception to this may be in those at high risk for the development of tumor lysis syndrome (e.g. patients with leukemia initiating chemotherapy).

30. Discuss treatment options for gout flares.

Medications most often used to treat acute flares include: **NSAIDs (full dose), oral colchicine, or glucocorticoids** (Table 44.1). Patients experiencing a severe flare (polyarticular or severe pain) may require combination therapy, understanding that the concomitant use of NSAIDs and oral glucocorticoids may be less desirable due to heightened potential for GI toxicity. Topical ice can also be used as an adjuvant. All NSAIDs demonstrate similar efficacy when given in anti-inflammatory doses. For acute flares, oral colchicine is dosed at 1.2 mg followed by 0.6 mg 1 hour later; this can be followed by prophylaxis dosing of 0.6 mg once or twice daily. Glucocorticoids can be administered by oral, intravenous, intramuscular, or intraarticular routes. Second-line options for the treatment of acute gout flare include IL-1 inhibition (anakinra or canakinumab) or ACTH. Urate-lowering therapy is typically deferred to intercritical periods once the acute flare has resolved, although ACR guidelines suggest it can be started during the acute flare time period as well.

31. What are the indications for chronic treatment of symptomatic hyperuricemia and how should this be managed?

Lifelong urate-lowering therapy (ULT) is indicated for gout patients characterized by:
- Frequent flares, often defined as more than two or three flares over a 1-year period
- Tophaceous gout

TABLE 44.1 Medications Used in the Treatment of Acute Gout Flare

NSAIDs	Full dose until resolution of flare; dosing variable based on NSAID chosen	Contraindicated in patients with moderate/severe CKD
Oral Colchicine*	1.2 mg PO followed by 0.6mg PO 1 hour later; continue 0.6mg daily or twice daily until flare resolution	Most effective within the first 36 hours of a flare. Contraindicated with significant renal or hepatic insufficiency. Avoid use with concomitant P450 3A4 and P-glycoprotein inhibitors including cyclosporine, clarithromycin/erythromycin, keto- and itraconazole, disulfiram, HIV protease inhibitors, diltiazem, verapamil, and grapefruit juice.
Intra-articular glucocorticoids (triamcinolone or methylprednisolone)	40–60 mg intraarticularly for large joints, 10–20 mg for small joints or bursae	Useful in treatment of 1–2 involved joints or bursae. Effective within the first 24 hours of an attack in 90% of patients.
Systemic glucocorticoids	Prednisone 0.5 mg/kg/d for 5–10 days without taper OR 2–5 days full dose then taper for 7–10 days OR triamcinolone 60 mg IM, can repeat once.	Rebound flare may occur if patient not given high enough dose or long enough course. May be used in patients with CKD.
IL-1 inhibitors	Canakinumab- 150 mg subcutaneous, single dose; may be repeated every 12 weeks. Anakinra (off-label)- 100 mg daily subcutaneous until symptom improvement (usually 3–5 days)	Reserved for when first line agents are ineffective or contraindicated.

CKD, chronic kidney disease; *HIV*, human immunodeficiency virus; *NSAID*, non-steroidal anti-inflammatory drug
*May consider use of colchicine in combination with NSAID or glucocorticoids for severe flare

- Chronic kidney disease
- Radiographic damage attributable to gout

Indications for xanthine oxidase inhibition versus uricosuric therapy, along with dosing information and side effect profiles, are discussed in Chapter 86. Xanthine oxidase inhibition (**allopurinol** or **febuxostat**) is considered to be first-line ULT, though both medications are equally efficacious when dosed optimally. The starting dose of allopurinol is 100 mg/day (with even lower initial doses with marked renal impairment) followed by gradual upward titration (often achieving daily doses >300 mg) to achieve a serum urate goal of <6 mg/dl. Dose titrations should be completed at regular (e.g., monthly) intervals to avoid 'treatment inertia'. This "start low and go slow" strategy can be used effectively in the vast majority of patients, even in patients with renal impairment provided regular monitoring is in place. HLA-B*5801 screening prior to the initiation of allopurinol should be considered for patients at increased risk of carrying this gene (e.g., individuals of Southeast Asian descent or Black/African-Americans), which carries a mortality risk approaching 20%. Febuxostat is typically initiated at a daily dose of 40 mg (urate lowering approximately equivalent to allopurinol 300 mg) and titrated upward after 2-3 weeks to 80 mg/day if the serum urate goal has not been achieved. Both febuxostat and allopurinol appear to be well tolerated in patients with moderate CKD. Probenecid is contraindicated in patients who have a history of nephrolithiasis, and lack efficacy in those with impaired renal function (GFR <50 ml/min). Pegloticase (a recombinant pegylated uricase dosed intravenously at two-week intervals) is approved for advanced gout that has proven refractory to other therapies (see Chapter 86). Although drug-related antigenicity has limited long-term use, concomitant administration of immunosuppressives such as methotrexate or mycophenolate mofetil has been shown to mitigate anti-drug antibody formation and improve the durability of pegloticase.

32. What drug–drug interactions complicate the use of xanthine oxidase inhibitors?

Mercaptopurine (MP) and its prodrug azathioprine are metabolized by xanthine oxidase. Thus, the concomitant use of MP or azathioprine with a xanthine oxidase inhibitor (allopurinol or febuxostat) can lead to increased immunosuppressive drug levels and life-threatening bone marrow toxicity. As a result, these combinations should be avoided when possible.

33. Gout flares can be precipitated with the initiation of ULT. How can this risk be minimized?

Anti-inflammatory prophylaxis is recommended to mitigate the risk of gout flares precipitated by ULT initiation. Importantly, ULT should not be stopped or reduced during a flare. Initiated concomitantly or prior to ULT, agents most commonly used in prophylaxis include low-dose NSAIDs (e.g., naproxen 250 mg twice daily) or oral colchicine (0.6 mg once or twice daily). In elderly patients or those with a GFR of 30 to 50 ml/min, colchicine doses may need to be reduced (0.6 mg/day or every other day) or avoided altogether with more advanced CKD (particularly as colchicine cannot be removed by dialysis). Low-dose glucocorticoid treatment (e.g., prednisone 5 to 10 mg/day) can be used for prophylaxis in those intolerant to or unable to take NSAIDs or colchicine. Although shown to be efficacious in prophylaxis with ULT initiation, the role of IL-1 inhibition is uncertain given poorly defined risk/benefit ratios. According to American College of Rheumatology (ACR) management guidelines, prophylaxis should be continued for at least 3–6 months after ULT initiation. Patients suffering from recurrent gout flares may require continued prophylaxis for more prolonged periods.

34. Outline the treat-to-target management strategy for gout.

The ACR and other subspecialty societies currently recommend a treat-to-target management strategy for gout, which includes ULT dose titration guided by serial serum urate measurements to achieve a target serum urate of <6.0 mg/dL, rather than a fixed-dose ULT strategy. Nonphysician providers (including nurses and pharmacists) may be important participants in the delivery of this treat-to-target strategy to improve patient adherence and outcomes.

35. Why is gout relatively common in organ transplant recipients? Are there special considerations in the management of gout in these patients?

Impaired renal function and therapy with cyclosporine or tacrolimus, which reduces urinary urate excretion, are likely factors. Polyarticular flares and early development of tophi have been reported. Treatment of flares and normalization of the hyperuricemia are often challenging. NSAIDs are relatively contraindicated in the setting of cyclosporine or tacrolimus therapy, or renal insufficiency; xanthine oxidase inhibitors are contraindicated with concurrent use of azathioprine/6-MP (see Question 32). Intra-articular or systemic glucocorticoids may be the safest treatment option for flares. Synovial fluid cultures should be performed routinely. Uricosurics are often ineffective in this setting as a result of impaired renal function. Finally, colchicine is relatively contraindicated in patients taking cyclosporine or tacrolimus due to rare cases of neuromyopathy that have been reported even in patients taking low-dose colchicine for brief periods.

ACKNOWLEDGMENT

The authors would like to acknowledge the contributions of Dr. Robert Janson, who was the author of this chapter in previous editions.

WEBSITES

https://www.rheumatology.org/I-Am-A/Patient-Caregiver/Diseases-Conditions/Gout
http://www.gouteducation.org

BIBLIOGRAPHY

Chen-Xu M, Yokose C, Rai SK, et al. Contemporary prevalence of gout and hyperuricemia in the United States and decadal trends: The National Health and Nutrition Examination Survey, 2007-2016. *Arthritis Rheumatol.* 2019;71(6):991–999.

Choi HK. A prescription for lifestyle change in patients with hyperuricemia and gout. *Curr Opin Rheumatol.* 2010;22:165–172.

Chowalloor PV, Siew TK, Keen HI. Imaging in gout: a review of the recent developments. *Ther Adv Musculoskelet Dis.* 2014;6:131–143.

Dalbeth N. Clinical features and treatment of gout. In: Firestein GS, ed. *Kelley & Firestein's Textbook of Rheumatology.* 11th ed. Philadelphia, PA: Elsevier; 2021:1710–1731.

FitzGerald JD, Dalbeth N, Mikuls T, et al. 2020 American College of Rheumatology guideline for the management of gout. *Arthritis Care Res (Hoboken).* 2020;72(6):744–760.

Keenan RT, Toprover M, Pillinger MH. Etiology and pathogenesis of hyperuricemia and gout. In: Firestein GS, Budd RC, Gabriel SE, Koretzky GA, McInnes IB, O'Dell JR, eds. *Kelley & Firestein's Textbook of Rheumatology.* 11th ed. Philadelphia, PA: Elsevier; 2021:1687–1709.

Merriman TR. An update on the genetic architecture of hyperuricemia and gout. *Arthritis Res Ther.* 2015;17:98.

Mikuls TR. Gout. *N Engl J Med.* 2022;387(20):1877–1887.

Mikuls TR. Urate-lowering therapy. In: Firestein GS, ed. *Kelley & Firestein's Textbook of Rheumatology.* 11th ed. Philadelphia, PA: Elsevier; 2021:1111–1124.

Terkeltaub RA, Furst DE, Bennett K, et al. High versus low dosing of oral colchicine for early acute gout. *Arthritis Rheum.* 2010;62:1060–1068.

CHAPTER 45

Calcium Pyrophosphate Deposition Disease

Itziar Quinzaños Alonso, MD

1. Calcium pyrophosphate deposition disease (CPPD) is a disease of the elderly, with onset and increasing frequency after the age of 50 years.
2. Patients younger than 55 years with chondrocalcinosis (CC) should be evaluated for a familial form or metabolic disease associated with CPPD.
3. Chronic CPPD should be considered in any elderly patient with symptoms suggesting seronegative rheumatoid arthritis (RA) or polymyalgia rheumatica.
4. Chronic CPPD should be considered in any patient with diffuse osteoarthritis (OA) in atypical joints such as the metacarpophalangeal joints (MCPs), wrists, elbows, and shoulders.
5. The mnemonic ABC (**A**lignment **B**lue **C**alcium) is useful for remembering the color of a CPPD crystal parallel to the first-order red compensator when viewing synovial fluid by polarized light microscopy.

1. What is calcium pyrophosphate dihydrate?

Calcium pyrophosphate dihydrate is a calcium salt ($Ca_2P_2O_7 \cdot 2H_2O$) that in crystalline form (called CPP crystals) is deposited in cartilage and other articular tissues, leading to a variety of clinical manifestations. CPPD is the preferred umbrella term for all presentations related to CPP crystal deposition. Other terms such as CPPDD/CPDD (calcium pyrophosphate dihydrate deposition disease) are the same as CPPD.

2. What factors predispose patients to CPPD development?

- Idiopathic (sporadic): the greatest risk factors are advancing age (odds ratio [OR] 2.25 for each decade over age 40) and primary OA (OR 2.66). Sex and obesity are not risk factors.
- Consequence of mechanical joint trauma or meniscectomy (OR 5.0).
- Familial predisposition: in young-onset CPPD. Mutations at two genetic loci have been described in familial forms of CPPD: CCAL1 (gain-of-function mutation at TNFRSF11B gene; chromosome 5p, gene that codes for osteoprotegerin) and CCAL2 (gain-of-function mutation at ANKH gene; chromosome 8q). These represent autosomal dominant forms of CPPD. Patients tend to present in their 20s and 30s and are more likely to have spinal involvement.
- Specific disease associations: primary hyperparathyroidism (OR 3.0), long-standing hypomagnesemia (OR 13.5), hypophosphatasia, and hemochromatosis. Other diseases have been associated with CPPD, but the evidence is not as strong. CPPD is thought less likely to coexist with RA (OR 0.18), but data in the literature are conflicting in this regard.
- Newer reported associations include low body mass index and low cortical bone mineral density.

3. Discuss the pathogenesis of CPPD crystal formation.

Fig. 45.1 shows factors that contribute to CPP deposition.

A high level of inorganic pyrophosphate (PPi) in cartilage is an important contributor to CPP crystal formation and is caused by:

- ANKH mutations: transport of more pyrophosphate from chondrocytes into cartilage. ANKH appears to be *over expressed* in patients with idiopathic CPPD disease and familial disease.
- Ectonucleotide pyrophosphatase/phosphodiesterase 1 (ENPP1) and ENPP3 *over expression*: increased levels of intracellular and extracellular pyrophosphate by hydrolyzing ATP. Specifically, ENPP1 is significant in generating inorganic pyrophosphate (PPi) within the extracellular cartilage matrix, mainly deriving it from extracellular ATP. Subsequent research has highlighted the extracellular process as more crucial in the pathophysiology of CPPD.

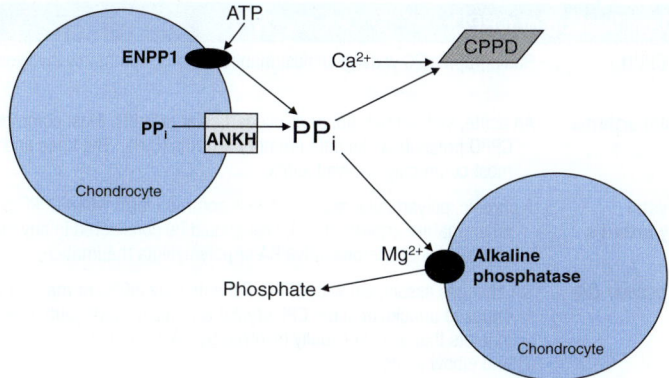

Fig. 45.1 Factors contributing to calcium pyrophosphate crystal deposition.

- Lack of tissue-nonspecific alkaline phosphatase (ALP), or *underactivity* (hypophosphatasia): the normal function of ALP is to break down PPi. When ALP function is abnormal, PPi levels increase. Magnesium is a cofactor for ALP, so hypomagnesemia lessens its activity. In addition, calcium (hyperparathyroidism), iron (hemochromatosis), and copper (Wilson disease) inhibit ALP.

Enhanced nucleation of CPP crystals in cartilage is also an important contributor to CPP crystal formation:

- Increased calcium concentrations (hyperparathyroidism) enhance crystal formation.
- Enhanced nucleation of CPP crystals due to increased iron (hemochromatosis) and copper (Wilson disease).
- Lack of inhibitors of nucleation: magnesium inhibits nucleation, so low levels contribute to crystal formation.
- Multiple changes in osteoarthritic cartilage composition (CILP, osteopontin) facilitate CPP crystal formation/deposition.

4. List the clinical presentations associated with CPPD.

CPPD-associated arthritis can present in a number of different ways; the diverse clinical presentations allow for organization in to subgroups listed in Table 45.1.

According to some estimates, CPPD-associated arthritis is the third most common cause of inflammatory arthritis, occurring in 4.5% of adult patients. It should be considered in the diagnosis of any acute or chronic mono-, oligo-, or polyarticular inflammatory or noninflammatory arthritis occurring in patients over the age of 55 years. If it occurs in a patient aged <55 years, then familial forms, certain metabolic diseases (hyperparathyroidism, hemochromatosis, hypomagnesemia, dialysis-dependent renal failure, others; see Question 22), and/or a history of joint trauma/meniscectomy need to be considered.

5. How common are CC and CPPD?

Cross-sectional studies show that 8% of community-dwelling individuals have CC on knee radiographs (with prevalence increasing to 14% if hand and pelvis films are performed as well; Fig. 45.2). CC is rare before age 55 and increases with age, with up to 30% of the population having CC on x-rays by the ninth decade of life. Asymptomatic CC is the most common clinical presentation of CPPD. In patients with CPPD, the most common sites of radiographic CC are the knees and triangular fibrocartilage of the wrists (>90%). Calcifications should be bilateral.

Comprehensive studies utilizing more sensitive imaging modalities such as ultrasound (US) are currently in progress, and may reveal a higher prevalence of radiographic disease than currently appreciated. Estimation of the true prevalence of CPPD has also been hampered by the historical absence of standardized classification criteria. The American College of Rheumatology (ACR) and the European Alliance of Associations for Rheumatology (EULAR) introduced classification criteria for symptomatic CPPD in 2023, which may provide more accurate estimates for the prevalence of symptomatic disease in the future (reference at end of chapter). A final

TABLE 45.1 Classification of CPPD

Asymptomatic CPPD (*lanthanic*)	Radiographic CC without clinical manifestations; commonly involves the knee.
Acute CPP crystal arthritis (*pseudogout*)	An acute, self-limited mono- or oligoarticular arthritis. Most common form when CPPD presents as an inflammatory arthritis (89%). The knee and wrist are the most commonly involved joints.
Chronic CPP crystal inflammatory arthritis (*pseudo-RA*)	A chronic, polyarticular arthritis. A less common form when CPPD presents as an inflammatory arthritis (11%). This should be considered in any elderly patient with new onset seronegative RA or polymyalgia rheumatica.
OA with CPPD (*pseudo-OA*)	OA changes associated with CPPD. Patients may (50%) or may not have superimposed attacks of acute CPP crystal arthritis (pseudogout). CPPD causes OA in joints that are not usually involved by OA, such as the MCPs and radiocarpal and elbow joints.
Other presentations	Tumoral CPP crystal deposition in periarticular and bony structures (*pseudotophaceous pattern*). Tendon deposits, most commonly in the Achilles, gastrocnemius and/or quadriceps tendons. Less common triceps and rotator cuff. *Pseudo-neuropathic pattern:* radiographic appearance is Charcot-like but the patient has normal pain perception. Cervical stenosis: from CPPD in the ligamentum flavum and/or transverse ligament of the atlas. Crowned dens: CPPD above the odontoid process can lead to acute neck pain and meningismus with crystal shedding. Axial involvement: intervertebral disc calcifications and sacroiliac joint involvement are more common in familial forms.

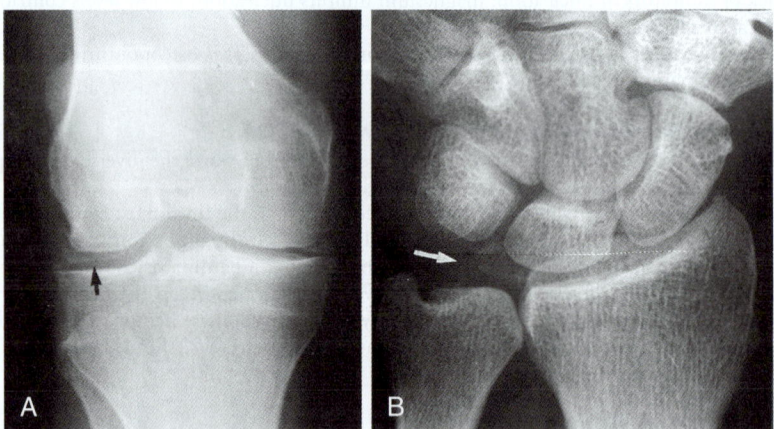

Fig. 45.2 (A) Chondrocalcinosis of the knee. (B) Triangular fibrocartilage complex of the wrist.

noteworthy consideration is the reported increase in CPPD prevalence in developed countries. This is thought to be propelled by increased life expectancy and factors contributing to hypomagnesemia, such as more common use of loop diuretics, proton pump inhibitors, calcineurin inhibitors, and post-surgical short bowel syndrome, all of which may impact worldwide prevalence moving forward.

6. Is all CC caused by CPP crystal deposition?

Calcium salts other than CPP, such as basic calcium phosphate (BCP), can appear as CC. For example, the calcification of intervertebral disc cartilage seen in ochronosis largely consists of calcium hydroxyapatite. Clinicians usually assume that certain radiographic patterns of CC, such as the triangular fibrocartilage complex in the wrist or the hyaline cartilage and menisci in the knees, are due to CPP deposition. However, this is not always the case and dystrophic calcifications comprising BCP deposition due to trauma can be seen in these areas, particularly if only found unilaterally.

7. Do all patients with CPPD have CC?

CPPD can cause arthritis without being seen as CC on x-rays. This can occur in up to 20% of patients with symptomatic CPPD. This is one reason why an acutely inflamed joint must be aspirated to identify the cause. An elderly patient who presents with an acutely inflamed knee could have gout or pseudogout as a cause of arthritis, even if the x-ray is normal, and can be accurately diagnosed only by aspirating the joint. The term **pyrophosphate arthropathy** has been used to describe structural damage to a joint associated with CPPD, with or without radiographic CC.

8. What is acute CPP crystal arthritis (pseudogout)? How does it present?

Acute CPP crystal arthritis (pseudogout) is an acute arthritis with rapid onset of pain and swelling. Physical exam reveals warmth, swelling with effusion, tenderness, and limited range of motion of the involved joint(s). Overlying erythema may simulate cellulitis. Occasionally systemic symptoms such as malaise and fever will also raise suspicion of infection (**pseudoseptic arthritis**). Attacks of pseudogout tend to be less painful and take longer to reach peak intensity than attacks of gout. Usually, only a single joint is affected, although oligo- and polyarticular pseudogout have been described. Large joints are affected more commonly than small joints, with the knee and wrist most frequently involved. Notably, the first metatarsophalangeal joint is rarely involved. Untreated pseudogout is self-limited, resolving within ≥7 to 10 days. Patients are typically asymptomatic between attacks.

9. Discuss the pathogenesis of acute CPP crystal arthritis (pseudogout).

Crystal shedding explains the occurrence of CPP crystals within the synovial fluid. These crystals may induce inflammation in several ways (Fig. 45.3).
- Engagement of toll-like receptor 2 in phagocytes and chondrocytes (with subsequent downstream activation of inflammatory pathways).
- Direct interaction with intracellular NALP-3, resulting in caspase-1 activation and emission of multiple cytokines.
- Release of neutrophil extracellular traps.
- Interaction with cell membranes causing nonspecific activation and release of prostaglandins, leukotrienes, and cytokines. Interleukin (IL)-8 is a potent neutrophil chemoattractant, which is critical in bringing more cells into the joint.

  Apart from inducing inflammation, CPP crystals have important direct catabolic effects on chondrocytes and synoviocytes via production of metalloproteinases, prostaglandins, and nitric oxide, altering the mechanical properties of cartilage.

10. How is acute CPP crystal arthritis diagnosed?

When a patient presents with an acute mono- or oligoarthritis, the critical and immediate diagnostic procedure is aspiration of the joint(s). The fluid obtained may appear yellow and cloudy, or

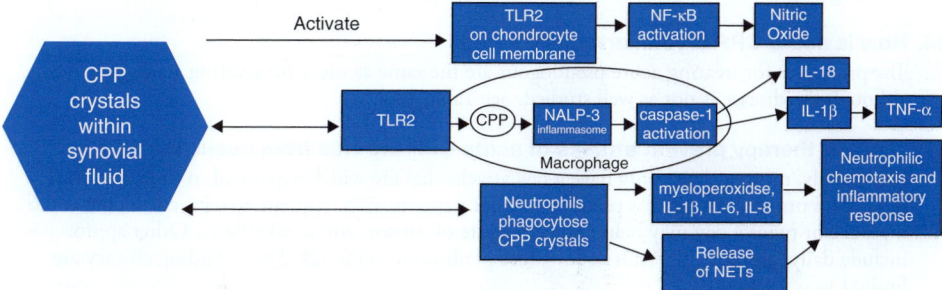

Fig. 45.3 Factors that contribute to calcium pyrophosphate crystal-induced inflammation. *CPP,* Calcium pyrophosphate; *IL,* interleukin; *TLR,* toll-like receptor; *TNF,* tumor necrosis factor; *NETs,* neutrophil extracellular traps.

even opaque and chalky because of suspended crystals. Synovial fluid is sent to the laboratory for a cell count and differential, as well as a Gram stain and bacterial culture. Synovial fluid leukocytosis with a predominance of polymorphonuclear leukocytes (PMNs) is present. A specimen of synovial fluid is also promptly analyzed for crystals by **polarized light microscopy.** The presence of **intracellular** CPP crystals confirms the diagnosis of pseudogout.

11. How is polarized light microscopy performed to definitively diagnose CPPD?

A drop of synovial fluid is placed on a clean microscope slide and covered with a cover slip. The slide is first examined under an ordinary light microscope, but the crystals are rarely visible. Therefore, a polarizer is typically needed to find CPP crystals, which appear as birefringent rhomboid or rectangular crystals with blunt or squared ends (see Chapter 7: Arthrocentesis, Synovial Fluid Analysis, and Synovial Biopsy). For a definitive diagnosis, a first-order red compensator is applied. CPP crystals are referred to as **weakly positively birefringent**. This means that CPP crystals appear blue when viewed under polarized light, with the long axis of the crystal parallel to the direction of slow vibration of light in the compensator.

12. What is a helpful mnemonic to remember how the crystals look under polarized light?

The mnemonic **ABC** (**A**ligned **B**lue **C**alcium) is useful: if the crystal is aligned with the red compensator and is blue, then it is CPP. CPP crystals lying with their long axes at right angles to the direction of slow vibration will appear yellow rather than blue. Observation of crystals inside a PMN, instead of floating free, helps to confirm that the CPP crystals are causing the arthritis.

13. What are the pitfalls to be wary of when diagnosing acute CPP crystal arthritis?

- **Septic arthritis** can coexist (in up to 1% of cases) with acute crystalline arthritis. Enzymes that degrade cartilage can be released into the joint (from the infecting bacteria or the PMNs). These enzymes are able to strip crystals from the structures in and around the joint, and an unwary clinician might miss a septic joint. This is why joint fluid should be sent for a Gram stain and culture on all arthrocentesis of acute arthritis.
- Pseudogout can present as **pseudoseptic arthritis**, an inflammatory arthritis that mimics septic arthritis; **Gram stain and cultures are persistently negative**. It is a diagnosis of exclusion.
- Although rare, it is possible for a patient to have simultaneous gout and pseudogout.
- Acute pseudogout in the wrist of an elderly person may cause carpal tunnel syndrome. Similarly, CPP deposition can cause cubital tunnel syndrome.
- Up to 20% of patients with pseudogout may not have CC on radiography. The synovial fluid must be examined for crystals.
- Acute pseudogout is frequently precipitated by an urgent medical illness, such as myocardial infarction or a surgical procedure. Fluid shifts with fluctuations in serum calcium levels may play a role in such attacks. An elderly hospitalized patient who complains of new joint pain should be investigated for pseudogout.
- Other potential precipitators of pseudogout: Intraarticular hyaluronate (especially in products with high concentrations of phosphate such as Synvisc) has been linked to subsequent acute CPP crystal arthritis in case reports. Other possible associations include the use of loop diuretics, granulocyte–macrophage colony-stimulating factor, and IV bisphosphonates.

14. How is acute CPP crystal arthritis treated?

The principles for treating acute pseudogout are the same as those for treating acute gout, although the disease is not as well studied. See Table 45.2.

15. Can any therapy prevent attacks of acute CPP arthritis from occurring?

Fortunately, most patients only have a few attacks that are widely separated in time, and thus require no prophylaxis against pseudogout. For patients with frequent attacks, colchicine at 0.6 mg once or twice a day may help reduce the rate of subsequent attacks/flares. Other approaches include daily low-dose NSAIDs or low-dose prednisone, although data regarding efficacy are limited.

TABLE 45.2 Treatment of Acute CPP Crystal Arthritis

TREATMENT	COMMENTS	DISADVANTAGES
Nonpharmacologic/aspiration	Ice packs, rest, and thorough aspiration of the affected joint may halt the attack	Usually insufficient for clinical relief Not feasible for polyarticular attacks
NSAIDs[a]	Prescribed at full antiinflammatory doses Consider prescribing with a gastric protection medication given affected patient population	Caution in elderly and patients with comorbid conditions: renal insufficiency, heart disease, peptic ulcer disease, etc.
Intraarticular steroids Long-acting preparations: e.g., 40 mg triamcinolone hexacetonide for large joints (knee), 10–20 mg for smaller joints (wrist)	Good option if avoiding NSAIDs Best method to provide prompt, complete relief of the attack with little risk of systemic adverse effects	Challenging in polyarticular attacks
Intramuscular steroids[a] 1 or 2 intramuscular injections of 60 mg triamcinolone acetonide	Useful in hospitalized patients with contraindications to NSAIDs and who decline an intraarticular injection	Systemic corticosteroid effects
Oral steroids[a,b] 40 mg of oral prednisone daily, which is tapered to zero in 10–14 days	Can be used if above therapy has failed or is contraindicated	Systemic corticosteroid effects
Adrenocorticotropic hormone[a] IV, IM, or SQ	Can be used in patients who do not respond to other therapies and have multiple comorbidities	Not FDA approved Very expensive
Colchicine[a,b] Load with 1.2 mg followed by 0.6 mg 1 hour later, can then be followed by 0.6 mg twice daily until the attack abates	Only use if glomerular filtration rate >50 mL/minute	Significant potential toxicity and drug interactions in the elderly population. Should be administered within 12–24 hours for optimal effectiveness.
IL-1 inhibitors[a] such as anakinra 100 mg subcutaneously daily for 3–5 days	Considered in the rare circumstance of treatment-resistant disease	Not FDA approved Expensive, quick onset of action

FDA, Food and Drug Administration; *IM*, intramuscular; *IV*, intravenous; *NSAIDs*, nonsteroidal anti-inflammatory drugs; *SQ*, subcutaneous.
[a]Polyarticular attacks of pseudogout can also be managed with these therapies.
[b]Newer data suggest that shorter courses of colchicine (1.5 mg on day 1 and 1 mg on Day 2) and prednisone (30 mg/day for 2 days) may be as effective as longer courses.

16. Can CPPD disease be confused with RA?

Yes, up to 5% of patients with CPPD arthritis have involvement of multiple joints, particularly the knees, wrists, and elbows, with chronic low-grade inflammation persisting for weeks or months (chronic CPP crystal arthritis, **pseudo-RA**). Joint involvement may be symmetric, and systemic symptoms such as fatigue or morning stiffness are present. Physical exam reveals synovial thickening, loss of joint motion, and flexion contractures. Inflammatory markers can be elevated. Up to 10% of CPPD patients will test positive for rheumatoid factor (RF) because of their age. If present, is usually a low titer. Higher RF titers, antibodies against cyclic citrullinated peptide, more widespread synovitis, involvement of the hands and feet, and characteristic erosions distinguish RA from pseudo-RA.

17. What steps should be taken to make the correct diagnosis and differentiate CPPD from RA?

Before making a diagnosis of seronegative RA in an elderly patient, or RA with only a low-titer positive RF, it is prudent to consider the possibility of CPPD by reviewing imaging (x-rays and ultrasound) and clinical features and through joint aspiration to examine the synovial fluid for crystals if necessary.

18. How do you treat chronic CPP crystal inflammatory arthritis?

NSAIDs, colchicine, and low-dose prednisone can be tried. If these are ineffective in controlling symptoms the following treatments may be considered:

- Hydroxychloroquine: one study supports its use, but has not been replicated
- Methotrexate: effective in observational studies but not randomized placebo-controlled trials
- IL-1 antagonists: a systematic review described a positive response in ~40% of patients with chronic CPP arthritis; an attempted RCT was aborted due to low recruitment, but initial results suggested it was as effective as prednisone with a faster onset of action
- IL-6 receptor blocker: one small open-label study and two case reports support its use

19. What features suggest that a patient has OA with CPPD rather than typical OA?

OA with CPPD (**pseudo-OA**) is seen in approximately half of patients diagnosed with symptomatic chronic CPPD-associated arthropathy. The pattern of joint involvement may be different from primary OA, the degree of articular damage may be more severe, and the disease course may be marked by intermittent episodes of inflammatory arthritis. Patients with CPPD presenting as pseudo-OA commonly have severe degenerative changes in the MCPs, radiocarpal joints, elbows, shoulders, and knees. Of these joints, only the knees are typically involved in primary OA. **Therefore, a patient with OA in atypical joints should be evaluated for CPPD.** Patients with pseudo-OA are treated with NSAIDs, analgesics, physical therapy, and joint surgery, similar to the therapy for primary OA.

20. What radiographic features in the knee suggest CPPD rather than typical primary OA?

The knee is the most common joint involved in CPPD. Certain radiographic features help in separating OA with CPPD from primary OA. In primary OA, the medial compartment of the knee is more commonly involved, resulting in varus changes. OA with CPPD is more likely to affect the lateral compartment, causing bilateral or unilateral valgus changes. Isolated patellofemoral OA, bilateral involvement, exuberant osteophytosis, and flexion contractures are also more common in OA with CPPD than in primary OA.

21. What is the best imaging modality to diagnose CPPD?

Plain radiography and ultrasonography (US) are the recommended imaging modalities. Computed tomography (CT) should be used if axial involvement is suspected. Radiographs (knee > wrist > symphysis pubis) typically show CC, but not always. Significant advancements have been made in standardizing US definitions for the diagnosis of CPPD, achieving high levels of diagnostic accuracy, particularly in detecting CPPD in the medial meniscus of the knee and utilizing targeted protocols during an acute flare (scanning two joints bilaterally plus the target joint showed an accuracy > 90% for the diagnosis in patients with acute mono/oligoarthritis). Nevertheless, the success of this modality is operator dependent and hence may not be widely applicable. Magnetic resonance imaging (MRI) is of little utility in this setting (insensitive to tissue calcification). Newer imaging technologies, such as advanced MRI techniques, diffraction-enhanced synchrotron imaging, and dual-energy CT, hold promise for the future.

22. Describe the appropriate laboratory workup in a patient with newly diagnosed CPPD.

Most cases of CPPD are sporadic or associated with normal aging. If the CPPD is severe or affects many joints, or the patient is younger than 50 years, it is reasonable to search for a metabolic cause. Evaluations must be individualized for persons older than 55 years, with hyperparathyroidism being a primary consideration. Recommended laboratory studies include:

- Calcium (rule out hyperparathyroidism).
- Phosphorus.
- Magnesium (rule out hypomagnesemia, usually from renal wasting—Gitelman's syndrome).
- ALP (rule out hypophosphatasia).
- Ferritin, iron, total iron-binding capacity (rule out hemochromatosis).
- Renal function.

23. What diagnostic tests are only warranted in special circumstances?

Tests for rare diseases, such as acromegaly or Wilson's disease, are only warranted if there are clinical features suggestive of these conditions. Hypothyroidism does not cause CPPD. However, initiation of thyroxine therapy in a hypothyroid patient with CPPD may precipitate a pseudogout attack; therefore, some clinicians elect to measure thyroid-stimulating hormone.

24. Does any treatment retard or reverse deposition of the CPP crystals causing the arthritis?

Unfortunately, there is no therapy to prevent deposition of CPP crystals or remove CPP deposits already present. Patients with an underlying disease such as primary hyperparathyroidism should have the disease treated. This may retard further CPP crystal deposition but will not resolve those already deposited. Some patients have been treated with the following:

- Magnesium: may be useful in patients with low magnesium levels. Has also been described in patients with normal levels because *in vitro* studies show that magnesium has inhibitory effects on CPP crystal nucleation and growth. *Note that loop and thiazide diuretics, proton pump inhibitors, and calcineurin inhibitors can cause hypomagnesemia.*
- Probenecid: it is postulated that probenecid lowers high PPi levels by blocking the ANKH anion channel. Though good theoretic rationale, this approach lacks evidence in the clinical setting.
- Phosphocitrate: lowers PPi levels, but needs to be given intravenously because of poor oral absorption. Evidence from animal studies and *in vitro* human fibroblast analyses, but no safety or clinical efficacy data in humans.
- Polyphosphates: dissolve synthetic crystals and crystals from human menisci without cell damage; these agents have not been tested *in vivo*.

BIBLIOGRAPHY

Abhishek A, Tedeschi SK, Pascart T, et al. The 2023 ACR/EULAR classification criteria for calcium pyrophosphate deposition disease. *Arthritis Rheumatol.* 2023;75(10):1703–1713.
Cipolletta E, Di Matteo A, Scanu A, et al. Biologics in the treatment of calcium pyrophosphate deposition disease: a systematic literature review. *Clin Exp Rheumatol.* 2020;38(5):1005–1007.
Cowley S, McCarthy G. Diagnosis and treatment of calcium pyrophosphate deposition (CPPD) disease: a review. *Open Access Rheumatol.* 2023;15:33–41.
Finckh A, McCarthy GM, Madigan A, et al. Methotrexate in chronic-recurrent calcium pyrophosphate deposition disease: no significant effect in a randomized crossover trial. *Arthritis Res Ther.* 2014;16:458.
Latourte A, Ea HK, Frazier A, et al. Tocilizumab in symptomatic calcium pyrophosphate deposition disease: a Pilot study. *Ann Rheum Dis.* 2020;79(8):1126–1128.
Mandl P, D'Agostino MA, Navarro-Compan V, et al. 2023 EULAR recommendations on imaging in diagnosis and management of crystal-induced arthropathies in clinical practice. *Ann Rheum Dis.* 2024;83:752–759.
Terkeltaub R, Firestein GS, Budd RC, et al. Calcium crystal disease: calcium pyrophosphate dihydrate and basic calcium. *Kelley and Firestein's Textbook of Rheumatology.* 11th ed. Philadelphia, PA: Elsevier; 2017:1732–1751.
Williams CJ, Rosenthal AK. Pathogenesis of calcium pyrophosphate deposition disease. *Best Pract Res Clin Rheumatol.* 2021;35(4):101718.
Zhang W, Doherty M, Bardin T, et al. European League Against Rheumatism recommendations for calcium pyrophosphate deposition. Part I: terminology and diagnosis. *Ann Rheum Dis.* 2011;70:563–570.

CHAPTER 46

Basic Calcium Phosphate and Other Crystalline Diseases

Elena Weinstein, MD

> **KEY POINTS**
>
> 1. Basic calcium phosphate (BCP) crystals can deposit in joints, muscles, and periarticular soft tissues and occur most commonly in the shoulder tendons/bursa.
> 2. BCP crystal deposits can remain asymptomatic or shed, causing acute calcific periarthritis.
> 3. BCP crystals are involved in the pathogenesis of large joint destructive arthritis such as Milwaukee shoulder syndrome and may contribute to osteoarthritis (OA) in other joints.

1. Are the crystals that cause gout and pseudogout the only crystals seen in synovial fluid?

Although monosodium urate crystals, which cause gout, and calcium pyrophosphate dihydrate (CPPD) crystals, which cause pseudogout, are the most commonly identified crystals in synovial fluid, many other crystals or particles may be encountered during polarized light microscopy. Some of these crystals cause disease and some are just interesting incidental findings (Box 46.1).

2. What are BCP crystals?

BCP crystals are a family of calcium-containing crystals including partially carbonate-substituted hydroxyapatite (HA), octacalcium phosphate, and tricalcium phosphate. The most abundant of these is HA. Collectively, these calcium-containing minerals are referred to as BCP. These minerals may be found in soft tissue and tendon calcifications and in some forms of arthritis, hence their relevance to rheumatology. Additionally, BCP crystals may also be found outside articular sites in the blood vessels, skin, and other structures.

3. What clinical syndromes are associated with BCP crystals?

BCP crystals are associated with a wide variety of clinical manifestations, including inflammation of joints and periarticular structures, osteoarthritis-like lesions, and a rapidly destructive arthritis. Two categories of musculoskeletal syndromes are of particular importance:

A) Calcific periarthritis
- Calcific deposits in tendons (chronic calcific tendinitis), bursae, joint capsules
- Acute calcific periarthritis

B) BCP-associated arthropathy
- Acute synovitis
- Destructive arthropathy (as seen in Milwaukee shoulder)
- Osteoarthritis with presence of BCP crystals (controversial, see Question 14)

BOX 46.1 Crystals and Particles Seen in Synovial Fluid

Monosodium Urate Crystals	Cholesterol crystals	Hemoglobin
Calcium pyrophosphate dihydrate crystals	Lipid droplets	Aluminum
Calcium hydroxyapatite crystals (and other basic calcium phosphate crystals)	Foreign organic matter (e.g., plant thorns)	Cystine
		Xanthine
Calcium oxalate crystals	Metallic fragments from prosthetic joints	Charcot–Leyden crystals
Injectable corticosteroid crystals	Immunoglobulin crystals in cryoglobulinemia	Amyloid

In addition, BCP crystals can result in subcutaneous/soft tissue calcifications:
- Connective tissue diseases: systemic sclerosis, dermatomyositis, systemic lupus erythematosus, mixed connective tissue disease
- Metastatic calcification: chronic renal failure with high calcium-phosphorous product (>70)
- Tumoral calcinosis

4. Describe the typical presentation of periarticular calcium deposits (calcific periarthritis).

BCP deposition is common in the shoulder, most commonly involving the rotator cuff tendons. Deposition within multiple areas of the shoulder is common, and 50% of cases are bilateral. Calcific periarthritis affects predominantly middle-aged women, most often on the dominant side. The supraspinatus tendon is most commonly involved followed by infraspinatus and subscapularis. Symptoms can range from asymptomatic to chronic smoldering pain to acute episodes of severe pain resulting from acute inflammation. Long-standing calcification can lead to adhesive capsulitis and sometimes tendon tears. Tendons around other joints may also be affected, including the hip, hand, foot, wrist, knee, and neck.

On radiographs, the calcific deposits can be dense and globular particularly when asymptomatic, or fragmented and fluffy in the setting of acute inflammation. Synovial fluid examination typically reveals <1000 WBC cells/mL^3. BCP crystals are not visible in regular light or polarizing microscopy due to their small size (20–100 nm) and lack of birefringence. Although clumps of BCP crystals can be seen with alizarin red staining, this is not specific for BCP as CPP crystals will also stain positive.

5. Why do the calcifications occur most commonly in the shoulder?

The supraspinatus tendon is prone to impingement. The tendon is poorly vascularized a few millimeters from its insertion into the humeral head. Therefore, its ability to recover from the repetitive trauma of impingement is poor at this site, resulting in ischemia and necrosis. This "critical zone" is prone to accumulating calcium salts (BCPs) causing calcific deposits in the tendon and bursa. Notably, other tendons that develop calcifications have a similar pathogenesis, with deposition at relatively avascular and traumatized sites in the tendon. Therefore, the calcification may be the result of chronic tendinitis as well as a driver of further tendon injury.

6. How is chronic calcific tendinitis treated?

Asymptomatic BCP deposits at periarticular sites require no therapy. Patients with symptomatic chronic calcific tendinitis (or bursitis) are managed conservatively, with physical therapy and non-steroidal anti-inflammatory drugs (NSAIDs). Local injections with a short-acting corticosteroid should be used sparingly because steroids may promote calcification in the long term. *Barbotage* refers to the use of a needle for repetitive aspiration and lavage to disrupt the local calcification, which may promote more rapid dissolution of the deposit by stimulating phagocytosis of the BCP crystals. Other therapies that have been described include treatment with high-energy extracorporeal shockwave therapy. Surgical or arthroscopic debridement of very large or severely symptomatic calcific deposits may be necessary. Pulsed ultrasound therapy has also been described for dissolving BCP crystals.

7. What is acute calcific periarthritis?

When BCP crystals are shed from a calcific deposit in tendons or other periarticular soft tissues, there is an intense local inflammatory reaction to the crystals similar to other crystalline arthritides. If this reaction occurs around a joint, the clinical picture is an acute arthritis with pain, warmth, loss of motion, and swelling. Constitutional symptoms such as fatigue and low-grade fever can occur. There may be elevated acute-phase reactants and peripheral white blood cell count. Plain radiographs may reveal the BCP deposit and thus identify the crystal causing the problem; of note, bone destruction is not seen (unlike the destructive BCP arthropathy, Milwaukee shoulder syndrome). Acute calcific periarthritis most commonly occurs in the shoulder and hip but has been described in other joints as well, including the hand and foot.

8. What is HA pseudopodagra? What is the crowned dens syndrome?

HA pseudopodagra is an *acute calcific periarthritis* occurring near the first metatarsophalangeal joint, causing podagra identical to that seen in gout. This presentation is more common in young women and with excessive foot pronation and repetitive trauma. The condition may be distinguished from gout according to the premenopausal status of the patient, the absence of monosodium urate crystals in synovial fluid, and characteristic calcifications around the joint on radiographs. Symptoms subside over several weeks, either spontaneously or with treatment. Interestingly, the calcific deposit may dissolve during the acute inflammatory episode, leading to disappearance of the calcification on follow-up x-rays. This can also occur in other joint areas (Fig. 46.1).

Crowned dens syndrome is an *acute calcific periarthritis* that can cause acute neck pain due to calcifications surrounding the odontoid process. These calcifications are most often due to CPP crystals but can occur with BCP crystals as well. The clinical picture varies widely from asymptomatic to severe pain with fever and elevated inflammatory markers. This condition occurs most commonly in the elderly and can present with fever and associated neurologic symptoms including headache and confusion. Calcifications are seen best on an open-mouth view of the odontoid process or a computed tomography (CT) scan of the area (more sensitive than radiograph). The characteristic pattern on CT is that of calcification surrounding the top and sides of the dens with a horseshoe or "crown"-like appearance.

9. Describe the treatment for acute calcific periarthritis.

Attacks of acute calcific periarthritis may be managed similarly to other crystalline arthritides. NSAIDs are commonly used as first-line therapy if there are no contraindications to their use. Aspiration of the joint and injection of a corticosteroid represent another expedient way to provide relief. Colchicine therapy is reportedly successful for acute calcific periarthritis, as well as IL-1 inhibition (small open-label case series of anakinra). Following the resolution of the acute attack, physical therapy can also be helpful to restore joint mobility and function.

10. Can BCP crystals cause inflammatory synovitis?

Acute attacks of arthritis due to BCP crystals in the knee and other joints have been described. The attacks resemble gout. A more chronic arthritis leading to erosive OA changes in the fingers has also been linked to BCP crystals. Unfortunately, these presentations are difficult to prove because of the difficulty in identifying BCP crystals in the synovial fluid.

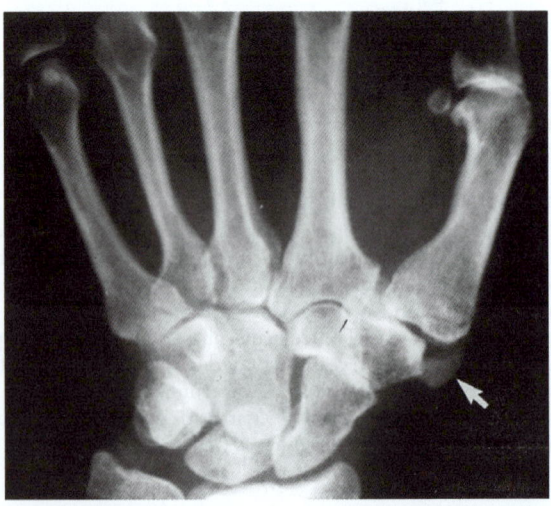

Fig. 46.1 Amorphous homogeneous deposits of basic calcium phosphate near the first carpometacarpal joint *(arrow).*

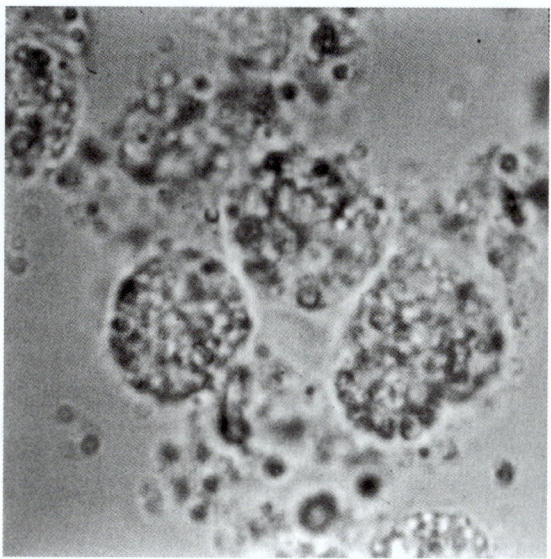

Fig. 46.2 Aggregates of basic calcium phosphate crystals seen in neutrophils under light microscopy.

11. How are BCP crystals identified if they are suspected of causing a joint problem?

Identification of BCP crystals is difficult. If characteristic calcifications are observed on plain radiographs or advanced imaging (such as CT scan or magnetic resonance imaging), it is often presumed that BCP is the cause of the symptoms. Aspiration of a calcific deposit may yield material that looks like toothpaste. BCP crystals are so small that individual crystals cannot be appreciated on plain microscopy; however, clumps of aggregated BCP crystals may be seen with an appearance described as stacked "shiny coins" (Fig. 46.2). Special stains, such as alizarin red, can confirm the presence of calcium in the aspirated material but are not specific for BCP. BCP crystals are not birefringent and are therefore not seen on polarized light microscopy. Precise crystal identification requires techniques such as transmission electron microscopy or x-ray diffraction, which are often available only in specialized centers or the research setting. Similarly, most clinical laboratories do not perform alizarin red staining due to the labor-intensive process for preparation of the dye. As a result, the history and supportive imaging findings remain the most powerful tools available to the clinician for diagnosis.

12. How does Milwaukee shoulder syndrome (apatite-associated arthropathy, rotator cuff tear arthropathy, or BCP-associated destructive arthropathy) present?

Milwaukee shoulder syndrome is a severe destructive arthritis of the glenohumeral joint with loss of the rotator cuff associated with the presence of BCP crystals (Fig. 46.3). It affects mostly elderly women and is usually bilateral. Unilateral disease typically occurs in the dominant shoulder, and in bilateral disease the dominant shoulder is usually more severely affected. Patients most often present with mild intermittent shoulder pain, worse with use and when lying on their side in bed. On exam, joint mobility can either be restricted or hypermobile, the latter due to instability seen when joint destruction is severe. Large joint effusions are common, and joint aspirates often reveal blood-tinged fluid with low leukocyte counts. BCP crystals are present in the joint fluid, and up to half of patients also have calcium pyrophosphate crystals. Early x-rays may show superior subluxation of the humeral head from the glenoid, suggestive of a rotator cuff tear. As the disease progresses, x-rays may show sclerosis and cyst formation, erosions, and ultimately, complete destruction of the glenohumeral joint.

BCP arthropathy can affect other joints as well, particularly the knees and hips. A loss of joint space in the lateral compartment in the knees distinguishes this from primary OA, similar to CPPD-associated arthropathy. Rapidly destructive arthritis of the finger due to BCP has been called the **Philadelphia finger**.

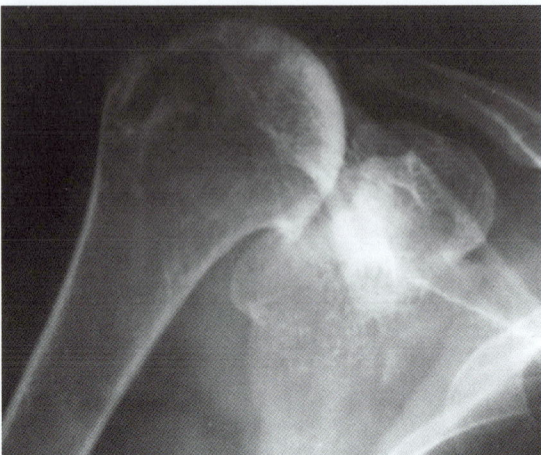

Fig. 46.3 Milwaukee shoulder. Note the upward migration of the humeral head indicating a rotator cuff tear.

13. How is Milwaukee shoulder syndrome treated?

Treatment options are limited, and treatment choice is primarily dictated by severity of symptoms. Some patients with mild symptoms do well with daily NSAIDs and/or analgesics. Local heat can be beneficial. If large effusions are present, repeated arthrocentesis may relieve symptoms. Intraarticular steroids can also be helpful at 2- to 3-month intervals. Some patients benefit from percutaneous joint lavage with saline, followed by steroid injection. Patients may benefit from joint protection (decreased joint usage) early in presentation, but physical therapy will be important to maintain range of motion and strengthen the surrounding muscles. Surgical intervention may be considered for advanced degenerative changes.

14. Do BCP crystals contribute to OA?

Intraarticular BCP crystals are found in up to 60% of patients with OA. Furthermore, their presence correlates with OA severity. Animal studies and *in vitro* experiments have shown numerous pathways through which BCP crystals may induce OA (including prostaglandin E_2, interleukin [IL]-1β, tumor necrosis factor α, and IL-6). Chondrocytes and other cells within the joint also respond to calcium crystals and may contribute to inflammation, cellular demise, and the breakdown of the matrix, all of which are crucial aspects of OA. Additional research showed that BCP crystals may promote osteoclast formation and subsequent bone remodeling. The clinical relevance of BCP crystals in OA remains uncertain, however, and research in this area is ongoing.

15. Describe the appearance and clinical presentation of other crystals in synovial fluid.

a. **Calcium oxalate crystals** are characteristically bipyramidal (or envelope-shaped) in appearance. They occur in effusions from patients with primary oxalosis or end-stage renal disease. Oxalosis can cause pathologic fractures and bone pain. Articular manifestations include acute inflammatory arthritis and tenosynovitis, especially of the feet.

b. **Cholesterol crystals** are found in synovial fluid from chronic joint effusions, usually rheumatoid arthritis. The crystals are square and plate-like with a single notched corner. Cholesterol crystals are beautifully birefringent, both positively and negatively. They do not cause inflammation. They are a sign of a chronic inflammatory effusion and form from the cholesterol in the cell membranes of neutrophils after they break down in the joint.

c. **Steroid crystals** in synovial fluid may be confused with CPPD crystals because they are often small, irregularly shaped or rectangular, and weakly birefringent. Careful polarized microscopy is necessary because steroid crystals may be positively or negatively birefringent (both types are often seen in the same field), whereas CPPD crystals are always weakly positively birefringent. The patient will also have a history of joint injection with corticosteroid, possibly weeks earlier. Patients sometimes do not volunteer this information, so a specific question about previous joint injections should be asked.

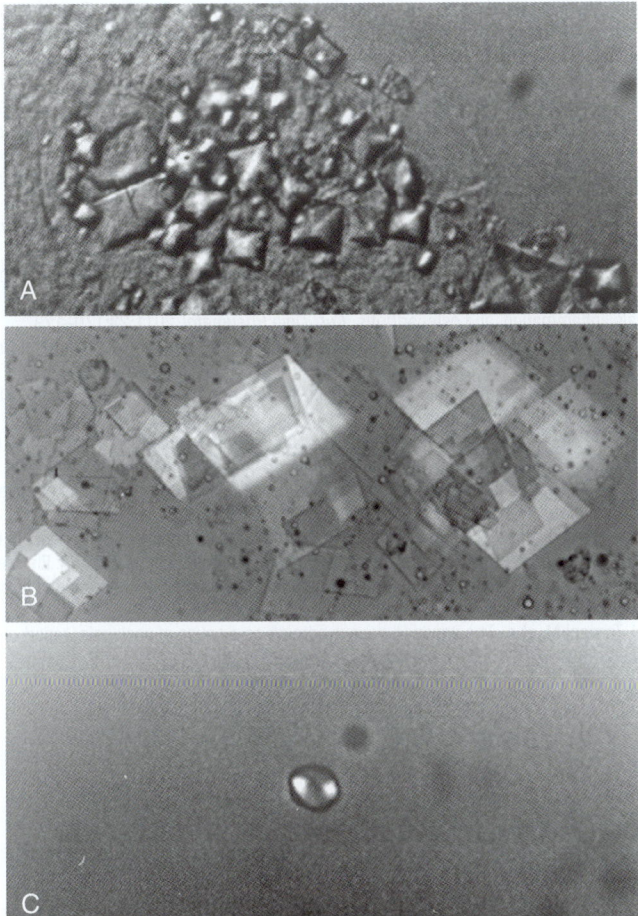

Fig. 46.4 Other synovial fluid crystals. (A) Calcium oxalate crystals have a characteristic bipyramidal shape under ordinary light micros-copy. (B) Plate-shaped cholesterol crystals are strongly birefringent when viewed under polarized light microscopy. These crystals were obtained from an aspirate of a knee effusion in a patient with rheumatoid arthritis. (C) Starch (talc) from examination gloves during slide preparation. (A, Courtesy The Upjohn Company. B, Ed Uthman, MD, pathologist. C, Courtesy The Upjohn Company.)

    d. **Talc (or starch) particles** from examination gloves are an artifact occurring during prepara-tion of synovial fluid slides. They resemble small beach balls when viewed under polarized light microscopy. This finding is mostly of historical interest, given powdered medical gloves are no longer commonly used in the clinical setting.

    e. **Lipid droplets** have a "Maltese cross" appearance under polarized light microscopy. Lipid droplets in synovial fluid may represent a subchondral fracture or may be seen occasionally in medical conditions including pancreatitis. Lipid droplets look like starch particles, although the size of starch particles is more variable.

    There are many other types of particles or contaminants that can appear in synovial fluid, such as glass fragments from coverslips and specks of cartilage, so all synovial fluids must be examined carefully (Fig. 46.4).

BIBLIOGRAPHY

Bernabei I, So A, Busso N, Nasi S. Cartilage calcification in osteoarthritis: mechanisms and clinical relevance. *Nat Rev Rheumatol.* 2023;19(1):10–27.

Dieppe PA, Crocker PR, Corke CF, Doyle DV, Huskisson EC, Willoughby DASOQ. Synovial fluid crystals. *J Med.* 1979;48(192):533.

Ea HK, Liote F. Advances in understanding calcium-containing crystal disease. *Curr Opin Rheumatol.* 2009;21:150–157.

Ecklund KJ, Lee TQ, Tibone J, Gupta R. Rotator cuff tear arthropathy. *J Am Acad Orthop Surg.* 2007;15:340–349.

Fam AG, Stein J. Hydroxyapatite pseudopodagra in young women. *J Rheumatol.* 1992;19:662–664.

Halverson PB, Carrera GF, McCarty DJ. Milwaukee shoulder syndrome: fifteen additional cases and a description of contributing factors. *Arch Intern Med.* 1990;150:677–682.

Hang-Korng E, Frederic L. Diagnosis and clinical manifestations of calcium pyrophosphate and basic calcium phosphate crystal deposition diseases. *Rheum Dis Clin North Am.* 2014;40:207–229.

MacMullan P, McMahon G, McCarthy G. Detection of basic calcium phosphate crystals in osteoarthritis. *Joint Bone Spine.* 2011;78:358–363.

Molloy Easmonn S, McCarthy Geraldine M. Hydroxyapatite deposition disease of the joint. *Curr Rheumatol Rep.* 2003;5:215–221.

Paul H, Reginato AJ, Schumacher HR. Alizarin red S staining as a screening test to detect calcium compounds in synovial fluid. *Arthritis Rheum.* 1983;26(2):191.

Rosenthal AK. Crystals, inflammation, and osteoarthritis. *Curr Opin Rheumatol.* 2011;23:170–173.

Rosenthal AK. Basic calcium phosphate crystal-associated musculoskeletal syndromes: an update. *Curr Opin Rheumatol.* 2018;30(2):168–172.

Schumacher HR, Chen LX. Other crystal-related arthropathies. In: Hochberg MC, Silman AJ, Smolen JS, et al. eds. *Rheumatology.* 5th ed. Philadelphia, PA: Mosby.

Schumacher HR, Reginato AJ. *Atlas of Synovial Fluid Analysis and Crystal Identification.* Philadelphia, PA: Lea & Febiger. 1991.

Stack J, McCarthy G. Basic calcium phosphate crystals and osteoarthritis pathogenesis: novel pathways and potential targets. *Curr Opin Rheumatol.* 2016;28(2):122–125.

Terkeltaub R. Calcium crystal diseases: calcium pyrophosphate dihydrate and basic calcium phosphate. In: Firestein GS, Budd RC, Gabriel SE, et al. eds. *Kelley's Textbook of Rheumatology.* 9th ed. Philadelphia, PA: Elsevier Saunders.

Whelan LC, Morgan MP, McCarthy GM. Basic calcium phosphate crystals as a unique therapeutic target in osteoarthritis. *Front Biosci.* 2005;10:530–541.

Wu DW, Reginato AJ, Torriani M, et al. The crowned dens syndrome as a cause of neck pain: report of two new cases and review of the literature. *Arthritis Rheum.* 2005;53:133–137.

CHAPTER 47

Endocrine-Associated Arthropathies

Jason R. Kolfenbach, MD

1. Which endocrine diseases have well-described rheumatologic manifestations associated with them?

DM	Hyperparathyroidism
Hypothyroidism	Acromegaly
Hyperthyroidism	Cushing's syndrome
Hypoparathyroidism	Hyperlipoproteinemia

DIABETES MELLITUS

2. What rheumatologic syndromes are more common in patients with DM?

- Intrinsic complications of DM.
    - Diabetic stiff hand syndrome (diabetic cheiroarthropathy).
    - Neuropathic arthropathy (Charcot joint) and diabetic osteolysis.
    - Diabetic amyotrophy.
    - Diabetic muscle infarction.
- Conditions with increased incidence in DM.
    - Adhesive capsulitis of the shoulder (frozen shoulder).
    - Calcific shoulder periarthritis (tendinitis).
    - Complex regional pain syndrome (shoulder-hand syndrome).
    - Flexor tenosynovitis of the hands (trigger fingers).
    - Dupuytren's contractures.
    - CTS.
    - Diffuse idiopathic skeletal hyperostosis (DISH).
    - Septic joint/osteomyelitis.

3. How does the diabetic stiff hand syndrome present?

This syndrome, also known as **diabetic cheiroarthropathy** ('cheiros' is the Greek word for hand)**,** presents with the insidious development of flexion contractures involving the small joints of the hands, commonly affecting the PIP and MCP joints, as well as the DIP and wrist locations.

This condition occurs in patients with type 1 or type 2 diabetes (estimated prevalence 10–20%) and correlates with disease duration, glucose control, and renal/retinal microvascular disease.

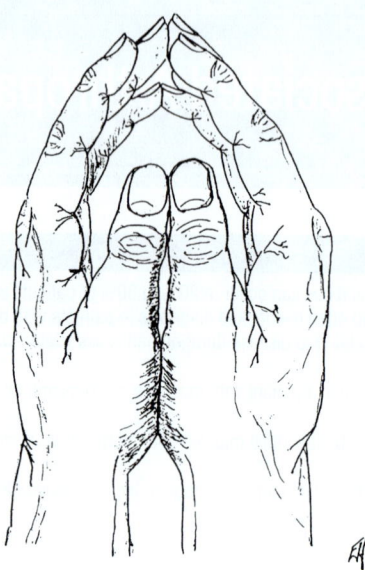

Fig. 47.1 Prayer sign in a patient with limited joint mobility due to diabetes mellitus.

The "prayer sign" observed on physical examination reflects the inability to fully extend the joints of the fingers (Fig. 47.1). These finger contractures are attributed to excessive glycosylation of dermal and periarticular collagen (impacting muscle, tendon, and joint capsule), decreased collagen degradation, and increased collagen hydration. Thickening and waxiness of the overlying skin are common, especially in the dorsum of the hands. As such, this condition can be confused with scleroderma. Laboratory serologies and hand radiographs are unremarkable. Importantly, the observed skin changes in diabetes can occur in the absence of limited joint mobility, and conversely, limited joint mobility in diabetes can occur in the absence of overlying skin abnormalities. Treatment is physical therapy and control of the underlying diabetes. Contractures usually progress slowly but rarely limit function significantly.

While hand involvement is most common, decreased range of motion at other joint locations can occur in the setting of diabetes as well, leading some to call this condition "limited joint mobility in diabetes" rather than diabetic stiff hand syndrome. Epidemiologic studies have shown a decreased prevalence of this condition over the past 40 years, presumably due to improved control of hyperglycemia in diabetics during that time period.

4. Discuss the relationship between Charcot joints and DM.

A Charcot joint occurs in <1% of all diabetics (both type 1 and type 2). It occurs in both men and women with equal frequency. More than two-thirds of patients are aged >40 years and have had long-standing (>10 years), poorly controlled diabetes complicated by a diabetic peripheral neuropathy. Patients present with relatively painless swelling and deformity of the joint. The foot (most commonly tarsometatarsal joints) and ankle are most commonly involved, although knee, hip, and spine involvement can occur as well. Occasionally it can be of sudden onset mimicking an infection. With progression of disease, the patient can develop "rocker bottom" feet due to midtarsal collapse. Skin over bony prominences can ulcerate and become infected without the patient's knowledge as a result of abnormal sensation resulting from the neuropathy.

Radiographs frequently show severe abnormalities characterized by **the 5 Ds:** destruction, density (increased), debris, disorganization, and dislocation (Fig. 47.2). The increased density and sharp margins of the bony debris can help distinguish a Charcot joint from infection. The exact pathophysiology is uncertain, but an autonomic neuropathy leading to increased blood flow, hyperemia, and osteoclastic resorption of bone is believed to be the primary mechanism, alongside repetitive microtrauma to a desensate foot. Treatment includes protected weight-bearing, soft casts, good

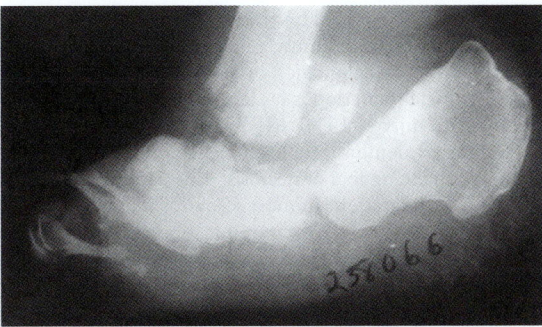

Fig. 47.2 Charcot joints of foot and ankle.

shoes, and aggressive treatment and prevention of skin ulcerations. Charcot joints, however, usually progress. There is no role for surgery (fusion, arthroplasty) other than amputation for severe cases. DM has replaced neurosyphilis as the most common cause of a Charcot joint.

5. What is diabetic osteolysis?

Diabetic osteolysis is a condition specifically occurring in diabetics. The osteolysis is characterized by osteoporosis and variable degrees of resorption of the distal metatarsal bones and proximal phalanges of the feet (a case report has described diabetic acro-osteolysis as well). Pain is variable. Radiographs have a characteristic "licked candy" appearance. The pathogenesis is unclear, although autonomic neuropathy has been postulated to play a role. The primary consideration in the differential diagnosis is osteomyelitis. Treatment is conservative and includes protected weight-bearing. The process may terminate at any stage and in some cases may completely resolve.

6. How does diabetic amyotrophy present? How is it different from diabetic muscle infarction?

Diabetic amyotrophy presents with severe pain and dysesthesia involving most commonly the proximal muscles of the pelvis and thigh. The paraspinal and shoulder girdle muscles can also be involved. Onset is commonly unilateral, but spread to the contralateral leg occurs in over 75% of patients. Anorexia, weight loss, and unsteady gait due to muscle wasting and weakness may be seen. The typical patient is a 50- to 60-year-old man with well-controlled, mild type 2 DM of several years' duration, although it can be the presenting sign of diabetes in up to 20% of cases. Usually, the patient has no evidence of diabetic retinopathy or nephropathy but may have a distal symmetric sensory neuropathy as well as signs of an autonomic neuropathy.

Laboratory evaluation is usually unremarkable except for an elevated cerebrospinal fluid protein. Electromyography (EMG)/nerve conduction velocity testing demonstrates changes compatible with neuropathy, and muscle biopsy shows muscle fiber atrophy without an inflammatory infiltrate. **The etiology is unclear but may be due to a vasculopathy affecting the lumbosacral plexus or femoral nerve.** Treatment is conservative and includes pain control (including agents such as gabapentin, tricyclic antidepressants, and pregabalin) and physical therapy. Studies examining nerve biopsy specimens have shown an inflammatory infiltrate within the blood vessel wall in roughly 50% of affected patients, suggesting a potential role for immunomodulating therapy. Conflicting data exist in the literature regarding the efficacy of intravenous immunoglobulin, corticosteroids, plasmapheresis, and cyclophosphamide, with lack of randomized controlled trial data for any immunosuppressive agent. Over 50% recover within 3 to 18 months, though recovery is often incomplete. Some patients have recurrent episodes.

Diabetic muscle infarction (spontaneous diabetic myonecrosis) is the spontaneous infarction of muscle. It occurs in patients with long-standing diabetes with multiple other microvascular complications (concurrent nephropathy in 75%; concurrent triad of nephropathy, retinopathy, and neuropathy in 45%). As such, it would be extremely uncommon for patients to present with diabetic muscle infarction as the first microvascular complication of diabetes. Patients present with acute onset of pain and swelling of thigh or calf muscles over a period of days to weeks.

Creatinine phosphokinase may be elevated but can be normal in 50–60% of patients. Clinical presentation, laboratory findings, and muscle magnetic resonance imaging (MRI) may help distinguish from infection/abscess, malignancy, or idiopathic inflammatory myositis (IIM). In contrast to IIM, diabetic muscle infarction is far less likely to involve symmetrical muscle groups (~10–20%) or the upper extremity (~15%). MRI with contrast (gadolinium) is the diagnostic imaging tool of choice and may demonstrate heterogeneous enhancement of the muscle surrounding low-signal, non enhancing foci of necrosis. This pattern, however, is not seen in all patients and is not specific for infarction. In most scenarios, the diagnosis can be made without the need for a muscle biopsy. In patients in whom infection cannot be excluded based on history, exam, laboratory, and imaging studies, a biopsy may be necessary. Unless there is remaining concern for a possible IIM (in which case excisional biopsy is preferred), an imaging-guided core biopsy should be sufficient to rule out infection, improve diagnostic confidence, and reduce the risk of post operative complications associated with excisional biopsy in this setting. The recurrence rate of diabetic muscle infarction is as high as 25–40% in some longitudinal series.

7. What is diabetic periarthritis of the shoulder?

Diabetic periarthritis of the shoulder is also known as **frozen shoulder** or **adhesive capsulitis**. It occurs in 10–33% of diabetics and is five times more common in diabetics than in nondiabetics. Patients present with diffuse soreness and global loss of motion of the shoulder, typically in the setting of long-standing diabetes. Up to 50% of patients have bilateral involvement, although the nondominant shoulder is frequently more severely involved. Laboratory studies and radiographs are unremarkable. Some patients may have **calcific (hydroxyapatite) periarthritis/tendinitis**, which is three times more common in diabetics than in nondiabetics and may increase the risk of developing a frozen shoulder. Treatment may include nonsteroidal anti-inflammatory drugs (NSAIDs), intraarticular steroids (weak data for efficacy), and physical therapy to improve range of motion. Efficacy data for manipulation under anesthesia are also weak. For unclear reasons, this syndrome may spontaneously remit after weeks to months.

8. The shoulder-hand syndrome can be a complication of a frozen shoulder. What is it?

When a frozen shoulder (with or without calcific periarthritis) is accompanied by vasomotor changes consistent with complex regional pain syndrome, it is known as shoulder-hand syndrome (see Chapter 64: Complex Regional Pain Syndrome).

9. How commonly does flexor tenosynovitis, DeQuervain tenosynovitis, or Dupuytren contracture occur in patients with DM?

Flexor tenosynovitis occurs in 5–33% of patients with diabetes. Women with long-standing diabetes are more commonly affected than men. Patients complain of aching and stiffness in the palmar aspect of the hand. Symptoms are worse in the morning. A "trigger" finger may occur as a result of an inflammatory nodule getting caught in the proximal pulley at the base of the finger. The thumb of the dominant hand is most commonly involved (75%), although multiple fingers on both hands can be affected. Laboratory findings and radiographs are unremarkable. Treatment includes NSAIDs, local steroid injections, and surgery.

    DeQuervain tenosynovitis occurs in 20% of patients with diabetes. Similar to flexor tenosynovitis, increased prevalence of this condition is thought secondary to a combination of microvascular disease affecting local nerves and blood vessels, glycosylation of proteins, and deposition of extracellular matrix proteins in the skin and periarticular structures.

    Dupuytren contracture occurs in 30–60% of patients with type 1 diabetes. Patients present with nodular thickening of the palmar fascia, leading to flexion contractures usually of the fourth and fifth digits. Patients usually have long-standing diabetes, although there is no association with control of the diabetes. The pathogenesis is thought to be due to contractile myofibroblasts producing increased collagen secondary to microvascular ischemia. Treatment includes NSAIDs, physical therapy, local steroid or collagenase injections, and rarely, surgical release.

10. What is the relationship between DM and CTS?

CTS commonly (20%) occurs in patients with diabetes. Patients present with numbness in the median nerve distribution. Nocturnal paresthesias, hand pain, and pain radiating to the elbow or shoulder (Valleix phenomenon) can also occur. Tinel and Phalen signs as well as Durkan pressure test may be positive. Thenar atrophy is a late sign and indicates muscle denervation. The neuropathy may be from extrinsic compression or due to microvascular disease causing vasa nervorum ischemia. Treatment includes splints, NSAIDs, local steroid injections into the carpal tunnel (relapse risk in diabetics with CTS higher than in nondiabetics, potentially due to higher rates of ischemic nerve injury rather than compressive), and surgical decompression. See Chapter 63 (Entrapment Neuropathies) for additional details on CTS.

11. What is DISH? How commonly does it occur in DM?

DISH is diffuse idiopathic skeletal hyperostosis, also known as Forestier disease. It occurs in up to 20% of patients with type 2 diabetes; patients are typically obese and aged over 50 years. Patients present with neck and back stiffness associated with loss of motion. Pain is not prominent. Radiographs are diagnostic and consist of at least four vertebrae fused together as a result of ossification of the anterior longitudinal ligament. Disc spaces, apophyseal joints, and sacroiliac joints are normal, helping separate it from osteoarthritis and axial spondylitis. Treatment typically consists of NSAIDs and physical therapy (see Chapter 50: Osteoarthritis).

12. What diabetes-associated complications can lead to symptoms that may mimic features of systemic sclerosis (SSc)?

- Diabetic stiff hand syndrome may result in flexion contracture of the fingers and indurated, thickened skin at the digits.
- Limited joint mobility (frozen shoulder, flexor tenosynovitis, Dupuytren contractures) and distal neuropathy may be confused with the tendon contractures and Raynaud phenomenon seen in SSc.
- Scleredema diabeticorum occurs primarily in patients with type 2 diabetes and is characterized by thickened, edematous areas of skin most commonly on the upper back and neck. This has also been called scleredema adultorum of Buschke, type 3.

13. Can any of the medications used to treat DM cause rheumatic manifestations?

- Thiazolidinediones (rosiglitazone, pioglitazone) and sodium-glucose cotransporter-2 inhibitors (canagliflozin, dapagliflozin, empagliflozin) have been associated with increased fractures and loss of bone density.
- Dipeptidyl peptidase-4 inhibitors (sitagliptin, saxagliptin, linagliptin, alogliptin) have been reported to cause severe arthralgias and myalgia. These symptoms were described in post-marketing data, suggesting a low prevalence of this potential side effect. Nonetheless, the Food and Drug Administration advises clinicians to monitor for joint and muscle symptoms during therapy.

THYROID DISEASE

14. Describe the arthropathy associated with severe hypothyroidism.

Myxedematous arthropathy typically affects the knee and hand joints. The patient presents with swelling and stiffness. Synovial thickening, ligamentous laxity, and effusions with a characteristic slow fluid wave (bulge sign) are common. The synovial fluid is noninflammatory, with an increased viscosity due to high hyaluronic acid levels resulting in a string sign of 1 to 2 feet instead of the normal 1 to 2 inches. Radiographs are typically normal.

Osteonecrosis can also occur (controversial). In adults, it typically involves the hip or tibial plateau. In children, abnormal epiphyseal ossification may occur, which can be confused with epiphyseal dysplasia or juvenile avascular necrosis (Legg–Calvé–Perthes disease) of the hip.

15. What other common rheumatologic syndromes are associated with hypothyroidism?

Think of **TRAP:**

T—Tunnel (carpal) syndrome (15% of hypothyroid patients; secondary to accumulation of glycosaminoglycans and subsequent edema within the carpal tunnel).

R—Raynaud phenomenon.

A—Aching muscles with findings indistinguishable from those of fibromyalgia (up to 30% of hypothyroid patients).

P—**P**roximal muscle weakness and stiffness with an elevated CK. Thyroid-stimulating hormone (TSH) should be very high (>20), and thyroxine (T4) low, in this setting if muscle symptoms are truly attributable to thyroid dysfunction.

Although chondrocalcinosis has also been ascribed to hypothyroidism, it probably does not occur more commonly than in age-matched controls.

16. What is the relationship between Hashimoto thyroiditis and other collagen vascular diseases?

Hashimoto thyroiditis occurs with increased frequency in several collagen vascular diseases. It has been described in systemic lupus erythematosus, Sjögren disease, and rheumatoid arthritis, as well as mixed connective tissue disease, SSc, and polymyositis. The coexistence of multiple autoimmune conditions is thought to occur due to shared genetic predisposition. The prevalence of HLA-B8, DR3, and DR5 is increased in patients with Hashimoto thyroiditis and several other autoimmune conditions commonly associated with this disease. Any patient with a collagen vascular disease should be followed closely for the development of hypothyroid symptoms. Alternatively, more than 50% of patients with Hashimoto thyroiditis may present with arthralgias and/or fibromyalgia-type symptoms, and antinuclear antibodies can be seen in 25% to 35% of patients, creating potential confusion with a primary rheumatic condition.

17. Which rheumatic problems occur in patients with hyperthyroidism?

- Osteoporosis—most common musculoskeletal manifestation.
- Painless proximal muscle weakness (70% of hyperthyroid patients)—more common in elderly patients with apathetic hyperthyroidism.
- Adhesive capsulitis of the shoulders (controversial)—especially in patients with proximal muscle weakness.
- Thyroid acropachy.

18. Describe thyroid acropachy.

Thyroid acropachy is a rare (1%) complication of Graves disease consisting of soft tissue swelling of the hands, digital clubbing, and periostitis, particularly involving the metacarpal and phalangeal bones. Radiographs are characteristic (Fig. 47.3). It is strongly associated with ophthalmopathy, cigarette use, and myxedema (common pretibial location; indurated, woody texture of skin

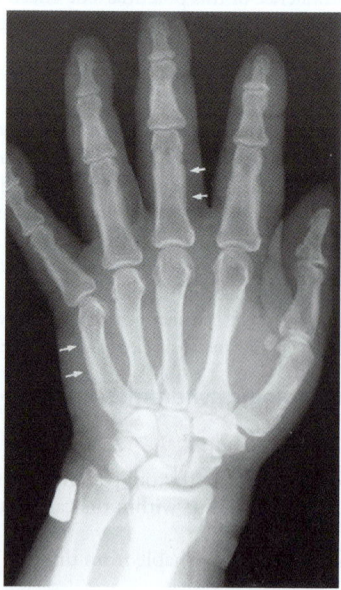

Fig. 47.3 Thyroid acropachy. Note the periosteal reaction along shafts of the metacarpals and phalanges (*arrows*).

with overlying nodules composed of hyaluronic acid that are ≥1 cm). The symptoms usually occur after the patient becomes euthyroid. Pain is variable but usually mild and does not tend to persist chronically. There is no effective therapy other than symptom control.

19. How do you differentiate hyperthyroid myopathy from the myopathies of hypothyroidism and idiopathic inflammatory myositis?

	TSH	T4	CK	Weakness	Biopsy
Inflammatory myositis	Normal	Normal	Increased	Mild-severe	Inflammation
Hypothyroidism	Increased	Decreased	Increased	Usually mild	Normal
Hyperthyroidism	Decreased	Increased	Normal	Usually mild	Normal

20. What medications used to treat hyperthyroidism can cause rheumatic syndromes?
- Propylthiouracil—can cause systemic vasculitis (perinuclear antineutrophil cytoplasmic antibody [ANCA]-positive) and/or drug-induced lupus syndrome. Similar to other drug-induced autoimmune syndromes, the prevalence of autoantibodies is substantially higher than development of clinical signs of autoimmunity.
- Methimazole—can cause a lupus-like syndrome. ANCA antibodies can develop in 10% to 15%, but rarely vasculitis. Reports of developing diabetes due to anti-insulin antibodies.

PARATHYROID DISEASE

21. List the rheumatic syndromes associated with primary hyperparathyroidism.
- Painless proximal muscle weakness with normal muscle enzymes but a neuropathic EMG.
- Chondrocalcinosis with pseudogout attacks usually owing to calcium pyrophosphate dihydrate crystals.
- Osteogenic synovitis due to subchondral bony collapse from thinning of bone (leading to osteoarthritis and subsequent reactive synovitis).
- Osteoporosis.
- Ectopic soft-tissue calcifications.
- Tendon ruptures.

22. What are the skeletal ramifications of hyperparathyroidism?
Osteitis fibrosa cystica represents the classic skeletal sequelae of prolonged advanced hyperparathyroidism from any cause. It most commonly occurs in patients with hyperparathyroidism associated with end-stage renal disease and is diagnosed by x-ray findings that are most prominent in the hands. **Subperiosteal resorption** with a blurring of the cortical margins on the radial side of the phalanges is seen, accompanied by a decrease in bone diameter and resorption of the tufts of the distal phalanges (Fig. 47.4). Diffuse osteopenia is common, and erosions may be seen in the joints of the hands, axial skeleton, and at the ends of the clavicles. Bone resorption may lead to reactive osteoid deposition at the vertebral sub-endplates resulting in sclerotic bands on spinal radiographs. The alternating sclerotic and radiolucent areas mimic the stripes of a rugby jersey (**rugger-jersey spine;** most common in secondary hyperparathyroidism). Discrete lytic lesions due to focal aggregates of osteoclastic giant cells and fibrous tissue with decomposing blood may occur and are known as **brown tumors** (more common in primary and tertiary hyperparathyroidism). Spinal compression fractures are common.

23. What is the relationship between chondrocalcinosis and primary hyperparathyroidism?
Up to 15% of patients with chondrocalcinosis will be found to have primary hyperparathyroidism. Conversely, over 50% of patients with long-standing primary hyperparathyroidism will have radiographic evidence of chondrocalcinosis.

24. What is the knuckle, knuckle, dimple, knuckle sign?
Patients with pseudo-hypoparathyroidism type Ia (PHP-1a; autosomal dominant Albright hereditary osteodystrophy) may have a skeletal deformity with a short fourth metacarpal. When they clench their hand to form a fist, a dimple appears where the fourth knuckle should be,

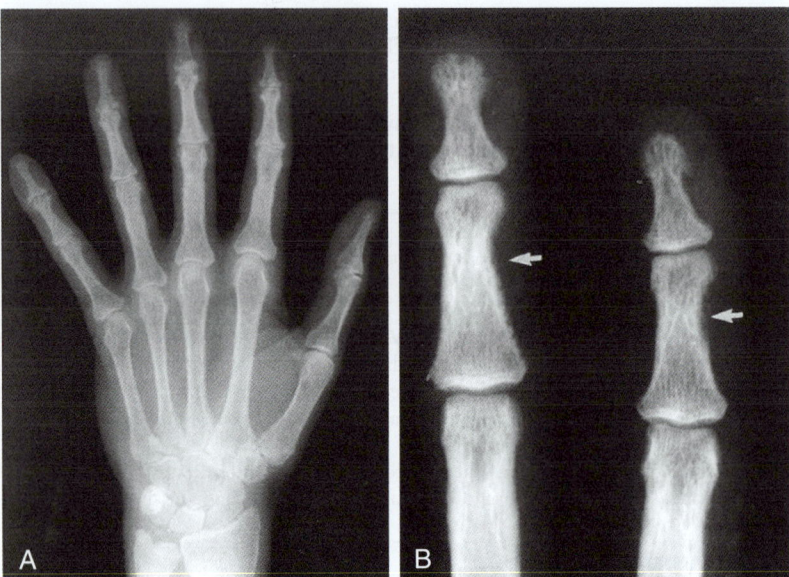

Fig. 47.4 (A) Radiograph of hand of a patient with hyperparathyroidism. (B) Close-up of phalanges demonstrating subperiosteal resorption *(arrows)*.

emphasizing the short fourth metacarpal bone. These patients have *resistance to parathyroid hormone* (low calcium, high phosphorous, high parathyroid hormone), short stature, obesity, ectopic calcifications around weight-bearing joints and paraspinal ligaments, and may have cognitive disabilities. It is due to a defect in GNAS1 resulting in PTH resistance. Patients with pseudo-PHP have similar clinical features to PHP-1a, including a short fourth metacarpal (and metatarsal) bone, but lack PTH resistance.

ACROMEGALY

25. How often does arthropathy occur in acromegaly?

It is common and may be seen in 30–70% of affected patients. Differences in the definition of arthropathy (symptom versus radiographic), disease activity and duration of acromegaly, and age differences among the study populations likely account for the wide variation in the literature. Degenerative disease is the most common articular manifestation, and crepitus on exam is the most common finding. The knees, shoulders, hips, lumbosacral, and cervical spine are the most frequent symptomatic areas, but the hands reveal the most characteristic radiographic changes. Clinical and radiographic changes occur due to excess growth hormone stimulating hepatocytes to produce somatomedin C (insulin-like growth factor), which affects osteocytes, chondrocytes, and fibroblasts.

26. List the radiographic findings in the hands of patients with acromegaly (Fig. 47.5).

Soft-tissue thickening	Deformation of epiphyses with squaring of phalanges
Enlarged terminal phalanx (spade-like)	Chondrocalcinosis (rare)
Increased joint/disc space	Periosteal apposition of tubular bones

27. What other rheumatologic syndromes may accompany acromegaly?

- CTS (up to 50% of patients).
- Proximal muscle weakness with normal EMG and normal muscle enzymes.
- Raynaud phenomenon (up to 33% of patients).

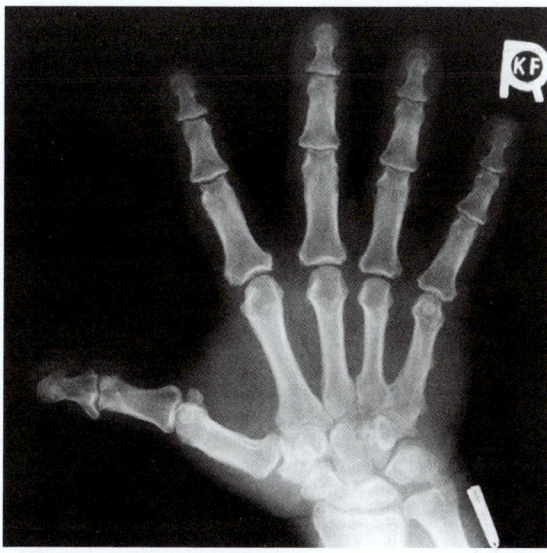

Fig. 47.5 Acromegaly of the hand.

- Chondrocalcinosis (rare).
- Vertebral fractures (increased risk despite normal or even increased bone mineral density).

CUSHING SYNDROME

28. List the rheumatic syndromes associated with excessive glucocorticoids

Proximal muscle weakness	Osteoporosis (all doses)
Osteonecrosis	Steroid withdrawal syndrome

29. Describe the myopathy seen with excessive glucocorticoids.

Proximal muscle weakness without muscle enzyme elevations can be seen in patients with Cushing syndrome or in patients receiving >10 mg of prednisone a day. EMG findings are usually normal or nonspecific. Muscle biopsy can show type 2b muscle fiber atrophy, which is nonspecific and can be seen with disuse atrophy. Patients should be treated with physical therapy, as muscle-strengthening exercises may delay the onset or improve this myopathy.

30. Which is more likely to cause osteonecrosis—endogenous Cushing or iatrogenic Cushing syndrome?

Iatrogenic Cushing (i.e., prednisone therapy) is much more likely than Cushing disease to cause osteonecrosis.

31. What is the steroid withdrawal syndrome?

This syndrome, sometimes called Slocumb syndrome, is characterized by myalgias, arthralgias, and lethargy following a rapid taper of glucocorticoids. Sometimes patients can develop noninflammatory joint effusions, particularly in the knees. Low-grade fevers occasionally occur. This withdrawal syndrome can be confused with reactivation of the primary disease for which the corticosteroids were used. Increasing the dose of glucocorticoids, tapering the steroids more slowly, and using NSAIDs can all help the symptoms.

FAMILIAL HYPERLIPOPROTEINEMIA

32. Describe the musculoskeletal disorders that have been associated with familial hyperlipoproteinemia.

- Type I, IV, V: gout is associated with the hypertriglyceridemia seen in these conditions. Type IV patients can have chronic arthralgias.
- Type II, III: tendinous xanthomas on digital extensor tendons and Achilles tendon. Achilles tendinitis can occur. Tuberous xanthomas on extensor surfaces (elbows, knees, hands) can mimic gouty tophi or rheumatoid nodules.
- Type II: episodic, acute, migratory inflammatory arthritis resembling acute rheumatic fever can occur in up to 50% of patients. Arthritis resolves in 2 weeks but frequently recurs. Cholesterol crystals are not found in the synovial fluid.
- Type III: osseous xanthomas in long bones can lead to pathologic fractures.

BIBLIOGRAPHY

Alsubheen SA, Faber K. The effectiveness of non-surgical interventions for managing adhesive capsulitis in patients with diabetes: a systematic review. *Arch Phys Med Rehabil.* 2019;100(2):350–365.

Anwar S, Gibofsky A. Musculoskeletal manifestations of thyroid disease. *Rheum Dis Clin North Am.* 2010;36:665–680.

Blazar PE, Floyd WE. Prognostic indicators for recurrent symptoms after a single corticosteroid injection for carpal tunnel syndrome. *J Bone Joint Surg Am.* 2015;97(19):1563–1570.

Fatourechi V, Ahmed DD. Thyroid acropachy: report of 40 patients treated at a single institution in a 26-year period. *J Clin Endocrinol Metab.* 2002;87(12):5435.

Fitzgibbons PG, Weiss APC. Hand manifestations of diabetes mellitus. *J Hand Surg.* 2008;33A:771–775.

Killinger Z, Payer J, Lazurova I, et al. Arthropathy in acromegaly. *Rheum Dis Clin North Am.* 2010;36:713–720.

Klemp P, Halland AM, Majoos FL, et al. Musculoskeletal manifestations of hyperlipidemia: a controlled study. *Ann Rheum Dis.* 1993;52:44–48.

Lebiedz-Odrobina D, Kay J. Rheumatic manifestations of diabetes mellitus. *Rheum Dis Clin North Am.* 2010;36: 681–699.

Mascolo A, Rafaniello C. Dipeptidyl peptidase (DPP)-4 Inhibitor-induced arthritis/arthralgia: a review of clinical cases. *Drug Saf.* 2016;39(5):401–407.

Merashli M, Chowdhury TA. Musculoskeletal manifestations of diabetes mellitus. *QJM An Int J Med.* 2015:853–857.

Misiorowski W, Bilezikian JP. Osteitis fibrosa cystica-a forgotten radiological feature of primary hyperparathyroidism. *Endocrine.* 2017;58(2):380–385.

Ormseth MJ, Sergent JS. Adrenal disorders in rheumatology. *Rheum Dis Clin North Am.* 2010;36:701–712.

Sattui SE, Markenson JA. Arthritis Accompanying Endocrine & Metabolic Disorders. *Kelley & Firestein's Textbook of Rheumatology.* 12th ed. Philadelphia, PA. Elsevier; 2025:2184–2196.

Taser F, Deger AN. Comparative histopathological evaluation of patients with diabetes, hypothyroidism and idiopathic carpal tunnel syndrome. *Turk Neurosurg.* 2017;27(6):991–997.

Wen HY, Schumacher Jr HR, Zhang LY. Parathyroid disease. *Rheum Dis Clin North Am.* 2010;36:647–664.

CHAPTER 48

Arthropathies Associated With Hematologic Diseases

Elizabeth D. Ferucci, MD, MPH

 KEY POINTS

1. If a fracture is suspected as a cause of hemarthrosis, evaluate the synovial fluid for fat droplets, which indicates release of bone marrow elements through bony disruption.
2. Joint aspiration is generally safe in patients on oral anticoagulation treatment and should be performed without delay if septic arthritis is possible.
3. If a symptomatic joint in a patient with hemophilia does not improve with factor replacement, consider infection.
4. Salmonella accounts for over 50% of osteomyelitis infections in patients with sickle cell disease (SCD).
5. Up to 40% of patients with SCD will experience osteonecrosis of the femoral or humeral head.

1. What is a hemarthrosis?

Hemarthrosis is defined as extravasation of blood into a joint's synovial cavity. The diagnosis may be readily apparent in the setting of hemophilia, but in other circumstances it is less clear. Streaks of blood, as opposed to the uniformly bloody fluid of a hemarthrosis, may be seen in the synovial fluid during routine arthrocentesis because of needle trauma to skin or other periarticular structures. Blood that appears in the synovial fluid at the end of an arthrocentesis is also typically because of trauma, particularly if the initial synovial fluid was not bloody. During an arthrocentesis, if frankly bloody fluid is seen initially on entering the joint, hemarthrosis must be suspected. The best option is to withdraw the needle and reenter the joint at another site. If the original arthrocentesis was traumatic, the synovial fluid obtained from the new site should become clear or be only blood-tinged. If diffusely bloody synovial fluid is seen again, hemarthrosis is likely. If you are still uncertain, check a hematocrit on the bloody synovial fluid. A hematocrit similar to peripheral blood is more likely from a traumatic arthrocentesis, whereas fluid from a hemarthrosis has a hematocrit less than peripheral blood. A synovial fluid hematocrit >10% will make the fluid appear grossly bloody.

2. Why is it important to accurately identify hemarthrosis?

A major concern with hemarthrosis is long-term joint damage owing to inflammation resulting from recurrent bleeding. This is of particular concern with syndromes such as hemophilia. In addition, fracture can cause hemarthrosis. As such, accurately identifying hemarthrosis and instituting appropriate treatment can reduce long-term joint-related disability.

3. What are the causes of hemarthrosis?

The causes of hemarthrosis are listed in Box 48.1.

4. What finding in the bloody synovial fluid may indicate that a fracture has caused the hemarthrosis?

A fracture may release blood and bone marrow elements including lipids into the synovial fluid. The synovial fluid may resemble "tomato soup." The fat globules released from the bone marrow may be seen floating at the top of the synovial fluid by bedside visualization of the fluid in the syringe or collection tube. If there are fat globules present in the synovial fluid identified either by direct visualization or by oil red O staining, a fracture should be suspected. Subtle fractures through bony endplates adjacent to joints may be difficult to see on plain radiography, and computed tomography or magnetic resonance imaging (MRI) may be necessary to identify the fracture.

BOX 48.1 Causes of Hemarthrosis

Trauma
Injury with or without fracture
Post-surgical postarthrocentesis

Bleeding disorders
Hemophilia
von Willebrand disease
Thrombocytopenia
Excessive anticoagulation
Thrombolytic therapy

Disorders of connective tissue
Ehlers–Danlos syndrome
Pseudoxanthoma elasticum

Tumors
Pigmented villonodular synovitis
Tumors metastatic to joints
Secondary tumors of synovium
Hemangiomas

Miscellaneous
Scurvy (vitamin C deficiency)
Sickle cell disease and other hemoglobinopathies
Myeloproliferative diseases with thrombocytosis
Munchausen's syndrome
Acute septic arthritis
Lyme disease
Arteriovenous fistula
Ruptured aneurysm
Charcot arthropathy
Gaucher's disease
Amyloid arthropathy
Acute or chronic crystalline arthritis (including hydroxy-apatite disease [e.g., Milwaukee shoulder])
Postdialysis

Note: Any condition causing intense inflammation will cause synovial vessels to be congested and friable, predisposing patients to hemarthrosis after seemingly insignificant trauma.

5. Is it safe to perform arthrocentesis when a patient has a prolonged prothrombin time (PT/INR) from warfarin therapy or is on anticoagulation with direct oral anticoagulants (DOACs)?

If a patient on oral anticoagulation therapy develops acute monoarthritis, diagnostic aspiration is warranted. It is suggested that joint aspiration is safe for patients on warfarin if the INR is <4.5, though systematic reviews have found that there is no specific cutoff and routine INR testing is not needed prior to joint aspiration. In addition, some suggest that reversal of anticoagulation is not necessary if the proper technique is carefully observed and an appropriately small-gauge needle is used. However, bleeding into the joint may occur following such arthrocentesis. Caution should be observed, particularly in large joints where it is difficult to apply direct pressure, such as the shoulder or knee. There are no published guidelines for reversal of anticoagulation before arthrocentesis. Importantly, if there is concern for post-procedure bleeding, the patient's joint should be observed after the procedure for 15–30 minutes to ensure that signs and symptoms of bleeding do not develop. While DOACs are held prior to elective surgery, similar to warfarin, there is no recommendation to hold DOACs or monitor levels prior to joint aspiration or injection. The available evidence suggests that joint aspirations in individuals on DOACs are safe.

6. What can be done for hemarthrosis in the setting of oral anticoagulation therapy?

Spontaneous hemarthrosis in the setting of warfarin therapy is uncommon and almost always occurs with an INR prolonged >2.5 times control and/or there is underlying joint damage from diseases such as osteoarthritis and rheumatoid arthritis. The knee is the most commonly affected joint. In the absence of underlying arthritis, spontaneous hemarthrosis is rare unless the INR is >5. Hemarthrosis is also uncommon with DOAC therapy and can be either spontaneous or post-traumatic.

For treatment, the affected joint is drained (for pain relief) and then rested. A mild compression bandage and ice may be applied and analgesia provided with acetaminophen or narcotics. Symptoms usually spontaneously subside without full reversal of anticoagulation. If the patient's underlying condition permits, complete reversal of anticoagulation may hasten recovery. Occasionally, an intraarticular injection of corticosteroids will be needed to control symptoms. Destructive arthritis from a single episode of hemarthrosis is rare; however, chronic joint destruction resulting from recurrent bleeding from warfarin therapy has been reported.

7. What rheumatologic problems can occur in patients with hemophilia?

- Acute hemarthrosis.
- Subacute or chronic arthropathy.
- End-stage arthropathy.
- Intramuscular or soft tissue hemorrhage (may cause pseudotumor or compartment syndrome).
- Subperiosteal hemorrhage (may cause bone pseudotumor).
- Septic arthritis.

8. How does acute hemarthrosis present in a patient with hemophilia?

Hemarthrosis is a common manifestation of Hemophilia A (factor VIII deficiency) and hemophilia B (factor IX deficiency). Prodromal symptoms of stiffness or warmth may occur in the affected joint. As the joint capsule distends, severe pain follows with swelling from effusion and decreased range of motion. The swelling will eventually tamponade the bleeding and the hemarthrosis will gradually resolve over days to weeks. Almost all patients with severe hemophilia (<1% of normal factor activity) and half of patients with moderate disease (1–5% factor activity) will have recurrent hemarthroses spontaneously or following minor trauma. Large joints (knees, elbows, ankles) are most commonly involved. If factor levels are >5% of normal, hemarthroses tend to be less frequent or occur following more significant trauma. Hemarthroses often first begin to occur in weight-bearing joints when a child is just learning to walk.

9. How do you treat acute hemarthrosis in a patient with hemophilia?

The mainstay of therapy for acute hemarthrosis in hemophilia is rapid replacement of deficient factors to achieve a level of ≥30%. A useful rule of thumb is that each international unit of virally inactivated plasma-derived or recombinant factor VIII (or IX) concentrate infused per kilogram of body weight causes a rise in factor levels by 2% or 2 IU/dL. In appropriate patients, factor replacement therapy can be promptly instituted by the family at the first symptoms of hemarthrosis to decrease the risks of sequelae. Factor concentrate is now screened for human immunodeficiency virus (HIV) and hepatitis B and C, making transmission of viral infections less of a risk for patients than in the past. Patient education and involvement are critical for the success of any treatment program. Other initial treatment consists of placing the joint at rest in as much extension as can be tolerated (to prevent contractures), with applications of ice packs and other local measures. Analgesics are given for pain. Mild compression bandaging may be useful. Some authors have advocated intraarticular glucocorticoids (GCs). Arthrocentesis, after appropriate factor replacement, may help relieve symptoms in selected patients. Once acute bleeding and pain are controlled, graded physical therapy to prevent muscle atrophy and contractures should be instituted.

10. When should septic arthritis be suspected if a patient with hemophilia develops acute monoarthritis?

The presence of blood in the joint can act as a culture medium. The presence of fever and/or if the pain of a suspected hemarthrosis fails to improve after factor replacement, concomitant septic arthritis must be suspected, and aspiration of the joint becomes mandatory. Notably, HIV infection in the setting of hemophilia is the most significant risk factor for septic arthritis. Any synovial fluid obtained on routine aspiration of a hemarthrosis should be submitted for Gram stain and culture. *Staphylococcus aureus* and *Streptococcus pneumoniae* are the most common organisms identified (Box 48.2).

BOX 48.2 Diagnostic Clues for Septic Arthritis Coexisting With Hemarthrosis

Failure of joint pain to resolve with factor replacement	Previous arthrocentesis in the same joint
Fever >38°C	Presence of arthroplasties
Peripheral leukocytosis	Underlying joint damage (chronic arthropathy)
HIV infection	Intravenous drug use

11. Do recurrent hemarthroses have any long-term consequences in patients with hemophilia?

As the patient approaches adulthood, acute hemarthroses become less frequent but chronic joint symptoms supervene. Recurrent hemarthroses lead to accumulation of hemosiderin in the joint lining tissues. The joint cartilage is degraded, and proliferative synovitis can develop, thought to occur due to local trauma as well as potentially locally generated inflammation. The end result is a chronically swollen joint, less painful than seen in acute hemarthroses, with decreased range of motion. Surrounding muscles become atrophic, and joint contracture is a frequent complication. Examination reveals bony enlargement, coarse crepitus, and deformity. Patients may be significantly disabled by chronic hemophilic arthropathy. The regular administration of factor replacement prophylactically has reduced the risk of developing subsequent chronic arthropathy. In hemophilia A, emicizumab (Hemlibra), the bispecific factor IXa- and factor X-directed monoclonal antibody, may be used for prophylactic therapy, avoiding the problems of risk of viral infections or inhibitor development that can occur with factor VIII replacement. Newer therapies that could potentially alter joint inflammation are also being evaluated.

12. Are there any characteristic radiographic findings in hemophilia?

Radiographs in acute hemarthrosis will be remarkable for soft tissue swelling, increased synovial density (iron deposition), and effusion. Chronic arthropathy of hemophilia may have both inflammatory (erosive) and degenerative features. Specific findings include proximal radial head enlargement, widening of the femoral and humeral intercondylar notches, talar flattening, and squaring of the inferior patella (Fig. 48.1). Point-of-care ultrasound is useful to detect early hemarthrosis but may not be as sensitive as MRI for other changes such as blood clots and synovial hypertrophy.

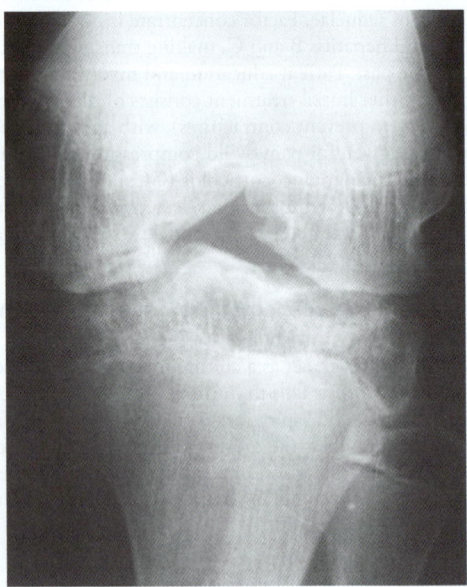

Fig. 48.1 Knee of a young patient with hemophilia. Note the degenerative and erosive changes of both femoral condyles and the tibial plateau.

13. What is the treatment of chronic hemophilic arthropathy?

The treatment principles for chronic hemophilic arthropathy are outlined in Box 48.3. Treatment programs must be individualized for each patient. Patients with complex arthropathy are frequently referred to specialized treatment centers.

BOX 48.3 Treatment Principles for Chronic Hemophilic Arthropathy

Prophylactic factor replacement therapy to prevent recurrences of hemarthrosis (factor goal >5%)
Non-weight-bearing rest periods to allow synovitis to regress
Physical therapy to improve joint stability and maintain muscle strength
Intraarticular glucocorticoids to reduce symptoms and recurrent hemarthroses
Nonacetylated salicylates or cox-2 specific inhibitors (celecoxib) for pain and swelling
Arthroscopic synovectomy for chronic synovitis unresponsive to conservative therapy
Total joint arthroplasty for end stage joint disease
Consider rifampicin chemical synoviorthesis (particularly small joints)
Consider radioisotope synovectomy (particularly if a factor inhibitor present) with P32 or 90-yttrium
Systemic and/or local anticytokine therapies are being evaluated

---

14. What rheumatologic manifestations can occur in patients with sickle cell disease (SCD)?

BOX 48.4 Rheumatologic Manifestations in Patients With Sickle Cell Disease

- Hand-foot syndrome (dactylitis)
- Bone infarction
- Osteonecrosis of bone
- Noninflammatory joint effusions adjacent to areas of bony crisis
- Chronic polyarthralgia
- Hyperuricemia and gout
- Hemarthrosis
- Septic arthritis
- Osteomyelitis
- Focal muscle necrosis
- Rhabdomyolysis

---

15. How does hand–foot syndrome present in a patient with SCD?

Hand–foot syndrome or sickle cell dactylitis is a problem typically seen in infants or children with SCD. Children present with bilateral acute pain and swelling diffusely in the fingers or toes, usually as a first manifestation of SCD. Fever and leukocytosis may accompany the dactylitis, but erythema typically does not. The etiology is thought to be local bone marrow ischemia. Subperiosteal new bone formation may be seen on radiographs of the metacarpal or metatarsal bones 2–5 weeks after the acute episode. Symptoms generally spontaneously subside in a few weeks.

16. What causes joint pain in patients with SCD?

Patients with SCD or less commonly the heterozygous state (sickle-β thalassemia, S-C, S-D disease) frequently experience polyarthralgias. Local sickling of cells leads to obstruction of the microcirculation and to bone infarctions. During painful crises, patients may experience chest, abdominal, back, muscle, and joint pain caused by microinfarctions. Diagnosis of SCD-related pain crisis is based on the patient's description of pain. Treatment of painful crises includes prompt parenteral opioids with or without nonsteroidal anti-inflammatory drugs. While hydration, oxygen, and red blood cell transfusions may be used, there are limited data to support their routine use. Hydroxyurea can reduce the frequency of painful crises and reduce mortality in SCD. Other musculoskeletal manifestations including painful large joint arthritis (usually the knees) often with noninflammatory synovial effusions lasting a few days to 3 weeks can also occur. These effusions are attributable to bone infarctions causing a "sympathetic" transudative effusion, which is typically unresponsive to intraarticular corticosteroids. Alternatively, some patients during an acute painful crisis will develop monoarticular or oligoarticular inflammatory arthritis that resolves within a week. Cultures and crystal examinations are negative. Finally, osteonecrosis of larger bones (frequently multifocal) such as the femoral or humeral head is seen in up to 40% of patients with SCD. Initially, radiographs may be normal. It may be difficult to distinguish among vaso-occlusive pain crisis, osteomyelitis, and osteonecrosis in some cases. MRI is the most sensitive method to detect both osteomyelitis and early osteonecrosis of the bone.

17. Name two characteristic radiographic findings that can be seen in the spine in patients with SCD.

Vertebral bodies can have a characteristic "Lincoln log" or H-shaped appearance owing to epiphyseal infarction from sickled cells causing endplate collapse. A second radiographic abnormality that may be observed is a central cup-like indentation ("codfish vertebrae") owing to osteoporotic weakness of the vertebrae caused by marrow expansion.

18. Can osteonecrosis of the femoral head be treated in the setting of SCD?

Treatment is challenging. An orthopedic surgeon should be consulted promptly. Radiographic staging can help guide initial treatment. Many patients may be managed conservatively at first, including being put on non-weight-bearing status along with pain management and physical therapy. Core decompression of the femoral head may be beneficial, though studies of its benefits in SCD are mixed. Prosthetic joint replacement is often the treatment when joint damage is advanced, although results are suboptimal. In a systematic review, total hip replacements for avascular necrosis of the femoral head in SCD had higher rates of surgical complications and revision rates than patients without SCD. Perioperative worsening of SCD is common and collaboration between specialists is recommended to optimize surgical outcomes.

19. Is gout seen frequently in SCD?

In children with SCD, hyperuricosuria without hyperuricemia occurs, probably as a result of increased red cell turnover associated with crises. Up to 40% of adult patients with SCD will have hyperuricemia caused by renal tubular damage with decreased uric acid excretion. However, gout is surprisingly uncommon. Occasionally gout may be seen; therefore, crystals should be looked for in joint effusions seen during SCD crisis.

20. What is the most common musculoskeletal infectious problem seen in SCD?

Osteomyelitis is seen much more frequently in SCD than in the general population. It is frequently multifocal. Because of functional asplenia, *Salmonella* infections account for 60% of osteomyelitis especially in children with SCD under 12 years of age. Fortunately, septic arthritis is less frequent but is usually caused by *S. aureus* or a gram-negative organism other than *Salmonella* when it occurs. The large proportion of gram-negative infections may be as a result of bacterial translocation across bowel mucosa that has been compromised by microinfarcts from sickling cells (Box 48.5).

BOX 48.5 Factors Predisposing Sickle Cell Disease Patients to Infection	
Functional asplenia with decreased clearance of bacteria	Decreased opsonization
Tissue damaged by crisis	Decreased interferon-γ production
Decreased neutrophil function at lower oxygen tensions	Increased risk of nosocomial infection

21. How does osteomyelitis present in SCD?

Presentation of osteomyelitis may be subtle, mimicking pain crisis or affecting multiple areas. Both pain crisis and osteomyelitis may present with bone pain, fever, and leukocytosis, and radiographs may be identical although patients with osteomyelitis have more severe symptoms. The patient's description of their pain and its similarity or not to prior pain crises may be helpful. Contrast-enhanced MRI can help differentiate between infection and infarction.

22. What is the management of suspected osteomyelitis in SCD?

The management of suspected osteomyelitis in SCD is similar to management of osteomyelitis in other patients, with the caveat that the causative organism is more likely to be *Salmonella*. There are no randomized trials to determine the antibiotic treatment approach. When possible, biopsy or aspiration should guide treatment, but empiric therapy can be prescribed. The optimal treatment duration is also not known, and a multidisciplinary treatment plan is recommended.

23. Do the other hemoglobinopathies have any rheumatologic manifestations?

Hemoglobin S-C disease and sickle-β thalassemia may develop similar manifestations to SCD, including hand–foot syndrome and gout. Osteonecrosis of bone has been reported in both conditions. Generally, rheumatologic manifestations are less common in these other hemoglobinopathies. There are case reports of osteonecrosis occurring in patients with sickle cell trait, but the incidence is the same as in age-matched controls with normal hemoglobin. Patients with β thalassemia major (Cooley's anemia) may develop arthropathy from marrow expansion, microfractures from osteoporosis, and scoliosis in patients surviving two decades. They do not get osteonecrosis. Chelation therapy with deferiprone (a second-line agent used to reduce iron overload from transfusions) can cause arthralgias in 20% of patients.

24. What are some rheumatic disease mimics associated with use of hydroxyurea?

Hydroxyurea is used in SCD to increase the levels of fetal hemoglobin; in addition, hydroxyurea is used for other hematologic conditions such as myelofibrosis and thrombocytosis. There are several rheumatic disease mimics associated with hydroxyurea, such as skin ulcers that are typically seen in the lower extremities and can mimic systemic vasculitis. Hydroxyurea has also been associated with development of a painful discoloration of the hands and feet (palmar-plantar erythrodysesthesia) that is also occasionally associated with blisters. It has also been associated with alopecia, and dermatomyositis-like and scleroderma-like syndromes. Treatment is typically withdrawal of hydroxyurea.

25. What autoimmune syndromes have been reported to occur in patients with a myelodysplastic syndrome (MDS)?

MDS is characterized by ineffective hematopoiesis, abnormal cell morphology, and propensity to develop acute leukemia. Autoimmunity and inflammation can occur in up to 25% of patients. The etiology is unclear but is possibly related to common pathways underlying both conditions. Autoimmune disorders reported in MDS include systemic vasculitis, connective tissue diseases, inflammatory polyarthritis, neutrophilic disorders (Sweet's syndrome or pyoderma gangrenosum), and other or unclassifiable autoimmune or inflammatory disorders. The recent discovery of the VEXAS syndrome may explain some of these clinical presentations (see Question 26). Some of these MDS patients (without VEXAS) improve considerably with glucocorticoids, which are often used in combination with conventional synthetic disease-modifying antirheumatic drugs (e.g., hydroxychloroquine, methotrexate) and occasionally biologics.

26. What are the rheumatologic manifestations of VEXAS syndrome?

VEXAS syndrome (acronym for **V**acuoles, **E**1 enzyme, **X**-linked, **A**utoinflammatory, **S**omatic) was reported in 2020 with mutation in the X-linked *UBA1* gene (encodes for ubiquitin-activating enzyme) as the underlying cause. Patients have a variety of hematologic manifestations that can include macrocytic anemia, vacuoles in myeloid and erythroid progenitor cells, thrombocytopenia, dysplastic bone marrow, and increased risk of hematologic malignancy including MDS. Rheumatologic manifestations reported in VEXAS include fever, vasculitis, chondritis (relapsing polychondritis), arthritis, alveolitis, uveitis/scleritis, and neutrophilic disorders (Sweet's syndrome). VEXAS may mimic or coexist with many rheumatologic conditions and should be included in the rheumatologist's differential diagnosis particularly in male patients over age 50 with autoinflammatory symptoms and an abnormal CBC with a high MCV >100fL and thrombocytopenia. The disease is refractory to most therapies and mortality is high. JAK inhibitors and allogeneic stem cell transplantation have had some success.

ACKNOWLEDGMENTS

The author would like to thank Dr. Kevin D. Deane (3rd and 4th editions) and Dr. Matthew T. Carpenter (1st and 2nd editions) for their contributions to this chapter in prior editions.

BIBLIOGRAPHY

Beck DB, Ferrada MA, Sikora KA, et al. Somatic mutations in UBA1 and severe adult-onset autoinflammatory disease. *N Engl J Med*. 2020;383:2628–2638.

Fassihi SC, Lee R, Quan T, Tran AA, Stake SN, Unger AS. Total hip arthroplasty in patients with sickle cell disease: a comprehensive systematic review. *J Arthroplasty*. 2020;35:2286–2295.

Gualtierotti R, Solimeno LP, Peyvandi F. Hemophilic arthropathy: current knowledge and future perspectives. *J Thromb Haemost*. 2021;19:2112–2121.

Hegeman EM, Bates T, Lynch T, Schmitz MR. Osteomyelitis in sickle cell anemia: does age predict risk of salmonella infection? *Pediatr Infect Dis J*. 2023;42:e262–e267.

Kavanagh PL, Fasipe TA, Wun T. Sickle cell disease: a review. *JAMA*. 2022;328:57–68.

Kotecha J, Gration B, Hunt BJ, Goodman AL, Malaiya R. The safety of continued oral anticoagulation therapy in joint injections and aspirations: a qualitative review of the current evidence. *J Clin Rheumatol*. 2022;28:223–228.

Marti-Carvajal A, Sola I, Agreda-Perez LH. Treatment for avascular necrosis of bone in people with sickle cell disease. *Cochrane Database Syst Rev*. 2019;12:CD004344.

Marti-Carvajal AJ, Agreda-Perez LH. Antibiotics for treating osteomyelitis in people with sickle cell disease. *Cochrane Database Syst Rev*. 2019;10:CD007175.

Seuser A, Djambas Khayat C, Negrier C, Sabbour A, Heijnen L. Evaluation of early musculoskeletal disease in patients with haemophilia: results from an expert consensus. *Blood Coagul Fibrinolysis*. 2018;29:509–520.

Tarar MY, Choo XY, Khan S. The risk of bleeding complications in intra-articular injections and arthrocentesis in patients on novel oral anticoagulants: a systematic review. *Cureus*. 2021;13:e17755.

Tarar MY, Malik RA, Charalambous CP. Bleeding complications in patients on warfarin undergoing joint injection/aspiration: systematic review and meta-analysis. *Rheumatol Int*. 2023;43:245–251.

Vanderhave KL, Perkins CA, Scannell B, Brighton BK. Orthopaedic manifestations of sickle cell disease. *J Am Acad Orthop Surg*. 2018;26:94–101.

Malignancy-Associated Rheumatic Disorders

Laura C. Cappelli, MD, MHS and Ami A. Shah, MD, MHS

CHAPTER 49

> **KEY POINTS**
>
> 1. The increased risk of lymphoma in rheumatoid arthritis, systemic lupus erythematosus, and Sjögren's syndrome is largely related to the disease activity of the rheumatic disease.
> 2. Unique autoantibodies associate with a significantly increased risk of concurrent malignancy in patients with new-onset idiopathic inflammatory myopathy (anti-transcription intermediary factor [TIF]-1 gamma or anti-nuclear matrix protein [NXP]-2) and systemic sclerosis (anti-RNA polymerase III).
> 3. When palmar fasciitis presents in a woman, consider ovarian carcinoma.
> 4. Leukocytoclastic vasculitis is the most common paraneoplastic vasculitis presentation.
> 5. Cancer therapies including immune checkpoint inhibitors can cause a variety of rheumatic syndromes.

1. What are the relationships between rheumatic disease and malignancy?

There are several important connections between autoimmune rheumatic diseases and malignancies. Rheumatic syndromes have been associated with increased risk for various malignancies; however, the types of associated cancer and strength of association vary by type of disease. Therefore, it is not recommended or cost effective to have an extensive search for occult malignancy with all rheumatic syndromes. Additionally, certain treatments for rheumatic disease may increase the risk for malignancy. Finally, immune checkpoint inhibitors, a type of cancer immunotherapy, can cause adverse events that are similar to rheumatic diseases.

2. What are potential mechanisms linking malignancy and rheumatic diseases or syndromes?

- Cancer secondary to rheumatic disease
  - Chronic inflammation or damage from rheumatic disease
  - Cytotoxic or biologic therapies
  - Inability to clear oncogenic infections
- Rheumatic disease or syndrome secondary to cancer
  - Direct tumor invasion of bones and joints.
  - Paraneoplastic rheumatic syndromes.
  - Rheumatic disease presenting concurrently with malignancy, potentially due to immune response to tumor antigens that are cross-reactive with normal tissues.
  - Worsening or development of rheumatic syndromes due to immune checkpoint inhibitor therapy used to treat malignancy.
  - Worsening or development of rheumatic syndromes due to chemotherapy used to treat malignancy.
  - Worsening or development of rheumatic syndromes due to radiation used to treat malignancy.
- Shared etiology
  - Common inciting exposure
  - Shared genetic susceptibility

3. What are the direct associations between musculoskeletal syndromes and malignancy?

Musculoskeletal symptoms can be directly related to pathologic mechanisms of the underlying tumor in metastatic disease, leukemia, lymphoma, and primary synovial and bone tumors. Bone metastases typically involve the long bones, spine, or pelvis and generally arise from breast, lung, and prostate more than kidney and thyroid neoplasms. The majority of skeletal metastases do not produce pain. Metastases or carcinomatous invasion of the synovium may rarely be the initial

489

manifestation of a malignancy. Large joints are most likely to be involved, with monoarthritis of the knee being the most common presentation. Metastases to joints distal to the elbows and knees are very rare and usually due to lung cancer. Severe joint pain, especially at night, with a noninflammatory (monoarticular predominance) or hemorrhagic joint effusion that rapidly reaccumulates after aspiration, should suggest carcinomatous invasion of the synovium. Synovial fluid cytology and/or synovial biopsy will be diagnostic.

4. Which malignancies are associated with preexisting CTD?

Malignancies associated with preexisting connective tissue diseases are outlined in Table 49.1.

5. Are autoantibodies related to the immune response to malignancy?

In DM/PM and systemic sclerosis, there are antibodies that are closely associated with malignancy in adults. Anti-TIF-1 gamma (anti-p155/140), anti-NXP-2 (anti-MJ; anti-p140), and anti-SAE autoantibodies in DM/PM and autoantibodies to RNA polymerase III and possibly anti-RNPC-3 in systemic sclerosis are associated with a higher risk of malignancy within a few years (before and after) of rheumatic disease onset. Prior studies have shown mutations in genes encoding autoantigens in tumors (e.g. TIF-1 gamma and RNA polymerase III) in patients with those autoantibodies and short-interval cancer. This indicates that the development of autoimmune disease in some patients may be related to an immune response to mutated tumor antigens that become cross-reactive.

TABLE 49.1 Preexisting CTD Associated With Malignancy

DISEASE (RISK)	MALIGNANCY	CLINICAL RISKS
Rheumatoid arthritis	Lymphoproliferative disorders (2–3 times increased risk) Lung cancer (1.5–2 times increased risk)	Longer disease duration, high disease activity, immunosuppression, Felty's syndrome
Systemic lupus erythematosus	Lymphoproliferative disorders (2–4 times increased risk) Cervical cancer	Adenopathy, ↑ spleen HPV-related
Discoid lupus	Squamous cell epithelioma	In plaques >20 years
Sjögren's syndrome	Lymphoproliferative disorders (15 times increased risk), hematologic malignancies	Palpable purpura, cutaneous ulcers, cryoglobulinemia, adenopathy, ↑ spleen, germinal centers MSG, low complement levels
Systemic sclerosis (1.4x)	Breast (within a short interval of SSc onset) Lung Hematologic Liver Bladder	Older age at onset, pulmonary fibrosis, Barrett's metaplasia, anti-RNA polymerase III antibodies
Dermatomyositis (3-7x)	Ovarian Oropharyngeal Breast Lung Colon	Older age, ulcerative skin lesions, anti-TIF1g, anti-NXP-2
Polymyositis (1.4-2x)	Ovarian Oropharyngeal Breast Lung Colon	PM < DM
ANCA vasculitis (1.6-2x)	Bladder cancer, lymphoproliferative disorders	Some due to cyclophosphamide
Eosinophilic fasciitis (10% have cancer)	Lymphoproliferative disorders	Aplastic anemia, thrombocytopenia

ANCA, Antineutrophil cytoplasmic antibody; *HPV*, human papillomavirus; *MSG*, minor salivary gland biopsy.

6. What are the risks for malignancy in patients with inflammatory myopathies and how should this risk be managed?

Patients with DM and PM have an increased risk (3–7 times for DM and 1.4–2 times for PM) for malignancy. The risk of malignancy is also increased in patients with amyopathic DM (normal levels of creatine phosphokinase, aldolase may be elevated). The diagnosis of a malignancy may precede, coincide with, or occur after DM/PM is diagnosed. The peak incidence of a cancer diagnosis is within the first year of PM/DM diagnosis. After 5 years, the malignancy risk decreases to near baseline. The most common malignancies are ovarian, lung, breast, colon, pancreas, bladder, hematopoietic/lymphoma, melanoma, esophageal, and cervix accounting for 70% of cases in Western populations, whereas nasopharyngeal malignancies are most common in Asian populations. Patients with antisynthetase antibodies, interstitial lung disease, inclusion body myositis, or children with DM rarely have an associated malignancy. Patients can be divided by risk according to their autoantibodies, age (>45 years), gender (male), presence of skin disease (particularly cutaneous ulcers), dysphagia, and resistance to immunosuppressive treatment. Cancer risk is increased in patients with antibodies to TIF-1 gamma (anti-p155/140), NXP-2 (anti-MJ/anti-p140), or SAE. All patients with myositis should update basic cancer screening as is age and sex appropriate per country of residence recommendations. For patients with moderate to high risk of malignancy, enhanced cancer screening at the time of diagnosis may include CT of the neck, thorax, abdomen and pelvis, cervical cancer screening, PSA, mammography, CA-125 blood test, pelvic ultrasound, fecal occult blood testing, colonoscopy, and SPEP/UPEP/free light chains. An FDG-PET/CT scan should be considered to screen for occult malignancy in patients with cancer-associated myositis-specific autoantibodies (e.g., anti-TIF-1 gamma, anti-NXP-2). Screening may be repeated 1 to 3 years from diagnosis in high-risk individuals. Other subsequent evaluations should be driven by the patient's risk factors and clinical symptoms.

7. How do you approach cancer screening for patients with systemic sclerosis?

Patients with systemic sclerosis and particular autoantibodies or clinical features have an increased risk of certain malignancies. For patients with RNA polymerase III antibodies and diffuse cutaneous involvement, there is an increased risk of breast, tongue, and prostate cancer, while those with anti-RNA pol III antibodies and limited skin involvement may have a higher risk of lung cancer. There are no high-quality data to guide screening strategies in these groups of patients, but grounding suspicion in known associations can be helpful when deciding to do additional imaging. There are other groups, like those with anti-centromere antibodies, who may have a lower risk for cancer than the general population and require only age- and sex-appropriate screening.

8. What is the risk of lymphoma in Sjogren's syndrome?

Non-Hodgkin's lymphoma can be increased as much as 15 times the rate of the general population in patients with Sjogren's syndrome. This is primarily driven by mucosa-associated lymphoid tissue (MALT lymphoma) but can be found in other body sites. As detailed in Table 49.1, certain clinical features like palpable purpura, cutaneous ulcers, cryoglobulinemia, adenopathy, and low complement are associated with higher risk of lymphoma.

9. Is polymyalgia rheumatica (PMR) a paraneoplastic syndrome?

The risk of malignancy in PMR has been debated previously. Contradictory findings were reported in earlier studies. Mainly relying on large databases, some authors report that for the first 6 to 12 months after diagnosis of PMR, the malignancy risk is increased. A population-based cohort found no difference in the cumulative risk of cancer in patients with PMR after 10 years of follow-up. In those with atypical symptoms for PMR (poor response to steroids, asymmetric involvement, adenopathy), an appropriate malignancy workup is recommended. For patients with typical PMR presentations, no malignancy evaluation is required beyond age- and sex-appropriate cancer screening.

10. What musculoskeletal paraneoplastic syndromes are associated with malignancy?

Musculoskeletal paraneoplastic syndromes that are associated with malignancies are outlined in Table 49.2.

TABLE 49.2 Musculoskeletal Paraneoplastic Syndrome Associated With Malignancy

PARANEOPLASTIC SYNDROME	MALIGNANCY	CLINICAL ASSOCIATION
Arthropathy		
Hypertrophic osteoarthropathy	Various types	Lung cancer (non-small cell) is most common
Amyloidosis	Multiple myeloma	25% of primary amyloidosis is associated with multiple myeloma
Secondary gout	Myeloproliferative disorders	Tumor lysis syndrome
Carcinomatous polyarthritis	Solid tumor or hematologic disorders	80% of women have breast cancer
Atypical polymyalgia rheumatica	Renal, lung, colon, myeloma	Unresponsive to corticosteroids after 6 months
Remitting seronegative symmetric synovitis with pitting edema (RS3PE) (16–30% have cancer)	Several tumors	Rapid onset wrist, hand arthritis with edema. May have fever. Poor response to prednisone
Vascular		
Vasculitis	Lymphoproliferative, various types	Cutaneous >> systemic vasculitis
Polyarteritis nodosa	Hairy-cell leukemia	Polyarteritis-like clinically and by arteriography
Digital necrosis	Solid, lymphoproliferative	Severe or asymmetric Raynaud's syndrome onset after the age of 50 years
Cryoglobulinemia	Plasma cell dyscrasias, non-Hodgkin's lymphoma	Purpura, digital ischemia, renal/pulmonary involvement
Cutaneous		
Sweet's syndrome	Leukemia (acute myeloid leukemia), others	Associated with malignancy in 15%
Palmar fasciitis and polyarthritis (80% have cancer)	Ovarian, breast, gastric, pancreatic	Progressive fibrosis and contractures
Panniculitis	Hematologic > pancreatic	Subcutaneous nodules and arthritis, eosinophilia
Erythromelalgia (<10% have cancer)	Myeloproliferative disorders	Severe burning pain, erythema, and warmth primarily in feet
Multicentric reticulohistiocytosis	Adenocarcinoma, ovarian, lung, others	Associated with malignancy in 30%
Miscellaneous		
Pyogenic arthritis	Colon cancer, multiple myeloma	Intestinal flora cultured, rare cause of primary septic arthritis
Antiphospholipid antibodies	Solid tumors, lymphoproliferative	Association with thrombosis is unclear
Oncogenic osteomalacia	Solid tumors; tumors of mesenchymal origin	Bone pain, muscle weakness low phosphorous, elevated FGF23 Octreotide scan to localize tumor

ANA, Antinuclear antibody; *EBV,* Epstein–Barr virus; *RNAP III,* RNA polymerase III.

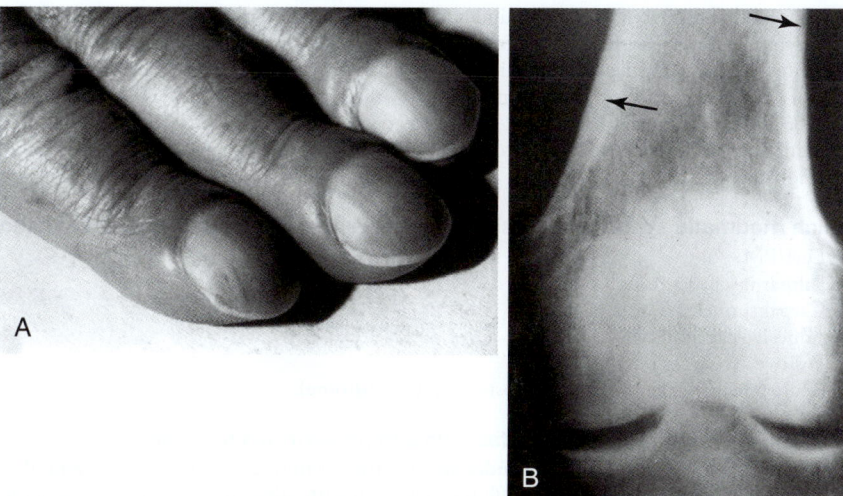

Fig. 49.1 (A) Clubbing of fingers. Soft tissue proliferation of the nail bed and distal tissues of the digits is seen. Usually, the nail makes an angle of 20 degrees or more with the projected line of the digit. When clubbing occurs, subungual proliferation causes diminution of the angle. (B) Roentgenogram of the knee shows subperiosteal new bone formation of the lower femoral shafts (*arrows*). New bone is separated from the old cortex by a radiolucent line (right); a later subperiosteal lesion is seen (left). (Copyright 2014 American College of Rheumatology. Used with permission.)

11. What is hypertrophic osteoarthropathy (HOA)?

HOA is a syndrome that includes (1) clubbing of fingers and toes, (2) periostitis of tubular bones, and (3) arthritis with a noninflammatory synovial fluid (Fig. 49.1). Primary HOA (pachydermo-periostosis) is autosomal dominant, appears during childhood mostly in males (M:F ratio, 9:1), and is characterized by clubbing, skin hypertrophy (pachyderma), coarse facial features, seborrhea, and hyperhidrosis. Secondary HOA may be limited to clubbing or include the full spectrum of symptoms. The generalized form is most often associated with intrathoracic malignant neoplasms in 90% of cases. It also occurs in patients with other malignancies, chronic infections (lung, sub-acute bacterial endocarditis, human immunodeficiency virus, others), cystic fibrosis, congenital cyanotic heart disease, inflammatory bowel disease, cirrhosis, Graves' disease, or on certain drugs (voriconazole). The clinical course of secondary HOA is determined by the underlying primary disease. Zoledronic acid can help symptoms, but successful treatment of the primary disease may lead to resolution of secondary HOA. Platelet/endothelial cell activation with the release of vascular endothelial growth factor and platelet-derived growth factor appears to play a key role in the etiology of HOA, which may be targets for future treatment.

12. What is paraneoplastic (carcinomatous) polyarthritis?

Polyarthritis rarely (<2%) presents in close temporal relationship (<1 year) to a diagnosis of cancer and may be associated with a variety of malignancies. Paraneoplastic polyarthritis should be strongly suspected in a patient with the following features: explosive onset of an asymmetric oligoarthritis or polyarthritis; late age of onset; predominant lower extremity involvement; sparing of the wrists and small hand joints; and absence of rheumatoid factor and anti-CCP, erosions, or rheumatoid nodules. Radiographs are normal and do not show periosteal reaction. Arthritis symptoms can improve with successful treatment of the malignancy.

13. Vasculitis occurs as a paraneoplastic syndrome with which malignancies?

Vasculitis rarely occurs in association with cancer. It is more likely to occur with lymphoproliferative or myeloproliferative disorder and may also be associated with solid tumors. Cutaneous leukocytoclastic vasculitis is the most frequent paraneoplastic presentation. Henoch–Schönlein purpura, medium-vessel vasculitis, and granulomatous vasculitis have been described. A polyarteritis nodosa-like vasculitis has been described most commonly in patients with hairy-cell leukemia and infrequently in other malignancies. Vasculitis may precede, coincide with, or follow the malignancy diagnosis.

A broad differential of vasculitis mimics including **Sweet's syndrome** and **VEXAS** (vacuoles, E1 enzyme, X-linked, autoinflammatory, somatic) should be considered. Sweet's syndrome is also known as acute febrile neutrophilic dermatosis and is associated with malignancy in 10% to 15% of patients. Sweet's is most commonly seen with acute myelogenous leukemia but has been described with many malignancies. In VEXAS, patients may have a variety of clinical findings reflecting the autoinflammatory syndrome; 30–50% of patients have an associated myelodysplastic syndrome.

14. Which rheumatic syndromes or signs have been described with ovarian carcinoma?
- DM/PM.
- Palmar fasciitis and polyarthritis.
- Carpal tunnel syndrome.
- Adhesive capsulitis.
- Positive ANA.
- Acute febrile neutrophilic dermatosis (Sweet's syndrome).

15. Describe the features of palmar fasciitis and polyarthritis syndrome.
Palmar fasciitis and polyarthritis syndrome (aka palmar fibromatosis) is most commonly associated with ovarian carcinoma, although it can be seen with other malignancies (breast, stomach, pancreas, lung, prostate, and colon). It is characterized by progressive, symmetric contractures of the digits, palmar fascia fibrosis, pain, and vasomotor instability similar to complex regional pain syndrome (CRPS). Symmetric polyarthritis can accompany the fibrosis. Progressive changes lead to a "woody hands" texture and appearance. Plantar fasciitis with lower extremity involvement can occur in some cases.

Histologic examination of the involved tissues reveals extensive fibrosis with increased fibroblast and mononuclear cell infiltration. There is no evidence of collagen deposition. Deposits of IgG in the palmar fascia and the presence of low-titer ANAs in some patients suggest an immunopathologic mechanism. Treatment response with chemotherapy, NSAIDs, corticosteroids, ganglionic blockade, and/or physical therapy is usually poor. Successful removal of the underlying tumor may result in dramatic clinical improvement of the palmar fasciitis syndrome.

16. What are the musculoskeletal features of leukemia and lymphoma?
Leukemia can present as a symmetric, asymmetric, or migratory polyarthritis or as bone pain. It can be the presenting manifestation in up to 6% of patients with childhood leukemia. Articular manifestations in acute leukemia occur in approximately 14% to 50% of children (acute lymphoblastic leukemia is most common) and 4% to 16% of adults. Joint pain typically involves the ankle, shoulder, or knee and has been attributed to leukemic synovial infiltration. Bone pain due to subperiosteal infiltration occurs in up to 50% of patients. Long bone pain is more common in children, whereas back pain is more common in adults. The joint and bone pain may be out of proportion to the clinical findings and may be nocturnal. Children may be initially diagnosed with juvenile idiopathic arthritis given the severity of the arthritic symptoms. Synovial effusions are uncommon, mildly inflammatory, and leukemic cells are rare. Hemorrhage into the joint can occur. Plain radiographs are normal in 50% at the onset of the bone pain, but bone scintigraphy will detect involvement early. Metaphyseal rarefaction and osteolytic lesions are characteristic radiographic findings. The diagnosis is confirmed by bone marrow and/or synovial biopsy. The joint or bone pain is optimally treated with systemic chemotherapy. Adults with acute myelogenous leukemia can mimic adult-onset Still's disease in their presentation.

Up to 25% of patients with non-Hodgkins lymphoma can have musculoskeletal symptoms, with bone pain being the most common. Lymphomatous arthritis is rare but should be suspected in patients with constitutional symptoms out of proportion to the severity of the arthritis. The diagnosis is confirmed by bone or synovial biopsy. Angioimmunoblastic T-cell lymphoma can be mistaken for an autoimmune disease. It typically presents with constitutional symptoms, fever, rash (maculopapular or urticarial), lymphadenopathy, and hepatosplenomegaly. Arthritis, vasculitis, Coombs-positive hemolytic anemia, and polyclonal gammopathy can also occur.

Notably, patients with hematologic malignancies can develop secondary gout, especially on initiation of chemotherapy. Septic arthritis can also occur. Consequently, all acute arthritic attacks should have the joint aspirated and the synovial fluid sent for cell count, crystals, Gram stain, and culture.

17. What is Schnitzler's syndrome?

Schnitzler's syndrome is an autoinflammatory disease that typically affects individuals over the age of 40 years. Patients typically present with a nonpruritic chronic recurring urticarial rash with individual lesions lasting 24–48 hours. Skin biopsy shows a neutrophilic dermal infiltrate. All patients have a monoclonal gammopathy, typically IgM-κ light-chain type. Other manifestations can include recurrent fever, bone or joint pain (55–75%), lymphadenopathy, and hepatosplenomegaly. A somatic mutation in *MYD88* L265P is found in 30% of patients, putting them at risk for developing lymphoplasmacytic lymphoma, which occurs in 15–20% of patients typically 10 years or more after disease onset. Interleukin-1 inhibitors have been successful in treating the autoinflammatory symptoms of Schnitzler's syndrome.

18. List immunomodulatory drugs used to treat CTD and their potential malignancies.

A list of immunomodulatory drugs used in the treatment of autoimmune rheumatic diseases and their association with malignancies is presented in Table 49.3.

19. Do biologic disease-modifying antirheumatic drugs (bDMARDs) or targeted synthetic DMARD (tsDMARDs) used to treat rheumatic diseases cause malignancy?

There were initial concerns about bDMARDs and increased risk of a variety of cancers. Now there have been large observational studies of tens of thousands of patients to assess risk. No increased risk was found for melanoma or lymphoma in patients with RA treated with TNF inhibitors versus those treated with other agents. Similarly, there seems to be no increased risk of cancer recurrence when patients with RA are treated with TNF inhibitors vs csDMARDs or rituximab.

A post-marketing study (ORAL Surveillance) has shown a possible increased risk of cancer for patients with RA treated with the JAK-inhibitor (JAK-i), tofacitinib, as compared to TNF-inhibitor therapy. A recent meta-analysis of all JAK-i trials (phase 2, 3, 4, long-term extension) across all clinical indications supported an increased cancer risk for JAK-i compared with anti-TNF therapy. However, JAK-i use was not significantly associated with any greater cancer risk than methotrexate, suggesting anti-TNF therapy may be protective rather than JAK-i causing cancer. Certainly, more studies across JAK-inhibitors are needed to evaluate this risk, but it is important

TABLE 49.3 Immunomodulatory Drugs/Agents Used in the Treatment of Rheumatic Diseases and Their Association With Malignancies

TREATMENT	MALIGNANCIES
Hydroxychloroquine	None
Sulfasalazine	None
Methotrexate	NMSC
Leflunomide	None
Azathioprine	Cutaneous squamous cell carcinoma
Cyclosporine	Risk for EBV-associated lymphoma; NMSC
JAK-inhibitors	Solid and hematologic cancers (controversial) NMSC
TNF-inhibitors	NMSC
Mycophenolate mofetil	Possible risk for lymphoproliferative disorders, NMSC
Cyclophosphamide (intravenous)	Small risk for lymphoma or bladder cancer
Cyclophosphamide (oral)	Bladder carcinoma (2–4 ×), non-Hodgkin's lymphoma, leukemia, NMSC

NMSC: non-melanoma skin cancer

information to consider and discuss this potential risk with patients as a part of shared decision making.

The risk for non-melanoma skin cancer is increased by treatment with several types of immunosuppression including TNF-inhibitors and JAK-inhibitors. Counseling about sun protection and having yearly skin examinations to evaluate for malignancy is important for these patients.

20. Can cancer therapies cause musculoskeletal syndromes?

- **Post-chemotherapy MSK symptoms:** myalgias and migratory arthralgias can occur in some patients 1 to 3 months after therapy for carcinoma of breast, ovary, or non-Hodgkin's lymphoma. This usually resolves within 1 year.
- **Aromatase inhibitors (AIs):** arthralgias and joint stiffness occur in up to 50% of breast cancer patients treated with aromatase inhibitors. Symptoms tend to occur within 1 to 3 months of starting therapy and commonly affect hands, wrists, and knees. Magnetic resonance imaging may show intraarticular fluid and tenosynovitis in the hands. NSAIDs are of limited benefit. Changing to an alternate AI may reduce the symptoms. Patients unable to tolerate an AI may be able to tolerate tamoxifen as an alternative, which can cause fewer musculoskeletal symptoms.
- **Bleomycin:** may cause Raynaud's and systemic sclerosis.
- **Taxanes:** can cause arthralgias, myalgias, and skin rash similar to subacute cutaneous lupus in breast cancer–treated patients.
- **Interferon-α:** can cause arthralgias, positive autoantibodies, systemic lupus erythematosus-like syndrome, and autoimmune thyroid disease.
- **Gemcitabine:** can cause systemic sclerosis-like illness with critical digital ischemia.
- **Hydroxyurea:** can cause a dermatomyositis-like rash.
- **Radiation:** head and neck radiation can cause xerostomia, which could be confused with Sjogren's syndrome. Radiation may also lead to fibrosing syndromes such as morphea. There has been concern that radiation could exacerbate systemic sclerosis given the association with morphea, but studies have shown that skin fibrosis has primarily been limited to the irradiated area rather than distant sites.

21. Describe how immune checkpoint inhibitors (ICIs) cause rheumatic symptoms.

ICIs are an increasingly used type of cancer immunotherapy. There are a wide variety of indications, and ICIs are being used in the adjuvant setting for earlier stage disease than previously. Immune checkpoints regulate the function of the immune system through inhibition of stimulation. Tumors activate checkpoints to decrease natural antitumor function. ICIs inhibit checkpoints (PD-1, PD-L1, CTLA-4, LAG-3) to enhance T-cell activity and promote the antitumor response. While ICIs have been effective anticancer therapy, overactivation of the immune system can lead to inflammatory syndromes called immune-related adverse events (irAEs) that can affect almost any organ (gastrointestinal, pulmonary, cardiac, dermatologic, endocrine, neurologic, and renal). Several rheumatic irAEs have been reported, including arthralgias, myalgias, inflammatory arthritis, vasculitis (including giant cell arteritis), sicca syndrome, myositis, PMR, eosinophilic fasciitis, sarcoidosis, and a scleroderma-like disease. These rheumatic syndromes can occur early or late in therapy, can be severe, may persist after ICI therapy is stopped, and often require immunosuppressive therapy including glucocorticoids, conventional synthetic DMARDs, bDMARDs (anti-TNF agents, tocilizumab), and/or intravenous immunoglobulin (IVIG). Patients with severe and persistent symptoms may require temporary or permanent cessation of the ICI. Treatment decisions require collaboration with the patient's oncologist. For moderate or severe events, corticosteroid therapy is the first line for most irAEs. Many trials of ICIs required prednisone dose to be <10 mg/day before administering ICIs so as not to interfere with the effectiveness of the therapy. If needed, the use of bDMARDs for a short time period does not appear to worsen the cancer or lessen its response to ICI therapy. Less is known about long-term therapy with immunosuppression. Importantly, patients with a preexisting rheumatic disease who develop cancer should not be denied ICI therapy outright because of concern for flare-up of the underlying disease. Rather, careful monitoring and multidisciplinary care and communication can lead to successful treatment of patients with preexisting autoimmune disease and cancer with ICI therapy.

ACKNOWLEDGMENT

The author would like to thank Dr. Jeanne Tofferi and Dr. Daniel Battafarano for their contributions to this chapter in the previous edition.

BIBLIOGRAPHY

Calabrese LH, Calabrese C, Cappelli LC. Rheumatic immune-related adverse events from cancer immunotherapy. *Nat Rev Rheumatol.* 2018;14:569–579.

Cappelli LC, Shah AA. The relationships between cancer and autoimmune rheumatic diseases. *Best Pract Res Clin Rheumatol.* 2020;34:101472.

Igusa T, Hummers LK, Visvanathan K, et al. Autoantibodies and scleroderma phenotype define subgroups at high-risk and low-risk for cancer. *Ann Rheum Dis.* 2018;77:1179–1186.

Joseph CG, Darrah E, Shah AA. Association of the autoimmune disease scleroderma with an immunologic response to cancer. *Science.* 2014;343:152–157.

Lin C-H, Huston DP. Collecting puzzle pieces. *N Engl J Med.* 2023;389:2189–2195.

Malcovati L. VEXAS: walking on the edge of malignancy. *Blood.* 2023;142:214–215.

Martinez-Lavin M, Vargas A, Rivera-Vinas M. Hypertrophic osteoarthropathy: a palindrome with a pathogenic connotation. *Curr Opin Rheumatol.* 2008;20:88–91.

Mecoli CA, Igusa T, Chen M, et al. Subsets of idiopathic inflammatory myositis enriched for contemporaneous cancer relative to the general population. *Arthritis Rheumatol.* 2023;75:620–629.

Mercer LK, Askling J, Raaschou P, et al. Risk of invasive melanoma in patients with rheumatoid arthritis treated with biologics: results from a collaborative project of 11 European biologic registers. *Ann Rheum Dis.* 2017;76:386–391.

Mercer LK, Galloway JB, Lunt M, et al. Risk of lymphoma in patients exposed to antitumour necrosis factor therapy: results from the British Society for Rheumatology Biologics Register for Rheumatoid Arthritis. *Ann Rheum Dis.* 2017;76:497–503.

Muller S, Hider S, Belcheret, et al. Is cancer associated with polymyalgia rheumatica? A cohort study in the general practice research database. *Ann Rheum Dis.* 2014;73:1769–1773.

Oldroyd AGS, Allard AB, Callen JP, et al. A systematic review and meta-analysis to inform cancer screening guidelines in idiopathic inflammatory myopathies. *Rheumatology (Oxford).* 2021;60:2615–2628.

Pinal-Fernandez I, Ferrer-Fabregas B, Trallero-Araguas E, et al. Malignancy and the risks of biologic therapy: current status. *Rheum Dis Clin North Am.* 2017;43:43–46.

Ramos-Casals M, Siso-Almirall A. Immune-related Adverse Events of Immune Checkpoint Inhibitors. *Ann Int Med.* 2024;177:ITC 17-32.

Russell MD, Stovin C, Alveyn E, et al. JAK inhibitors and the risk of malignancy: a meta-analysis across disease indications. *Ann Rheum Dis.* 2023;82:1059–1067.

Shah A, Casciola-Rose L, Rosen A. Cancer-induced autoimmunity in the rheumatic disease. *Arthritis Rheum.* 2015;67:317–326.

Ytterberg SR, Bhatt DL, Mikuls TR, et al. ORAL surveillance investigators. Cardiovascular and cancer risk with tofacitinib in rheumatoid arthritis. *N Engl J Med.* 2022;386:316–326.

FURTHER READING

Drug Safety information obtained from:Lexicomp Online. *Pediatric and Neonatal Lexi-Drugs Online*. Hudson, Ohio: Wolters Kluwer Clinical Drug Information, Inc.; 1978–2018 Accessed June 3, 2018.

CHAPTER 50

Osteoarthritis

Carly A. Wanglin, MD and Larry W. Moreland, MD

≫ KEY POINTS

1. Osteoarthritis (OA) is the most common articular disorder.
2. OA most commonly affects the distal interphalangeal (DIP) joints, proximal interphalangeal (PIP) joints, first carpometacarpal (CMC) joints, hips, knees, first metatarsophalangeal (MTP) joint, cervical spine, and lumbosacral spine.
3. OA is a clinical diagnosis based on radiographic findings and symptoms including dull joint pain, joint stiffness, bony enlargement, joint swelling, and/or joint instability.
4. OA is a complex disease to manage as no disease-modifying therapies exist.
5. The two major indications for joint replacement include pain unresponsive to medical therapy and loss of joint function.

---

1. What is osteoarthritis?

OA is a slowly progressive degenerative disease, often referred to as "wear and tear" arthritis. It begins as a preclinical condition and can become very advanced prior to symptom onset, as the affected cartilage is avascular and not innervated. Thus, the disease is heterogenous in its pathology and presentation, and predicting clinical trajectories is difficult. However, as the continuum of cellular change from pre-OA to severe OA progresses, patients typically experience joint pain and a loss of joint function.

2. What are the epidemiologic features of primary OA?

- More common with increasing age
- Relatively more common in men than in women aged <45 years and more common in women than men aged >45 years
- An estimated 20 to 30% of the adult population experience symptomatic OA in at least one joint
- Symptomatic knee OA in 7–17% and hip OA in 10% of those aged >45 years
- Radiographic knee, hip, and hand OA in 14–37%, 10%, and 35–45% of adults >45 years, respectively

PEARL: Radiographic OA is at least twice more common than symptomatic OA. Radiographic OA changes do not reliably correlate with OA symptoms.

3. What pathophysiology drives the development of OA?

The pathogenesis of OA is poorly understood. Repetitive trauma to articular cartilage may lead to damage and subsequent activation of the innate immune system (via release of damage-associated molecular patterns). This tends to occur in joints that bear excessive loads, such as lower extremity joints, or are used repetitively, like hand joints. Alternatively, OA may develop under normal loads if the underlying cartilage, bone, synovium, or supporting ligaments and muscles are abnormal (secondary OA; see Question 15).

4. What are the pathologic features of OA?

The following steps of pathologic progression explain the joint space narrowing, subchondral sclerosis, cysts/geodes, and osteophytes seen on radiographs in patients with OA (Fig. 50.1):

Early:
- Swelling of articular cartilage
- Loosening of collagen framework

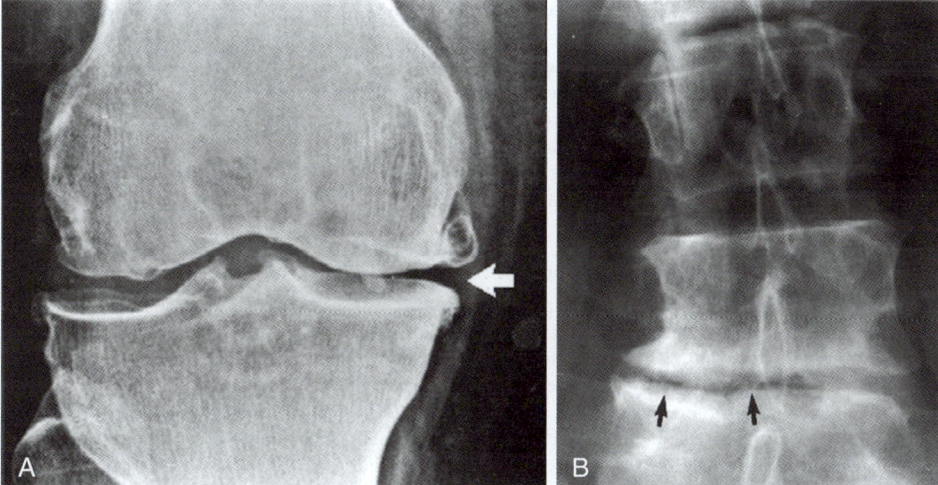

Fig. 50.1 (A) Radiograph of knee osteoarthritis showing sclerosis, cysts, osteophytes, and medial joint space narrowing *(arrow)*. (B) Anterior radiograph of the lumbar spine with disc disease/osteoarthritis. Note disc space narrowing, osteophytes, and vacuum sign *(arrows)*.

- Chondrocytes increase proteoglycan synthesis but also release more degradative enzymes
- Increased cartilage water content

Later:
- Degradative enzymes break down proteoglycan faster than it can be produced by chondrocytes, resulting in diminished proteoglycan content in cartilage
- Articular cartilage thins and softens (joint space narrowing on radiographs will be seen eventually), resulting in fissuring and cracking in cartilage
- Cartilage repair is attempted but inadequate
- Underlying bone is exposed, allowing synovial fluid to be forced into the bone by the weight and pressure across the joint. This shows up as subchondral cysts or geodes on radiographs.
- Remodeling and hypertrophy of the subchondral bone results in subchondral sclerosis and osteophyte ("spur") formation.

5. What are the clinical signs and symptoms of OA?

On history, patients describe dull joint pain that worsens with activity, stiffness after prolonged immobility (gelling), and/or a creaking, sandy or gritty sensation in the joints. On physical examination, crepitus, bony enlargement, and mild effusions (especially in the knees) may be noted. Joint instability and periarticular muscle atrophy are common.

6. How does OA differ from inflammatory arthritis?

Although there is some inflammation within and surrounding the joint space in OA, it is not a classic "inflammatory arthritis," as the arthritis is not driven by immune system overactivity. Inflammatory arthritis classically presents as red, hot, swollen joints, whereas joints with OA are often quite painful and may have a small effusion but do not typically develop the same degree of warmth and erythema. Inflammatory arthritis is often accompanied by signs and symptoms of systemic inflammation such as fatigue and cognitive dysfunction, which are absent in OA. Morning stiffness is brief (<30 minutes) in OA in comparison to stiffness due to inflammatory arthritis (which lasts >30 minutes). Of note, longstanding inflammatory arthritis can lead to secondary OA, and it is important to determine the etiology of a painful joint in this setting (ongoing inflammatory arthritis versus secondary OA) to ensure proper treatment.

7. What are the risk factors for the development of OA?

- Age: strongest risk factor associated with OA.
- Heredity: family risk studies estimate a 50% to 65% heritable component in primary OA.

- Sex: prevalence of OA increases in women after the age of 50 years.
- Obesity (see Question 8)
- Previous joint trauma: meniscal and ligament injuries as well as fractures can lead to altered joint biomechanics and articular incongruence leading to OA.
- Abnormal joint mechanics (e.g., excessive knee varus or valgus; hip dysplasia).
- Smoking (may contribute to degenerative disc disease).
- Certain occupations/sports causing repetitive high-impact loading: pneumatic drill operators (shoulders, elbows), ballet dancers (ankles), boxers (MCP joints), basketball players (knees, ankles), and others.

8. How does obesity predispose to OA?

Obesity is a risk factor for OA development for two reasons: (1) increased loads, especially over lower extremity joints; and (2) activation of proinflammatory cytokines. Studies of the knee show that the risk of knee OA increases by 36% for every 5 kg of weight gain. Conversely, it decreases by 50% for every 5 kg of weight loss in obese patients. Adipose tissue may serve as a source of proinflammatory cytokines, such as leptin, adiponectin, resistin, interleukin (IL)-1, IL-6, and tumor necrosis factor (TNF)-α that can further contribute to joint damage, even in non-weight-bearing joints. This may explain the increased risk for OA in women who have a higher percentage of adipose tissue and the association between obesity and non-weight-bearing DIP joints of the hands. The evidence for an association between obesity and OA is strongest for knee and hand OA.

9. Name the joints typically involved in primary (idiopathic) OA.

- DIP joints of the hands
- PIP joints of the hands
- First CMC joints of the hands
- Acromioclavicular joint of shoulder
- Hips
- Knees
- First MTP joints of the feet
- Facet (apophyseal) joints of the cervical spine and lumbosacral spine

10. Name joints not typically involved in primary OA.

- Wrists
- Elbows
- Shoulders (glenohumeral joint)
- Ankles
- MCP joints of the hands
- Second to fifth MTP joints of the feet

PEARL: Involvement of these atypical joints should prompt a search for inflammatory or secondary causes of OA (see Question 18).

11. Where do Heberden nodes and Bouchard nodes occur?

Bony articular nodules (osteophytes or "spurs") located on the DIP joints are called **Heberden** nodes, whereas those located on the PIP joints are called **Bouchard** nodes (Fig. 50.2). Both can occur on the fingers and toes. Palmar and lateral deviation of the distal phalanx as a result of these nodules is not uncommon. Heberden nodes are 10 times more frequent in women than in men. The tendency to develop Heberden nodes may be familial, with one estimate suggesting that a woman whose mother has Heberden nodes is twice as likely to develop similar joint changes as a woman without such a family history. The clinical importance of Heberden and Bouchard nodes is that they usually signify that the patient has primary nodal OA and does not have a secondary etiology for the OA.

12. Are laboratory studies helpful in evaluating OA?

Routine labs aren't recommended if clinical suspicion is high for OA based on history, lack of systemic symptoms, distribution of involved joints and physical exam. If the diagnosis is unclear or labs are ordered for other reasons, results that should be notably normal in OA include erythrocyte sedimentation rate (ESR), rheumatoid factor (RF) and anti-cyclic citrullinated peptide antibody (anti-CCP), and ANA.

If synovial fluid is evaluated, findings should include:

- Normal viscosity with good string sign
- Clear or yellow in color
- WBC <1000
- No crystals
- Negative culture

13. What are the classic radiographic findings in OA?

General abnormal findings

- Joint space narrowing that is nonuniform
- Osteophytes (bone spurs)
- Subchondral sclerosis
- Malalignment

Joint-specific abnormal findings

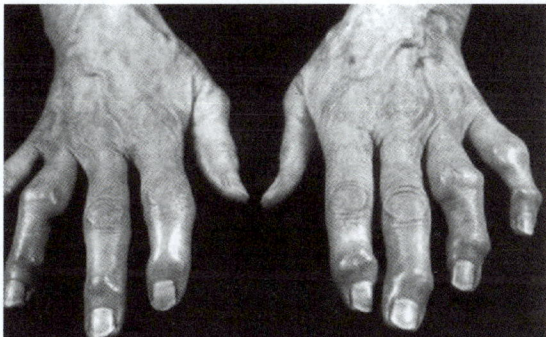

Fig. 50.2 Heberden (distal interphalangeal joints) nodes and Bouchard (proximal interphalangeal joints) nodes in a woman with osteoarthritis. (Copyright 2014 American College of Rheumatology. Used with permission.)

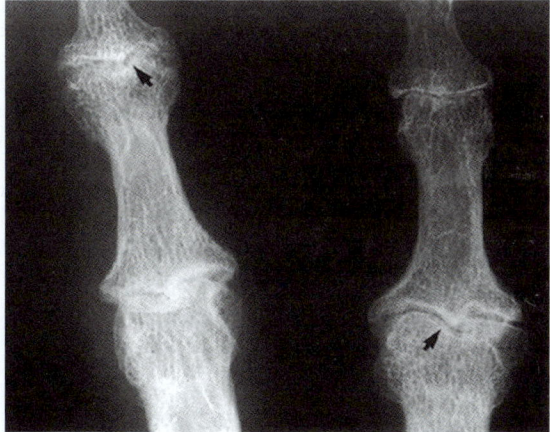

Fig. 50.3 Radiograph of the hands of a patient with erosive osteoarthritis of the distal and proximal interphalangeal joints. Note "gull wing" sign *(arrows)*, which is the hallmark of this disease.

- Hands – Heberden/Bouchard nodes (Fig. 50.2), Radiographs classically show the "gull wing" sign (Fig. 50.3), which is the hallmark of erosive OA.
- Spine – Vacuum sign in degenerative disc disease (a collection of nitrogen in a degenerated disc space).

Uninvolved aspects of radiographs:
- No ankylosis
- Normal bone mineralization
- Absence of calcifications in cartilage
- Absence of synovial-based marginal erosions

14. How is OA diagnosed?

Radiographic OA is at least twice more common than symptomatic OA. Therefore, OA identified on radiographs do not prove that OA is the cause of a patient's musculoskeletal pain or joint dysfunction. OA is diagnosed primarily based on clinical history and physical exam, though radiographs are helpful to confirm a diagnosis or for surgical planning if nearing need for joint replacement.

15. How is OA classified?

Primary, idiopathic OA
- Localized
- Hands (DIP, PIP, and first CMC joints): nodal OA
- Hands (DIP, PIP, and first CMC joints): EOA, inflammatory OA
- Feet (first MTP joint)
- Hip
- Knee
- Spine

Generalized (Kellgren syndrome)
Secondary OA

16. What is generalized OA?

Generalized OA is a variant of OA, sometimes called **Kellgren syndrome**, in which individuals have several affected joints in the typical distribution for OA. Although there is no universally accepted definition, most patients with generalized OA typically have four or more joint sites symmetrically involved. The most commonly involved joints are the hand interphalangeal joints (DIP and PIP joints) and first CMC joints, with the spine, knees, hips, and first MTP involved in descending frequency. The disease frequently manifests before the age of 40 to 50 years. Radiographic findings may be more severe than symptoms. Generalized OA may simply be a more widespread form of common OA, although some researchers have reported various associations with genetic polymorphisms or mutations that could contribute to more rapid cartilage degeneration.

17. What is secondary OA?

Secondary OA has the same clinical features as primary OA except that rather than its pathogenesis stemming from "wear and tear" or overuse, secondary OA has an identifiable etiologic risk factor in the affected joint(s). For that reason, secondary OA may have a different joint distribution, resulting in OA of the MCP joints, wrists, elbows, shoulders, ankles, and MTP joints. It may also lead to earlier onset of OA. A classic example is OA seen in the MCP joints of the hands in association with hemochromatosis (young patients) and calcium pyrophosphate (CPP) arthritis (older patients) or knee OA after anterior cruciate ligament (ACL) tear.

18. What are some common causes of secondary OA?

- Congenital disorders affecting the hips
  - Legg–Calvé–Perthes disease
  - Congenital hip dislocation
  - Slipped capital femoral epiphysis
  - Congenital shallow acetabulum
  - Femoroacetabular impingement (FAI)

- Dysplasias
  - Epiphyseal dysplasia
  - Spondyloepiphyseal dysplasia
- Mechanical features
  - Joint hypermobility syndromes
  - Leg length discrepancy
  - Varus/valgus deformity
  - Scoliosis
- Trauma
  - Anterior cruciate ligament tear
  - Meniscectomy (knee)
  - Fracture through joint
- Metabolic diseases
  - Hemochromatosis
  - Ochronosis
  - Gaucher's disease
  - Hemoglobinopathy
  - Crystal deposition disorders
- Endocrine disorders
  - Acromegaly
  - Hypothyroidism
  - Hyperparathyroidism
- Neuropathic joints
  - Diabetes mellitus
  - Syphilis
- Other
  - Any infectious or inflammatory arthropathy
  - Osteonecrosis
  - Paget disease
  - Kashin–Beck disease: osteochondropathy in China as a result of mycotoxins and selenium deficiency.

19. What is erosive OA?

Erosive OA (EOA), sometimes called **Crain disease**, is an aggressive subset (5–10%) of primary OA typically affecting the DIP, PIP, and first CMC joints bilaterally. EOA primarily occurs in Caucasian women aged 40 to 50 years and is rare in men. The first MTP joints are rarely involved. In EOA, there is a component of joint inflammation that is superimposed on the degenerative osteoarthritic symptoms. The clinical course of EOA usually waxes and wanes for up to 5 years with painful inflammatory "flares" leading to joint deformities. Radiographs are characteristic, showing osteophytes and central "erosions" with a hallmark "gull wing" or "inverted T" appearance (Fig. 50.3). Joint ankylosis occurs in 15% of cases. Decreased hand function is more common in patients with EOA than in those with typical nodal OA.

EOA is distinguished from rheumatoid arthritis in that it is not accompanied by systemic symptoms, does not involve the MCP joints, wrists, or second to fifth MTP joints, has a normal ESR and C-reactive protein, and negative RF and ANA.

20. What is the etiopathogenesis of EOA?

The etiology of EOA is unknown. There is a strong family history in 66% of patients. Genetic studies have reported an association of EOA with a particular IL-1 genotype on chromosome 2. Synovial biopsies reveal changes similar to RA with synovial hypertrophy and lymphocytic/neutrophilic infiltration. The centrally eroded cartilage is not caused by synovial pannus invasion. One theory is that cytokines such as IL-1 from the synovium may signal chondrocyte release of matrix metalloproteinases leading to cartilage destruction. This may be centrally accelerated where the cartilage is thinner. Another proposed etiology of EOA suggests a pathologic role of hydroxyapatite crystals and calcium pyrophosphate dihydrate (CPP) crystals.

21. Does running or jogging predispose to OA?

Previous joint injury and repetitive impact loading predispose to the development of OA, raising the question of whether runners are at increased risk for developing knee or hip OA. Although there is some disagreement in the literature, most of the present data suggest that in the absence of previous joint injury, recreational runners do not develop OA in the knee or hip at higher rates than others. However, highly competitive, elite runners may have an increased risk.

22. Does "cracking" one's knuckles lead to OA of the fingers?

The joint cavity is a potential space with a negative pressure compared with ambient atmospheric pressure. Joint synovial fluid acts as an adhesive seal that permits sliding motion between cartilage surfaces while effectively resisting distracting forces (due to surface tension). During knuckle cracking or popping, there is a fracture of this adhesive bond. A gas bubble is created within the joint, which cavitates with a cracking sound. This bubble of gas can require up to 30 minutes to dissolve before the synovial fluid adhesive bond can be reestablished and the joint "cracked" again. There are no data to support that it leads to OA of the finger joints. The evidence for this is a report by a physician who cracked the knuckles of his left hand twice a day for 50 years (36,500 times total) while not cracking the knuckles of his right hand. Symptom evaluation and radiographs showed that no arthritis developed in either hand.

23. What is manual labor metacarpal arthropathy syndrome?

Primary OA typically does not involve the MCP joints and its presence at this location should prompt an evaluation for secondary causes such as hemochromatosis and CPP arthritis. Rarely, OA of the MCP joints (worse in the dominant hand) has been described in male patients aged over 50 years who have engaged in heavy manual labor involving their hands for several decades (e.g., truck drivers, farmers, heavy machine operators). It is hypothesized that repetitive power gripping of both hands during heavy labor increases the articular surface load leading to MCP joint degeneration.

24. What is the relationship between FAI and OA?

Patients with femoroacetabular impingement (FAI) present with groin pain exacerbated by sitting or exercise. Hip flexion is limited to 90 degrees. There is limitation in hip internal rotation at the 90-degree flexed position, with pain at the end point of internal rotation (impingement sign). There may be a click or snap with hip rotation as a result of a labral or chondral lesion. The mechanism underlying FAI is that normal motion such as flexion results in abnormal contact between the femoral head or proximal femur at the head–neck junction, and the anterior rim of the acetabulum. This can lead to labral tears and early OA. Two types of FAI are recognized:

- **Cam impingement** is caused by any deformity of the proximal femur or femoral head resulting in an aspherical femoral head with loss of the normal femoral head–neck offset (pistol grip deformity). Flexion of the hip causes the abnormal femoral head to rotate into the acetabulum causing stress on the labrum and cartilage of the anterosuperior acetabular rim. A cross-table lateral radiograph, computed tomography scan, or magnetic resonance imaging (MRI) may show a cam deformity (so called because of its resemblance to a camshaft in an engine) at the femoral head–neck junction.
- **Pincer impingement** is caused by local or global overcoverage of the femoral head by the acetabulum. Hip flexion compresses the labrum against the acetabular rim cartilage. Radiographs show a deep acetabular socket (Fig. 50.4).

The treatment for FAI is surgical removal of bony factors contributing to abutment of the femoral head and/or neck with the acetabular ring.

25. Can pes planus cause knee OA?

Yes. Pes planus (flat feet) morphology with pronation causes rotational stress on the medial compartment of the knee leading to OA. In addition, the patella tracks laterally causing patellofemoral OA. Patients presenting with knee pain should have their foot morphology and gait analyzed. If pes planus is present, foot orthotics may help relieve the knee pain.

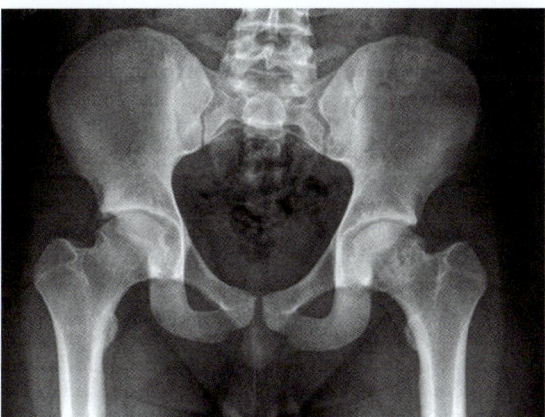

Fig. 50.4 Radiograph of the pelvis with bilateral cam deformities as well as a pincer deformity on the right causing femoroacetabular impingement.

26. What MRI findings in knee OA are associated with pain?

Bone marrow edema lesions under thinned cartilage correlate with pain. Notably, meniscal degenerative lesions are common but do not correlate with symptoms. This explains why knee arthroscopy to repair meniscal abnormalities rarely improves symptoms unless there are clear mechanical symptoms such as locking.

27. Why is primary OA of the ankle uncommon?

Primary OA of the ankle is nine times less common than OA of the knee or hip and usually a result of trauma (i.e., secondary OA). Because the weighted load (five times body weight when walking) on the ankle exceeds that of the knee (four times body weight) and hip (three times body weight), it is surprising that primary OA is so uncommon in the ankle. The reason for this is not entirely clear. However, there are clear anatomical and biomechanical differences between the ankle and the knee or the hip. For instance, the ankle is mainly a rolling joint with congruent surfaces at high load, whereas the knee joint is a mixture of sliding, rolling, and rotation with less congruent surfaces resulting in more stress on the knee cartilage. There are also differences in thickness and composition of ankle cartilage, which increases its tensile strength and gives it more resistance to catabolic cytokines such as IL-1β.

28. Can weather changes affect OA symptoms?

It is not uncommon to hear from a patient that they can predict changes in weather better than the weatherman based on flares of OA pain. Up to 66% of patients with OA claim to have increased pain when there are changes in barometric pressure and temperature. It is hypothesized that changes in barometric pressure and temperature increase stiffness of joints, which can heighten a nociceptive response. However, controlled trials are lacking, and large-scale utilization data do not show this association, so it remains controversial. Regardless, because changes in weather and barometric pressure occur everywhere, moving to a warm climate is unlikely to improve arthritis symptoms.

29. List the first line nonpharmacologic interventions for OA based on the site of OA.

- All joints
  - Patient education and self-management courses/books/websites
  - Occupational therapy, modification of activities of daily living
  - Topical lidocaine
  - Topical capsaicin (depletes nerve terminal of substance P, thereby decreasing pain)
  - Superficial heat and cold (including hot tubs)
  - Hydrotherapy
  - Unconventional: acupuncture (controversial)
  - Transcutaneous electrical nerve stimulator (controversial)

- Knees
  - Weight loss: every 1 lb (0.45 kg) lost results in a fourfold reduction in load per step on the knee. Weight loss of 5% results in 18% to 24% improvement in function in patients with knee OA.
  - Exercise for muscle strengthening/flexibility and aerobic conditioning
  - Medial taping of patella for patellofemoral disease.
  - Unloader/off-load knee brace or knee sleeve
  - Optimal footwear (athletic shoe) with shock-absorbing insoles: medial knee OA may be symptomatically improved, and progression potentially slowed by biomechanical interventions to unweight the knee. The use of clogs, dress shoes, and high heels increases medial compartment loading of the knee by 15% compared with flat shoes, flip flops, or bare feet.
- Hips
  - Foot orthotics: orthotics for pes planus/foot pronation to help knee and patellofemoral symptoms and heel lifts to alter forces causing pain in hip OA appear useful. However, in many clinical guidelines, lateral wedge insoles to unweight and help medial knee joint OA have not been shown to be beneficial (controversial).
  - Ambulatory aids (canes, crutches, walkers): cane can unload the hip by 25% to 40% if used in hand opposite the involved hip.
- Hands
  - Splinting for the CMCs
  - Paraffin baths
- Neck
  - Cervical collar
  - Cervical traction or distraction

Of note, pulsed electromagnetic fields and static magnets have not been shown to be effective in treating those with OA.

30. How would you initiate and advance pharmacologic treatment in a typical patient with OA?

No medication or intervention has been shown yet to stop or reverse the disease process underlying OA. Medications are used, therefore, to alleviate symptoms and increase function with the least toxicity. A reasonable approach to therapy is to start with **acetaminophen** 650 mg every 6 to 8 hours as needed (maximum total dose ≤3–4 g/day; ≤ 2 g/day if drink alcohol), which can decrease OA pain by approximately 30%. If unsuccessful, nonsteroidal anti-inflammatory drugs (NSAIDs) can be used. NSAIDs may be more effective than acetaminophen in treating localized inflammation especially in patients with a joint effusion. In these patients, using the smallest effective dose and duration and/or intermittent dosing is prudent if possible. Use of COX-2 inhibitors or addition of proton-pump inhibitors may help protect against gastrointestinal adverse effects. In patients who are considered high-risk for oral NSAID use, **topical NSAIDs**, **tramadol**, or **duloxetine** have resulted in a clinically relevant reduction in symptoms. Notably, there is no role for oral corticosteroids. However, in a single joint with an inflammatory component, **intraarticular corticosteroids** (see Chapter *82) can be helpful.

31. What is the role of exercise in OA therapy?

An individualized exercise program can play a significant role in improving the joint range of motion and function, and in reducing pain, in joints affected by OA. Several studies have shown that a supervised program of fitness walking results in the improvement of pain, and joint function. Other studies have shown that exercise can improve psychological well-being.

The ideal exercise should be one that minimizes weight-bearing but enables joint range of motion, muscle strengthening, and aerobic fitness. It is important that the individual selects an exercise program that is enjoyable, easily done, and possible to accomplish. Therefore, swimming can be an excellent option. When done in a warm pool, the individual can move affected joints, strengthen periarticular muscles, and improve cardiovascular fitness, all without bearing weight on diseased joints. Other good options include bicycling, walking, elliptical training, and cross-country skiing.

32. Are glucosamine and chondroitin effective in treating OA?

Glucosamine sulfate (or hydrochloride) and chondroitin sulfate (so-called nutraceuticals) are components of cartilage, and as such, have received attention as possibly beneficial supplements in OA. Pharmaceutically, they are classified as dietary supplements and as such are not regulated by the Food and Drug Administration (FDA). Consequently, compound amount, purity, long-term safety, and product labeling are not guaranteed. Absorption of both molecules also varies greatly between individuals. Published studies have shown conflicting results regarding the efficacy of glucosamine and chondroitin in OA and have largely not found them helpful in hip or knee OA, but there has been more support for use of chondroitin in hand OA and for use of glucosamine in TMJ OA. Specifically, the ACR and Arthritis Foundation strongly recommend against chondroitin for knee and hip OA, including combination products that include glucosamine and chondroitin sulfate, though they conditionally recommended chondroitin for hand OA.

33. What is viscosupplementation?

Viscosupplementation in OA consists of injecting hyaluronan (a glycosaminoglycan found in synovial fluid) into osteoarthritic joints. This theoretically allows for more viscous lubrication at low loads and shock absorbency at high loads. Hyaluronan may have chondroprotective (stimulates proteoglycan synthesis), antiinflammatory (scavenger sink for inflammatory mediators), and antinociceptive effects, which may explain its prolonged symptomatic benefit, even though the hyaluronan can only be detected for a few days (intraarticular half-life is 17–36 hours) in the joint after the injection. There are several different formulations with varying molecular weights, composition, side-effect profiles, and frequency of injections. None are superior to another. A direct comparison of viscosupplementation to intraarticular corticosteroids shows that they are relatively equivalent to each other for knee OA. However, the efficacy of viscosupplementation is highly controversial. Viscosupplementation is FDA approved only for the knee but has been used in the temporomandibular joint, shoulder, hip, and ankle.

34. What medications have been investigated for use in erosive OA (EOA)?

Multiple therapies have been used to control symptoms in patients with EOA. Topical and oral NSAIDs are typically tried first. Intraarticular steroid injections have proven effective in some patients. Because of the synovial inflammation resembling RA as well as theories on the potential role of IL-1 and/or crystalline disease in EOA pathogenesis, medications such as hydroxychloroquine, methotrexate, anti-TNF agents, and IL-1 antagonists have been tried with varying levels of success (the latter two therapies are generally considered cost-prohibitive given the equivocal efficacy data). Most of the EOA data exist in hand EOA, for which there are no currently available therapies that reliably prevent or delay disease progression, aside from one small RCT that found that adalimumab halted progression of joint damage but did not improve clinical symptoms.

35. List the indications for total joint replacement for OA of the hip or knee.

- Severe pain unresponsive to medical therapy. For example:
  - Consistently awakens from sleep as a result of pain
  - Cannot stand in one place for >20 to 30 minutes as a result of pain
- Loss of joint function. For example:
  - Cannot walk more than one block
  - Can't put on shoes and socks
  - Requiring a single-story house or apartment because of inability to climb stairs

36. What other therapies are being used or developed for OA?

Many compounds have been tried in OA, with little success. Ongoing research to find a disease-modifying OA drug remains a high priority, given the number of patients affected by OA. The following treatments do not have FDA approval, though show potential as effective OA treatments:

- **Autologous chondrocyte implantation.** Matrix-assisted autologous chondrocyte implantation has had promising results in initial clinical studies. More commonly utilized in younger patients with smaller cartilage defects.

- **Abrasion and microfracture surgery.** Microdrilling of subchondral bone releases autologous mesenchymal stem cells from the bone marrow that attempt to repair the osteoarthritic cartilage.
- **Injections of platelet-rich plasma (PRP).** PRP, defined as a volume of plasma with a platelet count above baseline. Venous blood is drawn from the patient and centrifuged to obtain PRP, which is then injected into the patient's joint. Theoretically, when the injected platelets degranulate, several factors are released, including transforming growth factor beta, platelet-derived growth factor, epidermal growth factor, and insulin-like growth factor. These factors may inhibit inflammation, offer chondroprotection, and increase cartilage synthetic activity. There is a lack of high-quality data supporting this practice at present.
- **Mesenchymal stem cell injections.** Intraarticular injection of mesenchymal stem cells has had inconsistent results thus far, with a need for higher-quality studies.
- **Genicular nerve block.** Cooled radiofrequency ablation (CRFA) of the branches of the genicular nerve (knee) has shown benefit in a randomized controlled trial compared with steroid injection. CRFA to other nerve sites has been evaluated in patients with sacroiliac and discogenic lumbar pain as well.

ACKNOWLEDGMENT

The authors wish to acknowledge Drs. Kumar Bharat and Scott Vogelgesang who were the authors of this chapter in the previous edition.

BIBLIOGRAPHY

Aitken D, Laslett LL, Pan F, et al. A randomised double-blind placebo-controlled crossover trial of HUMira (adalimumab) for erosive hand OsteoaRthritis—the HUMOR trial. *Osteoarthr Cartil*. 2018;26:880–887.

Avouac J, Vicaut E, Bardin T, et al. Efficacy of joint lavage in knee osteoarthritis: meta-analysis of randomized controlled studies. *Rheumatology*. 2010;49:334–340.

Banks SE. Erosive osteoarthritis: a current review of a clinical challenge. *Clin Rheumatol*. 2010;29:697–706.

Bannuru RR, Schmid CH, Kent DM, et al. Comparative effectiveness of pharmacologic interventions for knee osteoarthritis: a systematic review and network meta-analysis. *Ann Intern Med*. 2015;6(162):46–54.

Bellamy N, Campbell J, Robinson V, et al. Intraarticular corticosteroid for treatment of osteoarthritis of the knee. *Cochrane Database Syst Rev*. 2006;2:CD005328.

Bellamy N, Campbell J, Robinson V, et al. Viscosupplementation for the treatment of osteoarthritis of the knee. *Cochrane Database Syst Rev*. 2006;2:CD005321.

Clegg DO, Reda DJ, Harris CL, et al. Glucosamine, chondroitin sulfate and the two in combination for painful knee osteoarthritis. *N Engl J Med*. 2006;354:795–808.

Collins N, Crossley K, Beller E, et al. Foot orthoses and physiotherapy in the treatment of patellofemoral pain syndrome: randomized clinical trial. *Br J Sports Med*. 2009;43:169–171.

Davis T, Loudermilk E, DePalma M, et al. Prospective, multicenter, randomized, crossover clinical trialcomparing the safety and effectiveness of cooled radiofrequency ablation with corticosteroid injection in the management of knee pain from osteoarthritis. *Reg Anesth Pain Med*. 2018;43:84–91.

Englund M, Guermazi A, Gale D, et al. Incidental meniscal findings on knee MRI in middle-aged and elderly persons. *N Engl J Med*. 2008;359:1108–1115.

Favero M, Belluzzi E, Ortolan A, et al. Erosive hand osteoarthritis: latest findings and outlook. *Nat Rev Rheumatol*. 2022;18:171–183.

Felson DT, Niu J, Guermazi A, et al. Correlation of the development of knee pain with enlarging bone marrow lesions on magnetic resonance imaging. *Arthritis Rheum*. 2007;56:2986–2992.

Fernandes L, Hagen KB, Bijlsma JWJ, et al. EULAR recommendations for the non-pharmacological core management of hip and knee osteoarthritis. *Ann Rheum Dis*. 2013;72:1125–1135.

Katz JN, Arant KR, Loeser RF. Diagnosis and treatment of hip and knee osteoarthritis: a review. *JAMA*. 2021;325: 568–578.

Kolasinski SL, Neogi T, Hochberg MC, et al. 2019 American College of Rheumatology/Arthritis Foundation Guideline for the Management of Osteoarthritis of the Hand, Hip, and Knee. *Arthritis Rheumatol*. 2020;72:220–233.

Kraus VB, Jordan JM, Doherty M, et al. The genetics of generalized osteoarthritis (GOGO) study: study design and evaluation of osteoarthritis phenotypes. *Osteoarthritis Cartil*. 2007;15:120–127.

Kreuz PC, Kalkreuth RH, Niemeyer P, Uhl M, Erggelet C. Long-term clinical and MRI results of matrix-assisted chondrocyte implantation for articular cartilage defects of the knee. *Cartilage*. 2018;10:305–313.

Levy DM, Peterson KA, Vaught MS, Christian DR, Cole BJ. Injections for knee osteoarthritis: corticosteroids, viscosupplementation, platelet-rich plasma, and autologous stem cells. *Arthroscopy*. 2018;34:1730–1743.

McAlindon TE, LaValley MP, Harvey WF, et al. Effect of intra-articular triamcinolone vs saline on knee cartilage volume and pain in patients with knee osteoarthritis: a randomized clinical trial. *JAMA*. 2017;317:1967–1975.

Peck J, Slovek A, Miro P, et al. A comprehensive review of viscosupplementation in osteoarthritis of the knee. *Orthop Rev (Pavia)*. 2021;13(2):25549.

Puntillo F, Giglio M, Corriero A, et al. Unraveling the joints: a narrative review of osteoarthritis. *Eur Rev Med Pharmacol Sci*. 2024;28:4080–4104.

Roddy E, Zhang W, Doherty M. Aerobic walking and strengthening exercise for osteoarthritis of the knee? A systemic review. *Ann Rheum Dis*. 2005;64:544–548.

Shukla D, Sreedhar SK, Rastogi V. A comparative study of Botulinum Toxin A with Triamcinolone compared to triamcinolone alone in the treatment of osteoarthritis of knee. *Anesth Essays Res*. 2018;12:47–49.

Sibley JT. Weather and arthritis symptoms. *J Rheum*. 1985;12:707–710.

Sivakumar S, Sivakumar G, Sundramoorthy A. Effects of glucosamine in the temporomandibular joint osteoarthritis: a review. *Curr Rheumatol Rev*. 2024;20:373–378.

Sokolove J, Lepus CM. Role of inflammation in the pathogenesis of osteoarthritis. *Ther Adv Musculoskel Dis*. 2013;5:77–94.

Towheed TE, Maxwell L, Judd MG, et al. Acetaminophen for osteoarthritis. *Cochrane Database Syst Rev*. 2006;1:CD004257.

Unger DL. Does knuckle cracking lead to arthritis of the fingers? *Arthritis Rheum*. 1998;41:949–950.

Xing D, Wang Q. Mesenchymal stem cells injections for knee osteoarthritis: a systematic overview. *Rheumatol Int*. 2018;38:1399–1411.

FURTHER READING

https://www.ncbi.nlm.nih.gov/books/NBK482326/.

Metabolic Bone Disease

Michael T. McDermott, MD

1. What is osteoporosis?

Osteoporosis is a skeletal disorder characterized by compromised bone strength, predisposing to the development of fragility fractures. The diagnosis of osteoporosis is established by the presence of a fragility fracture, by low bone mass on bone mineral density (BMD) testing, or with the FRAX Risk Assessment tool. Bone strength is determined by both **bone mass** and **bone quality**.

2. What are fragility fractures?

Fragility fractures are those that occur spontaneously or following minimal trauma, defined as falling from a standing height or less. Vertebral, hip, and distal radius (Colles') fractures are the most characteristic, but osteoporosis predisposes to all types of fractures. Nearly 40% of women and 13% of men develop one or more osteoporotic fractures during their lifetime. Osteoporosis accounts for approximately 1.5 million fractures in the United States each year.

3. What are the complications of osteoporotic fragility fractures?

Vertebral fractures cause height loss, anterior kyphosis (dowager's hump), reduced pulmonary function (FVC decreases 9% for each vertebral fracture), and an increased mortality rate. Approximately one-third of all vertebral fractures are painful but two-thirds are asymptomatic. Hip fractures cause permanent disability in ~50% of people and a 20% excess mortality rate compared to the age-matched nonfracture population.

4. What factors contribute most to the risk of developing an osteoporotic fracture?

- Low BMD (twofold increased risk for every one standard deviation [T-score] decrease of BMD)
- Age (twofold increased risk for every decade of age above 60 years)
- Previous fragility fracture (fivefold increased risk for a previous fracture)
- Frequent falls
- Glucocorticoid use

5. How is the diagnosis of osteoporosis made?

Osteoporosis is diagnosed by any of the three criteria: a fragility fracture, low BMD, or high FRAX risk score.

Fragility Fracture Criteria
- A fragility fracture (previous or current) establishes a diagnosis of osteoporosis regardless of the BMD T-score.

Bone Densitometry Criteria
- BMD T-score ≤ -2.5 at any site indicates osteoporosis in people > age 50 years; the diagnostic T-score ranges are as follows:

T-score ≥ −1	Normal
T-score -1 to -2.5	Osteopenia
T-score ≤ −2.5	Osteoporosis

- In premenopausal women or men < age 50 years, a BMD **Z**-score ≤ -2.0 at the lowest skeletal site indicates low BMD for age.

FRAX Risk Assessment Criteria
- A FRAX 10-Year Risk Score: ≥3% for hip fracture or ≥20% for major osteoporosis fractures also diagnoses osteoporosis for drug-naïve people over age 40 with osteopenia by BMD testing.

6. How do you determine if a patient has had a previous vertebral fracture?

Back pain or tenderness are clues but may be absent, since two-thirds of vertebral fractures are asymptomatic. Height loss of >2 inches or dorsal kyphosis is highly suggestive clinical findings. Vertebral imagining with lateral spine films or DXA vertebral fracture assessment (VFA) is the most accurate way to detect existing vertebral fractures.

7. How is BMD currently measured?

Dual-energy x-ray absorptiometry (DXA) is the most accurate and widely used method in current practice. Radiation exposure is minimal with only 1–3 uSv/site compared with 50–100 uSv for one chest radiograph. BMD can also be measured by computed tomography (CT) (50 uSv) and ultrasound (US) (no radiation). Central densitometry measurements (spine and hip) are the best predictors of fracture risk and have the best precision for longitudinal monitoring. Peripheral densitometry measurements (heel, radius, hands) may be more widely available and less expensive but are less accurate.

8. What are the currently accepted indications for BMD measurement?

- Age ≥65 years (women); age ≥70 (men).
- Estrogen deficiency plus one risk factor for osteoporosis.
- Vertebral deformity, fracture, or osteopenia by x-ray.
- Primary hyperparathyroidism.
- Glucocorticoid therapy, ≥5 mg/day of prednisone for ≥3 months.
- Monitoring the response to an FDA-approved osteoporosis medication.

9. How do you read a bone densitometry report?

T-score: Number of standard deviations (SD) the person deviates from the mean BMD for young (30 years) normal subjects (peak bone mass). T-score is the best predictor of fracture risk (Fig 51.1).

Z-score: Number of SD the person deviates from the mean BMD for age-matched normal subjects. Z-score indicates if the BMD is appropriate for age. A low Z-score is predictive of an underlying secondary cause other than age or menopause.

Absolute BMD: Actual BMD in gm/cm^2. This value should be used to calculate changes in BMD during longitudinal follow-up.

10. What estimates of bone loss and fracture risk can be made from a person's BMD measurement by DXA?

T score	% Bone Loss*	Fracture Risk Increase
−1	12%	2-Fold
−2	24%	4-Fold
−3	36%	8-Fold
−4	48%	16-Fold

*Note: one must lose 30% of BMD to see osteopenia on a routine radiograph; this degree of loss suggests a T-score of −2.5.

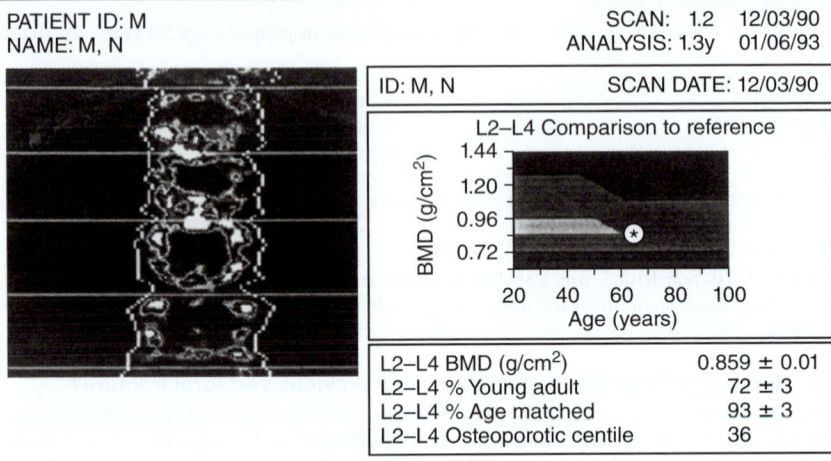

Fig 51.1 DXA scan report for lumbar spine.

REGION	BMD g/cm²	Young adult %	T	Age matched %	Z
L1	0.806	71	−2.70	95	−0.36
L2	0.834	70	−3.05	91	−0.72
L3	0.912	76	−2.40	99	−0.07
L4	0.831	69	−3.08	90	−0.74
L1–L2	0.820	71	−2.75	94	−0.41
L1–L3	0.854	73	−2.63	96	−0.30
L1–L4	0.847	72	−2.77	94	−0.44
L2–L3	0.876	73	−2.70	95	−0.37
L2–L4	0.859	72	−2.84	93	−0.51
L3–L4	0.869	72	−2.76	94	−0.42

PEARL: An older person is more likely to suffer a fracture than a younger person with the same T-score. This also applies to patients treated with GCs compared with a person who is not. Both age and GCs affect bone mass and bone microarchitecture putting patients at risk for fractures at a higher T-score.

11. How do you use the FRAX Risk Assessment tool?

The Fracture Risk Assessment (FRAX) tool (www.shef.ac.uk/FRAX/) is a free computer-based program developed by the World Health Organization (WHO). It uses clinical risk factors with or without femoral neck BMD to provide a 10-year absolute risk estimate for developing a hip or another major osteoporotic fracture. It is recommended for making treatment decisions in drug-naïve people over age 40 with *osteopenia* on BMD testing and without fragility fractures. Treatment is advised for those who have a 10-year risk ≥3% for hip fractures or ≥20% for major osteoporosis fractures.

12. What is a trabecular bone score and how is it used?

Trabecular bone score (TBS) is a newer technique developed to evaluate bone quality. TBS uses data from existing DXA lumbar spine images to produce a gray-level textural index that correlates well with fracture risk in postmenopausal women and in men aged ≥50 years. It can be used in conjunction with DXA to assist with decisions about initiation of osteoporosis therapy. The TBS can also be entered into the FRAX Risk Assessment tool. It should not be used alone and is not validated as a tool for monitoring therapy. TBS is particularly useful in disorders for which DXA alone significantly underestimates fracture risk, such as GIOP and diabetes mellitus.

13. What are the major risk factors for the development of osteoporosis?

Non-Modifiable	*Modifiable*
Advanced age	Low calcium intake
Race (Caucasian, Asian)	Low vitamin D intake
Female gender	Estrogen deficiency
Early menopause	Sedentary lifestyle
Slender build (<127 lb)	Cigarette smoking
Positive family history (hip fx)	Alcohol excess (>2 drinks/day)
Caffeine excess (>2 servings/day)	

PEARL: Mental disorders, use of antipsychotic or selective serotonin reuptake inhibitors (SSRI) medications, and hyponatremia are identified conditions that result in an increased fracture risk.

14. What other conditions must be considered as causes of low BMD?

Osteomalacia	Inflammatory Bowel Disease
Osteogenesis Imperfecta	Gastrectomy/bowel bypass surgery
Ehlers-Danlos syndrome	Primary Biliary Cirrhosis
Hyperparathyroidism	Multiple Myeloma
Hyperthyroidism	Rheumatoid Arthritis/SLE
Hyperprolactinemia	Ankylosing spondylitis
Alcoholism	Chronic Kidney Disease
Hypogonadism	Renal Tubular Acidosis
Cushing's Syndrome	Idiopathic Hypercalciuria
Eating/Exercise Disorders	Systemic Mastocytosis
Celiac Disease	High-Risk Medications*

*Glucocorticoids, excess thyroid hormone, anticonvulsants, heparin, lithium, SSRIs, aromatase inhibitors, premenopausal tamoxifen, leuprolide, and cyclosporine. Probable/Possible: Thiazolidinediones, proton pump inhibitors, excess vitamin A.

15. Outline a cost-effective evaluation to rule out other causes of low bone mass.

Calcium (albumin), phosphorous, creatinine, CO_2
Alkaline phosphatase
25 OH vitamin D
Testosterone (Men)
Thyroid Stimulating Hormone (TSH) (if clinically hyperthyroid)
Celiac disease antibody testing (if Caucasian with symptoms or low 25OH vit D level)
Urine (24 hours) calcium, sodium, creatinine
SPEP (if over age 50 with abnormal CBC)

PEARL: A patient needs a calcium (corrected for albumin level) x phosphorous product of ~24 to properly mineralize bone.
   Approximately one-third of women and two-thirds of men will have an abnormality detected with this evaluation. Therefore, this cost-effective evaluation is recommended for all osteoporosis patients. A low Z-score suggests that an underlying secondary cause (other than age or menopausal status) is even more likely to be present.

16. What are the most significant risk factors for frequent falls?

Frailty
Use of sedatives
Visual impairment
Cognitive impairment
Lower extremity disability
Obstacles to ambulation in the home

PEARL: The most predictive factor for a future fall is a previous fall within the past 6 months. Almost all hip fractures occur due to falls. Falls have been shown to predict fractures independently of the FRAX risk score.

17. How does osteoporosis differ in men?

Approximately 1–2 million men in the United States have osteoporosis. The diagnostic criteria are the same in men as in women (fragility fracture, T-score ≤ -2.5, FRAX risk scores). Nearly two-thirds of osteoporotic men have an identifiable secondary cause of bone loss, most often alcohol abuse, GC use, and hypogonadism, including GnRH analog use for prostate cancer. Treatment is generally the same in men as in women although testosterone replacement in hypogonadal men is an effective adjunctive strategy.

18. When should pharmacological therapy be initiated for osteoporosis (see chapter 87: Bone Strengthening Agents)?

Pharmacological therapy should be advised for any person who has osteoporosis by any of the 3 criteria discussed above (Question 5):
- History of vertebral, hip, wrist, or humerus fragility fracture
- T-Score ≤ −2.5
- FRAX Risk Score (10 Year) ≥3% for hip fracture or ≥20% for major osteoporosis fracture in drug-naïve people over age 40 with osteopenia by BMD testing.

19. How do glucocorticoids cause osteoporosis?

Glucocorticoids adversely affect both phases of bone remodeling leading to rapid bone loss. Bone formation is inhibited by accelerated osteoblast apoptosis and reduced new osteoblast development. Bone resorption is stimulated by decreased sex steroid levels and reduced production of osteoprotegerin, an endogenous bone resorption inhibitor. Osteocytes also undergo accelerated apoptosis.

PEARL: People on glucocorticoids fracture at higher/better BMD values (T-scores) than do people with other types of osteoporosis.

20. Define the fracture risk categories for glucocorticoid-induced osteoporosis.

Adults ≥40 Years of Age
- **Low Risk**
  - FRAX: MOF <10%, Hip Fracture <1%
  - BMD: T-score > −1.0
- **Moderate Risk**
  - FRAX: MOF 10–20%, Hip Fracture 1–3%
  - BMD: T-score −1.0 to −2.4
- **High Risk**
  - FRAX: MOF 20–30%, Hip Fracture 3–4.5%
  - BMD: T-score ≤ −2.5
- **Very High Risk**
  - FRAX: MOF >30%, Hip Fracture >4.5%
  - BMD: T-score ≤ −3.5, or
  - Prior osteoporosis fracture, or
  - GC dose ≥30 mg/day for >30 days or cumulative dose ≥5 g/year

Adults ≤40 Years of Age
- **Low Risk**
  - None of the above risk factors other than CG treatment
  - **Moderate Risk**
  - Ongoing CG treatment ≥7.5 mg/day for ≥6 months and BMD T-score < −3.0 OR significant bone loss compared to prior BMD (> least significant change)
- **High Risk**
  - Prior osteoporosis fracture, or
  - GC dose ≥30 mg/day for >30 days or cumulative dose ≥5 g/year

- **Very High Risk**
  - Prior osteoporosis fracture, or
  - GC dose ≥30 mg/day for >30 days or cumulative dose ≥5 g/year

Note: FRAX risk assessment must be adjusted if on GC:
FRAX GC Adjustment: If GC dose ≥7.5 mg/d, multiply MOF risk x 1.15 and hip fx risk x 1.2
*MOF: Major osteoporosis fracture.

21. How should people on glucocorticoids (GC) be assessed and monitored?

The 2022 recommendations of the American College of Rheumatology:

- Adults (≥18 years old) starting or continuing GC therapy (prednisone dose ≥2.5 mg/day or equivalent) for ≥3 months should have an initial clinical fracture risk assessment (fracture history, BMD, FRAX [age > 40 only], and lateral spine radiographs or VFA).
- Adults on chronic GC therapy (≥2.5 mg/day but <7.5 mg/day) at low fracture risk and not recommended to start osteoporosis (OP) medications, or moderate fracture risk who chose not to start OP medications, should have fracture risk repeated every 1–2 years.
- Adults on chronic GC therapy (≥2.5 mg/day) at moderate, high, or very high fracture risk and continuing OP medications ≥1 year should have fracture risk repeated every 1–2 years.

22. Which medications are recommended for prevention and treatment of glucocorticoid-induced osteoporosis (GIOP)?

The 2022 American College of Rheumatology (ACR) guidelines endorse bisphosphonates, denosumab, teriparatide, abaloparatide, romosozumab and raloxifene strongly, usually or conditionally (under specified circumstances) for GIOP prevention and treatment depending on the individualized fracture risk category (Question #20) based on age, FRAX, BMD, fracture history, and glucocorticoid (GC) dose. Adequate calcium and vitamin D intake and regular exercise, as tolerated, are recommended for all people treated with GC.

23. When should osteoporosis (OP) medications be considered in people over age 40 years who are taking glucocorticoid therapy?

The risk-stratified 2022 ACR recommendations for GIOP prevention and treatment in people over age 40 years are the following (see Question #20):

Low Fracture Risk: OP medications not recommended.

Moderate Fracture Risk: recommend for bisphosphonates, denosumab, teriparatide, abaloparatide, or raloxifene; conditionally recommend against romosozumab except in people intolerant of all other OP medications due to risk of myocardial infarction, stroke, or death.

High Fracture Risk: recommend for denosumab, teriparatide, or abaloparatide over bisphosphonates; recommend bisphosphonates over no treatment; conditionally recommend romosozumab or raloxifene in people intolerant of all other OP medications.

Very High Fracture Risk: conditionally recommend teriparatide or abaloparatide over anti-resorptive therapy; recommend denosumab or bisphosphonates over no treatment; conditionally recommend romosozumab or raloxifene in people intolerant of all other OP medications.

Receiving High-Dose GC (initial dose ≥ 30 mg/day for > 30 days or cumulative dose ≥ 5 g in 1 year): conditionally recommend teriparatide or abaloparatide over anti-resorptive therapy; strongly recommend oral bisphosphonates over no treatment; conditionally recommend IV bisphosphonates and denosumab over no treatment; conditionally recommend romosozumab or raloxifene in people intolerant of all other OP medications.

People with Organ Transplants, eGFR ≥ 35 ml/min, and No Evidence of Renal Osteodystrophy or Hyperparathyroidism: conditionally recommend expert evaluation for renal osteodystrophy in kidney transplant recipients; conditionally recommend bisphosphonates, denosumab, teriparatide, abaloparatide or raloxifene based on individual patient factors; conditionally recommend against romosozumab due to risk of myocardial infarction, stroke or death.

24. How do the 2022 ACR recommendations for GIOP prevention and treatment differ for people under the age of 40 years?

Moderate Fracture Risk: conditionally recommend bisphosphonates, denosumab, teriparatide or abaloparatide; conditionally recommend against romosozumab and raloxifene due to potential harmful effects.

25. How should you evaluate and manage people on intermittent pulses of IV GCs? How about inhaled GC therapy?

Guidelines for GIOP prevention/treatment in people receiving intermittent GC therapy are lacking. Those receiving ≥4 monthly IV pulses (1 g methylprednisolone equivalent) or high-dose oral pulses (prednisone ≥60 mg/d with taper over 2–4 weeks) within a 12-month period are at risk and should be considered for treatment. People on daily inhaled steroids (Advair 200 ug/d equivalent or higher dose) for a prolonged period can also lose significant BMD and should be periodically monitored.

26. Describe vitamin D metabolism and action.

Vitamin D exists in two natural forms: cholecalciferol (D3) and ergocalciferol (D2). Humans acquire vitamin D by two routes: endogenous synthesis in the skin during sunlight exposure (D3) and dietary intake (D2 and D3). Vitamin D from either source is converted in the liver by 25-hydroxylase to 25-hydroxy (OH) vitamin D and then by 1 alpha-hydroxylase in the kidney to 1,25-dihydroxy $(OH)_2$ vitamin D. The latter binds to intestinal vitamin D receptors to promote calcium and phosphorous absorption. PTH and hypophosphatemia are major inducers of 1 alpha-hydroxylase activity. As a person becomes vitamin D deficient and serum calcium decreases, PTH levels increase and induce the 1 alpha-hydroxylase enzyme to convert 25-OH vitamin D into 1,25 $(OH)_2$ vitamin D. Therefore, the 25-OH vitamin D level will decrease before the 1,25 $(OH)_2$ vitamin D level. **For this reason, measuring a 25-OH vitamin D level is the best measure of vitamin D stores.**

27. What causes osteomalacia?

Osteomalacia, which means "soft bones," results from impaired mineralization of bone matrix due to inadequate concentrations of serum phosphate and/or calcium, resulting in a low serum calcium x phosphate product (<24), or from a circulating inhibitor of mineralization.

Major Causes of Osteomalacia

Vitamin D deficiency
Low oral intake plus low sun exposure intake
Intestinal malabsorption
Abnormal vitamin D metabolism
Liver disease
Renal disease
Drugs (anticonvulsants, anti-tuberculous drugs, ketoconazole)
Hypophosphatemia
Low oral phosphate
Phosphate-binding antacids
Excess renal phosphate loss
Inhibitors of mineralization
Aluminum
Fluoride
Bisphosphonates
Hypophosphatasia

28. Describe the clinical features that are common to osteomalacia and rickets.

Osteomalacia/rickets causes pain and deformity in the long bones and pelvis. Laboratory features of osteomalacia due to vitamin D deficiency include low serum 25-OH vitamin D levels, low or low-normal serum calcium and phosphate, elevated alkaline phosphatase, elevated PTH, and low 24-hour urinary calcium excretion. Laboratory features of osteomalacia due to renal phosphate wasting (familial hypophosphatemic rickets/adult-onset vitamin D-resistant osteomalacia and oncogenic osteomalacia) include low serum phosphate, high alkaline phosphatase, high urinary phosphate (low tubular reabsorption of phosphate), and inappropriately normal or low 1,25 $(OH)_2$ vitamin D for the degree of hypophosphatemia.

Radiographs in adults may show characteristic pseudofractures (milkman's fractures, Looser's zones) where large arteries cross bones. Children may show changes in rickets (see question # 30). Bone biopsies show increased osteoid seams but with reduced hydroxyapatite deposition.

29. What causes acquired and congenital rickets?

Rickets results from impaired skeletal mineralization during childhood. Acquired rickets have the same etiologies as osteomalacia in adults. There are three main inherited disorders resulting in congenital rickets:

1. **Hypophosphatemic Rickets:** X-linked Hypophosphatemic Rickets (XLHR) results from inherited loss of function mutations in the PHEX gene, leading to increased bone expression of Fibroblast Growth Factor 23 (FGF 23) due to decreased FGF 23 proteolysis. Autosomal Dominant Hypophosphatemic Rickets (ADHR) results from activating mutations in the gene that encodes FGF 23, resulting in increased FGF 23 levels. FGF 23, the body's main phosphaturic factor, lowers serum phosphate by forming a ternary complex with the FGF 23 receptor and the Klotho protein to enhance renal phosphate loss through renal sodium-phosphate transporters; FGF 23 also reduces intestinal phosphate absorption by lowering serum 1,25 (OH)2 vitamin D levels through inhibition of renal 1-alpha hydroxylase and stimulation of renal 24 hydroxylase. This disorder was previously termed "Vitamin D-Dependent Rickets Type 1" because some patients partially respond to high-dose vitamin D therapy.

2. **Congenital 1-alpha-hydroxylase deficiency:** inactivating mutations of 1-alpha hydroxylase cause lifelong impairment of conversion of 25 OH vitamin D into 1,25 $(OH)_2$ vitamin D, resulting in chronic intestinal calcium and phosphate malabsorption. This disorder was previously termed "Vitamin D-Dependent Rickets Type 2" because some patients partially respond to high-dose vitamin D therapy.

3. **Congenital vitamin D resistance:** genetic mutations resulting in defective or absent vitamin D receptors cause impaired vitamin D action leading to chronic intestinal calcium and phosphate malabsorption. This disorder was previously termed "Vitamin D-Resistant Rickets" because high-dose vitamin D therapy is usually not beneficial.

30. What clinical manifestations are more specific for rickets and not osteomalacia?

Since rickets result from mineralization defects that occur during bone maturation, some clinical manifestations are distinct from those observed with osteomalacia in adults. Clinical features include bone pain, deformities, fractures, muscle weakness, and growth retardation. Laboratory findings are similar to those in osteomalacia. However, x-rays may show delayed opacification of the epiphyses, widened growth plates, widened and irregular metaphyses, and thin cortices with sparse, coarse trabeculae in the diaphyses. Deformities differ depending on the time of onset:

First Year of Life	After First Year of Life
Widened cranial sutures	Flared ends of long bones
Frontal bossing	Bowing of long bones
Craniotabes	Sabre shins
Rachitic rosary	Coxa vara
Harrison's groove	Genu varum
Flared wrists	Genu valgum

31. What is oncogenic osteomalacia?

Oncogenic (tumor-induced) osteomalacia is a rare cause of osteomalacia in adults and rickets in children. It is caused most commonly by benign (rarely malignant) endodermal or mesenchymal tumors that secrete FGF 23. FGF 23 inhibits phosphate transport in renal tubules and the renal 1-alpha hydroxylase enzyme; commercial FGF 23 assays are available.

Bone pain and myalgias are the most common presenting features. Laboratory findings include very low serum phosphate, high alkaline phosphatase, high urinary phosphate, a high

FGF 23 level, and low 1,25 (OH)$_2$ vitamin D. The tumors tend to be small and are best localized by Gallium-68 DOTA-Octreotate PET scanning. Surgical removal of the tumor is usually curative.

32. How are osteomalacia and rickets treated?

Etiology	Treatment
Nutritional Vitamin D Deficiency	Vitamin D, 5000 U/day until healing, then maintain 1000-2000 U/day
Malabsorption	Vitamin D, 50,000–100,000 U/day
Renal disease	Calcitriol, 0.25–1.0 mcg/day
Hypophosphatemic rickets	Calcitriol, 0.25–1.0 mcg/day, and oral phosphate
1 alpha-hydroxylase deficiency	Calcitriol, 0.25–1.0 mcg/day, and oral phosphate
Vitamin D resistance	Vitamin D, 100,000–200,000 U/day or calcitriol, 5–60 mcg/day, or IV calcium infusions

33. What is familial hyperphosphatemic tumoral calcinosis?

Familial hyperphosphatemic tumoral calcinosis results from inactivating mutations of the FGF 23 gene. FGF 23 normally acts through the FGF 23 receptor and co-receptor Klotho, to lower serum phosphorus by enhancing renal phosphate loss and reducing intestinal phosphate absorption by lowering serum 1,25 (OH)2 vitamin D levels through inhibition of renal 1 alpha-hydroxylase. Patients with this condition make insufficient amounts of functional FGF 23 and, as a result, develop painful ectopic calcifications and elevated serum phosphorus levels.

34. Discuss the causes and treatment of osteogenesis imperfecta (see Chapter 54).

Osteogenesis Imperfecta (OI) results from defective osteoblast function due most commonly. to mutations in genes that encode the alpha-1 and alpha-2 chains of type I collagen (COL1A1 and COL1A2). Autosomal recessive OI is caused by mutations in genes that encode proteins involved in type I collagen posttranslational modification (FKBP10, CRTAP, LEPRE1, PPIB) or other regulators of bone formation and homeostasis (SERPINH1, SERPINF1, SP7/OSX and IFITM5). OI varies in clinical features and severity. OI is best diagnosed with genetic testing.

Therapy goals are to prevent fractures, deformities, pain, and functional impairment. Data on the risks and benefits of pharmacologic therapy are scarce. Bisphosphonates are used for most forms of OI, but not type VI, in which bone mineralization is defective and bisphosphonates may be harmful. Anabolic therapy has also been used but its effects are dependent on the underlying mutation. People with OI are best managed in centers where there is experience treating this condition.

35. What is hypophosphatasia?

Hypophosphatasia results from inherited inactivating mutations of the gene that encodes the tissue nonspecific alkaline phosphatase isoenzyme (ALPL). The severity of the enzyme defect determines the clinical features, which vary from fetal demise to disabling pediatric forms to milder adult forms manifested by rickets or osteomalacia, dental abnormalities, multiple fractures, or just osteoporosis. Low serum alkaline phosphatase, elevated vitamin B6 or pyridoxal phosphate, and high urine phosphoethanolamine levels suggest the diagnosis, which can be confirmed with genetic testing. Recently, enzyme replacement, asfotase alpha, has become available for treatment of the more severe cases.

36. Define osteopetrosis.

Osteopetrosis (marble bone disease) results from defective osteoclast function. Mutations have been identified in the following genes: TCIRG1 (proton pump), CLCN7 (chloride channel), CAII (carbonic anhydrase II) and gl/gl (unknown function). Each of these abnormalities leads to the inability of osteoclasts to create an acidic environment in the resorption pit under its ruffled border that is needed for the dissociation of calcium hydroxyapatite from the bone matrix. The impaired bone resorption produces dense, chalky, fragile bones and bone marrow replacement. Skeletal x-rays show generalized osteosclerosis. The diagnosis is made by genetic testing. Bone marrow transplantation to provide normal osteoclasts may be needed in severe cases while high-dose calcitriol to stimulate osteoclasts can be effective in the milder forms.

BIBLIOGRAPHY

Bolton JM, Morin SN, Majumdar SR, et al. Association of mental disorders and related medication use with risk for major osteoporotic fractures. *JAMA Psychiatry*. 2017;74:641–648.

Buckley L, Humphrey MB. Glucocorticoid-induced bone disease. *New Engl J Med*. 2018;379:2547–2556.

Camacho PM, Petak SM, Binkley N, et al. American Association of Clinical Endocrinologists and American College of Endocrinology clinical practice guidelines for the diagnosis and treatment of postmenopausal osteoporosis—2016. *Endocrine Pract*. 2016;22(suppl. 4):1–42.

Carpenter TO, Imel EA, Holm IA, Jan de Beur SM, Insogna KL. A clinician's guide to X-linked hypophosphatemia. *J Bone Min Res*. 2011;26:1381–1388.

Carpenter TO. The expanding family of hypophosphatemic syndromes. *J Bone Min Res*. 2011;30:1–9.

Chong WH, Molinolo AA, Chen CC, Collins MT. Tumor-induced osteomalacia. *Endocr Relat Cancer*. 2011;18:R53–R77.

Damilakis J, Adams JE, Guglielmi G, Link TM. Radiation exposure in x-ray-based imaging techniques used in osteoporosis. *Eur Radiol*. 2010;20:2707–2714.

Drake MT, Murad MH, Mauck KF, et al. Clinical review. Risk factors for low bone mass-related fractures in men: a systemic review and meta-analysis. *J Clinical Endo Metab*. 2012;97:1861–1870.

Eastell R, Szulc P. Use of bone turnover markers in postmenopausal osteoporosis. Osteoporosis treatment: recent developments and ongoing challenges. *Lancet Diabetes Endocrinol*. 2017;5:908–923.

Ebeling PR, Nguyen HH, Aleksova J, et al. Secondary osteoporosis. *Endocr Rev*. 2022;43:240–313.

Florenzano P, Cipriani C, Roszko KL, et al. Approach to patients with hypophosphataemia. *Lancet Diabetes Endocrinol*. 2020;8:163–174.

Gattineni J. Inherited disorders of calcium and phosphate metabolism. *Curr Opin Pediatr*. 2014;26:215–222.

Harvey NC, Odén A, Orwoll E, et al. Falls predict fractures independently of FRAX probability: a meta-analysis of the osteoporotic fractures in men (MrOS) study. *J Bone Miner Res*. 2018;33:510–516.

Holick MF. Vitamin D deficiency. *N Engl J Med*. 2007;357:266–281.

Humphrey MB, Russell L, Danila MI, et al. 2022 American College of Rheumatology guideline for the prevention and treatment of glucocorticoid-induced osteoporosis. *Arthritis Rheumatol*. 2023;75:2405–2419.

Kinoshita Y, Fukumoto S. X linked hypophosphatemia and FGF-23 related hypophosphatemic diseases—prospect for new treatment. *Endocr Rev*. 2018;39:274–291.

Leboff MS, Greenspan SL, Insogna KL, et al. The clinician's guide to prevention and treatment of osteoporosis. *Osteoporosis Int*. 2022;33:2049–2102.

Licata AA, Binkley N, Petak SM, Camacho PM. Consensus statement by the American Association of Clinical Endocrinologists and American College of Endocrinology on the quality of DXA scans and reports. *Endocrine Pract*. 2018;24:220–229.

Lindsay R, Silverman SL, Cooper C, et al. Risk of new vertebral fracture in the year following a fracture. *JAMA*. 2001;285:320–323.

Marie PJ, Cohen-Solal M. The expanding life and functions of osteogenic cells: from simple bone-making cells to multifunctional cells and beyond. *J Bone Min Res*. 2018;33:199–210.

Mittan D, Lee S, Miller E, et al. Bone loss following hypogonadism in men with prostate cancer treated with GnRH analogs. *J Clin Endocrinol Metab*. 2002;87:3656–3661.

Palomo T, Vilaça T, Lazaretti-Castro M. Osteogenesis imperfecta: diagnosis and treatment. *Curr Opin Endocrinol Diabetes Obes*. 2017;24:381–388.

Rothman MS, Lewiecki EM, Miller PD. Bone density testing is the best way to monitor osteoporosis. *Am J Med*. 2017;130:1133–1134.

Ryan CS, Pefkov VI, Adler RA. Osteoporosis in men: the value of laboratory testing. *Osteoporosis Int*. 2011;22:1845–1853.

Shapiro JR, Lewiecki M. Hypophosphatasia in adults: clinical assessment and treatment considerations. *J Bone Min Res*. 2017;32:1977–1980.

Shevroja E, Reginster JY, Lamy O, et al. Update on the clinical use of trabecular bone score (TBS) in the management of osteoporosis: results of an expert group meeting. *Osteoporos Int*. 2023;34:1501–1529.

Targownik LE, Lix LM, Tetge CJ, Prior HJ, Leung S, Leslie W. Use of proton pump inhibitors and risk of osteoporosis-related fractures. *CMAJ*. 2008;179:319–326.

Walker MD, Shane E. Postmenopausal osteoporosis. *N Engl J Med*. 2023;389:1979–1991.

Whyte MP, Rockman-Greenberg C, Ozono K, et al. Asfotase alfa treatment improves survival for perinatal and infantile hypophosphatasia. *J Clin Endocrinol Metab*. 2016;101:334–342.

Wu CC, Econs MJ, DeMeglio LA, et al. Diagnosis and management of osteopetrosis: consensus guidelines from the osteopetrosis working group. *J Clin Endocrinol Metab*. 2017;102:3111–3121.

Zhou C, Fang L, Chen Y, Zhong J, Wang H, Xie P. Effect of selective serotonin reuptake inhibitors on bone mineral density: a systematic review and meta-analysis. *Osteoporos Int*. 2018;29:1243–1251.

WEBSITES

The National Osteoporosis Foundation
www.nof.org
NIH Osteoporosis and Related Bone Diseases - National Resource Center
www.osteo.org
American Society for Bone and Mineral Research
www.asbmr.org
Bones and Osteoporosis
www.bones-and-osteoporosis.com
International Society for Clinical Densitometry
www.iscd.org

CHAPTER 52

Paget Disease of Bone

Christine M. Swanson, MD, MCR, CCD

>> KEY POINTS

1. Paget disease of bone (PDB) is a chronic condition characterized by focal areas of abnormal osteoclasts that cause excessive bone resorption, followed by abnormal bone formation resulting in disorganized, weak bone.
2. PDB commonly presents as an incidental discovery of elevated alkaline phosphatase (ALP), or bone abnormality on a nonrelated imaging study.
3. Plain radiographs are used to diagnose PDB and nuclear medicine bone scans are used to evaluate the extent of disease.
4. The treatment of choice for PDB is intravenous (IV) zoledronate, and treatment is indicated in PDB patients with symptoms (e.g., bone pain), hypercalcemia, and those at high risk of developing complications from PDB or undergoing surgery at or near a pagetic site.
5. Osteoarthritis (OA) is common in PDB, in part due to pagetic involvement adjacent to joints and alterations in gait, force transmission, and stress on joints.

1. What is PDB?

PDB is a chronic disease characterized by abnormal bone remodeling in one or more bones. Pagetic osteoclasts (bone cells responsible for bone resorption) are abnormally large and overactive causing focal areas of excessive bone resorption. Compensatory increases in bone formation (by osteoblasts) at pagetic sites result in disorganized, structurally weaker bone that is often increased in size. Sir James Paget first described this condition in 1876 and referred to it as *osteitis deformans*; however, there is evidence that the condition existed in Western Europe during the Roman period. PDB can lead to bone pain, skeletal deformities, pseudofractures, and osteoarthritis, though many people with PDB are asymptomatic at diagnosis.

2. What causes PDB?

The cause of PDB is unknown and may have genetic and environmental influences. Mutations in the SQSTM1 gene, which encodes a protein that plays a role in osteoclast function, are seen in 40% to 50% of familial cases of PDB. Paramyxovirus infection has been proposed as a potential trigger for PDB as pagetic osteoclasts have been found to contain intranuclear structures resembling paramyxovirus nucleocapsids, though no virus has been cultured from pagetic osteoclasts. The incidence and severity of PDB are decreasing worldwide, and this may reflect changes in environmental contributions to PDB.

3. How does PDB typically present?

PDB is typically diagnosed when elevated ALP or an abnormal radiograph (x-ray) is found incidentally in patients being evaluated for other reasons. Symptoms depend on the site and extent of involvement. Up to 30% to 40% of patients are symptomatic at diagnosis with the most common symptom being bone pain (80%). Frequently bone pain develops later in the disease course. The pain is characterized as a deep and aching pain that occurs with rest or activity and is often worse at night. Other symptoms can include joint pain (50%) from secondary OA (most commonly of knee, hip, or spine), bone deformities (e.g., tibial bowing, skull thickening), neurologic complications due to neural compression from enlarging bone, and spontaneous fractures most commonly of the femur, tibia, and humerus.

4. Who is typically affected by PDB?

PDB prevalence increases with age. It typically affects older adults and is uncommon before the age of 40 years. Incidence of PDB also varies based on geography and sex. Men appear to be more commonly affected than women. PDB most commonly affects those of European descent and less commonly those of African and Asian descent. In the United States, PDB is estimated to affect 2% to 3% of the adult population over the age of 55 years.

5. How is PDB diagnosed?

PDB is a radiographic diagnosis and can be made with a plain x-ray. Typical findings of PDB on radiograph include focal osteolysis with sclerotic changes, thickening of the cortex, coarse trabecular pattern, and bone enlargement (Fig.52.1). ALP should be measured, which is often, though not always, elevated.

6. What is the differential diagnosis of PDB?

The differential for radiographic PDB may include chronic osteomyelitis, vertebral hemangioma, fibrous dysplasia, metaphyseal dysplasia (Engelmann disease), hyperostosis frontalis interna, familial expansile osteolysis, sternocostal clavicular hyperostosis, osteosarcoma, SAPHO syndrome (synovitis, acne, pustulosis, hyperostosis, osteitis), lymphoma, renal osteodystrophy, and metastatic cancer (e.g., prostate and breast cancer). Notably, PDB affecting the vertebrae and other bony sites tends to cause bony enlargement, which helps separate it from metastatic cancers. Elevated ALP can be seen in liver or biliary disease or any condition with increased bone turnover (e.g., osteomalacia, hyperparathyroidism, skeletal metastases).

7. Which bones are involved in PDB?

PDB may be monostotic (involvement of one bone) or more commonly (80%) polyostotic (involvement of two or more bones). It has a predilection for the axial skeleton but can affect

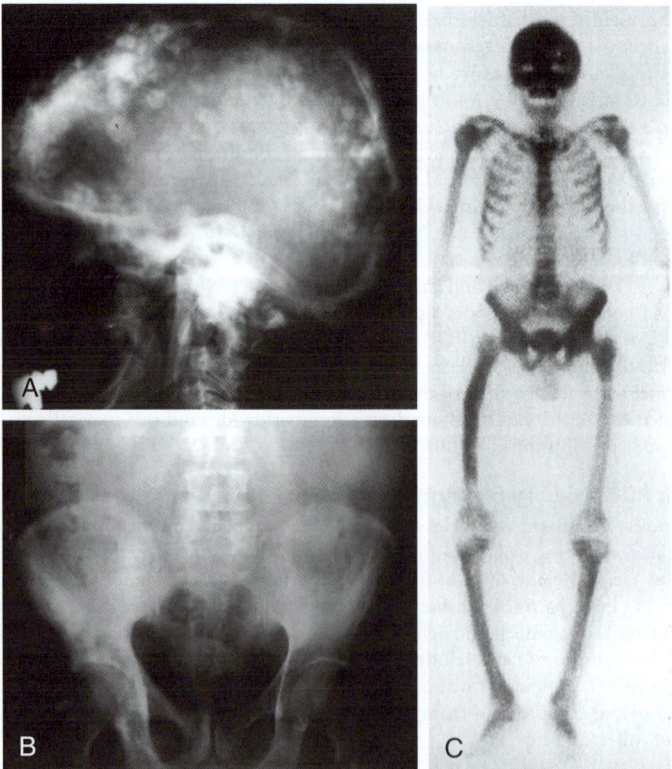

Fig. 52.1 The characteristic radiographic and scintigraphic findings seen in Paget's disease of bone. (A) A skull radiograph showing a thickened cranium with regions of dense sclerosis and osteopenia resulting in a "cotton wool" appearance. (B) A pelvic radiograph showing right hemipelvic loss of normal trabeculation, sclerosis, and cortical thickening, along with sclerosis of the iliopectineal line. (C) Full-body scintigraphy showing increased uptake in the skull, pelvis, lumbar spine, bilateral femurs with bowing of the right, tibias, scapula, and bilateral proximal humerus.

nearly any bone in the body. The most frequently involved bones are the pelvis (70%), femur (55%), lumbar spine (53%), skull (42%), and tibia (32%). Each individual pagetic site may progress or evolve over time; however, the number of skeletal sites involved is usually stable over time, and it is rare for new skeletal lesions to develop after diagnosis.

8. What are the typical histological and radiological appearances and triphasic progression of pagetic bone lesions?

PDB progresses through three phases. First, there is a focal increase in bone resorption due to increased osteoclast activity by numerous enlarged, often multinucleated osteoclasts **(lytic phase)**. Radiographic findings include bone loss, wedge-shaped areas of resorption in long bones (blade of grass), and circumscribed lytic lesions in the skull (osteoporosis circumscripta). Second, increased osteoblast activity and accelerated bone formation occur, resulting in disorganized collagen architecture (mosaic or woven, instead of the normal lamellar pattern) and a **mixed lytic/sclerotic phase.** This abnormal bone has impaired strength and is at higher risk for fracture. On x-ray, bones are enlarged and sclerotic. Additionally, bowing deformities, transverse linear radiolucencies ("pseudofractures"), and thickening of the calvarium (cotton wool) and iliopubic/ilioischial lines (brim sign) may be seen (Fig.52.1). Finally, in the third phase there is the **sclerotic phase** where there is reduced bone cell activity, areas of resorbed bone replaced by fibrous tissue, and persistence of abnormal bone architecture including enlarged, sclerotic bones. When atraumatic fractures of long bones occur, they typically are transverse (chalk stick) and not spiral, reflecting the weakened bony microarchitecture of pagetic woven bone.

9. Which laboratory tests should be obtained to evaluate and monitor PDB?

ALP, calcium, albumin, liver function tests, and 25-hydroxyvitamin D should be obtained in patients with suspected or known PDB. ALP can be within normal limits in those with limited, monostotic disease or during the initial osteolytic phase of PDB but rises during the osteoblastic phase and can correlate with disease activity. Measurement of ALP is the preferred assay in PDB. If liver disease is present or ALP is normal, other markers of bone formation (osteoblastic activity) such as bone-specific alkaline phosphatase (BSAP) or procollagen type I N-terminal propeptide (P1NP) can be checked. The elevated turnover marker can be followed over time every 6 to 12 months to assess a patient's response to treatment and/or PDB activity.

10. What imaging is recommended to determine the extent of skeletal involvement in PDB and for monitoring?

Plain x-rays are used to diagnose PDB, but the extent of PDB involvement is best measured by radionuclide bone scan (Fig. 52.1). Bone scan findings are nonspecific (e.g., may see false positives at osteoarthritic sites); however, it is the most sensitive exam for identifying PDB lesions. Early symptomatic lesions may be apparent on bone scan before x-ray changes, whereas burned-out pagetic lesions that are easily seen on x-ray may not have increased uptake on bone scan. It is recommended that patients with a newly diagnosed PDB have a bone scan during their initial evaluation, followed by x-rays of involved sites. Computed tomography (CT), magnetic resonance imaging (MRI), and positron emission tomography (PET) imaging are not routinely used in PDB.

11. What medications are available to treat PDB?

Adequate calcium and vitamin D are essential in PDB. Nitrogen-containing bisphosphonates (Table 52.1) are considered first-line therapy for treatment of PDB, as they target affected sites

TABLE 52.1 Bisphosphonates Used in the Treatment of Paget Disease of Bone

DRUG NAME	DOSAGE	DURATION
Zoledronate	5 mg IV (once, infused over 15–30 minutes)	N/A
Alendronate	40 mg/day orally	6 months
Risedronate	30 mg/day orally	2 months

and effectively suppress bone resorption by inhibiting osteoclasts. These medications include IV (zoledronic acid [zoledronate], pamidronate) and oral formulations (alendronate, risedronate). Calcitonin is less effective and not commonly used. There are case reports of denosumab being used in treatment of PDB; however, currently PDB is not an approved indication for denosumab. Additionally, there are significant risks with stopping denosumab without subsequent antiresorptive therapy (declining bone mineral density, increased risk of multiple vertebral compression fractures) (see Anastasilakis et al., *Journal of Clinical Medicine* 2021).

12. Which pharmacological agent is the treatment of choice for PDB?

Zoledronate, an IV infusion, is the treatment of choice for PDB because it has the fastest, most dramatic, and sustained effect on ALP and symptoms (pain, quality of life). After a single dose, 96% of patients normalize or have at least a 75% reduction in ALP levels at 6 months. Zoledronate is effective even in PDB patients who did not respond to previous treatment with other bisphosphonates. Sustained biochemical response to zoledronate may last for 6 years. Bisphosphonates are contraindicated in those with creatinine clearance <35 mL/minute.

13. What are the indications for treatment of PDB?

Bisphosphonate treatment should be considered for:
- Symptoms (e.g., bone pain that corresponds to a site of metabolically active PDB, bony deformity, high-output cardiac failure)
- Those at high risk of developing complications from PDB lesion (e.g., fracture in weight-bearing bones, headaches, nerve compression from involvement of the skull or spine, disease near major joints, hearing loss)
- Prior to orthopedic or elective surgery at or near a pagetic site to reduce hypervascularity and perioperative blood loss
- Hypercalcemia in the setting of immobilization.

14. What are the treatment goals in PDB?

Response to therapy is typically assessed with bone turnover markers. The preferred marker, ALP, normally decreases 1 to 2 weeks after zoledronate, reaching a nadir by 3 to 6 months. Bone resorption markers (e.g., serum collagen type 1 cross-linked C-telopeptide [CTX], urinary collagen type 1 cross-linked N-telopeptide [NTX]) fall more rapidly after treatment but are more expensive and cumbersome to obtain due to diurnal variation (e.g., must be drawn on fasting morning serum or second void morning urine, respectively). Other bone formation markers (e.g., P1NP, BSAP) may be trended if ALP cannot be used (e.g. liver disease). Sustained remission may be indicated by bone turnover markers in the lower half of the reference range, and retreatment may be considered if pagetic symptoms recur or bone turnover markers become elevated. There are no data to support that ALP normalization decreases risk of long-term complications; however, trials have been limited in size and duration.

15. What are the side effects of pharmacological therapy?

Bisphosphonates have been associated with a small increased risk of osteonecrosis of the jaw (particularly with invasive dental procedures and in cancer patients) and atypical (subtrochanteric) femoral fractures. Bisphosphonates can be nephrotoxic and are contraindicated in patients with impaired renal function (creatinine clearance < 35 mL/minute). Hypocalcemia can occur with bisphosphonate treatment, especially in those patients with vitamin D deficiency. Different formulations have specific side effects that should be considered. Oral formulations can cause esophagitis/dyspepsia. IV bisphosphonates (e.g., zoledronate) can cause a significant acute-phase response (fever, myalgias, arthralgia) lasting for 2 to 3 days after the infusion. Patients should be premedicated with acetaminophen before the infusion and optimization of vitamin D status prior to infusion may decrease the risk of an acute phase reaction in patients with PDB. Calcium and vitamin D should be supplemented daily to prevent secondary hyperparathyroidism and/or hypocalcemia.

16. What complications can arise in PDB?

Skeletal

Bone pain

Bone and joint deformities (bowing, frontal bossing)
Fractures (7% of patients)
Secondary osteoarthritis
Dental malocclusion

Neurologic

Deafness (auditory nerve entrapment or involvement of bones of inner ear; 13%)
Nerve entrapment (cranial nerves, spinal nerve roots)
Spinal stenosis (cauda equina syndrome)
Basilar invagination
Headaches, vertigo, tinnitus
Stroke (blood vessel compression)

Vascular

Hyperthermia
Vascular steal syndrome (external carotid blood flow to the skull at the expense of the brain)

Cardiac

High-output congestive heart failure (due to increased pagetic bone vascularity when over
   40% of skeleton involved)
Hypertension
Cardiomegaly
Angina

Malignancy

Osteogenic sarcomas (most commonly in humerus; 1%)
Fibrosarcomas, chondrosarcomas
Benign giant cell tumors

Metabolic

Hypercalcemia
Hypercalcuria
Nephrocalcinosis

17. What is the risk of osteosarcoma in a patient with PDB?

Transformation of a pagetic site to osteosarcoma has a poor prognosis but is quite rare, occurring in <1% of patients. Osteosarcoma should be suspected in PDB patients with increased bone pain and swelling, new mass, or new fracture at a pagetic site. MRI is useful in these instances to distinguish pagetic bone lesions from malignancies.

18. What other treatments should be considered for patients with complications from PDB?

Pain due to secondary OA in PDB may be effectively treated with traditional analgesics like acetaminophen or nonsteroidal antiinflammatory drugs. Medications such as gabapentin, pregabalin, and amitriptyline can be used if neuropathic pain is present. Other treatment modalities may include orthopedic surgery to correct bone deformities, address spinal canal stenosis, or treat pseudofractures. Canes and shoe lifts can be helpful for patients with limb deformities. It is also important for patients to have adequate calcium and vitamin D levels to avoid hypocalcemia, especially if planning for IV bisphosphonate treatment.

19. How does PDB contribute to OA risk?

OA is common in PDB and is present in 40% to 50% of patients. PDB commonly affects bone adjacent to joints and can contribute to OA by causing bony incongruencies. Bowing of long bones can increase the risk of OA as it alters gait and increases stress on joints via altered force transmission through the joint and premature loss of articular cartilage. Pagetic pain may cause people to favor their nonpagetic leg, which can contribute to OA development on the unaffected side.

20. How do you determine if the pain is due to pagetic bone pain or OA?

PDB and OA pain may both be described as "aching," and it is frequently difficult to distinguish which is causing symptoms in PDB patients. PDB pain is more likely to be present at rest. However, pain from both PDB and OA may worsen with weight bearing. Bisphosphonate treatment can be helpful in distinguishing the cause of pain as it will improve pagetic bone pain within 3 to 4 months, but not osteoarthritic pain. Alternatively, an injection of lidocaine into the affected joint (usually the hip) will transiently eliminate pain resulting from osteoarthritis but not PDB.

ACKNOWLEDGMENT

The author would like to acknowledge the contributions of Dr. David R. Finger and Dr. Matthew P. Wahl who authored this chapter in previous editions. CMS is supported by R01 HL151332.

BIBLIOGRAPHY

Banaganapalli B, Fallatah I, Alsubhi F, et al. Paget's disease: a review of the epidemiology, etiology, genetics and treatment. *Front Genet*. 2023;14:1131182.

Cundy T. Paget's disease of bone. *Metabolism*. 2018;80:5–14.

Gennari L, Rendina D, Falchetti A, Merlotti D. Paget's disease of bone. *Calcif Tissue Int*. 2019;104:483–500.

Hosking D, Lyles K, Brown JP, et al. Long-term control of bone turnover in Paget's disease with zoledronic acid and risedronate. *J Bone Miner Res*. 2007;22:142–148.

Langston AL, Campbell MK, Fraser WD, MacLennan GS, Selby PL, Ralston SH. PRISM Trial Group: randomized trial of intensive bisphosphonate treatment versus symptomatic management in Paget's disease of bone. *J Bone Miner Res*. 2010;25:20–31.

Mangham DC, Davie MW, Grimer RJ. Sarcoma arising in Paget's disease of bone: declining incidence and increasing age at presentation. *Bone*. 2009;44:431–436.

Mays S. Archaeological skeletons support a northwest European origin for Paget's disease of bone. *J Bone Miner Res*. 2010;25:1839–1841.

Merlotti D, Gennari L, Martini G, et al. Comparison of different intravenous bisphosphonate regimens for Paget's disease of bone. *J Bone Miner Res*. 2007;22:1510–1517.

Merlotti D, Rendina D, Cavati G, et al. Drug treatment strategies for Paget's disease: relieving pain and preventing progression. *Expert Opin Pharmacother*. 2023;24:715–727.

Merlotti D, Rendina D, Muscariello R, et al. Preventive role of vitamin D supplementation for acute phase reaction after bisphosphonate infusion in Paget's disease. *J Clin Endocrinol Metab*. 2020;105:e466–e476.

Paul Tuck S, Layfield R, Walker J, Mekkayil B, Francis R. Adult Paget's disease of bone: a review. *Rheumatology (Oxford)*. 2017;56:2050–2059.

Ralston SH. Clinical practice. Paget's disease of bone. *N Engl J Med*. 2013;368:644–650.

Ralston SH, Corral-Gudino L, Cooper C, et al. Diagnosis and management of Paget's disease of bone in adults: a clinical guideline. *J Bone Miner Res*. 2019;34:579–604.

Reid IR, Miller P, Lyles K, et al. Comparison of a single infusion of zoledronic acid with risedronate for Paget's disease. *N Engl J Med*. 2005;353:898–908.

Singer FR. The evaluation and treatment of Paget's disease of bone. *Best Pract Res Clin Rheumatol*. 2020;34:101506.

Singer FR, Bone 3rd HG, Hosking DJ, et al. Endocrine Society: Paget's disease of bone: an endocrine society clinical practice guideline. *J Clin Endocrinol Metab*. 2014;99:4408–4422.

Siris ES, Roodman GD. Paget's disease of bone. In: Rosen C, ed. *Primer on the Metabolic Bone Diseases and Disorders of Mineral Metabolism*. Hoboken, NJ: Wiley; 2012:335–343.

Tan A, Goodman K, Walker A, et al. Long-term randomized trial of intensive versus symptomatic management in Paget's disease of bone: the PRISM-EZ study. *J Bone Miner Res*. 2017;32:1165–1173.

FURTHER READING

https://www.bonehealthandosteoporosis.org/pagets/.

Osteonecrosis

Christopher C. Striebich, MD, PhD

1. List some synonyms for ON.

Avascular necrosis, aseptic necrosis, atraumatic necrosis, and ischemic necrosis.

2. How is ON defined?

ON refers to death of the cellular component of bone (osteocytes) and contiguous bone marrow resulting from ischemia. Although inciting factors for such ischemia are varied, their end results are clinically indistinguishable.

3. What skeletal regions are predisposed to developing ON?

Bones are most vulnerable in those areas having both limited vascular supply and restricted collateral circulation, which are areas that are also typically covered by articular cartilage. The area most frequently affected is the **femoral head.** At-risk areas include femoral head, carpal bones (scaphoid, lunate), humeral head, talus, femoral condyles, tarsal navicular, proximal tibia, and metatarsals.

4. Name some other common spontaneous ON syndromes.

- Scaphoid (Preiser's disease).
- Lunate (Kienböck's disease).
- Basal phalanges (Thiemann's disease).
- Capitulum of humerus (Panner's disease).
- Vertebral body (Kummell's disease).
- Femoral epiphysis (Legg–Calvé–Perthes).
- Tarsal navicular (Köhler's disease).
- Second metatarsal head (Freiberg's disease).

5. What is the etiology of this disorder?

The etiology of ON is most obvious and best understood in posttraumatic disruption of the arterial blood supply. Fractures of the femoral neck have been associated with ON in 15% of nondisplaced and 25% to 50% of displaced fractures. Hip dislocation causes ON in 10% to 25% of cases.

In ON cases that develop in the absence of trauma, various pathologic processes are capable of inducing hemostasis and, in turn, ischemia. Potential mechanisms include:

- Occlusion of blood vessels from sickled red blood cells, thrombophilia/coagulation disorders, and fat emboli (long bone fractures, fatty liver, hyperlipidemia)
- Bone marrow hypertrophy/infiltration and increased pressure in the bony compartment that compromises blood flow can occur in Gaucher's, leukemia, myeloproliferative disorders, and corticosteroids (fat hypertrophy).

- Bone marrow cellular toxicity and death because of external factors such as radiation, chemotherapy, and thermal injury.
- Genetic, epigenetic, and environmental factors as well as inflammatory pathways.

6. What clinical conditions are associated with ON?

The conditions associated with ON are shown in Box 53.1.

7. Briefly describe the pathogenesis of ON and the resulting symptoms.

Etiologic factors initiate hemostasis directly or trigger a cascade resulting in hemostasis. Histologic findings indicate that the final common pathway for the various inciting factors involves local intravascular coagulation and resultant tissue ischemia. The result is that of cancellous bone and bone marrow death. With subchondral cancellous bone death, collapse of the articular surface may or may not occur, depending on the extent of involvement.

Pain, the earliest symptom of ON, may occur in the early stages of involvement, before any radiographic changes are noted. This pain is likely to be the result of elevated intraosseous pressure because such pain can be relieved by decompression. In some individuals, no symptoms develop until the late stages of the disease process when collapse of the articular surface occurs and secondary degenerative changes develop. Others, in whom the area of infarction is small enough that collapse does not occur, may never develop symptoms. Radiographs in these patients reveal sclerotic areas often referred to as "bone islands" or "bone infarcts."

8. What are the epidemiologic features of ON?

- An estimated 10,000 to 30,000 new cases develop each year in the United States. Femoral head ON accounts for 10% of all total hip arthroplasties.

BOX 53.1 Conditions Associated with Osteonecrosis

Nontraumatic
Juvenile
Slipped capital femoral epiphysis
Legg–Calvé–Perthes

Adult
Corticosteroid administration
Alcohol use
Sickle cell anemia
Hemoglobinopathies (thalassemia, hemoglobin C disease)
Dysbaric osteonecrosis
Gaucher disease, Fabry disease
Radiotherapy/chemotherapy
Cushing disease
Diabetes mellitus
Hyperlipidemia
Hypercoagulable states/thrombophilia/disseminated intravascular coagulation
Pancreatitis
Pregnancy
Oral contraceptive use
Systemic lupus erythematosus, primary antiphospholipid syndrome, and other connective tissue disorders
Organ transplantation
Fat embolism
Severe acute respiratory syndrome
Carbon tetrachloride/lead poisoning
Tumor infiltration of marrow
Arteriosclerosis/vaso-occlusive disorders
Others: human immunodeficiency virus/highly active antiretroviral therapy, smoking, idiopathic

Traumatic
Fracture of the femoral neck
Fracture/dislocation of the hip
Hip trauma without fracture or dislocation
Hip surgery

- In cases of nontraumatic ON, corticosteroid and alcohol use may be responsible for 50% to 70% of cases; in up to 10% to 15% of cases, there is no identifiable risk factor (idiopathic).
- Males are affected more frequently than females at a ratio of approximately 8:1, possibly reflecting a higher incidence of trauma in males.
- Most cases develop in the <50-year-old age group. One exception to this observation is seen in ON of the knee (femoral condyles, proximal tibia), to which women over the age of 50 years are predisposed (female: male ratio of approximately 3:1).

9. What clinical features would lead to suspicion of this disorder?

The signs and symptoms stemming from ON are nonspecific. **Pain** is what leads affected individuals to seek medical evaluation. For the hip, which is the most commonly involved joint, pain is unilateral at onset and localizes to the groin, buttock, medial thigh, and medial aspect of the knee. Pain occurs with weight bearing but can be present at rest (66%) and at night (33%) because of elevated intraosseous pressure. Occasionally, knee pain is the major complaint in an individual with late-stage ON of the hip. Typically, morning stiffness is absent or of short duration (<1 hour), allowing differentiation from inflammatory monoarticular arthritides. Range of motion is not affected, except as limited by discomfort, until late degenerative changes develop. Although these findings are common to other potential etiologies, their occurrence in the setting of a patient with a predisposing risk (e.g., recent trauma, high-dose steroid use) should suggest underlying ON.

10. How much corticosteroid puts a patient at risk for ON?

Overall, 10% to 30% of patients on GCs develop ON. A previous review estimated a 4.6-fold increase in the rate of ON for every 10 mg/day increase in the mean daily dose of prednisone during the first 6 months of therapy. More recent reports suggest that the risk of ON is increased in patients who are on >20 mg/day of prednisone for over a month or receive >2 g total over 2 to 3 months.

The risk of ON increases by 5% for every 20-mg increase in prednisone dose taken for over one month. Although controversial, high-dose pulse corticosteroids alone (i.e., 1 g methyl-prednisolone monthly) do not increase risk unless followed by high-dose daily oral prednisone. Patients who smoke or have systemic lupus erythematosus (SLE), antiphospholipid antibodies, or rapidly develop profound Cushingoid features are particularly likely to develop ON.

11. How do corticosteroids cause ON?

GCs cause ON by both direct and indirect effects on cells. Direct effects include increased apoptosis of osteoblasts, osteocytes, and endothelial cells. Indirect effects include increased hypercoagulability, decreased angiogenesis, and modulated local vasoactive amine production, which can contribute to ischemia. Finally, increased intraosseous pressure because of adipogenesis and fat hypertrophy in the bone marrow can decrease blood flow to the area. However, because not all patients who receive steroids get ON, genetic factors are thought to play a role. Genetic differences in the affinity of GCs to bind to their receptors as well as the speed of metabolism of GCs to their inactive forms at the local tissue level may account for why less than half of GC-treated patients get ON.

12. How much alcohol intake does it take to be at risk for ON?

Overall, 2% to 5% of patients with alcohol use disorder will develop ON. It is estimated that a total of 150 L of 100% alcohol at a rate of 400 mL/week (i.e., one pint/week) increases the risk 9.8-fold for developing ON. The risk of ON increases with the amount of alcohol consumed weekly: 3-fold if <400 mL/week, 10-fold if 400 to 1000 mL/week, and 18-fold if >1000 mL/week. Susceptibility may be partly determined by genetics. Certain polymorphisms of alcohol-metabolizing enzymes may contribute to ON risk. Smoking also increases the risk.

13. What is the suspected cause of idiopathic ON?

ON without an identifiable cause accounts for 10% to 15% of all cases. Extensive analysis supports that many of these patients may have a hypercoagulable state as evidenced by elevated lipoprotein(a), low tissue plasminogen activator activity, and/or high plasminogen activator inhibitor levels. Others have been found to have high homocysteine levels, elevated antiphospho-lipid antibodies, low protein C or protein S levels, or the presence of Factor V Leiden.

14. Describe risk factors for the development of ON of the jaw.

Medications used to treat osteoporosis and other metabolic bone diseases have been associated with osteonecrosis of the jaw. Medication-related osteonecrosis of the jaw (MRONJ) has been seen with bisphosphonates (alendronate, zoledronic acid, and others), the RANKL inhibitor denosumab, as well as a variety of cancer therapeutics. The risk of developing MRONJ is higher in individuals receiving these therapies for the treatment of malignancies with osseous metastasis (≥2–5%) as opposed to osteoporosis (<0.15%) possibly due to the higher IV doses used. Increased risk is also seen with longer duration of treatment (>3 yrs). Other etiologies for osteonecrosis of the jaw have been identified, including many already described here for ON, as well as dentoal-veolar surgery.

15. What is spontaneous ON of the knee?

Spontaneous ON of the knee (SONK) is an idiopathic form of ON that affects primarily women (female:male = 3:1) over the age of 50 years. Patients present with knee pain. MRI shows lesions that tend to be small, with medial more than lateral femoral condyle involvement.

16. What is the role of plain radiographs in the diagnosis of ON?

Initially, plain films are normal. Later, a region of generalized osteopenia may develop (a non-specific finding). Eventually, after bone repair mechanisms have had time to work, a mottled appearance develops in the affected area because of the presence of "cysts" (regions of dead bone resorption) and contiguous sclerosis (regions of bone repair).

Early collapse of the cancellous bone beneath the subchondral plate is apparent as a pathogno-monic radiolucent line frequently referred to as the **crescent sign** (Fig. 53.1). Once in this stage, further collapse is almost inevitable, thus, it represents the earliest irreversible lesion of ON. Once the articular surface has collapsed and flattened, secondary degenerative changes develop, result-ing in joint space narrowing and secondary involvement of other bones within the articulation (e.g., acetabulum).

17. How good is MRI in the diagnosis of ON? What about other imaging studies?

Compared with other diagnostic studies, MRI has been found to have the highest sensitivity and best diagnostic accuracy, thus obviating invasive diagnostic procedures such as biopsy and bone marrow pressure determinations. Sensitivity and diagnostic accuracy appear to be 95% to 99%. The characteristic MRI finding is an area or **line of decreased signal** on both T1 and T2 images (Fig. 53.2). This area appears to correspond with the demarcation between live regenerating bone and necrotic tissue. In patients who cannot undergo an MRI, **radionuclide bone scanning** can

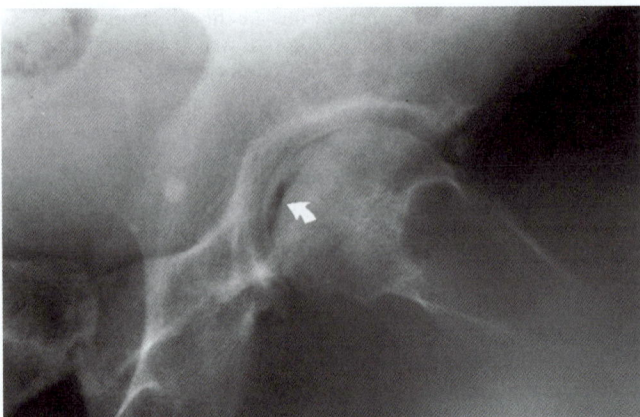

Fig. 53.1 A plain radiograph of the hip showing the crescent sign *(arrow)* of osteonecrosis.

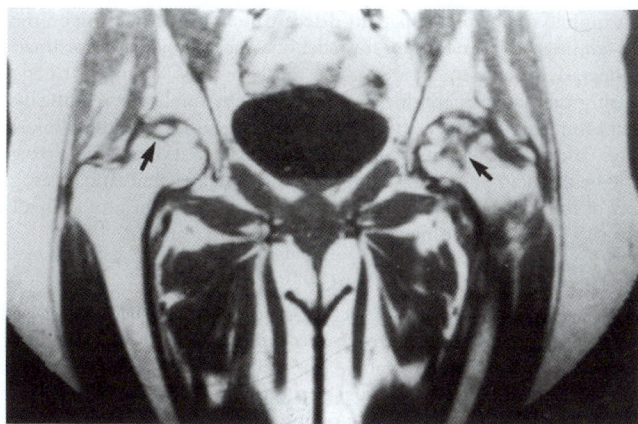

Fig. 53.2 Magnetic resonance imaging of bilateral hips showing necrotic bone *(arrows)* in both femoral heads consistent with osteonecrosis.

show a subchondral "cold spot" (avascular necrosis) surrounded by a "hot" area (donut sign) where there is increased osteoblastic activity at the interface with the necrotic bone. A computed tomography CT scan will show necrotic and reactive bone.

18. How often does ON occur in a bilateral fashion?

Approximately 50% of patients with symptomatic hip ON have asymptomatic disease in the contralateral hip at the time of initial presentation. Two-thirds of these asymptomatic hips will eventually progress to late-stage ON. Consequently, a bilateral hip MRI at the time of presentation is recommended. Similar frequencies would be expected in ON of the humeral head and knee. It is common to have multiple bony areas involved.

19. Describe the staging scheme for ON of the femoral head.

See Table 53.1.

20. Describe the medical management of ON.

The goal of treating ON is to prevent bony collapse and subsequent deformity. Thus, effective treatment is contingent upon diagnosis while ON is still in its early stages (stage II and less). Patients on GC should be tapered to the lowest possible dose. Recommended medical

TABLE 53.1 University of Pennsylvania (Steinberg) System of Staging of Osteonecrosis of the Femoral Head

STAGE	PLAIN RADIOGRAPHIC FINDINGS	MAGNETIC RESONANCE IMAGING[a]
0[b]	Normal	Normal
I	Normal	Abnormal
II	Osteopenia, bony sclerosis, cystic changes	Abnormal
III	Subchondral collapse ("crescent sign") without articular surface flattening	Abnormal
IV	Flattening of the articular surface without joint-space narrowing	Abnormal
V	Flattening of the articular surface with joint-space narrowing and/or acetabular involvement	Abnormal
VI	Advanced degenerative changes	Abnormal

[a]Each stage is further divided into three subclasses: A = small (<15% femoral head involvement, <2-mm depression of femoral head); B = moderate (15–30%, 2–4 mm); C = large (>30%, >4 mm) depending on the size of the lesion on magnetic resonance imaging.
[b]Stage 0 refers to an "at risk" asymptomatic, uninvolved hip in an individual with avascular necrosis on the contralateral side.

management is limited to having the patient **discontinue weight-bearing** on the affected side for 4–8 weeks and administering **analgesics** for relief of associated pain. Unfortunately, hip survival rates with nonoperative management are only in the 13% to 35% range for stage I–IV disease. Therefore, nonsurgical management does not change the natural course of the disease. Recently there have been promising reports with pharmacologic therapies including lipid-lowering drugs, bisphosphonates, and anticoagulants, which may be considered. Hyperbaric oxygen, pulsed electromagnetic field therapy, and extracorporeal shock therapy are being investigated. The best results with any of these therapies are achieved in patients where the area of involvement of the femoral head is ≤15% and do not involve the weight-bearing surface.

21. Describe the surgical management for ON.

In **early, reversible stages** of ON, several surgical procedures have been developed with the aim of preventing progression. Of these, **core decompression** of the femoral head has been most commonly performed and investigated. The rationale for this operation is that if increased intraosseous pressure can be relieved, vascular perfusion can then be enhanced and help prevent progression of the lesion. Several studies comparing core decompression with nonoperative management have shown favorable results, with success rates in the range of 47% to 84% for stage I to III disease. Core decompression has also shown some benefit when used to treat knee and humerus ON. **Vascularized fibula grafting** into the femoral head has been shown in several studies to be extremely promising, with 5-year hip survival rates of 81% to 89% for stage II to IV disease. However, there is a high complication rate (19%), so this procedure is a consideration only in medical communities in which a skilled surgeon with experience in this technique is available. In general, lesions <30% of the femoral head have the best results. Initial studies using **autologous mesenchymal stem cells** inserted into the femoral head after core decompression have shown encouraging results, but more research is needed.

In the **nonreversible stages** of ON (particularly stages V to VI), the goal of surgical intervention is to restore joint function and relieve associated pain. The effectiveness and reliability of **total hip arthroplasty** (replacement) have made earlier procedures attempting to achieve these goals obsolete.

22. Can ON be prevented?

Yes, to some extent. Modifiable risk factors can be manipulated, for example, steroid dose, alcohol intake, and control of diabetes and hyperlipidemia. As an example, the vast majority of cases of corticosteroid-related ON occur in patients who have received the equivalent of ≥20 mg of prednisone/day, especially for prolonged periods. In rheumatoid arthritis, where prednisone doses rarely exceed 10 mg/day, ON is uncommon. By contrast, in SLE, in which higher doses of steroids are frequently used, 30% to 50% of patients may develop some degree of ON. Early use of lipid-lowering drugs, bisphosphonates, antioxidants (vitamin E), and anticoagulants may be preventative.

23. What is bone marrow edema syndrome (BMES)?

BMES, also known as **transient osteoporosis,** is a self-limited transitory clinical entity characterized by pain, osteopenia on radiographs, and bone marrow edema on MRI. It most commonly involves the hip but can involve other lower extremity joints. This disorder typically affects women in the third trimester of pregnancy and middle-aged men. Usually, one hip is involved, but 40% to 80% can have bilateral involvement or involvement of other joints (knee, ankle, etc.). Symptoms last an average of 6 months. Up to 40% can have recurrences. Treatment is with analgesics and protective weight bearing. IV bisphosphonates have been used successfully and should be considered. Nifedipine, iloprost, and sympathetic nerve blockade have been used for pain relief. Vitamin D should be added if vitamin D levels are low. Core decompression is not indicated. **BMES differs from ON of the hip on MRI because it has both femoral head and femoral neck abnormalities, whereas ON only involves the femoral head**.

ACKNOWLEDGMENT

The author wishes to thank Dr. Robert T. Spencer for his contributions to this chapter in previous editions.

BIBLIOGRAPHY

Cohen-Rosenblum A, Cui Q. Osteonecrosis of the femoral head. *Orthop Clin North Am*. 2019;50:139–149.

Chang C, Greenspan A, Gershwin ME. The pathogenesis, diagnosis and clinical manifestations of steroid-induced osteo-necrosis. *J Autoimmun*. 2020;110:102460.

Chughtai M, Piuzzi NS, Khlopas A, et al. An evidence-based guide to the treatment of osteonecrosis of the femoral head. *Bone Joint J*. 2017;99-B(10):1267–1279.

Gadiwalla Y, Patel V. Osteonecrosis of the jaw unrelated to medication or radiotherapy. *Oral Surg Oral Med Oral Pathol Oral Radiol*. 2018;125:446–453.

Guo P, Gao F, Wang Y, et al. The use of anticoagulants for prevention and treatment of osteonecrosis of the femoral head: a systematic review. *Medicine (Baltimore)*. 2017;96:e6646.

Lai KA, Shen WJ, Yang CY, et al. The use of alendronate to prevent early collapse of the femoral head in patients with nontraumatic osteonecrosis. A randomized clinical study. *J Bone Joint Surg Am*. 2005;87:2155–2159.

Mont MA, Marker DR, Zywiel MG, et al. Osteonecrosis of the knee and related conditions. *J Am Acad Ortho Surg*. 2011;19:482–494.

Nevskaya T, Gamble MP, Pope JE. A meta-analysis of avascular necrosis in systemic lupus erythematosus: prevalence and risk factors. *Clin Exp Rheumatol*. 2017;35:700–710.

Patel S. Primary bone marrow oedema syndromes. *Rheumatology*. 2014;53:785–792.

Piuzzi NS, Chahla J, Jiandong H, et al. Analysis of cell therapies used in clinical trials for the treatment of osteonecrosis of the femoral head: a systematic review of the literature. *J Arthroplasty*. 2017;32:2612–2618.

Pritchett JW. Statin therapy decreases risk of osteonecrosis in patients receiving steroids. *Clin Orthop Relat Res*. 2001;386:173–178.

Rajpura A, Wright AC, Board TN. Medical management of osteonecrosis of the hip: a review. *Hip Int*. 2011;21:385–392.

Ruggiero SL, Dodson TB, Aghaloo T, Carlson ER, Ward BB, Kademani D. American Association of Oral and Maxillofacial Surgeons' Position Paper on Medication-Related Osteonecrosis of the Jaws-2022 update. *J Oral Maxillofac Surg*. 2022;80:920–943.

Shigemura T, Nakamura J, Kishida S, et al. Incidence of osteonecrosis associated with corticosteroid therapy among different underlying diseases: prospective MRI study. *Rheumatology*. 2011;50:2023–2028.

Zalavras CG, Lieberman JR. Osteonecrosis of the femoral head: evaluation and treatment. *J Am Acad Ortho Surg*. 2014;22:455–464.

FURTHER READING

http://www.orthoinfo.aaos.org.
https://medlineplus.gov/osteonecrosis.html.

CHAPTER 54

Heritable Connective Tissue Diseases

Alison M. Gizinski, MD

KEY POINTS

1. Osteogenesis imperfecta (OI) is classically a genetic defect of collagen type I causing "brittle bones," blue sclera, and abnormal teeth.
2. Ehlers–Danlos syndromes (EDS) are caused by multiple genetic defects of extracellular matrix (ECM) proteins causing joint hypermobility, skin hyperextensibility, and tissue fragility.
3. Marfan syndrome (MFS) is a genetic defect of fibrillin-1, leading to marfanoid habitus, aortic root dilatation, and an ectopic lens.

1. Discuss the characteristics of the heritable connective tissue diseases (HCTDs).

HCTDs are a heterogenous group of disorders that result from genetic defects that alter the quantity or structure of ECM proteins including collagens, fibrillins, elastin, and noncollagenous matrix proteins (tenascin, fibronectin, proteoglycans in the interstitial space, and integrins on cell surfaces). Depending on the ECM protein involved, one can predict which tissues are most likely to be affected including bone, cartilage, tendon, ligament, muscle, skin, eye, heart valves, blood vessels, and lung. There are over 450 well-characterized diseases. Although each is relatively rare, as a group they affect 1 in 5000 individuals. This chapter will discuss only the most common of these disorders.

2. Give the classification of HCTDs?

There are several different classifications that have been proposed. One classification is by the main collagenous structural property which has been altered.

- **Tensile HCTDs:** these disorders affect primarily type I or other (III, V) collagens, ECM proteins associated with these collagens, or elastin which are important for strength of bone, ligaments, tendons, skin, heart valves, and blood vessels. The disorders include: OI (collagen type I defect), EDS (collagen type I, III, or V defect; fibronectin defect, or enzyme deficiency), MFS (fibrillin-1 defect), congenital contractural arachnodactyly (CCA) (fibrillin-2 defect), pseudoxanthoma elasticum, cutis laxis, and supravalvular aortic stenosis (William syndrome caused by elastin gene deletion).
- **Compressive HCTDs:** these disorders affect multiple collagens and/or ECM proteins important for compression of cartilage and growth. Gene discovery has defined over 100 genes with various defects leading to abnormal collagens (types II, IX, X, XI), ECM proteins, defects in metabolic pathways (enzymes), defects in signal transduction and receptors, as well as others. The disorders include achondroplasias, epiphyseal chondrodysplasias (Stickler syndrome, spondyloepiphyseal dysplasia, and multiple epiphyseal dysplasia), metaphyseal chondrodysplasias, and others.
- **Barrier HCTDs:** these disorders affect type IV collagen (Alport syndrome) and type VII collagen (epidermolysis bullosa), which form barriers known as basement membranes.

TENSILE HEREDITARY CONNECTIVE TISSUE DISEASES

3. What is osteogenesis imperfecta (OI)? Which organs are involved, and why?

OI, also known as "brittle bone" disease, is a group of diseases defined by similar clinical manifestations (brittle bones and blue sclerae) occurring to various degrees with a similar etiology. It affects 1 in 20,000 individuals. The inheritance pattern and penetrance are variable. Most are autosomal dominant (AD), although some are autosomal recessive or due to sporadic mutations. Most patients with OI have an AD defect in one of the genes that encode type I collagen (COL1A1, COL1A2), which accounts for the structure and physical properties of bone. The genetic defects cause either low production (50% of normal) or abnormal quality (or both) of type I collagen which results in osteopenia and brittleness, leading to frequent fractures. Diminished type I collagen in the sclerae leads to translucency and apparent blueness, while in the teeth causes dentinogenesis imperfecta (opalescent teeth). Hearing loss, hypermobility, easy bruising, short stature, hernias, and excess sweating can also occur.

Clinical syndromes of brittle bone disease are variable. Affected individuals may experience *in utero* death from fractures, live birth with wormian bones, short stature, and multiple fractures, or live birth with mildly brittle bones and normal stature. The most severe forms of OI are typically spontaneous mutations or autosomal recessive (AR) genetic defects which affect proteins or enzymes that regulate type I collagen folding. Milder presentations are typically due to AD defects of one of the COL1A genes described earlier.

4. What is the Sillence classification of OI?

The original Sillence classification system grouped OI into four **clinical categories of severity (Types I-IV).** Based on discovery of other genetic defects and clinical presentations, Types V–XI have been subsequently added. Most forms can be classified clinically into mild, moderate, severe, and lethal.

Type I OI (mild): bone fragility, little or no deformity, normal stature, blue sclerae, osteopenia, and hearing loss in 50%, may (Type IA) or may not (Types IB/IC) have dentinogenesis imperfecta. Mutation of COL1A1 or COL1A2 gene causes underproduction (50%) of normal type I collagen and subsequent hypomineralization. T scores are often –2.5 to –4.0. Inheritance is AD.

Type II OI (usually lethal): multiple *in utero* fractures and blue or gray sclerae, *in utero*/neonatal death common. Inheritance is AD or AR, most with spontaneous mutations.

Type III OI (severe deforming): multiple fractures before age of 3 years, fractures heal with major skeletal deformities, triangular facies with frontal bossing, short stature, scoliosis, joint laxity, gray or blue sclerae, and hearing loss. Not usually ambulatory. Pulmonary insufficiency from thoracic deformity is a major cause of death before the age of 35 years. Usually results from a spontaneous mutation but can be AD or AR inheritance.

Type IV OI (moderate severity): variable short stature, variable bone fragility with a moderate number of fractures by the age of 10 years, wormian bones, normal (white) or gray sclerae, dentinogenesis imperfecta, some hearing loss, ambulatory. Inheritance is AD.

Type V OI (rare): similar to type IV but with hyperplastic callus formation post fracture (fracture risk moderate), normal sclera, limited pronation and supination at the forearm due to intramembranous bone formation. Mutation in IFITM5. Inheritance is AD.

Types VI-XI (rare): have moderate to severe skeletal manifestations and variable other manifestations. Inheritance is AR and involves mutations of various genes.

The diagnosis of OI is primarily clinical. Several laboratories will perform collagen biochemical and molecular (DNA sequencing) analysis from a skin biopsy, and NextGen Sequencing from whole blood is available from some laboratories as well. It is important to note that negative genetic testing does not rule out disease due to a false-negative rate of 10%, despite testing panels that may include 25 separate genes. Bisphosphonate therapy may be beneficial, especially intravenous pamidronate and zoledronic acid in Type I and Type II OI. Teriparatide and denosumab in adults with mild OI may be beneficial. Teriparatide is not considered safe for children due to osteosarcoma risk. Romosozumab, antibody to TGFβ, and gene therapy have shown promise in animal models. Clinical trials are ongoing. Corrective surgery, bracing, physical therapy, and continuous rehabilitative care are important.

5. What is the significance of increased joint mobility? How do you diagnose it?

Hyperflexible joints are common and do not necessarily indicate that someone has HCTD. Joint hypermobility decreases with age. Some studies suggest that 10% to 25% of the population may have hyperflexible joints, with 5% of people with hypermobility having symptoms. Symptoms from increased joint mobility can range from arthralgias to dislocation or injury. The diagnosis of EDS should be considered in patients with severe hypermobility and recurrent dislocations.

The **Beighton score** for joint laxity and hypermobility uses a simple nine-point system. A score of ≥5 indicates hypermobility on examination:

1. Hyperextension of the knee more than 10 degrees past 180 degrees. One point for each knee.
2. Hyperextension of the elbow more than 10 degrees past 180 degrees. One point for each elbow.

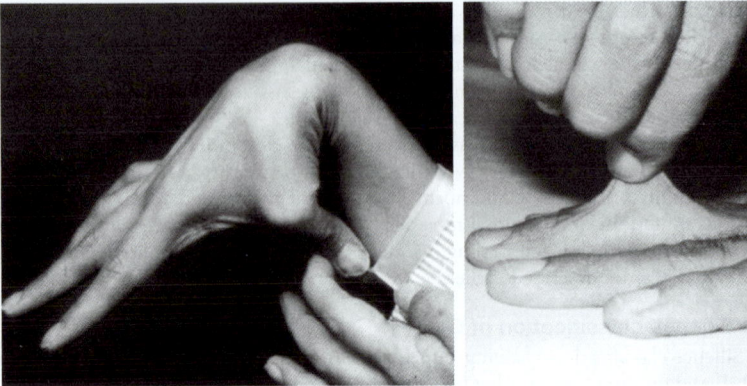

Fig. 54.1 Demonstration of the passive opposition of the thumb to the flexor aspect of the forearm in the Beighton score and skin hyperextenstibility greater than 1.5 cm at the dorsum of the hand.

3. Passive opposition of the thumb to the flexor aspect of the forearm. One point for each thumb. (see Fig. 54.1).
4. Passive extension of the little (fifth) finger beyond 90 degrees with the forearm flat on the table. One point for each little finger.
5. Forward trunk flexion (knees fully extended) so that the palms of the hands can be placed flat on the ground. One point.

6. Describe the clinical manifestations of EDS

The EDS are a group of uncommon connective tissue disorders resulting primarily in joint and skin laxity and arterial wall abnormalities. As a group (excluding hypermobile type), EDS affects 1 in 15,000 individuals. **Increased joint mobility** and **increased skin fragility and hyperextensibility** occur, though there is a wide variability in involvement. Hyperextensibility in patients with EDS may be greater in the small joints than large joints and may diminish with age. Skin hyperextensibility is defined as a capacity to stretch the skin 3 cm at the neck, elbows, and knees and 1.5 cm at the distal forearm or the dorsum of the hand (see Fig. 54.1). Skin laxity and fragility may manifest as easy bruisability, inability of stretched skin to return to normal, "cigarette paper" or "papyraceous-appearing" scars over the knees and other extensor surfaces, gaping wounds from minor trauma, or the inability of skin to retain sutures. Pes planus, pectus excavatum, and a high-arched palate can be present in all forms. Arteries may develop aneurysms or rupture because of elastic tissue laxity. There are several recognized clinical types of EDS. Most involve some abnormality in collagen synthesis or enzymatic modification of collagen. The 2017 International Classification of the EDS recognizes 13 types of EDS.

1. **Classical** (formerly classic EDS types I and II): hypermobility with joint dislocations, skin hyperextensibility, soft doughy skin, wide atrophic papyraceous scars, easy bruising ranging from mild to severe, and colluscoid pseudotumors of skin. Cervical insufficiency, uterine prolapse, scoliosis, and hernias can be seen. The most common genetic abnormality is a null allele for collagen type V (COL5A1 or COL5A2) and has AD inheritance. The classical type of EDS accounts for roughly 80% of EDS cases reported in the literature.
2. **Classical-like:** Skin hyperextensibility with velvety skin, joint hypermobility, easily bruised skin, and absence of atrophic scarring typify this category of EDS. Due to a mutation in the TNXB gene causing tenascin XB (ECM glycoprotein) deficiency. AR inheritance. Note that tenascin XB associates with type I collagen and is important for its stability and deposition.
3. **Cardiac-valvular:** severe progressive cardiac-valvular problems, skin hyperextensibility, atrophic scars, easy bruising, and joint hypermobility. COL1A2 mutations lead to lack of proα2-chain of type I collagen. AR inheritance.
4. **Hypermobile** (formerly EDS type III): **marked** hypermobility of large and small joints with soft skin but no scars. Much more common than other types of EDS, with a prevalence of 1 in 5000. Autonomic dysfunction including postural orthostatic tachycardia syndrome and postural acrocyanosis has been reported. Chronic joint pain, which may resemble

fibromyalgia, is common. Collagen/ECM protein defect unknown. Inheritance is suspected to be AD.

5. **Vascular** (formerly EDS IV): normal joint mobility, translucent skin with prominent venous pattern, marked bruising, aortic/arterial aneurysms, arterial rupture/dissections, rupture of uterus/bowel (sigmoid colon), and carotid-cavernous sinus fistula formation. Spontaneous hemopneumothorax and mitral valve prolapse can occur. No hyperelastic skin. Increased risk of maternal mortality during pregnancy. Surgery can be difficult due to friable arteries and organ tissue. Most commonly caused by various mutations in genes encoding for Type III collagen (COL3A1), which is found primarily in the skin, blood vessels, and walls of hollow viscera. AD inheritance.

6. **Kyphoscoliotic** (formerly EDS type VI): severe kyphoscoliosis with muscle hypotonia associated with joint laxity noted at birth, recurrent joint dislocation, and hyperextensible, fragile skin that develops gaping wounds with minor trauma and heals poorly. Unlike other EDS types, these patients have ocular fragility, blue sclerae, retinal detachment, glaucoma, and globe rupture that can lead to blindness. Most commonly due to mutations of the lysyl hydroxylase gene (PLOD1) results in deficiency of the enzyme. This enzyme is necessary for the conversion of lysyl residues to hydroxylysine on procollagen peptides, which is important for crosslinking and subsequent collagen stabilization. AR inheritance.

7. **Arthrochalasia** (formerly EDS VIIA and VIIB): significant hypermobility with large joint dislocations starting in newborn period (congenital hip dislocation), moderate skin hyper-extensibility and bruising, kyphoscoliosis, muscle hypotonia, frequent fractures, and short stature. Defect in type I collagen (COL1A1, COL1A2) involves lack of N-proteinase cleavage site, so type I collagen retains its N-terminal peptide resulting in abnormal collagen fibrils. AD inheritance.

8. **Dermatosparaxis** (formerly EDS VIIC): marked joint hypermobility, micrognathia, extremely fragile skin with bruising but no scars, sagging redundant skin, and blue sclerae. Large umbilical hernias are common. Short limbs, hands, and feet. Due to mutation in ADAMTS2 leading to a deficiency of procollagen N-propeptidase and abnormal type I collagen. AR inheritance.

9. **Brittle cornea syndrome:** thin cornea, early onset progressive keratoconus and keratoglobus, blue sclerae. Most commonly due to mutation in ZNF469, a zinc finger protein. AR Inheritance.

10. **Spondylodysplastic:** short stature, muscle hypotonia, bowing of limbs. Multiple gene mutations lead to glycosaminoglycan deficiency. AR inheritance.

11. **Musculocontractural:** Multiple congenital contractures, specific craniofacial features with broad forehead, micrognathia in infancy, protruding jaw in adolescence, low-set rotated ears, hyperextensible thin skin, atrophic skin, and organ fragility. Caused by a defect in the gene CHST14 (involved in glycosaminoglycan synthesis) or in the DSE gene. AR inheritance.

12. **Myopathic:** congenital muscle hypotonia and/or muscle atrophy, proximal joint contractures, hypermobility of distal joints. Defect involving COL12A1 gene for Type XII collagen. Inheritance is AR or AD.

13. **Periodontal** (formerly EDS VIII): severe periodontitis of childhood, lack of attached gingiva, pretibial plaques, joint hypermobility, and skin hyperextensibility. Gain of function mutations in C1R and C1S, involved in the classical pathway of complement. AD inheritance.

7. What are the Beighton (revised) diagnostic criteria for the joint hypermobility syndrome (JHS)?

Major criteria:
1. Beighton score of 4/9 or greater currently or historically (see Question 5).
2. Arthralgia for >3 months in four or more joints.

Minor criteria:
1. Beighton score of 1, 2, or 3/9 (0, 1, 2, or 3 if aged >50 years).
2. Arthralgia (≥3 months) in one to three joints or back pain (≥3 months), spondylosis, spondylolysis/spondylolisthesis.
3. Dislocation/subluxation in more than one joint, or in one joint on more than one occasion.
4. Three or more soft tissue lesions (epicondylitis, tenosynovitis, bursitis).
5. Marfanoid habitus.

6. Abnormal skin: striae, hyperextensibility, thin, papyraceous scarring.
7. Eye signs: drooping eyelids, myopia, or down-slanted palpebral fissures.
8. Varicose veins or hernia or uterine/rectal prolapse.

The JHS is diagnosed in the presence of two major criteria, or one major and two minor criteria, or four minor criteria. Note that major and minor criteria 1 are mutually exclusive as are major and minor criteria 2, since they are measuring the same manifestation.

8. Are JHS and EDS hypermobile type the same disease (controversial)?

The JHS has a familial predisposition and shows overlap with several HCTDs, most notably EDS hypermobile type. It is characterized by varying degrees of joint laxity without instability or disability and is an important cause of periarticular complaints. Arthralgias (hands, knees, and hips), knee effusions from patellar malalignment from laxity, daily headache from cervical spine hypermobility, and frequent ankle or wrist sprains are common. In addition to the clinical manifestations listed in the Beighton criteria, mitral valve prolapse and osteopenia (RR 1.8x) have been associated with JHS as well. Chronic fatigue, pain amplification (fibromyalgia-like), and dysautonomia have been reported more frequently in patients with JHS and EDS. The connective tissue defects responsible for JHS and EDS are unknown and hence the two cannot clearly be separated on a genetic basis. As such, some experts have suggested that JHS and EDS hypermobile type may represent a continuum. However, giving a patient the diagnosis of EDS may have adverse insurance implications whereas the diagnosis of JHS may not.

9. What are the revised Ghent criteria for the diagnosis of Marfan syndrome (MFS)?

MFS has an incidence of 1 in 3000 to 5000. The diagnosis can be difficult due to the multiple clinical manifestations. Diagnostic criteria have been established to help make a diagnosis. These criteria also call upon the clinician to rule out competing diagnoses such as Loey–Dietz syndrome, vascular EDS, and Shprintzen–Goldberg syndrome; therefore, referral to a medical geneticist should be considered.

Revised Ghent Criteria for Diagnosis of MFS
In the Absence of a Family History, Any One of the Following Gives the Diagnosis of MFS
Aortic root dilation[a] and/or dissection + ectopia lentis (bilateral upward)
Aortic root dilation[a] and/or dissection + fibrillin-1 gene (FBN1) mutation
Ectopia lentis and FBN1 mutation known to predispose to aortic root aneurysm/dissection
Aortic root dilation[a] and evidence of systemic features ($\geq$ 7 out of 20 points[b])
If a Family History of MFS in a First-Degree Relative, Any One of the Following Gives the Diagnosis of MFS
Ectopia lentis
Systemic features ($\geq$7 points)
Aortic root dilation[a] and/or dissection

---

[a]Dilation = aortic root diameter with Z-score $\geq$ 2 (calculators available on www.marfan.org)
[b]Systemic features include wrist and thumb sign (3 points); wrist or thumb sign (1 point); pectus deformity, carinatum (2 points) or excavatum (1 point) or chest asymmetry (1 point); hindfoot deformity (2 points); pes planus (1 point); pneumothorax (2 points); dural ectasia (2 points); protrusio acetabuli (2 points); reduced upper segment/lower segment ratio (<0.85) and increased arm span/height (>1.05) (1point); scoliosis or thoracolumbar kyphoscoliosis (1 point); reduced elbow extension <170 degrees (1 point); facial features (1 point); skin striae (1 point); myopia > 3 diopters (1 point); mitral valve prolapse (1 point).

10. What is the genetic defect in MFS, and how does it contribute to the clinical manifestations?

MFS is caused by mutations in the **fibrillin-1 gene** on chromosome 15. Over 3000 mutations of this gene have been reported. The predominant inheritance pattern is AD, although 25% of cases are due to sporadic mutations. Fibrillin-1 is produced by fibroblasts and forms a scaffold for the deposition of elastin. In addition to being a connective protein important in structural support for tissues, the fibrillin-1 protein also binds transforming growth factor β (TGF-β). Researchers now believe that the mutated fibrillin-1 cannot bind TGF-β resulting in excessive accumulation of TGF-β. Excess TGF-β can have deleterious effects on vascular smooth muscle development and the integrity of the ECM by binding to its receptor and upregulating TGF-β responsive genes

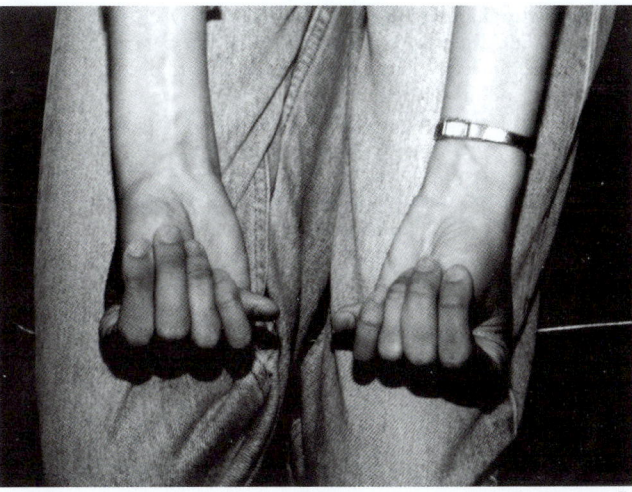

Fig. 54.2 Thumb sign: protrusion of the thumb past the hypothenar border when the hand is clenched in a fist.

such as those that regulate the production of matrix metalloproteinases (MMP-2 and MMP-9). The excess matrix metalloproteinases can interfere with tissue development and weaken the tissue. Therefore, organs that contain a lot of fibrillin-1 and elastin are most likely to be involved in MFS including the elastic walls of arteries (especially the aorta), heart valves, zonula fibers of the eye, ligaments, skin, and lung parenchyma.

11. Describe the phenotype and skeletal manifestations of MFS

Patients with MFS have a characteristic phenotype that is easily recognized: tall stature, long thin extremities (arm span/height ratio > 1.05 for white adults; may be lower in Asian and Afro-Caribbean), dolichostenomelia (abnormally low upper/lower body segment ratio of <0.85 for white adults and <0.78 for black adults compared with normal ratios of ≥0.93 for whites and ≥0.87 for blacks), and diminished subcutaneous fat. The lower segment is defined as the distance from the top of the symphysis pubis to the floor in the standing position, and the upper segment is the height minus the lower segment (of note, severe scoliosis may skew these measurements). Skeletal manifestations include arachnodactyly (spider digits), pectus excavatum or carinatum, loss of thoracic kyphosis, scoliosis (>20 degrees), reduced elbow extension (<170 degrees), and pes planus. Facial manifestations include dolichocephaly (long, narrow face) with a high-arched palate, malar hypoplasia, retrognathia, enophthalmos, and down slanting palpebral fissures.

12. How is arachnodactyly (spider digits) recognized?

- The **thumb sign,** or Steinberg's sign, is a protrusion of the entire distal phalanx past the hypothenar border when the hand is clenched in a fist (see Fig. 54.2).
- The **wrist sign,** or Walker–Murdoch sign, means that the top of the thumb overlaps the entire fingernail of the fifth finger when they encircle the wrist of the opposite hand.

13. Does the presence of arachnodactyly mean a patient has MFS? What is the differential diagnosis of arachnodactyly?

Arachnodactyly is present in about 90% of cases of MFS but is not diagnostic and may be seen in other diseases.

- **Loeys–Dietz syndrome** is an AD disease characterized by the triad of hypertelorism, bifid uvula/cleft palate, and arterial tortuosity with ascending aortic aneurysm or dissection. Thin, translucent, and velvety skin, easy bruising, and mild arachnodactyly can be seen.
- The **MASS phenotype** describes patients with **m**itral valve prolapse, myopia, borderline and nonprogressive **a**ortic root dilatation, **s**keletal findings, and **s**triae.

- **Congenital contractural arachnodactyly** (see Question 17).
- **Homocystinuria** is an AR disease caused by cystathionine beta synthase deficiency, characterized by tallness, arachnodactyly, lens dislocation (downward dislocation), spinal abnormalities, vascular thrombosis, and intellectual disability.
- Some patients with **mitral valve prolapse syndrome** may have associated aortic root dilation (commonly with Z-score <2.0), pectus excavatum, scoliosis and arachnodactyly.

14. Which MFS manifestations cause significant morbidity and mortality?

Ectopia lentis (upward dislocation) occurs in over half (50%–80%) of patients. Cardiovascular complications are multiple and common. Aneurysmal dilatation of the ascending aorta with dissection is the most common cause of death in patients. Mitral valve prolapse with regurgitation or aortic insufficiency is detectable in 60% to 70% of patients by echocardiography. Pulmonary manifestations include cystic disease and spontaneous pneumothorax. The primary cause of morbidity is skeletal disease of the spine. Thoracic kyphosis can lead to reduced lung capacity and pulmonary insufficiency. Scoliosis is a major management problem and may be rapidly progressive during adolescence, requiring surgery. Acetabuli protrusion can lead to accelerated hip osteoarthritis. Dural ectasia results from enlargement of the spinal canal due to vertebral bone enlargement (usually lumbosacral spine occurs in 67% of patients and can be a source of pain).

15. How is MFS managed?

Patients with clinical features consistent with MFS (see Question 9) should undergo counseling and genetic testing. Those found to have the genetic mutation should undergo aortic imaging to document aortic root size and monitor for dilation and/or dissection. Pregnancy is associated with increased cardiovascular risk, with progressive aortic dilatation and risk for dissection that occurs most frequently in the third trimester and early postpartum; hence, close monitoring is necessary. Annual ophthalmologic screening is recommended for detection of ectopia lentis, cataract, glaucoma, and retinal detachment. An orthopedic evaluation for spinal or peripheral joint conditions is recommended.

Preventative measures are taken to prevent and monitor for cardiovascular problems. B-adrenergic blockade and angiotensin receptor blockers (ARBs) have been used to slow dilatation of the aortic root. In addition to blocking angiotensin II, ARBs attenuate the effects of TGF-beta. The dose of beta blockers should be titrated to limit heart rate to <100 in adults and <110 in children following submaximal exercise (running up and down two flights of stairs). Addition of an ARB to beta blocker therapy as tolerated is recommended in patients with MFS with aortic aneurysm. Echocardiography is performed yearly to follow aortic dilatation; when the size exceeds 50% of normal (>45 mm) or shows a rapid change (≥0.5 cm/year), the frequency of screening is recommended at 6-month intervals. Echocardiography is also helpful in identifying the presence of mitral and aortic valvular disease. Patients with MFS should avoid contact sports, exercise to exhaustion, and isometric activities involving a valsalva maneuver. Elective surgery is indicated when aortic root diameter at the sinuses of valsalva approaches 50 mm. Fluoroquinolones should be avoided in MFS patients due to increasing the risk of aortic rupture.

16. What other genetic diseases should be considered in a patient with aortic aneurysm or dissection?

In general, the younger a person is in whom an aneurysm has been identified, the more likely the patient has a genetic cause. The following have been described (most are AD).

Diseases associated with defects in ECM proteins:
- Cutis laxa: mutations in elastin gene
- EDS vascular type: type III collagen
- EDS kyphoscoliosis type: lysyl hydroxylase deficiency
- Menkes syndrome: copper deficiency
- William syndrome: deletion of the elastin (ELN) locus
- Meester–Loeys syndrome: BGN gene mutation.

Diseases caused by matrix-cell signaling defects:
- MFS: Fibrillin-1 mutation
- Loeys–Dietz syndrome: Mutations in the TGFBR1, TGFBR2, SMAD3, TGFB2, or TGFB3 genes lead to defects in the transforming growth factor beta (TGF-β) pathway.
- Shprintzen–-Goldberg syndrome: SKI gene mutation

Diseases associated with intracellular protein defects:

- Familial aortic aneurysm: smooth muscle gene mutations (ACTA2, MYH11, myosin light chain kinase)
- Arterial tortuosity syndrome: glucose transporter 10 mutation (SLC2A10)
- Pseudoxanthoma elasticum: mutations in ABCC6 gene
- Homocystinuria: CBS gene mutation (cystathione beta synthase protein)
- Lujan syndrome, Ohdo syndrome: MED12 mutation.

First-degree relatives of patients with a gene mutation associated with aortic aneurysm and/or dissections should undergo counseling and genetic testing (large testing panels are available commercially through companies such as GeneDx).

17. What is congenital contractural arachnodactyly (CCA)?

CCA is an AD disease due to mutations of the **fibrillin-2 gene** on chromosome 5. Patients have a marfanoid habitus but unlike MFS have stiff joints, multiple contractures of large joints, "crumpled" ears, severe thoracic deformities, and no cardiac or eye abnormalities.

COMPRESSIVE HEREDITARY CONNECTIVE TISSUE DISEASES

18. What is the Stickler syndrome?

The **Stickler syndrome** is a relatively common (1 in 10,000) disease characterized by premature and severe osteoarthritis developing in the third decade. The diagnosis should be suspected in any young adult with degenerative hip arthritis or any infant with congenitally swollen joints (especially wrists). Other manifestations include myopia, retinal detachment, progressive sensorineural hearing loss, cleft palate, mandibular hypoplasia, and epiphyseal dysplasia. The disease may result from mutations in COL2A1, COL11A1, and COL11A2 (nonocular form). Patients with COL11A1 mutations have more severe eye involvement and hearing loss than patients with COL2A1 mutations. Mutations in the type XI collagen gene (COL11A2) result in a lack of collagen type XI in the vitreous humor of the eye. These patients do not have eye involvement but have severe hearing loss in addition to skeletal and joint manifestations.

BARRIER HEREDITARY CONNECTIVE TISSUE DISEASE

19. What is Alport syndrome?

Alport syndrome includes hereditary glomerulonephritis and deafness. Up to 85% of patients have mutations in the X chromosome COL4A5 gene, while 15% are AR or AD with defects in COL4A3 or COL4A4 genes. The defect is in a nonfibrillar basement membrane collagen (type IV collagen), which is an important component of the kidney basement membrane. Patients present with hematuria, sensorineural hearing loss, fleck retinopathy, and lenticonus. Proteinuria is treated with ACE inhibitors or ARBs. Patients frequently progress to renal failure.

BIBLIOGRAPHY

Beighton PH, Horan F. Orthopedic aspects of Ehlers-Danlos syndrome. *J Bone Joint Surg (Br)*. 1969;51:444–453.

Clinch J, Rogers VJ. Hypermobility syndrome. In: Hochberg MC, Gravallese EM, Smolen JS, van der Heijde D, Weinblatt E, Weisman MH, eds. *Rheumatology*. 8th ed. Philadelphia, PA: Elsevier; 2023:1902–1907.

Dwan K, Phillipi CA, Steiner RD, Basel D. Bisphosphonate therapy for osteogenesis imperfecta (review). *Cochrane Database Syst Rev*. 2014;7:CD005088.

Jovanovic M, Guterman-Ram G, Marini JC. Osteogenesis imperfecta: mechanisms and signaling pathways connecting classical and rare OI types. *Endocr Rev*. 2022;43:61–90.

Loeys BL, Dietz HC, Braverman AC, et al. The revised Ghent nosology for the Marfan syndrome. *J Med Genet*. 2010;47:476–485.

Malfait F, Francomano C, Byers P, et al. The 2017 international classification of the Ehlers-Danlos syndromes. *Am J Med Genet C Semin Med Genet*. 2017;175:8–26.

Marom R, Rabenhorst BM, Morello R. Osteogenesis imperfecta: an update on clinical features and therapies. *Eur J Endocrinol*. 2020;183:R95–R106.

Meester JAN, Verstraeten A, Schepers D, Alaerts M, Van Laer L, Loeys BL. Differences in manifestations of Marfan syndrome, Ehlers-Danlos syndrome, and Loeys-Dietz syndrome. *Ann Cardiothorac Surg*. 2017;6:582–594.

Syx D, De Wandele I, Rombaut L, Malfait F. Hypermobility, the Ehlers-Danlos syndromes and chronic pain. *Clin Exp Rheumatol*. 2017;107(5):116–122 suppl.

Wordsworth BP, Javaid MK. Heritable connective tissue disorders. In: Hochberg MC, Gravallese EM, Smolen JS, van der Heijde D, Weinblatt E, Weisman MH, eds. *Rheumatology*. 8th ed. Philadelphia, PA: Elsevier; 2023:1882–1901.

Yu C, Jeremy RW. Angiotensin, transforming growth factor B and aortic dilatation in Marfan syndrome: of mice and humans. *Int J Cardiol Heart Vasc*. 2018;18:71–80.

FURTHER READING

www.oif.org.
www.ehlers-danlos.com.
www.marfan.org-of interest, aortic root Z-score calculators are available through this website.
www.ncbi.nlm.nih.gov/gtr.

CHAPTER 55

Inborn Errors of Metabolism Affecting Connective Tissue

Jessica L. Bloom, MD, MSCS and Emily Shelkowitz, MD

 KEY POINTS

1. Consider homocystinuria in a patient with marfanoid habitus, stiff joints, intellectual disability, and thromboembolic events.
2. Lysosomal storage diseases may present with rheumatic manifestations resembling juvenile idiopathic arthritis, with attenuated forms presenting in adolescence or adulthood.
3. Suspect Fabry disease in a patient with fibromyalgia-like symptoms, acroparesthesias, angiokeratomas, and a paternal history of early-onset renal failure, myocardial infarctions, or strokes.

1. What categories of inborn errors of metabolism lead to connective tissue abnormalities?

Inborn errors of metabolism (IEM) are genetic (or inherited) disorders that typically arise from an enzyme deficiency that perturbs an aspect of cellular metabolism or organelle function. IEM are classified according to the specific aspect of metabolism (e.g., protein, carbohydrate, fat, metal, and purine/pyrimidine base metabolism) or specific organelle (e.g., lysosome, peroxisome, and mitochondria) that is affected. IEMs that affect the musculoskeletal system fall into six categories of metabolism: aminoacidopathies, purine disorders, disorders of metal metabolism, cholesterol synthesis disorders, lysosomal storage disorders (LSDs), and peroxisomal disorders (Fig. 55.1). LSDs are further classified by the type of storage material that accumulates and causes cellular damage such as mucopolysaccharidoses and sphingolipidoses.

2. What is the general approach to diagnosing inborn errors of metabolism?

Screening labs, enzymology testing, and molecular genetic sequencing are the three categories generally employed to investigate IEM. The approach may vary based on the clinician's level of suspicion, expertise, and access to resources.

- **Screening labs:** typically the least costly and more widely available. They assess for an end product deficiency (such as in Menkes disease) or abnormal elevations of metabolism intermediaries (such as homocystinuria or LSD). These principles are the basis of the expanded Recommended Uniform Newborn Screening Panel since the advent of tandem mass spectrometry technology in the early 2000s. As of 2024, homocystinuria is universally screened for while only some states screen for Hurler Syndrome, Fabry disease, and Gaucher disease. These have neither absolute sensitivity nor specificity and enzyme testing or molecular genetic testing must be utilized to confirm the diagnosis.
- **Enzymology testing:** involves the use of a specialized assay to measure enzyme activity levels and determine whether they are consistent with the established normal, carrier or affected ranges. Enzyme testing is not universally available for all disorders and may only be available in specific sample types, such as skin, muscle, and/or blood cells. Further, overlap may exist between the established ranges, leading to ambiguity when interpreting results. Nevertheless, enzyme testing remains the gold standard for many disorders and decreased enzyme activity levels are sufficient to make a diagnosis.
- **Molecular genetic testing:** has superseded the use of enzyme testing for many clinicians due to improved turnaround time and decreased costs. Single gene testing, panel testing, or broad genomic sequencing (such as exome or genome sequencing) may be considered. If considering a particular diagnosis, it is important to ensure that the study offers sufficient coverage of the genetic changes known to cause that disease (e.g., sequence variants versus exonic deletions or duplications). Still, certain areas within the genome and variant types remain challenging to capture; thus, if clinical suspicion remains high despite negative genetic testing, enzyme testing should be considered a second-tier test.

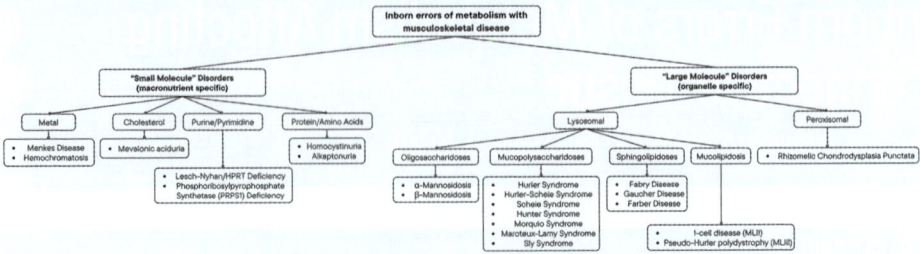

Fig 55.1 Categories of inborn errors of metabolism.

3. What is the biochemical basis of homocystinuria and why does the disease affect connective tissue? How is it diagnosed?

Homocystinuria refers to increased urinary excretion of homocystine, the oxidized form of homocysteine. The most common form, "Classic Homocystinuria," is caused by a deficiency of the cystathionine β-synthase (CBS) enzyme involved in the transsulfuration of homocysteine to cystathionine (Fig. 55.2). Cysteine, the amino acid deficient in homocystinuria, is necessary for proper crosslinking of structural proteins such as collagen and fibrillin in connective tissue and bone, the suspensory ligament of the eye, and the extracellular milieu of endothelial cells. Thus, altered collagen may be responsible for lens dislocation and osteoporosis, whereas altered proteins in the elastomeric complex or its substructure (fibrillin) may be responsible for the phenotypic similarity to Marfan syndrome.

Classic homocystinuria occurs in approximately 1 in 200,000 to 335,000 live births in the US. Other, less common forms of homocystinuria arise from defective remethylation of homocysteine to methionine caused by a deficiency of the B12-dependent methionine synthase enzyme or methylenetetrahydrofolate reductase (MTHFR). These may be distinguished by screening studies. For instance, an elevated total homocysteine level and methionine level should increase suspicion for classic homocystinuria. Molecular genetic testing is generally favored as CBS enzyme activity levels are only available in skin fibroblasts. Fewer than 5% of pathogenic variants are due to intragenic deletions or duplications that require other testing methodologies.

4. List the major clinical manifestations of classic homocystinuria

- Ectopia lentis (lens dislocated downward); hallmark finding. High myopia may be present in its absence.
- Thromboembolism (arterial and venous); the most common cause of mortality.
- Developmental delay, seizures, extrapyramidal signs (i.e., dystonia).
- Psychiatric concerns such as anxiety, depression, obsessive-compulsive behaviors, and personality disorders.
- Psychosis may be a presenting sign in adolescents.
- Marfanoid habitus with joint tightness (*not* joint laxity)
- Osteoporosis
- Severe premature atherosclerosis

Musculoskeletal findings include tall stature, arachnodactyly, dolichostenomelia, pes cavus, genu valgum, and chest wall (pectus)/spinal deformities. Generalized osteoporosis and joint tightening occur. Spinal osteoporosis occurs in up to two thirds of affected individuals by 15 years of age and is usually a combination of osteoporotic fractures, degenerative disc/joint disease, and scoliosis. Altered endothelial function from the cytotoxic effect of homocysteine and increased platelet activation are responsible for the thromboses and developmental delay.

> **PEARL:** Rule out homocystinuria in a patient with a Marfanoid habitus who has stiff joints and developmental delay.

5. What dietary changes and medications help treat homocystinuria?

Effective treatment requires early diagnosis. Vitamin B_6 is a cofactor for the CBS enzyme. Approximately half of individuals with classic homocystinuria carry genetic variants that are B6

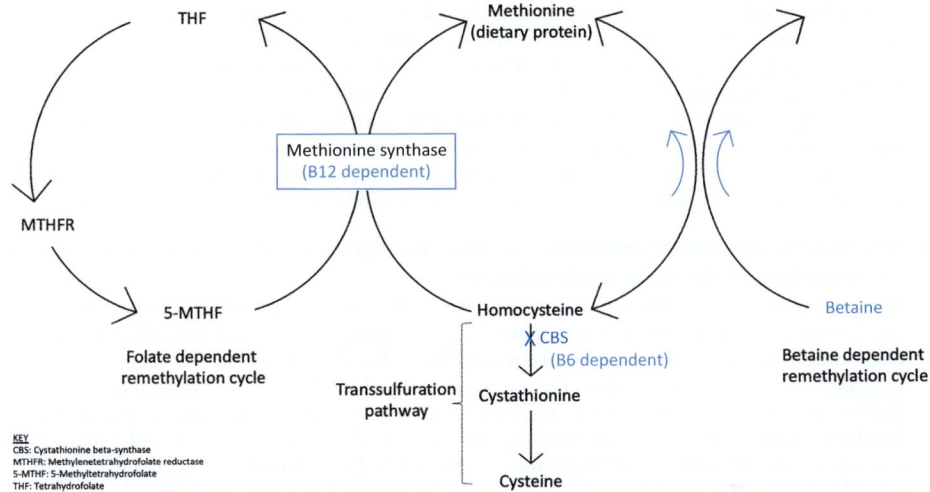

Fig 55.2 Homocysteine metabolic pathway. Methionine and Homocysteine Metabolism. Methionine is converted to homocysteine by a series of steps (not displayed). Typically, homocysteine is either converted back to methionine via the remethylation pathway or converted to cystathionine via Cystathionine Beta Synthase (CBS) as part of the transsulfuration pathway. A deficiency of CBS, as seen in Classic Homocystinuria, leads to elevated homocysteine levels, and to a lesser degree, elevated methionine levels and low cystathionine and cysteine levels. Elevated homocysteine levels may also be seen when the folate dependent remethylation cycle (displayed on the left-hand side of the figure) is not working optimally. This could be due to a primary enzyme deficiency, such as MTHFR deficiency, or a secondary enzyme deficiency as is the case in disorders of cobalamin (B_{12}) metabolism. The betaine-dependent remethylation cycle (displayed on the right-hand side of the figure) illustrates the rationale for betaine supplementation as a treatment option for individuals with homocystinuria.

responsive and respond to high doses of vitamin B_6 (300–600 mg/day of pyridoxine). They are able to maintain lower blood methionine and homocysteine levels and raise blood cysteine levels with monotherapy alone. Vitamin B_6 non-responders are treated with a low-protein, low-methionine diet. Betaine, which provides an alternative pathway for remethylating homocysteine back to methionine, is also prescribed. Folate and B12 (cofactors for remethylation enzymes) may be supplemented to enhance conversion of homocysteine to methionine (Fig. 55.2). CBS enzyme replacement therapy is undergoing clinical trials for classic homocystinuria. Long-term studies are needed, but vision, musculoskeletal, and neurocognitive outcomes are seemingly improved with early detection via newborn screening.

6. What is Menkes disease (kinky hair syndrome) and how does it affect connective tissue?

Menkes disease is a rare (1:100,000 live births) X-linked recessive disorder of copper metabolism in which malfunction of the ATPase-dependent transport of copper (*ATP7A* gene) results in poor copper intestinal absorption. This results in deficient activity of the copper-requiring metalloenzymes (e.g., lysyl hydroxylase) involved in collagen and elastin synthesis, thereby affecting connective tissue. Affected individuals may have highly extensible skin and joints, "sagging" cheeks/jowls, umbilical or inguinal hernias, bladder diverticula, and vascular tortuosities. Menkes disease typically presents with hypotonia, developmental delays, and seizures in early infancy with ensuing spasticity, reflex abnormalities, and intellectual disability. Canonical features include occipital horns (wedge-shaped calcifications at the site of sternocleidomastoid muscle attachment to the occipital bone) and pili torti (beaded, brittle, and sparse silver hair, aka "kinky hair"). Death and disability occur in early infancy if not treated with injectable copper supplementation, which does not reverse prior neurodegeneration.

7. What is the biochemical basis of lysosomal storage diseases (LSDs), and when should a rheumatologist consider it as a cause of musculoskeletal symptoms?

LSDs are inborn errors of metabolism characterized by excess accumulation of substrates in organs due to deficient lysosomal functioning. They are further stratified by the type of accumulating substrate, such as mucopolysaccharides (aka glycosaminoglycans or GAGs) in mucopolysaccharidoses and sphingosine-containing phospholipids in sphingolipidoses. Most LSDs range in presentation and severity depending on the amount of residual enzyme activity. The astute rheumatologist should be suspicious of childhood presentations of arthritis and musculoskeletal disease in which the patient has other unusual pathology (such as corneal clouding, developmental delay, frequent ENT infections, or early contractures) or of individuals with "attenuated" LSDs who lack classical systemic features but present with unexplained musculoskeletal pathology in adolescence or adulthood. A detailed family history may also direct care.

8. What are the skeletal manifestations of mucopolysaccharidoses (MPS) and the key distinguishing features for each subtype?

MPS are a major group of lysosomal storage diseases affecting 1 in 20,000 live births caused by the absence or malfunctioning of one of the 11 lysosomal enzymes needed to break down glycosaminoglycans (GAGs, formerly called mucopolysaccharides). As a result, catabolites of GAGs progressively deposit within various tissues, leading to skeletal dysplasia. Characteristic skeletal findings include short stature, joint contractures/stiff joints, carpal tunnel syndrome, and claw-hand deformity. Additional skeletal findings may include thick calvaria, an enlarged J-shaped sella turcica, a short and wide mandible, biconvex vertebral bodies, odontoid hypoplasia with atlantoaxial instability, short thick clavicles, coxa valga, V-shaped deformities of the distal ulna and radius, and short fingers with wide metacarpals and pointed proximal ends. Collectively, these skeletal changes are given the term "dysostosis multiplex." Depending on the subtype, individuals may also have intellectual disability, neurodegeneration, progressive skin thickening, corneal clouding, hearing loss, recurrent ENT infections, upper airway obstruction, cardiac disease, pulmonary hypertension, lung disease, and organomegaly.

Seven MPS subtypes have been identified (Table 55.1). All are autosomal recessive except for MPS II (Hunter syndrome), which is X-linked recessive. Hurler, Hunter, Morquio, Maroteaux-Lamy, and Sly syndromes (types I-H, II, IV, VI, VII) have short-trunk dwarfism, while attenuated forms (types I-HS, I-S, II, IVB, VI, VII) can have relatively normal stature. MPS can be diagnosed by urinary GAG fractionation, enzyme assays, and/or molecular genetics. While most forms present during the first years of life, some may present in adolescence or young adulthood.

9. What are the key features and skeletal manifestations of Gaucher disease?

Gaucher disease is a lysosomal storage disease caused by the accumulation of glucosylceramide within macrophages (i.e., Gaucher cells) due to biallelic variants in *GBA1* causing a deficiency of glucocerebrosidase. It affects 0.5–25 of every 100,000 live births. Type I (the non-neuropathic form) is the most common type with symptom onset typically in adolescence or adulthood. Prevalence is increased in the Ashkenazi Jewish population due to a common carrier variant. Splenomegaly with hypersplenism and pancytopenia are the most common presenting manifestations. Hepatomegaly occurs later, as does pulmonary involvement (interstitial lung disease, pulmonary hypertension). Skeletal involvement occurs in most patients, including long bone or hip/shoulder pain from osteonecrosis and bone infarctions, as well as back pain from osteoporosis with fractures. Bone crisis (10%) can cause acute pain and swelling and acute-phase reactant elevation. Radiographic abnormalities are seen in 80–95% of patients and include osteopenia, osteolytic lesions, bone infarcts with serpiginous osteosclerotic areas, distal femur deformity (Erlenmeyer flask), H-shaped vertebrae, and osteonecrosis of the femoral and humeral heads and femoral condyles. Historically, individuals underwent bone marrow biopsies to evaluate for hematologic malignancies that ultimately demonstrated Gaucher cells. Now, if suspected, enzyme testing in circulating lymphocytes or genetic testing is commonly pursued to avoid more invasive diagnostic procedures.

10. What manifestations of Farber disease may cause someone to present to a rheumatologist?

Farber disease is an extremely rare lysosomal storage disease caused by a variant in the ASAH1 gene that codes for the acid ceramidase enzyme. Autosomal recessive inheritance leads to a deficiency of the enzyme and accumulation of ceramide in lysosomes. Although life expectancy is quite limited (most often due to lung disease), affected individuals may get subcutaneous nodules and painful, swollen joints with contractures. Individuals also get hepatosplenomegaly,

TABLE 55.1 Mucopolysaccharidoses Affecting the Skeletal System

MPS SUBTYPE	GENE	INHERITANCE	DEFICIENT ENZYME
MPS I	IDUA	Autosomal recessive	Alpha-L-iduronidase
Hurler:	Developmental delay (with or without regression), coarse facies, corneal clouding, hearing loss, recurrent ENT infections, cardiopulmonary disease, dysostosis multiplex, hepato-splenomegaly. Severe.		
Hurler-Scheie:	Intermediate phenotype.		
Scheie:	Hip dysplasia, joint stiffness, valvular disease, corneal clouding. Attenuated. Normal intelligence, JIA mimic		
MPS II	IDS	X-linked	Iduronate sulfatase
Hunter:	Similar to MPSI. Neurodegeneration and development of contractures are often early and progressive features. Distinguishing features are the absence of corneal clouding and inheritance (only affects XY males).		
MPS IV	GALNS, GLB1	Autosomal recessive	N-acetylgalac-tosamine-6-sulfatase, beta-galactosi-dase
Morquio syndrome:	Short stature, pectus carinatum, odontoid hypoplasia with cervical spine instability, kypho-scoliosis, joint laxity, genu valgum, cardiopulmonary disease, corneal clouding, cataracts. Joint laxity, less corading, and normal intellect are distinguishing features. Type B (caused by biallelic changes in *GLB1*) can have attenuated forms.		
MPS VI	ARSB	Autosomal recessive	N-acetylgalac-tosamine-4-sulfatase (arylsulfatase B)
Maroteaux–Lamy:	Similar to MPSI, but neuropsychiatric differences are less striking and may be static rather than progressive.		
MPS VII	GUSB	Autosomal recessive	Beta-glucuronidase
Sly Syndrome:	May be difficult to distinguish from MPSI. Neurologic regression is less common.		

nephropathy, systemic inflammation, osteoporosis, hoarse voice, and central nervous system disease. There is no current treatment.

11. What inborn error of metabolism mimics fibromyalgia?

Fabry disease, an X-linked lysosomal storage disease, is caused by a deficiency of the lysosomal enzyme, α-galactosidase A (α-Gal A), which causes glycosphingolipids to accumulate in lysosomes. While most males develop symptoms during childhood, some may have a milder course and/or later-onset phenotype. The classic disease has an incidence of 1 in 40,000 individuals, but milder forms are underrecognized in both males and females. Accumulation of globotriao-sylceramide within vascular, dorsal root ganglia, and autonomic nervous system cells leads to neurologic manifestations including small-fiber peripheral neuropathy (e.g. burning of palms and soles and decreased temperature perceptibility), irritable bowel syndrome–like symptoms, and ischemic strokes. As a result of the discomfort, males and heterozygous females may present similarly to someone with fibromyalgia. Progressive cardiac, cerebrovascular, and/or renal disease can also develop and are major causes of morbidity and mortality. Diagnosis should be suspected in any patient with a paternal family history of early-onset renal failure. Patients should be examined for characteristic ocular stigmata (cornea verticillata) and dermal signs (angiokeratomas). The diagnosis is confirmed in males by genetic testing or α-Gal A activity in plasma or peripheral leukocytes. By contrast, enzyme activity levels may be normal in females, and therefore genetic testing is required. Early diagnosis and treatment are important.

12. What are the general approaches to treatment for lysosomal storage disorders?

Multidisciplinary teamwork is a mainstay of treatment for all lysosomal storage disorders (LSDs). Subspeciality referrals and surveillance studies may be necessary for disease-specific risks. Disease-modifying therapies are available in some forms, though nearly all have limited tissue penetration and differing abilities to reverse and treat existing cellular damage. Therapies for many neuronopathic LSDs are still palliative due to poor penetrance across the blood–brain barrier. Fortunately, the landscape is rapidly changing. Up-to-date information regarding emerging therapies can be accessed via clinicaltrials.gov. Basic therapy types include substrate reduction, chaperone, enzyme replacement, and gene therapies, all of which are costly and place significant burdens on patients, families, and payers.

Substrate reduction therapies reduce the amount of substrate that is synthesized and later subject to ineffective clearance/catabolism. As of 2024, two oral substrate reduction therapies, cerdelga (eliglustat) and zavesca (miglustat), are available for adults with Gaucher disease. *Chaperone therapies* stabilize the misfolded enzyme that is not working properly. Consequently, not all variants are amenable to chaperone therapies. As of 2024, the oral chaperone therapy galafold (migalastat) is approved for adults with Fabry disease. *Enzyme replacement therapies* replace the deficient enzyme via recurrent intravenous infusions. As of 2024, enzyme replacement therapies are available for MPSI, MPSII, MPSIV, MPSVI, MPSVII, Gaucher disease, and Fabry disease and are FDA approved for the treatment of children and adults. *Gene therapies* alter the genetic code and recover the function of a deficient protein/enzyme. As of 2024, multiple gene therapies are in preclinical and clinical studies. None are FDA approved for the treatment of LSD.

Hematopoietic stem cell transplant may be considered for severe forms of MPSI to treat central nervous system manifestations. The benefit is thought to arise from the new IDUA enzyme capable of accessing various sites of cellular storage, including the central nervous system, due to the replacement of IDUA-deficient macrophages with marrow-derived donor macrophages. It is not widely accepted in other LSD due to a lack of demonstrated efficacy.

ACKNOWLEDGMENTS

Thank you to Dr. Sterling West for his work on this chapter in prior editions.

BIBLIOGRAPHY

Biegstraaten M, Cox TM, Belmatoug N, et al. Management goals for type 1 Gaucher disease: an expert consensus document from the European working group on Gaucher disease. *Blood Cells Mol Dis*. 2018;68:203–208.

Costi S, Caporali RF, Marino A. Mucopolysaccharidosis: what pediatric rheumatologists and orthopedics need to know. *Diagnostics (Basel)*. 2022;13:75.

Foster HE, Rabinovich CE. *Musculoskeletal Manifestations of Systemic Disease. Textbook of Pediatric Rheumatology*. 8th ed. Philadelphia, PA:Elsevier; 2021:691–701.

Germain DP, Altarescu G, Barriales-Villa R, et al. An expert consensus on practical clinical recommendations and guidance for patients with classic Fabry disease. *Mol Genet Metab*. 2022;137(1–2):49–61.

Germain DP, Fouilhoux A, Decramer S, et al. Consensus recommendations for diagnosis, management, and treatment of Fabry disease in paediatric patients. *Clin Genet*. 2019;96:107–117.

Gerrard A, Dawson C. Homocystinuria diagnosis and management: it is not all classical. *J Clin Pathol*. 2022;75:744–750.

Grabowski GA, Mistry PK. Therapies for lysosomal storage diseases: principles, practice, and prospects for refinements based on evolving science. *Mol Genet Metab*. 2022;137:81–91.

Huemer M, Diodato D, Schwahn B, et al. Guidelines for diagnosis and management of the cobalamin-related remethylation disorders cblC, cblD, cblE, cblF, cblG, cblJ and MTHFR deficiency. *J Inherit Metab Dis*. 2017;40:21–48.

James RA, Sigh-Grewal D, Lee SJ, et al. Lysosomal storage disorders: a review of musculoskeletal features. *J Paed Child Health*. 2016;52:262–271.

Loret A, Jacob C, Mammou S, et al. Joint manifestations revealing inborn metabolic diseases in adults: a narrative review. *Orphanet J Rare Dis*. 2023;18:239.

Manger B, Mengel E, Schaefer RM. Rheumatologic aspects of lysosomal storage diseases. *Clin Rheumatol*. 2007;26:335–341.

Michels H, Mengel E. Lysosomal storage diseases as differential diagnoses to rheumatic disorders. *Curr Opin Rheumatol*. 2008;20:76–81.

Morishita K, Petty RE. Musculoskeletal manifestations of mucopolysaccharidoses. *Rheumatology.* 2011;50(Suppl 5):v19–v25.

Ojha R, Prasad AN. Menkes disease: what a multidisciplinary approach can do. *J Multidiscip Healthc.* 2016;9:371–385.

Pastores GM, Meere PA. Musculoskeletal complications associated with lysosomal storage disorders: Gaucher disease and Hurler-Scheie syndrome (mucopolysaccharidosis type I). *Curr Opin Rheumatol.* 2005;17:70–78.

Singh S, Ojodu J, Kemper AR, Lam WKK, Grosse SD. Implementation of newborn screening for conditions in the United States first recommended during 2010–2018. *Int J Neonatal Screen.* 2023;9:20.

Stirnemann J, Belmatoug N, Camou F, et al. A review of Gaucher disease pathophysiology, clinical presentation and treatments. *Int J Mol Sci.* 2017;18:441.

Thümler A, Miebach E, Lampe C, et al. Clinical characteristics of adults with slowly progressing mucopolysaccharidosis VI: a case series. *J Inherit Metab Dis.* 2012;35:1071–1079.

Vairo FPE, Chwal BC, Perini S, et al. A systematic review and evidence-based guideline for diagnosis and treatment of Menkes disease. *Mol Genet Metab.* 2019;126:6–13.

Weinreb NJ, Goker-Alpan O, Kishnani PS, et al. The diagnosis and management of Gaucher disease in pediatric patients: where do we go from here? *Mol Genet Metab.* 2022;136:4–21.

FURTHER READING

GeneReviews (https://www.ncbi.nlm.nih.gov/books/NBK1116/).

National Center for Biotechnology Information (www.ncbi.nlm.nih.gov).

National Organization for Rare Disorders (www.rarediseases.org).

Newborn Screening Information Center (newbornscreening.hrsa.gov).

CHAPTER 56

Storage and Deposition Diseases

Kathleen Jo Corbin, MD, MHS

> **KEY POINTS**
>
> 1. Musculoskeletal symptoms can be the presenting manifestation in up to 33% of patients with hemochromatosis.
> 2. Arthritis associated with hemochromatosis commonly affects the hands, especially the second and third metacarpophalangeal joints bilaterally.
> 3. Wilson disease should be considered in patients with the triad of liver disease, neurologic disease, and destructive polyarticular arthritis.
> 4. Ochronotic arthropathy associated with alkaptonuria commonly causes severe lumbar spine osteoarthritis with disc space calcifications and vacuum discs.

HEREDITARY HEMOCHROMATOSIS

1. What is hereditary hemochromatosis (HHC)?

Hereditary hemochromatosis is a genetic disorder of iron metabolism in which excess gastrointestinal iron absorption results in iron deposition in tissues, ultimately causing tissue damage. In HHC, genetic mutations result in abnormal regulation of hepcidin, which leads to hyperabsorption of iron. In the typical Western diet, approximately 1 mg of iron is absorbed per day. In HHC, iron absorption can be as high as 2–4 mg per day. Accumulation of iron in tissues may lead to development of reactive oxygen species, causing tissue damage.

2. What is the pattern of inheritance for HHC?

HHC is an autosomal recessive condition (Types 1–3) with variable penetrance resulting from mutations in one of several genes involved in regulation of iron homeostasis:

- **Classic/HFE-related HHC (type 1):** Mutations in the *HFE* gene, located on chromosome 6, result in hepcidin deficiency and are responsible for most cases of HHC (approximately 80% of cases in the United States). The two most common variants in *HFE* are C282YA and H63D. Over 80% of patients with type 1 HHC are homozygous for the C282Y gene mutation. Patients with type 1 HHC who are not homozygous for C282Y (i.e. compound heterozygotes or homozygous for other *HFE* mutations) typically have milder disease which tends to occur only when an associated comorbidity exists (e.g., alcoholism). Recent screening studies suggest that the *HFE* gene occurs in up to 5% of whites. Frequency of mutations causing HHC is highest in white individuals of northwestern European descent. The global prevalence of *HFE* mutation is 1.9%, making this one of the most commonly inherited metabolic diseases.
- **Juvenile HHC (type 2):** Mutations in the hemojuvelin (*HJV*) gene on chromosome 1 (type 2a) or the hepcidin antimicrobial peptide (*HAMP*) gene on chromosome 19 (type 2b) lead to HHC in individuals younger than 30 years. Prevalence of Juvenile HHC is very low and is seen in both white and non-white individuals.
- **Transferrin receptor-2 gene (type 3):** due to mutation in *TFR2* gene on chromosome 7. Autosomal recessive disorder that is seen both in whites and non-whites. Its onset is at 30–40 years.
- **Ferroportin gene (type 4):** due to mutation in *SLC40A1* (*FPN1*) gene on chromosome 2. Autosomal dominant disease that is seen both in whites and non-whites. Its onset is at 10–80 years.

3. Describe the typical clinical presentation of classic (type 1) HHC.

HHC typically presents with organ toxicity due to tissue iron deposition. Symptoms usually develop between ages 40–60 years. Males tend to have the onset of symptoms at an earlier age, in part due to physiologic blood loss due to menstruation in females. The most commonly affected organ is the liver, as it is the principal site of normal iron storage. Affected individuals can present with elevated liver transaminases, hepatomegaly (95%), and hepatic fibrosis that can progress to cirrhosis. Risk of hepatocellular carcinoma in patients with HHC is increased (20x) in patients with hepatic fibrosis. Other common manifestations include skin hyperpigmentation (50%), diabetes mellitus, hypogonadism/decreased libido (20–40%), and arthropathy (40–80%). Cardiac involvement, including dilated cardiomyopathy, heart failure, and conduction abnormalities, is present in approximately 30% of patients and is a principal cause of death in untreated patients. Constitutional symptoms including fatigue, generalized pain, and weakness are also common. Patients can have increased susceptibility to infections, particularly due to *Vibrio vulnificus* from uncooked seafood (sepsis) and *Yersinia enterocolitica* (septic arthritis), is observed because of enhanced bacterial virulence and impaired macrophage clearance caused by iron overload.

4. What are the musculoskeletal manifestations of classic (type 1) HHC?

Arthropathy is reported in 40–80% of patients with HHC, which includes arthralgias, arthritis, and chondrocalcinosis. The mechanisms of arthropathy are unclear but may be due to iron deposition in cartilage. Arthralgia is often an early symptom in HHC and can affect any joint.

Arthritis can be the initial presentation in up to 33% of patients with HHC. Small joints of the hands, especially metacarpophalangeal (MCP) joints, are commonly involved, which may resemble rheumatoid arthritis. In particular, a destructive inflammatory arthritis of the MCPs of the second and third fingers is commonly described in patients with HHC, leading to limited flexion of the second and third MCPs referred to as the "iron salute." Radiographs show osteoarthritis-like changes with sclerotic margins, joint-space narrowing, and hook-like osteophyte formation at the MCPs (Fig. 56.1). Chondrocalcinosis due to calcium pyrophosphate deposition (CPPD) is common in patients with HHC, particularly in the knees, wrists, and hips.

PEARL: Rule out hemochromatosis in any young (< 40–50 years) white male who is presenting with "seronegative rheumatoid arthritis."

5. What is the cause of osteopenia / osteoporosis in classic (type 1) HHC?

Possible causes of decreased bone density in HHC include direct inhibition of bone formation due to iron deposition in the synovium, hypogonadotropic hypogonadism from pituitary iron infiltration, and altered vitamin D metabolism due to hepatic cirrhosis.

6. How is a diagnosis of classic (type 1) HHC made?

In the fasting state, transferrin saturation greater than 60% in males or 50% in females, along with elevated serum ferritin greater than twice the upper limit of normal is 95% sensitive and 85% specific for diagnosis of hemochromatosis. Genetic testing is recommended for all patients with transferrin saturation ≥45% and ferritin >200 µg/L, especially if there is a family history of HHC. A diagnosis of HHC is clear for individuals with iron overload and homozygous *HFE* C282Y mutation. Additional evaluations (e.g. liver biopsy) may be indicated in patients with iron overload but who lack homozygosity in *HFE* C282Y.

A definitive diagnosis can be made by direct measurement of iron in a liver biopsy. However, iron overload can also be evaluated with MRI of the liver, heart, or both, and may be preferable as a noninvasive approach. Synovial biopsies in HHC patients with arthritis show iron deposition in synovial lining cells with electron microscopy confirming the iron being located predominantly in the type B cells. This pattern of iron deposition is different from that seen in other diseases such as rheumatoid arthritis, osteoarthritis, pigmented villonodular synovitis, and hemophilia where iron is deposited primarily in the synovial stroma.

7. What are the treatments for classic (type 1) HHC?

Removal of excess iron is typically done via phlebotomy, usually once a week after diagnosis, until target serum ferritin levels (50–100 ng/mL) are achieved. Maintenance phlebotomy is usually required every 3–4 months to maintain normal serum ferritin levels. Alternatives to phlebotomy include iron chelation and erythocytapheresis, which are rarely used.

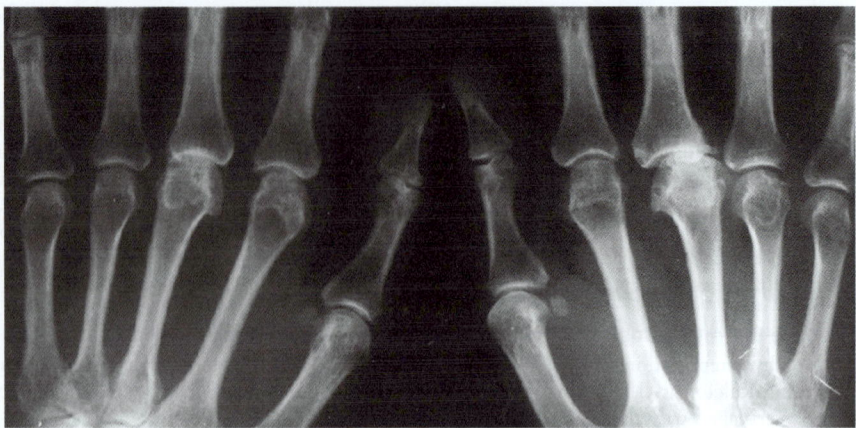

Fig. 56.1 Hand radiographs for a patient with hemochromatosis. Note the degenerative arthritis of the metacarpophalangeal joints with hook-like osteophytes.

Life expectancy of symptomatic patients is extended considerably by removal of excess iron stores (90% 5-year survival versus 33% survival without therapy). Hepatomegaly, liver function studies, and skin pigmentation all improve, and cardiac function stabilizes or improves with phlebotomy. Diabetes mellitus improves in approximately 50% of cases. Phlebotomy has little effect on hypogonadism or arthropathy. Hepatic fibrosis may improve, but cirrhosis is irreversible. Hepatocellular carcinoma, a late sequela in one-third of those who develop hepatic cirrhosis, is not diminished by phlebotomy and is a major cause (30–45%) of death even in treated individuals. Because the life expectancy of homozygotes diagnosed and treated before the development of cirrhosis is the same as that of the general population, the importance of family screening and early therapy cannot be overemphasized.

WILSON DISEASE

8. What is Wilson disease and its pattern of inheritance?

Wilson disease, also called hepatolenticular degeneration, is a genetic disorder of copper metabolism in which copper accumulates in the liver, brain, and other tissues due to decreased excretion of biliary copper. Wilson disease is an autosomal recessive condition resulting from mutations in *ATP7B* on chromosome 13, which encodes a copper transport protein. More than 500 mutations in ATP7B have been identified, but the most common mutation H1069Q accounts for 30 to 60% of cases. Most patients are compound heterozygotes.

9. Describe the typical clinical presentation of Wilson disease.

Clinical presentation of Wilson disease can be highly variable. Patients can present from early childhood through adulthood. Common manifestations include the following:
- **Liver disease:** Liver disease is the initial presentation in 50% of cases, as the liver is a major site of copper accumulation. Abnormal liver transaminases are seen in over 95% of cases. Clinical presentation can range from abdominal pain and acute hepatitis to fulminant liver failure and cirrhosis.
- **Neuropsychiatric disease:** The most common neurologic manifestations include tremors, rigidity, and dystonia. Dysarthria and ataxia are also common. Psychiatric symptoms including mood disorders, psychosis, and personality changes occur in up to 33% of cases.
- **Ocular disease:** Kayser–Fleischer rings are golden-brown rings caused by granular deposits of copper in the cornea. They are present in 95% of patients with neurologic disease and 50 to 60% of patients with liver disease.

Less common manifestations of Wilson disease include musculoskeletal symptoms, kidney disease (Fanconi syndrome), hemolytic anemia (Coombs negative), infertility in females, and sexual dysfunction in males.

10. **What are the musculoskeletal manifestations of Wilson disease?**

Musculoskeletal manifestations occur in 50% of patients with Wilson disease but are rarely the presenting symptom. Destructive symmetric arthritis, particularly affecting the large joints such as knees and hips, can also involve the spine, hands (MCPs), wrists, elbows, and shoulders. Chondrocalcinosis can also occur. Radiographic changes can mimic those of osteoarthritis including joint space narrowing, osteophyte formation, and subchondral sclerosis. Osteoporosis or osteomalacia may be present as a result of Fanconi syndrome or renal tubular acidosis, both of which are common in Wilson disease.

11. **How is a diagnosis of Wilson disease made?**

The diagnosis of Wilson disease can be made in patients with Kayser-Fleischer rings and decreased serum ceruloplasmin (<200 mg/L) or elevated urinary copper excretion. Liver biopsy and genetic testing for *ATP7B* mutations can confirm the diagnosis.

12. **What are the treatments for Wilson disease?**

Copper chelating agents such as penicillamine and trientine are used for symptomatic and asymptomatic patients. Oral zinc therapy is used in asymptomatic patients, as zinc interferes with enteral absorption of copper, and has been shown to prevent development of symptomatic liver disease. Patients with Wilson disease are also advised to avoid foods rich in copper such as organ meats, nuts, chocolate, mushrooms, and shellfish.

ALKAPTONURIA (OCHRONOSIS)

13. **What is alkaptonuria and its pattern of inheritance?**

Alkaptonuria is a genetic disorder of tyrosine catabolism that results in elevated levels of homogentisic acid (HGA), which polymerizes and forms a pigment that deposits in connective tissues throughout the body (ochronosis). Alkaptonuria is an autosomal recessive condition resulting from mutations in the *HGD* gene on chromosome 3, which cause deficiency of homogentisic acid dioxygenase. Alkaptonuria, which was first described in 1902, was the first human disease that demonstrated the Mendelian principle of inheritance of an autosomal recessive trait.

14. **Describe the typical clinical presentation of alkaptonuria.**

The most common clinical manifestations of alkaptonuria are as follows:
- Urine that becomes dark (bark brown or black) if left standing. This can be observed in affected babies with dark-stained diapers.
- Abnormal brown or blue pigmentation is most visible in the cartilage of the ears and sclerae and can be seen in the skin axillae and inguinal areas as well.
- Ochronotic arthritis, caused by pigment deposition in the large joints and spine.
  Other clinical manifestations include kidney stones and cardiac involvement (coronary artery and aortic valve calcification). Notably, patients who take minocycline can have pigmentary changes in the skin and cartilage resembling ochronosis. Patients who take hydroxychloroquine can have skin hyperpigmentation.

15. **What are the musculoskeletal manifestations of alkaptonuria?**

Ochronotic arthritis typically presents in the third decade of life or later. Pigment deposition in cartilage causes tissue to become stiff and brittle and is cytotoxic to chondrocytes, resulting in osteoarthritis. The most common site involved is the spine, especially the lumbosacral region, followed by the knees, hips, and shoulders. Patients develop pain, stiffness, and range-of-motion limitations in the back and joints. Abnormal calcification and ossification occur, including ankylosis of the spine. Synovial fluid may have a characteristic ground-pepper appearance caused by pigmented cartilage fragments. Many patients with ochronotic arthritis require joint replacement.

16. **What are the characteristic radiographic findings for ochronotic arthritis?**

Lumbosacral radiographs show premature degenerative changes, ligamentous calcifications that can resemble ankylosing spondylitis, dense wafer-like calcifications of the intervertebral discs, vacuum discs, and narrowing of the intervertebral spaces (Fig. 56.2). Lack of involvement of sacroiliac joints can help distinguish ochronotic arthritis from axial spondyloarthritis/ankylosing

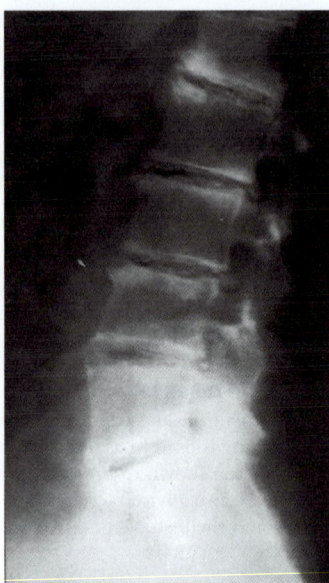

Fig. 56.2 Lateral radiograph of the spine in a patient with ochronosis. Note the vertebral disc-space calcification at multiple levels.

spondylitis. The radiographic appearance of the large peripheral joints in ochronotic arthritis is virtually indistinguishable from that in primary osteoarthritis.

17. How is a diagnosis of alkaptonuria made?

Although the darkening of urine can be observed in diapers of infants, less than 25% of patients with alkaptonuria are diagnosed before 1 year of age. Diagnosis typically occurs in the third decade of life. Diagnosis is confirmed by elevated HGA levels in urine and genetic testing for *HGD* mutations.

18. What are the treatments for alkaptonuria?

There are no currently approved treatments for alkaptonuria. Dietary restriction of tyrosine and phenylalanine reduces the excretion of homogentisic acid, but with unclear clinical effect. Nitisinone (Orfadin) is currently under investigation for the treatment of alkaptonuria and prevention of ochronosis. This drug inhibits the enzyme 4-hydroxyphenylpyruvic acid dioxygenase which produces homogentisic acid. Of note, a 2011 trial reported that nitisinone was not effective once arthritis was established. Treatment of ochronotic arthritis is therefore similar to that of primary osteoarthritis including exercise/physical therapy, NSAIDs, and intra-articular steroids.

ACKNOWLEDGMENT

The author would like to acknowledge the contributions of Dr. Sterling G. West, who was the author of this chapter in the previous edition.

BIBLIOGRAPHY

Balaban B, Taskaynatan M, Yasar E, et al. Ochronotic spondyloarthropathy: spinal involvement resembling ankylosing spondylitis. *Clin Rheumatol.* 2006;25:598–601.

Carroll GJ, Breidahl WH, Olynyk JK. Characteristics of the arthropathy described in hereditary hemochromatosis. *Arthritis Care Res.* 2012;64:9–14.

European Association for Study of Liver. EASL clinical practice guidelines: Wilson's disease. *J Hepatol.* 2012;56:671–685.

Hunter T, Gordon D, Ogryzlo MA. The ground pepper sign of synovial fluid: a new diagnostic feature of ochronosis. *J Rheumatol.* 1974;1:45–53.

Kowdley KV, Brown KE, Ahn J, et al. ACG clinical guideline: hereditary hemochromatosis. *Am J Gastroenterol*. 2019;114:1202–1218.

Loret A, Jacob C, Mammou S, et al. Joint manifestations revealing inborn metabolic diseases in adults: a narrative review. *Orphanet J Rare Dis*. 2023;18:239.

Mannoni A, Selvi E, Lorenzini S, et al. Alkaptonuria, ochronosis, and ochronotic arthropathy. *Semin Arthritis Rheum*. 2004;33:239–248.

Olynyk JK, Ramm GA. Hemochromatosis. *N Engl J Med*. 2022;387:2159–2170.

Perry MB, Suwannarat P, Furst GP, et al. Musculoskeletal findings and disability in alkaptonuria. *J Rheumatol*. 2006;33:2280–2285.

Ranganath LR, Milan AM, Hughes AT, et al. Suitability of nitisinone in alkaptonuria 1 (ssSONIA 1). *Ann Rheum Dis*. 2016;75:362–367.

Roberts EA, Schilsky ML. Current and emerging issues in Wilson's disease. *N Engl J Med*. 2023;389:922–938.

Suwannarat P, Phornphutkul C, Bernardini I, Turner M, Gahl WA. Minocycline-induced hyperpigmentation masquerading as alkaptonuria in individuals with joint pain. *Arthritis Rheuma*. 2004;50:3698–3701.

Wu K, Bauer E, Myung G, Fang MA. Musculoskeletal manifestations of alkaptonuria: a case report and literature review. *Eur J Rheumatol Inflamm*. 2018;6:98–101.

FURTHER READING

http://rarediseases.info.nih.gov/GARD.

CHAPTER 57

Rheumatologic Manifestations of the Primary Immunodeficiency Syndromes

Tho Truong, MD

> ### KEY POINTS
>
> 1. The most common disease-defining features of primary immunodeficiency (PI) are recurrent infection and tissue-threatening autoimmunity.
> 2. Mutations in genes affecting signaling proteins involved in upregulating or downregulating the immune response, and immune cell number or function, can lead to immune dysregulation causing both immunodeficiency and autoimmunity.
> 3. Common variable immunodeficiency (CVID) may present in early adulthood as large and medium joint inflammatory polyarthritis; significant hypogammaglobulinemia may not present until later.
> 4. Early complement protein (C1, C4, and C2) deficiencies are associated with autoimmune diseases, whereas late (C5 to C8) deficiencies are associated with infections with Neisseria.
> 5. Understanding the genetic basis of PI syndromes may lead to a better understanding of potential infection- and autoimmune-related adverse events when disease-modifying antirheumatic drugs (DMARDs) or biologics are used to treat rheumatic or oncologic disease.

1. Why are the primary immunodeficiency (PI) syndromes of concern in rheumatology?

PI syndromes are phenotypes of inborn errors of immunity (IEI) that result in immune dysregulation that may present as features of rheumatologic disease. At least 485 IEIs to date have been established; this includes 55 novel monogenic defects and 1 autoimmune phenocopy. Over a third of IEI phenotypes include autoimmune manifestations with organ-threatening disease, such as autoimmune endocrinopathies, autoimmune cytopenia (autoimmune hemolytic anemia [AHA], idiopathic thrombocytopenia [ITP]), lymphocytic or granulomatous lung or gastrointestinal (GI) tract disease, or disease meeting American College of Rheumatology or European League Against Rheumatism classification criteria for rheumatoid arthritis (RA) (CVID, lipopolysaccharide-responsive and beige-like anchor protein [LRBA] deficiency, cytotoxic T-lymphocyte-associated protein 4 [CTLA4] haploinsufficiency) or systemic lupus erythematosus (SLE) (TREX1; C4, PRKCD, and FasL deficiencies). Many of the identified genes associated with PI syndromes predispose individuals not only to immune dysregulation leading to autoimmunity but also to severe infection; treatment is therefore caveated, and knowledge of specific immune defects can be helpful in choosing the most appropriate management.

2. What are some of the proposed mechanisms for autoimmunity found in PI disorders? What are some PI disorders with autoimmune manifestations?

Pathogenic mechanisms that have been proposed and are being studied include (Table 57.1):
- Defects in central and peripheral tolerance
- Impairment of apoptosis of autoreactive T cells
- Diminished T-regulatory cell (Treg) number and/or function. One important recent discovery is the recognition of the role of "checkpoint" regulatory molecules, such as CTLA4, that influence antigen recognition and development of Treg cells.
- Mutations in genes involved in signaling cascades which play a downregulatory role in inflammation. Since the last edition, the understanding of activated PI3 kinase delta syndrome (APDS) has grown and has been more widely identified.
- Persistent inflammation due to frequent, recurrent, or chronic infections, which results in cell death and a larger than usual burden of cellular debris, leading to decreased clearance of self-antigens and immune complexes.

Coexistence of certain PI and autoimmunity also may be coincidental rather than causal. However, in most PI syndromes with autoimmunity for which a genetic basis has been delineated, the mechanism for autoimmunity can be explained by the genetic defect, which is demonstrated in functional studies of the gene product.

TABLE 57.1 Examples of PI Syndromes With Associated Autoimmune Manifestations

ASSOCIATED GENETIC DEFECT(S)	SYNDROME(S) W/AUTOIMMUNE PROBLEMS	AFFECTED IMMUNITY
AIRE	APECED	T cell subset development
FOXP3	IPEX	and tolerance
RAG1, RAG2	CVID, CID, SCID	
RAG1, RAG2, DCLRE1C	Omenn syndrome	
CTLA4, LRBA	CVID, CID, hCTLA4	Lymphocyte signaling pathway
PI3K	CVID, CID	
PKC-δ	CVID, CID, ALPS, SLE	
DOCK8	DOCK8 syndrome	
LAT	CID, SCID	
JAK and STAT family	CMC and hyper IgE syndrome	
CD40L	Hyper-IgM	
Complement protein genes	SLE	Complement pathway
CASP10, CASP8, FAS, FASL,	ALPS	Abnormal resolution of inflammation
TNFSF6, TNFRSF6		
ACP5	SPENCD	Interferon signaling pathway
TMEM173	SAVI	

AIRE, autoimmune regulator; *APECED*, autoimmune polyendocrinopathy-candidiasis-ectodermal dystrophy; *FOXP3*, forkhead box P3; *IPEX*, immunodysregulation polyendocrinopathy enteropathy X-linked; *RAG1, RAG2*, recombination activating gene 1, (and 2); *DCLRE1C*, Cross-Link Repair 1C, gene encoding "Artemis" protein; *CVID*, common variable immunodeficiency; *(S)CID*, (Severe) Combined Immunodeficiency; *CTLA4*, cytotoxic T-lymphocyte associated protein 4 (also called CD152 or cluster of differentiation 152); *LRBA*, lipopolysaccharide-responsive and beige-like anchor protein; *PI3K*, phosphoinositide 3-kinase; *PKC-d*, protein kinase C delta; *DOCK 8*, dedicator of cytokinesis 8; *LAT*, linker for activation of T cells; *JAK STAT*, Janus kinase, signal transducer and activator of transcription protein; *CD40L*, cluster of differentiation 40 ligand (also called CD154); *ALPS*, autoimmune lymphoproliferative syndrome; *SLE*, systemic lupus erythematosus; *CMC*, chronic mucocutaneous candidiasis; *CASP8 and 10*, caspase 8, 10; *FAS(L)*, FS=7 associated surface antigen (ligand), also called CD95 or apoptosis antigen 1 or APO-1; *TNFSF6*, tumor necrosis factor superfamily member 6; *TNFRSF6*, tumor necrosis factor superfamily receptor member 6; *ACP5*, acid phosphatase 5 (encodes tartrate resistant acid phosphatase (TRAP) protein; *TMEM173*, transmembrane protein 173; *SPENCD*, spondyloenchondrodysplasia with immune dysregulation; *SAVI*, STING (stimulator of interferon genes) – associated vasculopathy.

3. Which components of the immune system are involved in the PI syndromes?

All components (B cell, T cell/natural killer [NK] cell, phagocytes, complement system) of the immune system (see Chapter 4) have been shown to be affected in various PI syndromes. Humoral (antibody) immunodeficiencies constitute the majority of PIs. Many humoral (B cell) immunodeficiencies occur in combination with T-cell deficiencies due to the dependence of antibody development on normal T-cell function as well as shared genes involved in both T-cell and B-cell development. Some of the more recently recognized disorders involve mutations in components of the innate immune system, mutations that involve genes that control fundamental cellular development (DOCK8) or metabolic functions. The individual PI syndromes may be due to dysfunction of a single component of the immune system, such as C4 deficiency, or dysfunction of multiple components, such as impairment of B-cell, T-cell, and phagocyte function in certain severe combined immunodeficiencies (SCIDs).

4. What are the clinical features which should raise suspicion for PI syndromes?

Any child with two or more sinopulmonary infections within 1 year, four or more ear infections within 1 year, or two or more deep skin or organ infections including septicemia should be evaluated for a PI disorder. The first test to get is a complete blood count with differential. Physical exam findings in children may include dysmorphic facial features such as low-set ears and stigmata of developmental delay. Adults with recurrent respiratory tract infections, especially any community-acquired types of pneumonia or unexplained chronic diarrhea, should be screened for low quantitative immunoglobulins of all classes (IgG, IgM, IgA, and IgE). Cytopenias occur in both children and adults with PI syndromes. Adults may have a normal exam, or abnormalities such as absent tonsils (with no history of tonsillectomy), hepatosplenomegaly, synovitis, petechiae, pallor, and/or abnormal breath or bowel sounds.

5. **The types of recurrent infections in a particular patient offer a clue to the underlying PI syndrome. Which microorganisms are responsible for recurrent infections in B-cell immunodeficiency syndromes?**

Microbial cultures are important to determine if a patient truly has recurring infections, and if so, with which organism(s). More often than not, symptoms of frequent upper respiratory tract infections in adults may be due to uncontrolled allergic rhinosinusitis, asthma, or chronic aspiration rather than true infections. The risk of infection is also elevated in patients with these more common illnesses. In B-cell immunodeficiency, such as X-linked (Bruton's) agammaglobulinemia (XLA), inadequate immunoglobulin production leads to recurrent infection with extracellular, encapsulated, pyogenic bacteria, particularly *Streptococcus pneumoniae, Haemophilus influenzae,* and *Moraxella catharralis.* These organisms typically cause acute and chronic infections of the upper (sinusitis, otitis, bronchitis) and lower (pneumonia) respiratory tracts, meningitis, and bacteremia. GI infections (*Giardia, Cryptosporidium, C. difficile,* and norovirus) are also increased.

6. **What laboratory tests are performed to evaluate the integrity of the humoral immune system (B-cell function)?**

A simple initial screen for hypogammaglobulinemia is to subtract the albumin from the total protein and see if it is <1.5 g/dL. A reasonable screen for the evaluation of B-cell function is to determine the serum IgA level and perform inexpensive *in vivo* functional tests. If all these tests are normal, clinically significant B-cell dysfunction may be reasonably excluded. If IgE is normal, a class-switching defect is unlikely. If any of these tests are abnormal, further testing to characterize B cell development and referral to clinical immunology is appropriate (Table 57.2). As with rheumatologic evaluations, further testing to diagnose a disease requires objective evidence for tissue or end-organ involvement.

7. **Which organisms are responsible for infections in primary T-cell immunodeficiency, such as thymic hypoplasia (DiGeorge syndrome)?**

- Viruses (e.g., herpes viruses).
- Intracellular bacteria (e.g., mycobacteria).
- Fungi (e.g., *Candida* species).
- Other (*Pneumocystis jirovecii*).

Primary T-cell immunodeficiency usually manifests during infancy and results in inadequate cell-mediated immunity, leading to infections similar to those encountered in patients with HIV infection, the prototypic acquired T-cell immunodeficiency state. CD4+ helper T cells (Th2 subset) interact with B cells to facilitate immunoglobulin class switching and productive antibody response to most protein antigens. CD4+ T cells (Th1 subset) and CD8+ cytotoxic T cells play a key role in detecting and eradicating intracellular organisms such as viral, fungal, mycobacterial, and pneumocystis. Treg cells (CD4+ CD25+ FOXP3+ T_{REG}) are important in peripheral tolerance and absence of these cells leads to early-onset autoimmunity. Recently, the Th17 subset of CD4+ T helper cells has been shown to be important in controlling superficial fungal infections. Patients with cellular defects (STAT1/3) or 1L-17 mutations develop severe chronic mucocutaneous candidiasis.

8. **What laboratory tests can be used to evaluate the integrity of the cellular immune system (T-cell function)?**

A reasonable screening evaluation of T-cell function is to determine the absolute lymphocyte count and perform a Candida skin test (Table 57.3). If these are both normal, clinically significant T-cell dysfunction may be excluded. If the Candida skin test is negative, negative delayed-type skin testing with at least four other antigens is necessary to demonstrate that T-cell function is inadequate. If these screening tests are abnormal, more sophisticated in vitro tests may be necessary to define the underlying PI disorder. HIV testing should be performed as part of the screening evaluation to exclude this acquired T-cell disorder.

TABLE 57.2 Laboratory Evaluation of B-cell Function

CATEGORY	SPECIFIC TESTS	COMMENTS
In vivo functional tests (routine screening tests)	Isohemagglutinin titers (anti-blood group A and B)	Naturally occurring; predominantly IgM
	Diphtheria and tetanus booster immunization	Serum antibodies assayed prior to and 2 weeks later; assesses capacity to synthesize IgG antibodies against protein antigens.
	Pneumococcal immunization	Serum antibodies assayed prior to and 3 weeks later; assesses capacity to synthesize antibodies against polysaccharide antigens. Currently, no formal consensus on the reference ranges for normal.
Immunoglobulin quantitation	IgM, IgG, IgA levels	Various immunoassays may be used; readily available
	IgG subclass, IgE levels	ELISA and RIA available (expensive)
In vitro tests (expensive)	Peripheral blood total B cells	Flow cytometry, CD19+ B cell numbers
	B cell subsets	Class-switched memory B cells (CD27+$^+$IgD-) versus non-switched memory B cells (CD27+$^+$IgD+) and immature or transitional B cells
Genetic testing BTK (XLA), CVID, CID with monogenetic cause	In vitro immunoglobulin synthesis	Peripheral blood mononuclear cells stimulated in vitro with pokeweed mitogen (not frequently done for clinical decisions)

ELISA, enzyme-linked immunosorbent assay; *RIA*, radioimmunoassay.

TABLE 57.3 Laboratory Evaluation of T-cell Function

CATEGORY	SPECIFIC TESTS	COMMENTS
In vivo functional tests	*Candida* skin test	Examine degree of induration 48–72 hours later
(skin testing for delayed-type hypersensitivity) (routine screening tests)	PPD, *Trichophyton*, mumps, tetanus/diphtheria toxoid, keyhole-limpet hemocyanin	If *Candida* skin test is negative, testing with at least four of these antigens must be performed to determine if cell-mediated immunity is inadequate
Absolute lymphocyte count (routine screening test)	Determine from total WBC count and % lymphocytes	Severe cell-mediated immunity disorder unlikely in setting of normal lymphocyte count
In vitro tests (expensive)	Quantitation of: Total T cells, CD4$^+$ cells, CD8$^+$ cells, NK cells	Specific monoclonal antibodies may be used.
	Lymphocyte blastic transformation	Assessment of radiolabeled thymidine uptake following stimulation with lectins (such as PHA), specific antigen (such as *Candida*), or one-way mixed lymphocyte reaction
	Quantitate ability of T cells to synthesize IL-2 and IL-2 receptors (CD25)	These and lymphocyte blastic transformation assay are indicators of successful T-cell activation

IL, interleukin; *PHA*, phytohemagglutinin; *PPD*, purified protein derivative (for tuberculosis); *WBC*, white blood cell.

9. What infections are characteristic of an abnormality of phagocytic cells?

Phagocytic cell dysfunction can be from defects in neutrophil numbers (e.g., congenital or cyclic neutropenia), adherence (e.g., leukocyte adhesion deficiency 1 [LAD-1]), chemotaxis, degranulation (e.g., Chediak–Higashi), microbial killing (e.g., chronic granulomatous disease), or from defects in monocyte numbers (congenital) or macrophage dysfunction (e.g., defect in interferon-γ receptor or interleukin (IL)-12 signaling). Patients with absence of pus at sites of infection and poor wound healing have defects in neutrophil numbers, adhesion, or chemotaxis. Patients with neutrophil defects of microbial killing present with lymphadenitis and visceral or perirectal abscesses with granuloma formation caused by low-virulence gram-negative organisms, such as *E. coli*, *Serratia*, or *Klebsiella*. Other patients will have gingivitis and skin infections or furunculosis with *Staphylococcus* species or *Pseudomonas*. Patients with macrophage defects have frequent mycobacterial infections.

10. How is neutrophil function measured?

The standard neutrophil tests include assessment of numbers, examination of the neutrophils for giant granules on peripheral smear (Chediak–Higashi), and a test for measurement of oxidative burst (chronic granulomatous disease). Flow cytometry-based dihydrorhodamine 123 assay is better than the nitroblue tetrazolium test for assessing neutrophil oxidative burst. If those are normal, testing for adherence problems such as LAD-1 deficiency (measure CD11a, CD11b, CD18), chemotaxis defects, specific granule (lactoferrin) deficiency, and phagocytosis defects can be undertaken.

11. What are the infectious manifestations of homozygous complement deficient states?

The complement deficiencies can be divided into those of the classical pathway (C1–C9), alternative complement pathway (factors B, D, and P), the mannose-binding lectin (MBL) pathway and their associated proteases (MASP-1 and MASP-2), and the complement regulatory proteins (C1INH, factor H, factor I, MCP). Deficiency of C3 or MBL is associated with recurrent blood-borne infections with encapsulated bacteria including *S. pneumoniae* and *H. influenza*. Deficiencies of components of the membrane attack complex (C5–C9) or alternative complement pathway factors are associated with recurrent *Neisseria* infections, (both *N. meningitidis* and *N. gonorrhoeae*). C6 deficiency is most common. **Patients with recurrent bouts of Neisserial infections, particularly when systemic, should be evaluated for the presence of a complement deficiency.** All patients should be immunized with the conjugate meningococcal vaccine. Use of prophylactic antibiotics is controversial due to the risk of causing antibiotic-resistant strains of *Neisseria*.

12. How do you screen for homozygous complement and MBL deficiency?

In the general population, complement deficiencies are uncommon whereas up to 3% can have MBL deficiency. The **total hemolytic complement assay (CH_{50})** assesses the integrity of the classic pathway of complement activation. Patient's serum is added to a standardized suspension of sheep red blood cells (RBCs) coated with rabbit antibody. These "immune complexes" allow activation of the classic pathway, resulting in lysis of the sheep RBC. The CH_{50} is the reciprocal of the serum dilution that lyses 50% of the sheep RBC. Because specific deficiencies that lead to rheumatologic manifestations are usually in the classical, rather than the alternative pathway, CH_{50} is the ideal inexpensive screening test. Homozygous deficiency of a complement component in the classical pathway results in a CH_{50} of 0; individual complement levels may then be determined by immunoassay. Complement component deficiencies of the classical pathway have an autosomal recessive pattern of inheritance. If the CH_{50} is normal, the alternative pathway function should be tested with the AH_{50} and MBL should be measured since deficiency in these components can be associated with severe infections.

13. Which PI syndromes are most commonly associated with autoimmune phenomena?

- Selective IgA deficiency, CVID, XLA, and hyper-IgM syndrome are the B-cell immunodeficiency syndromes commonly associated with autoimmune phenomena.
- Absence of certain complement components (C1, C2, and C4) is also associated with autoimmune phenomena, particularly SLE.
- Chronic granulomatous disease, a primary disorder of neutrophils in which there is diminished oxidative burst, is associated with the presence of antinuclear antibody (ANA) and a malar-like rash in female carriers (but less commonly, SLE) and inflammatory bowel disease.
- SCID, Omenn syndrome (Rag 1and 2 defects), APECED, i.e., autoimmune polyendocrinopathy-candidiasis-ectodermal dystrophy (AIRE defect), IPEX (Foxp3 defect), autoimmune lymphoproliferative syndrome (FAS defect), and Wiskott–Aldrich syndrome (WASp defect) have T-cell and immune tolerance defects and can have autoimmune cytopenias (AIHA, ITP), autoimmune enteropathy, arthritis, other organ-specific immune-mediated damage, and/or

atopic (eczema) features as part of their presentations. PIs affecting CD8 and NK cell cytotoxicity such as perforin deficiency are at risk of developing hemophagocytic syndrome (Table 57.1).

14. What are the rheumatologic manifestations of X-linked (Bruton's) agammaglobulinemia (XLA)?

XLA is a rare disorder characterized by absent or near-absent levels of serum IgG, IgM, and IgA and by abnormal in vivo B-cell functional tests due to a defect within the Bruton's tyrosine kinase (BTK) gene, resulting in abnormal function of this signal transduction protein, which is normally present within B cells at all stages of development. This results in characteristic cellular abnormalities, such as failure of maturation of the B-cell line and absence of B cells. Arthritis occurs in approximately 20% of patients, with half of these cases due to infection with the typical pyogenic bacteria. Furthermore, patients appear vulnerable to infections with enterovirus and *Mycoplasma*.

There are cases of arthritis in XLA in which an infectious agent cannot be detected despite rigorous evaluation. Our clinical experience with patients with agammaglobulinemia or hypogammaglobulinemia and arthritis is that they much more commonly have aseptic arthritis (either inflammatory or degenerative in nature) or arthralgias without arthritis. However, atypical organisms such as *Ureaplasma urealyticum* and *Mycoplasma* species organisms have been reported in patients with PI syndromes who present with a more "subacute" clinical picture (pain and persistent joint swelling but no diminished range of motion, joint is not hot or red). In these cases, a trial of doxycycline or a macrolide has been suggested, though the duration of therapy is unclear (Table 57.4).

15. What are autoimmune problems associated with selective IgA deficiency?

- Systemic autoimmune disorders (SLE, SLE-spectrum of disease [undifferentiated connective tissue disease], RA, juvenile idiopathic arthritis, Sjogren's, dermatomyositis, vasculitis, etc.) occur in 7% to 36% of patients (four times increased risk).
- Organ-specific autoimmune disorders (diabetes mellitus type I, myasthenia gravis, psoriatic arthritis, inflammatory bowel disease, autoimmune cytopenias, autoimmune endocrinopathies, autoimmune hepatitis, etc.).

IgA deficiency is the most common immunodeficiency with a prevalence of 1/333 to 1/700 in Caucasians. Of these, 20% are familial. It is characterized by absent (<5 mg/dL) levels of serum and secretory IgA, accompanied by normal levels of serum IgG and IgM. Cell-mediated immunity is intact. It is usually asymptomatic, and there are no specific treatments for IgA deficiency, other than to avoid IgA-containing blood products or medications. It may be useful in raising clinical suspicion for one of the autoimmune diseases earlier.

16. List the autoantibodies seen in patients with selective IgA deficiency without clinically expressed autoimmune disease.

Rheumatoid factor and ANA are most consistently observed. Other autoantibodies that may be present include antibodies against double-stranded and single-stranded DNA, cardiolipin, thyroglobulin, thyroid microsomes, smooth muscle, gastric parietal cell, striated muscle, acetylcholine receptor, and bile canaliculi. IgG and IgE autoantibodies against IgA occur in 40% to 60%

TABLE 57.4 Rheumatologic Manifestations of X-linked Agammaglobulinemia

MANIFESTATION	COMMENTS
Septic arthritis	Occurs in 10% of patients
Extracellular, encapsulated bacteria (*S. pneumoniae*, *H. influenzae*), *S. aureus*	
Mycoplasma, particularly *Ureaplasma urealyticum*	
Enteroviruses, particularly echovirus and coxsackie virus	
Aseptic, possibly autoimmune, arthritis	Usually mono- or oligoarticular; involves large joints; rarely destructive; rheumatoid factor and ANA absent. Occurs in 10% of patients.
Dermatomyositis-like syndrome associated with progressive enterovirus (ECHO) CNS infection	Presents with rash and muscle weakness.

of patients, which puts them at risk for severe reactions to blood transfusions and intravenous immunoglobulin (IVIG) therapy.

17. What is CVID and describe the rheumatologic manifestations of CVID and how these manifestations are diagnosed?

CVID is a heterogeneous group of immunodeficiency disorders characterized by quantitative IgG levels less than two standard deviations below the mean for the patient's age, low IgA or IgM levels, and poor specific antibody response to vaccinations. Clinically, patients present with recurrent respiratory tract infections and not uncommonly, aseptic arthritis (30%), cytopenias (ITP in ~20%, AHA, pernicious anemia), and granulomatous (sarcoid-like) or lymphocytic interstitial lung and/or GI disease (5%–10%). Other organ-specific autoimmunity can occur in the liver (autoimmune hepatitis), endocrine (thyroiditis, diabetes), and skin (psoriasis, vitiligo). Septic arthritis with bacteria (extracellular and/or encapsulated) or Mycoplasma (particularly *U. urealyticum*) can also occur.

More single-gene defects have been associated with PI syndromes within nonconsanguineous families who have presented with a CVID phenotype (hCTLA4, LRBA, PIK3, ICOS, CD19, TACI, BAFF-R). However, the majority of patients with the CVID phenotype who have been sequenced do not have a monogenetic explanation for their condition. Since the diagnosis of CVID requires a significant deficiency in circulating IgG, IgG-based serologic tests are unreliable and not used to definitely diagnose autoimmune manifestations. As with rheumatologic evaluation for rheumatic diseases, diagnosis is based on a history which would raise concern for inflammatory arthritis or end-organ damage. Clinical examination may reveal synovitis, alopecia, rashes/vitiligo, focal weakness, hepatosplenomegaly, pulmonary crackles, and so on. Arthritis in CVID most commonly involves large- and medium-sized joints, although involvement of proximal interphalangeal and metacarpophalangeal joints have been also reported. Rheumatoid nodules are not common, though erosions and periarticular osteopenia have been reported. While arthralgias may respond somewhat to IVIG therapy, true arthritis with synovitis on exam responds to the same oral DMARDs (hydroxychloroquine, methotrexate, azathioprine, sulfasalazine) used in the treatment of seronegative RA. While biologics may raise the risk of infection in patients, tumor necrosis factor (TNF)-blockade and rituximab have been successfully used in patients with more aggressive (erosive or refractory to oral DMARDs) arthritis as well as granulomatous (infliximab, rituximab) or lymphocytic interstitial lung disease (rituximab in conjunction with azathioprine or mycophenolate mofetil).

18. What is the hyper-IgM syndrome?

The hyper-IgM immunodeficiency syndrome (type 1) is characterized by extremely low levels of IgG, IgA, and IgE and either a normal or markedly elevated concentration of polyclonal IgM. Patients develop both recurrent pyogenic infections and opportunistic infections like *P. jirovecii* pneumonia. There is also an increased frequency of autoimmune disorders (autoimmune cytopenias, arthritis, nephritis) and malignancy (lymphoma, tumors of the GI tract). The defect causing this x-linked syndrome is an abnormal gene resulting in a defective CD40 ligand (CD 154) on the surface of activated CD4+ T cells. This mutation results in the failure of T cells to interact with CD40 on B cells. This lack of B-cell signaling by T cells results in the B cell failing to undergo isotype switching and producing only IgM. Two other types (2 and 3) of this syndrome have different genetic defects and inheritance patterns. Other mutations that affect immune globulin isotype switching and result in laboratory abnormalities that are similar to those seen in patients with defective expression of CD40L are inherited in an autosomal recessive manner and include mutations in genes for CD40, NFκB essential modulator (NEMO), activated cytidine deaminase (AID), and uracil deglycosylase (UNG).

19. Discuss the therapy for XLA, CVID/PIs with clinically significant hypogammaglobulinemia, and selective IgG deficiency (can have normal quantitative IgG levels but lack specific vaccine responses); what must be considered if patients also have IgA deficiency?

IVIG is usually administered in a dose of 200 to 600 mg/kg every month to maintain trough IgG levels of 500 to 800 mg/dL, and then is adjusted for clinical response (less frequent or severe infection). Prophylactic antibiotics are controversial due to the evolution of resistant organisms.

IVIG should not be administered in patients with IgA deficiency since many patients have autoantibodies against IgA, including IgE anti-IgA, which may result in severe, occasionally fatal anaphylaxis. These patients should ideally receive blood products obtained from other patients with IgA deficiency.

20. How are organ- or tissue-threatening autoimmune problems treated in patients with PI syndrome?

In general, autoimmunity that is organ-threatening should be treated, and the options for treatment are generally the same as for immunocompetent patients. Rigorous exclusion of infection, to the extent that is practically possible, and closer follow-up of the PI syndrome patient, is required. Patients with IgG deficiency as part of their PI syndrome should concomitantly be treated with adequate IgG replacement. While arthralgias may respond somewhat to IVIG therapy, our experience is that true synovitis on exam responds to the same oral DMARDs (hydroxychloroquine, methotrexate, azathioprine, sulfasalazine) used in the treatment of seronegative RA. Biologics should be used with extreme caution only if oral DMARDs fail. In patients with CVID or combined T and B immunodeficiency (CID), TNF-blockade and abatacept, have been successfully used in patients for more aggressive (erosive or refractory to oral DMARDs) arthritis as well as in granulomatous lung and GI disease (infliximab, rituximab) or lymphocytic interstitial lung disease (rituximab in conjunction with azathioprine or mycophenolate mofetil). Rapamycin has also been used in CVID, CID, and SCID patients with lymphocytic end-organ disease (lung, liver). CVID or CID syndromes with arthritis, lung, liver, CNS, and/or GI tract underlying CTLA haploinsufficiency or LRBA deficiency may respond well to abatacept, although norovirus and *Legionella pneumophila* infection were reported in this population. John Cunningham (JC) virus infection, cytomegalovirus, and hepatitis B reactivation have been described with use of rituximab therapy, but patients are at a lower risk if on sufficient IVIG replacement. High-dose IVIG given as 1–2 g/kg divided over 3–4 days has also been used successfully in patients with PI syndrome and inflammatory arthritis or SLE-like disease, including dermatomyositis. This can be an option if immunosuppressive therapies need to be avoided.

21. What are the rheumatologic manifestations of homozygous complement deficient states?

Deficiencies of the early components of the classic pathway (C1, C4, and C2) are associated with immune complex disease, particularly SLE or lupus-like glomerulonephritis. Dermatomyositis, vasculitis, and others have also been described. This may be due to impaired clearance of apoptotic cells, inability to maintain circulating immune complexes in a soluble state, and/or inability to remove circulating immune complexes. The reported prevalence of SLE is 93% with C1q, 75% with C4, and 33% with C2 deficiency. C2 deficiency is the most common complement deficiency (1 in 20,000 individuals).

Factor H deficiency as well as polymorphisms have been associated with atypical (diarrhea-negative) hemolytic-uremic syndrome and glomerulonephritis. A similar syndrome may occur with factor I and MCP defects. These patients may be helped by treatment with eculizumab (Soliris). Since factor H deficiency can also lead to secondary C3 deficiency, patients may be at increased risk for infections.

ACKNOWLEDGMENT

The author would like to thank Drs Sterling West and Mark Malyak for their contributions to this chapter in previous editions.

BIBLIOGRAPHY

Bousfiha A, Moundir A, Tangye SG, et al. The 2022 update of IUIS phenotypical classification for human inborn errors of immunity. *J Clin Immunol.* 2022;42:1508–1520.

Borgaert DJA, Dullaers MK, Lambrect BN, et al. Genes associated with common variable immune deficiency: one diagnosis to rule them all? *J Med Genet.* 2016;53:575–590.

Costagliola G, Cappelli S, Consolini R. Autoimmunity in primary immunodeficiency disorders: an updated review on pathogenic and clinical implications. *J Clin Med.* 2021;10:4729.

Dimitriades VR, Sorensen R. Rheumatologic manifestations of primary immunodeficiency diseases. *Clin Rheumatol.* 2016;35:843–850.

Goyal R, Bulua AC, Nikolov NP, et al. Rheumatologic and autoimmune manifestations of primary immunodeficiency disorders. *Curr Opin Rheumatol.* 2009;21:78–84.

Notarangelo LD. Primary immunodeficiencies. *J Allergy Clin Immunol.* 2010;125:S182–S194.

Schmidt RE, Grimbacher B, Witte T. Autoimmunity and primary immunodeficiency: two sides of the same coin? *Nat Rev Rheumatol.* 2018;14:7–18.

Subbarayan A, Colarusso G, Hughes SM, et al. Clinical features that identify children with primary immunodeficiency diseases. *Pediatrics.* 2011;127:810–816.

Singh A, Joshi V, Jindal AK, Mathew B, Rawat A. An updated review on activated PI3 kinase delta syndrome (APDS). *Genes Dis.* 2019;7:67–74.

Torgerson TR. Immunodeficiency diseases with rheumatic manifestations. *Pediatr Clin North Am.* 2012;59:493–507.

FURTHER READING

www.primaryimmune.org.
www.nichd.nih.gov/health/topics/primaryimmunodeficiency.cfm.
www.info4pi.org.

CHAPTER 58

Skeletal Dysplasias

Lisa Zickuhr, MD, MHPE

KEY POINTS

1. A skeletal dysplasia should be considered in any patient with premature osteoarthritis and/or disproportionate short stature.
2. Hypophosphatasia may mimic rickets and osteomalacia and is associated with low alkaline phosphatase (ALP) levels. Adults with milder disease frequently have a history of poorly healing metatarsal stress fractures.

1. What exactly is a skeletal dysplasia?

Dysplasia is a term literally meaning abnormal growth. Applied to the skeletal system, the term encompasses a heterogenous group of >450 conditions in which abnormalities affect developing bone or cartilage and are broadly grouped under the heading of skeletal dysplasias or **osteochondrodysplasias.** Although each individual syndrome is rare, collectively the overall incidence is 1 in 5000 births. These dysplasias are heritable and can range in severity from lethal to mere radiologic curiosities. The genetic cause has been identified for at least 350 of these disorders. Early identification allows initiation of treatment and genetic counseling.

2. How do skeletal dysplasias most commonly present?

Skeletal dysplasias can be diagnosed as early as during fetal development, when ultrasonography reveals reduced limb growth or other developmental abnormalities. Oftentimes, pediatricians identify infants born with head and facial dysmorphisms, disproportionate growth of the upper and lower limbs, or extra-articular irregularities affecting any organ system. Young children should prompt evaluation for skeletal dysplasia if their growth rate suddenly declines, as some skeletal dysplasias appear during early childhood. Patients with skeletal dysplasias most often present to the rheumatologist with early-onset osteoarthritis or early-onset metabolic bone disease, usually with a familial history suggesting an underlying genetic cause.

3. How do clinicians diagnose skeletal dysplasias?

A thorough history and physical examination lay the foundation for diagnosing skeletal dysplasias. Clinicians should inquire about growth history (e.g., when short stature was first identified, changes in growth rate), joint pain, history of fractures, extra-articular manifestations (e.g., respiratory symptoms, history of kidney disorders, or hearing, vision, or cognitive abnormalities), and family history while examining for growth parameters (e.g., height, head circumference, upper:lower limb segment ratio, arm span), cranial malformations (e.g., frontal bossing, facial dysmorphism), and other skeletal dysmorphisms (e.g, pectus excavatum, scoliosis, lordosis). Clinicians considering a diagnosis of skeletal dysplasia should proceed with a skeletal survey to identify radiographic features consistent with a specific or family of conditions. Skeletal surveys are most informative during childhood before the growth plates, or **physes**, fuse and should be performed serially to monitor for progression or new development of findings. Lastly, genetic testing helps establish the diagnosis. Together, clinical, radiographic, and genetic data contribute to the diagnosis of skeletal dysplasias.

4. How are the skeletal dysplasias classified?

By international consensus, these disorders are formally classified into 46 groups based on clinical manifestations, radiographic findings, or causative genetic mutation (Table 58.1). It is useful and practical, however, to group these disorders according to where the most prominent abnormalities in growth occur. The mnemonic **EMPD** ("empty") can help broadly group these syndromes.

TABLE 58.1 Classification of Skeletal Dysplasias

GROUP NO.	GROUP NAME	GROUP NO.	GROUP NAME
1.	FGFR3 chondrodysplasia group	2.	Type 2 collagen group
3.	Type II collagen group	4.	Sulfation disorders group
5.	Perlecan group	6.	Aggrecan group
7.	Filamin group and related disorders	8.	TRPV4 group
9.	Ciliopathies with major skeletal involvement	10.	MED and pseudoachondroplasia group
11.	Metaphyseal dysplasias	12.	SMD
13.	SE(M)D	14.	Severe spondylodysplastic dysplasias
15.	Acromelic dysplasias	16.	Acromesomelic dysplasias
17.	Mesomelic and rhizomesomelic dysplasias	18.	Campomelic dysplasia and related disorders
19.	Slender bone dysplasia group	20.	Dysplasias with multiple joint dislocations
21.	CDP group	22.	Neonatal osteosclerotic dysplasias
23.	Oseteopetrosis and related disorders	24.	Other sclerosing bone disorders
25.	Osteogenesis imperfect and decreased bone density group	26.	Abnormal mineralization group
27.	Lysosomal storage diseases with skeletal involvement (dysostosis multiplex group)	28.	Osteolysis group
29.	Disorganized development of skeletal components group	30.	Overgrowth syndromes with skeletal development
31.	Genetic inflammatory / rheumatoid-like osteoarthropathies	32.	Cleidocranial dysplasia and related disorders
33.	Craniosynostosis syndromes	34.	Dysostoses with predominant craniofacial involvement
35.	Dysostoses with predominant vertebral with or without costal involvement	36.	Patellar dysostoses
37.	Brachydactylies (without extraskeletal manifestations)	38.	Brachydactylies (with extraskeletal manifestations)
39.	Limb hypoplasia: reduction defects group	40.	Extrodactyly with and without other manifestations
41.	Polydactyly-syndactyly-triphalangism group	42.	Defects in joint formation and synostoses

CDP, Chondrodysplasia punctate; *FGFR3*, fibroblast growth factor receptor 3; *MED*, multiple epiphyseal dysplasia; *SE(M)D*, spondyloepi(meta)physeal dysplasias; *SMD*, spondylometaphyseal dysplasias; *TRPV4*, transient receptor potential cation channel subfamily V member 4.
Taken from Zankl A, Briggs M, Bateman JF. Skeletal dysplasias. In: Thakker RV, ed. *Genetics of Bone Biology and Skeletal Disease*. London, United Kingdom: Elsevier; 2018:469–480.

E—**E**piphyseal dysplasias: the epiphysis is at the end of tubular bone and is formed as a secondary site of ossification. Normal development of the epiphysis is required if the joint surface is to be normal.

M—**M**etaphyseal dysplasias: the metaphysis is the wider part of a tubular bone between the diaphysis and physis.

P—**P**hyseal dysplasias: the physis, or epiphyseal cartilage plate, separates the metaphysis from the epiphysis during growth. It is the primary site responsible for elongation of tubular bones.

D—**D**iaphyseal dysplasia: the diaphysis is the shaft of a long or tubular bone. It is composed of the spongiosa and cortex and is covered with periosteum.

These disorders can be further differentiated depending on whether the spine is involved: spondyloepiphyseal dysplasia (SED), spondylometaphyseal dysplasia, or spondyloepimetaphyseal dysplasia (Fig. 58.1).

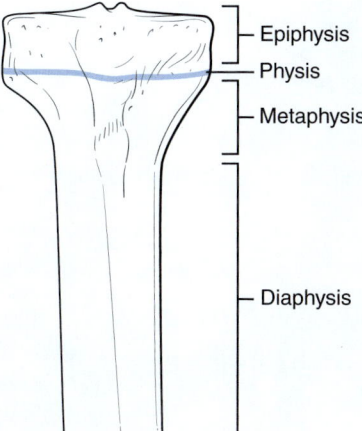

Fig. 58.1 Parts of long bone.

5. **What are the distinguishing features of the epiphyseal dysplasias?**

Epiphyseal dysplasia is characterized by abnormal ossification of the developing epiphysis. The resulting morphologic abnormalities of the ossification centers are used to differentiate the various subtypes within this category. The most important epiphyseal dysplasias from a rheumatologic standpoint are multiple epiphyseal dysplasia (MED) and SED.

6. **How does a patient with MED present clinically? How is MED treated?**

MED is primarily a group of autosomal dominant disorders (75% of cases) affecting 1 in 20,000 individuals. Identified gene abnormalities and associated proteins include COL9A1, COL9A2, COL9A3 (collagen 9 α-1, 2, and 3 chains), COMP (cartilage oligomeric matrix protein) and MATN3 (matrilin 3). An autosomal recessive variant (25% of cases) due to a mutation of the sulfate transporter gene (SLC26A2) has also been reported. Usually, the patient complains of symmetric joint pain in the hips, knees, wrists, and shoulders as a result of precocious osteoarthritis. Limitation in range of motion of affected joints is frequent. The spine is usually spared. Radiographs reveal irregular, flattened, small epiphyseal ossification centers during childhood and a deformed articular surface after physeal closure. The long bones of the legs and arms are most prominently affected. Adult stature is generally diminished and is proportionate to the severity of involvement. Early disabling degenerative arthritis is a common end result. Symptoms usually occur before adolescence but may not become apparent until early adulthood, especially in the autosomal recessive variant which causes less severe epiphyseal deformity. Treatment of patients with MED includes medications to help relieve symptoms and surgery to correct deformities in children and total joint replacement in adults.

7. **What other conditions can be confused with MED?**

Inflammatory arthritis: The pain and symmetry of involvement are sometimes mistaken for inflammatory arthritis. On closer evaluation, the absence of signs and symptoms of inflammation usually suffices to rule out this condition.

Hypothyroidism: Occult hypothyroidism can lead to developmental skeletal abnormalities that may closely resemble some of the hereditary epiphyseal dysplasias. Thyroid function should always be checked when a diagnosis of epiphyseal dysplasia is being considered.

Juvenile osteochondrosis: These disorders, including Legg–Calvé–Perthes disease, may have a radiographic appearance similar to epiphyseal dysplasia but are usually limited to a single joint.

8. **Describe the radiographic abnormalities typical for SED.**

The SEDs are a diverse group of disorders linked by the radiographic findings of marked **platyspondyly** (short flat vertebrae) in association with abnormalities of **epiphyseal ossification.** Severe abnormalities in the epiphyses of long bones also occur. Spinal and long bone

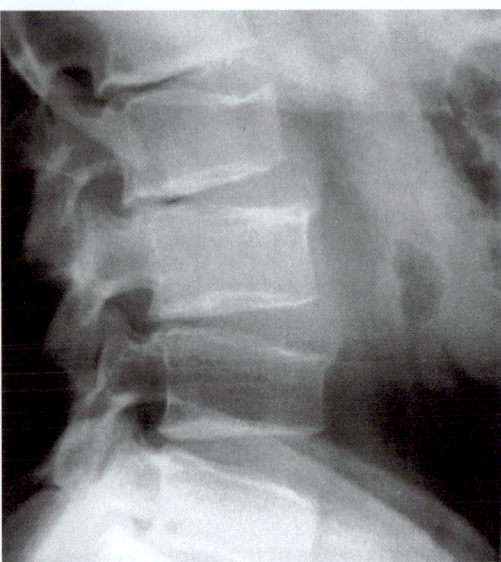

Fig. 58.2　Spondyloepiphyseal dysplasia.

abnormalities often result in dwarfism with severe osteoarthritis. Genetic studies have linked this to abnormalities in the collagen type 2 gene (*COL2A1*) (Fig. 58.2).

9. **SED tarda and SED tarda with progressive arthropathy can sometimes be confused with juvenile idiopathic arthritis (JIA). Why?**

   Both of these X-linked recessive disorders are accompanied by enlargement of the ends of the tubular bones in the hands, which may be mistaken for JIA on visual inspection. Radiographic evaluation inevitably leads to the correct diagnosis.

10. **What abnormality characterizes the metaphyseal dysplasias?**

    These dysplasias are characterized by a failure either to form or to absorb the spongiosa of developing bone. Important disorders from a rheumatologic standpoint within this category of dysplasias include the hypophosphatasias. Severe forms of hypophosphatasia have an autosomal recessive inheritance and occur in 1 in 100,000 live births. Milder forms that may present in adulthood are more common and have a variable inheritance pattern.

11. **What is the primary differential diagnosis in the hypophosphatasias?**

    The hypophosphatasias may look like **rickets** in children and **osteomalacia** in adults. Subtle radiographic findings may allow the distinction to be made, but the diagnosis of hypophosphatasia is ultimately based on the findings of an exceptionally low serum ALP in conjunction with high serum levels of inorganic pyrophosphate (PPi) and pyridoxal-5'-phosphate and high urine phosphorylethanolamine levels. Mutations of *ALPL* on chromosome 1, which codes for tissue-nonspecific ALP (TNSALP), are responsible for this disease. These mutations lead to low levels of tissue ALP leading to less cleavage of PPi. The accumulation of PPi inhibits hydroxyapatite crystal formation. It also leads to excessive calcium deposits in the form of chondrocalcinosis, nephrolithiasis, nephrocalcinosis, and calcified muscle and ligaments. Consideration of hypophosphatasia is warranted in any case of suspected rickets or osteomalacia, especially in patients with early loss of deciduous teeth. Many adult patients present with poorly healing metatarsal stress fractures. Asfotase alfa (Strensiq), TNSALP enzyme replacement therapy for young patients with severe hypophosphatasia, has redirected the prognosis of severe cases from palliative to a treatable, chronic condition. Adults with mild disease may be misdiagnosed with osteoporosis. Bisphosphonate therapy is contraindicated and will further weaken bone density and increase the risk of fractures, including atypical femoral fractures.

PEARL: Consider hypophosphatasia in any patient with poorly healing metatarsal stress fractures who has a low serum ALP level.

12. One of the most common skeletal dysplasias is considered a physeal dysplasia and leads to dwarfism. Name this syndrome.

Achondroplasia is one of the most common skeletal dysplasia, occurring in 1 in 25,000 live births. This physeal dysplasia is transmitted as an autosomal dominant trait, although spontaneous mutations are probably responsible for most cases (80%). Mutations have been identified in the fibroblast growth factor receptor 3 (*FGFR3*) gene. This mutated receptor is constitutively active leading to shortened bones. Achondroplasia is considered a disproportionate dwarfism with rhizomelic (shorter proximal compared with distal) short limbs, macrocephaly with prominent frontal bossing, and some midface hypoplasia. An exaggerated lumbar lordosis is usually seen as well as flexion contractures at the elbows and hips. Intelligence is normal. Mean adult height is approximately 52 inches in men and 49 inches in women. Rheumatologic complaints may stem from a narrowed spinal canal (cervical and lumbar) with symptoms of spinal stenosis or from ligamentous laxity of the knees, leading to complaints of pain and premature degenerative disease. Treatment is symptomatic.

13. Where is the abnormality of bone formation found in the diaphyseal dysplasias?

Diaphyseal dysplasias result from abnormal formation of endosteal or periosteal bone. These dysplasias can be subclassified as hyperplasias or hypoplasias. Osteogenesis imperfecta is considered a hypoplastic diaphyseal dysplasia (see Chapter 54: Heritable Connective Tissue Disease).

14. A 21-year-old man complains of lower leg pain and swelling that has been gradually increasing. An X-ray is obtained (Fig. 58.3). What is this disorder?

Melorheostosis, a nonhereditary idiopathic diaphyseal hyperplasia. Clinically, the patient complains of joint pain with onset usually in late childhood or early adulthood. Decreased range of motion, joint contracture or ankylosis, growth disturbances, foot deformities, and dystrophic

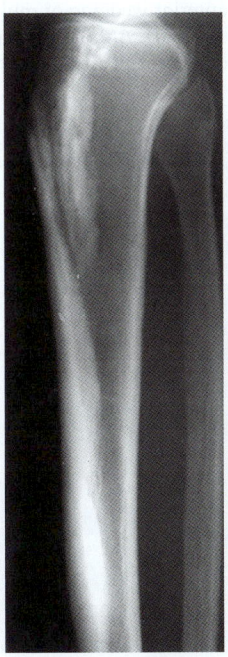

Fig. 58.3 Melorheostosis.

skin, muscle, and soft tissue changes overlying affected bone are other features of this unusual disorder. The x-ray is characteristic and reveals dense, wavy, periosteal bony excrescences, which have been described as resembling wax flowing down the side of a candle. The etiology is unknown.

15. **Another diaphyseal hyperplasia has radiographic and clinical features in common with hypertrophic osteoarthropathy, including clubbing of the digits, painful swollen joints, and periosteal bony apposition, but it is also associated with thickened, wrinkled elephant-like skin. Name this disorder.**

    Pachydermoperiostosis (Touraine–Solente–Gole syndrome). A literal translation of the term describes the major clinical manifestations of the disorder, which include digital clubbing, thickening of the skin of the face and folds in the scalp, excessive sweating of hands and feet, and periostitis. It can mimic acromegaly. It usually begins at puberty and progresses over the next 10 years. The genetic mutation responsible involves *HPGD* on chromosome 4, which encodes 15-hydroxyprostaglandin dehydrogenase and is responsible for prostaglandin degradation. The mutation leads to a lack of enzyme function resulting in persistently elevated prostaglandin E_2 levels. A similar syndrome has also been reported in patients with a deficiency of a solute carrier involved in prostaglandin transport caused by mutations in the *SLCO2A1* gene. Treatment is with nonsteroidal antiinflammatory drugs to block prostaglandin production.

16. **A 15-year-old boy complains of thoracic back pain with no clear history of trauma. The pain is worse with activity, improves with rest, and is not associated with significant morning stiffness. Physical exam is remarkable only for a hint of increased thoracic kyphosis with some lower thoracic tenderness to palpation in the midline and mild paravertebral muscle spasm. Workup reveals a normal erythrocyte sedimentation rate, serum chemistries, and complete blood count. An X-ray report lists that the findings are most consistent with Scheuermann's disease. What is that?**

    Vertebral osteochondritis, or Scheuermann's disease, is a developmental abnormality of ossification of the endplates of vertebrae seen most often in the thoracic spine but also seen in the thoracolumbar and lumbar regions. It occurs during adolescence and is symptomatic in up to 60% of those affected, although it may also be found by chance on plain spine or chest x-rays requested for other reasons. The x-ray shows anterior wedging of multiple vertebrae with Schmorl's nodes and irregular vertebral endplates (Fig. 58.4). Although the pathogenesis is uncertain, a hereditary weakening of the vertebral endplates present in affected patients is believed to allow disc material

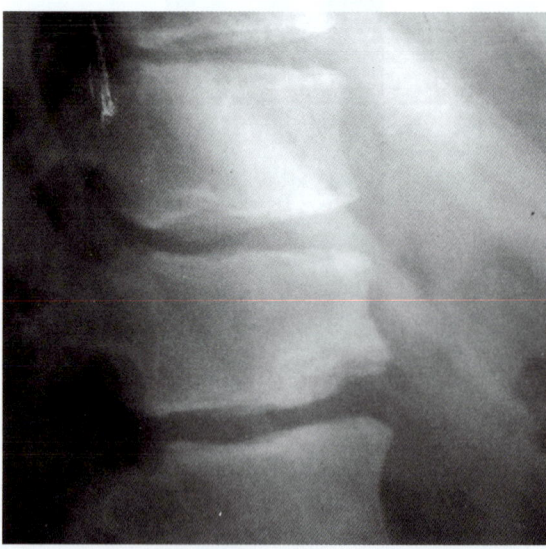

Fig. 58.4 A radiograph of the spine showing irregular vertebral endplates in a patient with Scheuermann's disease.

to encroach into the vertebral bodies. This then leads to abnormal growth and the x-ray changes described. Therapy is usually symptomatic and aimed at minimizing the tendency toward kyphosis. Occasionally, surgical intervention is required.

17. **A newborn girl has a reproducible "click" as you flex and abduct her right hip (Ortolani's sign). You suspect that the child may have congenital dislocation of the hip. How can you verify this suspicion? What do you tell the parents?**

Congenital hip dislocation or dysplasia is screened for shortly after birth using physical exam maneuvers, such as Ortolani's sign, and by inducing dislocation and reduction of an unstable hip (Barlow's sign). Plain films may not be easily interpretable in the first weeks of life, and modalities such as ultrasound, computed tomography, or magnetic resonance imaging generally offer better sensitivity. Congenital hip dysplasia has an excellent prognosis if recognized soon after birth. Treatment usually involves splinting the legs in abduction, thus allowing the shallow acetabulum to fully contain the femoral head. If the diagnosis is missed, however, later therapy is often much more involved and may require extensive orthopedic surgery. If left untreated, this condition leads to premature osteoarthritis and may require early total hip replacement (Fig. 58.5).

18. **An 18-year-old man presents with a history of multiple fractures and progressive joint pain. He was a healthy child until age 9, when he dislocated his left hip and his growth trajectory slowed. He developed additional joint pain with degenerative changes noted on imaging, eventually requiring bilateral hip replacements in his teens. Physical examination reveals short stature, scoliosis of the spine, shortened limbs, joint laxity, and corneal clouding. X-rays of the lumbar spine show hook-shaped vertebra. Laboratory testing demonstrates deficient activity of the N-acetylgalactosamine-6-sulfate sulfatase (GALNS) enzyme. Name this disorder.**

The patient has **mucopolysaccharidosis type IVA**, also known as Morquio syndrome. The mucopolysaccharidoses are a family of genetic metabolic disorders that affect lysosomal storage, causing abnormal storage of glycosaminoglycans that affect bones, connective tissues, and internal organs (see Chapter 55: Inborn Errors of Metabolism Affecting Connective Tissue). Mucopolysaccharidosis type IVA occurs when a deficiency in GALNS enzymatic activity impairs the degradation of heparan sulfate and chondroitin-6-sulfate, leading to their accumulation in cartilage, ligaments,

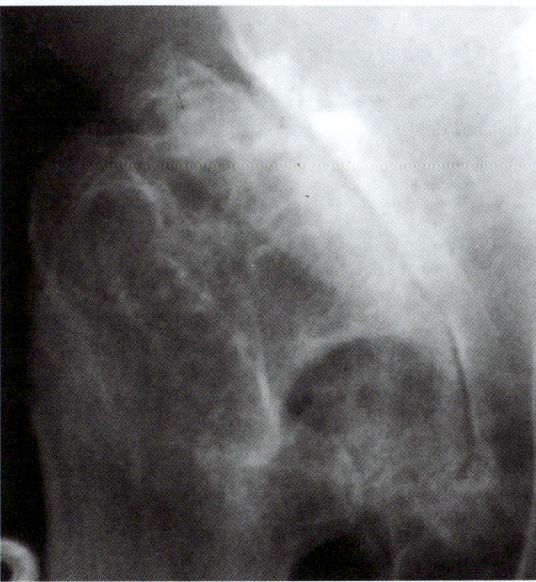

Fig. 58.5 A hip radiograph from an adult with congenital hip dysplasia that was not treated during childhood. Note severe degenerative changes, shallow acetabulum, and malformed femoral head.

cornea, and other extracellular matrices. Common clinical manifestations include joint sub-luxations (especially of the hips), early-onset degenerative arthritis, and short stature as well as clouded corneas, regurgitant or stenotic heart valves, and obstructive airway disease. Vertebral bodies adopt a hook shape at the anterior aspect. Manifestations compound over time with further accumulation of mucopolysaccharides, and the diagnosis is confirmed with reduced GALNS enzymatic activity. Treatment focuses on supportive care and enzyme replacement therapy with recent data suggesting benefit from hematopoietic stem cell therapy.

ACKNOWLEDGMENT

The author would like to thank Dr. Sterling West for his contribution to this chapter in the previous edition.

BIBLIOGRAPHY

Alanay Y, Rimoin DL. Osteochondrodysplasias. In: Rosen CJ, ed. *Primer on the Metabolic Bone Diseases and Disorders of Mineral Metabolism*. 8th ed. Washington, DC: American Society for Bone and Mineral Research; 2013:794–804.

Anthony S, Mark R, Shakun W, Masini M. Multiple epiphyseal dysplasia. *J Am Acad Ortho Surg*. 2015;23:164–172.

Castori M, Sinibaldi L, Mingarelli R, et al. Pachydermoperiostosis: an update. *Clin Genet*. 2005;68:477–486.

Cho SY, DK Jin. Guidelines for genetic skeletal dysplasias for pediatricians. *Ann Pediatr Endocrinol Metab*. 2015;20:187–191.

Handa A, Grigelioniene G, Nishimura G. Skeletal dysplasia families: a stepwise approach to diagnosis. *Radiographics*. 2023;43:e220067.

Kotwal A, Clarke BL. Melorheostosis: a rare sclerosing bone dysplasia. *Curr Osteoporosis Rep*. 2017;15:335–342.

Krakow D, Rimoin DL. The skeletal dysplasias. *Gen Med*. 2010;12:327–341.

Mortier GR, Cohn DH, Cormier-Daire V, et al. Nosology and classification of genetic skeletal disorders: 2019 revision. *Am J Med Genet A*. 2019;179:2393–2419.

Padash S, Obaid H, Henderson RDE, et al. A pictorial review of the radiographic skeletal findings in Morquio syndrome (mucopolysaccharidosis type IV). *Pediatr Radiol*. 2023;53:971–983.

Reis FS, Lazaretti-Castro M. Hypophosphatasia: from birth to adulthood. *Arch Endocrinol Metab*. 2023;67(5):e000626.

Smith R, Wordsworth P. *Clinical and Biochemical Disorders of the Skeleton*. 2nd ed. Oxford: Oxford University Press; 2016.

Supradeeptha C, Shandilya SM, Vikram Reddy K, Satyaprasad J. Pachydermoperiostosis—a case report of complete form and literature review. *J Clin Ortho Trauma*. 2014;5:27–32.

Tsirikos AI, Jain AK. Scheuermann's kyphosis: current controversies. *J Bone Joint Surgery Br*. 2011;93:857–864.

Zankl A, Briggs M, Bateman JF. Skeletal dysplasias. In: Thakker RV, ed. *Genetics of Bone Biology and Skeletal Disease*. London, United Kingdom: Elsevier; 2018:469–480.

FURTHER READING

http://www.isds.ch.
http://www.rarediseases.info.nih.gov/GARD.

Approach for the Patient With Neck and Low Back Pain

Kristina Barber, MD, Lindsay Burke, MD, and Jason Friedrich, MD

The lower back is at the crossroads where the psyche (mind) meets the soma (body).

— Voltaire (1694–1778)

KEY POINTS

1. Acute, nonspecific low back pain (LBP) is exceedingly common, generally self-limited, and typically only requires conservative care.
2. Screening for red flags will allow for identification of concerning etiologies of neck and back pain which require further workup and imaging.
3. Generally, imaging should only be ordered if red flags are identified or if it will change the plan of care.
4. Providers should identify patients at risk for progression from acute/subacute to chronic pain, provide education, and consider multimodal and multispecialty treatments for modifiable risk factors.

1. List the rheumatic disorders commonly involving the neck (Table 59.1).

TABLE 59.1 Common Rheumatic Disorders Involving the Neck

DISORDER	FEATURE
Rheumatoid arthritis (RA)	C1–C2 (atlantoaxial) subluxation due to pannus formation, cranial settling
Juvenile idiopathic arthritis	C2–C3 fusion, C1–C2 subluxation, fusion of apophyseal joints
Axial spondyloarthritis (axial SpA)	Ankylosis, C5–C6 fracture, C1–C2 subluxation
Diffuse idiopathic skeletal hyperostosis (DISH)	Anterior longitudinal ligament ossification, stiffness
Osteoarthritis	C5–C7 spondylosis
Polymyositis	Flexor muscle weakness
Polymyalgia rheumatica	Pain and stiffness
Fibromyalgia	Widespread myofascial pain

2. What are the most common causes of neck pain?

- Mechanical pain: This describes position and posture-related musculoskeletal pain. Assessment of posture and discussion of daily ergonomics can be helpful in identifying triggers and improving symptoms.
- Cervical disc herniation: The most common levels of cervical disc herniation are **C5-6 and C6-7**. Patients may present with neck pain in isolation or may report radicular symptoms. A neurologic exam to evaluate for weakness, sensation, or reflex changes can discern if true radiculopathy exists. Hyperreflexia with positive Hoffman sign and/or imbalance with tandem gait may suggest secondary cervical myelopathy.
- Cervical spondylosis: This diagnosis refers to degenerative changes in the cervical spine involving the anterior column (vertebral bodies, intervertebral discs) or posterior column (facet joints). There is poor correlation between radiographic findings and presence of symptoms.
- Whiplash Associated Disorder: This refers to neck pain resulting from traumatic rapid acceleration/deceleration or flexion/extension of the cervical spine. Often patients will describe this injury after a rear-end motor vehicle collision. This mechanism leads to muscular strain and

ligamentous disruption which is termed myofascial pain. Additionally, the cervical facet joint capsules may be sprained. Typically, cervical x-rays are unremarkable. Whiplash-associated disorder generally has a positive prognosis, but up to 50% of patients report ongoing pain, and 16% report resultant long-term functional disability. Severity of post-injury pain, co-morbid mood disorder, catastrophizing, fear-avoidance behaviors, and legal factors all predict prolonged symptomatology. Advanced imaging is typically not necessary unless patients have ongoing pain despite a robust course of at least six weeks of conservative care including physical therapy.

3. Describe a basic cervical spine examination.

Alignment and posture of the cervical spine should be assessed first. Common deviations include a head forward (anterocollis) and shoulder protracted posture or straightening of the expected cervical lordosis. Active range of motion is then tested including cervical flexion, extension, side-bend, and rotation. Note side-to-side differences and whether pain is elicited on the ipsilateral or contralateral side. The occipital protuberance, occipital condyles, midline cervical spine (spinous processes, interspinous ligaments), and cervical paraspinal as well as upper shoulder and periscapular musculature should be palpated. Muscular pain may reflect primary myofascial pain or be referred from underlying cervical spine pathology.

4. What are the special tests for the cervical spine?

If there is concern for cervical radiculopathy the following tests can be utilized.

- **Spurling Test:** The patient extends and rotates their head to the ipsilateral side then the provider applies an axial load to the top of the head. If this reproduces pain or sensory changes in a cervical dermatomal pattern, then it is positive. Sensitivity 50–95% and specificity 86–94%.
- **Shoulder Abduction Relief test (or Bakody sign):** This maneuver, when positive, leads to relief of pain with ipsilateral shoulder abduction and subsequent placement of the ipsilateral hand on the head. Sensitivity 45–55% and specificity 85%.
- **Upper limb tension test (ULTT):** While supine, the examiner abducts the patient's shoulder to 110 degrees, externally rotates the shoulder to 90 degrees, supinates the forearm, extends the wrist and fingers, and slowly extends at the elbow while the patient contralaterally flexes the neck. Reproduction of pain or symptoms into the ipsilateral arm is positive. The test is designed to put stress on the nerve by elongating it, analogous to the straight-leg raise in the lumber spine. Sensitivity 50% and specificity 86%.

5. How do you test strength and sensation as part of the cervical spine exam (Table 59.2)?

TABLE 59.2 Upper Extremity Sensorimotor Neurologic Exam

NERVE[a]	MOTOR ACTION[b]	MUSCLES INVOLVED[b]	SENSORY TESTING (LIGHT/SHARP TOUCH)
C4	Shoulder abduction	Deltoid	Over the acromioclavicular joint
C5	Shoulder abduction, elbow flexion	Deltoid, biceps, brachialis, brachioradialis	Lateral upper arm, extending distally to lateral antecubital fossa
C6	Elbow flexion, wrist extension	Biceps, wrist extensors	Dorsal thumb
C7	Elbow extension, wrist flexion, finger extension	Triceps, wrist flexors, finger extensors	Dorsal aspect of middle finger
C8	Finger flexion	Finger flexors	Dorsal aspect of the little finger
T1	Finger adduction & abduction	Palmar (finger adductors) & dorsal (finger abductors) interossei	Medial upper arm, extending distally to medial antecubital fossa

[a]The approximate distribution of cervical nerve impingement: C5 (5% of cases), C6 (35%), C7 (35%), C8 (25%), T1 (rare)
[b]Attributing specific motor actions and muscle involvement to a specific cervical level is often difficult, since innervation usually occurs by two or more nerve roots.

6. List the reflexes to evaluate as part of the cervical spine exam (Table 59.3).

TABLE 59.3 Upper Extremity Reflexes

REFLEX	NEUROLOGIC LEVEL	DESCRIPTION
Biceps	C5	Hyperreflexia indicates a central nervous system lesion. Hyporeflexia indicates a lesion from the cervical nerve roots distally.
Brachioradialis	C6	As above
Triceps	C7	As above
Hoffman's sign	Cervical spinal cord or brain	The provider stabilizes the patient's middle finger just proximal to the DIP, and then exerts a downward 'flick' to the distal finger/nail. A positive sign is characterized by flexion and adduction of the thumb and flexion of the index finger. Sign of hyperreflexia indicative of a CNS lesion in the cervical spinal cord or brain.
Clonus	Central nervous system	The provider rapidly dorsiflexes a patient's ankle and feels for plantarflexion beats. Indicative of a spinal cord or brain lesion.

7. Describe features of cervical myelopathy and cervical radiculopathy (Table 59.4).

TABLE 59.4 Differing Symptoms and Signs of Cervical Myelopathy and Radiculopathy

	CERVICAL MYELOPATHY	CERVICAL RADICULOPATHY
Description	Chronic compression of the cervical spinal cord	Compression of the cervical nerve root
Etiology	Degenerative secondary to uncovertebral or facet hypertrophy, degenerative disc disease, ligamentum flavum hypertrophy Cervical listhesis leading to central canal narrowing Acute cervical disc herniation causing central canal stenosis	Degenerative secondary to cervical degenerative disc disease with disc height loss, uncovertebral or facet arthropathy Cervical listhesis, especially with instability Acute disc herniation
Presenting Symptoms	Neck pain, hand and foot paresthesias, ataxia, fine motor/coordination deficits, bladder urgency or incontinence	Neck pain, cervical dermatomal arm or hand pain or sensory loss, upper extremity weakness
Physical Exam Findings	Hyperreflexia, positive Hoffman's sign, imbalance with tandem gait	Decreased cervical range of motion, specific cervical myotomal weakness, specific cervical dermatomal sensation change, focal hyporeflexia, positive Spurling, Bakody, or upper limb tension test

8. What categories should the differential diagnosis for low back pain (LBP) include?

- Mechanical: myofascial, posture-related, discogenic, facetogenic, sacroiliac joint, degenerative pain.
- Traumatic: fractures, facet joint capsule or ligamentous sprains.
- Neuropathic: lumbosacral radiculopathy, spinal stenosis with neurogenic claudication, conus medullaris and cauda equina syndrome.
- Inflammatory: axial SpA.
- Infiltrative: cancer, infectious (osteomyelitis, abscess, and discitis).
- Referred: intraabdominal pathology (e.g., abdominal aortic aneurysm, nephrolithiasis).
- Psychosocial: mood disorder related, somatization, secondary gain.
- Nociplastic: chronic pain syndrome, fibromyalgia.

9. Outline the suggestive signs, symptoms, and initial evaluation and management plans for the various etiologies of LBP (Table 59.5).

TABLE 59.5 Presenting Features & Recommended Evaluation for Common Causes of Low Back Pain

DIAGNOSIS	SPECIFIC FEATURE	SPECIFIC WORKUP OR TREATMENT
Myofascial Pain	Improves with myofascial techniques like massage, heat, and topical medications	De-medicalization, physical therapy, graded exercise, TENS unit
Malignancy	Nocturnal pain, constitutional symptoms (e.g. fever, weight loss)	Advanced imaging (lumbar spine MRI with and without contrast; possible lumbar CT), age-appropriate cancer screening, referral to oncology as appropriate
Infection	Fevers, chills, leukocytosis, nocturnal pain, history of intravenous drug use or spine intervention	CBC, CRP, lumbar spine MRI with and without contrast
Spondyloarthritis	Morning stiffness more than 60 minutes	CRP, HLA-B27 (limited sensitivity/specificity), lumbar spine and SI x-rays (consider MRI without contrast if x-ray is nonrevealing)
Compression fracture	Focal bony tenderness, history of osteopenia, osteoporosis	Lumbar x-ray, consider lumbar spine MRI without contrast if assessing for chronicity of compression fracture. DEXA scan to assess bone density.
Spondylosis	Morning stiffness less than 30 minutes	Lumbar x-ray, referral to physical therapy
Lumbar stenosis with neurogenic claudication	Leg heaviness or pain with ambulation or activity. Improvement with forward flexion (positive shopping cart sign) or sitting	Lumbar x-ray to assess for listhesis, lumbar spine MRI without contrast
Psychosocial	History of mood disorder, fear avoidance, catastrophizing	Validated screening tools include: • Patient health questionnaire (PHQ) 9 • Fear avoidance belief questionnaire (FABQ) • Pain catastrophizing scale (PCS) • Treat with graded exercise, education (on pain transmission), pain psychology techniques.

10. List the key elements from the history in a patient with LBP (Table 59.6).

TABLE 59.6 Key Historical Elements in Patients With Low Back Pain

O	Onset	When did the pain begin? Was there an inciting event or trauma?
L	Location	Where does the pain start? Does it radiate? What distribution?
D	Duration	How long has the pain been present?
C	Character	Aching, dull, stabbing, cramping, burning, tingling? Numeric rating scale (0-10/10)
A	Aggravating factors	What makes the pain worse?
R	Relieving factors	What makes the pain better?
T	Treatments to date	Medications, modalities, therapies, bracing.
S	Surgeries or interventions to date	Surgeries, injections, other procedures

11. What are the potential pain generators of mechanical LBP?

Mechanical pain can be categorized as anterior column, posterior column, sacroiliac joint related, myofascial, or multifactorial (mixed). Anterior column pain stems from structural changes to the intervertebral disc, vertebral end plate, or the vertebral body. Posterior column pain results from structural changes to the facet joints, pars interarticularis, or lamina. Patients with sacroiliac joint pain typically present with a chief complaint of low back and buttock pain. Lastly, the overlying soft tissues can also cause pain especially in response to asymmetric, atypical load or poor posture.

12. List the red flag signs and symptoms that may prompt further investigation in a patient presenting with LBP (Table 59.7).

TABLE 59.7 Potential Red Flag Features[a,b] in Patients Presenting With LBP	
PATIENT FACTORS	**SIGNS & SYMPTOMS**
Age greater than 50 years	Bowel or bladder incontinence
Immunosuppression	Saddle anesthesia (sensory loss)
History of malignancy	Fixed neurologic change (weakness, sensory deficit)
Chronic steroid use	Nocturnal pain (or pain unable to be relieved with rest or position changes)
History of trauma	Fevers and chills
History of intravenous drug use	Unexplained weight loss
	Morning stiffness greater than 60 minutes in a patient age less than 40 years
	Symptoms present greater than 6 weeks

[a]Most LBP is mechanical in nature and typically improves over 2–6 weeks. As such, the presence of red flag features may not be associated with worrisome pathology in the subacute setting (<3 months).
[b]Obtaining imaging studies and additional work-up in every patient with red flag features is controversial and may lead to costly evaluations for a common condition. As such, clinical judgement should be used on a case-by-case basis.

13. What is sciatica?

Sciatica is a colloquial, nonspecific term used to describe pain radiating from the back into the leg(s). Since this is a generalized term, a provider should clarify a patient's actual distribution of pain. Pain radiating into the buttock and legs is generally due to: a) referral from the lumbar disc, facet, or sacroiliac joint, or b) lumbar radiculopathy. A true sciatic nerve compression by the piriformis muscle (piriformis syndrome) occurs in <0.5% of cases.

14. What are the components of a basic lumbar spine exam?

Inspection: evaluate standing posture looking for scoliosis, anterior pelvic tilt, pelvic obliquity
Range of motion: assess lumbar flexion, extension, side bend, and rotation; note any pain
Palpation: assess for tenderness along the lumbar spinous processes or interspinous ligament,
    lumbar paraspinal musculature, and sacroiliac joints (posterior superior iliac spine)
Neurologic exam (see Tables 59.8 and 59.9)

15. Compare and contrast true lumbar radiculopathy with lumbar radicular-pattern pain. What tests can be used to assess each on physical exam?

When a patient presents with pain radiating into the leg, it is important to discern if it is true radiculopathy or radicular-pattern pain. True radiculopathy necessitates an objective neurologic deficit in the distribution of the nerve root affected (weakness, sensory alteration, or diminished reflex). When the neurologic exam is intact, the condition is called radicular-pattern pain or radiculitis. This may be secondary to chemical irritation or inflammation that generates pain in the distribution of the nerve root, but without mechanical compression causing axonal or myelin injury. Both conditions can lead to significant pain and positive neural tension signs on exam (See Table 59.10).

TABLE 59.8 Lower Extremity Sensorimotor Exam

NERVE[a]	MOTOR ACTION	MUSCLES INVOLVED	SENSORY TESTING (LIGHT TOUCH)
L2	Hip flexion	Rectus femoris, iliopsoas	Proximal medial thigh
L3	Knee extension	Vastus medialis, intermedius, vastus lateralis, sartorius, rectus femoris	Medial thigh just proximal to the medial joint line
L4	Foot dorsiflexion	Tibialis anterior, extensor digitorum longus	Medial malleolus
L5	Great toe extension	Extensor hallucis longus	Webspace between the great toe and second toe
S1	Foot plantarflexion	Gastrocnemius, soleus, tibialis posterior, plantaris	Posterolateral calcaneus

[a]The approximate distribution of lumbar nerve impingement: L1-3 (rare), L4 (5% of cases), L5 (67%), S1 (28%)

TABLE 59.9 Lower Extremity Reflexes

REFLEX	NEUROLOGIC LEVEL	DESCRIPTION
Patella	L3, L4	Hyperreflexia indicates a CNS lesion. Hyporeflexia indicates a lesion from the cervical nerve roots distally.
Medial Hamstring	L5	As above
Achilles	S1, S2	As above

TABLE 59.10 Lumbar Neural Tension Tests

TEST	NERVE ROOTS	DESCRIPTION	POSITIVE RESPONSE	SENSITIVITY	SPEC.
Slump	L4-S1	Patient seated with affected leg fully extended. They then flex their neck and slump forward.	Reproduction of pain, paresthesia in their typical distribution	84%	83%
Straight leg raise	L4-S1	Patient is supine. The examiner raises the ipsilateral leg to greater than 40 degrees and dorsiflexes the foot.	Reproduction of pain, paresthesia in their typical distribution	52%	89%
Crossed straight leg	L4-S1	Patient is supine. The examiner raises the contralateral leg to 40 degrees and dorsiflexes the foot.	Reproduction of pain, paresthesia in their typical distribution	28%	90%
Femoral nerve stretch	L1-3	Patient is prone. The examiner flexes the knee to 90 degrees then raises the thigh off the exam table.	Reproduction of pain, paresthesia in their typical distribution	40-100%	83%

16. **How are the sacroiliac joints assessed on exam?**

The sacroiliac joints are complex diarthrodial joints with overlying anterior and posterior ligamentous complexes. Most cases of sacroiliac joint pain are mechanical secondary to side-to-side imbalance with alteration in overlying ligamentous complex or intraarticular changes. Inflammatory changes secondary to rheumatic disease are less common. Imaging does not improve diagnostic yield unless an inflammatory etiology is in question. MRI showing symmetrical and bilateral T2 hyperintensity of the joints can be seen with axial SpA. The gold standard for diagnosing sacro-iliac joint pain is with intraarticular anesthetic injection; however, this is not typically necessary. Specific physical exam maneuvers to provoke the sacroiliac joints can be performed as described below. The diagnosis is supported if at least three tests reproduce the patient's typical back or buttock pain.

- Fortin finger test: Patient localizes pain (with their finger) to the sacroiliac joint (~1cm infero-medial to posterior superior iliac spine)
- Thigh thrust test: With the patient supine, the examiner flexes the ipsilateral knee and hip to 90 degrees. Then a downward or posteriorly directed force is applied through the knee and hip.
- Patrick test: With the patient supine, the examiner flexes the ipsilateral leg to 90 degrees at the hip and knee. The examiner then externally rotates the leg and places the heel onto the contra-lateral thigh (Fig. 4 position, with the leg flexed, abducted, and externally rotated [FABER]). Downward gentle pressure is applied on the ipsilateral knee while stabilizing the contralateral anterior iliac crest. Pain arising from the contralateral pelvis is suggestive of sacroiliac joint pain.
- Gaenslen test: The patient lays supine at the edge of the exam table and allows the ipsilateral leg to fall off the side of the table. The contralateral leg is then flexed into the chest. Ipsilateral back or buttock pain is positive (the maneuver can also elicit contralateral SI pain).
- Sacral thrust test: While the patient is prone, the examiner applies an anteriorly directed thrust over the sacrum.
- Compression test: While the patient is side-lying, the examiner applies a downward force over the iliac crest.
- Distraction test: While the patient is supine, the examiner applies posterolateral pressure over the bilateral anterior superior iliac spines.

The Schober test can assess lumbosacral range of motion in patients with suspected axial SpA. A description of this maneuver and additional exam measurements carried out in axial SpA can be found in Chapter 33: Axial Spondyloarthritis.

17. What are "Waddell's signs"?

If there is concern that a component of the patient's presentation of back pain is psychosomatic or secondary to malingering, specific exam findings called Waddell's signs can be utilized. To evalu-ate for nonorganic features, Waddell and colleagues reported eight distinguishing signs which are described below. Patients satisfying three or more of Waddell's signs may have a nonanatomic cause for their LBP.

- Superficial tenderness—Tenderness to light touch over a wide area of the lumbar skin.
- Nonanatomic tenderness—tenderness over a wide area which crosses over nonanatomic boundaries and is not localized to a specific structure
- Axial loading— report of LBP when applying an axial force on the top of the patient's head
- Simulated rotation—when the shoulders and pelvis are rotated in unison <30 degrees (e.g. acetabular rotation test) in either direction, the structures in the back are not stressed. If the patient reports pain with this maneuver, the test is considered positive.
- Distracted straight-leg raise—Reported pain during supine straight leg raise test, but no pain with seated leg extension while examiner distracts the patient.
- Regional sensory change—stocking-glove distribution of sensory change rather than following a dermatomal pattern.
- Regional weakness—"breakaway weakness" or cogwheeling with strength testing (with normal muscle strength), not explained on a neuroanatomical basis.
- Overreaction—disproportionate or exaggerated pain response (grimacing, tremor, verbalization) to a stimulus that is not reproduced when the same stimulus is given again at a later time.

18. What is lumbar spinal stenosis?

Lumbar spinal stenosis describes narrowing of the either the central canal, lateral recess, or neu-roforamen of the lumbar spine. Often the term is used to signify central canal narrowing alone. This typically occurs as a result of disc herniation or degenerative change, facet arthropathy, or ligamentum hypertrophy. Lumbar spondylolisthesis can also cause stenosis. Patients may develop spinal stenosis in the setting of ankylosing spondylitis, DISH, RA, or congenital malformations such as spina bifida. Patients with central lumbar stenosis can present with pain, paresthesia, or heaviness in the legs with ambulation that improves with forward flexion and sitting. This is called neurogenic claudication. Improvement in walking tolerance with leaning forward on a cart, or the ability to exert leg muscles comfortably in a seated position (e.g. bike), can help differentiate neurogenic claudication from vascular claudication.

19. What is cauda equina syndrome?

Cauda equina syndrome is a neurologic sequela secondary to compression of the central lumbosacral canal. Symptoms include bilateral lower extremity weakness, perineal sensory loss (saddle anesthesia), and bowel and bladder dysfunction or incontinence. This can happen acutely from a disc herniation or trauma. It can also result from progression of chronic degenerative changes. Less commonly, ankylosing spondylitis or malignancy can cause cauda equina syndrome. Patients with acute cauda equina syndrome require an emergent evaluation with MRI and a neurosurgical consultation for decompression.

20. Define spondylosis, spondylitis, spondylolysis, and spondylolisthesis.

- **Spondylosis** refers to degenerative changes in the spine including degenerative disc disease, vertebral endplate changes, and arthropathy of the facet joints. The C5 to C7 and L3 to L5 vertebral segments are most commonly affected.
- **Spondylitis** describes inflammatory mediated changes in the spine from rheumatic conditions (e.g. axial SpA). Vertebral enthesitis leading to syndesmophytes often occurs. Affected patients are typically younger than 45 years of age.
- **Spondylolysis** refers to a defect in the pars interarticularis (the bone connecting the superior and inferior articular processes of the vertebrae). Typically, the defect is at the L5 level and can be unilateral or bilateral. Pars defects can be congenital, traumatic, or the result of hyperextension leading to a stress fracture (often in the developing bone of a child). Many patients with spondylolysis are asymptomatic; however, they are at risk to develop a spondylolisthesis.
- **Spondylolisthesis** refers to the translation of one vertebral segment on another. Anterolisthesis is the forward translation of one vertebral segment in relation to the vertebral segment below, whereas retrolisthesis is the posterior displacement of a vertebral body relative to the one below. Spondylolisthesis is graded on a scale from I-IV and is classified as dynamic or stable using flexion and extension radiographs. Grades III & IV, and unstable spondylolistheses warrant surgical evaluation.

21. What are the indications for obtaining a lumbosacral spine radiograph in a patient with LBP?

Imaging studies are indicated if the patient presents with any of the aforementioned red flag findings, neurologic deficit, or is recalcitrant to initial treatment. For patients presenting with acute to subacute nonspecific LBP without any of those features, lumbar radiographs are unnecessary. Ordering unnecessary imaging studies increases healthcare costs and can lead to potentially unnecessary invasive treatments.

22. When is it appropriate to order advanced imaging in the workup of a patient with LBP?

Advanced imaging can be pursued in patients with red flag symptoms, when symptoms are refractory to conservative management (at least six weeks), when there is clinical suspicion for cancer, infection, potentially progressive neurological injury, or as a component of procedural planning. Lumbosacral MRI is the advanced imaging test of choice as it visualizes the soft tissue structures of the spine in detail. CT without contrast is helpful in evaluating lumbar spine hardware or bony changes. If an MRI is desired but the patient has a contraindication, CT myelogram can be ordered to visualize the spinal cord and nerve roots. Occasionally an MRI or CT of the sacroiliac joints is needed to diagnose early axial SpA. As always, imaging studies must be interpreted in conjunction with the clinical presentation as many "abnormal" findings are present in asymptomatic individuals.

23. When should electrodiagnostic evaluation be ordered for a patient with LBP?

Electrodiagnostic assessment includes nerve conduction studies (NCS) and electromyography (EMG). Electrodiagnostic evaluation is considered an extension of the physical exam and may be ordered when radiculopathy or peripheral neuropathy is suspected, and alternative diagnostic strategies are equivocal. Electrodiagnostic testing only evaluates for peripheral nerve injury and is not helpful in the assessment of central nervous system processes. If the severity of neural injury needs to be assessed or a provider needs to differentiate between lumbosacral radiculopathy and other peripheral nerve injury, electrodiagnostic assessment is useful. The test is most useful if performed at least six weeks after the onset of symptoms as this allows time for Wallerian degeneration to occur, which leads to more definitive findings.

24. When should surgery be advised for a patient with radicular symptoms due to a herniated disc?

Given that most patients presenting with acute disc herniation and radicular symptoms improve with conservative therapy, surgical referral is not uniformly needed. Patients should be referred for surgical evaluation if they have progressive weakness or nonimproving radiculopathy and have failed a trial of conservative therapy for at least six weeks. Patients with incapacitating pain or an increasing neurologic deficit may be considered for earlier referral. Surgical outcomes are more favorable for patients who experience radicular pain rather than isolated axial pain.

25. What diagnostic tests are used to evaluate for lumbar radiculopathy?

Clinical exam, including the neurological exam, is the most useful diagnostic method for detecting lumbar radiculopathy. Many asymptomatic patients will have pathology identified on imaging studies. For example, 25% to 50% of individuals without LBP will have a disc bulge or protrusion at one or more lumbar disc levels on advanced imaging. As such, when imaging is used, close clinical correlation is needed. Commonly used diagnostic tests are shown in Table 59.11 below. Diagnostic accuracy is lower for radicular-pattern pain without objective signs of radiculopathy on exam.

26. What exercises are beneficial for patients with mechanical LBP?

A multimodal approach to pain management is most efficacious for treatment of mechanical LBP. Exercises aimed at core strengthening and spinal stabilization provide additional support to protect the spine and prevent re-injury. Individualized exercise regimens under the guidance of physical therapy are recommended. In general, returning to gentle aerobic exercise as soon as possible after injury is encouraged. Proper lifting mechanics should be emphasized.

27. What are the clinical recommendations for a patient with acute mechanical LBP?

Reassurance should be provided to the patient that acute, mechanical back pain is typically self-limited and not dangerous. Patients should return to their desired activities and work as soon as possible. Graded return to sport or activity may be necessary starting with consistent low-impact aerobic exercise. Bed rest will lead to deconditioning and development of more stiffness and myofascial pain. Patients can be referred to physical therapy to develop a home exercise program focused on return to activity, range of motion, and core strengthening and stabilization. Recurrent episodes of LBP are common and secondary prevention strategies should be emphasized, such as ergonomics, exercise, weight and stress management, pain education, and coping strategies.

TABLE 59.11 Diagnostic Tests for Suspected Lumbar Radiculopathy

	SENSITIVITY (%)	SPECIFICITY (%)
Electromyography	70–90[a]	90
CT	92	88
Myelography	90	87
MRI	93	92

[a]Sensitivity drops to 40% if no evidence of motor weakness on physical exam.

28. What pharmacologic strategies can be used in the treatment of acute mechanical LBP?

Acetaminophen, nonsteroidal anti-inflammatory drugs (NSAIDs), skeletal muscle relaxants, and topical anesthetics may be beneficial in providing symptomatic relief. Opioid analgesics should generally be avoided due to potential for dependence, abuse, and risk for hyperalgesia (neurologically enhanced pain sensitivity).

29. What is the prognosis of patients with mechanical LBP?

Up to 84% of individuals will develop back pain during their life. Despite the number of people affected, the episode-specific prognosis is very good. Within one week of an acute episode, 50% of patients have symptomatic improvement; 75% will improve after one month; and 87% improve at three months. However, up to 70% of patients have recurrent pain within the year and secondary prevention strategies are needed in most patients to reduce recurrences.

30. How can a provider identify risk factors for progression from acute pain to chronic pain syndrome?

Most people will experience at least one episode of back pain during their lifetime typically with no specific identified structural etiology (nonspecific LBP). While most episodes are self-limited, improving by 3 months, 4–25% of patients develop chronic nonspecific LBP. Predictive factors for progression to chronic pain include female sex, higher BMI, prior episode of LBP, higher baseline pain score or reported functional deficit at presentation, occupation involving heavy lifting, work-related injury, history of psychiatric diagnosis (anxiety, PTSD, depression), catastrophizing, and fear avoidance behaviors. While many factors are not modifiable, earlier identification of patients at risk for progression is important as they may require more frequent follow up and a more functional restoration approach including addressing mood disorder, modifications or light duty at work, and additional reassurance that movement is safe and not causing structural damage even if it is painful. Validated screening tools are available for early identification of patients more likely to develop chronic back pain, such as the STarT Back Screening Tool.

ACKNOWLEDGMENT

The authors would like to thank Drs. Richard Meehan and Jason Kolfenbach for their contributions to this chapter in previous editions.

BIBLIOGRAPHY

Alagingi NK. Chronic neck pain and postural rehabilitation: a literature review. *J Bodyw Mov Ther*. 2022;32:201–206.

Kazeminasab S, Nejadghaderi SA, Amiri P, et al. Neck pain: global epidemiology, trends and risk factors. *BMC Musculoskelet Disord*. 2022;23(1):26.

Nieminen LK, Pyysalo LM, Kankaanpää MJ. Prognostic factors for pain chronicity in low back pain: a systematic review. *Pain Rep*. 2021;6(1):e919.

Ou-Yang DC, York PJ, Kleck CJ, et al. Diagnosis and management of sacroiliac joint dysfunction. *J Bone Joint Surg Am*. 2017;99(23):2027–2036.

Siempis T, Tsakiris C, Anastasia Z, et al. Radiological assessment and surgical management of cervical spine involvement in patients with rheumatoid arthritis. *Rheumatol Int*. 2023;43(2):195–208.

Walsh JA, Magrey M. Clinical manifestations and diagnosis of axial spondyloarthritis. *J Clin Rheumatol*. 2021;27(8):e547–e560.

Will JS, Bury DC, Miller JA. Mechanical low back pain. *Am Fam Phys*. 2018;98(7):421–428.

Zaina F, Côté P, Cancelliere C, et al. A systematic review of clinical practice guidelines for persons with non-specific low back pain with and without radiculopathy: identification of best evidence for rehabilitation to develop the WHO's package of interventions for rehabilitation. *Arch Phys Med Rehabil*. 2023;104(11):1913–1927.

CHAPTER 60

Fibromyalgia

Guiset Carvajal, MD

"I get irritated with people who don't believe fibromyalgia is real … Chronic pain is no joke. And it's every day waking up not knowing how you're going to feel."

—Stefani Germanotta (Lady Gaga), diagnosed with fibromyalgia

 KEY POINTS

1. Fibromyalgia (FM) is a chronic noninflammatory, nonautoimmune central afferent processing disorder leading to diffuse pain syndrome as well as other symptoms.
2. Similar to patients with other chronic pain disorders, functional magnetic resonance imaging (fMRI) shows expanded receptive fields for central pain perception and emotional modulation in patients with FM.
3. The most effective drugs for FM syndrome (FMS) are tricyclic agents (TCAs), dual reuptake inhibitors, and anticonvulsants that downregulate sensory processing.
4. Opioids and corticosteroids are not effective in the treatment of FM and should be avoided.
5. Patient education, physical activity/exercise, and cognitive behavioral therapy (CBT) are important pillars of therapy alongside adjunctive medical therapy.

CLINICAL FEATURES

1. What is FM?

FM is a chronic (>3 months), noninflammatory, nonautoimmune central afferent processing disorder leading to diffuse pain syndrome. The core symptoms typically include widespread pain, fatigue, stiffness, sleep disturbance, cognitive problems (fibrofog), and mood disorder (depression, anxiety, or both). Physical examination and pathologic investigation reveal no evidence of articular, osseous, or soft tissue inflammation. Patients may have tender points on exam both above and below the waist; these tender points are neither sufficiently sensitive nor specific for FM; therefore, formal diagnosis is no longer reliant on their presence. FM may occur alone (primary FM) or may be associated with several other disorders (secondary FM). In primary FM, laboratory results and radiographs are normal.

In 2016, a revision was made to the diagnostic criteria initially proposed in 2010. FM may now be diagnosed in adults when all of the following criteria are met:
- Widespread pain index (WPI) ≥7 and a symptom severity scale (SSS) score ≥5, or WPI = 4–6 and SSS score ≥9.
- Presence of *generalized pain*, located in ≥4 body regions (upper and lower bilateral extremities and axial region). Of note, jaw, chest and abdominal pain are not included in this definition of generalized pain.
- Symptoms present for at least 3 months.

Per the criteria, a diagnosis of FM is valid irrespective of the presence of concurrent diagnoses such as rheumatoid arthritis or systemic lupus erythematosus, which can also cause pain. Indeed, the prevalence of FM in these conditions is higher than in the general population. Similarly, a diagnosis of FM does not exclude the presence of other clinically important illnesses.

The **WPI** is the number of areas in which the patient has had pain over the last week. There are 19 areas (bilateral temporomandibular joint [TMJ, 2], shoulder [2], upper arm [2], lower arm [2], hip [2], upper leg [2], lower leg [2], neck [1], chest [1], abdomen [1], upper back [1], lower back [1]), therefore 19 is the maximum score. Tender points are no longer part of the criteria since patients (especially men) can have FM without characteristic tender points. The **SSS score** includes assessment of symptom severity in three items over the past week. The three items are (1) fatigue, (2) waking from sleep unrefreshed, and (3) cognitive disturbances. Each is subjectively scored for severity using a Likert score (0 = none, 1 = mild, 2 = moderate, and 3 = severe) and added together (score range 0–9). In addition, the patient should be assessed for the presence of the following symptoms over the prior 6 months: headaches, pain or cramping in the lower abdomen, and depression. The presence of each of these 3 items (score range 0–3) should be added to the score above for a final SSS score (range 0–12). The WPI and SSS scores can be summed to generate the **fibromyalgia severity (FS) scale** (also known as the polysymptomatic distress (PSD) scale).

2. What are tender points and trigger scores, and how are they different?

In normal individuals (and in patients with FM), there exist specific regions on the surface anatomy that are more sensitive to applied pressure than other sites. These areas are primarily at musculotendinous junctions and not at tendon insertion sites into bone. FM is a disorder of generalized pain amplification, and thus these regions may be exceedingly tender and are referred to as **tender points.** Historically, tender points were integral to the diagnosis of FM. The initial American College of Rheumatology criteria for diagnosis of FM (1990) included the presence of pain in at least 11 of 18 specific tender points upon palpation. This criterion was removed in later revisions (2010 and 2016) due to its limitations and the recognition of FM as a widespread pain syndrome. Clinicians may still choose to perform examination of classic tender points to elicit discomfort suggestive of abnormal pain processing. The amount of point pressure utilized to elicit tender points is 4 kg/cm2 (enough pressure to blanch your distal thumbnail).

In contrast to FM, regional myofascial pain syndrome is a localized form of pain characterized by the presence of a **trigger point.** Upon palpation of the trigger point, severe local tenderness and radiation of pain into characteristic regions are elicited. Though the discomfort of myofascial pain syndrome remains regional, it is usually more widespread than bursitis or tendinitis. Regional myofascial pain syndrome most commonly involves the unilateral lower back, neck, shoulder, or hip region.

3. List some other symptoms that commonly occur in patients with FM.

Fatigue (90%).
Nonrestorative sleep (75%).
Arthralgias/myalgias/stiffness (80%).
Mood disturbance (75%).
Cognitive dysfunction (20–30%).
Muscle spasms/paresthesias (20–30%).

4. List some other conditions that are felt to be central pain sensitivity syndromes that commonly coexist in patients with FM.

Tension/migraine headache (50–60%).
Irritable bowel syndrome (IBS, 40%).
Restless legs/periodic limb movement syndrome (15%).
Urinary frequency/urgency (including interstitial cystitis).
Primary dysmenorrhea/chronic pelvic pain/urethral syndrome.
TMJ disorders.
Hypersensitivity and multiple chemical sensitivity syndrome (odors, bright lights, loud noises, medications).

5. Discuss the sleep disorder associated with FM.

Sleep disorders are a prevalent and clinically significant aspect of FM. The relationship between sleep disturbance and FM is complex and bidirectional, indicating that poor sleep can exacerbate FM symptoms, and FM can in turn lead to sleep difficulties.

Non–rapid eye movement (REM) sleep progresses through four stages that can be identified by electroencephalography. Quiet wakefulness with closed eyes is characterized by alpha-waves (8–13 Hz), whereas alert wakefulness with eyes open and bright lights is characterized by beta-waves (14–25 Hz). Non-REM stage I sleep is a transition from wakefulness and is associated with predominantly theta-wave activity (4–7 Hz). As deeper sleep is reached, the frequency of brain waves slows further, so that by non-REM stage IV sleep, delta-waves (<4 Hz) account for >50% of brain wave activity. It is delta-wave, or non-REM stage IV sleep, that is responsible for restful and restorative sleep.

The sleep disturbance associated with FM, termed alpha-delta sleep, is characterized by disruption of delta-wave sleep by frequent alpha-wave intrusion, such that non-REM stage IV sleep is significantly reduced. This sleep pattern is not specific for FM and may be present during periods of emotional stress, in chronic painful conditions such as rheumatoid arthritis (RA) and osteoarthritis, in sleep apnea syndrome, and in some otherwise normal individuals. Alpha-delta sleep is clinically associated with nonrestorative sleep.

PEARL: An evaluation for sleep apnea should be considered in all patients with suspected FM, even in the absence of traditional risk factors such as obesity. Clinicians should inquire about snoring habits and nonrestorative sleep, measure neck circumference (increased risk noted at >17 inches in men and >16 inches in women) and perform an oral examination to assess if the tongue obstructs the view of the posterior pharynx. These assessments can aid in identifying sleep apnea, which may coexist with FM and exacerbate symptoms.

6. Who generally develops FM and at what age?

FM affects 3% to 6% of the adult population in the United States. Higher prevalence is reported in **females**, who represent 70% to 90% of those diagnosed. The condition typically manifests between **30 and 55 years of age**, although it can occur in individuals ranging from children to the elderly. FM incidence increases following trauma, infections, and among individuals with inflammatory arthritis (see Question 8).

PEARL: New-onset FM-like symptoms in a patient older than 55 to 60 years may suggest an underlying etiology such as infection, neoplasia, or arthritis, rather than primary FM.

7. What variables contribute to a patient's predisposition to developing FM?

The etiology of FM is unknown. However, several variables may contribute to a patient's predisposition to developing FM as well as the severity of the symptoms:
- **Biologic variables**
  Inheritance: genetic polymorphisms have been reported in the COMT enzyme, serotonin transporter and receptor, and the dopamine, β2-adrenergic, glutamate and cannabinoid receptor genes.
  Female sex: young and middle-aged females are most at risk.
  Sleep architecture abnormalities.
  Neuroendocrine response to stress: attenuated corticotropin-releasing hormone and insulin-like growth factor-1 (somatomedin C) response.
  Autonomic dysregulation: postural orthostasis and tachycardia syndrome.
- **Environmental and sociocultural variables**
  Early life developmental experiences: sexual or physical abuse in childhood.
  Family variables: spousal and family support systems.
  Work variables: job satisfaction.
  Sedentary lifestyle and obesity.
- **Psychologic variables**
  Personality traits: perfectionist or self-sacrificing personalities are common.
  Catastrophizing and negative beliefs: belief that pain cannot be controlled.
  Hypervigilance and preoccupation with pain (which may interfere with therapy).
  Low self-efficacy and defective coping mechanisms.
  Depression, anxiety, and post-traumatic stress disorder (PTSD) are often comorbid with FM, suggesting a bidirectional relationship.

8. What are the recognized triggers for FM?

Psychological stress and trauma: chronic psychological stress and traumatic events (including early life trauma such as sexual or physical abuse) and catastrophic events leading to posttraumatic stress disorder (PTSD).

Acute trauma, especially involving the neck and upper body (e.g. cervical whiplash).
Infections: Epstein–Barr virus, parvovirus, Lyme, hepatitis C.
Sleep apnea.
Coexisting rheumatic disease: secondary FM prevalence in RA, SLE, and psoriatic arthritis
~20%; prevalence in ankylosing spondylitis (AS) ~10–12%.
Only a minority of patients experiencing one of these triggers develop a widespread pain
syndrome, suggesting a biochemical predisposition.

9. What other conditions should be considered in a patient presenting with FM-like symptoms?

- Rheumatologic: RA, SLE, systemic sclerosis, Sjogren disease, polymyositis, polymyalgia rheumatica, spondyloarthritis.
- Endocrine and nutritional disorders: hypothyroidism, adrenal insufficiency, hyperparathyroidism, osteomalacia, vitamin D deficiency, iron deficiency anemia.
- Myopathy: metabolic, statin-induced, myotonic dystrophy.
- Gastrointestinal: celiac, hemochromatosis, inflammatory bowel disease.
- Infections: subacute bacterial endocarditis, Lyme disease, hepatitis C, human immunodeficiency virus, parvovirus, brucellosis.
- Neurologic: multiple sclerosis, myasthenia, peripheral neuropathy, small fiber neuropathy.
- Malignancy: certain cancers may rarely present with widespread pain and fatigue.
- Sleep disorders: sleep apnea and restless legs syndrome.
- Psychiatric: major depression, substance abuse, eating disorders, somatoform disorders (see Question 10)
- Others: Chiari malformation, Fabry disease, chronic fatigue syndrome (also known as myalgic encephalomyelitis, or systemic exertion intolerance syndrome).

10. Which psychological disorders are sometimes confused with FM? Why?

Functional psychiatric disorders, such as somatoform disorders, often result in symptoms
identical to those of FM. The term functional suggests that the syndrome has no organic basis
and is due to purely psychologic factors. It is conceivable that in some patients with FM, the
condition originates as a functional disorder and subsequently the objective clinical, sleep, and
neurotransmitter abnormalities become manifest as a result of neuro-psycho-immuno-endocrine
interrelationships. Thus, while a functional psychiatric disorder could in theory precipitate FM in
some patients, *FM itself is not a functional disorder in that organic pathophysiologic mechanisms have
been identified as the etiology of symptoms.*

Organic psychiatric disorders, notably major depressive disorder (MDD) and anxiety
disorder, coexist in up to 75% of patients with FM. Furthermore, many patients diagnosed with
MDD experience symptoms of sleep disturbance, fatigue, and musculoskeletal pain. Given these
overlapping features, it can be difficult (if not impossible) for a clinician to distinguish between
FM and MDD at the initial encounter, and in roughly three-fourths of patients with FM, both
conditions will be present.

Finally, the **anxiety** and **mild depression** often present in FM may be a psychologic response
to concerns regarding financial and personal independence in the setting of chronic pain and disability. This association may be present in any chronic pain or debilitating syndrome.

11. Outline an evaluation of a patient with suspected FM?

- **History:** pain severity (typically described as deep and aching) and location; timing of symptom onset; fatigue severity; sleep disturbances, snoring and other symptoms of sleep apnea; mood disturbances, cognitive dysfunction; paresthesias, hypersensitivity (odors, bright lights, loud noises), other central sensitivity syndromes (see Question 4), and triggers (see Question 8). Family history of central sensitivity syndromes: first-degree relatives are eight times more likely to have FM.
- **Physical examination:** evaluation for tender points and allodynia; careful examination of the joints and sites of enthesis to identify primary inflammatory conditions; muscle strength testing and neurologic exam. Patients may also exhibit signs of fatigue, discomfort, and pain behavior during examination.

- **Laboratory examination:** complete blood count, complete metabolic panel, C-reactive protein, creatine phosphokinase, thyroid-stimulating hormone, 25-hydroxy vitamin D (to identify non-FM contributors to symptomatology). Rheumatoid factor or antinuclear antibody testing is unnecessary unless there is objective joint swelling or laboratory abnormalities suggesting inflammation.

12. How can the pain of FM be distinguished from the pain of widespread arthritis? Why is this important?

Patients with FM generally have diffuse deep aching pain that may be perceived to originate within joints, muscles, or both; thus, it may be confused with a diffuse arthritis syndrome such as RA or spondyloarthritis. Pain involving the axial skeleton is nearly universally present in FM, with patients experiencing lower back, cervical spine, and/or thoracic spine pain. Patients with FM also commonly experience bilateral pain in the upper and lower extremities. True arthritis can be excluded by the physical examination. The joint exam in primary FM reveals **absence** of effusion, synovial proliferation, deformity, and warmth. In addition, the presence of tenderness on exam consistently outside of anatomic joint locations is helpful in distinguishing this disorder from a diffuse arthritis syndrome.

FM may occur alone (primary FM) or may coexist with numerous other medical syndromes, including rheumatic disease (20% of patients with RA and SLE can have secondary FM). Therefore, the presence of an arthritis syndrome does not exclude the presence of coexistent FM, and vice versa. In these cases, the diagnosis of superimposed FM may be considered if subjective pain and constitutional symptoms exceed that expected for the degree of objective arthritis as determined by physical examination, radiographs, and laboratory tests. The presence of diffuse tender points may also suggest the diagnosis of coexistent FM.

The importance of recognizing the existence of secondary FM in patients with an underlying inflammatory arthritis is two-fold: a) to **avoid** unnecessary escalation of immunosuppressive therapy, and b) to appropriately address the primary symptom driver (counseling and therapeutic intervention for FM). The evaluation of patients with RA or SLE who have secondary FM may be challenging, as these patients may have tenderness with joint palpation due to central sensitization and generalized pain magnification rather than active inflammatory disease. This may mislead the physician, prompting inappropriate escalation in therapy. Therefore, in patients with an inflammatory arthritis who have secondary FM, the presence of swollen joints, limitation of range of motion, and abnormal inflammatory markers may be more important than the presence of tender joints on exam. Similarly, evidence has shown that several disease activity measurements can be adversely influenced by conditions such as FM, osteoarthritis, and depression and should be interpreted with caution in these settings.

PATHOPHYSIOLOGY

13. Describe the ascending pain pathways. Discuss the concept of peripheral and central sensitization in chronic pain syndromes.

Sensory fibers (nociceptor afferents) that transmit pain sensations innervate all the body tissues. There are two types of sensory fibers—myelinated **A-delta (δ)** and unmyelinated **C fibers.** These fibers have free nerve endings containing nociceptors that respond to noxious stimuli. There are specific nociceptors for mechanical, thermal, and chemical stimuli. Another receptor **(polymodal receptor)** responds to more than one stimulus and is only found on C fibers. Aδ fibers are rapidly conducting and respond mostly to mechanical and thermal stimuli. C fiber afferents conduct more slowly and produce perceptions of dull, aching, or burning pain.

These nociceptor afferents (first-order neurons) enter the spinal cord via dorsal roots and terminate in the dorsal horn of the spinal cord. These afferents release excitatory neurotransmitters that activate second-order neurons. The Aδ sensory neurons mainly release glutamate that binds to the N-methyl-D-aspartate (NMDA) receptor on second-order neurons that cross the cord and ascend in the neospinothalamic (lateral spinothalamic) tract and terminate in the ventroposterior basal nuclei of the thalamus. From there, the neural input is relayed to the somatosensory cortex which is important for sensory discrimination, location, and anticipation of the pain. The C fiber sensory neurons release substance P and other neurotransmitters that stimulate second-order

ASCENDING PAIN PATHWAYS   DESCENDING ANALGESIC PATHWAY

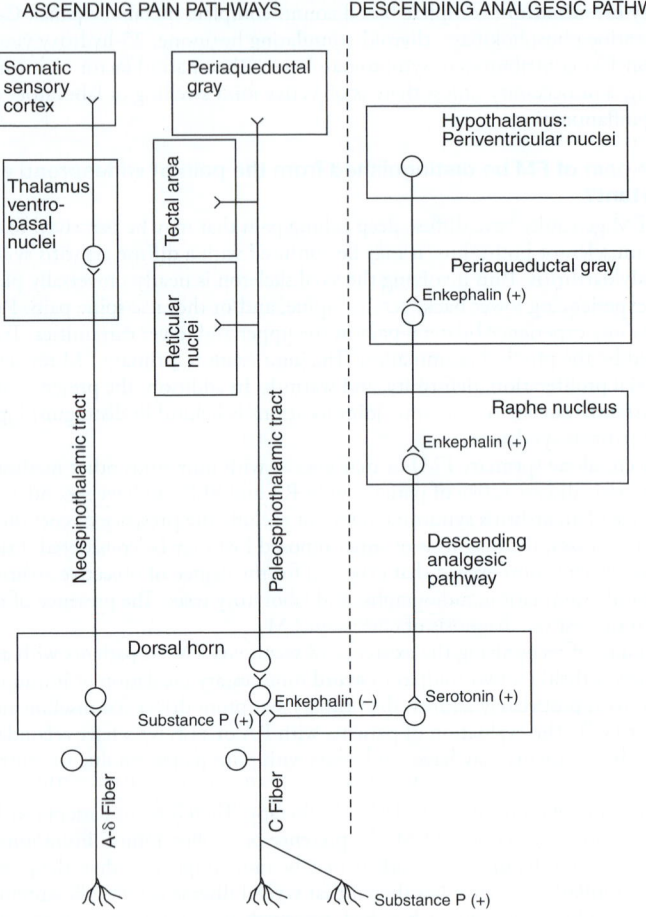

Fig. 60.1 Pain pathways.

neurons in the dorsal horn of the spinal cord. Also located in this area are the wide dynamic range (WDR) neurons that are stimulated by both noxious and non-noxious stimuli transmitted from the periphery by C fibers with polymodal nociceptors. The second-order neurons including the WDR neurons ascend in the paleospinothalamic tracts that terminate in the thalamus (anterior spinothalamic tract), periaqueductal gray (PAG) and reticular formation/nuclei (spinoreticular tract), and the medullary and tectal areas (spinotectal tract; Fig. 60.1).

From the thalamus, PAG, and other gray matter areas, third-order neurons transmit to other areas of the brain and spinal cord. Spinothalamic projections facilitate nociceptive input to the insular cortex, which has interconnections with the amygdala, prefrontal cortex, and anterior cingulate cortex. These regions form a network involved in emotional, cognitive, and autonomic responses to pain. In addition, there are interconnections with the hypothalamus that are involved in stress and autonomic responses. Finally, stimulation of the PAG, hypothalamus, and other areas is important in activation of the **descending analgesia pathway.**

The concept of peripheral and central sensitization is important for an understanding of widespread chronic pain conditions such as FM. With continuous and prolonged noxious stimulation (e.g., whiplash injury), peripheral polymodal C fibers and nearby silent nociceptive neurons that were previously unresponsive to stimulation now become responsive. The nociceptors begin to initiate signals spontaneously so that non-noxious stimuli are now perceived as noxious due to lowered pain threshold **(peripheral sensitization)**. The result of peripheral sensitization causes a greater and more persistent barrage of nerve impulses to the dorsal root of the spinal cord. Release of substance P by C fibers sensitizes second-order neurons, including WDR neurons, to neurotransmitters, such as glutamate. The enhanced and persistent glutamate effect on second-order neurons can result in physiologic changes in the nerves so they become hyperexcitable. This is called **windup.** These hyperexcitable second-order neurons transmit excessively to the brain areas described earlier, resulting in expanded receptive fields, increased interconnectivity, and increased blood flow to the stimulated areas. The ability to expand the receptive field is called **neuroplasticity** and occurs more easily in younger brains, which may explain why painful events early in life are particularly likely to trigger FM. Due to these physiologic changes, **central sensitization** occurs so that the individual feels pain at a lower threshold and with increased intensity.

14. **What abnormalities in the central nervous system (CNS) have been implicated in FM?**

Most investigators believe that the pathophysiology of FM is due to central sensitization within the CNS, manifesting as amplified pain perception. Thus, physical stresses to the musculoskeletal system that in the normal individual are perceived as nontender touch, position sense and nontender temperature sensation are perceived as pain in the patient with FM. It appears that the pain threshold is lower in patients with FM. The underlying abnormalities within the CNS leading to amplified pain perception are not completely understood, but a number of specific abnormalities have been observed in the afferent pain processing areas of the CNS in some patients with FM:
   - Increased excitability of dorsal horn nuclei due to abnormal **windup:** increased levels of substance P, nerve growth factor, glutamate, and aspartate measured in cerebrospinal fluid (CSF) of patients with FM
   - Expanded receptive fields for central pain perception **(central sensitization):** fMRI shows expanded fields in the insula, anterior cingulate cortex, and somatosensory cortex.
   - Abnormalities within the descending analgesia system: **decreased** levels of pain **inhibitory neurotransmitters** (antinociceptive) including norepinephrine, serotonin, and dopamine in the CSF of patients with FM
   - Suppression of normal activity of dopamine-releasing neurons in limbic system.
   Note: the levels of opioids are increased in the CSF of patients with FM; this may explain why narcotics have not proven to be effective in controlling the widespread pain typical of FM.

15. **Do FM patients have any abnormalities on brain imaging to support a central mechanism for their amplified pain perception?**

Brain MRIs are normal in FM patients. However, functional imaging studies using single-photon emission computed tomography (SPECT) scans and fMRI have shown decreased regional cerebral blood flow to the thalamus and caudate nucleus in FM patients compared with healthy individuals. The caudate nucleus and thalamus signal noxious stimuli, and decreased blood flow to these areas has been demonstrated in other chronic pain disorders. One explanation for these findings is that the widespread pain in FM activates inhibitory mechanisms in an attempt to reduce the evoked activity in the thalamus and decrease pain processing. With reduced activity, the thalamus needs less blood flow. An alternative explanation is that it takes less stimulation of the thalamus to induce pain in patients with FM, or that patients with FM have decreased gray matter density in the thalamus. The reduced blood flow to the caudate may indicate an abnormal dopaminergic system, which is important in pain modulation, pleasure perception, and motivational responses.

fMRI has also shown increased blood flow, connectivity, and activity in the insula, anterior cingulate cortex, and primary and secondary somatosensory cortices in response to painful stimuli. These are all areas that are involved with pain perception and emotional modulation from any cause of chronic pain. These findings on fMRI support a physiologic basis causing an FM patient's increased perception of pain.

16. **Discuss the descending analgesia pathway and its potential role in the pathophysiology of FM.**

The descending analgesia system (also called the descending noxious inhibitory control [DNIC] pathway) is a physiologic mechanism by which the transmission of pain is inhibited at the dorsal horn and other locations within the CNS (Fig. 60.1). Projections from the origin of this pathway within the hypothalamus and PAG, utilizing enkephalin as a neurotransmitter, reach the raphe magnus nucleus within the pons and medulla. The raphe nucleus sends projections into the dorsal horn, utilizing serotonin as a neurotransmitter, where they stimulate interneurons whose neurotransmitter is again enkephalin. These axons innervate the presynaptic region of incoming pain fibers, leading to the presynaptic inhibition of transmission of painful sensation to second-order pain fibers, most likely through the inhibition of calcium channels. Another part of the DNIC pathways is the locus coeruleus located in the pons. Upon stimulation by ascending pain fibers, the locus coeruleus is activated and sends projections utilizing norepinephrine as a neurotransmitter to the cortex, brainstem, and spinal cord. This results in increased alertness and sympathetic activity and decreased pain sensation and parasympathetic activity.

The implication of the descending analgesia system in the pathophysiology of FM has been suggested by studies that have demonstrated **decreased serotonin** or serotonin availability within the CNS. Additionally, metabolites of **norepinephrine and dopamine are decreased** in the CSF of patients with FM. This is important because there are norepinephrine-mediated pain inhibitory pathways that descend to the spinal cord and dopamine-mediated pain inhibitory pathways in the CNS that may be abnormal in FM patients.

APPROACH TO TREATMENT

17. List the major components of therapy for FM.

- Patient education and support.
- Nonpharmacologic therapies: physical therapy, CBT, occupational therapy.
- Lifestyle modification: regular exercise, stress management, sleep hygiene.
- Pharmacologic therapies: analgesics, antidepressants, anticonvulsants.
- Treatment of associated conditions: mood disorders, sleep disturbance, IBS, migraines, etc.

A multidisciplinary approach to the treatment of this disorder that incorporates patient education, emphasizes patient self-management techniques, and establishes incremental goals for functionality and relief of symptoms can achieve meaningful results.

18. What key principles of chronic disease management should clinicians follow to optimize patient outcomes in FM?

1. **Team-based care is necessary for meaningful improvement.**

   Utilize a multidisciplinary team as well as local resources like patient support groups, warm water exercise facilities and educational programs. Incorporate specialists from other fields to treat comorbid conditions such as psychiatric disease, IBS, and migraines. Online resources and additional reading materials may be helpful to facilitate self-care. Some studies have shown efficacy of online CBT, which may improve access to this treatment modality.

2. **Disease management should be viewed as a marathon, not a sprint**.

   Several symptoms may be present simultaneously at the initial (or subsequent) visit. Focus should be placed on one or two of the most pressing symptoms or functional impairments. With medical therapies and prescriptions for physical activity, "start low and go slow" (many patients with FM experience medication sensitivity/intolerance). For some patients, the goal of pain relief can become all-encompassing and can hinder efforts to address functional impairments (e.g., inability to engage in physical activity due to severe pain). Addressing analgesia in such patients is important but should be coupled with education and CBT focused on pain tolerance and advancement of physical activity in the setting of pain.

3. **The patient has important responsibilities in disease management**.

   The role of the patient should be clearly outlined through specific expectations regarding activity, sleep hygiene, and self-management. Consider writing recommendations as prescriptions to emphasize their importance in relation to pharmacologic therapy.

4. **The management of FM can be a cyclical process**.

   Ongoing therapy frequently requires repeated efforts on patient education as well as continued discussion on evolving patient goals and management of expectations.

5. **It is important to recognize that symptom relief does not reside inside a pill bottle**. Evidence suggests that nonpharmacologic therapies offer a higher degree of impact than medication therapy, with data on **physical activity and exercise** being the most robust. Medicine is a very useful tool in the treatment of FM, but represents only one facet of therapy and does not supplant the need for a multimodal approach to treatment. Emphasizing this fact with patients may help establish realistic expectations for drug therapy, reduce frustration, and increase participation in nonpharmacologic management.

6. **No single therapy is completely effective for FM, and treatment approaches differ from patient to patient** depending on the predominant symptom.

19. List important points regarding the disease process that should be emphasized in patient education programs.

1. The Legitimacy of FM: Emphasize that FM is a well-recognized medical condition, and address misconceptions that have unfortunately resulted in many patients' chronic symptoms being labeled as purely psychologic in nature.

2. Pathophysiology and Disease Comorbidities: Educate patients on FM's underlying mechanisms and associated conditions. This can reassure patients of a unifying diagnosis and provide insight in to subsequent strategies for symptom control.

3. Primary FM is neither life- nor organ-threatening: Clarify that FM's symptoms, while significant, are not indicative of life-threatening conditions like cancer or severe arthritis (unless FM is secondary to one of these disorders).

4. Importance of Self-Management: Highlight the importance of patient-led management strategies including exercise, sleep hygiene, engaging in CBT, and seeking support networks. Emphasize goal-setting and self-monitoring to enhance control over the disease.

5. Chronic Nature of FM: FM is a chronic illness. Similar to other chronic medical conditions such as heart disease, it can be managed through lifestyle modification and medicine, but not cured.

6. Set Realistic Treatment Goals: Encourage realistic expectations for treatment, focusing on improved functionality and symptom relief rather than complete eradication of symptoms.

Websites providing opportunities for patient education and online CBT are listed at the end of this chapter.

20. What is the goal of physical activity programs in FM patients?

Exercise improves muscle conditioning, which may lead to less muscle microtrauma and interrupt the positive feedback loop. Aerobic exercise can enhance mental health, improve cognitive function, prevent physical deconditioning, improve restorative sleep, and increase endogenous endorphins within the CNS. Because patients with FM often experience severe postexercise pain, the intensity of exercise should initially be low and gradually increased as tolerated. Initial attempts in some patients may only include gentle stretching and limited daily walking. Exercise should be nonimpact, such as swimming, water aerobics, walking with proper footwear, or bicycling. Some patients find group exercise programs including Tai Chi and yoga to be beneficial, and evidence in the literature supports their use. Physical therapy consultation may be helpful in designing the optimal exercise program for a particular patient. Ultimately, the primary goal of activity programs is to improve overall health and quality of life.

21. What medications are Food and Drug Administration (FDA) approved for treatment of FM? How do you choose which one to use?

Three medications are FDA approved for treatment of FM:

- **Dual reuptake inhibitors (serotonin-norepinephrine reuptake inhibitors [SNRI]):** increase serotonin and norepinephrine at synapses in the descending analgesia pathways.
  Duloxetine (Cymbalta): start 20 to 30 mg in the morning with food. Titrate monthly up to 60 mg/day (evidence is less clear on higher doses).
  Milnacipran (Savella): start 12.5 mg in the morning with food. Increase by 12.5 mg every 3 to 7 days to effect. Typical dose: 50 mg twice a day (BID; doses of 100 mg BID have been described).
- **Anticonvulsant (α2-δ ligands):** bind to ligand on voltage-gated calcium channels letting less calcium in, which decreases the release of excitatory neurotransmitters (glutamate, substance P).

Pregabalin (Lyrica): start 50 mg with food before bed. After 1 week, increase to 50 mg BID and titrate dose to effect. Typical dose: 75 to 150 mg BID (max dose 225 mg BID).

One of these three may be more beneficial than the others depending on the associated FM-related symptoms:

- Duloxetine: consider in FM patients with depressed mood and fatigue or osteoarthritis of the back or knees.
- Milnacipran: consider in FM patients with cognitive dysfunction (fibrofog) and fatigue.
- Pregabalin: consider in FM patients with profound sleep disturbance and/or neuropathic pain symptoms.

22. What other medications have shown effectiveness in therapy for FM?

Patients often cannot afford or insurance may deny the use of FDA-approved medications to treat FM. Several other medications can be used.

1. **SNRI: Venlaxafine** (Effexor) is an SNRI shown to be beneficial in FM. It could be used in someone who cannot afford duloxetine or milnacipran which are also SNRIs. Venlaxafine is often started at 37.5 mg in the morning with food and increased weekly to effect or max dose of 375 mg daily (typical dosing: 75–150 mg BID). There is an extended release form that can be used once a day starting at 37.5 mg and titrated weekly to effect or max dose of 225 mg daily.

2. **TCAs:** Low-dose TCAs administered before bedtime have been objectively demonstrated to improve the sleep disturbance, pain, and tender points in a proportion of patients with FM. An example of such a regimen is the administration of **amitriptyline** at a dosage of 10 to 25 mg 1 to 3 hours prior to bedtime. This dose may be increased by 10 to 25 mg increments at 2-week intervals; the usual effective dose is 25 to 100 mg daily.

   Adverse effects are common and are due to the TCA's anticholinergic and antihistamine activities. They include morning drowsiness, dry mouth, and constipation. If amitriptyline causes too many side effects, other TCAs can be tried.

	Sedative	Anticholinergic
Amitriptyline (Elavil, Endep)	++++	++++
Imipramine (Tofranil)	+++	+++
Doxepin (Sinequan)	+++	+++
Nortriptyline (Pamelor)	++	+
Desipramine (Norpramin)	+	+

   As shown, the secondary amines (nortriptyline, desipramine) may be better tolerated but are less strong than the tertiary amines. In addition, amitriptyline and imipramine are most likely to cause orthostatic hypotension and cardiac toxicity (arrhythmias), although others may also cause these problems. **Cyclobenzaprine** (Flexeril) also acts as a weak TCA-like drug in FM. It is commonly used to treat muscular stiffness, and low-dose therapy has been studied as an augment to sleep disturbance as well. Dosing typically starts at 5 to 10 mg at bedtime (QHS). Daytime dosing may be added. Maximum daily dose is 30 mg.

   Although the mechanism of action of TCAs in FM treatment remains unclear, the small dosages used and the rapid onset of action suggest that it is not due to the treatment of underlying depression. Since TCAs inhibit the reuptake of serotonin (and norepinephrine) at synaptic junctions, it is hypothesized that the greater availability of serotonin may be responsible for improved stage IV sleep in addition to providing a central analgesic effect through potentiation of the descending analgesic pathways. TCAs may also have an effect on CNS endorphins as well as on peripheral pain receptors.

3. **Anticonvulsants: Gabapentin** (Neurontin) can be used as a less expensive substitute for pregabalin. Dosing is often started low since patients with FM often experience general drug intolerance. A common approach would start at 100 to 300 mg QHS. If 300 mg QHS is tolerated, a morning dose can be added and titrated to effect. Typical dosing: 300 to 600 mg thrice a day (TID; maximum dose 1200 mg TID).

4. **Analgesia. Tramadol** (Ultram) has been shown to help reduce pain in patients with FM. The analgesic effect of tramadol is most likely due to its SNRI effect and not due to its weak binding to the mu opioid receptor. In fact, opioids are not effective in FM and should be avoided.

Likewise, **acetaminophen** and nonsteroidal anti-inflammatory drugs **(NSAIDs)** are **not** effective for analgesia unless the patient also has associated pain due to osteoarthritis.

5. **Other "niche" therapies:** Other medications have been tried depending on the associated symptoms:
   - **Selective serotonin reuptake inhibitors (SSRIs)**: may be used to treat associated depression.
   - **Modafinil (Provigil):** has been described in noncontrolled, retrospective series to treat fatigue. Dose varies between 50 to 200 mg BID. Armodafinil (Nuvigil) can also be used.
   - **Trazodone** (Desyrel): may help sleep disturbances. Start 25 mg QHS and titrate weekly to effect. Maximum dose is 200 mg QHS.
   - **Ropinirole** (Requip): a dopamine (D3) receptor agonist that can help restless leg syndrome. Start 0.25 mg 1 to 3 hours before bed and titrate to effect or max dose 4 mg QHS.
   - **Naltrexone:** trials have shown that low-dose naltrexone (4.5 mg daily) improves pain and mood in 30% of FM patients. It does not improve fatigue or sleep. The mechanism of action is unclear but is postulated to be due to the ability of low-dose naltrexone to attenuate the production of proinflammatory cytokines and neurotoxic superoxides via suppressive effects on CNS microglia cells. Low doses do not affect the mu opioid receptors.

The potential benefit of psychedelic medicines, such as psilocybin and ketamine, are being studied in the treatment of FM. These treatments are considered investigational and hence are not part of the typical treatment algorithm for FM.

23. What medications have been shown to be ineffective in patients with FM?

Opioids, corticosteroids, NSAIDs, benzodiazepines, nonbenzodiazepine hypnotics, guaifenesin, S-Adenosylmethionine, melatonin, magnesium, and DHEA are not effective and should be avoided.

24. List some of the potential side effects from medications used to treat FM.

- All SNRIs may increase risk for suicidal ideation upon initiation.
- Many of the drugs (SNRIs, SSRIs, tramadol, others) can increase the chance of developing **serotonin syndrome** when used together or at high doses. Pregabalin and gabapentin do not increase this risk. Potential drug interactions need to be checked and the patient monitored. Patients who develop hyperreflexia on these medications are most at risk.
- SNRIs, milnacipran: nausea, vomiting which are lessened by giving it with food. Insomnia, dizziness, high BP, and liver and renal dysfunction can occur.
- Pregabalin, gabapentin, TCAs: fatigue, somnolence, dizziness, weight gain, dry mouth, hyponatremia (TCAs).
- Tramadol: fatigue, somnolence, dizziness, nausea, headache, high BP, and liver and renal dysfunction.

25. What is the prognosis for FM?

The prognosis for FM varies widely among individuals and is influenced by a range of factors, including the severity of symptoms, comorbid conditions, and the effectiveness of the treatment plan. Outcome studies suggest that the majority of patients continue to experience symptoms despite specific treatment. Overall, about 30% to 40% of patients will have 40% to 50% relief of their pain. However, this is an average response as some patients get excellent symptom relief, whereas some get none. The number of patients needed to treat to get a 30% reduction in pain and other symptoms varies between 7 and 19 patients, which is cost-effective. A sympathetic patient–physician interaction and an organized approach to therapy that includes nonpharmacologic intervention and patient self-management techniques will commonly lead to meaningful improvement in many patients.

26. What is the impact of FM on the patient and society?

The disease impact of FM is not trivial and is comparable to RA. On an average, a patient with FM sees the doctor three to four times more often than the general population (17 versus 4 visits/year). This contributes to high direct medical costs. In addition, patients with FM miss ~15 to 20 days of work annually, contributing to high indirect costs. Furthermore, it is estimated that as many as 25% of patients with FM in the United States receive some form of disability or injury compensation. This highlights not only the personal health challenges faced by patients, but also the broader economic implications for society.

ACKNOWLEDGMENT

The author would like to acknowledge the contribution of Dr. Jason Kolfenbach who was the author of this chapter in the previous edition.

BIBLIOGRAPHY

Ablin JN, Buskila D. Update on the genetics of the fibromyalgia syndrome. *Best Pract Res Clin Rheumatol.* 2015;29(1):20–28.

Arnold LM, Clauw DJ. A framework for fibromyalgia management for primary care providers. *Mayo Clin Proc.* 2012;87(5):488–496.

Arnold LM. Strategies for managing fibromyalgia. *Am J Med.* 2009;122:S31–S43.

Clauw DJ, Arnold LM, McCarberg BH. The science of fibromyalgia. *Mayo Clin Proc.* 2011;86(9):907–911.

Duffield SJ, Miller N. Concomitant fibromyalgia complicating chronic inflammatory arthritis: a systematic review and meta-analysis. *Rheumatology (Oxford).* 2018;57(8):1453–1460.

Fitzcharles MA. Fibromyalgia: evolving concepts over time. *CMAJ.* 2013;185(13):E645–E651.

Huser W, Bernardy K, Arnold B, et al. Efficacy of multicomponent treatment in fibromyalgia syndrome: a meta-analysis of randomized controlled clinical trials. *Arthritis Rheum.* 2009;61:216–224.

Lyes M, Yang KH, Castellanos J, Furnish T. Microdosing psilocybin for chronic pain: a case series. *Pain.* 2023;164(4):698–702.

Moldofsky H. The significance of dysfunctions of the sleeping/waking brain to the pathogenesis and treatment of fibromyalgia syndrome. *Rheum Dis Clin North Am.* 2009;35:275–283.

Nahin RL, Boineau R. Evidence-based evaluation of complementary health approaches for pain management in the United States. *Mayo Clin Proc.* 2016;91(9):1292–1306.

Pamfil C, Choy EHS. Functional MRI in rheumatic diseases with a focus on fibromyalgia. *Clin Exp Rheumatol.* 2018;36(suppl 114):82–85 (5).

Pastrak M, Abd-Elsayed A, Ma F, Vrooman B, Visnjevac O. Systematic review of the use of intravenous ketamine for fibromyalgia. *Ochsner J.* 2021;21(4):387–394.

Traynor LM, Thiessen CN, Traynor AP. Pharmacotherapy of fibromyalgia. *Am J Health Syst Pharm.* 2011;68:1307–1319.

Williams DA, Clauw DJ. Internet-enhanced management of fibromyalgia: a randomized controlled trial. Pain. 151(3):694–702.

Wolfe F, Clauw DJ, Fitzcharles MA, et al. 2016 revisions to the 2010/2011 fibromyalgia diagnostic criteria. *Semin Arthritis Rheum.* 2016;46(3):319–329.

Yunus MB. Central sensitivity syndromes: a new paradigm and group nosology for fibromyalgia and overlapping conditions, and the related issue of disease versus illness. *Semin Arthritis Rheum.* 2008;37:339–352.

WEBSITES

https://fibroguide.med.umich.edu/ (on-line modules aimed at patient education and self-help; Dr. Daniel Clauw, University of Michigan)

www.fmaware.org (National Fibromyalgia Association website)

www.fibrocenter.com (pharmaceutical industry sponsored site)

https://moodgym.com.au/ (on-line CBT option; annual prescription of $27; small randomized study using this platform showed improvement compared to usual therapy; additional studies evaluating on-line CBT have demonstrated effectiveness in FM as well)

CHAPTER 61

Regional Musculoskeletal Disorders

Bharat Kumar, MD, MMEd

1. What is bursitis?

- Bursitis is the condition that occurs when a bursa becomes inflamed.
- A bursa is a sac with a potential space that makes it easier for one tissue to glide over another. They are often located near, and sometimes communicate with joints.
- There are approximately 160 bursae in the body, but only a few of them become clinically affected.
- Most bursae differentiate during development, but new ones may form (sometimes referred to as adventitial bursae) in response to irritation, inflammation, or trauma.
- On ultrasound, normal bursa appears to be compressible and anechoic (black). When inflamed, they may appear more distended (less compressible) and potentially more echogenic (lighter in color) due to debris, blood, or purulent material.

2. What are the differences between tendinitis, tendinosis, and tenosynovitis?

- **Tendinitis** is an acute, subacute, or chronic inflammation of the tendon associated with vascular disruption, which may be caused by tendon trauma, crystal deposition (especially basic calcium phosphate crystals), or infection, among other causes. On ultrasound, there is increased spacing of fibrillar lines and reduced echogenicity (darker) due to swelling.
- **Tendinosis (tendinopathy)** is intratendinous atrophy and degeneration that is often associated with chronic tendinitis. Tendinosis can lead to partial or complete tendon rupture. Findings on ultrasound are similar to tendinitis but doppler signals are not expected.
- **Tenosynovitis** is inflammation of the paratendon, which is the outermost sheath that is lined in some instances by a synovial membrane (e.g., tendons of the thumb involved in De Quervain tenosynovitis). It may or may not coexist with tendinitis. On ultrasound, fluid can be found within the tendon sheath.

Most of these conditions can be classified as "overuse" syndromes. Aging can decrease the integrity of the tendon, making it more prone to injury and incomplete healing.

3. How can bursitis, tendinitis, tendinopathy, and other regional musculoskeletal syndromes be treated?

- **Identify, modify, and avoid the precipitating movements or actions:** bursitis and tendinitis are frequently caused by repetitive motions or movements (e.g., baseball pitchers often develop bicipital tendinitis).
- Rest the affected area: however, intermittent gentle range of motion needs to be maintained, or the joint capsule may contract or "freeze."
- Anti-inflammatory or analgesic medications: nonsteroidal anti-inflammatory drugs (NSAIDs) probably have a more important role than just analgesia.
- Splinting of the affected area can prevent further overuse

- Superficial heat and cold.
- Range of motion/flexibility and muscle strengthening exercises. Supervised physical therapy is instrumental in ensuring proper patient education and adherence to optimal technique.
- Ambulatory aids (cane, crutches, or walker).
- Local corticosteroid injections may provide short-term relief but also may predispose to tendon rupture, especially in the Achilles tendon. Ultrasound-guided injections may help improve the accuracy of injecting steroids in small spaces.
- Surgery (bursectomy, tenosynovectomy, reattachment of ruptured tendons).
  Data is inconsistent regarding the use of extracorporeal shock wave therapy (ESWT), ionto-phoresis, polarized light, therapeutic ultrasound, or low-level laser therapy.

4. Name the three most common nonarticular causes of shoulder pain.
- Impingement syndrome.
- Subacromial bursitis.
- Bicipital tendinitis.

5. Describe the shoulder impingement syndrome. How does it occur?
The shoulder impingement syndrome is a chronic, painful condition of the shoulder that results from an encroachment of the tendons of the rotator cuff (most commonly the supraspinatus), most commonly experienced during shoulder abduction.

In the normal functioning shoulder, the rotator cuff serves as a dynamic stabilizer. Its principal function lies in humeral head depression during shoulder abduction. The rotator cuff also assists with early abduction (0–30 degrees) as well as with internal and external rotation. When the rotator cuff is inflamed secondary to chronic, repetitive microtrauma, or due to acute posttraumatic tendon strain, it becomes relatively ineffective at shoulder depression, a characteristic called reflex inhibition. Consequently, the humeral head moves closer to the coracoacromial arch (superior translation) during the contraction of the deltoid muscle as seen with shoulder abduction. With increased superior translation of the humeral head, there is impingement of the tendons on the coracoacromial arch, which leads to tendon inflammation and increased reflex inhibition. This is the **vicious cycle of impingement** and can lead to rotator cuff tears or decreased motion to avoid pain with resultant adhesive capsulitis (frozen shoulder; Fig. 61.1).

6. What are the three stages of shoulder impingement syndrome?
- Stage I usually occurs under 25 years of age and is characterized by tendon hemorrhage and edema.
- Stage II usually occurs between 25 and 40 years and is characterized by tendinitis and fibrosis of the subacromial bursa.
- Stage III usually occurs over 40 years of age and is characterized by tears of the rotator cuff and bicipital tendon.
  Stages I and II are reversible with appropriate treatment.

7. How does the impingement syndrome present clinically?
- Pain with active shoulder movement (patient moves arm), especially flexion (between 60 and 120 degrees), abduction and internal rotation.
- Much less or no pain with passive movement (examiner moves arm).
- Absence of swelling, redness, or warmth at shoulder joint.
- Radiographically, the space between the humeral head and inferior surface of the acromion may be <8 mm.

8. What tests are done to isolate individual rotator cuff tendons that can become inflamed and cause shoulder pain?
- **Jobe test (empty can test):** this maneuver isolates the supraspinatus, which is commonly involved in impingement syndrome. The patient places the arm in 90 degrees of abduction, 30 degrees of forward flexion, and internal rotation with the elbow extended and the arm rotated so that the thumb is pointing to the floor. The examiner pushes down on the arm as the patient resists this pressure. This will cause a worsening of the pain if the supraspinatus is involved, with a sensitivity of 86% and specificity of 50%. Further confirmation of

IMPINGEMENT CYCLE

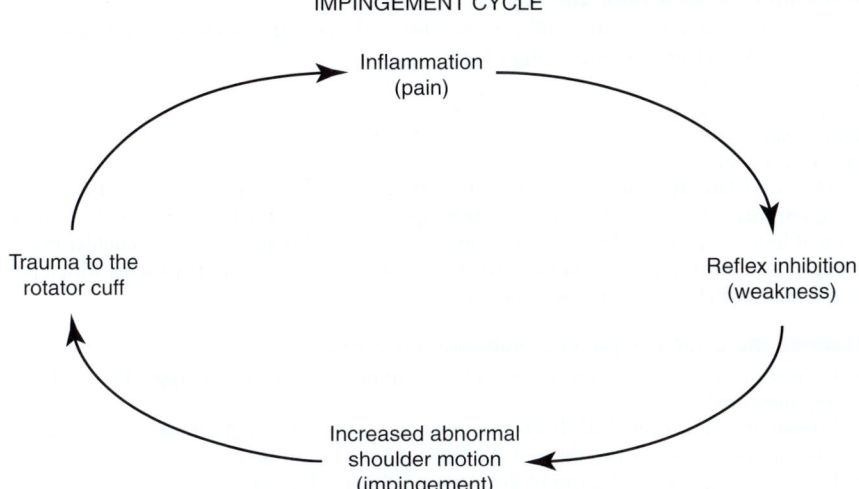

Fig. 61.1 The vicious cycle in the impingement syndrome.

supraspinatus pathology is obtained when the Jobe test is repeated, but this time the shoulder is in external rotation (thumb pointing up), which should cause *less* pain.
- **Infraspinatus isolation test:** this maneuver places strain on the infraspinatus and teres minor tendons. The arms are placed at the patient's side with elbows at the waist flexed to 90 degrees and 45 degrees of internal rotation. Shoulder external rotation is resisted, and the test is positive if this results in pain.
- **Gerber push with force test (lift-off test):** this maneuver isolates the subscapularis tendon. The patient's shoulder is placed passively in internal rotation and slight extension by placing the hand behind the back, 5 to 10 cm from the belt line, with the palm facing outward and the elbow flexed at 90 degrees. The examiner pushes the palm toward the patient's back while the patient resists. The test is positive if this results in pain or weakness is elicited.

9. What are the Neer and Hawkins–Kennedy impingement tests?

In the right clinical context, these are provocative maneuvers that are sensitive (80–90%) for impingement but not very specific (30–50%). The Neer test causes pain when the patient's shoulder is flexed forward maximally by the examiner, while the arm is internally rotated (palm down) and the shoulder is stabilized. The Hawkins–Kennedy test reinforces a positive Neer impingement test. The examiner puts the shoulder into 90 degrees of forward flexion and flexes the elbow to 90 degrees. The arm is internally rotated as if the patient is emptying a can of soda in front of themselves. Both these maneuvers compress the greater tuberosity of the humerus against the anterior acromion (Neer test) or coracoacromial ligament (Hawkins–Kennedy test) and elicit discomfort in patients who have a rotator cuff tear or impingement.

10. What is the impingement sign?

The impingement sign is considered "positive" and the diagnosis supported when an injection of local anesthetic (10 mL of 1% plain lidocaine) into the subacromial space ameliorates the pain caused by the Jobe, Neer, and Hawkins–Kennedy tests.

11. How is the impingement syndrome treated?

The mainstays of management are physical therapy and anti-inflammatory medications. Regaining full shoulder motion and rotator cuff strength are the therapy goals. Inflammation in the tendons is treated with oral NSAIDs or a local injection of corticosteroid. Nonoperative management should be pursued for at least 6 months before consideration of surgical decompression, unless a full-thickness rotator cuff tear is present.

12. How common are rotator cuff tears?

The incidence of **partial** rotator cuff tears increases with age and can result from trauma or tendon degeneration from chronic impingement:

Age 40 years: 33%
Age 50 years: 55%
Age 60 years: 65%
Age 70 years: 80%

Most are relatively asymptomatic and 30–50% are bilateral. Weakness may be demonstrated on supraspinatus testing (50% sensitivity, 60% specificity). Full thickness tears are less common (25% of individuals aged >60 years) and should be suspected in patients with shoulder muscle atrophy, those who "hike" the shoulder when asked to lift the arm, and in patients with a positive drop arm test (30% sensitivity, 90% specificity).

13. Describe the clinical aspects of subacromial bursitis.

- Unusual for it to occur in the absence of the impingement syndrome (typically secondary to impingement).
- Primary inflammation of the bursa may occur as a result of crystal deposition or infection.
- Clinical findings similar to those of the impingement syndrome.
- Focal tenderness when the area of the bursa is palpated (Fig. 61.2).

14. Describe the clinical aspects of bicipital tendinitis.

- Anterior shoulder pain.
- Pain worsened with active shoulder movement.
- Positive Yergason's maneuver and/or Speed's test.
- Less pain with passive movement.
- Absence of swelling, redness, or warmth at shoulder joint.

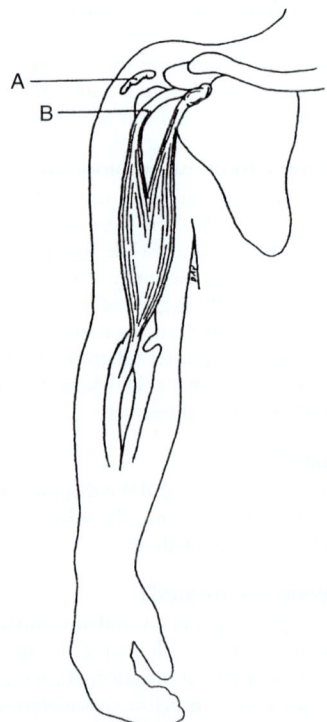

Fig. 61.2 Shoulder anatomy. (A) Subacromial bursa. (B) Biceps tendon, long head. *Illustrations by Debra Vogelgesang.*

- Focal tenderness when area overlying long head of biceps tendon is palpated (Fig. 61.2).
- Frequently accompanies the impingement syndrome (relatively uncommon as a clinically isolated syndrome).

15. What are Yergason's maneuver and Speed's tests?
- **Yergason's maneuver**—pain in the area of the long head of the biceps tendon (LHBT) is elicited by resisted supination of the forearm when the elbow is held at the side and flexed to 90 degrees. This is a difficult test to perform and interpret.
- **Speed's test**—the patient's elbow is extended, forearm supinated (palm up), and humerus flexed forward 60 to 90 degrees. Pain in the area of the biceps tendon is elicited by downward resistance applied to the forward-flexed arm (63% sensitivity, 35% specificity).

16. What is a "frozen shoulder"?
Also called **adhesive capsulitis** or pericapsulitis, frozen shoulder can occur after **any** cause of shoulder pain that leads an affected individual to limit the motion of the shoulder because of pain. Patients with diabetes are particularly prone to develop this condition. With little movement, the shoulder joint capsule and surrounding structures contract, making the range of motion physically restricted in addition to being painful. Examination reveals at least 50% reduction in both active and passive range of motion. Arthrography shows decreased volume of the joint capsule. It is rarely seen before the age of 40 years. The process typically has three phases:
- Phase I: increasing pain and stiffness for 2 to 9 months
- Phase II: substantial stiffness but less pain for 4 to 12 months
- Phase III: pain resolves and function is gradually restored over 5 to 26 months.

While many patients experience improvement in pain and function, complete symptom resolution is uncommon. Options for short-term management are limited by poor data on efficacy. NSAIDs and analgesics are reasonable options for control of pain and may be coupled with gentle range of motion exercises at home. Other modalities with unclear efficacy include corticosteroid injection, supervised physical therapy, and surgical intervention.

17. List three causes of nonarticular elbow pain.
- Lateral epicondylitis (tennis elbow).
- Medial epicondylitis (golfer's/bowler's elbow).
- Olecranon bursitis.

18. List the clinical features of lateral epicondylitis.
- Lateral elbow pain, especially with motions such as turning a screwdriver, shaking hands, or hitting backhand in tennis.
- Incidence is 1% to 3% of the general population. Smoking, repetitive movement for >2 hours/day, or lifting loads >20 kg are risk factors.
- Pain is worsened with **extension** of the wrist, especially against resistance, when the elbow is in full extension.
- Pain, swelling, and warmth may be present at the common origin of the extensor carpi ulnaris, extensor carpi radialis longus and brevis, and extensor digitorum (Fig. 61.3).

19. List the clinical characteristics of medial epicondylitis.
- Medial elbow pain (much less common than lateral epicondylitis).
- Pain is worsened with **flexion** of the wrist, especially against resistance, when the elbow is in full extension.
- Pain, swelling, and warmth may be present at the origin of flexor carpi ulnaris, flexor carpi radialis, and pronator teres (Fig. 61.3).

20. Beyond physical therapy, ice, and NSAIDs, how is epicondylitis treated?
- Counterforce brace or strap placed 10 cm distal to the joint line.
- Physical therapy, including eccentric exercise (e.g., flexbar, or use of an elastic band for resistance) and additional flexibility and strengthening modalities

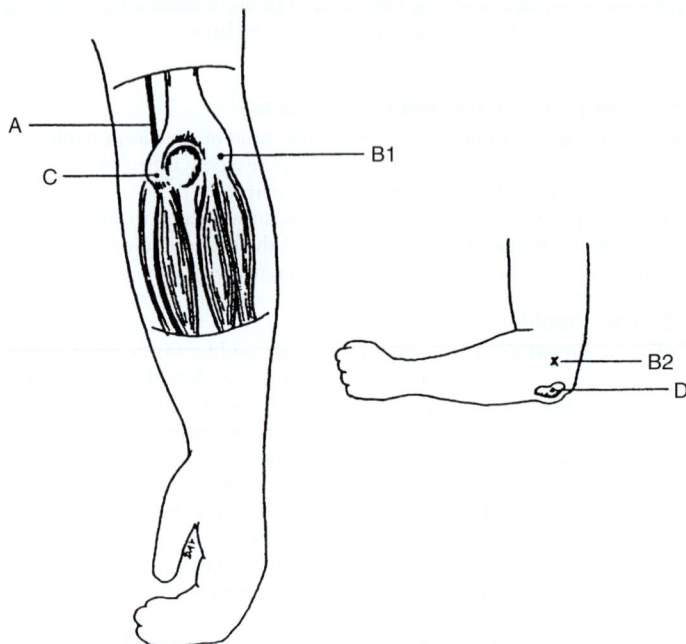

Fig. 61.3 Elbow anatomy. (A) Ulnar nerve. (B1 and B2) Lateral epicondyle. (C) Medial epicondyle. (D) Olecranon bursa. *Illustrations by Debra Vogelgesang.*

- Local corticosteroid injection (controversial): many experts feel that epicondylitis is a degenerative tendinopathy and not an inflammatory lesion; studies suggest that steroid injections help symptoms in the short term but actually make long-term recovery worse.
- Occasionally, splinting the wrist to prevent flexion and extension can help (**caution:** the splint should be removed two to three times a day to allow wrist movement).
- Less than 5% to 10% will need surgical debridement after 6 months of conservative therapy.

21. Describe the clinical features of olecranon bursitis.
- Pain, swelling, and warmth at the location of the olecranon bursa on the extensor surface of the elbow (Fig. 61.3).
- Typically elbow extension is normal, but flexion may be limited.
- Can be secondary to trauma, rheumatoid arthritis (RA), crystalline arthropathies (gout, calcium pyrophosphate dihydrate deposition disease), dialysis, or infection (frequently caused by a break in the surrounding skin).

22. What is De Quervain stenosing tenosynovitis?
- Tendinitis involving the abductor pollicis longus (APL) and extensor pollicis brevis (EPB) tendons.
- Most frequently described as pain at the base of the thumb.
- APL/EPB tendons form the palmar side of the anatomic snuffbox.
- A positive Finkelstein maneuver supports the diagnosis (see Question 23).

23. What physical examination tests are performed to diagnose De Quervain stenosing tenosynovitis?
- **Finkelstein (Eichhoff) maneuver:** the patient touches the thumb to the base of the fifth finger, then wraps the other fingers around the thumb and abducts of the wrist (the fist moves toward the ulnar side) eliciting pain (sensitivity 89%, specificity 14%).

- **Wrist hyperflexion and abduction of the thumb (WHAT) test:** the patient fully flexes his/her wrist and keeps his/her thumb fully extended and abducted while the examiner applies a gradually increasing resistance against abduction of the thumb, causing pain (sensitivity 99%, specificity 29%).

24. Beyond NSAIDs, ice, and avoiding precipitating maneuvers, how is De Quervain tenosynovitis treated?

- Splint for the thumb and wrist called a **forearm-based thumb spica splint.**
- Local corticosteroid injections may be considered, preferably guided by ultrasonography.
- Surgical release if conservative therapy fails.

25. What is the intersection syndrome?

This is a common overuse syndrome at the distal forearm that results from inflammation at the point where the APL/EPB tendons cross over the extensor carpi radialis longus and extensor carpi radialis brevis tendons in the wrist. This condition is often seen in laborers who perform repetitive dorsiflexion of the wrist or in athletes such as rowers. The area of inflammation is 6 to 8 cm proximal to the radial styloid. There may be swelling and crepitus with active wrist extension.

26. What is greater trochanteric pain syndrome (GTPS)?

GTPS is a common condition causing pain in the lateral aspect of the pelvis. Although commonly called trochanteric bursitis, bursitis on imaging is only present in about 20% of patients. Rather, gluteus medius and minimus tendinopathy, and iliotibial band (ITB) thickening (typically in the region of the entheses of the gluteal muscle insertions), are much more common. Some authors have likened GTPS to rotator cuff tendinopathy in the shoulder, with bursitis involved in a minority of cases and representing a secondary process. Pain is exacerbated by lying on the affected side, walking, climbing stairs, rising from a seated position, and external rotation and abduction of the hip. With significant gluteus medius pathology, the patient may have a positive Trendelenburg test and significant weakness or inability to complete a single repetition of the single-leg mini squat test where the patient squats on the affected leg to 60 degrees.

Initial therapy consists of NSAIDs and physical therapy. ITB tightness may contribute to symptoms in GTPS and can be evaluated by the **Ober test** (see Chapter 5: History and Physical Examination). ITB stretches and myofascial release through the use of a foam roller may be beneficial. Similarly, physical therapy aimed at stretching and strengthening the gluteus medius and minimus muscles should be considered. Local corticosteroid injection can be helpful in many patients despite the low prevalence of documented bursitis on imaging. Failure to respond to initial therapy may suggest a leg length discrepancy (leading to gait abnormalities), gluteus tendon rupture/tear, or hallux rigidus, and evaluations for these conditions should be initiated.

27. What does a "snapping hip" mean?

Snapping hip is characterized by a snapping sensation as hip tendons move over bony prominences. The most common site is the ITB snapping over the greater trochanter, usually with walking or rotation of the hip (**ITB syndrome**). Patients may subsequently develop trochanteric bursitis. Patients usually have a positive Ober test suggesting ITB tightness or contracture. Additional conditions associated with a snapping sensation at the hip include: gluteal tendon snapping over the greater trochanter, and *internal hip etiologies* such as iliopsoas tendons snapping over the iliopectineal eminence, acetabular labral tear, or intra-articular loose bodies.

28. What is "weaver's bottom"?

- Also called ischial bursitis.
- Bursa lies superficial to the ischial tuberosity.
- Can be caused by prolonged sitting on hard surfaces, especially in thin individuals.

29. What is prepatellar bursitis ("housemaid's knee")?

- Pain, swelling, and warmth in the prepatellar bursa (Fig. 61.4).
- Caused by repetitive trauma or overuse, such as kneeling on a hard surface.
- Can be affected in patients with gout.
- Can become infected, especially after breaks in the skin.

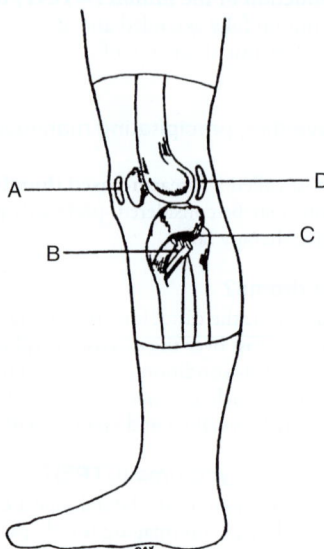

Fig. 61.4 Knee anatomy. (A) Prepatellar bursa. (B) Conjoined tendons. (C) Anserine bursa. (D) Posterior fossa (where Baker's cyst will be felt). *Illustrations by Debra Vogelgesang.*

30. What is pes anserine bursitis?

Inflammation of the pes anserine ("goose's foot") bursa located at the medial aspect of the knee approximately 6 cm below the anteromedial joint line. The bursa (Fig. 61.4) lies between the conjoined tendons of the sartorius/gracilis/semitendinosus muscles and the medial collateral ligament. It is frequently described as knee pain, but it is typically noticed when lying on one's side in bed when the knees are opposed. **Pain is worsened by going upstairs.** It is more common in patients with obesity, valgus knee deformities, and pes planus.

31. What is a Baker cyst?

Also called a **popliteal cyst,** this is swelling in the popliteal fossa with minimal tenderness (Fig. 61.4). Its proposed cause in some individuals involves a communication between the semimembranosus/gastrocnemius bursa and the knee joint. Some have postulated a one-way valve effect in which synovial fluid moves from the knee to the bursa. Baker cysts can occur secondary to any process that produces synovial fluid. A ruptured cyst can occasionally dissect down the calf and be confused with deep venous thrombosis. Ecchymoses inferior to the medial malleolus of the ankle (crescent sign) is characteristic.

32. Name five causes of heel pain.

- Achilles enthesitis.
- Achilles tendinitis.
- Retrocalcaneal (Achilles) bursitis.
- Plantar fasciitis.
- Heel fat pad atrophy.

33. What is enthesitis?

An **enthesis** is the place where a tendon or ligament attaches to a bone. These areas can become inflamed (enthesitis) in spondyloarthritis (SpA; e.g. reactive arthritis and other members of the SpA family). Achilles enthesitis is a cause of heel pain and is characterized by swelling, warmth, and pain where the Achilles tendon inserts into the calcaneus (Fig. 61.5).

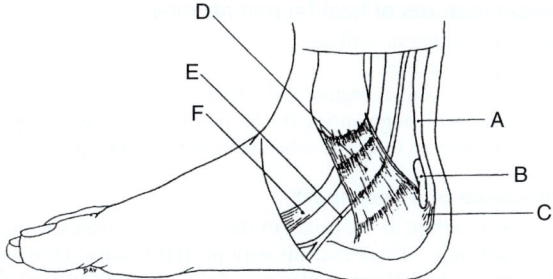

Fig. 61.5 Medial ankle and foot anatomy. (A) Achilles tendon. (B) Achilles bursa. (C) Achilles enthesis. (D) Flexor retinaculum. (E) Posterior tibial nerve. (F) Posterior tibial tendon. *Illustrations by Debra Vogelgesang.*

34. Describe the clinical features of Achilles tendinitis.
- Heel pain, sometimes described as posterior leg pain, worsening with dorsiflexion.
- Area of most tenderness is 2 to 3 cm proximal to the attachment to the calcaneus (Fig. 61.5).
- Tendon may be swollen with thickening, especially 2 to 3 cm proximal to the insertion.
- May rupture spontaneously.
  Sudden onset of pain during dorsiflexion
  Audible pop or snap
  Positive Thompson test

35. How is the Thompson test performed?
The patient kneels on a chair with the feet extending back over the edge. As the examiner squeezes and pushes the calf toward the knee, normaly plantarflexion of the foot should be seen; however, in Achilles tendon rupture, there will be no movement.

36. How does retrocalcaneal (Achilles) bursitis present clinically?
- Heel pain.
- Fullness or swelling proximal and anterior to the attachment of the Achilles tendon to the calcaneus (Fig. 61.5).
- Pain on palpation of the bursa.

37. Describe the clinical features of plantar fasciitis.
Some may describe heel pain, but most affected individuals complain of pain along the plantar surface of the foot. The pain is worsened by pressure on the bottom of the foot (i.e., walking, running, palpation). **It is also worse with the first steps taken after getting out of bed in the morning.** There is tenderness at the attachment site of the plantar fascia to the inferior aspect of the calcaneus. Predisposing factors include obesity, pes planus, pes cavus, short Achilles tendon, and standing/running on hard surfaces.

38. How is plantar fasciitis treated?
- Initial therapy:
  Heel cup or other heel cushioning: consider custom orthotics if foot abnormalities are present.
  NSAIDs.
  Stretching exercises of the plantar fascia and Achilles tendon; "soda can roll" with foot.
  Reduce weight-bearing exercise.
- If no improvement after approximately 2 to 3 months, continue the plan above and add:
  Night splint: holds the foot in minimal dorsiflexion while sleeping
  Consider a local corticosteroid injection.
- If no improvement after approximately 6 to 12 months of conservative therapy, consider a referral for surgery (<10% of patients).

39. What are the clinical features of heel fat pad atrophy?
- Pain with prolonged standing or walking.
- Pain with initial weight-bearing.
- Tenderness in the central, plantar region of the heel.
- Tenderness is improved with augmenting the fat pad (simultaneously squeezing the medial and lateral sides of the heel to force the subcutaneous tissue in a plantar direction).

40. What is the significance of a heel spur?
A heel spur (osteophyte) develops at the origin of the flexor brevis muscle just superior to the plantar fascia in approximately 50% of patients with plantar fasciitis. However, the spur is not a source of pain and is present in 20% of similar-age adults who do not have plantar fasciitis.

41. What is posterior tibial tendinitis?
Inflammation of the posterior tibial tendon and its synovial sheath. Pain is located more prominently on the medial side of the ankle. The pain and swelling are localized to the path of the posterior tibial tendon (Fig. 61.5), with increased pain on resisted foot inversion.

42. What are some clinical features of dysfunction or rupture of the posterior tibial tendon?
- **Acquired pes planus**—also called a flat foot, in which the normal contour of the longitudinal arch becomes flattened.
- **"Too many toes" sign**—caused by hindfoot valgus and forefoot abduction. When the foot is viewed from behind the heel, you can see more toes over the lateral side of the affected foot than on the unaffected side.
- **"Heel-rise" sign**—the inability to rise to the ball of the affected foot while lifting the unaffected foot.

BIBLIOGRAPHY
Bisset L, Paungmali A, Vicenzino B, et al. A systemic review and meta-analysis of clinical trials on physical interventions for lateral epicondylalgia. *Br J Sports Med*. 2005;39:411.

Charles R, Fang L, Zhu R, et al. The effectiveness of shockwave therapy on patellar tendinopathy, Achilles tendinopathy, and plantar fasciitis: a systematic review and meta-analysis. *Front Immunol*. 2023;14:1193835.

Ciccotti MC, Schwartz MA, Ciccotti MG. Diagnosis and treatment of medial epicondylitis of the elbow. *Clin Sports Med*. 2004;23:693–705.

Cole C, Seto C, Gazewood J. Plantar fasciitis: evidenced-based review of diagnosis and therapy. *Am Fam Physician*. 2005;72:2237.

Coombes BK, Bisset L, Brooks P, et al. Effect of corticosteroid injection, physiotherapy, or both on clinical outcomes in patients with unilateral lateral epicondylalgia: a randomized controlled trial. *JAMA*. 2013;309:461–469.

Gomoll AH, Katz JN, Warner JJ, et al. Rotator cuff disorders: recognition and management among patients with shoulder pain. *Arthritis Rheum*. 2004;50:3751–3761.

Koester MC, George MS, Kuhn JE. Shoulder impingement syndrome. *Am J Med*. 2005;118:452–455.

Levine WN, Kashyap CP, Bak SF, et al. Nonoperative management of idiopathic adhesive capsulitis. *J Shoulder Elbow Surg*. 2007;16:569–573.

Long SS, Surrey DE, Nazarian LN. Sonography of greater trochanteric pain syndrome and the rarity of primary bursitis. *AJR Am J Roentgenol*. 2013;201:1083–1086.

Muir JJ, Curtiss HM, Hollman J, et al. The accuracy of ultrasound-guided and palpation-guided peroneal tendon sheath injections. *Am J Phys Med Rehabil*. 2011;90(7):564–571.

Murrell GA, Walton JR. Diagnosis of rotator cuff tears. *Lancet*. 2001;357:769–770.

Rennie WJ, Saifuddin A. Pes anserine bursitis: incidence in symptomatic knees and clinical presentation. *Skeletal Radio*. 2005;34:395.

Richie CA, Briner WW. Corticosteroid injection for treatment of de Quervain's tenosynovitis: a pooled quantitative literature evaluation. *J Am Board Fam Pract*. 2003;16:102.

Shiri R, Viikari-Juntura E, Varonen H, Heliövaara M. Prevalence and determinants of lateral and medial epicondylitis: a population study. *Am J Epidemiol*. 2006;164:1065.

Silva L, Andreu JL, Munoz P, et al. Accuracy of physical examination in subacromial impingement syndrome. *Rheumatology*. 2008;47:679–683.

CHAPTER 62

Sports Medicine and Occupational Injuries

Bradley Changstrom, MD and Jack Spittler, MD

≫ KEY POINTS

1. The shoulder relies on tendons and ligaments for movement and stability. These are subjected to tremendous stress leading to injury, particularly in overhead athletes.
2. Strains and sprains are acute injuries and generally resolve faster than overuse injuries, which require significant rehabilitation to allow for healing.
3. Most sports-related or occupational-related injuries can be initially managed with rest, nonsteroidal anti-inflammatory drugs (NSAIDs), and physical therapy.
4. Abnormal body position and mechanics contribute to the majority of recreational or occupational injuries and must be corrected as part of the treatment plan.

1. What is a ligament sprain and how is severity determined?

A **sprain** is an acute, traumatic injury to a **ligament.** There are three grades of sprains:
- First-degree—mild pain due to tearing less than one-third of ligamentous fibers, <5 mm laxity.
- Second-degree—moderate pain and swelling, one-third to two-thirds of fibers of ligament torn, 5 to 10 mm laxity.
- Third-degree—often no or minimal pain from a complete rupture of the ligament, causing joint instability.

2. How are sprains treated?

The initial focus of **grade 1 and grade 2 sprains** is usually RICE (Rest, Ice, Compression, Elevation) therapy; however, evidence supporting this approach is limited. Oral or topical NSAIDs may be a useful adjunct in the acute phase to reduce pain. Evidence favors early motion and functional support (bracing or taping) for lower grade sprains, especially the ankle. Neuromuscular and proprioceptive training programs are safe, effective interventions that should be implemented as soon as pain allows. Orthobiologics (e.g., platelet-rich plasma, stem cell treatments, etc.) may be considered to augment healing; however, data are very limited in this regard. **Grade 3** injury treatment is more complicated and may involve surgical repair depending on the type and extent of the injury.

3. What are the differences between tendinopathy, tendinosis, and tendinitis?

Tendinopathy is an umbrella term for the spectrum of changes that occur in a damaged or diseased tendon. These changes may contribute to pain and reduced function. Normal tendon is composed of highly organized collagen fibers. In contrast, abnormal tendons have fragmented collagen, disorganized collagen bundles, accumulation of glycosaminoglycans, and increased microvasculature, which lead to adverse changes in the material properties of the tendon. **Tendinitis** reflects acute inflammation in the tendon, either from an initial injury or a "flare-up" of an existing, chronic injury. Microscopically, local tissue breakdown occurs with tissue lysis, lymphocytic infiltration, and blood extravasation. When these issues become chronic (**tendinosis**), histologic features show no inflammatory cell invasion at the site of the lesion and the normal tissue is replaced by angiofibroblastic, hyperplastic tissue.

4. How does treatment differ for tendinitis and tendinosis?

As **tendinitis is an acute problem**, treatment is focused on reducing pain and inflammation. RICE therapy, NSAIDs, and physical therapy are mainstays of treatment. Other treatment adjuncts may include low-level laser, therapeutic ultrasound, and corticosteroid injection. For **chronic tendinosis**, treatment shifts toward disrupting the hyperplastic, diseased tendon in hopes of restoring more normal collagen fibers, fiber arrangement, and ultimately tendon function.

Eccentric training and loading programs have shown beneficial effects in chronic tendinosis. Other adjuncts (often more invasive) include extracorporeal shockwave therapy (ESWT), platelet-rich plasma (PRP) injection, needle fenestration/prolotherapy, percutaneous tenotomy, and stem cell therapy. The evidence behind these treatments is limited but improving with time. Orthotics, splinting, braces, or taping may be used to facilitate protected motion for a tendinopathy diagnosis.

5. List some common sites of tendinopathy/fasciopathy occurring in athletes and manual laborers.

Plantar fascia
Achilles tendon (see Chapter 61: Regional Musculoskeletal Disorders)
Patellar tendon
Posterior tibialis tendon (see Chapter 61: Regional Musculoskeletal Disorders)
De Quervain (extensor pollicus brevis, abductor pollicus longus) tendons
Lateral epicondyle (tennis elbow)
Medial epicondyle (golfer's elbow)
Rotator cuff tendons (see Chapter 61: Regional Musculoskeletal Disorders)
Biceps (long head) tendon (see Chapter 61: Regional Musculoskeletal Disorders)
Gluteal (medius, minimus) tendons

6. How common is shoulder pain in athletes and manual laborers?

Shoulder pain affects all ages (older people more than young adults) and is present in 18–26% of adults at any point in time. It is the third most common musculoskeletal complaint for which a patient seeks care. It is most common in workers whose jobs involve repetitive, forceful, overhead work, lifting heavy loads, and vibration. The majority of symptoms are related to the rotator cuff. See Chapter 61 for a more comprehensive discussion of common shoulder problems.

7. What is tennis elbow?

Tennis elbow, better termed **lateral epicondylopathy,** is usually an overuse syndrome that presents with lateral elbow pain. Few patients who have symptoms of this disorder have actually acquired it through playing tennis, but it is generally seen in those performing activities that require repetitive wrist extension and forearm supination. The differential diagnosis of lateral elbow pain also includes elbow arthritis, focal chondral injury in the elbow joint, nerve compression of the radial or posterior interosseous nerve, and cervical spondylosis with radiculopathy. It is primarily a degenerative process resulting from microtearing involving the origin of the extensor carpi radialis (ECR) muscles. The healing of the tendinous origin is impaired by chronic overuse and becomes symptomatic. On exam, pain is generally most pronounced with resisted wrist extension, and specifically with extension of the middle finger (as this maneuver tests the most commonly involved muscle, which inserts onto the dorsal aspect of the third metacarpal). Initial treatment is universally conservative and can include an elbow **counterforce brace** over the proximal forearm, a wrist extension brace to off-load the ECR brevis, NSAIDs, and a home exercise or physical therapy program of **stretching and eccentric strengthening**. Corticosteroid delivered via injections or iontophoresis remains controversial but may be beneficial in the acute period (e.g., 6–8 weeks) for pain relief. Steroids, however, increase the risk of long-term, chronic tendinosis. The condition is generally self-limited, with 90% of patients experiencing resolution of their symptoms in 12 to 18 months. For chronic, refractory tendinosis treatment, ESWT, PRP injections, needle fenestration/prolotherapy, or percutaneous tenotomy treatments may be utilized.

8. What is golfer's elbow?

Golfer's elbow, better termed **medial epicondylopathy,** results from an overuse injury and subsequent degeneration of the tendinous origin of the flexor pronator muscle mass at the elbow. In golfers, this area is placed under valgus stress at the top of a backswing in golfing and proceeds through the downswing until impact with the ball. The condition is also found in approximately 4–8% of workers in an occupational setting. Pain is elicited over the elbow's medial epicondyle and is increased with resisted wrist flexion and forearm pronation. Management includes rest, ice, NSAIDs, counterforce brace or splinting, and physical therapy. Just as in lateral epicondylitis, corticosteroid injections are controversial with evidence for short-term improvement but potential tendon weakening in the long term. For chronic, refractory tendinosis treatment, ESWT, PRP injections, needle fenestration/prolotherapy, or percutaneous tenotomy treatments may be utilized. Providers must be aware of the location of the ulnar nerve during injections in order to avoid any iatrogenic injury. As such, ultrasound may be used to guide needle placement during procedures.

9. How do you test for rotator cuff tendinopathy?

The four rotator cuff tendons are the supraspinatus, infraspinatus, teres minor, and subscapularis (SITS). Each of these tendons can be isolated by certain examination manuevers. The supraspinatus is tested by the **empty can test** (see Chapter 61 for a full description of these exam manuevers). Weakness and/or pain with resistance can indicate tendinopathy or tear. The infraspinatus and teres minor sit together in the posterior shoulder. Pain and/or weakness with **resisted external rotation** indicates pathology. Finally, the subscapularis tendon is the largest rotator cuff tendon and is the key to shoulder strength when weight lifting and internally rotating the arm. Weight lifters, tennis players, and swimmers are more likely to injure this muscle. The subscapularis is tested by the **liftoff test**.

10. What is a superior labrum anterior-to-posterior (SLAP) lesion?

SLAP lesions involve an injury to the superior glenoid labrum and the biceps anchor complex. The glenoid labrum is a cartilaginous lining of the glenoid (shoulder "socket"), which serves to deepen the glenoid resulting in increased stability of the shoulder. Injuries to the labrum that result in fraying or tears are often seen in overhead-throwing athletes. Symptoms may include a deep shoulder ache and painful popping or catching in the shoulder with overhead activities. Provocative tests are designed to elicit pain when the lesion is compressed and include the O'Brien active compression test, the crank test, and the clunk test. All have poor sensitivity and specificity. Magnetic resonance imaging (MRI) is the gold standard for diagnosis, with a sensitivity/specificity of over 90% in detecting SLAP lesions. Nonsurgical care includes NSAIDs, physical therapy, and rest followed by gradual return to activity. If nonsurgical therapy fails, surgical arthroscopy for diagnosis and repair may be considered.

11. What is a stinger (burner) injury?

The **stinger** is a well-known injury in football, resulting from forced deviation of the neck away from the inferiorly pulled ipsilateral shoulder. This occurs when tackling, blocking, or ground contact results in a traction injury to the cervical nerve roots, brachial plexus, or peripheral nerves. It can also occur in the workplace from a similar load to the head and neck, such as an object falling from above. The result is significant unilateral shoulder and arm "burning" pain involving the lateral aspect of the entire upper extremity. Motor weakness of the involved C5 and C6 root innervated muscles (deltoid, supraspinatus, biceps) is commonly associated. Stingers should be managed by rest and avoidance of sports participation or manual labor until pain has resolved and normal strength has returned. "Recurrent stingers" should be evaluated for cervical spinal stenosis, as this condition increases the risk of damage to the spinal cord during contact sports and activities.

12. How common are hip injuries in the athletic population?

Hip injuries make up 6% of all athletic injuries, with an increasing prevalence due to improvements in recognition and diagnosis. Recognition of these injuries (including strains, fractures, and impingement) is important, as their sequelae can have a lasting impact on an athlete's or manual laborer's career. Prompt identification and treatment in the acute setting may prevent long-term consequences. Because the hip joint is stabilized by multiple layers of protective anatomy, and supports six to eight times an individual's weight, injury is often the result of a great deal of force such as an impact or quick change in direction.

13. What is a hip pointer?

A **hip pointer** refers to a contusion of the iliac crest that occurs most often in contact sports including rugby, football, and ice hockey and makes up approximately 11% of hip injuries. This can also occur from a direct blow in the workplace. Physical exam reveals acute pain, swelling, and hematoma over the iliac crest that coincides with a history of impact to the area. Frequently, the individual will have difficulty weight-bearing. Treatment includes ice, analgesics, and a supervised stretching program with return to sport/occupation when symptoms allow.

14. What is a sports hernia?

A **sports hernia** is a general term for pain that localizes to the inguinal area of an athlete (or laborer) without evidence of a definite herniation. Confusion surrounds this diagnosis because physicians may use different terminology to describe this injury, including 'athletic pubalgia,' 'core muscle injury,' 'osteitis pubis,' or 'groin pain syndrome in the athlete.' Anatomically it is ill-defined and is attributed to tension placed on the inguinal structures including the rectus abdominis-adductor longus aponeurosis and the pubic tubercle or pubic symphysis, causing tearing and eliciting pain. The most commonly cited mechanism is increased tension in the groin due to high levels of twisting, turning, sprinting, or kicking. Physical examination findings are subtle, showing a dilated and tender superficial inguinal ring in the absence of a hernia and a tender pubic tubercle where the conjoined tendon inserts. A resisted situp may elicit pain at the pubic crest. Radiographs of the hip and pelvis are important to evaluate the osseous structures and rule out other causes of pain. MRI remains the primary tool in diagnosis. Conservative treatment including formal physical therapy should be attempted for up to 6 months. If unsuccessful, laparoscopic surgical repair (with possible nerve decompression) may be warranted.

15. How do swimmer's knee, jumper's knee, and runner's knee differ from each other?

Swimmer's knee (breaststroker's knee) is medial knee pain resulting from the valgus stress placed on the knee by the kick used in swimming the breaststroke. This usually results in a chronic strain of the medial collateral ligament (MCL).

Jumper's knee is an accepted term for **patellar tendinopathy.** It is common in high jumpers and volleyball or basketball players. This injury is characterized by pain at the inferior pole of the patella at its attachment to the patellar tendon. It occurs as a result of repetitive stress whose frequency of occurrence exceeds the body's rate of natural repair or healing.

Runner's knee is more correctly called **patellofemoral syndrome.** It presents as anterior knee pain, generally worsened by stairs and caused by dynamic valgus rather than any structural pathology of the cartilage. It is common in runners and more often found in women than men. Pain is caused by compression of nerve fibers in the retinaculum or in the subchondral bone of the patella, or from a secondary synovitis. This is one of the most common causes of knee pain.

16. List the differential diagnosis for anterior knee pain.

Historically there have been many catch-all terms for patients with anterior knee pain, but as research has progressed, the differential diagnosis has become more extensive.

Chondromalacia patellae	Symptomatic plica of the knee
Patellar malalignment or tracking abnormality	Fat pad syndrome (Hoffa disease)
Quadricep or patella tendinopathy	Bursitis, infrapatellar/prepatellar
Tight iliotibial band (ITB)	Pes anserine bursitis
Meniscal pathology	Blunt trauma, occult fracture
Osteochondritis dissecans (patella)	Referred pain from hip or lumbosacral spine

17. What common muscle imbalance can give rise to anterior knee pain?

Patellar maltracking resulting from a relative **weakness of the vastus medialis portion of the quadriceps and weakness of the hip abductors**. This maltracking leads to increased pressure on the patella and pain. With time, it can lead to chondromalacia. Tenderness over the medial patellar facet as an examination maneuver has the highest sensitivity for the diagnosis of patellofemoral pain. It is common in young adults and responds to directed strengthening of the quadriceps and hip abductors. Adjunctive modalities of oral NSAIDs and patellar centralizing bracing or taping can also be effective.

Other common conditions that affect the patella and give rise to anterior knee pain are true patellar malalignment, limb malrotation, and tendinopathy. Physicians should also evaluate the patient for pes planus with foot pronation to see if this is contributing to patellar maltracking. If present, foot orthotics can help the anterior knee pain.

18. **What physical examination tests are most sensitive and specific for the diagnosis of an anterior cruciate ligament injury (ACL)?**

The ACL is a crucial ligamentous stabilizer of the knee. A tear results from a twisting (valgus) or hyperextension injury. Greater than 50% of ACL ruptures are accompanied by a meniscal tear. Overall, female athletes are 2 to 10 times more likely to sustain an ACL injury than male athletes depending on the sport. This may be due to multiple factors including anatomy, hormones, and neuromuscular imbalance.

The best-known test for ACL deficiency is the **anterior drawer sign.** It is performed with the patient supine and the knee flexed to 90 degrees. With the hamstrings relaxed, the examiner grasps the proximal tibia with both hands and attempts to slide the tibia anteriorly while simultaneously stabilizing the patient's leg (can be accomplished by sitting on the foot). The degree of tibial translation is compared with the uninjured knee. This is a subjective test with the least sensitivity of all the tests for an ACL tear.

The most sensitive test is the **Lachman test.** With the thigh supported, muscles relaxed, and the femur stabilized by one of the examiner's hands, the knee is placed in 20 to 30 degrees of flexion, and the proximal tibia is then translated anteriorly by the examiner's other hand. ACL-deficient knees exhibit increased translation and a soft or absent endpoint as compared with the opposite, uninjured knee.

The most specific test is the **pivot shift test.** It is performed by applying a valgus and internal rotation force on the tibia with the knee in full extension and hip abducted 10 to 20 degrees. The knee is then gently flexed. A clunk of tibial rotation is appreciated as the knee passes 20 to 40 degrees of flexion. This must be compared with the opposite side. The appreciable clunk occurs when the tibia, which is abnormally subluxated (anterior and internally rotated), is pulled back into its normal position by the secondary restraints.

19. **How will a meniscal tear present, and is there a single best test for diagnosis?**

The meniscus functions as a cushion between the femur and tibia on the medial and lateral sides of the knee. It is well suited to compression but tears when subjected to shear stress with a turning or twisting motion. The blood supply of the inner two-thirds of the meniscus is limited, leading to poor healing of injured tissue and a typical course of chronic recurring symptoms. The torn tissue may create a mechanical block to the free motion of the knee, which will symptomatically manifest as clicking, popping, and locking, and is associated with pain and swelling at the joint line. These symptoms correlate, but often unreliably, to an audible/palpable pop with flexion/extension of the knee with the patient supine (**McMurray test**) and prone (**Apley test**) on physical examination. Joint line tenderness is one of the best clinical signs of a meniscal tear, but all of these tests should be combined with the history, as the presentation of a meniscal tear can be confused with patellofemoral pathology, particularly in the absence of a single precipitating event. MRI or arthroscopy reliably confirms diagnosis, and the problem is most efficiently remedied by arthroscopic repair or partial meniscectomy. Chronic degenerative meniscal tears can oftentimes be treated with physical therapy alone.

20. **What is the "terrible triad" of knee injury?**

An ACL tear, complete medial collateral ligament tear, accompanied by a meniscal tear. This combination is almost always a result of sporting activities, particularly a valgus impact to the knee with the foot firmly planted. The knee in these injuries exhibits a markedly positive anterior drawer test, a positive Lachman test and pivot shift test, and marked valgus angulation with applied stress in full extension. The knee will be stable to varus stress testing because the lateral collateral ligament and posterior cruciate ligament remain intact. Effusion from hemarthrosis may be mild secondary to medial capsular tearing, which allows the traumatic bleeding to exit the knee joint. Suspicion of an injury of this magnitude should lead to the prompt referral to an orthopedic surgeon and for advanced imaging (noncontrast MRI).

21. **What is the difference between a low ankle sprain and high ankle sprain?**

Ankle sprains are a very common injury in athletes and those in the workforce. The most common sprain is a low ankle sprain resulting from an inversion injury. The lateral ligaments (anterior talofibular and calcaneofibular) are the most commonly involved. An injury to the anterior tibiofibular syndesmosis is referred to as a "high ankle sprain" and is more severe and requires more time for recovery. Eversion injuries are less common but involve injury to the medial deltoid ligament. The goal of treatment is to prevent chronic pain and instability. Initially patients are treated with ice, NSAIDs, and a brace. When the patient can bear weight without increased pain (2–4 weeks), exercises are started to increase strength and prevent chronic instability.

22. Name two lower extremity tendons susceptible to overuse injuries occurring in runners.

- Achilles tendinopathy (see Chapter 61: Regional Musculoskeletal Disorders).
- Posterior tibialis tendinopathy (see Chapter 61: Regional Musculoskeletal Disorders).

23. What is the best treatment for acute rupture of the Achilles tendon?

Acute Achilles tendon rupture usually results from a forced contraction of the gastrocnemius muscle against resistance, which occurs either during sports participation or from a fall. It is not rare, and these are not subtle injuries. The patient usually has symptoms of pain, most notable in walking, and weakness in the pushoff phase of gait. A positive **Thompson test** is common, oftentimes with a palpable defect in the tendon.

The best treatment remains controversial. Options include closed treatment with placement in a long or short leg cast with the foot in equinus (plantar-flexed by gravity). Many long-term studies have compared surgical with nonsurgical treatment. The healing rate is excellent with both techniques. Some studies do show earlier and better restoration of calf strength with surgical intervention. Therefore, selection of the best treatment option is individualized, with age, activity level, patient and surgeon-specific factors, and experience as guiding parameters.

24. What is a "turf toe"?

Turf toe is a sprain of the plantar capsule ligament complex of the first metatarsophalangeal joint. It more commonly occurs on artificial turf and results from a hyperextension injury. Hyperflexion and valgus injuries to this toe can cause similar symptoms. Treatment includes rest, taping of the toe to restrict dorsiflexion, and stiffening of the sole of the shoe to prevent motion. Without proper therapy, hallux rigidus can result.

25. What is the most sensitive test for the diagnosis of a bone stress injury (stress reaction/stress fracture)?

A bone stress injury (stress reaction or stress fracture) is an overuse injury that occurs when periosteal resorption exceeds bone formation. The history is generally consistent with a recent increase in the level of training, followed by the insidious onset of pain. Patients at high risk of low bone density can develop bone stress injuries in the setting of relatively normal activity. The tibia is the most common site for bone stress injuries in runners (30%), but other areas can be affected depending on the activity or sport. Examination often reveals a focal area of tenderness along the bone. Percussion of the bone away from the site can cause pain at the fracture. The pain is increased if a vibrating 128-Hz tuning fork is placed on the site (75% sensitivity).

Plain radiographs are often negative. There is a large spectrum of bone stress injuries, and radiographs typically only show higher grade injuries. **MRI has the best sensitivity** to detect bone stress injuries and can help grade injury severity. Bone scans are uncommonly used for diagnosis, unless a patient has a contraindication to an MRI. Bone stress injuries that occur in high-risk locations (defined as an area with poor blood supply like the navicular, or areas under tension like the anterior tibia) should be referred to a specialist as they are more likely to progress to delayed union fractures or nonunion fractures, and may ultimately need surgical management.

26. What are the risk factors for recurrent bone stress injuries (stress reaction/stress fracture)?

Athletes with bone stress injuries should be questioned about symptoms consistent with '**relative energy deficiency in sport**' (REDs; the female and male 'athlete triad' are subsets of REDs). This may include a history of eating disorders or disordered eating, amenorrhea or fertility issues in women, sexual dysfunction in men, or a history of recurrent bone stress injuries. Patients with the risk factors described above should be referred for specialty evaluation, which may include nutrition consultation, sports psychology, endocrinology, and primary care sports medicine or orthopedics (due to the high risk of recurrent bone stress injuries and other complications).

Patients who have other risk factors for low bone density can also develop bone stress injuries. This includes patients with inflammatory arthritis, malabsorption, and chronic steroid use, among others. A dual-energy x-ray absorptiometry (DEXA) scan should be considered in patients with recurrent bone stress injuries or insufficiency fractures.

27. What are some hand injuries that can occur in athletes?

1. **Mallet finger.** Extensor tendon avulsion with or without fracture involving the distal interphalangeal (DIP) joint. The athlete cannot extend the DIP joint.
2. **Jersey finger.** Avulsion of the flexor digitorum profundus tendon causing inability to flex the DIP joint. Usually occurs from grabbing a jersey when tackling in football.
3. **Gamekeeper's or skier's thumb.** Rupture of the ulnar collateral ligament of the first metacarpophalangeal (MCP) joint. Frequent skiing injury.
4. **Boxer's knuckle.** Longitudinal tear of the extensor digitorum communis tendon or sagittal bands overlying the metacarpal head (usually the third MCP). Results in extensor weakness of the affected finger, and at times, painful extensor tendon subluxation.

28. How common are occupational overuse injuries?

Repetitive movements for prolonged periods of time can lead to overuse injuries in several professions, resulting in work-related disability and costing billions of dollars. Common injuries include bicipital tendinitis, rotator cuff tendonitis, carpal tunnel syndrome, and De Quervain tendinitis. For example, 10–20% of musicians, typists, keypunch/calculator/cash register operators, and assembly line workers will experience a repetitive strain syndrome. An analysis of surgeons and interventional physicians showed that the most common work-related overuse injuries in this population included degenerative cervical spine disease, rotator cuff pathology, degenerative lumbar spine disease, and carpal tunnel syndrome. Early diagnosis and preventative measures are key to decreasing the incidence of these injuries. It should be noted that there is much controversy and debate over the scientific evidence supporting the relationship between cumulative trauma/repetitive strain disorders and many occupations.

29. What occupations are associated with osteoarthritis?

Several occupations can cause stress and trauma to joints, leading to early osteoarthritis. This most likely occurs in joints that have been previously injured, have an abnormal joint alignment, or are unstable as a result of ligamentous injury. Examples include ballet dancers (ankle, feet); farmers (hips, knees); miners (elbow/knees/spine), riveters, or metalworkers (elbows); pneumatic tool operators (upper extremity joints); coal miners (knees); and cotton mill workers (hands). The relationship between osteoarthritis and sporting activities is less clear, owing to repeated joint injuries in addition to repetitive loading.

30. What medications are useful in occupational or sports-related injuries (and when should they be used)?

NSAIDs can be effective in reducing initial pain and swelling in acute injuries. More prolonged use is recommended for chronic overuse conditions; however, patients should be monitored closely for side effects. Corticosteroid injections for chronic conditions are not definitive treatment but can be used to facilitate rehabilitation. Injections should be performed by experienced clinicians who are familiar with their side effects. Corticosteroids can increase the rate of collagen degradation, decrease new collagen formation, lower tendon tensile strength, and lead to tendon rupture if the procedure is performed incorrectly or too often.

31. How can injuries be prevented?

Part of the responsibility of the physician is to educate the athlete or worker on how to prevent further injury. Just treating the acute or chronic injury is not enough. Emphasis should be placed on the importance of a dynamic warm-up before activities. Healthcare providers should also draw attention to the importance of stretching and range-of-motion exercises, which are typically more effective after the muscles have 'warmed up' through activity. Other measures include recommendations for limiting pitches in high school pitchers (varies by age), instructing female athletes in how to pivot, jump, and land to prevent ACL injuries, or having an ergonomic evaluation of a patient's worksite.

ACKNOWLEDGMENT

The authors would like to acknowledge the contributions of Drs. Donald Eckhoff, Rebecca Griffith and Armando Vidal, who were the authors of this chapter in previous editions.

BIBLIOGRAPHY

Amin NH, Kumar NS, Schickendantz MS. Medial epicondylitis: evaluation and management. *J Am Acad Orthop Surg*. 2015;23(6):348–355.

Chen ET, Borg-Stein J, McInnis KC. Ankle sprains: evaluation, rehabilitation, and prevention. *Curr Sports Med Rep*. 2019;18(6):217–223 JunErratum in: Curr Sports Med Rep. 2019 Aug;18(8):310.

Cheung EC, Boguszewski DV, Joshi NB, et al. Anatomic factors that may predispose female athletes to anterior cruciate ligament injury. *Curr Sports Med Rep*. 2015;14(5):368–372.

Crossley KM, Callaghan MJ. Patellofemoral pain. *Br J Sports Med*. 2016;50(4):247–250.

Egger AC, Berkowitz MJ. Achilles tendon injuries. *Curr Rev Musculoskelet Med*. 2017;10(1):72–80.

Epstein S, Sparer EH, Tran BN, et al. Prevalence of work-related musculoskeletal disorders among surgeons and interventionalists: a systematic review and meta-analysis. *JAMA Surg*. 2018;153(2):e174947.

Flato R, Passanante GJ, Skalski MR, et al. The iliotibial tract: imaging, anatomy, injuries, and other pathology. *Skeletal Radiol*. 2017;46(5):605–622.

Forlizzi JM, Ward MB, Whalen J, et al. Core muscle injury: evaluation and treatment in the athlete. *Am J Sports Med*. 2023;51(4):1087–1095.

Fredericson M, Bergman AG, Hoffman KL, et al. Tibial stress reaction in runners. Correlation of clinical symptoms and scintigraphy with a new magnetic resonance imaging grading system. *Am J Sports Med*. 1995;23:472–481.

George E, Harris AH, Dragoo JL, et al. Incidence and risk factors for turf toe injuries in intercollegiate football: data from the National Collegiate Athletic Association Injury surveillance System. *Foot Ankle Int*. 2014;35(2):108–115.

Hall M, Anderson J. Hip pointers. *Clin Sports Med*. 2013;32(2):325–330.

Hopkins JN, Brown W, Lee CA. Sports hernia: definition, evaluation, and treatment. *JBJS Rev*. 2017;5(9):e6.

Hunt KJ, Phisitkul P, Pirolo J, et al. High ankle sprains and syndesmotic injuries in athletes. *J Am Acad Orthop Surg*. 2015;23(11):661–673.

Iqbal ZA, Alghadir AH. Cumulative trauma disorders: a review. *J Back Musculoskelet Rehabil*. 2017;30(4):663–666.

Kasitinon D, Li WX, Wang EXS, et al. Physical examination and patellofemoral pain syndrome: an updated review. *Curr Rev Musculoskelet Med*. 2021;14:406–412.

Lynch TS, Bedi A, Larson CM. Athletic hip injuries. *J Am Acad Orthop Surg*. 2017;25(4):269–279.

Makhmalbaf H, Moradi A, Ganji S, et al. Accuracy of Lachman and anterior drawer tests for anterior cruciate ligament injuries. *Arch Bone Joint Surg*. 2013;1(2):94–97.

Millar NL, Silbernagel KG, Thorborg K, et al. Tendinopathy. *Nat Rev Dis Primers*. 2021;7(1):1 Jan 7Erratum in: *Nat Rev Dis Primers*. 2021 Feb 3;7(1):10.

Morelli KM, Brown LB, Warren GL. Effect of NSAID on recovery from acute skeletal muscle injury: a systematic review and meta-analysis. *Am J Sports Med*. 2017;46(1):224–233.

Mountjoy M, Ackerman KE, Bailey DM, et al. 2023 International Olympic Committee's (IOC) consensus statement on Relative Energy Deficiency in Sport (REDs). *Br J Sports Med*. 2023;57(17):1073–1097.

Pulos N, Kakar S. Hand and wrist injuries: common problems and solutions. *Clin Sports Med*. 2018;37(2):217–243.

Roos KG, Marshall SW, Kerr ZY, et al. Epidemiology of overuse injuries in collegiate and high school athletics in the United States. *Am J Sports Med*. 2015;43(7):1790–1797.

Saunier J, Chapurlat R. Stress fracture in athletes. *Joint Bone Spine*. 2018;85(3):307–310.

Shah S, Thomas AC, Noone JM, et al. Incidence and cost of ankle sprains in United States Emergency Departments. *Sports Health*. 2016;8(6):547–552.

Smucny M, Kolmodin J, Saluan P. Shoulder and elbow injuries in the adolescent athlete. *Sports Med Arthrosc Rev*. 2016;24(4):188–194.

Weber S, Chahal J. Management of rotator cuff injuries. *J Am Acad Orthop Surg*. 2020;28(5):e193–e201.

Wolf JM. Lateral epicondylitis. *N Engl J Med*. 2023;388(25):2371–2377.

FURTHER READING

https://orthoinfo.aaos.org/.
https://www.sportsmedtoday.com.

CHAPTER 63

Entrapment Neuropathies

Lisa Davis, MD, MsCS

 KEY POINTS

1. Entrapment neuropathies occur due to compression of nerves in a narrow anatomic path, or due to compression and/or traction, which causes ischemia and damage to the axon, connective tissue, and the nerve itself.
2. Carpal tunnel syndrome (CTS) is the most common entrapment neuropathy.
3. Knowledge of anatomy and predisposing factors is necessary for the accurate diagnosis of entrapment neuropathies.
4. Most entrapment neuropathies of short duration can be treated conservatively.

1. What are the patterns of pain and nerve damage, and how does this help with the diagnosis of the condition?

Pain falls into three broad categories: **nociceptive pain** (pain due to tissue disease or damage**), neuropathic pain** (pain caused by disease or damage to the somatosensory system), and **mixed pain** (the coexistence of both nociceptive and neuropathic pain). Damage to nerves should be further categorized by the pattern of distribution— peripheral or central, symmetric or asymmetric, large or small fibers; small fiber neuropathies can be further divided into somatic fibers, autonomic fibers, or both. Additionally, the temporality of the damage (acute or insidious) and whether the damage affects sensory function, motor function, or both should be noted. By assessing the patterns and distributions of temporality, pain, and malfunction, the diagnosis can be narrowed and the appropriate treatment prescribed.

2. What are entrapment neuropathies, and how do they occur?

Entrapment neuropathies are classically defined as occurring due to external compression of a peripheral nerve within a narrow anatomic path. However, the definition of entrapment neuropathies has since been expanded to encompass damage due to other forms of compression. For example, metabolically compromised nerves (such as from diabetes, hypothyroidism, or alcoholism) are more vulnerable to external compression, not only in narrow anatomic paths. Entrapment neuropathy injuries result from compression and/or traction, causing ischemia and damage to the axon, connective tissue, and the nerve itself. Nerve damage is characterized by physiologic slowing, demyelination, and remyelination. Entrapment neuropathies occur in peripheral nerves, are typically asymmetric, occur in large fibers, may occur acutely or insidiously, and may impact sensory and/or motor fibers.

3. What are the classifications of nerve injuries and what are the typical findings?

Seddon was the first to classify nerve injuries into three categories based on the presence of demyelination and the extent of damage to the axons and other connective tissues. This classification was expanded by Sunderland (Table 63.1). The mildest form of damage, **neurapraxia** (*neur-* meaning "nerve" and *-apraxia* from Greek meaning "the total or partial loss of the ability to perform coordinated movements"), can occur from mild compression or from mild traction to the nerve. This results in focal, segmental demyelination without damage to the axon or to connective tissues of the nerve. Neurapraxia can result in conduction slowing and gain of function symptoms. If the compression continues or the traction injury is more severe, **axonotmesis** (*axono-* meaning "axon" and *-tmesis* from Latin and Greek meaning "to cut") may occur. This results in damage to the axon with focal demyelination, while the nerve's connective tissues are maintained. Axonotmesis will result in loss of function symptoms. If the injury is severe enough, **neurotmesis** (meaning transection of the nerve) may occur.

TABLE 63.1 Classification of Nerve Injury

SEDDON	SUNDERLAND	INJURY TYPE	PATHOLOGY FINDINGS	EMG FINDINGS	DURATION OF SYMPTOMS/ PROGNOSIS
Neurapraxia	Grade I	Mild compression or traction resulting in transient ischemia or paranodal demyelination	Focal, segmental demyelination without damage to axons or connective tissues	Decrease in conduction velocity. No denervation on EMG. Focal demyelination confirmed by nerve conduction preservation below the injury	Transient; recovery in a few weeks
Axonotmesis	Grade II		Axon is damaged, but endoneurium is intact		
Axonotmesis	Grade III	Closed crush or traction injury	Axon and endoneurium are damaged, but epineurium is intact.	Denervation seen on EMG.	Recovery is slow, occurring in a proximal to distal pattern. Requires months and may be incomplete
Axonotmesis	Grade IV		Axon, endoneurium, and epineurium are damaged, but the epineurium is intact.		
Neurotmesis	Grade V	Closed crush injury, severe traction, or laceration	The nerve is transected	Denervation seen on EMG. Nerve conduction is not seen below the lesion	Prognosis is poor without surgical intervention

4. Describe characteristic clinical features of entrapment neuropathies.

Gain of function in entrapment neuropathies results in abnormal excitability or reduced inhibition of the peripheral nerve. Symptoms may include:

- Paresthesia
- Spontaneous pain
- Hyperalgesia
- Allodynia

Loss of function indicates reduced impulse conduction; symptoms may include:

- Hypoesthesia or anesthesia
- Muscle weakness and atrophy are late findings and indicate denervation.

Other important points:

- Symptoms are typically worse at night (often due to lack of distraction and poor positioning)
- Symptoms are often unilateral, except for idiopathic CTS
- Swelling or vasomotor abnormalities are absent

- While these symptoms of entrapment neuropathies may occur in specific patterns associated with the nerve affected, there is evidence that symptoms may occur outside of the nerve distribution. This may be due to neuroinflammation in peripheral nerve injuries caused by immune cells recruited to the site and/or by the large variability and overlap of dermatomes in individuals.

5. Do entrapment neuropathies occur in rheumatoid arthritis (RA)?

Inflammation and swelling of synovium, bursae, ligaments, or tendon sheaths can cause pressure on adjacent nerves. Entrapment neuropathies have been reported to occur in nearly half of patients with chronic RA at some point in their lifetime. There does not appear to be any correlation with duration of disease, positive rheumatoid factor, level of acute-phase reactants, functional class, or extra-articular disease. CTS occurs with a reported frequency of 23–69% in RA. Entrapment neuropathies can occur in all causes of inflammatory arthritis (e.g., psoriatic arthritis).

6. What are some other etiologies that should be considered when evaluating entrapment neuropathies?

- Polyneuropathies
- Radiculopathies
- Plexopathies
- Complex regional pain syndrome (CRPS)
- Mononeuritis multiplex: due to diabetes, vasculitis, amyloidosis
- Infectious etiologies: due to Lyme disease (*Borrelia burgdorferi*), leprosy (*Mycobacterium leprae* or *Mycobacterium lepromatosis*)
- Inflammatory etiology: *Lewis–Sumner syndrome* (also known as multifocal acquired demyelinating sensory and motor neuropathy, an inflammatory condition that leads to demyelination of the nerves in the upper extremities), *multifocal motor neuropathy with conduction block* (a variant of chronic inflammatory demyelinating polyneuropathy with subacute onset of asymmetric weakness without sensory symptoms), *sensory perineuritis* (a pure sensory form of mononeuritis multiplex with focal thickening of the perineurium, often associated with systemic diseases), *Parsonage-Turner Syndrome/Brachial Plexitis* (thought to be an inflammatory syndrome affecting long thoracic nerve)
- Hereditary etiology: Charcot-Marie-Tooth types 1 and 2, Hereditary neuropathy with liability to pressure palsies

7. How are entrapment neuropathies usually diagnosed?

The presence of characteristic symptoms (peripheral nerve involvement in a certain distribution with sensory and/or motor symptoms) along with provocative maneuvers (e.g., Tinel sign) is usually adequate to support the diagnosis. Electrodiagnostic studies (nerve conduction velocities and electromyography) are often used to confirm and localize the site of entrapment, although this study can be normal in 10–25% of patients who have a definite entrapment neuropathy.

8. When are electrodiagnostic studies indicated?

- When the diagnosis is uncertain; however, clinical suspicion should take precedence as even those with clinically apparent entrapment neuropathies can have normal electrodiagnostic studies.
- To exclude radiculopathy or polyneuropathy
- To follow the course of patients being treated conservatively
- Before surgery

9. What are some common entrapment neuropathies? (see Table 63.2)

- Median nerve entrapment: carpal tunnel syndrome (CTS), anterior interosseous nerve (AIN) syndrome, pronator teres syndrome (PTS)
- Ulnar nerve entrapment: cubital tunnel syndrome (CuTS), Guyon's canal syndrome (GCS)/ulnar tunnel syndrome/handlebar palsy
- Thoracic outlet syndrome (TOS)

TABLE 63.2 Common Entrapment Neuropathies

ENTRAPMENT NEUROPATHY	NERVE INVOLVED	STRUCTURES INVOLVED	COMMON CAUSES/ PREDISPOSED INDIVIDUALS	SYMPTOMS
Carpal tunnel syndrome	Median nerve	Carpal tunnel	Occupation with high levels of repetition and force, metabolically compromised nerves, swelling, synovitis	Sensory or mixed
Anterior interosseus nerve syndrome	Median nerve: anterior interosseus nerve branch	Pronator teres	Trauma, muscle variations	Motor
Pronator teres syndrome	Median nerve	Pronator teres	Those with repetitive grasping and pronating movements such as carpenters, tennis players	Sensory, motor, or mixed
Cubital tunnel syndrome	Ulnar nerve	Cubital tunnel	Trauma, truck drivers, prolonged phone-to-ear use	Mixed
Guyon's canal syndrome/ ulnar tunnel syndrome/ handlebar palsy	Ulnar nerve	Guyon's canal or ulnar tunnel	Trauma, cyclists, basketball players, golf players, racket sports players	Sensory, motor, or mixed
Thoracic outlet syndrome	Brachial plexus	Thoracic outlet	Cervical rib, muscle abnormalities, congenital bands, clavicular fracture, sports with repetitive overhead movements	Mixed
Crutch palsy	Radial nerve	Axilla	Improper use of crutches	Mixed
Saturday night palsy	Radial nerve	Radial groove of the humerus	Inebriation, improper placement in anesthesia	Motor or mixed
Posterior interosseous nerve syndrome	Radial nerve: posterior interosseous nerve branch	Elbow	Trauma, violin players	Motor or mixed
Suprascapular nerve entrapment	Suprascapular nerve	Suprascapular notch	Ganglion cysts, scapular injury, carrying heavy loads on the shoulder	Mixed
Meralgia paresthetica /lateral femoral cutaneous syndrome	Lateral femoral cutaneous nerve		Obesity/tight clothes, trauma	Sensory
Sciatic compression neuropathy	Sciatic nerve	Multiple sites within the pelvis and gluteal compartment	Overuse (running, cycling), oversized wallet in the back pocket ("fat wallet syndrome"), weak gluteal muscles	Mixed

TABLE 63.2 Common Entrapment Neuropathies—cont'd

ENTRAPMENT NEUROPATHY	NERVE INVOLVED	STRUCTURES INVOLVED	COMMON CAUSES/ PREDISPOSED INDIVIDUALS	SYMPTOMS
Common fibular nerve palsy / peroneal nerve palsy	Common fibular (peroneal) nerve	Fibular head	Prolonged immobilization, habitual leg crossing	Motor or mixed
Tarsal tunnel syndrome	Tibial nerve	Tarsal tunnel	Valgus deformity, inflammatory arthritis, hypermobility	Mixed
Interdigital neuropathy/Morton's neuroma	Interdigital plantar nerve	Transverse metatarsal ligament	Hallux valgus deformities, tight-fitting shoes, high heels	Sensory

- Radial nerve entrapment: crutch palsy, Saturday night palsy, posterior interosseous nerve (PIN) palsy
- Suprascapular nerve (SSN) entrapment
- Meralgia paresthetica (MP)/lateral femoral cutaneous syndrome
- Sciatic compression neuropathy
- Common fibular nerve (CFN) palsy/peroneal nerve palsy
- Tarsal tunnel syndrome (TTS)
- Interdigital neuropathy/Morton's neuroma

10. What is carpal tunnel syndrome (CTS)?

CTS is easily the most common entrapment neuropathy, with a prevalence of 0.2% to 1%. Nine flexor tendons and the median nerve pass through the carpal tunnel, which is narrowest at its mid-portion. CTS occurs when the median nerve is compressed by the flexor retinaculum/ transverse carpal ligament at the wrist, producing characteristic nocturnal dysesthesias (70%), but occasionally progressing to sensory loss and weakness of thumb abduction (motor function) (Fig. 63.1). Pain can radiate into the proximal arm (40%). This condition is bilateral in half of patients and occurs with increased frequency in occupations associated with high levels of repetition and force (meatpackers, shellfish packing, and musicians). Additionally, patients with more metabolically compromised nerves (diabetics, alcoholics) or those experiencing more swelling (pregnancy) or synovitis (RA) are at increased risk.

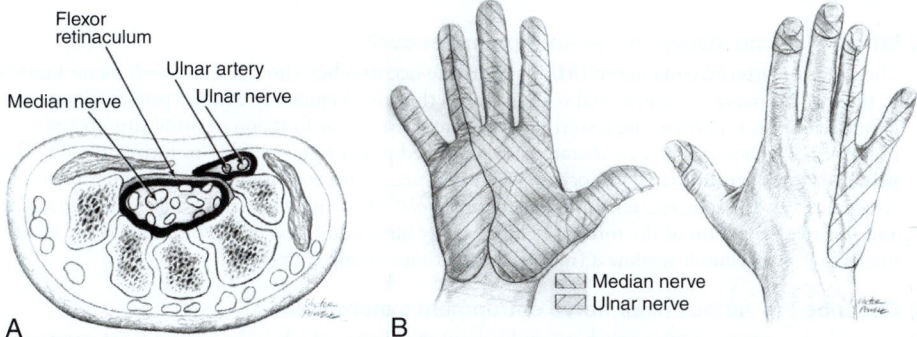

Fig. 63.1 (A) Wrist anatomy showing the median nerve through the carpal tunnel in close proximity to Guyon's canal, where the ulnar nerve passes. (B) Median and ulnar nerve sensory distributions. (Illustration by Victor Powell.)

11. Describe physical examination signs indicative of CTS. How do they compare with other diagnostic testing?

In CTS, numbness commonly affects the index, middle, and radial sides of the ring finger. The thumb is less often symptomatic. A positive Tinel sign occurs when tapping the nerve at the site of entrapment produces pain and dysesthesias radiating into the sensory distribution of the nerve distally. (A point of clarification—a positive Tinel sign may be obtained at many sites of entrapment; it is not limited to the carpal tunnel.) In CTS, this test has a pooled sensitivity of 50% and specificity of 77%. Phalen test is positive when passive wrist flexion to 90 degrees for one minute produces or worsens paresthesias in the median nerve distribution. It has a pooled sensitivity of 68% and specificity of 73% for CTS. The direct median nerve compression test is positive when pain and paresthesias occur within 30 seconds of pressure exerted over the carpal tunnel by the examiner's thumb. The "volar hot dog" (swelling at the wrist on the ulnar side of the palmaris longus tendon) has been reported in over 90% of patients with CTS. In addition to provocative maneuvers, two-point discrimination (sensitivity 25%, specificity 90%), grip strength, and thenar muscle function and atrophy should be examined. Electrodiagnostic studies have a sensitivity of 85% and specificity of 95% for CTS. Ultrasonography and magnetic resonance imaging (MRI) can be useful in patients with equivocal electrodiagnostic studies.

12. List some diseases associated with CTS.

Use the mnemonic **PRAGMATIC.**
Pregnancy (20%)
RA (any inflammatory arthritis)
Acromegaly
Glucose (diabetes)
Mechanical (overuse, occupational)
Amyloid
Thyroid (myxedema)
Infection (tuberculosis, fungal)
Crystals (gout, pseudogout)

13. What are the treatment options for CTS?

Nonsurgical therapy consists of avoidance of repetitive wrist motion, cock-up wrist splints at night (and for work), along with anti-inflammatory medications. Ergonomic evaluation of the patient's workplace may be beneficial. In patients with less than six months of symptoms, a local corticosteroid injection results in excellent short-term relief in 80% of cases. Indications for **surgical therapy** (sectioning of the transverse carpal ligament) include failure of conservative therapy, lifestyle-limiting symptoms, and muscle weakness or atrophy. Long-term surgical results are favorable in over 75% of patients. Complete recovery of nerve function occurs only if surgery is performed before evidence of denervation on electromyography/nerve conduction velocity.

14. Where else can median nerve entrapment occur?

The **anterior interosseous nerve (AIN) syndrome** occurs when this nerve, a *purely motor* branch of the median nerve, is compressed 6 cm distal to the lateral epicondyle in the pronator teres. While sensation is normal, the resulting loss/decrease of motor function of distal thumb and index finger flexion produces a characteristic flattened pinch sign (inability to form an "O"). The **pronator teres syndrome (PTS)** occurs when the median nerve is compressed by the pronator teres muscle at the forearm, resulting in proximal volar forearm pain that is worsened by grasping and resistive pronation of the forearm. Patients may have numbness of the thumb and the index finger (sensory), thumb weakness (motor), and writer's cramp (mixed).

15. Describe the various ulnar nerve entrapment syndromes.

Ulnar nerve compression at (or above and below) the elbow, which is the second most common entrapment neuropathy of the upper extremity, can occur from external pressure at the medial epicondylar groove (due to synovitis, osteophytes, anesthetized patients with prolonged resting of the elbow on a flat surface), flexion dislocation, and/or compression at the aponeurosis of the flexor carpi ulnaris (Osborne's ligament), the so-called cubital tunnel (Fig. 63.2). **Cubital tunnel**

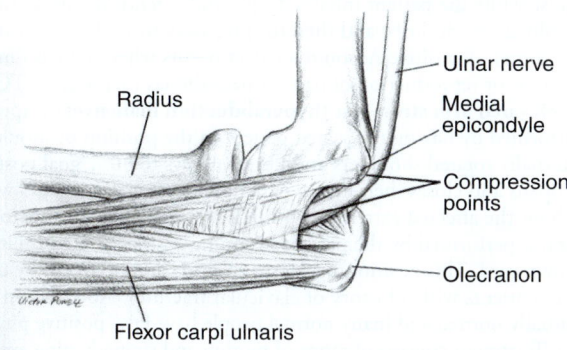

Radius

Ulnar nerve

Medial epicondyle

Compression points

Olecranon

Flexor carpi ulnaris

Fig. 63.2 Anatomy of the ulnar nerve at the elbow showing sites of common entrapment at the medial epicondyle and the cubital tunnel. (Illustration by Victor Powell.)

syndrome (CuTS) results in paresthesias in an ulnar nerve distribution (the little finger and ulnar side of the ring finger), weakness in grasping and pinching, catching the little finger on the edge of the pants' pocket when putting the hand into the pocket (weak interossei and finger adduction), and hypothenar atrophy. The most sensitive provocative test for CuTS (91%) is direct pressure over the ulnar nerve posterior to the medial epicondyle while the elbow is in flexion. Other provocative tests include Tinel sign over the cubital tunnel and the elbow flexion test (where the elbow is held in full flexion and the wrist is extended, and a positive test is paresthesia/pain while in this position for one minute or less). Therapy consists of avoidance of prolonged elbow flexion, local steroid injections (in RA), and surgical release in severe cases. A patient may develop ulnar neuropathy months to years after trauma to the cubital tunnel (usually after an elbow fracture), which is referred to as **tardy ulnar palsy**.

Guyon canal syndrome, ulnar tunnel syndrome, or "handlebar palsy" occurs when the ulnar nerve is compressed near or in Guyon's canal (also known as the ulnar tunnel), which is a space formed by the pisiform bone and the hook of the hamate at the wrist (Fig. 63.1). As the ulnar nerve passes through Guyon's canal, it splits into the deep motor branch (which innervates the majority of the medial intrinsic hand muscles) and the superficial sensory branch (which innervates the palmar surface of digit five and the medial side of digit four). Depending upon where the nerve compression occurs (zone 1 is proximal to the bifurcation of the nerve, zone 2 surrounds the deep motor branch, and zone 3 surrounds the superficial sensory branch), the clinical presentation can be mixed, purely motor, or purely sensory, respectively. Direct pressure over Guyon's canal causes paresthesias.

16. What is thoracic outlet syndrome (TOS)?

TOS, which is often difficult to diagnose, can occur from neurologic (95% of cases) or vascular (5% of cases) compression (arterial or venous). TOS is most likely to occur in patients who have had trauma (clavicular fracture), repetitive strain injury (poor ergonomics at desk worksite), sports-related activities (overhead sports such as baseball pitchers, swimmers, volleyball, etc.), or anatomic abnormalities (cervical rib, Pancoast tumor). **Neurogenic TOS** occurs when there is brachial plexus impingement from a cervical rib (35%), fibrous tissue bands, scalene muscles, or an elongated transverse process of C7. Symptoms of neurogenic TOS include neck pain, arm pain, paresthesias, sensory loss in the ulnar distribution over the hand and forearm, hand weakness, arm weakness, and shoulder weakness. **Arterial TOS** occurs when compression of the subclavian artery results in ischemic symptoms, including pain, pallor, claudication, paresthesias, and coldness. **Venous TOS** results in severe upper extremity edema, cyanosis, and deep upper extremity pain. Paget–Schroetter syndrome is form of venous TOS caused by thrombosis of the subclavian vein.

Provocative tests for neurogenic TOS have variable sensitivity and specificity and should be used for diagnosis with caution. The **Adson maneuver** is performed with the patient in a sitting position with their elbow fully extended and the shoulder in 30° of abduction. The examiner palpates the radial pulse while the patient inhales deeply and extends the neck, turning the head to the side being examined (cervical rib) and then turning away from the side being examined (scalenus anticus syndrome). A positive Adson maneuver occurs when there is diminution of the radial pulse (arterial TOS) or reproduction of pain or paresthesias (neurogenic TOS). Another provocation test, the **elevated arm stress test (hyperabduction maneuver)** is specific for neurogenic TOS and is performed by having the seated patient in the position of shoulder abduction to 90°, with fully externally rotated shoulders and flexed elbows to 90° ("goal post arms"). The patient then rapidly opens and closes their fists; a patient with neurogenic TOS will have rapid onset of pain throughout the affected extremity within 20–30 seconds. The **costoclavicular maneuver** is another test performed by the patient assuming an exaggerated military posture with shoulder back and downward. This positioning causes compression between the clavicle and first rib (may be positive in patients with a history of clavicular fracture). Note that in TOS, electrodiagnostic studies are usually normal and many normal people have false-positive physical examination provocation tests. Treatment consists of range of motion and strengthening exercises to improve posture, avoidance of hyperabduction, botulinum toxin injections, and surgery for those patients with severe, refractory symptoms (cervical rib or fibrous band resection).

17. How does radial nerve entrapment occur?

The radial nerve runs in the posterior compartment of the spiral groove of the humerus, and then wraps anteriorly to the distal aspect of the humerus. At the elbow, the radial nerve divides into a deep motor branch (the posterior interosseus nerve, PIN) and a superficial sensory branch. Improper positioning during anesthesia, sleeping (or lying) on the arm, or improperly fitting crutches can result in prolonged compression of the nerve along its pathway. Compression in the axilla results in **crutch palsy,** while compression at the posterior upper arm (at the spiral groove) results in **Saturday night palsy**. It is classically described as an intoxicated patient falling asleep with the arm outstretched on the arm of a chair and resulting in acute weakness of the wrist and finger extensors (wrist drop and finger drop). Weakness is often severe, with up to one-third having complete paralysis; most patients recover after two to three months. Sensory symptoms are less common than weakness. The **PIN,** a motor branch of the radial nerve, can be impinged at the elbow (e.g. RA synovitis) resulting in finger extension weakness and partial weakness of wrist extension. There may be sensory loss in the dorsal lateral hand.

18. How does a patient with suprascapular nerve (SSN) entrapment present?

The **SSN** innervates the supraspinatus and infraspinatus muscles. The nerve can become compressed in the suprascapular notch usually from carrying heavy loads on the shoulder. Patients have pain over the posterior and lateral shoulder with weakness on abduction and external rotation of the shoulder. Atrophy of the supraspinatus muscle can occur. Electromyography can confirm the diagnosis. Physical therapy, local corticosteroid injection, or surgical decompression can be helpful.

19. What is meralgia paresthetica?

Meralgia (Greek for "pain in the thigh") **paresthetica** results when the lateral femoral cutaneous nerve of the thigh, a sensory nerve, is compressed at the inguinal ligament just medial to the anterior superior iliac spine. This syndrome results in burning pain and dysesthesia over the anterolateral thigh (Fig. 63.3). Direct pressure of the nerve where it exits the pelvis can increase symptoms. Common causes include obesity, pregnancy, trauma, surgical injury (appendectomy or inguinal herniorrhaphy), tight-fitting clothing (belts), and diabetes mellitus. This syndrome is usually self-limiting, and treatment is conservative, involving weight loss, avoidance of tight clothing, and occasional local steroid injections at the site of compression.

20. Describe sciatic compression neuropathy.

The sciatic nerve is the longest nerve in humans, and injury can occur at multiple sites along its course. **Sciatic compression neuropathy (SCN)** is characterized by pain and/or dysesthesias in the buttock, hip, and posterior thigh caused by compression of the sciatic nerve. Within the pelvis, sciatic neuropathy may occur due to surgeries, vaginal birth, neoplasms, etc. At the level of the gluteal compartment, the sciatic nerve can be trapped by the piriformis muscle (piriformis syndrome), gluteal contractures, hamstring muscles, vascular lesions, fibrovascular lesions (from

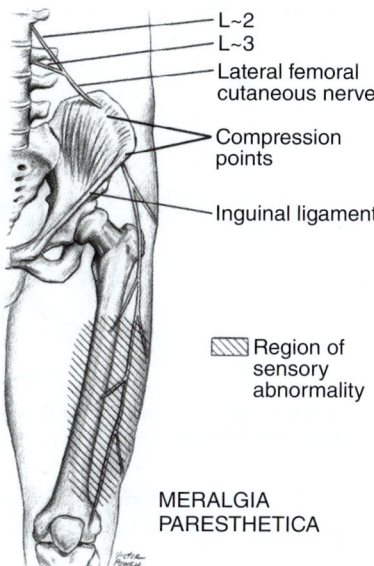

L~2
L~3
Lateral femoral
cutaneous nerve

Compression
points

Inguinal ligament

Region of
sensory
abnormality

MERALGIA
PARESTHETICA

Fig. 63.3 Anatomy of the lateral femoral cutaneous nerve. The inguinal ligament and the anterior superior iliac spine are the most likely points of entrapment. (Illustration by Victor Powell.)

trauma), and space-occupying lesions. **Piriformis syndrome** may arise from overuse injury (running, bicycling), weak gluteal muscles, and compression by an oversized wallet ("fat wallet syndrome"). Symptoms include pain over the buttocks (50–95%) radiating down the back of the leg and aggravation of pain with sitting (39–97%). It occurs more commonly in women and is usually precipitated by trauma. Physical examination reveals external tenderness over the greater sciatic notch (59–92%) and buttock pain on resisted hip abduction and external rotation when the patient is seated (32–74%). With the patient supine, buttock pain with hip flexion, adduction, and internal rotation (FAIR) is also seen along with the tenderness of the piriformis muscle on rectal or vaginal examination. Physical therapy (lateral stretching and strengthening), nonsteroidal anti-inflammatory drugs, local steroid injections, and botulinum toxin injections can be beneficial. Nerve compression from a herniated disc or facet arthropathy may cause symptoms similar to SCN and should always be ruled out.

21. Which nerve is most likely to be compressed in a patient with a painless foot drop?

The common fibular nerve (CFN), is also known as the peroneal nerve. **CFN palsy** usually occurs following compression over the head of the fibula from prolonged leg crossing, squatting, leg casts, and braces. The distal lateral leg often has decreased sensation and decreased foot eversion (superficial peroneal nerve) and dorsiflexion (deep peroneal nerve; footdrop) is affected because the lesion occurs proximally in the common peroneal nerve.

22. Describe tarsal tunnel syndrome.

The **tarsal tunnel syndrome** occurs when the posterior tibial nerve is compressed at the flexor retinaculum, located posterior and inferior to the medial malleolus (Fig. 63.4). Patients often have a burning dysesthesia of the toes and sole of the foot that extends proximally to the medial malleolus and is often improved by walking. A positive Tinel sign (obtained by percussing posterior to the medial malleolus) and a positive tourniquet test (applying pressure over the flexor retinaculum) will often reproduce the symptoms. Holding the ankle for 10 seconds in dorsiflexion and eversion will also exacerbate symptoms. This occurs more often in women and is associated with trauma, fracture, valgus deformity, hypermobility, inflammatory arthritis (up to 25%

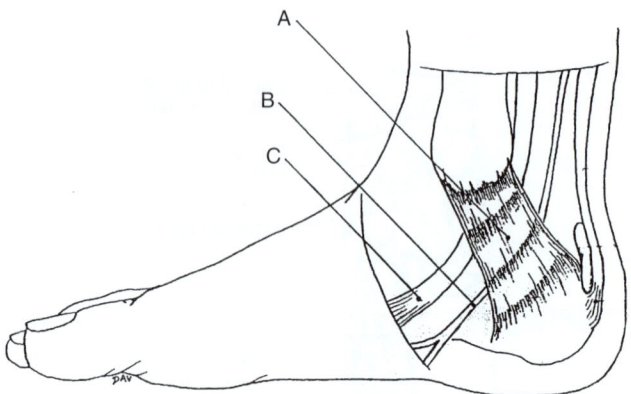

Fig. 63.4 Diagram showing the posterior tibial nerve (B) and posterior tibialis tendon (C) as they descend inferior to the medial malleolus and underneath the flexor retinaculum (A). (Illustration by Debra Vogelgesang.)

of patients with RA), diabetes, and occupational factors. Treatment consists of anti-inflammatory medications, local steroid injection, and orthotics. Surgical release is indicated when conservative measures fail.

23. What is Morton's neuroma?

Morton's neuroma is perineural fibrosis of the interdigital plantar nerve caused by entrapment of the nerve most commonly by the transverse metatarsal ligament, usually located between the third and fourth or second and third metatarsal heads. This occurs more commonly in people who wear tight-fitting shoes or high heels. Patients complain of dysesthesias between the two toes and state that they feel like they are walking on a marble or wrinkled sock. Metatarsal compression may cause a palpable click **(Mulder click)** as the neuroma is forced downward, where it may be felt on the plantar surface. Ultrasound and MRI can confirm the diagnosis. Treatment consists of wearing more supportive shoes, padding the metatarsal heads, and local steroid injections. Surgical removal is done if conservative therapy fails.

ACKNOWLEDGMENT

The author would like to acknowledge the contributions of Dr. David R. Finger, who was the author of this chapter in a previous edition.

BIBLIOGRAPHY

Baron R, Binder A, Wasner G. Neuropathic pain: diagnosis, pathophysiological mechanisms, and treatment. *Lancet Neurol*. 2010;9:807–826.
Dy CJ, Mackinnon SE. Ulnar neuropathy: evaluation and management. *Curr Rev Musculoskelet Med*. 2016;9:178–184.
Faktorovich S, Filatov A, Rizvi Z. Common compression neuropathies. *Clin Geriatr Med*. 2021;37:241–252.
Gilchrist JM, Dandapat S. Neuromuscular mimics of entrapment neuropathies of upper extremities. *Hand*. 2020;15:599–607.
Manoharan D, Sudhakaran D, Goyal A, Srivastava DN, Ansari MT. Clinico-radiological review of peripheral entrapment neuropathies—part 1 upper limb. *Eur J Radiol*. 2020;131:109234.
Manoharan D, Sudhakaran D, Goyal A, Srivastava DN, Ansari MT. Clinico-radiological review of peripheral entrapment neuropathies—part 2 lower limb. *Eur J Radiol*. 2021;135:109482.
Menorca RMG, Fussell TS, Elfar JC. Nerve physiology. Mechanisms of injury and recovery. *Hand Clin*. 2013;29:317–330.
Panther EJ, Reintgen CD, Cueto RJ, Hao KA, Chim H, King JJ. Thoracic outlet syndrome: a review. *J Shoulder Elb Surg*. 2022;31:e545–e561.
Schmid AB, Fundaun J, Tampin B. Entrapment neuropathies: a contemporary approach to pathophysiology, clinical assessment, and management. *Pain Rep*. 2020;5:e829.

FURTHER READING

www.orthoinfo.aaos.org.

CHAPTER 64

Complex Regional Pain Syndrome

Kyle D. Maier, MD

"The greatest evil is physical pain."

St Augustine (354–430 CE)

1. What is Complex Regional Pain Syndrome?

Complex Regional Pain Syndrome (CRPS) is a poorly understood set of chronic pain disorders defined by pain that is out of proportion in time or severity to an inciting (typically traumatic) event. It has a prevalence of around 5–25 cases per 100,000 person-years. It is characterized by the development of persistent **regional** inflammatory changes, autonomic dysfunction, allodynia and hyperalgesia, and edema in a non-dermatomal distribution — most often in an extremity and following a specific insult. The syndrome demonstrates variable progression over time.

2. What is the history of CRPS?

CRPS has been described since at least the 16th century when French battlefield surgeon Ambrose Pare reported a syndrome of burning pain after peripheral nerve injury suffered by King Charles IX. Dr. Silas Mitchell, a US Army physician, further characterized this condition in 1864 and developed the name "causalgia" to describe it. It was not until 1994 that the International Association for the Study of Pain (IASP) developed the current designation. In 2003, the Budapest Clinical Diagnostic Criteria were developed due to the perceived oversensitivity of the 1994 IASP diagnostic criteria (and possible "overdiagnosis" of the syndrome). It has been called by many names, as outlined below.

Causalgia (now CRPS II)	Shoulder–hand syndrome	Acute atrophy of bone
Reflex dystrophy	Sudeck's atrophy	Reflex sympathetic dystrophy (now CRPS I)
Transient osteoporosis	Algodystrophy	Algoneurodystrophy
Posttraumatic osteoporosis		

3. What is the suspected pathogenesis of CRPS?

CRPS is thought to be a disorder with multiple potential etiologies. It is characterized chiefly by **peripheral nervous system** changes in response to an inciting/traumatic event, followed by **central nervous system sensitization, autonomic dysfunction, and inflammatory changes**. There is evidence of a possible genetic predisposition (certain HLA haplotypes, as well as increased predilection among siblings, have been described) in addition to psychologic factors that may influence disease development.

Initially, nociceptive sensitization occurs in response to an inciting event, driven by local release of pro-inflammatory mediators like TNF-alpha and prostaglandin E2. This, in turn, leads to a decrease in the depolarization threshold in nearby nerves. Furthermore, Aδ and polymodal C nociceptive fibers, which travel to the spinal cord, cause a release of excitatory amino

623

acids (glutamate, asaparagine) that subsequently act on N-methyl-D-aspartate (NMDA) receptors within the dorsal horn of the spinal cord. Further release of inflammatory neuropeptides, substance P, and calcitonin gene-related peptide (CGRP), increases the susceptibility of nerve firing within the dorsal horn and contributes to chronic pain sensation and synaptic plasticity. There is contemporaneous linking of these nerves and signaling peptides with the autonomic nervous system, which may help explain the autonomic symptoms seen in the condition. Over time, structural CNS changes and chronic CNS sensitization may take place. This has effects beyond allodynia/hyperalgesia, as symptoms may extend to impaired motor function, and/or limb neglect.

Immunologic influences are likely, with noted increases in neuropeptides and pro-inflammatory mediators, as described above. The exact role (and timing) of these mediators in disease pathogenesis is poorly understood. Some studies have also suggested a possible role for IgG autoantibodies against the autonomic nervous system in CRPS, but further research is necessary to delineate whether this is important in clinical practice.

Pearl: CRPS is a poorly understood condition with a pathophysiologic basis involving **inflammatory** and **neuropathic** mechanisms, leading to **sustained hyperexcitation** in sensory, motor, and autonomic nerves.

4. What are the signs and symptoms of CRPS?
- Pain and swelling in an extremity
- Trophic cutaneous changes in the same extremity (increased/decreased hair growth, nail changes/pitting, skin tone changes and atrophy)
- Vasomotor instability (edema, sweating changes, temperature changes)
- Motor weakness/dysfunction or sensory disorders of the limb, including proximal joints (weakness, limited range of motion, dystonia, light-touch sensitivity, allodynia)

The pain of CRPS is often described as **burning, or stabbing, severe pain involving a generalized (non-dermatomal) area** like the hand or foot. **Allodynia** (pain from a typically non-noxious stimulation) and **hyperpathia** (prolonged pain after stimulation) are commonly seen. **Temperature changes** including atypical warmth (or coolness) with unusual sweating (or conversely, xerosis) can be seen in the area. Trophic changes like subcutaneous **atrophy** or loss of hair are often seen later during the evolution of the condition, as well as development of flexion contractures or abnormal muscular activity (dystonia).

Pearl: Bilateral extremity, truncal, and facial CRPS are highly controversial diagnoses and are **extremely seldom described** (should prompt strong consideration of an alternative etiology)

5. What are the typical demographic characteristics of CRPS? How do pediatric patients and adult patients differ?
Adult CRPS occurs more often in women than in men (~3:1). It is most common between the ages of 40 to 60 years old. Incidence is between 5 and 26 cases per 100,000 per year. It is generally thought to involve the upper extremity more often than lower, and type I CRPS is significantly more common than type II.

Childhood CRPS is more common in girls and Caucasians. It is unusual in young children (<7 years) and typically seen in the early teens. It is possible that CRPS is underreported in children, as pediatric CRPS often lacks some of the more characteristic features seen in adults (lower rates of inciting trauma, higher rate of lower extremity involvement). The disease course is typically more benign in children, with better response to therapeutic intervention than adults.

6. How is CRPS diagnosed?
Diagnosis of CRPS is clinical, and no single serologic or radiographic test fully distinguishes it. The Budapest criteria were created in 2003 to better discriminate CRPS and non-CRPS neuropathic pain. The IASP formally adopted revised CRPS clinical diagnostic criteria in 2012 (updated again in 2019), which are largely based on the original Budapest criteria (Table 64.1).

TABLE 64.1 IASP Diagnostic Criteria for CRPS (also known as the Budapest criteria)	
All of the following must be present: Continuing pain disproportionate to any inciting event One physical exam sign in two of the categories below *at the time of examination* One symptom in three of the categories below No other diagnosis better explains the patient's presentation	
Category	**Signs/Symptoms**
Sensory	Symptoms: Reported hyperesthesia, allodynia Signs: Evidence of allodynia to light touch, deep pressure, hyperalgesia to pinprick
Vasomotor	Symptoms: Reported temperature asymmetry, skin color changes, skin color asymmetry Signs: Evidence of the above, asymmetry of temperature >1 C
Sudomotor/Edema	Symptoms: Reported edema or sweating changes or asymmetry Signs: Evidence of the above
Motor/Trophic	Symptoms: Reported decreased range of motion, weakness, tremor, dystonia, trophic changes of hair/nails/skin Signs: Evidence of the above
Note: The above criteria have a sensitivity of 85% and specificity of 69% for the diagnosis of CRPS. If a patient has one symptom from all four symptom categories and one sign from two of the four sign categories, the sensitivity is 70% and specificity is 94%.	

7. How is CRPS categorized?

CRPS has been historically categorized into two types:

- **CRPS type I** – formerly Reflex Sympathetic Dystrophy, 90% of cases – occurs without a prior specific peripheral nerve injury.
- **CRPS type II** – formerly causalgia, 10% of cases – occurs with a known peripheral nerve injury.

  More recently, some clinicians have begun describing CRPS as "cold CRPS" or "warm CRPS". This designation is based on clinical phenotype, with the "warm" subtype more commonly reported at symptom onset. In addition, recent IASP consensus meetings have proposed the term "CRPS with remission of some features" for patients who no longer meet full criteria for the disorder, but suffer from continued symptoms.

8. What are known precipitating and predisposing factors for the development of CRPS?

Around 75% of the time, there is a clear precipitating factor prior to the development of CRPS. **Fractures involving the upper extremities**—especially antebrachial fractures—appear to be high risk. Higher-energy injuries, fracture severity, requirement of surgical correction, and prolonged general anesthesia, are all associated with disease development. Interestingly, time under regional anesthesia is not associated with risk. See Tables 64.2 & 64.3 for additional details.

9. When does CRPS typically develop after an inciting event?

CRPS typically begins **within 4–6 weeks** after an inciting event. In 80% or more of cases, symptom onset is within 12 weeks. Notably, 5–7% develop CRPS in the **contralateral/nontraumatized limb** in the course of their disease.

10. What are the stages of CRPS?

The existence of discrete progressive stages of CRPS is somewhat controversial due to the diagnostic uncertainty regarding this condition, as well as lack of evidence for clear *sequential* progression in studies to date. Historically, three stages of CRPS have been described as outlined below (see Figure 64.1 as well).

Stage 1 (acute stage)—lasts **6–12 months**

- Classic symptoms as per IASP criteria: pain, swelling, color change
- Painful movement and tendency for disuse of affected limb
- Early osteoporosis on x-rays

TABLE 64.2 Precipitating Factors for CRPS	
Trauma (common cause)	Chemical burns
Fractures (common cause)	Electrical burns
Lacerations	Postherpetic neuralgia
Crush injuries	Cervical spine pathology
Contusions	Subcutaneous injections
Sprains (common cause)	Drugs (barbiturates)
Immobilization in a cast	Malignancies (ovarian)
Myocardial infarctions	Pregnancy
Strokes and other central nervous system (CNS) injury (common cause)	**Peripheral nerve diseases** (common cause)
Pleuropulmonary diseases	Emotional stress
Surgery, especially carpal tunnel release and foot surgery (common causes)	

TABLE 64.3 Predisposing Factors for CRPS	
Diabetes mellitus	Neurovegetative dystonia
Hyperparathyroidism	Hypertriglyceridemia
Hyperthyroidism	Alcohol and/or tobacco use disorder
Multiple sclerosis	Chronic low back pain
Use of angiotensin-converting enzyme (ACE) inhibitors	Psychological factors: history of PTSD, anxiety, or catastrophizing; emotional trauma or life stressors concurrent to inciting event

Stage 2 (dystrophic stage)—lasts **additional 1–2 years**
- Persistent pain
- Swelling gives way to brawny, hard edema
- Subcutaneous tissue and intrinsic muscles begin to atrophy
- Cooler extremity, which may be mottled or cyanotic
- Progression of osteoporosis

Stage 3 (atrophic stage)—persisting additional years
- Pain may remain constant or slowly diminish
- Extremity becomes stiff due to persistent disuse
- Periarticular thickening of the skin is seen
- Skin becomes smooth, glossy, and drawn. Nails become brittle
- May see muscle spasm, dystonia, and tremor
- Osteoporosis progresses further, sometimes with pathologic fractures
- Bony ankylosis has been described

A fourth stage (psychological stage) has been further characterized, involving loss of job, unnecessary surgery, orthostatic hypotension or hypertension, neurodermatitis, and depression. Most patients will not fit neatly in to any particular stage, and fluctuation between stages can occur. Earlier stages are generally felt to be more responsive to treatment. The time in which a patient experiences a given stage is also variable.

11. How should you evaluate a patient with a tender and swollen limb in which you may suspect CRPS? What should the differential diagnosis include?

For any patient presenting with a single painful extremity with swelling, color change, and severe pain, careful examination of the affected limb is necessary. Information should be gathered on the distribution of involvement, presence of allodynia/hyperalgesia, visible rash or other skin changes,

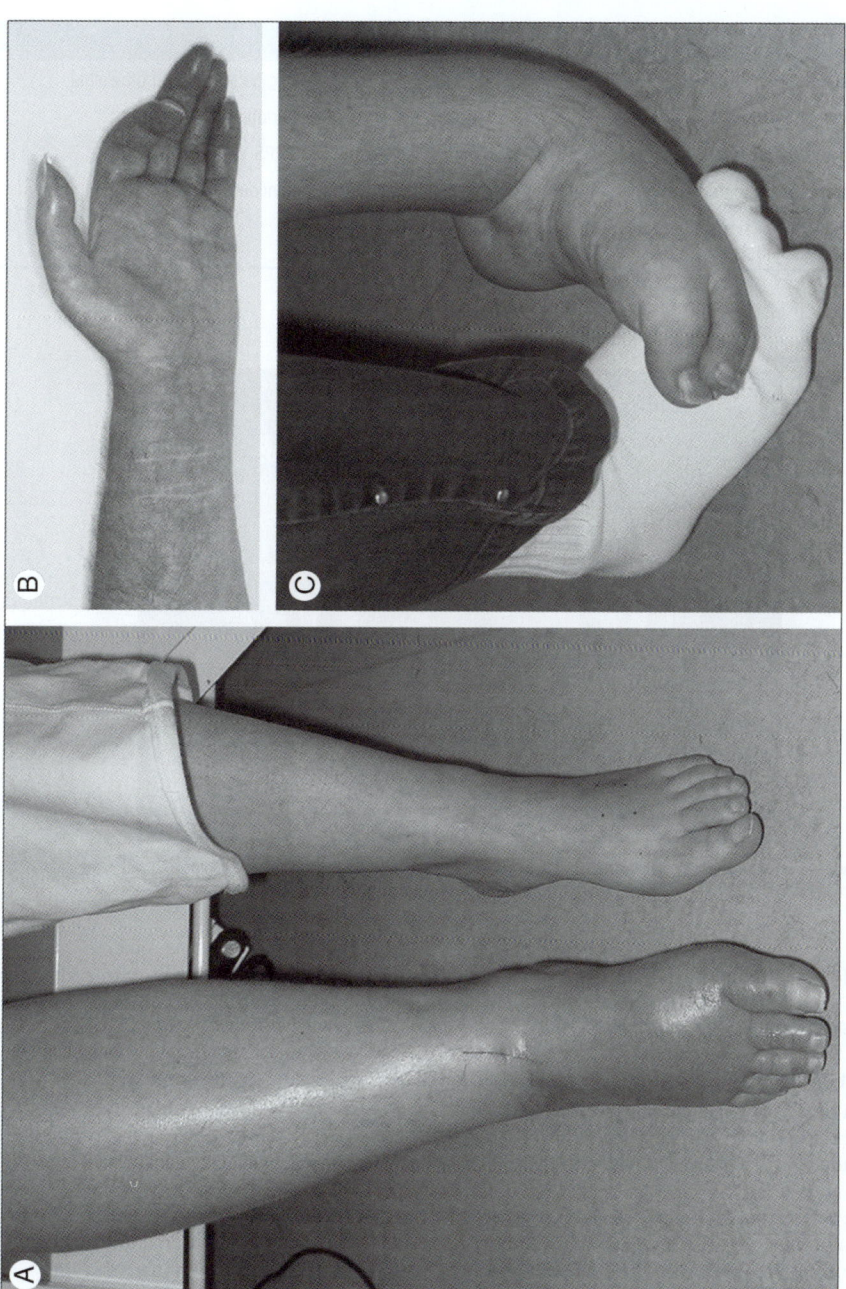

Fig. 64.1 Clinical photographs highlighting various stages of CRPS. (A) The acute phase, with warmth and erythema of the right lower extremity. (B) The "cold" form of CRPS in stage 2, with noted skin atrophy and mottled distal discoloration. 1C highlights the dystonia sometimes evident in later stages of CRPS. (From Marinus J, Moseley GL, Birklein F, et al. Clinical features and pathophysiology of complex regional pain syndrome. *Lancet Neurol.* 2011;10(7):637–648. https://doi.org/10.1016/S1474-4422(11)70106-5)

TABLE 64.4 Differential Diagnosis for a Painful, Swollen Limb		
Inflammatory arthritis	Malignancy	Angioedema/Erythromelalgia
Cellulitis/osteomyelitis	Fracture	Peripheral neuropathy
Compartment syndrome	Systemic sclerosis	CRPS
Deep venous thrombosis	Osteonecrosis	Pancoast tumor
Venous insufficiency syndromes, including lipodermatosclerosis		

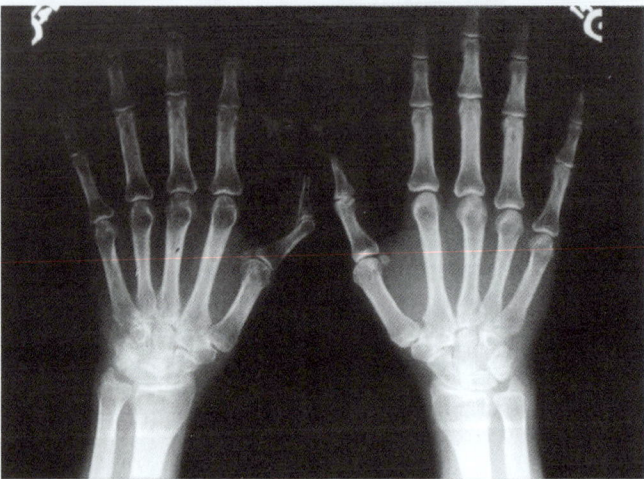

Fig. 64.2 Radiograph of the hands showing CRPS of left hand. Note marked periarticular osteoporosis compared with right hand (Sudeck's atrophy).

and documentation of the sensory exam. A complete history and exam is necessary to evaluate for other areas of potential involvement outside of the presenting complaint, and to properly narrow the differential (Table 64.4).

12. What radiographic studies can be used in CRPS and what do they show?

Plain film x-ray—soft tissue swelling and regional patchy or mottled osteopenia can be seen, particularly in comparison to the contralateral side (see Fig 64.2). This pattern was first described by Sudeck in 1900 and is often referred to as **Sudeck's atrophy.** Importantly, it is only seen in <50% of patients.

Bone Scintigraphy / triple phase bone scan (TPBS)—most helpful within the first five months of symptom onset. A negative bone scan does not exclude the diagnosis, but an abnormal bone scan may predict improved responsiveness to corticosteroid and/or bisphosphonate therapy.

- In stage 1, 80% will demonstrate abnormalities, particularly increased blood velocity and blood pooling with early and delayed hyperfixation. A quantitative increase in radiotracer uptake (ipsilateral >1.32 compared to contralateral) in the third phase of the bone scan in joints distal to trauma is characteristic.
- In stage 2, there is normalization of blood velocity and blood pooling, but a persistence of early and delayed hyperfixation. Bone scan is interpreted as abnormal approximately 50% of the time in this stage
- In stage 3, there is reduced blood velocity and blood pooling, and a minority of patients will continue to have early and delayed hyperfixation.

CT/MRI—there is no clear role for computed tomography or magnetic resonance imaging to confirm or rule out a diagnosis of CRPS. These modalities may be helpful to evaluate for other musculoskeletal disorders that may be confused with CRPS.

13. What other diagnostic testing can be performed in the initial evaluation of CRPS?

Autonomic testing (resting sweat output, resting skin temperature, quantitative sudomotor axon reflex test) can provide objective evidence of dysautonomia, but obtaining the studies is often clinically impractical. Stress thermography with cold exposure is sometimes useful as a screening test.

Electromyography (EMG) has shown some validity in the evaluation of CRPS (particularly in patients with myoclonus, as somewhat distinct changes can be seen in that setting).

Musculoskeletal ultrasonography has been described to demonstrate myoglobular distortion in CRPS patients that is clinically distinct from other forms of chronic neuropathic pain, but this is still an area of ongoing research.

Regional sympathetic nerve block (stellate ganglion or lumbar sympathetic nerve) may lead to transient relief of symptoms in CRPS, but does not fully confirm the diagnosis.

14. What therapies have the best evidence for treatment of CRPS? What other therapeutic modalities have been used?

The evidence for treatment of CRPS suggests that earlier interventions are the most efficacious. Of these, the following have the strongest evidence base:

- Physical therapy
- Corticosteroids
- Calcitonin
- IV bisphosphonates
- Cognitive behavioral therapy
- Spinal cord or dorsal root ganglion stimulation
- Sympathetic nerve block, potentially sympathectomy (though controversial per Cochrane review)
- IV ketamine

Many other treatments have varying levels of support for use (see Table 64.5).

15. Outline an appropriate approach to multimodal therapy for CRPS.

- All patients should be treated with a multidisciplinary or interdisciplinary approach, often involving physical therapy (PT), pain management, behavioral health, primary care, orthopedic surgery, and/or rheumatology.
- All patients should be educated on the nature of the disease, and recognition that treatments are not expected nor proven to "cure" the disease but may help manage symptoms and improve outcomes.
- All patients should undergo evaluation and receive guidance from PT and/or occupational therapy (OT) throughout the disease course. This should be tailored to symptom severity at the time of the evaluation, and modified as the disease progresses. During the earlier, acute stage, when pain is often significant even at rest, programs should be less aggressive (e.g. involve skin desensitization or gentle passive mobilization). As the pain becomes more tolerable, PT can progress to active isometric strengthening and eventually isotonic training.
- All patients should be offered counseling services and psychologic support
- Patients with **early CRPS** (within 3–6 months of symptom onset) with active pain and swelling, particularly with positive bone scintigraphy, **should be treated with prednisone** (60–80mg a day for 2 weeks, with taper over the following 4 weeks). Corticosteroids can modulate the effect of inflammatory neuropeptides
- Patients should be offered analgesic therapy, potentially including opioids, NSAIDs, topical lidocaine, TCAs, gabapentinoids, SSRIs, SNRIs, and/or carbamazepine. The choice of agent should depend on severity of pain and quality/description of pain. Development of a small fiber neuropathy can be seen, and these patients may benefit from treatment aimed at reducing nerve pain transmission.
- Depending on pain severity (i.e. if pain is severe both at rest and with movement), more aggressive therapy can be instituted early. At any given time, it is not possible for a clinician to know if a patient's pain is more (or less) sympathetically mediated. Nonetheless, patients

TABLE 64.5 Summary of Treatments for CRPS

CATEGORY	TREATMENT
Stimulation of inhibitory neurons	• Spinal cord stimulation
Physical therapy modalities	• Massage, counterirritants • Graded motor imagery, mirror therapy, pain exposure therapy • Ultrasound • Electroacupuncture • Transcutaneous nerve stimulators
Anti-inflammatory agents	• Nonsteroidal anti-inflammatory drugs (NSAIDs) • Ketorolac in an intravenous (IV) regional block • Oral corticosteroids (IV is impractical, intrathecal ineffective) • Intravenous immunoglobulin (proven ineffective after 1 year of symptoms) • Mycophenolate, plasma exchange, low-dose naltrexone, and an epidermal growth factor inhibitor (cetuximab) are all being studied for this indication
Sympathetic Nerve Blocks	• Lidocaine, mepivacaine, bupivacaine, etc., injected into sympathetic ganglion (brachial plexus, stellate ganglion) • Bier block with IV guanethidine, bretylium, reserpine (depletes norepinephrine) (not very effective and rarely used) • Oral β-blockers (not very effective) • Epidural clonidine • Prazosin, phenoxybenzamine, terazosin (α-1 adrenergic blockers) • IV phentolamine (α-1 adrenergic blocker) • Oral, patch, or epidural clonidine • Sympathectomy (surgical) • Injection of opioid into sympathetic ganglion
Depletion of peripheral nerve substance P	• Topical capsaicin
Anticonvulsants	• Phenytoin • Carbamazepine • Gabapentin and pregabalin (high dose) • Valproic acid
Anti-osteoporotic therapy	• IV bisphosphonates (pamidronate 1 mg/kg) • High dose (40 mg/day) or normal dose (70 mg/week) oral alendronate • Calcitonin (rarely used, but reasonable outcomes)
Treatment of Dystonia	• Intrathecal baclofen (GABA agonist) • Local botulinum toxin injections
Psychological therapy	• Establish rapport with the patient, provide emotional support, assess for depression, and treat with psychotherapy and medications if indicated • Thermal biofeedback, relaxation training, alcohol and tobacco cessation • Cognitive behavioral therapy
Various other therapies	• IV lidocaine and 5% lidoderm patches (sodium channel blocking agents) • IV ketamine (block NMDA receptor) • Amantadine (similar to ketamine) • Stop ACE inhibitors • Tricyclic antidepressants and serotonin and norepinephrine reuptake inhibitors • Calcium channel blockers • Topical Dimethyl sulfoxide • Topical lidocaine • Cannabinoids • Repetitive transcranial magnetic stimulation (in trials) • As an absolute last resort, amputations have been considered, controversially, but have demonstrated improved pain outcomes in some patients.

with CRPS often demonstrate more severe autonomic dysfunction early in the disease course, and in these patients, sympathetic nerve block may be effective. Up to 50% of patients with symptoms lasting less than 1 year can improve with this therapy. However, **repeated nerve blocks do not improve or prolong the analgesic effect**, and failure to respond to this therapy suggests additional CNS sensitization.
- In prolonged (>12 months) or treatment-resistant illness, the following therapies can be considered:
  - Epidural spinal cord stimulators can reduce pain in 50% of patients.
  - Dorsal root ganglion stimulators have demonstrated better treatment response (>60% of patients) than traditional dorsal column spinal cord stimulators.
  - IV ketamine (delivered as either inpatient or outpatient infusion therapy) has shown promising results in improvement of pain.
  - Sympathectomy has shown potential benefit, particularly if there is at least partial response to initial sympathetic nerve blocks.

16. How can you intervene to potentially prevent development/redevelopment of CRPS?

While data are sparse, intervention for patients at higher risk for development of CRPS (high-risk surgeries/trauma, history of CRPS) has demonstrated some benefit. Vitamin C 500 mg administered daily for 50 days is a low-risk intervention that may reduce development of CRPS in patients with wrist fractures or lower limb injuries. Administration of alphalipoic acid has also shown therapeutic potential in both treatment and prevention of CRPS in experimental murine models. Perioperative stellate ganglion block, or IV mannitol, may reduce the recurrence rate of CRPS.

17. What is the prognosis for CRPS?

As noted previously, all therapies are more effective when introduced early (<2–3 months of onset). Up to 85% of adults improve within the first year, but only 30% are symptom-free within 5 years. Two to three percent have a relapsing course. In children, 95% or more experience symptom resolution within the first year.

ACKNOWLEDGMENT

The author wishes to thank Dr. Sterling West for his contributions to this chapter in the previous edition.

BIBLIOGRAPHY

Barrett MJ, Barnett PJL. Complex regional pain type 1. *Pediatr Emer Care*. 2016;32:185–191.
Duong S, Bravo D, Todd KJ, et al. Treatment of complex regional pain syndrome: an updated systemic review and narrative synthesis. *Can J Anaesth*. 2018;65:658.
Ferraro MC, Cashin AG, Wand BM, et al. Interventions for treating pain and disability in adults with complex regional pain syndrome: an overview of systematic reviews. *Cochrane Database Syst Rev*. 2023;6(6):CD009416.
Harden RN, McCabe CS, Goebel A, et al. Complex regional pain syndrome: practical diagnostic and treatment guidelines. *Pain Med*. 2022;23(Suppl 1):S1–S53.
Kachko L, Efrat R, Ben Ami S, et al. Complex regional pain syndromes in children and adolescents. *Pediatr Int*. 2008;50:523–527.
Kauer H, Muhleman M, Balon HR. Complex regional pain syndrome diagnosed with triple-phase bone scanning. *J Nucl Med Technol*. 2017;45:243–244.
Lii TR, Singh V. Ketamine for complex regional pain syndrome: a narrative review highlighting dosing practices and treatment response. *Anesthesiol Clin*. 2023;41(2):357–369.
Neumeister MW, Romanelli MR. Complex regional pain syndrome. *Clin Plast Surg*. 2020;47(2):305–310.
O'Connell NE, Wand BM, Gibson W, et al. Local anaesthetic sympathetic blockade for complex regional pain syndrome. *Cochrane Database Syst Rev*. 2016;7:CD004598.
Okumo T, Takayama Y, Maruyama K, et al. Senso-immunologic prospects for complex regional pain syndrome treatment. *Front Immunol*. 2022;12:786511.
Ott S, Maihofner C. Signs and symptoms in 1,043 patients with complex regional pain syndrome. *J Pain*. 2018;19:599.
Rodrigues P, Cassanego GB, Peres DS, et al. Alpha-lipoic acid reduces nociception by reducing oxidative stress and neuroinflammation in a model of complex regional pain syndrome type I in mice. *Behav Brain Res*. 2024;459:114790.

Shafiee E, MacDermid J, Packham T, et al. The Effectiveness of rehabilitation interventions on pain and disability for complex regional pain syndrome: a systematic review and meta-analysis. *Clin J Pain*. 2023;39(2):91–105.

Shim H, Rose J, Halle S, et al. Complex regional pain syndrome: a narrative review for the practising clinician. *Br J Anaesth*. 2019;123(2):e424–e433.

Smart KM, Wand BM, O'Connell NE. Physiotherapy for pain and disability in adults with complex regional pain syndrome (CRPS) types I and II. *Cochrane Database Syst Rev*. 2016;2:CD010853.

van den Berg C, de Bree PN, Huygen FJPM, et al. Glucocorticoid treatment in patients with complex regional pain syndrome: a systematic review. *Eur J Pain*. 2022;26(10):2009–2035.

FURTHER READING

www.rsds.org.

Benign and Malignant Tumors of Joints and Synovium

Alison M. Gizinski, MD

 KEY POINTS

1. The majority of mass lesions in the joints are benign.
2. The most common benign joint neoplasms are tenosynovial giant cell tumors (TGCTs) and synovial chondromatosis. Both are best diagnosed by magnetic resonance imaging (MRI) followed by biopsy.
3. The most common malignant tumor of the joint is synovial sarcoma.
4. A benign or malignant neoplasm of the joint should be considered in any patient with nontraumatic hemarthrosis.

---

1. **Why should practicing physicians be concerned with tumors that affect the joints and synovium?**

   Benign and malignant neoplasms affecting articular and periarticular structures may mimic inflammatory arthritis. Awareness of these conditions is crucial to prevent diagnostic delays and to avoid the initiation of ineffective and/or inappropriate therapy. Fortunately, primary neoplasms of the joint are rare.

2. **A young adult presents with a solitary, painless mass adjacent to a finger joint that has been slowly enlarging. What tumor is suggested by this scenario?**

   This presentation would be typical for a **localized tenosynovial giant cell tumor (TGCT) of the tendon sheath.** This benign condition, which occurs with a slightly increased predilection for females, is second only to the ganglion as a source of localized swelling in the hand and wrist. It occurs less frequently (3–10%) in the ankle and foot. These nodular lesions usually occur in association with a tendon sheath (formerly called giant cell tumor of tendon sheath). Excision is curative and recurrences are rare.

3. **TGCT exists in three forms: diffuse, localized, and localized TGCT of tendon sheath. How do these forms differ?**

   - **TGCT of joints and tendon sheaths, diffuse type** [also called **pigmented villonodular synovitis** pigmented villonodular synovitis (PVNS)]: the entire synovium of an affected joint or tendon sheath is involved. It affects individuals in their 30s and 40s with equal sex distribution. Grossly, the synovium is red-brown to mottled orange-yellow and prolific with coarse villi, finer fronds, and diffuse nodularity resembling an Angora rug. It is almost always monoarticular. The most common locations include the knee (80%), hip (15%), and ankle. Swelling and effusion accompanied by moderate discomfort, decreased range of motion, and increased warmth to palpation are typical. Pain is frequently less than anticipated for the degree of swelling.
   - **Localized TGCT of the joint** (also called benign giant cell synovioma or localized nodular synovitis): involves only a portion of a synovial surface in a joint, and the lesion is often pedunculated. It presents with symptoms similar to a loose body. It tends not to be as darkly pigmented and has less villous proliferation than is seen in the diffuse form.
   - **Localized TGCT of the tendon sheath** (also called giant cell tumor of the tendon sheath or fibroxanthoma of the tendon sheath) has been discussed in Question 2 earlier. Histologically, all three forms of villonodular synovitis are remarkably similar.

   TGCT is characterized by synovial hypertrophy and hyperplasia with hemosiderin deposition. Hyperplasia results from the proliferation of multinucleated giant cells and synovial fibroblasts, or synoviocytes with accumulation of mononuclear cells. Several genetic and chromosomal alterations have been identified in TGCT. Only a few cells in TGCT have one of these abnormalities. Some cells are aneuploid and exhibit trisomy 5 and/or 7, which can contribute to synovial proliferation. A small percentage (15%) of TGCT cells have a specific translocation between chromosomes 1p13 and 2q35 in which the gene coding for colony-stimulating factor-1 (CSF-1), also called macrophage colony-stimulating factor 1, is fused to the collagen VI alpha-3 gene. These cells overexpress CSF-1. Many of the remaining cells in the tumor are inflammatory cells (most CD68$^+$ macrophages) recruited into the tumor because they contain the receptor for CSF-1. Bleeding into the synovium causes the hemosiderin deposition.

4. What does the synovial fluid analysis reveal in the diffuse type of TGCT (PVNS)?

Typically, the fluid is brown or grossly **hemorrhagic.** This finding on joint aspiration should raise diffuse TGCT as a diagnostic consideration. However, up to 50% of patients will not have a hemorrhagic synovial fluid. Additionally, similar hemorrhagic fluid can be seen in trauma, Charcot joint, bleeding disorders, synovial hemangiomas, metastasis to joints, sickle cell disease, and Ehlers–Danlos syndrome.

5. What are the characteristic radiographic findings in a patient with the diffuse type of TGCT (PVNS)?

Plain radiographs are usually nonspecific, except for mild increased density of the soft tissue of the joint due to blood and hemosiderin deposits. The tumor may invade into the bone causing cysts or scalloped erosive changes with sclerotic borders with preserved joint space until late in the disease course. The erosive changes can mimic gout or tuberculosis. The MRI appearance of TGCT is diagnostic in most cases. Nodules with sufficient hemosiderin appear dark on both T1- and T2-weighted images. Characteristic blooming artifact can be seen on gradient-echo imaging sequences due to hemosiderin deposition.

6. Describe the histologic characteristics of TGCT.

Grossly, the synovium looks like a tan to red-brown "shaggy carpet." Microscopically, TGCT is distinctive. It is characterized by a dense cellular infiltrate composed of synovial cell hyperplasia with surface and subsynovial invasion of mitotically active cells with eosinophilic cytoplasm. Other invading cells are fibroblasts, lipid-laden macrophages (xanthoma cells), hemosiderin-containing macrophages, and scattered, frequent, multinucleated giant cells. Although TGCT is locally aggressive, it rarely metastasizes.

7. How is TGCT treated?

Surgical treatment with complete synovectomy is standard either via open or arthroscopic approaches. Recurrences, particularly in diffuse type TGCT (PVNS), occur in 20% to 40%. Intraarticular installation of radioisotopes or low-dose external beam radiation is used in refractory cases. Total joint arthroplasty may be necessary for cure. In inoperable cases or where operation would be morbid, tyrosine kinase inhibitors (pexidartinib) with activity against CSF-1 receptor and monoclonal antibodies targeting CSF-1 or the CSF-1 receptor may be useful. Clinical trials are ongoing.

8. What is synovial chondromatosis and how does it present?

Synovial chondromatosis is characterized by the development of multiple foci of cartilaginous metaplasia (neoplasia) via unknown etiology in the synovial membranes of joints and rarely of tendon sheaths or bursae. These foci form nodules that may be invaded by blood vessels leading to endochondral ossification (termed osteochondromatosis). The chondral nodules in the synovial membrane of joints are frequently released as free bodies **(joint mice)** into the joint space. It most commonly affects men in their 30s to 50s. It is almost always monoarticular affecting the knee (70%) more than the hip (20%), shoulder, ankle, elbow, or other joints. Clinically, there is an increasingly limited range of motion with crepitus and often with unexpected locking. Effusions, pain, and stiffness commonly occur. Over time the loose bodies may cause mechanical wear on joint surfaces leading to cartilage degeneration.

9. How is synovial chondromatosis diagnosed?

Radiograph may be diagnostic if the chondroid bodies are calcified (66%) resembling a calcified mulberry or popcorn (Fig. 65.1). MRI will show nodules of cartilage in the synovium which are

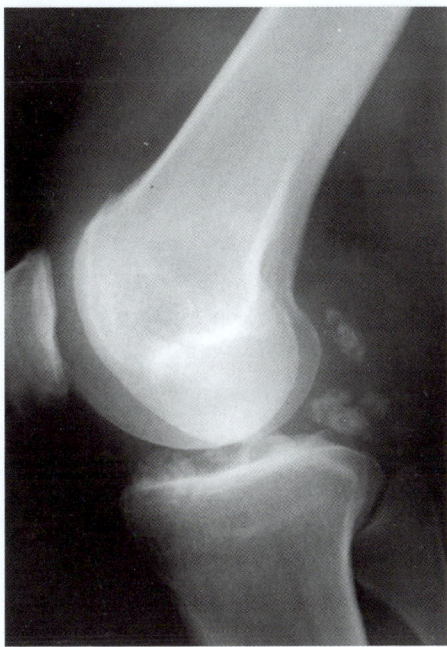

Fig. 65.1 Synovial chondromatosis of the knee demonstrating multiple, calcified chondroid bodies.

dark on T1-weighted images and bright (white) on T2-weighted images due to water content in the hyaline cartilage. Loose bodies can be seen. Arthroscopic biopsy is diagnostic if performed.

10. How is synovial chondromatosis managed?

Treatment is via synovectomy and removal of all the loose bodies if mechanical symptoms are present. Recurrences occur in up to 11%. Though considered benign, this condition can result in extensive local joint destruction if left untreated. Synovial chondromatosis never metastasizes but may rarely undergo malignant transformation into **synovial chondrosarcoma** (up to 6% of patients). Histologic identification of malignant transformation can be exceedingly difficult.

11. What other benign tumor-like lesions can involve the joints?

- **Lipomas** may occur within the joint capsule or synovium, but true intraarticular lesions are rare.
- **Lipoma arborescens** is a diffuse increase in subsynovial fat causing chronic effusions usually in the suprapatellar portion of the knee.
- **Chondroma** is an isolated mass of benign cartilage, usually in the knee.
- **Hemangiomas** are unusual intraarticular lesions that occur most frequently in the joints of children and young adults. The knee is the most common site. Recurrent hemarthrosis may occur. Diagnosis can be made by computed tomography, MRI, or angiography.
- **Osteoid osteomas,** when occurring within the joint, have less of the "classic" pattern of nocturnal pain relieved by nonsteroidal anti-inflammatory drugs and tend to involute spontaneously after 5 to 10 years.

12. What is the most common primary malignant neoplasm involving the joint?

Synovial sarcoma. This tumor constitutes 5% to 10% of all soft tissue sarcomas. It is a highly malignant neoplasm and generally occurs in the lower extremities (70%) of young people, with peak age of occurrence being 15 to 29 years. The tumor usually arises in the periarticular tissues of the knee or ankle. Only 10% of these malignancies arise directly within the joint itself.

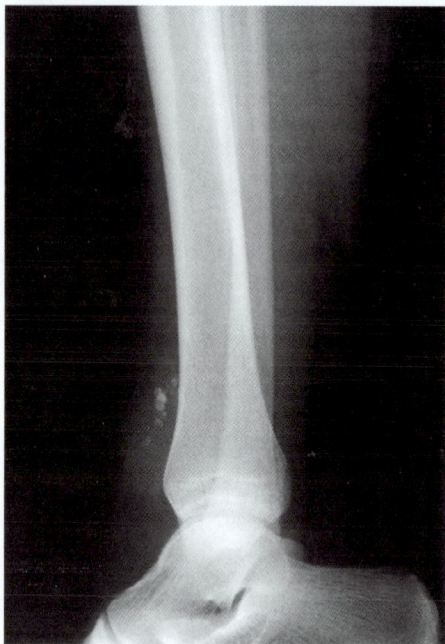

Fig. 65.2 Synovial sarcoma adjacent to the ankle. Note the speckled calcifications.

13. How does synovial sarcoma present clinically?

A slowly growing, often minimally symptomatic mass adjacent to the joint is the typical presentation. Pain is reported by about 50% of patients. Soft tissue calcification on plain radiograph occurs in 30% to 50% of the patients with a fine, stippled or dense appearance (Fig. 65.2). This finding serves to provide a clue as to the underlying diagnosis. MRI is the imaging procedure of choice since it defines the extent of the lesion.

14. What is the cell of origin for synovial sarcoma?

The histology of this tumor may be **biphasic,** in which epithelial cells arranged in clusters, tubules, and acini are interspersed in a spindle-cell stroma; or **monophasic,** in which either the epithelial or spindle cells predominate. Other morphologic types are recognized. Behavioral features include calcifying, ossifying, and poorly differentiated types. Though this tumor is called synovial sarcoma, ultrastructural and immunohistochemical studies have implicated an epithelial origin. The majority (>90%) of synovial sarcomas are characterized by a translocation which fuses the SS18 gene on chromosome 18 to either SSX1, SSX2, or SSX4 on chromosome X. The SS18-SSX fusion protein binds to the BAF complex and displaces the tumor suppressor BAF47. The modified BAF complex leads to activation of the transcription factor, Sox2, which is necessary for proliferation of the synovial sarcoma. Detection of the translocation in tumor cells using an SS18 probe is important for confirming the diagnosis and determining the prognosis of a synovial sarcoma.

15. How is synovial sarcoma treated? What is the prognosis?

Treatment involves an aggressive combination of radical surgery, radiation therapy, and chemotherapy. Prognosis depends in large part on tumor stage at the time of discovery, age of patient (<25 years old do better), sex (females have a survival advantage), and whether or not the tumor

BOX 65.1 Five-Year Survival in Synovial Sarcoma by Stage	
All tumors	60%
Localized	76%
Regional	56%
Distant	11%

is poorly differentiated (Box 65.1). The cause of death in progressive disease is usually due to extensive pulmonary metastasis. Other common sites of metastasis include regional lymph nodes, bones, liver, skin, and brain.

16. Clear-cell sarcoma is a rare highly malignant tumor of tendons, ligaments, and fascial aponeuroses. It usually presents as a slowly growing mass about the foot. What is its association with a malignancy more commonly thought of as a skin cancer?

There are multiple lines of evidence suggesting that clear-cell sarcoma is a representation of **malignant melanoma.** This evidence includes an immunohistochemical staining pattern with S-100 and HMB-45, which are considered specific for melanoma, evidence of melanin by special staining, and the presence of characteristic premelanosomes by electron microscopy. However, unlike melanoma, clear cell sarcomas demonstrate a translocation between chromosomes 12 and 22 causing an *EWSR1/ATF1* gene fusion. Treatment consists of surgical excision, radiation, and chemotherapy. Prognosis is generally poor (5YS=47-59%).

17. In which malignant diseases can joint involvement occur as a secondary feature?
- Metastatic carcinoma.
- Lymphoma/myeloma.
- Leukemic infiltration (12–65% of children and 4–13% of adults with leukemia).
- Contiguous spread of adjacent bone sarcomas.

18. What is the "classic" presentation of carcinoma metastatic to a joint?
- Advanced lung, gastrointestinal, or breast cancer is the most common etiology.
- Involvement is usually monoarticular, with the knee being the most common site.
- Effusion is often hemorrhagic.
- Synovial fluid cytology reveals the malignancy in approximately 50% of cases.

BIBLIOGRAPHY

Brahmi M, Vinceneux A, Cassier PA. Current systemic treatment options for tenosynovial giant cell tumor/pigmented villonodular synovitis: targeting the CSF1/CSF1R axis. *Curr Treat Opt Oncol.* 2016;17:10.

Gazendam AM, Popovic S, Munir S, et al. Synovial sarcoma: a clinical review. *Curr Oncol.* 2021;28:1909–1920.

Habusta SF, Mabrouk A, Tuck JA. Synovial chondromatosis. *StatPearls.* Treasure Island (FL): StatPearls Publishing; 2024.

Kerr DA, Rosenberg AE. Tumors and tumor-like lesions of joints and related structures. In: Firestein GS, Budd RC, Gabriel SE, Koretzky GA, McInnes IB, O'Dell JR, eds. *Firestein & Kelley's Textbook of Rheumatology.* 11th ed. Philadelphia, PA: Elsevier; 2021:2167–2188.

Murphey MD, Rhee JH, Lewis RB, et al. Pigmented villonodular synovitis: radiologic-pathologic correlation. *Radiographics.* 2008;28:1493.

Noailees T, Brulefert K, Briand S, et al. Giant cell tumor of tendon sheath: open surgery or arthroscopic synovectomy? A systematic review of the literature. *OTSR.* 2017;103:809–814.

Robert M, Farese H, Miossec P. Update on tenosynovial giant cell tumor, an inflammatory arthritis with neoplastic features. *Front Immunol.* 2022;13:820046.

WEBSITES

http://www.cancer.gov.

CHAPTER 66

Common Bony Lesions: Radiographic Features

Mary K. Lowry, MD

1. How should a bone lesion be characterized radiographically?

Bone lesions should not be defined radiographically as malignant or benign, but rather as aggressive or nonaggressive. Some malignant lesions can have a nonaggressive appearance, and many benign lesions (osteomyelitis, Langerhans cell histiocytosis of bone) can have a very aggressive appearance. There are a number of criteria that should be assessed when evaluating a bony lesion.

a. **Demographics:** Patient demographics, particularly age, play a significant role in developing a differential diagnosis of bone lesions. Benign lesions make up the majority of bone lesions in younger patients (less than 30 years old) with the exception of Ewings sarcoma and osteosarcoma, the most common malignant lesions in this age group. In patients older than 30 years, malignant lesions are more prevalent, with metastases, multiple myeloma, and chondrosarcoma being the most encountered. When evaluating bone lesions, it is imperative to take into consideration the age of the patient before forming a differential diagnosis.

b. **Location:** The location of the lesion within the bone and skeleton is helpful as specific lesions have a propensity to affect certain locations in the skeleton.

　i. **Skeletal location:** Bone tumors demonstrate a propensity for a certain location in the skeleton. Whether the lesion lies in the axial skeleton (skull, spine, and pelvis) or appendicular skeletal or a flat (iliac bone) or long bone (humerus) may assist in narrowing the differential diagnosis.

　ii. **Longitudinal osseous location:** A lesion's location in the bone as it relates to the diaphysis, metaphysis, or epiphysis of long bones is important for narrowing a differential diagnosis. Special consideration should be given to epiphyseal equivalents (patella) and flat bones (pelvis, ribs) and epiphyseal or metaphyseal equivalents (around apophyses or in flat bones that form by membranous ossification). Most common tumor sites (Table 66.1):

　　• **Epiphysis:** chondroblastoma, clear-cell chondrosarcoma, giant cell tumor (GCT), aneurysmal bone cyst (ABC). Of note, GCT and ABC usually arise from the metaphysis and extend into the epiphysis.

　　• **Metaphysis:** osteosarcoma, chondrosarcoma, GCT, chondromyxoid fibroma, enchondroma, nonossifying fibroma (NOF), ABC (long bones).

　　• **Diaphysis:** Ewings sarcoma, osteoid osteoma, osteoblastoma, enchondroma (phalanges), fibrous dysplasia (FD).

　iii. **Axial location:** The lesion's location within axial plane of the bone should be defined as central intramedullary, eccentric intramedullary, cortically based, or surface (periosteal)-centered.

c. **Zone of transition:** Refers to the transition zone or perimeter between the lesion and the adjacent uninvolved bone. The zone of transition should only be characterized on radiograph and should not be applied to CT or MR images. The zone of transition is classified as:

　i. **Narrow:** well-defined margins that can be easily traced. This is a nonaggressive feature.

　ii. **Wide or ill-defined:** poorly defined margins, not easily traceable. This is an aggressive feature.

TABLE 66.1 Types of Tumor by Osseous Location

EPIPHYSEAL	METAPHYSEAL	DIAPHYSEAL
Chondroblastoma	Osteosarcoma	Ewings sarcoma
Clear-cell chondrosarcoma	Chondrosarcoma	Osteoid osteoma
Giant cell tumor[a]	Giant cell tumor	Osteoblastoma
Aneurysmal bone cyst[a]	Chondromyxoid fibroma	Enchondroma (phalanges)
	Enchondroma	Fibrous dysplasia

[a]Begin in the metaphysis and extend to the epiphysis.

   d. **Pattern of bone destruction:** the pattern of bone replacement should be assessed and characterized as:
     i. **Geographic:** well-defined lesion of the bone. Geographic lesions have a narrow zone of transition by definition. This is a nonaggressive feature.
     ii. **Blastic or sclerotic:** densely sclerotic lesion of bone. Can be aggressive or nonaggressive.
     iii. **Permeative:** ill-defined bony destruction with a wide zone of transition, a "moth-eaten" appearance. This is an aggressive feature.
     iv. **Bubbly:** multilocular lucencies/septations, with or without an expansile appearance. This is usually a nonaggressive feature.
   e. **Presence of matrix:** This is one of the most critical and difficult decisions in the radiographic assessment of a bone lesion. The confident presence of matrix can narrow the differential markedly. If present, matrix falls into one of the following categories (Table 66.2):
     i. **Clear or cystic** (Fig. 66.1)
     ii. **Fibrous:** uniform intermediate density described as "ground-glass" in appearance. Lesions producing fibrous matrix are usually (but not always) nonaggressive (Fig. 66.2).
     iii. **Chondroid:** punctate matrix described as "rings and arcs" or "Cs and Js." Usually density equal or greater than of cortical bone and well defined. Can be associated with either aggressive or nonaggressive lesions (Fig. 66.3).
     iv. **Osteoid:** amorphous, fluffy, cloudy appearing matrix, usually less dense than cortical bone and often with smudged, ill-defined margins in aggressive lesions. Osteoid matrix can be immature and fluffy with a smudged/ill-defined margin favoring an aggressive lesion (arrow) or can be more mature, resembling bone, and favor a nonaggressive lesion (Fig. 66.4).
   f. **Periosteal reaction:** The bones' response to an insult is to lay down new bone and form a protective callous. The periosteum is a remarkable combination of tissues that has progenitor cells ready to differentiate into osteoblasts and chondroblasts. This allows the rapid formation of new bone, producing the radiographically visible periosteal reaction. Pathologic processes that are aggressive and rapidly growing produce a periosteal reaction indicative of ongoing attempts to wall off the expanding lesion. Periosteal reactions can be described in one of four typical patterns:
     i. **Smooth:** Favors a nonaggressive, slow-growing, or reactive process allowing the formation of solid callous/periosteal new bone (Fig. 66.5). Smooth periosteal reaction uniformly affecting the tibial and fibula (arrows) is often seen with chronic vascular insufficiency.

TABLE 66.2 Types of Nonaggressive Primary Bone Tumors by Matrix Appearance

CLEAR	FIBROUS	CHONDROID	OSTEOID
Unicameral bone cyst	Fibroxanthoma	Enchondroma	Osteoma
Aneurysmal bone cyst	Fibrous dysplasia	Osteochondroma	Osteoid osteoma
Giant cell tumor		Chondroblastoma	Osteoblastoma
Eosinophilic granuloma		Chondromyxoid fibroma	

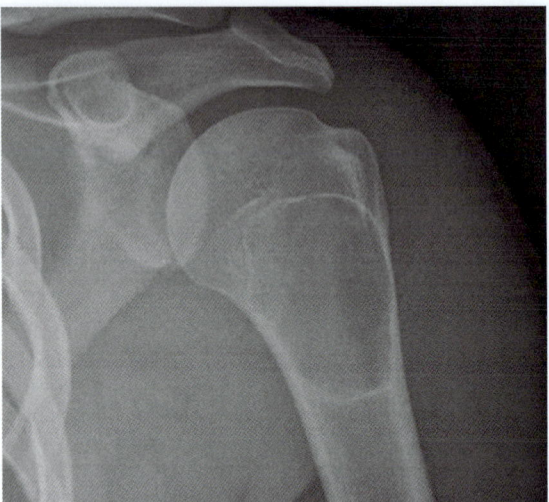

Fig. 66.1 Lesion with clear or cystic matrix.

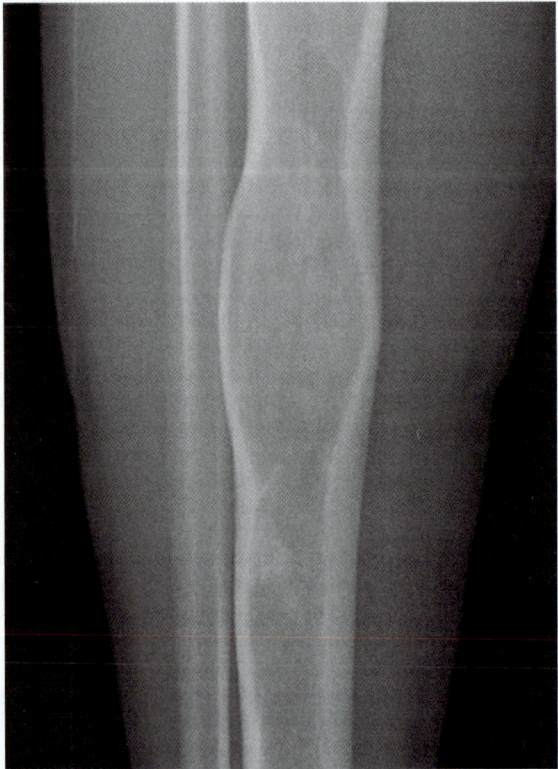

Fig. 66.2 Lesion with fibrous matrix.

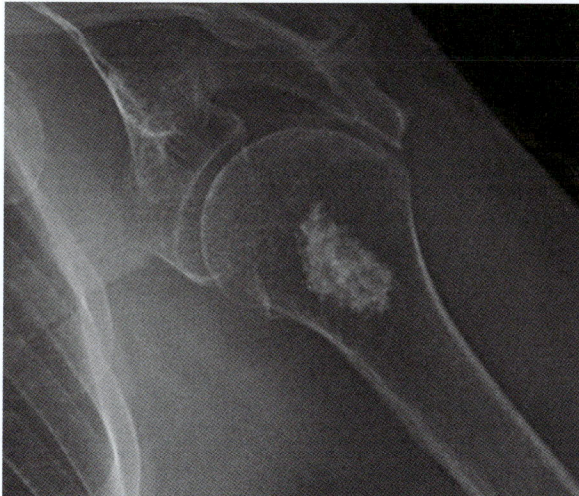

Fig. 66.3 Lesion with chondroid matrix.

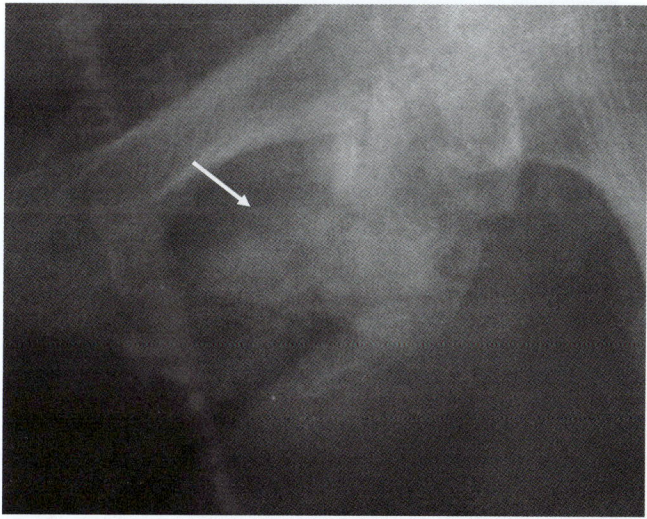

Fig. 66.4 Lesion with osteoid matrix.

ii. **Lamellated (onion skin):** Layers of periosteal new bone laid down on one another. Indicative of an aggressive or fast-growing lesion as the new periosteal layers are not allowed sufficient time to mature before another is laid down on top (Fig. 66.6).

iii. **Codman's triangle:** A very aggressive appearance, indicative of osseous soft tissue mass expanding at such a rate that the adjacent margin of periosteal new bone is lifted up, forming a triangle with the underlying cortex (Fig. 66.7).

iv. **Perpendicular:** Hair-on-end periosteal reaction is highly associated with aggressive lesions.

v. **Sun burst:** The most aggressive form of periosteal reaction is seen exclusively in very aggressive lesions. The appearance is that of divergent strings of periosteum extending from the margin of the bone. This characteristic has classically been described in osteosarcoma (Fig. 66.8).

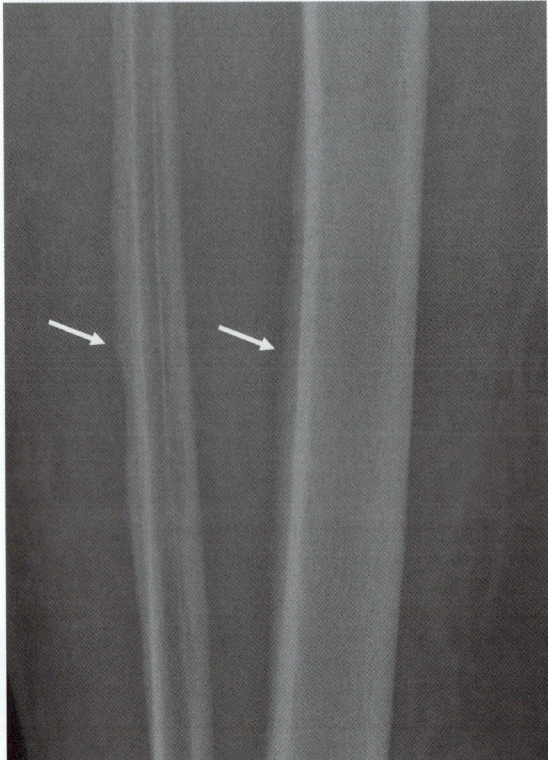

Fig. 66.5 Lesion with smooth periosteal reaction.

g. **Presence or absence of a soft tissue mass/cortical breakthrough:** Visible cortical break-through and/or soft tissue mass are the hallmarks of an aggressive lesion of bone. Despite reasonable assumption to the contrary, a large soft tissue may be present in the absence of profound cortical disruption. This feature is common in small round blue cell tumors (lymphoma and Ewings sarcoma) in which tumor cells characteristically spread through cortical tunnels, resulting in an appearance of intact cortex with a large surrounding soft-tissue mass.

h. **Polyostotic versus monostotic:** This alters the differential significantly. Primary bone lesions are rarely polyostotic; therefore, the presence of multiple bone lesions favors secondary processes such as metastatic disease or myeloma. Whole body bone scan, positron emission tomography–computed tomography (PET-CT), or whole-body magnetic resonance imaging (MRI) may help clarify this issue.

2. **A 22-year-old man presents with an ankle injury after inversion. Incidental osseous finding in the distal femur demonstrates a cortically based bubbly, mildly expansile lesion of bone with a narrow zone of transition and sclerotic margins located in the metaphysis of the tibia. No internal matrix (Fig. 66.9 a & b). What bone lesion is this?**

Nonossifying fibroma (NOF). The term *NOF* is commonly used interchangeably with **fibrous cortical defect** or **fibroxanthoma.** NOF is common (30–40%) in children and adolescents. As the skeleton matures, these lesions typically ossify with in-filling of bone and can often remain radiographically visible as a sclerotic focus or linear thickening along the metaphyseal cortex. This late-stage sclerosis yields the confusing descriptive name of an "ossifying" NOF. The characteristic well-marginated nonaggressive appearance and eccentric cortical- and metaphyseal-based location all suggest the appropriate and reassuring diagnosis. These lesions can be reliably diagnosed by imaging and should not be biopsied.

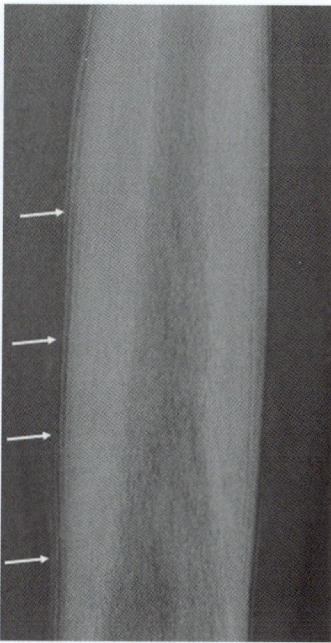

Fig. 66.6 Lesion with lamellated periosteal reaction.

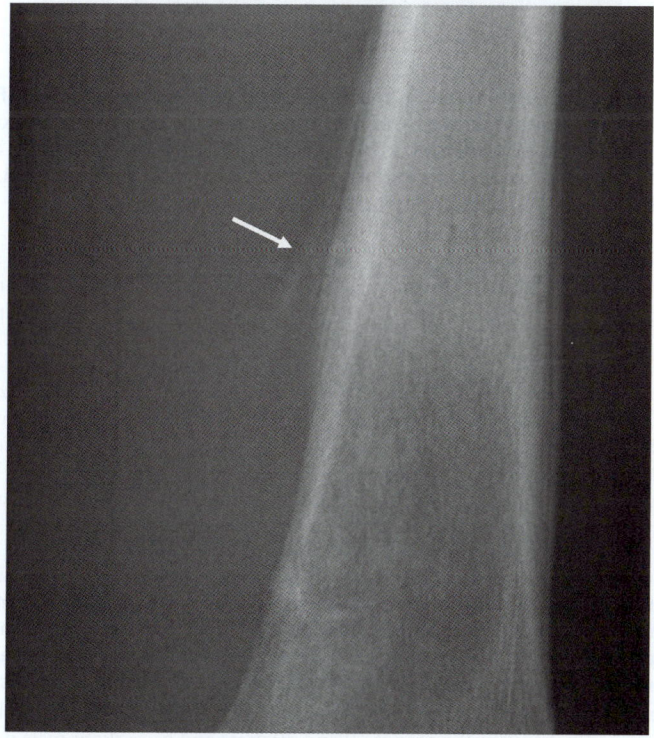

Fig. 66.7 Lesion with Codman's triangle.

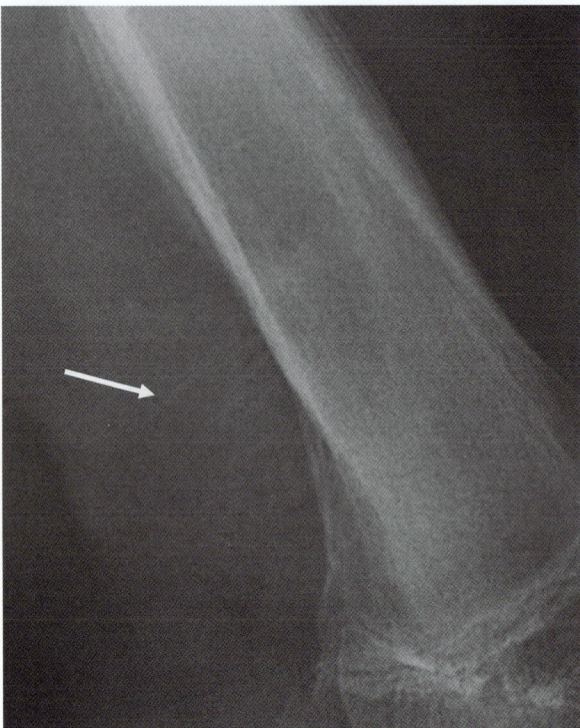

Fig. 66.8 Lesion with sunburst periosteal reaction.

3. **A 6-year-old boy fell while playing and presented with acute arm pain (Fig. 66.10). Radiographs demonstrate a well-defined radiolucent lesion of the proximal humeral diaphysis, with a narrow sclerotic zone of transition and linear density in the dependent portion (arrow). An angulated pathologic fracture is present through the center of the lesion. What bone lesion is this?**

Unicameral (simple) bone cyst (UBC). A true fluid-filled cystic lesion within the central medullary canal of the metaphysis of long bones. The pathognomonic feature of UBC is a thin linear horizontal fragment, or "fallen fragment", that often occurs with pathologic fracture (arrow). The fallen fragment is important in that it confirms the singular fluid-filled cavity present only in UBCs. UBCs generally occur in the long tubular bones, especially the proximal ends of the humerus (50–60%) and femur (30%), and may represent a disturbance of growth at the physeal plate rather than a true neoplasm. These are asymptomatic lesions unless traumatized. Pathologic fracture of a UBC can lead to in-filling of the lesion with healing bone. Surgical intervention, either with surgical curettage and bone packing, steroid injection, or injection of cement or ablative material, may be pursued to prevent a multiplicity of pathologic fractures and subsequent bone deformity and shortening. On radiographs, a favorable response is noted by a decrease in lesion size and an increase in radiodensity with adjacent cortical thickening.

4. **A 20-year-old male presents with worsening non-traumatic left arm pain (Fig 66.11A and B). Radiographs demonstrate an ill-defined lesion occupying the mid-diaphysis of the humerus. Aggressive features include cortical destruction, permeative narrow zone of transition, cortical destruction, lamellated periosteal reaction (arrow), and probable associated soft tissue mass. What bone lesion is this?**

Ewings sarcoma. Primary bone lesion of childhood is made up of small, round, blue cells. This lesion typically occurs between the ages of 10 and 20 years and has a slight male predilection. Radiographs suggest the diagnosis through the classic meta-diaphyseal location and permeative

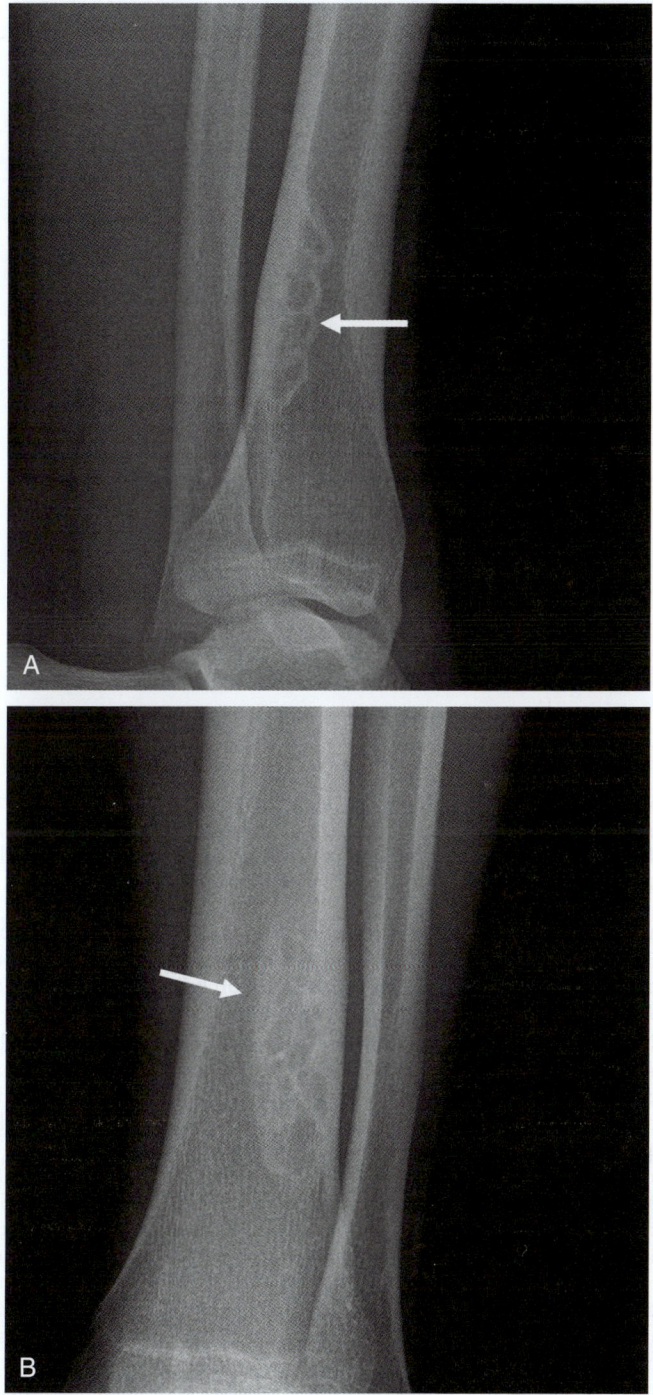

Fig. 66.9 (**A**) Nonossifying fibroma (NOF); (**B**) Nonossifying fibroma (NOF).

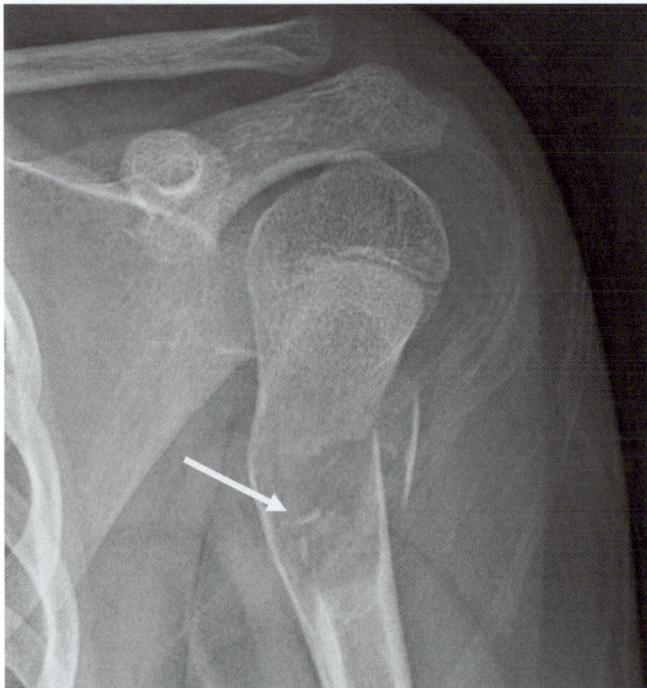

Fig. 66.10 Unicameral bone cyst.

pattern of bone involvement. In addition to the long bones, which make up 60% of the lesions, the flat bones (pelvis, scapula, ribs) and spine may also be affected in 40%. The small round blue cells that make up the lesion have a propensity to seep out of small cortical channels, creating large peri-osseous soft tissue masses often with little detectable cortical destruction.

5. **A 32-year-old male presents with chronic posterior leg pain following long athletic practices. Radiographs demonstrate a well-defined pedunculated lesion arising from the posterior tibia with medullary continuation with the metaphysis (Fig. 66.12 A and B). What bone lesion does this represent?**

Osteochondroma. This lesion, also known as an "exostosis," is the most common bone tumor and is more accurately described as a developmental lesion rather than a tumor. This osseous excrescence often arises from the metaphyseal region of a long tubular bone, with the lower extremity most commonly affected (femur/tibia 50%). This lesion can be pedunculated or sessile in morphology but always demonstrates the pathognomonic medullary continuity. Pedunculated osteochondromas typically grow to point away from the adjacent joint, differentiating them from entheses at the tendinous insertions. These tumors may be singular or multiple and affect all age groups, typically presenting by the first or second decade of life. Osteochondromas are usually asymptomatic but can cause symptoms when they are associated with mechanical irritation of the adjacent soft tissues, nerve impingement, or adventitial bursitis.

All osteochondromas have a cartilage cap, although this is typically thin. This cartilage cap is important in that it provides the source of malignant degeneration and can be assessed accurately by MRI or ultrasound. A cartilage cap of >1.5 cm in skeletally mature patients and >3 cm in immature patients is suspicious for malignant transformation and should be treated surgically. Malignant transformation is suggested radiographically by the presence of bony erosions at the distal tip of the lesion, by new or increased chondroid matrix, or by the resorption/disappearance of previously seen chondroid matrix.

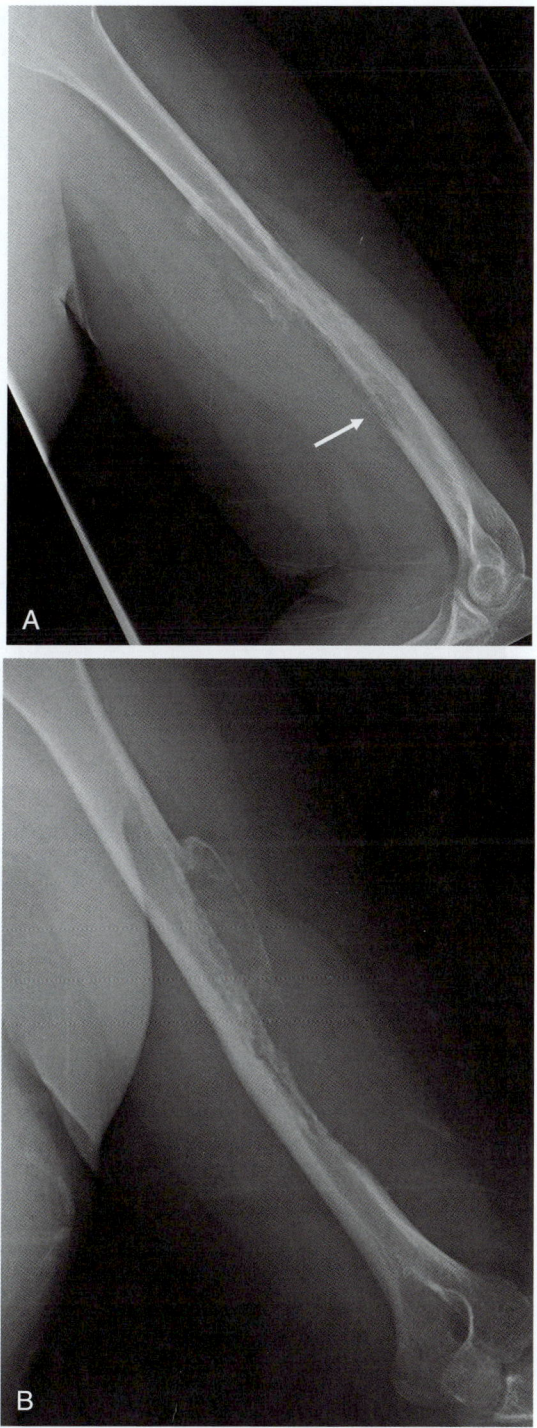

Fig. 66.11 (**A**) Ewings sarcoma; (**B**) Ewings sarcoma.

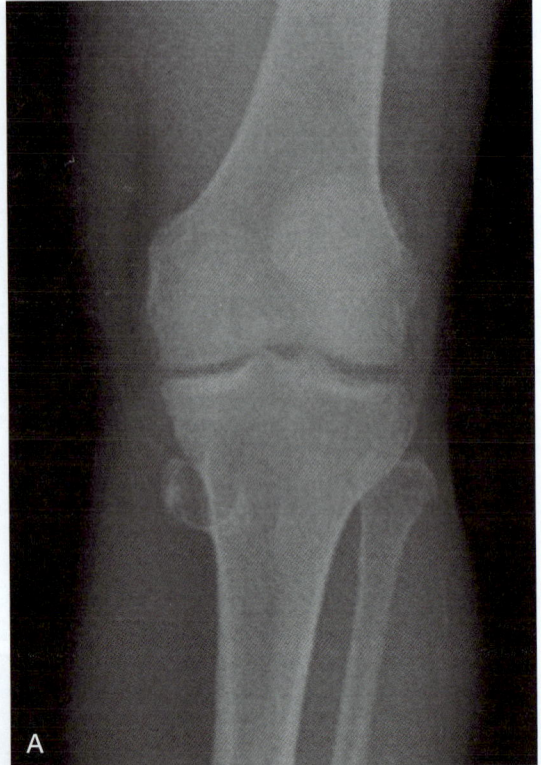

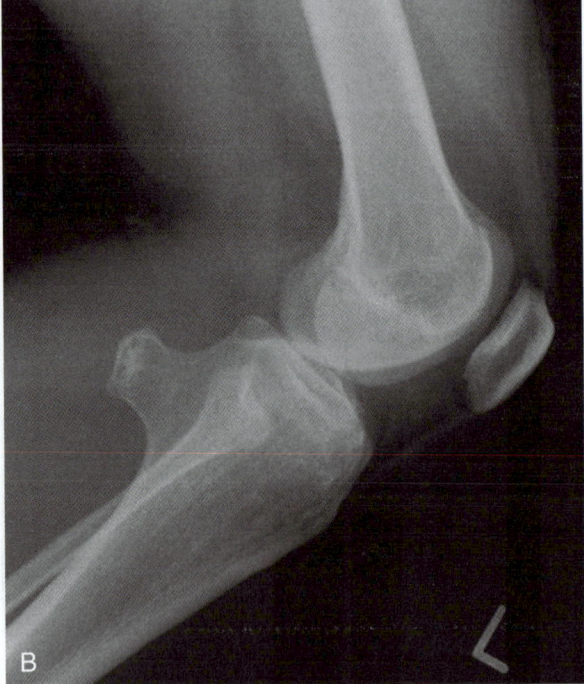

Fig. 66.12 (**A**) Osteochondroma; (**B**) Osteochondroma.

Growth of a known osteochondroma after skeletal maturity is reached, new or worsening pain, or a palpable new soft-tissue mass overlying an osteochondroma can all indicate malignant transformation and should be investigated with MRI. The incidence of malignant transformation to chondrosarcoma is rare, ranging from 1% in solitary osteochondromas to 5% in cases of autosomal dominant **multiple hereditary exostoses.** Axial or central lesions, such as in the spine or flat bones, degenerate at a greater frequency than appendicular-based lesions.

6. **A 17-year-old male presents with left hip pain, greater at night, and relieved with aspirin. Radiographs demonstrate a cortically based lucent nidus (white arrow) in the left femoral neck with profound asymmetric cortical thickening (black arrow) along the proximal femoral shaft (Fig. 66.13). What might this lesion be?**

   Osteoid osteoma. Benign but painful bone-forming lesions typically occur in young patients aged 10 to 35 years. The ovoid, sharply marginated, radiolucent center or nidus measuring <2 cm with a wide zone of adjacent reactive sclerosis is pathognomonic of this lesion. Osteoid osteomas are classically cortically based and are commonly seen in the long bones of the appendicular skeleton, with the femoral neck being the most common location. Over 90% of patients with this lesion complain of nighttime pain relieved by aspirin. CT scan is the imaging modality of choice for demonstrating the nidus, as the subtle lucency may be occult on radiographs. Image-guided thermal ablation of the lesion has replaced surgical excision as the treatment of choice. Approximately 30% of patients treated percutaneously for osteoid osteoma will require a second ablation to achieve complete relief.

7. **A 44-year-old female presents with pain in the wrist. Radiographs show an eccentric, mildly expansile, lytic lesion in the distal radius that extends to the articular surface and demonstrates a wide zone of transition. The cortex is thinned with questionable breakthrough at the ulnar margin (Fig. 66.14). What lesion is this?**

   Giant cell tumor (GCT). These tumors tend to occur in the skeletally mature individual after physeal closure. Although they originate in the metaphysis of the bone, they commonly extend to a subarticular location within the epiphysis, a defining feature of this lesion. GCT of bone typically occurs in young adults with a peak incidence between 20 and 30 years and is most commonly found in the distal femur or proximal tibia (50–70%). The vast majority of GCTs are histologically benign, with approximately 5% deemed malignant. Despite their benign histologic pattern, GCTs can be locally very aggressive and destructive. Wide resection is typically curative, but given the subarticular location of GCT, joint-sparing surgery is typically performed with local resection and curettage with bone graft or cementation. The recurrence rate after local excision

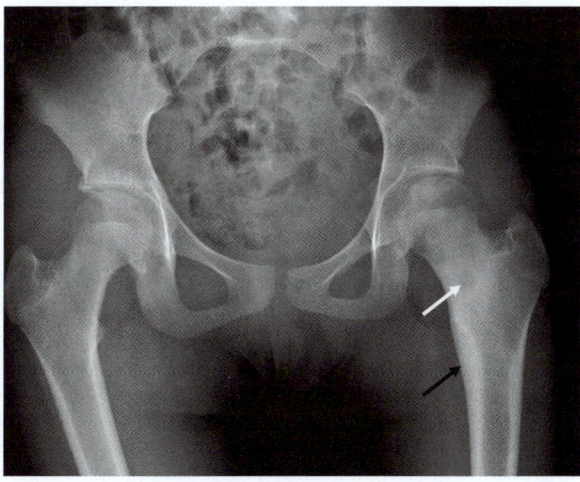

Fig. 66.13 Osteoid osteoma.

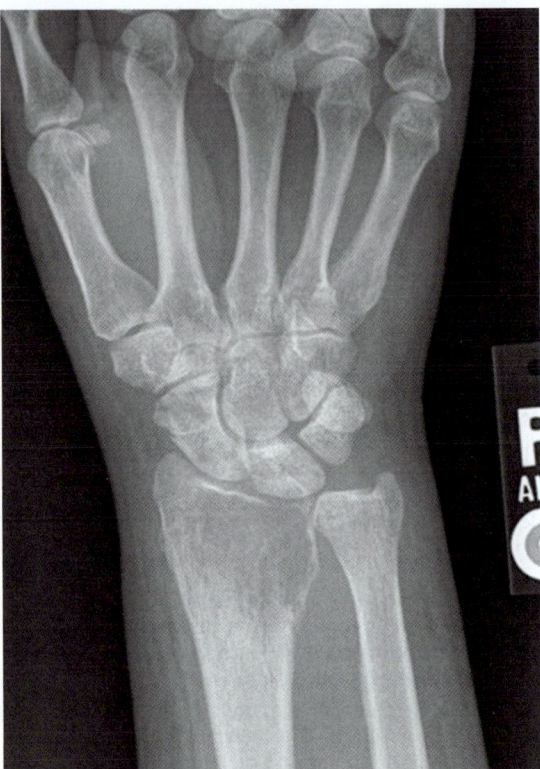

Fig. 66.14 Giant cell tumor.

is quite variable, ranging from 25% to 60%. GCT is one of the few tumors that can produce benign metastases, most frequently to the lung.

8. **A 10-year-old boy presents with progressively worsening upper arm pain and restricted shoulder motion. Radiographs demonstrate a lucent lesion in the epiphysis of the proximal humerus, respecting the margin of the adjacent open physis (Fig. 66.15). What is the most likely diagnosis?**
   Chondroblastoma is a rare benign chondrogenic neoplasm that occurs most often in the skel-etally immature patient and classically involves the epiphyses of long bones but may also be found in the talus, calcaneus, patella, or pelvic bones. Radiographic features include an eccentric lucent lesion with a smooth geographic contour defined by a thin, sometimes indistinct peripheral sclerosis. It is one of the few primary bone lesions that arise in the epiphysis. Internal chondroid matrix can help make the diagnosis but is only seen in about half of the cases. Chondroblastomas are benign lesions, and treatment typically consists of surgical curettage and grafting. Percutane-ous radiofrequency ablation has also been shown to be effective in some cases.

9. **A 60-year-old woman has a painless lucent lesion in the proximal phalanx of the long finger as seen on the radiograph (Fig. 66.16). What bone lesion is this?**
   Enchondroma. This well-circumscribed, geographic lesion arises eccentrically within the diaphysis of the phalanx. The lobulated contour is characteristic of cartilaginous lesions, as are the punctate, sharply defined calcifications (arrow). Endosteal erosion and bulging of the cortex are common. Enchondromas are the most common, nonaggressive lesions of the hands. Greater than 50% of enchondromas occur in the diaphyses of the short, tubular bones of the hands and feet. The remaining occur most often in the metaphyses of the long tubular bones. In the fingers and toes, enchondromas are more often lytic in nature with few punctate areas of internal matrix.

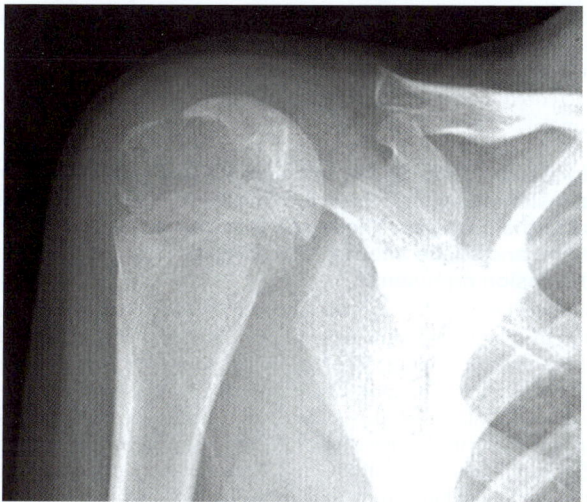

Fig. 66.15 Chondroblastoma.

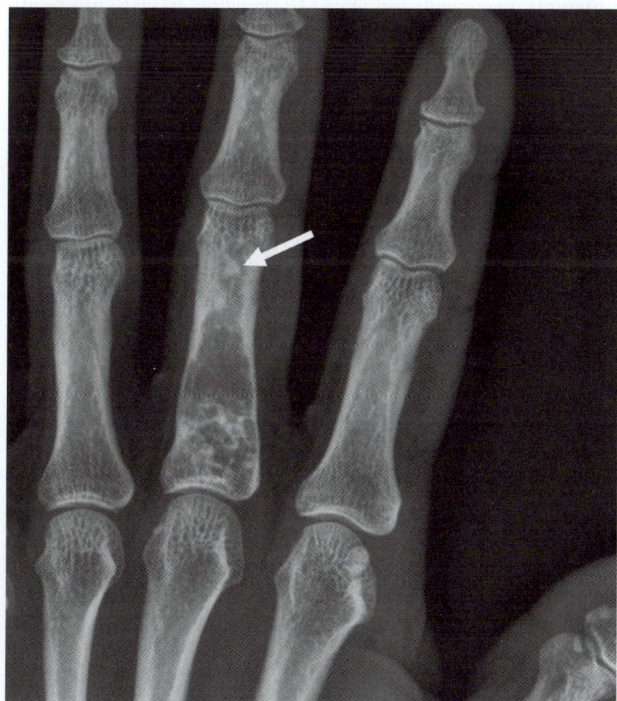

Fig. 66.16 Enchondroma.

This is in contrast to the typical enchondroma of the proximal appendicular skeleton, which more often demonstrates ring and arc intra-lesional chondroid matrix. Malignant transformation occurs in 1% of solitary enchondromas, usually arising in lesions of the long, tubular, or flat bones, and is not a valid concern in phalangeal enchondromas.

Enchondromatosis (Ollier disease) is a rare, nonhereditary disorder consisting of widespread involvement of predominantly one side of the body with multiple, asymmetrically distributed enchondromas. Often, there is associated shortening and deformity of the long bones affected. Malignant transformation of an individual lesion in Ollier disease is common, occurring in one-third to one-half of patients. **Maffucci syndrome** is a rare, congenital disorder of mesodermal dysplasia characterized by enchondromatosis and soft-tissue hemangiomas. Malignant transformation is common.

10. **A 43-year-old man presents with thigh pain. Radiograph of the femur demonstrates an incidental lesion occupying the entire medullary canal of the femur from the femoral neck to the condyles. The lesion is mixed lytic and sclerotic with a slightly expansile nature and subtle internal ground glass opacity (Fig. 66.17 A and B). What does this bone lesion represent?**

Fibrous dysplasia (FD). This lesion classically presents as a nonaggressive, mixed-density fibro-osseous lesion in the diaphysis and metaphysis of long bones. The "ground-glass" internal matrix is characteristic of fibrous components. These nonaggressive, ground-glass density, long lesions of bone are classic for FD. Histologically, FD represents a fibroosseous lesion, in which normal bone is replaced by abnormal fibrous tissue within an abnormally arranged trabecular pattern. About 20% to 25% of patients with FD have multiple sites of involvement. The femur and tibia, skull and mandible, and ribs are commonly affected. **McCune-Albright syndrome** is identified by the triad of polyostotic, predominantly unilateral FD, café-au-lait macular lesions with irregular "coast of Maine" margins, and endocrine dysfunction, particularly precocious puberty. This disease is due to a mutation of the gene, GNAS1, on chromosome 20 that is involved in G-protein signaling and prevents downregulation of cAMP signaling. **Mazabraud syndrome** is characterized by polyostotic FD with multiple intramuscular myxomatous lesions and usually presents in middle-aged women.

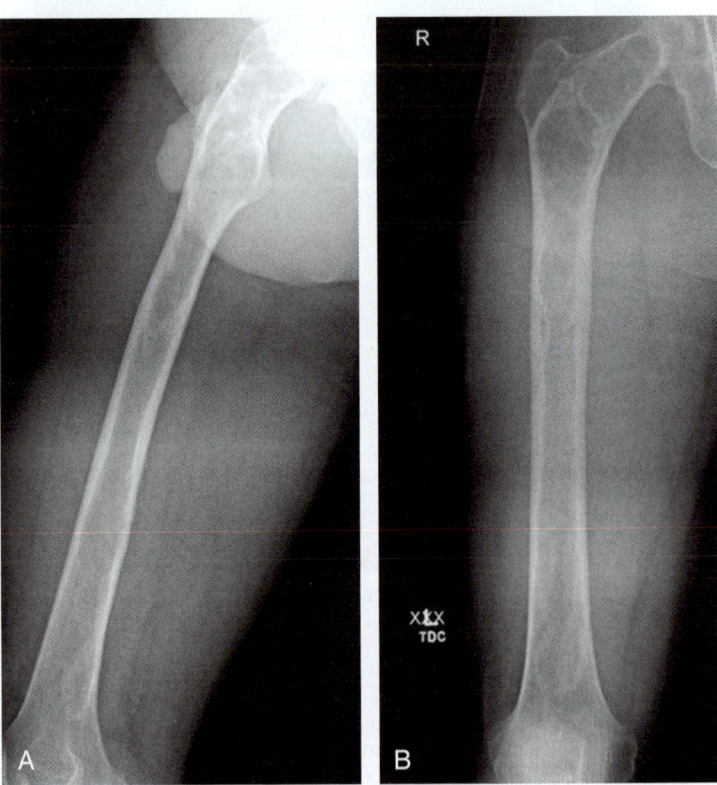

Fig. 66.17 **(A)** Fibrous dysplasia; **(B)** Fibrous dysplasia.

11. **A 17-year-old male presents with worsening atraumatic pain and swelling around the knee (Fig. 66.18 A and B). Radiographs demonstrate a mixed-density lesion in the distal femoral metaphysis with central foci of cloud-like osteoid matrix (black arrow). Aggressive features include cortical disruption, a wide zone of transition, Codman's triangle of periosteal reaction (arrowheads), and sunburst periosteal reaction (white arrows). What is the diagnosis of concern in this patient?**

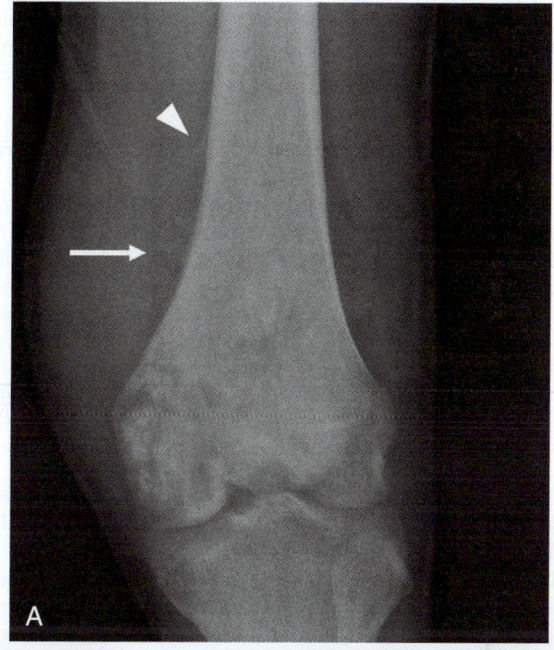

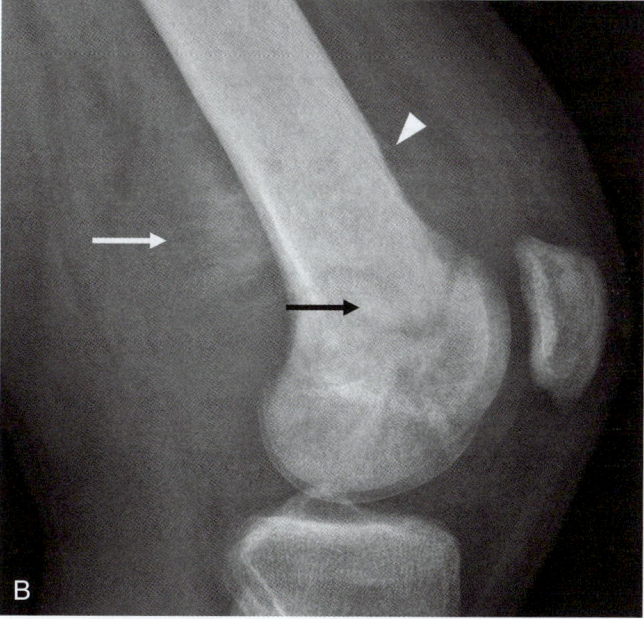

Fig. 66.18 (**A**) Osteosarcoma. (**B**) Osteosarcoma.

Osteosarcoma. This is the second most common primary bone tumor, accounting for 20% of malignant bone lesions, and is the most common bone tumor in children. Osteosarcoma may be seen in primary and secondary forms. Primary osteosarcoma is a tumor of childhood, most commonly affecting patients aged 10 to 30 years. The propensity for involvement of the young is thought to be related to the hyperactivity of growth centers seen in adolescence. Secondary osteosarcoma is seen in the elderly as a response to prior radiation therapy or as malignant transformation of benign lesions such as Paget disease of bone. The vast majority (80%) of osteosarcomas occur centrally within the medullary canal of long appendicular bones, but surface osteosarcomas (e.g., parosteal and periosteal osteosarcomas) also occur. Radiographically, osteosarcomas are defined by medullary and cortical bone destruction, a wide zone of transition, and aggressive periosteal reaction. The presence of cloud-like osseous matrix is variable and may or may not be present.

12. **A 6-year-old boy presents with arm pain after a fall. A radiograph shows a large geographic lucent lesion with cortical thinning and medullary expansion. Pathologic fracture is evidenced by cortical buckle and discontinuity (arrow) through the center of the lesion (Fig. 66.19 A and B). What bone lesion does this represent?**
Aneurysmal bone cyst (ABC). This osteolytic lesion is a tumor of childhood that often presents before physeal closure. The expansile nature of ABCs is thought to be caused by local alterations in hemodynamics (i.e., venous obstruction and/or arteriovenous fistulas), which result in blood-filled cavities creating the characteristic fluid-fluid levels on MRI. ABCs may develop *de novo* or form as a response to prior trauma or insult from preexisting lesions. About 60% to 70% of ABCs occur within the long tubular bones, usually originating from the metaphysis. These cysts also have a predilection for the posterior elements of the vertebral bodies, where they can be difficult to distinguish from other nonaggressive lesions that occur in this location (e.g., osteoblastomas and GCTs).

13. **A 20-year-old boy with head pain shows a single, lytic, "punched-out" lesion on a skull film (Fig. 66.20). What lesion is this?**
Eosinophilic granuloma (EG). The exquisitely well-circumscribed, "punched-out" lesion in the skull with a clear matrix is characteristic of EG. Often, the margin appears beveled secondary to involvement of both the inner and outer tables of the calvarium. In the mandible, the loss of supporting bone results in the appearance of "floating teeth." When the metaphysis or diaphysis of the long bones is affected, the lesion is associated with both endosteal scalloping and extensive, thick, laminated periosteal reaction. EG is also one of the causes of a complete collapse of a vertebral body, a condition known as vertebra plana. Plain film remains the modality of choice for documentation of EG lesions as 30% to 35% of lesions have no uptake of radionuclide on bone scan and up to 10% result in "cold" areas of abnormally decreased uptake. Lesions can be monostotic or polyostotic.

    Langerhans cell histiocytosis (Histiocytosis X) is a group of diseases caused by the clonal proliferation of Langerhans cells, which are epidermal dendritic cells. An activating mutation of the BRAF gene is commonly found. When it is unifocal and involves only bone without extraskeletal involvement, it is called EG. When it is multifocal with both bone and visceral involvement, it is called Letterer-Siwe or Hand–Christian–Schüller disease, depending on the presentation. **Letterer-Siwe disease** is marked by rapid dissemination and a poor prognosis. It tends to appear in children aged <2 to 3 years, causing bone lesions, hepatosplenomegaly, and occasionally "honeycomb" interstitial lung disease. With chemotherapy, the 5-year survival rate is only 50%. **Hand–Christian–Schüller disease** is associated with the chronic dissemination of osseous lesions, fever, and skin lesions usually in the scalp and ears. Peak onset is 3 to 10 years old. Up to 50% of cases involve the pituitary stalk, leading to diabetes insipidus. The characteristic triad is bone lesions, diabetes insipidus, and exophthalmos. About 10% to 30% of cases are fatal.

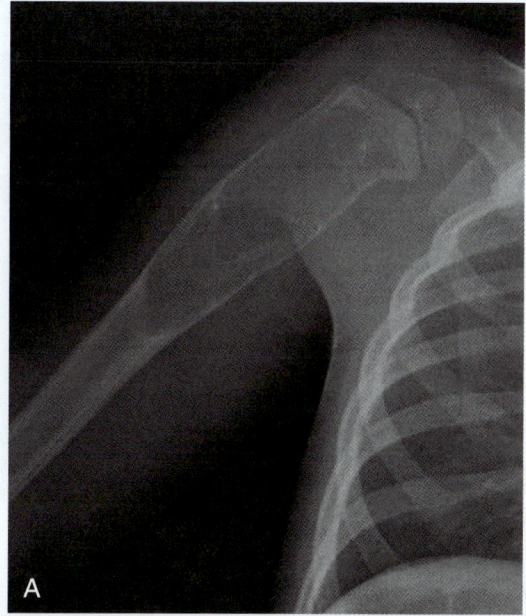

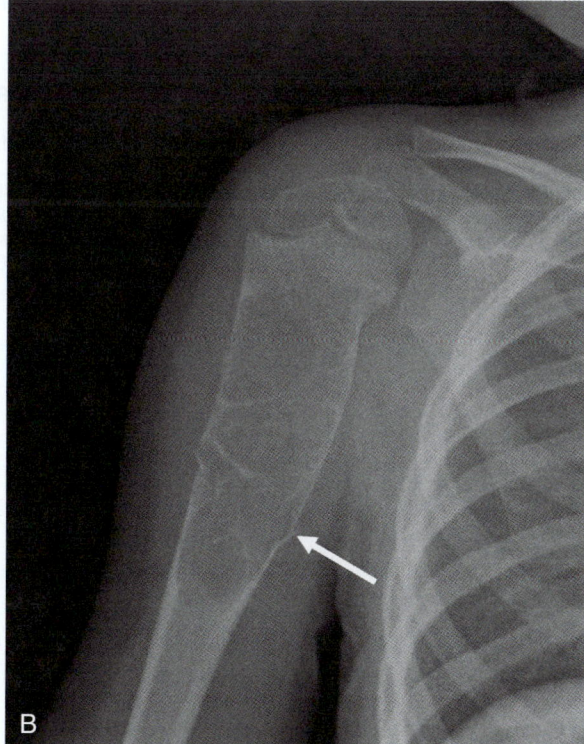

Fig. 66.19 (**A**) Aneurysmal bone cyst (ABC); (**B**) Aneurysmal bone cyst (ABC).

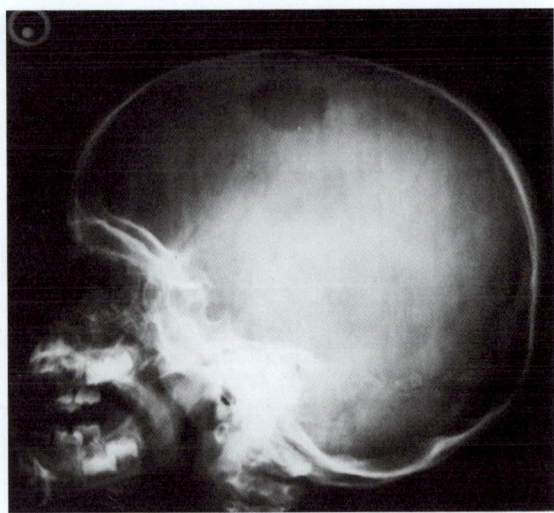

Fig. 66.20 Eosinophilic granuloma (EG).

ACKNOWLEDGMENT

The author would like to thank Dr. Brian Petersen for his contributions to the previous editions of this chapter.

BIBLIOGRAPHY

Berquist TH, Dalinka MK, Alazraki N, et al. Bone tumors: American College of Radiology— ACR appropriateness criteria. *Radiology.* 2000;215(suppl):261–264.
Gonzalez-Huete A, Salgado-Parente A, Suevos-Ballesteros C, et al. Radiographic evaluation of bone tumors. *Radiographics.* 2023;43(11):e230048.
Hudson TM. *Radiologic-Pathologic Correlation of Musculoskeletal Lesions.* Baltimore, MD: Williams & Wilkins; 1987.
Miller T. Bone tumor and tumor-like conditions: analysis with conventional radiography. *Radiology.* 2008;246:662–674.
Resnick D, Kransdorf MJ. *Bone and Joint Imaging.* 3rd ed. Philadelphia, PA: Elsevier Saunders; 2005.
Resnick D. *Diagnosis of Bone and Joint Disorders.* 4th ed. Philadelphia, PA: WB Saunders; 2002.

FURTHER READING

www.bonetumor.org.
www.radiopedia.org.

Approach to the Child With Joint Pain

Eileen C. Rife, MD and Randy Q. Cron, MD, PhD

  KEY POINTS

1. A limp in a child is pathologic until proven otherwise.
2. Malignancy is more likely than systemic juvenile idiopathic arthritis (sJIA) in any child who has fever, a painful arthritis, an elevated lactate dehydrogenase (LDH) level, and/or a low platelet count.
3. Neck, back, or bone pain in a young child is never normal and demands an extensive workup.

1. What is the differential diagnosis of joint pain in childhood?

There are at least 110 illnesses associated with arthritis or related musculoskeletal syndromes in childhood. The broad differential diagnosis can be remembered with the mnemonic **PRIME BONE PAIN:**

P—Pharmacologic: serum sickness; medication side effects (i.e., quinolones), drug-induced lupus.

R—Rheumatologic: JIA; systemic lupus erythematosus (SLE); Sjogren disease; systemic sclerosis; mixed connective tissue disease (MCTD); vasculitis; dermatomyositis; sarcoidosis.

I—Infectious/post-infectious: a) bacterial (osteomyelitis, discitis, septic arthritis, rheumatic fever, tuberculosis, Lyme, Kingella), b) viral ("toxic/transient" synovitis, human immunodeficiency virus, hepatitis B/C, parvovirus, Epstein–Barr virus, herpes virus), c) reactive arthritis

M—Metabolic/genetic: mucopolysaccharidoses; mucolipidoses; heritable collagen disorders (i.e., Marfan).

E—Episodic: autoinflammatory syndromes (FMF, HIDS, TRAPS, CAPS, BLAU, PAPA, DIRA). See Chapter 79: Familial Autoinflammatory Syndromes.

B—Blood: sickle cell anemia; hemophilia; disrupted blood supply/avascular necrosis (i.e., Legg–Calvé–Perthes).

O—Orthopedic: chondromalacia patellae; Osgood–Schlatter disease; osteochondritis dissecans; slipped capital femoral epiphysis (SCFE).

N—Neoplastic: neuroblastoma; leukemia; lymphoma; bone tumors; pigmented villonodular synovitis; metastases; Langerhans histiocytosis.

E—Endocrine: hypercortisolism; hypothyroidism; rickets; diabetes mellitus.

P—Pain: Amplified musculoskeletal pain syndrome (AMPS)/fibromyalgia; complex regional pain syndrome (CRPS); conversion disorder.

A—Accidental/trauma; foreign body (i.e., thorn synovitis).

I—Inflammatory: inflammatory bowel disease; chronic nonbacterial osteomyelitis (CNO).

N—"Normal variants": growing pains; hypermobility.

2. What are the characteristics of an organic versus a nonorganic etiology for joint pain?

Organic	Nonorganic (functional)
Occurs day and night	Occurs toward the end of the day or at night (in the case of "growing pains")
Occurs during weekends and on vacation	Occurs primarily on school days
Severe enough to interrupt play and other pleasant activities	Child is typically able to carry out normal daily activities
Located in joint	Between joints, fascial regions, or widespread
Child limps or refuses to walk	Child has unusual gait, inconsistent
Description fits with logical anatomic explanation	Description is illogical, often dramatically stated, and not aligned with known anatomic or physical process

3. **What are the historical clues of an organic versus a nonorganic etiology for joint pain?**

Organic: Signs of systemic illness, including weight loss, malaise, fatigue, fever, night sweats, rash, diarrhea.

Nonorganic: Isolated pain in an otherwise healthy child. May have a history of concomitant depression or anxiety. Can occur in the setting of chronic disease, but pain amplified beyond that expected with usual disease process. Often many missed days of school for pain.

4. **List the physical signs that suggest an inflammatory cause for joint pain.**

Point tenderness.

Redness.

Swelling.

Limitation of movement of affected extremity secondary to pain or anatomic restriction.

Objective muscle weakness or atrophy.

Signs of systemic illness: fever, rash, lymphadenopathy, and organomegaly.

5. **Which laboratory tests are helpful in differentiating causes of joint pain? See Table 67.1.**

TABLE 67.1 Laboratory and Imaging Evaluations to Help Differentiate Causes of Joint Pain

TEST	CONDITIONS IN WHICH TEST MAY BE HELPFUL
Complete blood count, with differential	Leukemia (if blasts on smear)
	Infections in bones, joints, muscles
	Systemic connective tissue diseases
Sedimentation rate	Infections
	Systemic connective tissue diseases
	Inflammatory bowel disease
	Tumors
Radiographs	Bone tumors, malignant and benign
	Osteomyelitis (chronic)
	Discitis (late)
	Fractures
	Scoliosis
	Rickets
	Slipped capital femoral epiphysis
	Legg–Calvé–Perthes disease
	Leukemia (leukemic lines on x-ray)
MRI or other advanced imaging (bone scan, CT, PET)	Osteomyelitis (acute and chronic)
	Discitis
	Osteoid osteoma
	Malignancies (leukemia, bone tumors, and metastases)
	Infarction of bone
	Complex regional pain syndrome
Muscle enzymes	Inflammatory muscle disease
	Muscular dystrophy
	Rhabdomyolysis

Abbreviations: MRI = magnetic resonance imaging; CT = computed tomography; PET = positron emission tomography. Adapted from Cassidy JE, et al. *Textbook of Pediatric Rheumatology.* 6th ed. Philadelphia PA: WB Saunders; 2011.

TABLE 67.2 Causes of Acute and Chronic Monoarthritis	
Acute Monoarticular	Undifferentiated JIA (early) Infection/Post infectious: • Septic arthritis • Reactive Arthritis (particularly joints of the lower extremities) • Lyme (particularly the knee) Trauma or foreign body synovitis Sarcoid (polyarticular of the lower extremities more common) Gout (in pediatric patients think familial variants) Malignancy (bone tumors/sarcomas/localized lesions)
Chronic Monoarticular	Oligoarticular JIA Infectious/post-infectious: • Lyme (particularly the knee) • Tuberculosis/mycobacterial • Fungal Malignancy: (PVNS, bone tumors/sarcomas/localized lesions) Sarcoid (particularly the ankles and knees) Foreign body synovitis Avascular necrosis Hemarthrosis Synovial chondromatosis Internal derangements Lipomatosis arborescens

JIA, juvenile idiopathic arthritis; *PVNS*, pigmented villonodular synovitis.

6. How does the number of affected joints help in sorting through the differential diagnosis of arthritis?

Factors helpful in assessing the etiology of arthritis are the duration of the disease at the time the child is evaluated, the sex and age of the child, and the onset type and pattern of joint involvement. The differential diagnosis of polyarthritis is considerably different from that of monoarthritis or oligoarthritis (Tables 67.2 & 67.3). JIA is the most common cause of chronic monoarthritis, particularly in girls under the age of 5.

7. How does the diurnal variation in joint pain aid in diagnosis?

Stiffness and pain on range of motion (ROM) immediately upon arising and after periods of inactivity ("gelling") are classic findings for the inflammatory arthritides. Morning stiffness typically improves with heat and ROM exercises. The duration of morning stiffness is an excellent gauge of the severity of the arthritis and the efficacy of therapy. In contrast, mechanical joint pain worsens over the course of the day and with activity. Nighttime pain and/or awakening with pain are red flags for neoplasia. Alternatively, isolated nighttime pain may be attributable to "growing pains" in an otherwise healthy child.

8. In which conditions are the affected joints erythematous?

Septic arthritis, rheumatic fever, foreign body synovitis, and neoplasia. Erythematous joints are very rare in JIA and in most other rheumatic conditions. They should be a "red flag" for the above diagnoses. The arthritis of rheumatic fever is typically characterized by its migratory nature and by pain that is often out of proportion to the severity of findings on joint examination (e.g., degree of swelling). The arthritis that occurs in rheumatic fever is highly responsive to nonsteroidal anti-inflammatory drug (NSAID) therapy.

TABLE 67.3 Causes of Acute and Chronic Polyarthritis	
Acute Polyarticular	JIA: • SJIA • Early polyarticular JIA (RF+ or RF-) • Early juvenile psoriatic arthritis • Early inflammatory bowel disease/enteropathic Early CTD: • SLE • MCTD • Sjogren's disease • Systemic Sclerosis • Juvenile dermatomyositis Infection/post-infection: • Reactive arthritis (particularly large joints) • Rheumatic fever • Septic • Gonococcal arthritis • Lyme • Infective endocarditis • Viral-associated (parvovirus, EBV, HIV, COVID) Malignancy: • Acute leukemia (ALL and AML) • Neuroblastoma • Langerhans histiocytosis • Metastatic lesions • Lymphoma Gout (in pediatric patients, think familial variants) Sarcoidosis (particularly, the knees and ankles) Systemic vasculitis Autoinflammatory syndromes (predominately episodic)
Chronic Polyarticular	JIA Polyarticular: • sJIA • JIA (RF+ or RF-) • Juvenile psoriatic arthritis • Inflammatory bowel disease-associated/enteropathic CTD: • SLE • MCTD • Sjogren's disease • Systemic sclerosis • Juvenile Dermatomyositis Infectious: • Tuberculosis/mycobacterial • Fungal • Lyme (rare to be polyarticular) Mucopolysaccharidosis Sarcoidosis Pseudorheumatoid dysplasia Systemic vasculitis

ERA, enthesitis-related arthritis; *JIA*, juvenile idiopathic arthritis; *MCTD*, mixed connective tissue disease; *PVNS*, pigmented villonodular synovitis; *RF*, rheumatoid factor; *SLE*, systemic lupus erythematosus; *sJIA*, systemic JIA; *ALL*, acute lymphoblastic leukemia; *AML*, acute myeloid leukemia; *HIV*, human immunodeficiency syndrome; *EBV*, Epstein-Barr Virus.

9. In a child with a swollen joint, how is the joint fluid helpful in determining the etiology of joint pain? See Table 67.4.

TABLE 67.4 Typical Joint Fluid Findings in Arthritis[a]

GROUP/CONDITION	WBC COUNT (/ML)	PMN (%)	MISCELLANEOUS FINDINGS
Noninflammatory			
Normal	<200	<25	—
Traumatic	<2000	<25	Debris
Inflammatory			
SLE	5000–10,000	10–25	LE cells
Rheumatic fever	5000–10,000	10–50	—
JIA	10,000–20,000	-	-
Reactive arthritis	10,000–20,000	-	Reiter cells
Infectious			
Tuberculous arthritis	25,000	50–60	Acid-fast bacteria[b]
Septic arthritis	50,000–300,000	>75	Low glucose, bacteria

JIA, juvenile idiopathic arthritis; *LE,* lupus erythematosus; *SLE,* systemic lupus erythematosus; *PMN,* polymorphonuclear neutrophils; *WBC,* white blood cell.
[a]These are guidelines and some inflammatory arthritides like JIA can have a synovial fluid WBC count >100,000/mL (pseudoseptic). Crystal-induced synovitis is rare in childhood apart from genetic (familial hyperuricemia, FMF), neoplastic (leukemia), enzymatic (Lesch-Nyhan), and nephropathic origins.
[b]Yield in synovial fluid often low; synovial biopsy should be considered, particularly if tuberculosis is high on the differential.
Adapted from Petty RE, et al. *Textbook of Pediatric Rheumatology.* 8th ed. Philadelphia, PA: Elsevier; 2021.

10. How is leg length assessed in a child? Why is the affected leg often longer in a child with oligoarticular JIA?

Leg length is measured from the anterior superior iliac spine to the medial malleolus. In a child with a joint contracture, the functional leg length may be shorter than the actual leg length, and therefore both must be measured. Leg length discrepancy (LLD) reflects a chronic disease process. The affected leg is often longer in a child with chronic arthritis, particularly arthritis affecting the knee. This is a result of increased blood flow to the joint in response to localized inflammation and cytokine release. The increased blood flow may lead to development of a "macroepiphysis". Affected children may have an abnormal gait and correction with a lift (on the bottom of the shoe of the shorter leg) is recommended when the LLD is >2cm. The shorter, unaffected leg will usually "catch up" to the affected leg and may overgrow the affected leg, since the epiphysis of the inflamed joint will undergo accelerated fusion. Muscle bulk of the thigh or the calf may be reduced in the affected leg and will rarely "catch up" to that of the unaffected leg, particularly if the arthritis onset was at <6 years of age.

11. What are "red flags" for neoplasia as the etiology of joint pain?

- Limb bone pain.
- Joint redness.
- Fever, weight loss, night sweats.
- Nighttime pain.
- Adenopathy.

Limb bone pain as an independent variable is strongly associated with cancer, followed by weight loss, thrombocytopenia, monoarticular hip involvement, and male sex. Factors independently associated with JIA include the following: morning stiffness, joint swelling, and involvement of the small joints of the hands.

Malignancy must be considered in any child in whom a diagnosis of sJIA is entertained, as the classic features of SJIA (i.e., fever, rash, and arthritis) are commonly seen in malignancy. Malignant infiltration of bone or synovium may mimic polyarthritis. In addition, joint effusions occur in children with malignancy, possibly owing to antigen–antibody complex deposition producing a serum sickness-like picture. This may also be responsible for the tremendous inflammatory response (high erythrocyte sedimentation rate [ESR] and anemia) seen in some children with malignancy —again mimicking sJIA.

Acute leukemia can cause polyarthritis and should be suspected in children with an elevated ESR with thrombocytopenia. Other frequent laboratory abnormalities include an elevated LDH (>2x upper limit of normal), anemia, elevated uric acid, and abnormal peripheral blood smear. Notably, the white blood cell (WBC) count and differential may initially be normal. Blasts on blood smears may be a later finding.

Radiographs of affected joints demonstrating epiphyseal leukemic (growth arrest) lines and/or advanced imaging may be helpful in diagnosis. Examples of advanced imaging include whole-body bone scan, positron emission tomography (PET)/computed tomography (CT), PET/magnetic resonance imaging (MRI), or MRI of clinically affected sites. Bone marrow examination is recommended prior to initiation of high-dose corticosteroid therapy for sJIA in cases where the diagnosis is unclear, since inappropriate use of corticosteroids in malignancy can delay diagnosis, mask high-risk features, and adversely affect prognosis.

12. What neoplasms are most likely to have musculoskeletal complaints upon presentation in childhood?

- Acute leukemia (acute lymphoblastic leukemia, acute myeloid leukemia)—consider in any child with "painful" JIA. Accounts for roughly one-third of all childhood malignancies, and musculoskeletal pain is a presenting symptom in >30% of cases.
- Neuroblastoma—patients may have systemic symptoms and ~20% have musculoskeletal complaints. A majority (>80%) of cases occur in children <5 years old.
- Ewing sarcoma and other malignant bone tumors or soft-tissue sarcomas—may present with localized pain or swelling, or a monoarthritis-like presentation.
- Lymphoma.
- Langerhans histiocytosis.

13. Describe the characteristics of childhood pain syndromes: primary fibromyalgia, complex regional pain syndrome (CRPS) type 1, "growing pains." See Table 67.5.

TABLE 67.5 Demographic, Clinical, and Laboratory Features of Childhood Pain Syndromes

	AMPS/FIBROMYALGIA	CRPS	GROWING PAINS
Age at onset	Adolescence	Late childhood and adolescence	4–12 years
Sex ratio	Female > male	Female > male	Equal
Symptoms	Widespread musculoskeletal pain (>3 months)	Exquisite superficial and deep pain in the distal part of an extremity	Deep aching, cramping pain in thigh or calf
	All day, most days	Daily, exacerbated by passive or active movement	Usually in evening or during the night
	More generalized	Typically affects one region	Bilateral
	Other possible symptoms: headache, abdominal pain, dizziness, TMJ pain, fatigue, paresthesias, disturbed sleep patterns.	Other possible symptoms: Skin color changes, swelling, hair changes, temperature changes in affected region.	
Signs	Widespread tender areas, often at characteristic sites (especially neck and back)	Pain (superficial or deep), sensory abnormalities (i.e., hyperesthesia), motor/trophic changes, sudomotor/edema (i.e., sweating), vasomotor (i.e., skin mottling, temperature changes). Guarding of affected region.	Physical exam normal
Investigations	Labs, imaging normal	Possible osteoporosis and bone scan abnormalities	Labs, imaging normal

AMPS, amplified musculoskeletal pain syndrome; *CRPS*, complex regional pain syndrome.

14. How does CRPS in childhood differ from adult CRPS?

- Less likely to have an antecedent triggering event i.e., trauma, surgery, illness.
- Lower extremity predominance in children versus upper extremities in adults.
- Marked female predominance in children as compared to adults.
- Few neurologic symptoms or chronic trophic changes observed in children.
- Psychosocial and personality factors may play a more prominent role in children.
- Excellent response to conservative measures with physical and occupational therapy, and counseling.

15. Describe the characteristics of common nonrheumatic knee pain syndromes in childhood: Patellofemoral pain syndrome and Osgood–Schlatter disease. See Table 67.6.

TABLE 67.6 Clinical and Laboratory Features of Osgood-Schlatter Disease and Patellofemoral Pain Syndrome

	PATELLOFEMORAL PAIN SYNDROME	OSGOOD–SCHLATTER
Age at onset	Adolescence	Adolescence
Sex ratio	Female > male	Male > female
Symptoms	Gradual or acute onset exertional knee pain, worse with flexion, running, squatting, stairs	Gradual onset pain over tibial tubercle exacerbated by exercise, squatting, flexion, stairs, kneeling
	Bilateral common	Bilateral in 25–50%
Signs	Poorly localized with patellar palpation; pain with resisted quadriceps contraction and patellar compression; rare effusion.	Point tenderness and swelling over attachment of patellar tendon
Investigations	Typically normal laboratory and imaging. Clinical diagnosis.	Radiographs with soft tissue swelling, enlarged (sometimes fragmented) tibial tubercle

16. What are the causes of hip pain in childhood?

1. Inflammatory
   - JIA (primarily enthesitis-related arthritis [ERA]/juvenile spondyloarthritis [JSpA]).
   - Chronic nonbacterial osteomyelitis (CNO; femur, pelvis).
   - Transient Synovitis.
2. Neoplastic
   - Generalized (i.e., leukemia)
   - Local/benign (i.e. osteoid osteoma)
   - Malignant (i.e. Ewing sarcoma).
3. Infectious/post-infectious
   - Septic arthritis.
   - Lyme disease.
   - Rheumatic fever.
   - Reactive arthritis.
   - Psoas abscess.
   - Discitis.
   - Osteomyelitis (femur, pelvis).
4. Mechanical/trauma/orthopedic
   - Slipped capital femoral epiphysis (SCFE)
   - Trochanteric bursitis.
   - Iliac apophysitis.
   - Protrusion acetabuli.
   - Avascular necrosis (AVN) (i.e., Legg–Calvé–Perthes disease).

> **PEARL:** Arthritis of the hip joint is **rare at the onset of oligoarticular JIA**. In a young child presenting with arthritis of the hip, consider septic or malignant etiologies first.

- The presence of (1) fever (≥38.5°C); (2) WBC count >12,000/µL; (3) ESR ≥40 mm/hour; (4) C-reactive protein ≥20 mg/L; and (5) inability to bear weight predicts **septic arthritis** to be more likely than transient synovitis of the hip.
- Transient synovitis of the hip may cause severe pain, but the process is self-limited —lasting only a few weeks —and laboratory/radiologic studies are typically normal.
- In the absence of systemic symptoms, congenital dislocation can also be considered.
- In older children and adolescents, **AVN** and **SCFE** should be considered.
- In older children, **ERA/JSpA** may present with unilateral or bilateral hip involvement, although distal joints are affected more commonly than proximal joints.
- Be aware that hip pain may rarely be referred to the knee— although it is more typically localized to the mid-anterior groin.

17. What are some causes of back pain in childhood?

Back and neck pain are relatively rare complaints in young children (as opposed to adolescents and adults) and should be taken seriously. Discitis is a rare cause of back pain in younger children with peak incidence around 1–3 years. It is generally considered an infection of intervertebral disc spaces caused by various pathogens (e.g., viruses, *Staphylococcus aureus, Kingella kingae*), although bacteria and viruses are seldom recovered by aspiration, and disc biopsies are not necessary for diagnosis. Fever, refusal to walk, unusual posturing (tripoding), stiffness, and point tenderness over the lumbar region are characteristic findings. The ESR is usually elevated. Plain radiographs may show disc-space narrowing, although usually not until late in the disease. MRI and Tc-99m bone scans are more sensitive at the time of presentation.

Malignancy (e.g., metastases, primary bone tumors, or leukemia) should be considered in the differential. ERA/JSpA is also a possibility, although, JSpA generally presents as peripheral arthritis (75% of children at presentation), with back complaints (pain, stiffness, or limitation of motion of the lumbosacral spine or sacroiliac joints) only reported by 25% of affected children prior to the third decade.

Chronic nonbacterial osteomyelitis and spondylolysis (with or without spondylolisthesis) can cause chronic back pain with a waxing/waning course. Scheuermann disease, or rarely herniation of an intervertebral disc, can result in chronic pain in the lower thoracic or lumbar region.

18. Which over-the-counter medications and NSAIDs are used to treat arthritis in childhood?

Owing to the concern of possible Reye syndrome, salicylates are rarely used, especially during influenza season or varicella outbreaks (Kawasaki syndrome being a notable exception). NSAIDs are available in liquid formulation (naproxen, ibuprofen, meloxicam, and indomethacin), which are easier to administer to children aged <5 years. Celebrex capsules can be opened, and the liquid dispensed if pills are an issue in young children. Naproxen, tolmetin, meloxicam, ibuprofen, and celecoxib are FDA-approved for patients with JIA. Indomethacin is FDA-approved for JIA patients aged >14 years.

ACKNOWLEDGMENT

The authors and editor thank Terri H. Finkel, MD, PhD, Esi Morgan, MD, MSCE, and Courtney Crayne, MD, MSPH for their contributions to this chapter in previous editions.

BIBLIOGRAPHY

Charles B, Alyssa L. Complex regional pain syndromes in children and adolescents. *Anesthesiology.* 2005;102:252–255.

Civino A, Alighieri G, Prete E, et al. Musculoskeletal manifestations of childhood cancer and differential diagnosis with juvenile idiopathic arthritis (ONCOREUM): a multicentre, cross-sectional study. *Lancet Rheumatol.* 2021;3:e507–e516.

Fernandez M, Carrol CL, Baker CJ. Discitis and vertebral osteomyelitis in children: an 18-year review. *Pediatrics.* 2000;105:1299–1304.

Gonçalves M, Terreri MT, Barbosa CM, Len CA, Lee L, Hilário MO. Diagnosis of malignancies in children with musculoskeletal complaints. *Sao Paulo Med J.* 2005(1):21–23.

Houghton KM. Review for the generalist: evaluation of anterior knee pain. *Pediatr Rheumatol Online J.* 2007;5:8.

Junnila JL, Cartwright VW. Chronic musculoskeletal pain in children: part I. Initial evaluation. *Am Fam Physician.* 2009;74:115–122.

Junnila JL, Cartwright VW. Chronic musculoskeletal pain in children: part II. Rheumatic causes. *Am Fam Physician.* 2006;74:293–300.

Kamper SJ, Henschke N, Hestbaek L, et al. Musculoskeletal pain in children and adolescents. *Braz J Phys Ther.* 2016;20(3):275–284.

King S, Chambers CT, Huguet A, et al. The epidemiology of chronic pain in children and adolescents revisited: a systematic review. *Pain.* 2011;152:2729–2738.

Onel KB, Horton DB, Lovell DJ, et al. 2021 American College of Rheumatology Guideline for the Treatment of Juvenile Idiopathic Arthritis: Therapeutic Approaches for Oligoarthritis, Temporomandibular Joint Arthritis, and Systemic Juvenile Idiopathic Arthritis. *Arthritis Rheumatol.* 2022;74(4):553–569.

Pavone V, Vescio A, Valenti F, et al. Growing pains: what do we know about etiology? A systematic review. *World J Orthop.* 2019;10(4):192–205.

Petty RE, Laxer RM, Wedderburn LR. *Textbook of Pediatric Rheumatology.* 8th ed. Philadelphia, PA: Elsevier; 2021.

Sherry D, Malleson P. The idiopathic musculoskeletal syndromes in childhood. *Rheum Dis Clin North Am.* 2002;28:669–685.

Sultan J, Hughes PJ. Septic arthritis or transient synovitis of the hip in children: the value of clinical prediction algorithms. *J Bone Joint Surg Br.* 2010;92:1289–1293.

FURTHER READING

http://www.arthritis.org/conditions-treatments/disease-center/juvenile-arthritis.
https://www.carragroup.org.
http://www.printo.it/pediatric-rheumatology/.
http://www.ped-rheum.com.
http://www.stopchildhoodpain.org/.

CHAPTER 68

Juvenile Idiopathic Arthritis

Megan L. Curran, MD and Joel Brian Shirley, DO

> ## ⟩⟩ KEY POINTS
>
> 1. Juvenile idiopathic arthritis (JIA) consists of several subgroups with different clinical characteristics, pathogenesis, and responses to therapy.
> 2. Systemic JIA (sJIA) symptoms include quotidian fever, rash, and arthritis, which respond best to interleukin (IL)-1 and IL-6 inhibition.
> 3. Oligoarticular JIA is characterized by young age of onset, female predominance, positive antinuclear antibody (ANA), and chronic anterior uveitis.
> 4. Polyarticular JIA with a positive rheumatoid factor (RF) resembles adult seropositive rheumatoid arthritis (RA).
> 5. ANA positivity, female sex, and age <7 years at time of diagnosis increase the risk of chronic uveitis regardless of the JIA subgroup.
> 6. Enthesitis-related arthritis (ERA) is characterized by lower extremity enthesitis and/or arthritis, predominantly male sex, human leukocyte antigen-B27 (HLA-B27), acute anterior uveitis, and sometimes the insidious development of sacroiliitis (which may require MRI to identify as x-rays are insensitive for early disease).

1. Based on the International League of Associations for Rheumatology (ILAR) classification, what are the main types of JIA? What percentage of JIA does each comprise?

JIA is a group of childhood arthritides with complex etiologies involving genetic, autoimmune and environmental factors, beginning before the age of 16 years and lasting at least 6 weeks. Prevalence is highest in age ≥12 years, non-Hispanic Black or African American children and adolescents, those with anxiety or depression, those who are physically inactive, are overweight or have a heart condition, or live in a food-insecure or smoking household.

Worldwide prevalence varies depending on diagnostic criteria used, JIA subtype queried, and populations studied. Prevalence estimates across Europe and North America vary between 3.8 and–400/100,000 children, with a pooled prevalence of 30/100,000 using ILAR criteria. A US national survey found approximately 220,000 children and adolescents had some form of arthritis in the period between 2017 and 2021, only slightly less common than diabetes (approximately 350,000) and epilepsy (approximately 450,00).

The ILAR JIA subgroups are:
- Systemic JIA (10% of all JIA)
- Oligoarthritis (50%)
- Polyarthritis, RF-positive (3%)
- Polyarthritis, RF-negative (20%)
- Psoriatic arthritis (7%)
- ERA/juvenile spondyloarthritis (5–10%), likely underrecognized
- Undifferentiated arthritis (10–15%): patients who meet criteria for more than one subgroup or exclusion criteria for all subgroups

2. In the differential diagnosis of arthritis in childhood, what is the significance of a migratory versus additive pattern of onset?

A **migratory pattern**—where one arthritic joint improves as another becomes inflamed—is seen classically in rheumatic fever and gonococcal arthritis, but can also be seen in arthritis associated with Lyme disease, lupus, and other viral infections. An **additive pattern**—in which initial swollen joints remain persistently inflamed while others become swollen—is characteristic of JIA, post-streptococcal reactive arthritis, psoriatic arthritis, and sarcoidosis.

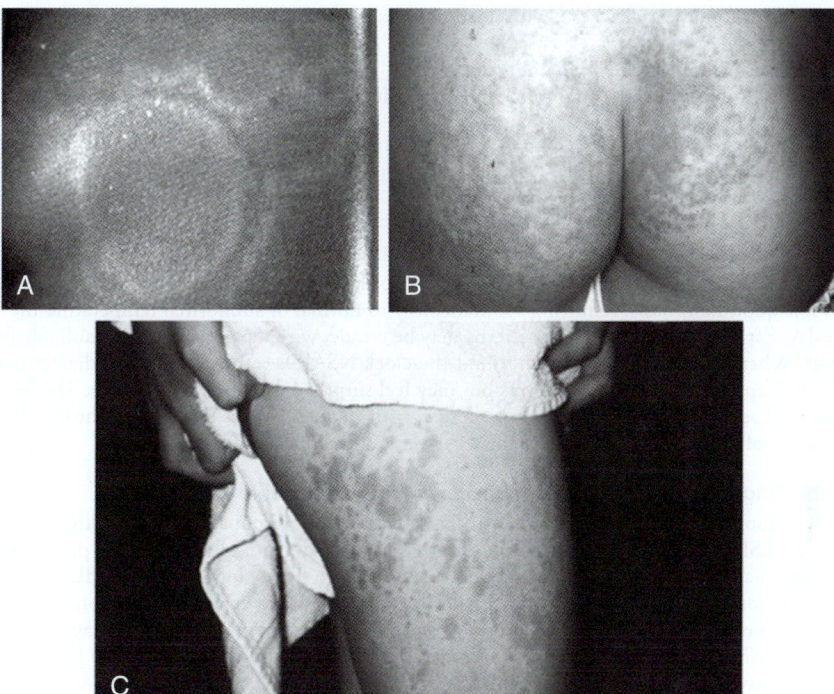

Fig. 68.1   (A) Erythema marginatum. (B) IgA vasculitis (Henoch–Schönlein purpura). (C) Systemic juvenile idiopathic arthritis (JIA).

3. Which rashes are specific to causes of juvenile arthritis?

Erythema marginatum is a nonpruritic macular rash with a serpiginous erythematous border. The rash is pathognomonic of acute rheumatic fever and is one of the five major criteria. It appears in the acute phase of illness along with carditis and arthritis and may remain for many weeks thereafter.

Lower extremity purpura is characteristic of IgA vasculitis (Henoch–Schönlein purpura). It appears in crops, from small petechiae to large ecchymoses, and is prominent in dependent or pressure-bearing surfaces. This rash usually precedes other common manifestations (joint swelling and abdominal pain). It self-resolves within 4 weeks for most children.

Evanescent macules are seen in 80% of patients with sJIA. The rash coincides with febrile episodes and disappears within a few hours without residua. It is migratory, commonly appearing on the trunk and extremities. On light-toned skin, the color is characteristically described as salmon-pink but can vary on different skin tones. Macules are less than 5 mm, although larger macules with central clearing may be present. In older patients, the rash can appear urticarial and may be pruritic. Lesions may be elicited by rubbing or scratching the skin (Koebner phenomenon or dermatographism) or by heat (hot bath or a warm washcloth on the skin) (Fig. 68.1).

4. What are the demographic and clinical characteristics of sJIA?

Systemic JIA is a diagnosis of exclusion, characterized by arthritis, fever, elevated inflammatory markers, and rash. Arthritis may be absent at first, and joint involvement can vary from minimal arthritis to polyarthritis. Infections, malignancies, and Kawasaki disease may present similarly.

- Peak age of onset: 1 to 5 years
- Sex ratio: equal
- ILAR classification criteria for sJIA:
  - Arthritis in one or more joints

- Fever for at least 2 weeks, with documentation of a quotidian pattern for at least 3 days (see Question #5)
- One or more of the following:
  - Evanescent rash, often more apparent when the patient is febrile (see Question #3)
  - Generalized lymphadenopathy
  - Hepatomegaly and/or splenomegaly
  - Serositis (pleural, pericardial, and/or peritoneal; 10% of patients)

5. Two fever patterns are represented below (Fig 68.2) that may aid in the diagnosis of a fever of unknown origin (FUO). Which is characteristic of sJIA?

The sJIA fever pattern occurs with spikes to 39°C or higher on a daily (quotidian) or twice daily (double quotidian) basis, remitting spontaneously to normal or subnormal temperature the rest of the day. Early in the course, fever patterns may be erratic, with a pattern indistinguishable from sepsis. When erratic, treatment with round-the-clock NSAIDs can elicit the quotidian pattern. Children appear quite ill during fevers but may feel surprisingly well when afebrile. The fever pattern of sepsis, in contrast, may be perpetual, with frequent spikes throughout the day. Upon initiation of appropriate antibiotics, the fever curve should become less persistent.

6. In the diagnosis of FUO, what laboratory tests are specific for sJIA?

None. Laboratory tests demonstrate a striking inflammatory response, typically with highly elevated ESR and CRP. Significant leukocytosis, even to leukemoid levels, is often present with a left shift (bandemia). There may be moderate anemia with hemoglobin 7 to 10 g/dL. Thrombocytosis is common. Because leukocytosis and thrombocytosis are expected in sJIA, normal, low, or falling values should increase the clinician's suspicion for development of macrophage activation syndrome (MAS; see Question #8). While elevated liver transaminases and ferritin levels are common in active sJIA, significant elevation can be a sign of MAS. Creatinine kinase, ANA, and RF are typically normal or negative in patients with sJIA.

7. What is the differential diagnosis for sJIA?

- Any infection
  - Infections causing quotidian fevers: endocarditis, bartonella, brucellosis, mycoplasma, malaria, and tuberculosis.
- Kawasaki disease
- Castleman disease
- Kikuchi–Fujimoto disease
- Serum sickness
- Malignancy (acute lymphoblastic leukemia)
- Primary hemophagocytic lymphohistiocytosis (HLH)
- Other childhood rheumatic diseases: systemic lupus erythematosus, anti-neutrophil cytoplasmic antibody (ANCA) associated vasculitis, polyarteritis nodosa, sarcoidosis
- Autoinflammatory diseases: cryopyrin-associated periodic syndromes, tumor necrosis factor (TNF) receptor-associated periodic fever syndrome, and familial Mediterranean fever

8. What is the most feared life-threatening complication seen in sJIA?

Macrophage activation syndrome (MAS). MAS is a form of hemophagocytic lymphohistiocytosis occurring secondary to a rheumatologic condition. MAS is caused by excessive activation and expansion of macrophages and T cells, resulting in an overwhelming inflammatory reaction. It is

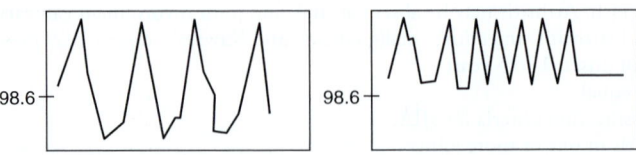

Fig. 68.2 The fever pattern of systemic juvenile idiopathic arthritis (JIA) (*left*) compared with bacterial sepsis (*right*).

commonly associated with infectious triggers, including Epstein-Barr virus, or flare of an underlying rheumatologic condition.

MAS occurs in up to 10% of sJIA patients. The most common manifestations are persistently high fevers, hepatosplenomegaly, lymphadenopathy, severe cytopenias, liver dysfunction, hypertriglyceridemia, encephalopathy including seizures and coma, and coagulopathy (elevated prothrombin time and partial thromboplastin time because of low fibrinogen). If untreated, MAS can lead to multiorgan failure and eventually death.

MAS should be considered in any sJIA patient who develops a precipitous decrease in ESR (due to fibrinogen consumption), decrease in leukocyte and platelet counts, liver dysfunction, and hypertriglyceridemia. Ferritin levels >3,000 to 10,000 ng/mL can be seen and fibrin degradation products are increased. Soluble IL-2 receptor alpha (sCD25) reflecting activated T cells and soluble CD163 reflecting activated macrophages are increased in MAS. Biopsies can, but do not always, show macrophages (CD163+) exhibiting hemophagocytosis in the bone marrow, lymph nodes, or liver. Importantly, some patients develop MAS during their initial sJIA presentation, even before arthritis is present. A febrile patient with known or suspected sJIA is classified as having MAS if the following criteria are met: ferritin >684 ng/mL and any two of the following: platelet count <182 × 10⁹/L, aspartate aminotransferase >48 units/L, triglycerides >156 mg/dL, fibrinogen <361 mg/dL.

9. **What is the current therapy for sJIA? What is the prognosis?**

Recommendations for the treatment of sJIA have been defined by the 2021 American College of Rheumatology (ACR) Guideline for the Treatment of JIA. A reasonable approach to therapy for sJIA with or without MAS is outlined in Figure 68.3.

sJIA course may proceed as monophasic (approximately 40%), polycyclic (periods of remission interspersed with flares; approximately 10%), or persistent disease (approximately 50%). Systemic features (fever, rash, pericarditis) tend to subside over months to years, but some patients develop progressive and recalcitrant arthritis. During periods of active disease, linear growth is delayed. Pulmonary disease may complicate sJIA and/or its treatment and can confer poor prognosis. Long-term follow-up studies from the early 2000s reported remission in approximately one-third of patients; newer studies suggest that targeted biologic treatments may improve patient outcomes and reduce glucocorticoid side-effect burden.

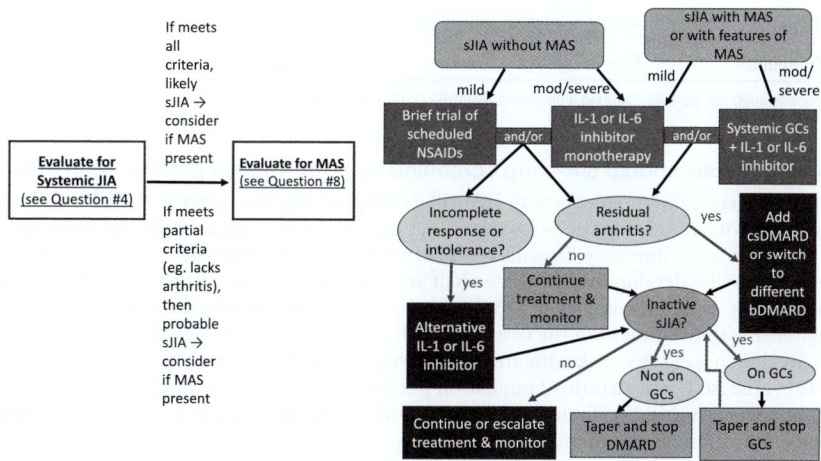

Fig. 68.3 Diagnosis and suggested pharmacologic management of systemic juvenile idiopathic arthritis with and without macrophage activation syndrome, modified from 2021 American College of Rheumatology Guidelines for pharmacologic management *sJIA*, systemic juvenile idiopathic arthritis; *MAS*, macrophage activation syndrome; *NSAID*, nonsteroidal anti-inflammatory drug; *csDMARD*, conventional synthetic DMARD (generally methotrexate); *bDMARD*, biologic DMARD; *GC*, glucocorticoid

10. What are the demographics and clinical characteristics of oligoarticular JIA?

Oligoarticular JIA, defined as the involvement of one to four joints during the first 6 months of disease, is the most common subcategory of JIA in North America/Europe. There is no adult equivalent diagnosis. It most commonly presents as asymmetric knee arthritis; presentation can be subtle with limp and minimal pain. The most commonly involved joints are the knees, then ankles, and then wrists. Finger involvement should raise concern for psoriatic arthritis. Hip and back pain are unusual; a child with hip or back pain needs workup for causes other than JIA.

- Peak age of onset: 1–3 years old
- Sex ratio: female > male 3:1
- Two subgroups of arthritis defined after 6 months:
  - **Persistent:** never more than one to four joints involved
  - **Extended:** more than four joints involved after the first 6 months of disease. This develops in 30–50% of patients, especially those with symmetric joint involvement, wrist or ankle involvement, and an elevated ESR at onset.
- Laboratory abnormalities: ANA is positive in 65% of cases in low to moderate titer (1:160 to 1:640) and is more commonly positive in young girls. RF is negative, white blood cell count is normal, and acute-phase reactants are only mildly elevated. Fever, iron-deficiency anemia, or significantly elevated ESR/C-reactive protein (CRP) should prompt workup for septic arthritis, inflammatory bowel disease arthritis, or malignancy.
- **Chronic nongranulomatous anterior uveitis:** Uveitis is a serious complication of JIA that is often asymptomatic. It can lead to ocular damage and blindness if not identified and adequately treated. Uveitis can precede arthritis in 10% of cases. If there is any suspicion of oligoarticular JIA in a patient under the age of 7, a rapid slit-lamp exam is strongly recommended to promptly identify and treat uveitis.

11. What types of anterior uveitis are associated with JIA (Table 68.1)?

TABLE 68.1 Anterior Uveitis in Juvenile Idiopathic Arthritis

	ACUTE UVEITIS	CHRONIC UVEITIS
Disease association	Spondyloarthritis (enthesitis-related arthritis)	Oligoarticular JIA, polyarticular RF negative JIA, psoriatic JIA
Lab markers	HLA-B27 antigen	Positive ANA
Symptoms	Painful, red, photophobic eye	None
Complications	Few	Synechiae, cataract, glaucoma, band keratopathy

ANA, antinuclear antibody; HLA-B27, human leukocyte antigen-B27; JIA, juvenile idiopathic arthritis.

12. How frequently should slit-lamp screening be performed in patients with JIA?

Approximately 20% of patients with JIA will develop uveitis. Frequency is related to JIA subtype. ANA positivity and young age (<7 years old) at the time of JIA diagnosis are the strongest risk factors. Uveitis is commonly detected at the first screening ophthalmology or optometry exam. Of JIA patients who develop uveitis, almost half are diagnosed with uveitis shortly before, around the same time as, or shortly after their JIA diagnosis. Of JIA patients who develop uveitis, 90% are diagnosed with uveitis within the first 4 years, thus representing the highest risk period. Uveitis activity does not always track with arthritis activity: it may manifest when arthritis is in remission. In 2019, the ACR and Arthritis Foundation published updated guidelines for the screening of JIA-associated uveitis. See Table 68.2. These guidelines do not apply to a child with established uveitis, for whom regular monitoring is required.

TABLE 68.2 Recommended Screening Frequency for Uveitis in Patients With JIA, Modified From 2019 ACR/Arthritis Foundation Recommendations

JIA CATEGORY	RISK DETERMINATION	SCREENING FREQUENCY
Oligoarthritis RF negative polyarthritis Psoriatic arthritis Undifferentiated JIA	High risk = meet all three of the following: 1. ANA positive 2. JIA age of onset <7 years 3. Disease duration ≤4 years	Screen every 3 months
	Low or moderate risk = meet one of the following: 1. ANA negative 2. JIA age of onset ≥7 years 3. Disease duration >4 years	Screen every 6–12 months
Systemic JIA, RF positive polyarthritis, enthesitis-related arthritis	Low or moderate risk	Screen every 6–12 months

ANA, antinuclear antibody; *JIA*, juvenile idiopathic arthritis; *RF*, rheumatoid factor.

13. A patient presents with poorly localized leg pain sufficient to interrupt sleep and cause a limp. Which malignancies must be considered in the differential diagnosis?

Malignant bone tumors, Langerhans cell histiocytosis, leukemias, soft tissue sarcomas, and neuroblastomas are the most common neoplasms that cause musculoskeletal symptoms. They can present as limb or joint pain or swelling. In a study of patients with leukemia, 20% had arthralgia and another 20% had arthritis at diagnosis. Presentations include mono or oligoarticular (up to 4) joint involvement, hip and/or knee involvement, night sweats, weight loss and fevers. Laboratory abnormalities including cytopenias, especially thrombocytopenia, elevated ESR, CRP, lactate dehydrogenase or uric acid, should prompt imaging. Blood smear analysis and bone marrow biopsy should be considered.

14. What is the treatment and prognosis for oligoarticular JIA?

Patients with oligoarticular JIA are commonly treated with nonsteroidal anti-inflammatory drugs (NSAIDs) and intraarticular steroids. Lidocaine anesthetic can be used to numb the skin prior to intraarticular steroid injection or mixed directly with the injectable steroid. Oral or subcutaneous methotrexate is added if arthritis does not fully respond to joint injection. A TNF-α inhibitor is added if arthritis persists despite methotrexate.

Long-term outcome for patients with oligoarticular JIA is likely better compared to other JIA subtypes; studies show up to 50% of patients achieve remission off medication, though arthritis can recur years after onset. Chronic sequelae include leg length discrepancy (affected limb can be longer or shorter), joint contractures, and ocular damage from uveitis.

15. Compare RF-negative with RF-positive polyarthritis

The clinical features of RF-negative and RF-positive polyarticular JIA are outlined in Table 68.3. The RF-negative polyarthritis subgroup includes patients with significant clinical heterogeneity. Two groups of interest within this subgroup include:

- **ANA-positive girls aged <7 years:** Resemble oligoarticular JIA, except more than 4 joints are involved in the first 6 months of diagnosis. Clinical characteristics include asymmetric onset of arthritis and higher risk of developing chronic uveitis, similar to that seen in extended oligoarthritis patients.
- **ANA-negative children aged >7 to 9 years:** Clinical characteristics include symmetric polyarthritis similar (but not as severe) to RF-positive polyarticular JIA. The arthritis seen in these children, as well as children with RF-positive polyarthritis, is similar to adult RA with both large and small joint involvement. However, they have more hip, shoulder, C-spine, and distal interphalangeal joint involvement than adults. Radiographic changes distinguishing these two pediatric groups from adult RA include fusion of the carpal bones, micrognathia from temporomandibular joint arthritis, and fusion of C-spine apophyseal (facet) joints.

TABLE 68.3 Comparison Between RF-Negative and RF-Positive Polyarticular JIA

	RF-NEGATIVE	RF-POSITIVE
Peak age of onset (years)	1–3; 9–14	>12
Sex ratio, female:male	3:1 younger; 10:1 older	4:1–13:1
Joint disease	Insidious and progressive Fewer affected joints Asymmetric, larger joints TMJ disease common	More rapid onset Greater number of affected joints Symmetric small joints of hands and fingers (ulnar drift, swan neck, and boutonniere deformities)
Serologies	ANA (50%), ACPA rare	ANA (55%), ACPA (>60%)
Extraarticular manifestations	Chronic anterior uveitis (15–20%)	Rheumatoid nodules (30%), vasculitis, rheumatoid-associated lung disease, Felty syndrome (all rare)

ACPA, anticitrullinated protein antibodies; *ANA,* antinuclear antibody; *HLA,* human leukocyte antigen; *TMJ:* temporomandibular joint; *RA,* rheumatoid arthritis; *RF,* rheumatoid factor.

16. List the treatments used in the polyarticular subgroup of JIA.

As evidence has amassed, JIA treatment guidelines have become more emphatic about early treatment of polyarticular JIA with medications other than NSAIDs. Patients with low disease activity at diagnosis can be treated with NSAIDs and intraarticular steroids, but initial treatment with a conventional synthetic disease-modifying antirheumatic drug (csDMARD), generally methotrexate, is strongly recommended over NSAID monotherapy. Patients with moderate to high disease activity at diagnosis should be started on methotrexate, and a biologic drug (generally a TNF-α inhibitor, abatacept or tocilizumab) should be added if inadequate response after 6-12 weeks. Biologics may be considered for initial therapy in patients with high disease activity or poor prognostic features like high-risk joint involvement (c-spine, wrist, hip) or erosive changes. Tofacitinib, a Janus kinase (JAK) inhibitor in the targeted synthetic DMARD category (tsDMARD), is approved for use in patients aged ≥2 years with poor response to TNF-α inhibition. TNF-α and JAK inhibitors can be used alone or with methotrexate.

csDMARDs:
- Methotrexate: Start at 10–15 mg/m^2 per week. Can be given orally or subcutaneously (SQ). Usual SQ maximum dose is 25 mg/week. SQ formulation allows greater absorption. Children require and tolerate higher doses than adults owing to differences in metabolism.
- Leflunomide: <20 kg (10 mg every other day, orally), 20–40 kg (10 mg daily, orally); >40 kg (20 mg daily, orally).

Biologic DMARDs
- Etanercept (TNF-α inhibitor): 0.8 mg/kg per week SQ weekly (max 50 mg weekly).
- Adalimumab (TNF-α inhibitor): 10kg to <15kg (10mg SQ every 2 weeks); 15mg to <30kg (20 mg SQ every 2 weeks); >30 kg (40 mg SQ every 2 weeks).
- Infliximab (TNF-α inhibitor): 5 mg/kg intravenously (IV) at 0, 2, 6 weeks and then every 4–8 weeks.
- Tocilizumab (IL-6 inhibitor): IV:<30 kg (10 mg/kg IV every 4 weeks); >30 kg (8 mg/kg IV every 4 weeks). SQ injection injection: <30kg (162mg SQ every 3 weeks); >30kg (162mg SQ every 2 weeks).
- Abatacept (CTLA4 fusion protein that prevents T cell co-stimulation; for use in patients ≥6 years): IV: 10 mg/kg (max 1000 mg) at 0, 2, 6 weeks, then every 4 weeks. SQ injection: 10–25 kg (50 mg SQ once weekly); 25–50 kg (87.5 mg SQ once weekly); >50 kg (125 mg SQ once weekly).
- Rituximab: 750 mg/m^2 (max 1000 mg) IV at 0 and 2 weeks. Used in refractory RF+ polyarticular disease.

tsDMARDs:
- Tofacitinib (JAK inhibitor): 10-20 kg (3.2 mg twice daily, orally); 20-40 kg (4 mg twice daily, orally); >40 kg (5 mg twice daily, orally). Used for polyarticular-course JIA in patients ≥2 years old with inadequate response or intolerance to ≥ 1 TNF inhibitor.

17. What are the demographic and clinical characteristics of juvenile psoriatic arthritis?

- Peak age of onset: bimodal, 2 to 4 years, and mid-to-late childhood
- Sex ratio: younger cohort is more female predominant, and older-onset patients have equal sex distribution
- Diagnosis based on presence of psoriasis and arthritis or arthritis, and two of the following three features:
  - Dactylitis (swelling of entire digit due to tenosynovitis and arthritis)
  - Nail pitting (minimum two pits on more than one nail) or onycholysis
  - Psoriasis in a first-degree relative
- Arthritis patterns can include oligoarticular, polyarticular, or axial arthritis (sacroiliitis and enthesitis)
- The younger patient cohort tends to be similar to oligoarticular JIA, with female predominance, ANA positivity, and increased risk for anterior uveitis, but differs in having more dactylitis, finger, toe, and wrist involvement
- Treatment is similar to oligoarticular, polyarticular, or ERA subgroups of JIA depending on presentation and severity

18. What are the demographic and clinical manifestations of the ERA subgroup of JIA?

The ERA subgroup includes patients with inflammation predominantly affecting lower extremity joints and entheses. Arthritis may eventually affect the sacroiliac (SI) joints and spine, though SI and spine involvement are rare at disease onset. Other spondyloarthritis-related conditions such as psoriatic arthritis, reactive arthritis, and inflammatory bowel disease-associated arthritis share features of ERA but are not formally included in the ILAR subgroup.

- Peak age of onset: 10 to 13 years
- Sex ratio: male > female 7:1
- Genetics: HLA-B27 positive in 60% to 80% depending on ethnicity
- The hallmark of the ERA subgroup is the presence of **enthesitis** (inflammation at sites of tendon/ligament insertion into bone). The most common sites are patellar tendon, Achilles tendon, plantar fascia insertions into calcaneus and metatarsal heads, greater trochanter, and tibial tuberosity (may mimic Osgood–Schlatter disease).
- Most frequent joints are the knee, ankle, and midfoot (tarsitis)
  - Axial involvement is infrequent at disease onset but likely underappreciated. Sacroiliitis may not be appreciated on x-ray, but noncontrast MRI is more sensitive for detection. Up to 40% will develop ankylosing spondylitis within 10 years of onset. Risk factors for sacroiliitis or spondylitis are HLA-B27 presence, family history of ankylosing spondylitis, male sex, hip arthritis, tarsitis, higher number of inflamed entheses, and higher number of arthritic joints at disease onset.
- Extraarticular manifestations:
  - Uveitis: **acute anterior uveitis** in 3–7% of patients (see Question #11). Cardiovascular: aortic insufficiency can rarely occur.
- Laboratory: ESR elevated; ANA and RF negative.
- Treatment: tailored to predominant manifestations. NSAIDs, intraarticular steroid injections, sulfasalazine, and methotrexate are commonly used for peripheral disease, with use of TNF-α inhibitors if disease is refractory. TNF-α inhibitors are indicated when axial disease is present. JAK inhibitors and biologic drugs targeting IL-17 and IL-12/23 pathways are approved for adult spondyloarthritis and for pediatric patients of varying ages with psoriatic arthritis and ERA.
- Reactive arthritis and inflammatory bowel disease-associated arthritis can occur and resemble their adult counterparts. Because children may have few abdominal symptoms, inflammatory bowel disease should be in the differential diagnosis for any child with iron-deficiency anemia, weight loss, and arthritis.

19. In a child with JIA, what is the risk that a sibling will develop the same illness?

One population-based study found that a sibling of a patient with JIA is ~10 times more likely to be diagnosed with JIA than a child whose sibling does not have JIA. Given the background prevalence of JIA in the general population, this equates to an absolute risk of ~1.5 cases per 100.

Familial and genome-wide association studies estimate the genetic contribution to JIA is 13–32%; other contributors are gene-environment interactions and environmental factors that induce epigenetic changes, modulate the immune system, or change the microbiome.

20. School-aged children with JIA have legal rights to therapeutic resources in school. What are they?

Two federal laws support educational and school environment needs for students with juvenile arthritis. The Individuals with Disabilities Education Act (IDEA) ensures that children with disabilities have the same opportunities as all children and applies from preschool through high school. This includes support services like transportation, mobility services, and therapies (speech, physical and occupational). Section 504 of the Rehabilitation Act requires public school districts to provide reasonable accommodations and modifications for students up to age 22 with certain disabilities.

ACKNOWLEDGMENT

The authors would like to thank Drs. J. Roger Hollister and Jamie Lai for their contributions to this chapter in previous editions.

BIBLIOGRAPHY

Angeles-Han ST, Lo MS, Henderson LA, et al. Juvenile idiopathic arthritis disease-specific and uveitis subcommittee of the childhood arthritis rheumatology and research alliance. Childhood arthritis and rheumatology research alliance consensus treatment plans for juvenile idiopathic arthritis-associated and idiopathic chronic anterior uveitis. *Arthritis Care Res (Hoboken)*. 2019;71(4):482–491.

Brix N, Hasle H, Rosthøj S, et al. Characteristics of children with acute lymphoblastic leukemia presenting with arthropathy. *Clin Rheumatol*. 2018;37(9):2455–2463.

Civino A, Alighieri G, Prete E, et al. Musculoskeletal manifestations of childhood cancer and differential diagnosis with juvenile idiopathic arthritis (ONCOREUM): a multicentre, cross-sectional study. *Lancet Rheumatol*. 2021;3(7):e507–e516.

Flato B, Lien G, Smerdel-Ramoya A, et al. Juvenile psoriatic arthritis longterm outcome and differentiation from other subtypes of juvenile idiopathic arthritis. *J Rheumatol*. 2009;36:642–650.

Grevich S, Shenoi S. Update on the management of systemic juvenile idiopathic arthritis and role of IL-1 and IL-6 inhibition. *Adolesc Health Med Ther*. 2017;8:125–135.

Hersh AO, Prahalad S. Immunogenetics of juvenile idiopathic arthritis: a comprehensive review. *J Autoimmun*. 2015;64:113–124.

Martini A, Lovell DJ, Albani S, et al. Juvenile idiopathic arthritis. *Nat Rev Dis Primers*. 2022;8(1):5.

Onel K, Rumsey DG, Shenoi S. Juvenile idiopathic arthritis treatment updates. *Rheum Dis Clin North Am*. 2021;47(4):545–563.

Onel KB, Horton DB, Lovell DJ, et al. 2021 American College of Rheumatology guideline for the treatment of juvenile idiopathic arthritis: therapeutic approaches for oligoarthritis, temporomandibular joint arthritis, and systemic juvenile idiopathic arthritis. *Arthritis Care Res (Hoboken)*. 2022;74(4):521–537.

Petty RE, Laxer RM, Lindsley CB, et al. *Textbook of Pediatric Rheumatology*. 8th ed. Philadelphia, PA: Elsevier; 2021.

Ravelli A, Minoia F, Davì S, et al. 2016 classification criteria for macrophage activation syndrome complicating systemic juvenile idiopathic arthritis: a European League Against Rheumatism/American College of Rheumatology/Paediatric Rheumatology International Trials Organisation Collaborative Initiative. *Ann Rheum Dis*. 2016;75(3):481–489.

Ringold S, ST Angeles-Han, Beukelman T, et al. 2019 American College of Rheumatology/Arthritis Foundation guideline for the treatment of juvenile idiopathic arthritis: therapeutic approaches for non-systemic polyarthritis, sacroiliitis, and enthesitis. *Arthritis Rheumatol*. 2019;71(6):846–863.

Juvenile Systemic Connective Tissue Diseases and Vasculitides

Eileen C. Rife, MD, MPH and Randy Q. Cron, MD, PhD

Children are not just little adults, but adults can sure be big babies.

—Anonymous

> ## » KEY POINTS
>
> 1. Childhood-onset systemic lupus erythematosus (SLE) is more severe at presentation than adult-onset SLE with more organ damage, higher disease activity, increased medication burden, and higher mortality rates.
> 2. Inflammatory myositis in childhood is almost always dermatomyositis.
> 3. Immunoglobulin A vasculitis (IgAv), formerly called Henoch–Schoenlein purpura (HSP), is the most common small-vessel vasculitis in childhood.
> 4. Juvenile localized scleroderma (JLS) is the predominant childhood form of scleroderma, and it typically responds to early, aggressive immunomodulatory therapy. JLS is a distinct entity from systemic sclerosis (SSc), which is rare in pediatric patients.

1. What are the childhood-onset systemic connective tissue diseases?

SLE, juvenile dermatomyositis (JDM), mixed connective tissue disease (MCTD), undifferentiated connected tissue disease (UCTD), SSc, Sjögren disease (SjD).

2. Discuss the epidemiology of childhood-onset SLE (cSLE).

SLE is the most common connective tissue disease (CTD) of childhood. The proportion of all patients with SLE showing symptoms before 18 years of age is between 15% and 20%. In childhood, the disease generally occurs after age 10 (60%) and rarely before age 5 (5%). The gender distribution of cSLE is roughly 5:1 (female: male) before the age of 12 years. The gender distribution during adolescence is similar to the adult population, 9:1-10:1. The discrepancy in gender distribution is thought to be attributable to hormone changes in adolescence. cSLE rates are higher in non-Caucasian children. Roughly 10% of affected patients have a first-degree relative with SLE, and there is a 20-fold increased risk in siblings. Concordance in monozygous twins is around 25–60%.

3. What classification criteria are used in childhood-onset SLE?

The classification criteria for adult SLE are also used for cSLE. The most recent criteria set forth by the American College of Rheumatology (ACR) and the European Alliance of Associations for Rheumatology (EULAR) were published in 2019. These are not diagnostic criteria, but rather were created to define relatively homogeneous patient populations for inclusion in clinical trials. These criteria are often extrapolated to pediatric populations, and display higher sensitivity (~85%) than previous criteria when a cut-off score of ≥10 is used. The specificity in pediatric patients is ~70–80%. Using a cutoff score ≥13 results in higher specificity and positive predictive value. An ANA titer ≥ 1:80 is required at baseline prior to application of the criteria to a specific patient. Of note, younger pediatric patients display less ANA positivity at diagnosis, which underscores the caution in using these criteria for diagnostic purposes.

4. What are the clinical manifestations of SLE? How commonly do they occur?

SLE is a complex autoimmune disease characterized by upregulation of both the innate and adaptive immune system, with resultant multi-organ involvement. An easy way to remember the complex array of systemic manifestations of SLE is to think from head to toe (Table 69.1).

TABLE 69.1 Systemic Manifestations of Systemic Lupus Erythematosus

General (90%)	Malaise, weight loss, fever
Skin (55–70%)	Malar rash/photosensitivity, discoid lupus, vasculitic lesions, alopecia
Brain (25%)	Headache, psychosis, chorea, seizures, neuropathy, cerebrovascular accident, transverse myelitis
Eye (3–30%)	Cotton-wool spots, retinitis, episcleritis, iritis (rarely)
Mouth (20–50%)	Oral ulcers (hard palate, typically painless)
Chest (15–20%)	Pleuritis, pneumonitis, pulmonary hemorrhage, shrinking lung syndrome
Heart (15–20%)	Pericarditis, myocarditis, Libman–Sacks endocarditis
Digestive system (25–40%)	Hepatosplenomegaly, mesenteric arteritis, colitis, hepatitis, pancreatitis
Kidneys (>50%)	Glomerulonephritis, nephrotic syndrome, hypertension
Extremities (60–80%)	Arthralgia or arthritis, myalgia or myositis, RP, thrombophlebitis, aseptic necrosis

PEARL: A child with SLE who develops psychosis while on prednisone is much more likely to have neuropsychiatric lupus than steroid psychosis (which is very rare in childhood). Avascular necrosis as a result of steroid usage rarely occurs in children aged <14 years.

PEARL: Discoid lesions are more likely to be accompanied by additional systemic manifestations of SLE in pediatric patients compared to adults, where isolated discoid lupus is more common.

5. **How do the antinuclear antibody (ANA) pattern and titer aid in the diagnosis and management of SLE?**

ANAs are present in the sera of almost all children with active SLE. In fact, the absence of ANAs, particularly at the time of symptomatic disease, should prompt consideration of an alternative diagnosis. The average ANA titer in individuals with SLE is 1:320, although in active disease it may be considerably higher (>1:1280). Changes in the ANA titer do not indicate disease activity and are not followed subsequent to diagnosis. By contrast, the anti-double-stranded DNA (anti-dsDNA) antibody titer, which is found in >80% of patients, often correlates with disease activity. The "rim" pattern on the ANA, in which fluorescence rims the nuclear membrane, is pathognomonic of SLE, although rarely seen. The "homogeneous" pattern, in which fluorescence uniformly coats the nucleus, is the pattern most commonly seen in SLE. The "speckled" pattern is the least specific and is common in MCTD and Sjögren disease.

The ANA is a highly subjective test, and the pattern and titer vary greatly among laboratories. Low titer positive results occur in 5–20% of healthy individuals. Several studies suggest that the most common pattern amongst healthy individuals (at low titer) is the dense finely speckled pattern. False-negative results are rare, but if you are convinced of the diagnosis of SLE, the ANA should be repeated in a different laboratory and/or at a future date. Additional reasons an ANA may be negative in a patient with SLE include: lab error, a non–nuclear antibody pattern (i.e. cytoplasmic pattern), or prozone (hook) effect.

6. **How does the ANA profile aid in the diagnosis and management of SLE and related childhood-onset CTDs?**

A negative ANA profile does not completely rule out any of the childhood-onset CTDs; but a positive ANA profile can be helpful in making a specific diagnosis (Table 69.2). Anti-dsDNA and anti-Smith (anti-Sm) antibodies are both specific for SLE. High titers of anti-ribonucleoprotein antibodies are suggestive of MCTD, and anti-Ro (SS-A) and/or anti-La (SS-B) antibodies are commonly seen with SjD. Anti-Ro/SS-A antibodies are also frequently positive with SLE. Anti-histone antibodies may be present in both drug-induced lupus and SLE. Of note, a positive ANA is rarely present with systemic juvenile idiopathic arthritis (sJIA, also known as Still's disease) or ANCA vasculitis.

TABLE 69.2 Anti–Nuclear Antibody Subtypes in Juvenile Systemic Connective Tissue Disease

	ACTIVE SLE	MCTD	SSC	PRIMARY SJÖGREN	JIA (POLY)
ANA	99%	100%	80–97%	>70%	40–50%
Anti-native DNA	60%	Neg	Neg	Neg	Neg
Anti-Sm	30%	Neg	Neg	Neg	Neg
Anti-RNP	30%	>95% titer >1:10,000	Common (low titer)	Rare	Rare
Anti-centromere	Rare	Rare	7–8%	Neg	Neg
Anti-topoisomerase I (Scl-70)	Rare	Rare	20–30%	Neg	Neg
Anti-Ro (SS-A)	30%	Rare	Rare	70%	Rare
Anti-La (SS-B)	15%	Rare	Rare	60%	Rare

ANA, antinuclear antibody; *anti-RNP,* anti-ribonucleoprotein; *anti-Sm,* anti-Smith antibody; *JIA,* juvenile idiopathic arthritis; *MCTD,* mixed connective tissue disease; *SLE,* systemic lupus erythematosus; *SSc,* systemic sclerosis/scleroderma.

7. Which other autoantibodies (other than ANA and ANA profile) can be helpful in the diagnosis of systemic childhood-onset CTD?

Antibodies reactive with Scl-70 are not typically measured in the standard ANA profile but are found in 15% to 20% of individuals with SSc. Myositis-associated (e.g. anti-ro/SS-A) and myositis-specific antibodies (MSAs) are found in distinct subsets of children with JDM. If present, their clinical associations are often similar to adults, such as anti-Jo-1and anti-MDA5 identifying those children at increased risk for developing interstitial lung disease. There are a few notable differences between pediatric autoantibody associations compared to adults:

• anti-HMG-CoA Reductase antibody is not associated with statin therapy in children.
• anti-TIF1γ antibody is not associated with malignancy in children.
• anti-NXP2 antibody is not associated with malignancy in children.

While not autoantibodies, low levels of complement (e.g., C3, C4) are frequently found in newly diagnosed SLE and the laboratory results return quicker than an ANA and ANA profile of antibodies.

Vasculitic syndromes associated with the presence of antineutrophil cytoplasmic antibodies (ANCA, cytoplasmic or perinuclear) are granulomatosis with polyangiitis (GPA), microscopic polyangiitis (MPA), eosinophilic granulomatosis with polyangiitis (EGPA), and crescentic glomerulonephritis. Rheumatoid factor (RF) is frequently positive in SjD and MCTD.

8. Describe the management of children with SLE.

General
• Counseling, education.
• Adequate rest.
• Use of sunscreen.
• Immunizations, especially pneumococcal.
• Management of infection.
• Avoiding triggers (e.g. UV exposure).
• Hydroxychloroquine.
• Glucocorticoids (GC): note that children metabolize GC faster than adults, and larger relative doses are typically used in children.
• Nonsteroidal anti-inflammatory drugs (NSAIDs): for musculoskeletal symptoms (caution if renal or cardiac disease is present).
• Immunosuppressive medications: mycophenolate mofetil; azathioprine; methotrexate (typically prescribed for inflammatory arthritis; caution if renal insufficiency); cyclophosphamide;

calcineurin inhibitors: cyclosporine and tacrolimus (caution with renal disease and hypertension), voclosporin (off-label, not approved in pediatrics).
- Biologic therapy: anti-B-cell therapy: rituximab, belimumab; type 1 interferon receptor antibody (anifrolumab): off-label, approved in adults; interleukin-1 inhibition: off-label use of anakinra for MAS complicating SLE or rilonacept for recurrent pericarditis; complement inhibitors (e.g. eculizumab): for use in atypical hemolytic uremic syndromes (aHUS) or complement-mediated thrombotic microangiopathy (TMA) syndromes.
- Plasmapheresis: indicated for thrombotic thrombocytopenic purpura, catastrophic antiphospholipid syndrome (CAPS), transverse myelitis, neuromyelitis optica.
- Intravenous immunoglobulin (IVIG): used for CAPS, macrophage activation syndrome (MAS), immune hemolytic anemia/thrombocytopenia, and iatrogenic hypogammaglobulinemia (e.g. repeated rituximab dosing).

9. Discuss the pathophysiology of neonatal lupus (NL).

NL is associated with the transplacental passage of maternal anti-Ro/SS-A and anti-La/SS-B IgG antibodies. One or more clinical manifestations of NL occur in 25% to 30% of infants whose mothers have antibodies, regardless of underlying maternal disease. The most frequent abnormalities include: photosensitive rash (lesions of discoid lupus or subacute cutaneous lupus), hepatic dysfunction, neutropenia, and thrombocytopenia. Congenital heart block (CHB) is of greatest concern and identified most often between 18 and 26 weeks of gestation. It is highly associated with anti-Ro/SS-A antibodies (especially anti-Ro52). The cutaneous, hepatic, and hematologic manifestations are transient, generally resolving within 2 to 6 months after delivery, whereas heart block (typically third degree) is often permanent and commonly requires a pacemaker. The overall risk of CHB is 2%, but increases to 18% in anti-Ro/SS-A-positive mothers with a previous child with CHB. Mothers with these antibodies are screened with weekly fetal echocardiograms/obstetric ultrasounds starting at 16 weeks gestation through 26 weeks. Development of first-degree heart block (controversial), second-degree heart block, pericardial effusion or cardiomyopathy in the fetus may be treated with fluorinated steroids that cross the placenta (dexamethasone, betamethasone). The use of IVIG in this setting has also been described in the literature. There is no clear evidence that third-degree heart block can be reversed with medications, but some experts in the field will still attempt treatment and concurrent non-conduction endpoints may still be amenable to therapy. Infants with third-degree heart block will require a pacemaker in most cases. Fetal mortality is 20% in those who develop CHB and cardiomyopathy (fetal hydrops) *in utero*. Hydroxychloroquine may reduce the risk of NL and is prescribed during pregnancy for all SLE patients unless contraindications exist. Current guidelines from the ACR recommend use of hydroxychloroquine in all anti-Ro/SS-A-positive patients during pregnancy in an attempt to prevent NL and CHB in the fetus.

10. What is the differential diagnosis of Sjögren disease (SjD) in childhood?

SjD is characterized by dry eyes (keratoconjunctivitis sicca), dry mouth, carious teeth, parotitis and other glandular enlargement. It is important to differentiate SjD from benign recurrent parotid swelling, acquired immunodeficiency syndrome, sarcoidosis, IgG4 syndrome, tuberculosis, lymphoma, severe malnutrition, and mumps. Salivary gland biopsy of the lip can be helpful as a diagnostic tool. SjD is less frequent in children than adults, but can be severe with multi-organ involvement including the central nervous system (e.g., transverse myelitis).

11. What forms of systemic vasculitis occur in childhood?

The most common small-vessel vasculitis in childhood is **IgA vasculitis** (IgAv), formerly called Henoch Schoenlein Purpura (HSP). **ANCA-associated vasculitis** (GPA, MPA, EGPA) can occur in children and may present initially by mimicking IgAv. **Primary central nervous system (CNS) vasculitis** may involve small or medium-sized vessels of the brain and spinal cord. Small-vessel vasculitis can also occur secondary to an underlying primary CTD including systemic JIA, JDM, and SLE. Small-vessel vasculitis can also be seen with inflammatory bowel disease, particularly Crohn's disease.

Polyarteritis nodosa (PAN) can occur in childhood (5% of cases) and is characterized by rash, fever, weight loss, and cutaneous nodules. Life-threatening renal, gastrointestinal, cardiac, and CNS complications can occur, but lung involvement is rare. **Cutaneous PAN** is reported in both the adult and pediatric literature. **Kawasaki disease** uniquely affects the pediatric population and is discussed in detail in the next chapter (Chapter 70: Kawasaki disease).

Large-vessel vasculitis is rare in childhood, with **Takayasu arteritis** making up the greatest proportion of cases. Up to 30% of Takayasu arteritis cases occur in childhood, typically developing in adolescent females.

12. What is the classic tetrad of IgA vasculitis in children?

- Palpable purpura.
- Colicky abdominal pain.
- Arthralgia or arthritis.
- Renal disease.

IgAv is a small vessel leukocytoclastic vasculitis primarily affecting children between the ages of 3 and 15 years. It is the most common vasculitis of childhood and rare in adults. The mean age at presentation is 6–7 years, and the male-to-female ratio is ~1.5:1. Approximately one-half of children have a history of preceding upper respiratory tract infection, with a variety of organisms identified (particularly streptococcus). Purpura is the most common initial manifestation, but can be preceded by arthritis, edema, testicular swelling and abdominal pain. Renal disease is generally mild, occurring in 40% to 50% of cases, and often coincides with vasculitis onset (or within the first 2 months). Laboratory abnormalities include an elevated erythrocyte sedimentation rate (ESR; >50%) and elevated serum IgA (37%). Complement levels are typically normal. Over 95% of children with IgAv have a self-limiting course lasting 2 to 6 weeks. Recurrence occurs in 33% of patients overall, with 20% recurring within the first year. Children with renal disease and those over 8 years of age are more likely to have recurrence. Up to 5% of children will suffer persistent purpura with or without persistent renal disease. In patients who have renal involvement, 30% develop renal insufficiency, and 5% progress to renal failure.

13. List the clinical manifestations of IgA vasculitis. See Table 69.3.

TABLE 69.3 Clinical Manifestations of IgAv

	% AT ONSET	% POST ONSET	NOTES
Purpura	50–100	100	Normal platelet count
Edema	10–20	20–50	Painful, scrotal edema (13%)
Arthritis	25–70	60–84	Large joints
GI	20-30	50	Intussusception (2.3–3.5%), volvulus (<1%), ileal infarction
Renal	15	21–54	Renal failure (2%)
GU	2	12–16	Scrotal involvement in boys 2–38%
Pulmonary	?	?	Abnormal CO diffusion in 5%, mild interstitial changes on CXR without symptoms
Hemorrhage	?	Rare	Fatal
CNS	?	Very rare	Headache, encephalitis, seizures

CNS, central nervous system; *GI*, gastrointestinal; *GU*, genitourinary. Adapted from Petty RE, Laxer RM, Lindsley CB, Wedderburn L, Fuhlbrigge RC, Mellins ED. *Textbook of Pediatric Rheumatology*. 8th ed. Philadelphia, PA: Elsevier; 2021.

14. How is the diagnosis confirmed? What role does IgA play in the pathogenesis?

In the appropriate clinical setting, a skin biopsy with direct immunofluorescence showing a leukocytoclastic vasculitis with **predominantly IgA vessel wall deposition** is diagnostic of IgAv. However, IgAv is considered a clinical diagnosis, and biopsy is not required in all cases. Several hypotheses describing the role of IgA antibodies in disease pathogenesis have been described in the literature.

- IgAv often occurs following a reported upper respiratory tract infection. It can also occur in the setting of ANCA-associated vasculitis, spondyloarthritis, and inflammatory bowel disease (most often Crohn's disease). Each of these clinical scenarios involves inflammation at mucosal surfaces, where IgA plays a role in mucosal immunity.

- In patients with IgAv, serum IgA1 has been shown to be galactose-deficient at the hinge region O-linked glycan. This predisposes the antibody to form immune complexes with IgG (IgA–IgG immune complexes) that subsequently deposit in tissues.
- IgA anticardiolipin antibodies may also be involved in the pathogenesis.

15. **What clinical features of IgAv at disease onset are associated with poor prognosis? See Table 69.4.**

TABLE 69.4 Poor Prognostic Factors at Onset of IgA Vasculitis

MANIFESTATION	COMMENT
Melena	7.5-fold increase in renal disease
Persistent rash for 2–3 months	Associated with glomerulonephritis
Hematuria with proteinuria >1 g/day	15% Progress to renal insufficiency
Nephrosis with renal insufficiency	50% Renal insufficiency in 10 years

Adapted from Petty RE, Laxer RM, Lindsley CB, Wedderburn L, Fuhlbrigge RC, Mellins ED. *Textbook of Pediatric Rheumatology*. 8th ed. Philadelphia, PA: Elsevier; 2021.

16. **How should IgA Vasculitis be treated?**
- Arthritis responds to NSAIDs.
- Edema responds to steroids.
- Abdominal pain with a positive test for blood in stool should be treated with steroids.
- Evaluate for and treat infection (e.g., group A β-hemolytic Streptococci, *Helicobacter pylori*).
- Recurrent skin purpura may respond to dapsone.
- Aggressive treatment (high-dose or IV pulse corticosteroids) for children with poor prognostic signs including severe organ involvement.
- Severe nephritis: high-dose IV pulse methylprednisolone plus azathioprine or cyclophosphamide; angiotensin-converting enzyme inhibitors for proteinuria.
- Recurrent hospitalizations for chronic IgAv with GI manifestations may benefit from B-cell depletion with rituximab.

PEARL: Corticosteroid therapy helps arthritic and abdominal symptoms but may not prevent nephritis or subsequent recurrences.

17. **Which enzyme deficiency has been associated with some cases of childhood-onset PAN?**

Childhood-onset PAN is a systemic necrotizing vasculitis affecting small- and medium-sized arteries causing arterial aneurysms and ischemia leading to multisystem organ dysfunction. A subset of patients with childhood-onset (and young adult) PAN has been associated with **adenosine deaminase 2 deficiency (DADA2)**. This enzyme deficiency is caused by one of over 60 reported loss-of-function mutations of the CECR1 gene, and is inherited as an autosomal recessive trait. One-half of reported cases have presented before the age of 5, with 70–80% presenting before 18 years of age. Patients present with a vasculopathy ranging from livedo reticularis to a life-threatening vasculitis affecting multiple organs. Particularly common manifestations include fever (60%), livedo reticularis (50%) or other rashes (70% overall), hemorrhagic and/or ischemic strokes (66%), and peripheral nervous system involvement (60%). Other organs (intestine, liver, and kidney) can be involved. The spectrum of disease manifestations in patients with DADA2 extends beyond vasculitis/vasculopathy, and may include: a) evidence of immunodeficiency (hypogammaglobulinemia in 25%), b) hematologic abnormalities (including severe cytopenias), c) hepatosplenomegaly (30%) and generalized lymphadenopathy (10%), and d) symptoms consistent with an autoinflammatory syndrome.

The pathogenesis of how DADA2 leads to a vasculopathy is unclear. ADA2 acts as a growth factor important in endothelial cell and hematopoietic cell development. Furthermore, this enzyme induces monocyte proliferation and macrophage differentiation. Patients with DADA2 have an increase in M1 (proinflammatory) macrophages. Treatment of DADA2-associated PAN is markedly different than classic PAN. Antitumor necrosis factor agents are considered first-line therapy for patients with vasculitis/vasculopathy, whereas traditional immunosuppressives (e.g., cyclophosphamide) are ineffective. Notably, relapses are common when therapy is discontinued. Allogeneic hematopoietic stem cell transplantation has been successful in treatment-resistant cases, especially in patients with a predominant hematologic phenotype.

18. Describe the epidemiology and clinical manifestations of a child presenting with juvenile dermatomyositis (JDM).

JDM is an immune-mediated vasculitis that presents with an inflammatory myositis and a characteristic skin rash. The peak age of onset is 7.5 years with 25% occurring in children less than 4 years of age. Females are affected at two to five-fold the rate of males. Symmetric muscle weakness of the proximal musculature (limbs, girdle, neck) is prominent (80–100% of patients). The Gower maneuver is often abnormal, and the child will be unable to do a sit-up as a result of weakness. The head may hang back as the child is lifted from a lying position, owing to weakness of the neck flexors. Several characteristic skin findings may be seen on exam. Edema of the eyelids and face, with a heliotrope or mauvish rash around the eyes, is present in 75% of cases. Deep red patches, known as Gottron papules, are present over the extensor surfaces of the finger joints, elbows, knees, and ankle joints in 66–95% of cases. These patches may ulcerate as a result of vasculitis. Telangiectasias may be found around the eyelids, and capillary dilatation and dropout can be found around nailfolds and gum margins. GI manifestations include dysphagia (18–44%) and intestinal vasculitis causing abdominal pain, lower GI bleeding, and bowel perforation. Arthralgia or arthritis may occur (20–60%), sometimes with swelling and contractures of the fingers resulting from tenosynovitis. The most common lung finding is a decreased carbon monoxide diffusing capacity in 50% of patients. Cardiac involvement is rare. Treatment of JDM with the combination of GCs plus other immunomodulating therapy (e.g., methotrexate and intravenous immunoglobulin) is more effective than GCs alone.

19. How can the muscle weakness of JDM be differentiated from that of other causes of weakness?

The muscle weakness of JDM predominantly involves the proximal musculature, and in general, the involvement is symmetric. The child gives a history of difficulty in climbing stairs or riding a bicycle over the course of several weeks. Symptoms are subacute or chronic and progressive. Symptoms that are acute in onset, intermittent, or exercise-related should prompt consideration of a different diagnosis. Some of the maneuvers detailed in the previous question (e.g., Gower maneuver) can discriminate true muscle weakness from, for example, inanition. The palate and swallowing musculature may be weak in JDM and manifest with choking, cough, or aspiration pneumonia. Serum muscle enzymes are often elevated, but not to the degree seen in the muscular dystrophies. Assays for all muscle-derived enzymes are required (aldolase, creatine kinase, aspartate aminotransferase, and lactate dehydrogenase) as only one may be elevated in any given patient. ANA is positive in 10% to 85% of patients. Myositis-specific antibodies (MSA) are found in 66% of patients. The most common MSAs are anti-p155/140 (TIF-1λ; 20–30%), anti-NXP2 (MJ; 15–25%), and anti-Mi2 (5–10%). In patients who have symptoms such as a "classic" skin rash, muscle weakness, and elevated muscle enzymes, the diagnosis can be made clinically. Subclinical dysphagia or swallowing dysfunction can be assessed with a swallow study. A magnetic resonance imaging (MRI) scan of shoulder or thigh muscles can preclude the need for electromyography (EMG) and/or muscle biopsy if short tau inversion recovery (STIR) or T2-weighted images of the muscle shows increased signal, indicative of muscle edema and inflammation. In atypical cases, an EMG may be necessary, and MRI can determine the best site for biopsy. EMG will show spontaneous fibrillations, increased insertional activity, and small muscle unit action potentials. The muscle biopsy will show inflammation and/or fiber necrosis, perifascicular atrophy, and small-vessel vasculitis.

20. How is JDM different from adult dermatomyositis or polymyositis?

In children:
- Dermatomyositis is distinguished by being a generalized vasculitis.

- Polymyositis is exceedingly rare in childhood. In a child with progressive weakness, other muscle diseases are more likely than polymyositis.
- Unlike adults, malignancy is rarely associated with childhood dermatomyositis (see Question 7, above, regarding discussion of MSA antibodies).

21. Can a patient have just skin involvement and no muscle disease in JDM?

While uncommon, patients with clinically amyopathic JDM can have skin involvement without muscle disease. Over the course of two years, 25% to 30% of patients will develop muscle involvement.

22. What chronic sequelae can be seen in patients with JDM?

- In severe chronic JDM, nodules resulting from subcutaneous calcinosis may occur (up to 40%). This is more common in patients with anti-NXP2 (MJ) antibodies. Mobility may be impaired if calcinotic lesions involve the joints or musculature. Infections can occur where calcinosis breaks through the skin. The strongest factor associated with calcinosis development in JDM is disease duration, followed closely by delayed diagnosis, male gender, and black race.
- Partial or generalized lipodystrophy develops in 30% to 40% of patients with JDM. The face is frequently involved. It is often associated with metabolic syndrome, insulin resistance, hirsutism, clitoromegaly, and acanthosis nigricans. This is more common in patients with anti-p155/140 (TIF-1λ) antibody.
- Interstitial lung disease (ILD) is a rare, severe manifestation of JDM which is more common in patients with anti-MDA5 antibody or anti-aminoacyl-tRNA synthetases.

23. Discuss the causes of Raynaud phenomenon (RP) in children.

The environmental triggers of RP in children are similar to those described in adults. The most common triggers include cold temperatures, exercise, medications, and emotional stress. *Primary RP* (also called Raynaud disease) is a term used when there is no definable underlying cause for symptoms (idiopathic). Primary RP is much less common in children than adults; as such, an evaluation for secondary causes (SLE, SSc, DM, among others) should be conducted.

RP should be distinguished from normal vasomotor instability, particularly in young girls. It should also be distinguished from acrocyanosis, a vasospastic disorder of persistent coldness and bluish discoloration of the hands and feet. Patients with RP associated with digital ulcers, nailfold capillary abnormalities, and/or an ANA with a nucleolar or centromere pattern are more likely to have (or to develop) a systemic CTD and have secondary RP. RP occurs at high frequency (80–90%) in children with MCTD or SSc.

24. Describe the types of scleroderma that occur in childhood.

Scleroderma is characterized by abnormally increased collagen deposition in the skin and occasionally the internal organs.

- **Juvenile localized scleroderma** (JLS) is a separate entity from Juvenile Systemic Sclerosis (JSSc), and is ten times more common than SSc during childhood. JLS is characterized by cutaneous involvement and occasional extension into the underlying connective tissue or musculature. In severe cases, the underlying bony structures may be involved. The most recent classification criteria (the 2006 Padua criteria) divide JLS into five subtypes: linear, circumscribed (plaque) morphea, generalized morphea, pansclerotic (deep) morphea, and mixed morphea. JLS may occur anywhere on the body, including the face, forehead, and scalp (*en coup de sabre*). Facial involvement can also be progressive and associated with hemifacial atrophy (Parry–Romberg syndrome) or may include ipsilateral CNS involvement. ANA (50%), RF (10–25%), and hypergammaglobulinemia can be seen. Arthritis may be a manifestation in the RF+ patients. Seizures and uveitis can be seen as part of the Parry–Romberg syndrome or *en coup de sabre*, depending on the depth of involvement. For severe or progressive disease, treatment includes high-dose IV methylprednisolone followed by prednisone with taper over 3 to 6 months. Methotrexate is coadministered with steroids and continued for at least two years. There is a 30% recurrence rate after discontinuation of methotrexate.
- **Juvenile Systemic Sclerosis** (JSSc) typically presents with skin changes including induration, tightening, or atrophy, as well as Raynaud's phenomenon. Other manifestations include: calcinosis, myositis, arthritis, GI dysmotility, tendon friction rubs (diffuse subset), abnormal

nailfold capillaroscopy (with dropout, tortuous dilated loops or distorted architecture) and telangiectasias. JSSc can generally be classified into four subsets: diffuse cutaneous SSc (dcSSc), limited cutaneous SSc (lcSSc), systemic sclerosis-sine scleroderma, and overlap syndrome. JSSc is rare before the age of 16. It is one of the most severe conditions in pediatric rheumatology, with an estimated 5-year mortality of 7.5%.

25. List some infections and immune disorders that can mimic childhood CTD.

- **Acute rheumatic fever:** Rare before the age of 4 years. Severely painful, migratory polyarthritis with fever (see Chapter 43: Acute Rheumatic Fever and Post-Streptococcal Arthritis).
- **Parvovirus infection:** Young children get erythema infectiosum ("slapped cheeks"). Older children and adults can get fever (50%), polyarthritis, and rash. Can mimic systemic or polyarticular JIA. IgM anti-parvovirus antibodies can be negative for the first 2 to 3 weeks, but polymerase chain reaction (PCR) for parvovirus B19 DNA will be positive. Arthritis can last over 4 months (50%) (See Chapter 40: Viral Arthritides).
- **Epstein–Barr virus infection:** Can mimic SLE. Monospot is negative in children aged <4 years. Diagnose with IgM antibodies to viral capsid antigen and negative antibodies to Epstein–Barr nuclear antigen during initial acute infection. EBV viral load as detected by PCR can also be useful diagnostically.
- **Immunodeficiency:** Humoral and combined immunodeficiency can present as infections including septic joints. Echovirus can cause myositis and mycoplasma can cause chronic monoarticular arthritis. Consider immunodeficiency in any child with history of two or more previous bacterial pneumonias (see Chapter 57: Rheumatologic Manifestations of the Primary Immunodeficiency Syndromes).
- **Lyme disease:** Can mimic oligoarticular JIA. May start out as a migratory arthritis and/or cause morphea-like lesions (see Chapter 38: Lyme Disease).
- **Human immunodeficiency virus infection:** Can present as muscle, skin, or joint problems in children. Generalized adenopathy, fever of unknown origin with organomegaly, and thrombocytopenia are other presentations (see Chapter 41: HIV-associated Rheumatic Syndromes).
- **Additional infectious mimickers:** Cytomegalovirus, syphilis
- **Immune-mediated and neoplastic mimickers:** multicentric Castleman disease, sarcoidosis, IgG4-related disease, Autoimmune Lymphoproliferative Syndrome (ALPS), and malignancy (e.g. angioimmunoblastic T-cell lymphoma).

26. What bowel disease is most likely to present with arthritis and systemic symptoms?

Up to 20% of children with Crohn disease have arthritis, which is usually mono- or oligoarticular. Children will not volunteer information about their bowel habits, so they must be asked. Furthermore, some children with arthritis due to Crohn disease will not have bowel symptoms or a positive stool guaiac. Consequently, inflammatory bowel disease needs to be considered in any child with arthritis, weight loss, halt in linear growth, iron-deficiency anemia, and elevated ESR. A stool fecal calprotectin test can be helpful in these cases.

ACKNOWLEDGMENT

The authors and editor thank Terri H. Finkel, MD, PhD, Esi M. Morgan, MD, MSCE, and Courtney Crayne, MD, MSPH for their contributions to this chapter in previous editions.

BIBLIOGRAPHY

Boros CA, Lythgoe HM, Wedderburn LR, et al. Connective tissue diseases in childhood. In: Hochberg MC, Gravallese EM, Smolen JS et al, eds. *Rheumatology*. 7th ed. Philadelphia, PA: Elsevier; 2019:916–923.

Charras A, Smith E, Hedrich CM. Systemic lupus erythematosus in children and young people. *Curr Rheumatol Rep.* 2021;23:20.

Jauhola O, Ronkainen J, Koskimies O, et al. Renal manifestations of HSP in a 6 month prospective study of 223 children. *Arch Dis Child.* 2010;95:877–882.

Livingston B, Bonner A, Pope J. Differences in clinical manifestations between childhood-onset lupus and adult-onset lupus: a meta-analysis. *Lupus.* 2011;20:1345–1355.

Lundberg IE, Tjärnlund A, Bottai M, et al. 2017 European League Against Rheumatism/American College of Rheumatology classification criteria for adult and juvenile idiopathic inflammatory myopathies and their major subgroups. *Ann Rheum Dis.* 2017;76:1955–1964.

Mariz HA, Saito EI, Barbosa SH, et al. Pattern on the antinuclear antibody-HEp-2 test is a critical parameter for discriminating antinuclear antibody-positive healthy individuals and patients with autoimmune rheumatic diseases. *Arthritis Rheum.* 2011;63:191–200.

Martini G, Vittadello F, Kasapçopur O, et al. Factors affecting survival in juvenile systemic sclerosis. *Rheumatology (Oxford).* 2009;48:119–122.

Meyts I, Aksentijevich I. Deficiency of adenosine deaminase 2 (DADA2): update on the phenotypes, genetics, pathogenesis, and treatment. *J Clin Immunol.* 2018;38:569–578.

Mina R, Brunner HI. Pediatric lupus—are there differences in presentation, genetics, response to therapy, and damage accrual compared with adult lupus? *Rheum Dis Clin North Am.* 2010;36:53–80.

Petty RE, Laxer RM, Lindsley CB, et al. *Textbook of Pediatric Rheumatology.* 8th ed. Philadelphia, PA: Elsevier; 2021.

Sammaritano LR, Bermas BL, Chakravarty EE, et al. 2020 American College of Rheumatology guideline for the management of reproductive health in rheumatic and musculoskeletal diseases. *Arthritis Rheumatol.* 2020;72(4):529–556.

Wahren-Herelenius M, Sonesson SE, Clowse ME. Neonatal lupus erythematosus. In: Wallace DJ, Hahn BH, eds. *Dubois' Lupus Erythematosus and Related Syndromes.* 8th ed. Philadelphia, PA: Elsevier Saunders; 2013:464–472.

Zulian F, Woo P, Athreya BH, et al. The Pediatric Rheumatology European Society/American College of Rheumatology/European League against Rheumatism provisional classification criteria for juvenile systemic sclerosis. *Arthritis Rheum.* 2007;57:203–212.

FURTHER READING

http://www.lupus.org/.
https://www.carragroup.org.
http://www.myositis.org.
http://www.scleroderma.org/medical/juvenile.shtm.

CHAPTER 70

Kawasaki Disease

Lyndsey D. Cole, MD and Katharine F. Moore, MD

≫ KEY POINTS

1. Kawasaki disease (KD) is the most common vasculitis and cause of acquired heart disease in children.
2. Consider KD in any child, especially those <5 years, presenting with high fevers ≥5 days and one or more of the following: conjunctivitis, rash, mucous membrane changes, hand/foot redness/swelling, and unilateral cervical lymphadenopathy.
3. Consider KD in the differential diagnosis of any infant under the age of 6 months with fever for ≥7 days without a source.
4. When considering KD, a careful history is essential. Some manifestations of KD may be transient but still count toward fulfilling the diagnostic criteria.
5. Incomplete KD not meeting full diagnostic criteria does exist, and treatment should be promptly initiated when this is suspected.
6. Intravenous immunoglobulin (IVIG) and aspirin are the gold-standard first-line therapies for KD.

---

1. What is KD?

KD is an acute, self-limited, febrile illness of childhood characterized by systemic inflammation of the medium-sized arteries in multiple organs and tissues, most notably the coronary arteries. KD leads to the development of coronary artery aneurysms in up to 25% of untreated cases and 5% of treated patients; for infants under 6 months, the risk is closer to 50%. KD is the leading cause of acquired heart disease in children in the developed world.

2. What are the diagnostic criteria for KD?

Fever or a history of fever is a necessary component in the clinical criteria for KD. Exceptions include young infants in whom fever may be low grade or unrecognized, or patients diagnosed late in the illness whose parents did not recognize fever during the acute phase. Fever is usually high grade (>38.5°C), unresponsive to antibiotics, poorly responsive to antipyretics, and lasts an average of 1–3 weeks.

The diagnostic criteria for complete KD are:

Fever for ≥5 consecutive days, with at least four of the following[a]:

1. **Conjunctivitis (>90%):** bilateral bulbar nonexudative conjunctivitis, often with limbic sparing
2. **Oral changes (90%):** erythema, fissuring, cracking, or bleeding of lips; diffuse oropharyngeal erythema without exudate; and/or "strawberry" tongue
3. **Cervical lymphadenopathy (25–70%):** one or more enlarged nodes in the anterior cervical triangle, usually unilateral and sometimes painful
4. **Rash (70–90%):** erythematous, usually a diffuse maculopapular eruption; erythroderma, erythema multiforme-like, urticarial, scarlatiniform, and micropustular eruptions can also be seen; typically involves the trunk and extremities, and there may be accentuation in the groin (50%); bullous, vesicular, and petechial rashes are not seen in KD.
5. **Extremity changes (60–85%):** often the last manifestation to occur; erythema of palms and soles with firm and sometimes painful edema of the hands and feet; desquamation of the fingers and toes begins in the periungual area usually 2–3 weeks after fever onset; desquamation may also involve the palms and soles.

---

[a]If all of the clinical criteria are present, the diagnosis can be made on Day 4 of fever. With a classic presentation, experienced clinicians may make the diagnosis at Day 3 of fever. In many patients, clinical criteria appear sequentially over time. A history of any of the clinical criteria count toward diagnosis even if not present at the time the diagnosis is made.

3. **What if a patient presents with ≥5 days of fever but does not have enough clinical criteria to meet the case definition of KD? Does incomplete KD exist?**

Yes, "incomplete KD" does exist. The clinical case definition of KD does not identify all children with the disease, and 10–25% of patients with KD do not fulfill diagnostic criteria at diagnosis. This is particularly true for infants aged <6 months who may present with only fever. The American Heart Association has published an algorithm for the evaluation of children with suspected incomplete KD. Using this algorithm, children with fever for ≥5 days and at least two clinical diagnostic criteria, or infants with fever for ≥7 days without an alternative diagnosis, should have C-reactive protein (CRP) and erythrocyte sedimentation rate (ESR) obtained. If CRP >3.0 mg/dL and/or ESR >40 mm/hour, then supplementary laboratory studies and echocardiogram (echo) should be performed. Supplementary lab criteria include: anemia for age, white blood cell (WBC) count ≥15,000/mm^3, platelets ≥450,000/mm^3, albumin ≤3 g/dL, elevated alanine aminotransferase, and urine WBC ≥10/HPF. If three or more of the supplementary lab criteria are identified and/or the echo has positive findings, then a diagnosis of KD should be made and the patient should be treated (see Question #7 for a list of positive echo findings).

4. **What epidemiologic facts are known about KD?**
   - KD affects predominantly, but not exclusively, young children. Majority (75%) of children are aged <5 years.
   - Male: female ratio is 1.5:1.
   - The highest relative risk (17×) is in Asian children, especially those with Japanese ancestry.
   - The incidence is approximately 2% in siblings and 13% in identical twins.
   - Recurrence rate is ~3%.
   - It is most common in winter and early spring in North America.
   - Local outbreaks and epidemics of KD have been reported.
   - Most common vasculitis of childhood (previously called infantile polyarteritis nodosa).
   - Rarely occurs in adults with or without coexistent human immunodeficiency virus.

5. **What other clinical symptoms or conditions may be seen in the acute phase of the illness?**
   - **Musculoskeletal:** arthritis or arthralgia may involve large and/or small joints (7.5–25%). Usually short-lived. Synovial fluid WBC count can be >100,000/mm^3.
   - **Cardiovascular:** myocarditis, pericarditis, shock, aneurysms of medium-sized arteries (20–25%), aortic root enlargement.
   - **Ocular:** anterior uveitis (up to 80%)
   - **Respiratory:** cough (30%), hoarseness.
   - **Gastrointestinal:** vomiting and diarrhea with abdominal pain (40–60%), pancreatitis, hepatitis (30–40%), gallbladder hydrops.
   - **Genitourinary:** urethritis, sterile pyuria.
   - **Nervous system:** extreme irritability (50%), aseptic meningitis, facial nerve palsy, sensorineural hearing loss (<1%).
   - **Skin:** inflammation at previous BCG immunization site (characteristic).
   - **Systemic:** macrophage activation syndrome (MAS).

6. **Is there a diagnostic laboratory test for KD?**

There is no single diagnostic test for KD. Laboratory tests show findings of acute inflammation including elevated ESR, CRP, WBC (generally with neutrophilic predominance), and platelet count. The platelet count typically rises after the seventh day of illness and may exceed 10^6/mm^3. Other lab findings commonly seen include anemia for age, eosinophilia, elevated liver enzymes (AST, ALT, GGT), and sterile pyuria. Any patient with KD who develops thrombocytopenia, highly elevated liver enzymes, high triglycerides, and/or extreme hyperferritinemia should be evaluated for MAS.

7. **What is the role of echo in the diagnosis of KD?**

Data suggest that 80% of children with KD who ultimately develop coronary artery lesions (Z-score ≥2 to <2. 5 = dilation; Z-score ≥2.5 = aneurysm) will have them present at the time of diagnosis. In general, **an abnormal echo can be used to support the diagnosis of KD, but a normal echo cannot be used to rule out KD**. A Z-score ≥2.5 in the LAD or RCA has very high specificity for the diagnosis of KD, but lacks sensitivity. Similarly, without a Z-score of ≥2.5, an echo is also considered positive for the diagnosis of KD if three or more of the following are met: Z-score of the LAD or RCA between 2 to 2.5; decreased left ventricular function; mitral regurgitation; or pericardial effusion.

8. Which other diseases need to be considered in the differential diagnosis of KD?
- Staphylococcal and streptococcal toxin-mediated disease: scarlet fever, toxic shock.
- Viral infections: measles, adenovirus, enterovirus, Epstein–Barr virus, multisystem inflammatory syndrome in children (MIS-C) (see Question #15)
- Drug hypersensitivity reactions: Stevens–Johnson syndrome.
- Rheumatologic: other medium-vessel vasculitides; systemic-onset juvenile idiopathic arthritis.
- Other (with appropriate epidemiologic risk factors): leptospirosis, Rickettsial infections, mercury intoxication.

9. What causes KD?
The cause of KD is unknown. Current data suggest that the disease results from an immune response to a classic antigen in genetically susceptible individuals. It is not uncommon for patients with KD to have a concurrent viral illness at the time of diagnosis. Numerous infectious pathogens have been proposed as etiologic agents, yet none have been proven. The two most active lines of investigation suggest infection with a novel RNA virus via the respiratory tract or transport of an agent in tropospheric winds that initiates the immunologic cascade of KD when inhaled. Epidemiology, genome-wide association studies and linkage analysis have provided evidence that there is genetic susceptibility to KD and disease outcomes. In particular, the genes FCγR2a, caspase 3, human leukocyte antigen class II, B-cell lymphoid kinase, inositol 1,4,5-trisphosphate kinase C, and CD40 have been implicated. Histologically, KD is a neutrophilic non-granulomatous panmural necrotizing vasculitis of the medium-sized arteries, accompanied by intimal hyperplasia.

10. What is the initial treatment of KD?
Intravenous immune globulin (IVIG) at a dose of 2 g/kg given over 10–12 hours is the standard-of-care initial treatment for acute KD. This is more effective in preventing persistent coronary artery aneurysms if given within the first 10 days after disease onset. IVIG is given in conjunction with high-dose aspirin (30–50 or 80–100 mg/kg per day in four divided doses). Once the fever has resolved, the dose of aspirin is decreased to a single oral dose of 3–5 mg/kg per day for its antiplatelet effect. In those who do not develop coronary artery abnormalities, the aspirin can be discontinued 6 weeks after treatment initiation and when the ESR, CRP, and platelet counts have normalized.

11. Are there patients with KD who might benefit from more aggressive initial therapy?
Approximately 10–35% of patients with KD fail to respond to the initial IVIG dose or develop recrudescent fever. These patients are characterized as IVIG-resistant and are at high risk for developing coronary artery aneurysms, requiring additional therapy to interrupt the inflammatory process. There have been many efforts to prospectively identify patients with a high likelihood of IVIG resistance or who are at risk for developing coronary artery aneurysms. Researchers from Japan have developed successful scoring systems to predict IVIG resistance, and intensified therapy with prednisolone and IVIG in these high-risk patients was shown to improve coronary artery outcomes. Unfortunately, these scoring systems have shown low sensitivity in multiethnic US populations.

The 2021 KD Treatment Guidelines from the American College of Rheumatology (ACR) and the Vasculitis Foundation (VF) give a conditional recommendation for using IVIG with adjunctive glucocorticoids as initial therapy, over IVIG alone, for patients at high risk of IVIG resistance or developing coronary artery aneurysms. High-risk patients were defined as those with a Z-score of ≥2.5 for the LAD or RCA, or age <6 months. Corticosteroids are given over a 2–3-week tapering course. Use of non-glucocorticoid immunosuppressive agents with IVIG in high-risk patients was given a conditional recommendation as well, although currently there is more data supporting the use of glucocorticoids over non-glucocorticoids.

12. How do you treat patients with KD who also show signs of MAS?

MAS is a life-threatening cytokine storm that can occur in many inflammatory conditions including KD. For patients with KD and suspected MAS, it is crucial to initiate IVIG for KD in parallel with aggressively treating MAS, as both conditions are associated with high morbidity and mortality. MAS treatment typically involves anakinra and glucocorticoids, and timely initiation of therapy is crucial for improving chances of survival.

13. What is the treatment for patients with KD who are resistant to initial IVIG therapy?

IVIG resistance is defined as fever that occurs from 36 hours to 7 days after the end of the IVIG infusion. Ten to thirty-five percent of patients with KD are IVIG-resistant. The 2021 ACR/VF treatment guidelines include the following:

- For patients with acute KD and persistent fevers after initial treatment with IVIG, a second course of IVIG is conditionally recommended over the use of glucocorticoids
- For patients with acute KD and persistent fevers after repeated treatment with IVIG, either nonglucocorticoid immunosuppressive therapy or glucocorticoids may be used.

The authors of these guidelines acknowledge the lack of comparative treatment studies, and their conditional recommendations are influenced by the current standard of care. Standardized clinical pathways for specific therapies may vary by institution. Options for therapy in IVIG-resistant patients include administration of a second dose of IVIG (2 g/kg), infliximab (5–10 mg/kg), or corticosteroids (2 mg/kg/day tapering over 15 days, or high-dose "pulse" dosing at 20–30 mg/kg intravenously for 3 days with or without a subsequent taper of oral prednisone). For patients with refractory KD who fail to respond to a second course of IVIG, infliximab, and/or steroids, other therapies to consider include anakinra, cyclosporine, cyclophosphamide, or plasma exchange.

14. What is the appropriate follow-up for patients with KD after discharge from the hospital?

Patients without coronary artery lesions should be seen by a pediatric cardiologist and repeat echo obtained approximately 1–2 weeks and 6 weeks after discharge from the hospital. If the echo remains normal at 6 weeks, patients may discontinue thromboprophylaxis with aspirin. Patients should also be seen at 1-year follow-up for repeat echo and lipid profile testing. Some experts recommend follow-up every 5 years thereafter with exercise stress testing and lipid profile testing. General heart-healthy lifestyle counseling should be provided at all visits. For patients with coronary artery lesions, closer follow-up with cardiology is indicated. Thromboprophylaxis with aspirin, clopidogrel, warfarin, and/or low-molecular-weight heparin is decided based on the size and location of the coronary artery lesions as well as the presence or absence of thrombosis. Medical therapies with β-blockers, angiotensin-converting enzyme inhibitors, and statins may also need to be considered.

15. What is the long-term outcome of patients with a history of KD?

The majority of coronary artery lesions will normalize in size by 1 year after diagnosis. However, despite normalization of internal luminal size, the arterial wall architecture and function may remain abnormal in some patients, which may lead to stenosis and occlusion over time. Long-term follow-up data on KD patients is currently lacking. Patients with persistent lesions are at continued high risk for thrombosis and myocardial infarction.

16. What is multisystem inflammatory syndrome in children (MIS-C)?

MIS-C is a hyperinflammatory febrile illness associated with preceding SARS-CoV-2 infection characterized by multiorgan dysfunction, which has overlapping features with KD. It was first described in 2020 during the COVID-19 pandemic. Onset of MIS-C typically occurs 2–6 weeks after SARS-CoV-2 infection; the infection itself is frequently mild or asymptomatic. Cases of

MIS-C peaked 1–2 months after previous peaks in SARS-CoV-2 cases, and are now less common. The CDC 2023 case definition of MIS-C requires the following:

Patient <21 years old without a more likely diagnosis who has all five of the following:

1. Fever
2. Severity of illness requiring hospitalization or resulting in death
3. Evidence of systemic inflammation with CRP ≥3 mg/dL
4. New onset manifestations in two or more categories:
   * Cardiac: left ventricular ejection fraction <55%, coronary artery abnormalities, or elevated troponin
   * Mucocutaneous: rash, inflammation of oral mucosa, conjunctivitis, or erythema/edema of hands or feet
   * Shock
   * Gastrointestinal: abdominal pain, vomiting or diarrhea
   * Hematologic: thrombocytopenia or lymphopenia
5. Confirmed laboratory evidence of SARS-CoV-2 infection

17. How does MIS-C differ from KD in diagnosis and treatment?

Distinguishing between MIS-C and KD is not always possible. Compared to patients with KD, those with MIS-C tend to have an older average age, more rapid clinical decompensation with higher prevalence of left ventricular dysfunction/shock, less frequent coronary artery aneurysms, more prominent GI symptoms, and lab findings of thrombocytopenia, hyponatremia, and lymphopenia. ACR guidelines for treatment of MIS-C recommend initial treatment with IVIG 2 g/kg (may require slower administration due to risk of fluid overload in patients with cardiac dysfunction) and IV methylprednisolone 1–2 mg/kg/day. Some institutions have also used infliximab + IVIG as initial therapy.

ACKNOWLEDGMENT

The authors would like to acknowledge the contributions of Dr. Samuel Dominguez and Dr. Marsha Anderson, who were the coauthors of this chapter in the previous edition.

BIBLIOGRAPHY

Bratincsak A, Reddy VD, Purohit PJ, et al. Coronary artery dilation in acute Kawasaki disease and acute illnesses associated with fever. *Pediatr Infect Dis J.* 2012;31(9):924–926.

Dominguez SR, Anderson MS, El-Adawy M, et al. Preventing coronary artery abnormalities: a need for earlier diagnosis and treatment of Kawasaki disease. *Pediatr Infect Dis J.* 2012;31(12):1217–1220.

Fraison JB, Sève P, Dauphin C. Kawasaki disease in adults: Observations in France and literature review. *Autoimmun Rev.* 2016;15(3):242–249.

Gorelik M, Chung SA, Ardalan K, et al. 2021 American College of Rheumatology/Vasculitis Foundation guideline for the management of Kawasaki disease. *Arthritis Care Res (Hoboken).* 2022;74(4):538–548.

Ha KS, Jang G, Lee J, et al. Incomplete clinical manifestation as a risk factor for coronary artery abnormalities in Kawasaki's disease: a metaanalysis. *Eur J Pediatr.* 2013;172:343–349.

Henderson LA, Canna SW, Friedman KG, et al. American College of Rheumatology clinical guidance for Multisystem Inflammatory syndrome in children associated with SARS-CoV-2 and hyperinflammation in pediatric COVID-19: version 3. *Arthritis Rheumatol.* 2022;74(4):e1–e20.

Kawasaki T, Kosaki F, Okawa S, et al. A new infantile acute febrile mucocutaneous lymph node syndrome (MLNS) prevailing in Japan. *Pediatrics.* 1974;54:271–276.

Kobayashi T, Saji T, Otani T, et al. Efficacy of immunoglobulin plus prednisone for prevention of coronary artery abnormalities in severe Kawasaki disease (RAISE study): a randomised, open-label, blinded-endpoints trial. *Lancet.* 2012;379:1613.

McCrindle BW, Rowley AH, Newburger JW, et al. Diagnosis, treatment, and long-term management of Kawasaki disease: a scientific statement for health professionals from the American Heart Association. *Circulation.* 2017;135(17):e927–e999.

Rowley AH. Kawasaki disease: novel insights into etiology and genetic susceptibility. *Ann Rev Med.* 2011;62:69–77.

Tremoulet AH, Best BM, Song S, et al. Resistance to intravenous immunoglobulin in children with Kawasaki disease. *J Pediatr.* 2008;153:117–121.

Tremoulet AH, Jain S, Jaggi P, et al. Infliximab for intensification of primary therapy for Kawasaki disease: a phase 3 randomized, double-blind, placebo-controlled trial. *Lancet.* 2014;383(9930):1731–1738.

Turnier JL, Anderson MS, Heizer HR, et al. Concurrent respiratory viruses and Kawasaki disease. *Pediatrics.* 2015;136(3):e609–e614.

Yellen ES, Gauvreau K, Takahashi M, et al. Performance of 2004 American Heart Association recommendations for treatment of Kawasaki disease. *Pediatrics.* 2010;125:e234–e241.

Genetic Muscle Diseases: Metabolic and Other Genetic Muscle Disorders

Matthew Wicklund, MD

Sickness is a place, more instructive than a long trip to Europe, and it is a place where there's no company, where nobody can follow.

–Flannery O'Connor (1925–1963)

KEY POINTS

1. Muscle cramps, pain, or myoglobinuria brought on by exercise suggests a metabolic myopathy.
2. Muscle symptoms with short bursts of high-intensity exercise and the second wind phenomenon are characteristic of one of the glycogen storage diseases, of which McArdle disease is most common.
3. Muscle symptoms with prolonged low-intensity exercise and/or prolonged fasting suggest a disorder of fatty acid oxidation, of which CPT II deficiency is most common.
4. Elevated resting serum lactate or growth differentiation factor 15 (GDF-15) levels and/or ragged red fibers on muscle biopsy are characteristics of mitochondrial myopathies.
5. The most common metabolic myopathies associated with myoglobinuria are CPT II deficiency and McArdle disease.
6. The most common myopathies confused with polymyositis are acid maltase deficiency (Pompe disease) and the limb-girdle muscular dystrophies.
7. Children presenting with a muscle disease without rash almost always have a metabolic or other genetic myopathy and not primary polymyositis.
8. If your evaluation for a metabolic myopathy does not yield an answer, reconsider a metabolic presentation of a muscular dystrophy or RYR1-associated myopathy.
9. Genetic testing is now the first step in evaluation of cases suspected to be metabolic myopathies.

1. What is the relative prevalence of genetic muscle diseases?

The combined prevalence of genetic muscle disease is estimated to be a minimum prevalence of ~80/100,000. Metabolic myopathies comprise ~5/100,000, while mitochondrial myopathies are thought to involve another ~5/100,000. The remainder of genetic muscle diseases consists of the following disorders: dystrophinopathies (Duchenne and Becker muscular dystrophies along with symptomatic female dystrophinopathy gene carriers) at ~12/100,000; myotonic dystrophies (type 1 and type 2) at ~30/100,000; facioscapulohumeral muscular dystrophy at ~12/100,000; limb-girdle muscular dystrophies at ~8/100,000; and the remainder of genetic muscle diseases encompass ~8/100,000. One should always bear in mind the full spectrum of disorders presenting with symptoms related to muscles.

2. What are metabolic myopathies?

Metabolic myopathies are conditions that have in common abnormalities in muscle energy metabolism that result in skeletal muscle dysfunction. **Primary metabolic myopathies** are associated with biochemical defects that affect the ability of the muscle fibers to maintain adequate levels of adenosine triphosphate (ATP). The three main categories of primary metabolic myopathies are glycogen storage diseases, fatty acid oxidation defects, and mitochondrial cytopathies, due to respiratory chain impairment. Since enzyme defects often are partial, metabolic myopathies may manifest from infancy through adulthood. **Secondary metabolic myopathies** are attributed to various endocrine and electrolyte abnormalities.

Metabolic myopathies can be divided into two groups based on clinical presentation: (1) the acute form manifesting repeated episodes of myalgias, exercise intolerance, hyperkalemia, contractures, rhabdomyolysis and myoglobinuria with a normal examination between episodes;

and (2) the progressive form with proximal and axial muscle weakness, and often accompanied by involvement of other organ systems such as liver, heart, endocrine, or the peripheral or central nervous system.

3. Which conditions are considered primary metabolic myopathies?

(Most common disorders in bold)

A. Disorders of glycolysis/glycogenolysis (Eponym, GSD, gene)
- **Acid maltase deficiency** (Pompe disease, 2, *GAA*)
- Debrancher enzyme deficiency (Cori or Forbes disease, 3, *AGL*)
- Branching enzyme deficiency (Andersen disease, 4, *GBE1*)
- **Myophosphorylase deficiency** (McArdle's disease, 5, *PYGM*)
- Phosphofructokinase deficiency (Tarui's disease, 7, *PKFM*)
- Phosphorylase b kinase deficiency
  - α subunit (9D, *PHKA1*)
  - β subunit (9B, *PHKB*)
- Phosphoglycerate mutase deficiency (10, *PGAM2*)
- Lactate dehydrogenase deficiency (11, *LDHA*)
- Aldolase A deficiency (12, *ALDOA*)
- β-enolase deficiency (13, *ENO3*)
- Phosphoglucomutase deficiency (14, *PGM1*)
- Glycogenin-1 deficiency (15, *GYG1*)
- Glycogen synthase 1 deficiency (0, *GYS1*)
- RBCK1 E3 ubiquitin ligase deficiency (*RBCK1*)
- Phosphoglycerate kinase deficiency (*PGK1*)

B. *Disorders of fatty acid oxidation*
- Primary carnitine deficiency (CD) syndromes
  - Carnitine acetyltransferase deficiency (*CRAT*)
  - **Carnitine palmitoyltransferase II deficiency (*CPT2*)**
  - Multiple acyl-CoA dehydrogenase deficiency (*ETFA, ETFB, ETFDH*)
- Secondary carnitine deficiency syndromes
  - Acyl-CoA dehydrogenase deficiencies
    - Short chain (*HADH*)
    - Medium chain (*ACADM*)
    - Very long chain (*ACADVL*)
    - Trifunctional protein deficiency (*LCHAD*)
- Lipin-1 deficiency (*LPIN1*)

C. *Mitochondrial myopathies*
- Electron transport chain protein deficiency
- Multiple AcylCoA dehydrogenase deficiency (Complex I-IV mutations)
- Mitochondrial ATP synthase deficiency (Complex V mutations)
- Coenzyme Q10 gene mutation

4. What are secondary causes of metabolic myopathies?

A. *Endocrine myopathies*
- Acromegaly
- Carcinoid syndrome
- Cushing's and Addison's diseases
- Hyper- and hypothyroidism
- Hyperaldosteronism
- Hyperparathyroidism

B. *Metabolic-nutritional myopathies*
- Hepatic failure
- Malabsorption and periodic paralysis
- Uremia
- Vitamin D deficiency

C. *Electrolyte disorders*
- Elevated or decreased levels of sodium, potassium, or calcium
- Hypomagnesemia
- Hypophosphatemia

D. *Genetic muscle diseases* (e.g., muscular dystrophies)
- Dystrophinopathies (Duchenne & Becker muscular dystrophies)
- Limb girdle muscular dystrophies (LGMD 1C, 2A, 2B, 2C-E, 2I, 2L, 2T)
- RYR1-related myopathies

5. What is the source of energy for muscle contraction?

Hydrolysis of ATP. Intracellular concentrations of ATP are maintained by the action of enzymes such as creatine kinase, adenylate cyclase, and myoadenylate deaminase. The energy to replenish ATP after it is consumed during muscle contraction is provided by intermediary metabolism of carbohydrates and lipids by pathways of glycolysis, the Krebs cycle, β-oxidation, and oxidative phosphorylation.

6. How does ATP provide the energy for muscle contraction?

The immediate source of energy for skeletal muscle during work is found in preformed organic compounds containing high-energy phosphates, such as ATP and creatine phosphate. Creatine kinase (CK or CPK) helps maintain intracellular ATP concentrations by catalyzing the reversible transphosphorylation of creatine and adenine nucleotides and by modulating changes in cytosolic ATP concentrations.

At rest, when there is excess ATP, the terminal phosphate of ATP is transferred to creatine, forming creatine phosphate (CrP) and adenosine diphosphate (ADP) in a reaction catalyzed by CK. The CrP serves as a reservoir of high-energy phosphate. With muscle activity and ATP utilization, CK catalyzes the transfer of those phosphates from CrP to rapidly restore ATP levels to normal. The stores of CrP are sufficient to allow the re-phosphorylation of ADP to ATP for only a few minutes of exercise.

Thus, CK along with its products, creatine, and creatine phosphate, serve as a shuttle mechanism for energy transport between mitochondria, where ATP is generated by oxidative metabolism (Krebs' cycle and respiratory/cytochrome chain), and the myofibrils, where ATP is consumed during muscle contraction and relaxation. (see Fig 71.1.)

7. What is the role of carbohydrate metabolism during muscle work?

Glycogen, the major storage form of carbohydrate, is the major source of ATP generation when physical activity is of short duration and high intensity (lifting heavy weight) or when anaerobic conditions exist (running sprints).

Glycogen is mobilized to form glucose-6-phosphate (G-6-P) by glycogenolysis in a process started by the enzyme <u>myophosphorylase</u>. Glucose and glucose-6-phosphate are metabolized through a series of reactions in the glycolytic pathway to pyruvate. Under aerobic conditions, pyruvate enters the Krebs' (TCA) cycle and is metabolized to carbon dioxide and water. Under aerobic conditions, a net of 36 molecules of ATP is generated for each molecule of glucose. However, under anaerobic conditions, pyruvate is converted to lactate and does not enter the Krebs cycle. Under these conditions, only two molecules of ATP are generated for each glucose

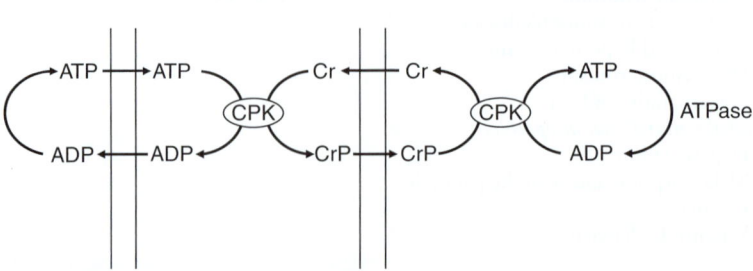

Fig. 71.1 ATP production in muscles. *ADP*, adenosine diphosphate; *ATP*, adenosine triphosphate; *ATPase*, adenosine triphosphatase; *CPK*, creatine phosphokinase; *Cr*, creatine; *CrP*, creatine phosphate.

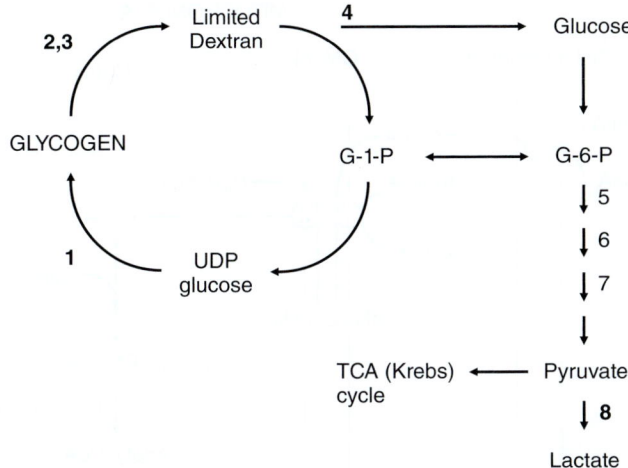

Fig. 71.2 Carbohydrate metabolism. Catalyst enzymes: (1) brancher enzyme; (2) phosphorylase b kinase; (3) myophosphorylase; (4) debrancher enzyme; (5) phosphofructokinase; (6) phosphoglycerate kinase; (7) phosphoglycerate mutase; (8) lactate dehydrogenase; (9) (not shown), acid maltase, which catalzes release of glucose from glycogen and maltase in lysosomes.

molecule. Anaerobic glycogenolysis can supply energy to muscle for only several minutes until the muscle fatigues, whereas there are sufficient muscle glycogen stores to supply energy for up to 90 minutes under aerobic conditions (see Fig 71.2).

8. What is the role of lipid metabolism during muscle work?

Lipids, especially long-chain fatty acids, constitute the major substrate for energy production (ATP) during fasting intervals, at rest, and with muscular activities of low intensity and long duration (more than 40–50 min).

Long-chain fatty acids (LCFA) from adipose tissues move through the bloodstream bound to albumin. These, plus medium and small chain fatty acids, move across endothelial cells and into muscle fibers, where they are available for energy production, storage, or synthesis into membrane components. To be processed for energy, the free fatty acid must enter the mitochondria. Short and medium-chain fatty acids cross freely into the mitochondria. Long-chain fatty acids must combine with carnitine to enter the inner mitochondrial matrix. The combination of long-chain fatty acids with carnitine and their release into the mitochondrial matrix are catalyzed by carnitine palmitoyltransferase (CPT) I and CPT II, respectively (1 and 2 in the diagram), which are located on the inner mitochondrial membrane (IM). Once in the mitochondria, the fatty acids are converted to their respective coenzyme A (CoA) esters and sequentially shortened by the process of β-oxidation, which release acetyl CoA that then enters the tricarboxylic acid (TCA, Krebs') cycle. CPT deficiency, trifunctional protein deficiency, and very long-chain acyl-CoA dehydrogenase deficiency are the most common fatty acid oxidation defect disorders (see Fig 71.3).

9. How do disorders of glycogen and glucose metabolism present clinically?

Patients who develop muscle cramps, spasms, and/or myoglobinuria with short bursts of high-intensity exercise (weightlifting or sprinting) may have a defect of glycogen metabolism known as a glycogen storage disease (GSD). There are 16 types of GSD (glycogenoses, types 0–15) with eleven having muscle symptoms. Most are autosomal recessive. Mostly, these patients are well at rest and perform low-intensity exercise without difficulty, because free fatty acids are the major source of energy under these conditions. The enzymatic block that interferes with the use of carbohydrates to generate ATP causes problems only when exercise reaches a level that produces anaerobic conditions. Typically, the patient starts exercising and within a few minutes the muscle fatigues (patients describe this as "hitting the wall"). In some cases (McArdle's and Tarui's diseases), continued exertion can result in improved exercise tolerance, referred to as the "**second wind**" phenomenon. However, in many patients if they continue exercising, the muscle becomes painful and may develop a firm cramp. This can result in muscle damage and myoglobinuria.

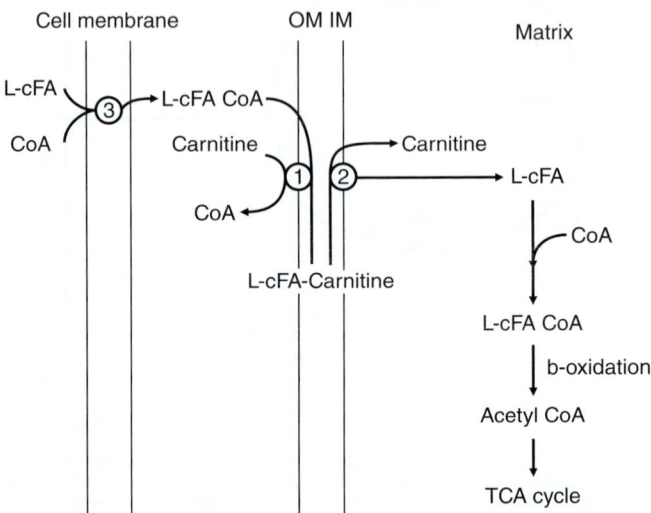

Fig. 71.3 Fatty acid metabolism. *CoA*, coenzyme A; *IM*, inner mitochondrial membrane; *L-cFA*, long-chain fatty acid; *OM*, outer mitochondrial membrane; *TCA*, tricarboxylic acid.

Over time, four of the GSDs (acid maltase deficiency, aldolase A deficiency, branching enzyme deficiency, and debrancher deficiency) may result in fixed weakness.

10. Describe the clinical presentation seen in myophosphorylase deficiency (McArdle's disease; glycogenosis type V).

McArdle's disease is one of the two most common GSDs. Its inheritance is autosomal recessive and due to pathogenic variants in *PYGM*, the gene for myophosphorylase. It is a common cause of recurrent rhabdomyolysis and myoglobinuria, second only to CPT deficiency among the metabolic myopathies. Myophosphorylase degrades glycogen to glucose-1-phosphate and hence is important in calling up stored energy for muscle use. The cardinal manifestation of this deficiency is exercise intolerance associated with pain, fatigue, cramps, and/or weakness. The degree of intolerance varies among affected individuals. Symptoms generally follow activities of high intensity and short duration. Symptoms should resolve with rest. In fact, at rest, affected individuals function well and adjust their activities to a level below their threshold for symptoms. Some individuals experience the "second wind" phenomenon, which is a marked improvement in exercise tolerance about 10 minutes into aerobic exercise involving large muscle masses (jogging or cycling). For unknown reasons, severe cramps and myoglobinuria are rare before adolescence. An elevated CK at rest is common. Forearm exercise testing is usually diagnostic, showing a flat venous lactate curve. Definitive diagnosis requires genetic testing or histochemical and biochemical testing on muscle biopsy showing enzyme deficiency. Careful and progressive exercise training, low-dose creatine monohydrate, and pre-exercise sucrose or glucose may improve exercise performance and tolerance in patients with this condition.

11. How does phosphofructokinase deficiency (Tarui's disease; glycogenosis type VII) present?

The clinical manifestations of phosphofructokinase (fructose-6-phosphate to fructose-1, 6-phosphate) deficiency can be identical to those of McArdle's disease. However, glucose or sucrose intake before exercise may exacerbate muscle symptoms. The second wind phenomenon is less common, and exercise intolerance is likely to be associated with nausea and vomiting. About one-third of affected persons develop myoglobinuria, and most have elevated CK at rest. The disease can also cause *hemolytic anemia*.

PEARL: Consider this diagnosis in any patient with exercised-induced muscle symptoms, elevated CK, and hemolytic anemia.

12. How does acid maltase deficiency (Pompe disease; glycogenosis type II) present?

Acid maltase deficiency is one of the two most common GSDs. It is caused by one of >200 pathogenic variants in the gene that codes for the intra-lysosomal enzyme acid alpha-glucosidase (GAA) that catalyzes the release of glucose from maltose, oligosaccharide, and glycogen in lysosomes. Its deficiency is transmitted by autosomal recessive inheritance and produces three different clinical syndromes depending on the severity of the enzyme deficiency.

1. The infantile form causes symptoms of muscle weakness, hypotonia, and congestive heart failure that begin shortly after birth and previously progressed to death within the first 2 years of life.
2. The childhood and juvenile forms present in the first two decades with progressive proximal muscle weakness. Death was previously from respiratory failure and occurred before 30 years of age.
3. The adult form presents in the third to seventh decades of life with insidious, painless limb-girdle weakness, and elevated CK. The respiratory muscles are usually affected and 30% present with respiratory failure. This form is frequently misdiagnosed as polymyositis or limb-girdle muscular dystrophy. Muscle biopsy reveals diagnostic findings in only two-thirds of cases. Typical histologic changes involve muscle fibers with vacuoles filled with periodic acid-Schiff positive material and stain intensely for acid phosphatase, another lysosomal enzyme. EMG shows myopathic changes, electrical irritability, and brief myotonic discharges without clinical evidence of myotonia. Definitive diagnosis is confirmed through genetic testing or decreased GAA enzyme activity in blood. Therapy requires enzyme replacement therapy with alglucosidase alpha (Lumizyme), avalglucosidase alpha (Nexviazyme), or cipaglucosidase alpha-atga (Pombiliti) with miglustat (Opfolda).

PEARL: Consider this diagnosis in any patient suspected of muscle disease with significant respiratory insufficiency.

13. How do disorders of lipid metabolism present clinically?

In patients with disorders of lipid metabolism, symptoms such as muscle pain, stiffness/tightness, or myoglobinuria are usually induced by events such as prolonged low-intensity exercise (hiking, soccer), prolonged fasting, infection, general anesthesia, exposure to cold, and low-carbohydrate, high-fat diets. The heart, skeletal muscle, and liver depend on fatty acid oxidation for energy. Metabolic blocks in fatty acid oxidation result in accumulation of abnormal amounts of fatty acid in those tissues, leading to cardiomyopathy, weakness, and fatty liver. An increasing number of neurologic diseases have been associated with defects in fatty acid metabolism. Many of them cause abnormalities in the CNS.

Few disorders of lipid metabolism present as isolated exercise intolerance without other organ involvement. Primary muscle carnitine deficiency and CPT II deficiency are the two that can present predominantly muscle manifestations. In contrast to patients with glycogen metabolic defects, patients with these lipid metabolism defects often do not experience muscle cramps. They do not have the second wind phenomenon. CK levels at rest and the EMG are usually normal or only show mild abnormalities.

14. What is the syndrome of carnitine palmitoyl transferase (CPT) deficiency?

CPT II deficiency is an autosomal recessive disorder characterized by attacks of exertional myalgias and myoglobinuria (80%). Patients, most of whom are male, experience no difficulty with short bursts of strenuous activity. Indeed, the favorite recreational sport of the patient is often weightlifting. When prolonged exercise is demanded, particularly in the fasting state (when the body is dependent on fatty acid metabolism as a source of energy), muscle pain, fatigue, and myoglobinuria may occur. Patients do not experience the "second wind phenomenon." CPT II deficiency is the most common genetic metabolic myopathy causing recurrent rhabdomyolysis. The resultant myoglobinuria can cause renal failure. Diagnosis is made by genetic testing or measuring CPT activity in biopsied muscle. Treatment consists of education about avoidance of prolonged strenuous exercise and fasting. Interestingly, careful and progressive exercise training in the fed state increases exercise tolerance. Carbohydrates before and during exercise and a high carbohydrate diet may improve exercise tolerance. Triheptanoin (Dojolvi), a synthetic medium odd-chain (C7) triglyceride consisting of three odd-chain, 7-carbon-length fatty acids, is available commercially as a treatment to reduce muscle symptoms.

15. What are mitochondrial myopathies (MM)?

These are a clinically and biochemically heterogeneous group of disorders with abnormalities in the number, size, structure, and function of mitochondria. As a group, they are the most common cause of a genetic metabolic myopathy. However, most present with symptoms other than myopathy (stroke, encephalopathy). The most typical morphologic change on muscle biopsy is the **ragged red fiber**, a distorted-appearing muscle fiber that contains large peripheral and intermyofibrillar aggregates of abnormal mitochondria. On a muscle biopsy, these appear as red deposits on modified Gomori trichrome staining. Many MM are attributed to defects in the 37 genes of the mitochondrial genome, which are maternally inherited. However, nuclear DNA also contains hundreds of genes producing proteins vital to mitochondrial structure and function. Diagnosis of mitochondrial disorders occurs via genetic testing of the mitochondrial genome along with those nuclear genes associated with mitochondrial function. Muscle biopsy histology and mitochondrial respiratory chain enzyme activity in muscle tissue can prove helpful or confirmatory in some cases.

Syndromes associated with abnormalities of mitochondria have a variety of clinical manifestations and are thus often called mitochondrial cytopathies. Many present multisystem problems with involvement of the CNS, heart, and skeletal muscle. The skeletal muscle involvement is manifested by progressive proximal muscle weakness, external ophthalmoplegia, ptosis, and exercise intolerance due to premature fatigue out of proportion to weakness. Mild activity, such as walking up one flight of stairs, can cause symptoms that resolve with a short rest, but recur with activity. Patients complain of heaviness or burning in muscles, but most often do not have cramps. Serum creatine kinase levels may be normal to moderately elevated. Lactate levels are elevated at rest (~65% of cases) or with trivial exercise.

Treatment for mitochondrial myopathies often involves treatment with a mitochondrial cocktail, dietary supplementation with creatine monohydrate (0.1 gm/kg/d), coenzyme Q10 (5–15 mg/kg/d), and vitamin E (5–15 mg/kg/d). If carnitine levels are low, then treatment with L-carnitine (330 mg, 1–3 capsules up to three times daily) can be tried. Patients with multiple Acyl-CoA dehydrogenase deficiency (MADD) often demonstrate dramatic improvement with riboflavin (100 mg daily). Nearly all patients with MM improve mildly with gradually increased aerobic exercise.

16. How do you clinically evaluate patients with suspected metabolic muscle disease?

The evaluation begins with a careful history and thorough physical exam. The problem of diagnosing metabolic myopathies is confounded because at rest, patients are usually asymptomatic and have normal physical findings. The importance of the physical exam is to pick up any additional multisystem abnormalities which might indicate a mitochondrial myopathy. Patients with metabolic myopathies typically present with one of the following:

- Metabolic myopathies presenting with exercise intolerance, severe prolonged cramps, and **red-wine or cola-colored urine** (indicating myoglobinuria). If symptoms occur during strenuous brief exercise, then a glycogen storage disorder is most likely (e.g., McArdle disease), since glycogen is the main source of energy during brief exercise. If symptoms (usually myalgias and myoglobinuria without cramps) occur only after prolonged exercise and are worse during illness or fasting, then a lipid storage disorder (e.g., CPT II deficiency) is more likely, since free fatty acids are the most important source of fuel during prolonged exercise.
- Metabolic myopathies that present with progressive muscle weakness indistinguishable from limb-girdle muscular dystrophies or inflammatory myopathies include acid maltase, branching enzyme, debrancher, aldolase A, and carnitine deficiencies.

17. How are metabolic myopathies diagnosed?

Genetic testing is now the first line of investigation for metabolic myopathies. Once a detailed history and physical examination is completed, and a metabolic myopathy (or other myopathy) is suspected, panel, exome, or genome sequencing is the next step. If a definitive diagnosis does not stem from genetic testing, then further evaluations including laboratory testing and electro-diagnostic studies are warranted. Increased levels of CK, aldolase, transaminases, lactate dehydrogenase, carnitine, potassium, phosphorous, creatinine, lactate, ammonia, and myoglobin may be observed in the blood of patients depending on the metabolic myopathy. Of these, CK is the most sensitive. Levels are generally normal except for patients with McArdle disease (myophosphorylase deficiency).

The electromyogram (EMG) is useful in excluding a neuropathic process, demonstrating myopathic changes, and may delineate an optimal site for a muscle biopsy. Elevated muscle enzymes and myopathic changes on EMG are variable and nondiagnostic. A normal EMG does **not** exclude a metabolic myopathy. MRI has been used to identify patterns of muscle involvement and as a guide for muscle biopsy. Magnetic resonance spectroscopy is a tool useful for in vivo evaluation of muscle energetics. In the evaluation of patients with metabolic muscle disease, when genetic testing results are negative or of undetermined significance, **muscle biopsy** can provide important diagnostic information (including enzyme analysis on muscle tissue).

Metabolic myopathy specialists have moved to a genetic testing first approach. The cost of genetic testing has plummeted, while the availability, speed of processing, and sheer number of genes tested have increased. Genetic testing is more cost effective, faster, and less invasive. This genetics first diagnostic stratagem still may require clinicians to circle back to ancillary testing to clarify variants of undetermined significance.

18. What is the forearm exercise test? How is it performed?

The forearm exercise test (FET) is a nonspecific tool used in individuals suspected of having myophosphorylase deficiency or a block anywhere along the glycogenolytic or glycolytic pathway. This test exploits the abnormal biochemistry that results in the absence of those enzymes. Normal muscle generates lactate from the degradation of glycogen when it exercises. With defects in glycolysis or glycogenolysis, pyruvate is not produced under anaerobic conditions, and thus no lactate can be generated by lactate dehydrogenase. In addition, ammonia, inosine, and hypoxanthine concentrations increase significantly. A protocol for forearm exercise testing follows:
1. A blood sample for analysis of baseline lactate, ammonia, and pyruvate levels is drawn through an indwelling catheter in an antecubital vein, preferably placed without use of a tourniquet.
2. In the past, a sphygmomanometer cuff was placed on the upper arm of the side with the indwelling catheter and inflated to at least 20 mmHg above systolic pressure. However, the blood pressure cuff is not necessary, and can lead to forearm rhabdomyolysis and compartment syndrome, especially in patients with McArdle disease.
3. The subject rhythmically squeezes a tennis ball, or similar object, at maximal intensity for 14 seconds followed by a one-second reprieve, for a total of 60 seconds. After the 60 seconds of exercise, additional venous samples for lactate and ammonia are obtained at 1, 2, 4, 6, and 10 minutes thereafter. Pyruvate can be drawn at 2 and 4 minutes after exercise. As they are drawn, the blood vials should be placed on ice and immediately transported to the laboratory and processed.

In normal individuals, lactate and ammonia increase at least 2.5 times baseline values in the first two samples after exercise and then gradually decrease toward baseline. The major reason for a false-positive result is insufficient work by the subject while exercising. This should be suspected if both lactate and ammonia fail to rise. If lactate (and pyruvate) does not rise but ammonia does, the patient may have a defect in glycolysis, such as McArdle's disease. If pyruvate rises but lactate does not, the patient has LDH-m subunit deficiency. In CPT II deficiency both lactate and ammonium rise appropriately.

19. Why is muscle biopsy a valuable diagnostic tool in the evaluation of metabolic myopathies?

Muscle biopsy for routine histologic, histochemical, and ultrastructural analysis (electron microscopy) is helpful in evaluating a suspected metabolic myopathy, primarily because it helps rule out other conditions that can cause muscle dysfunction and allows testing for deficiencies or absence of specific glycolytic pathway enzymes. However, biopsy should be the ultimate step in the clinical evaluation, done only if a diagnosis has not been made via history, examination, genetic testing, laboratory testing (including FET), and EMG. Specific enzymes can be tested in muscle tissue by immunohistochemistry. The most important studies are listed below:

Stain	Condition
Periodic acid-Schiff	Glycogen storage diseases
Sudan black or Oil red O	Lipid storage diseases
Gomori	Mitochondrial myopathy
Acid phosphatase	Acid maltase deficiency
Specific enzymes:	Myophosphorylase
	Phosphofructokinase
	Lactate dehydrogenase

20. **What is the approach to evaluation and management of a patient with rhabdomyolysis and myoglobinuria?**

There is no agreed-upon definition of the level of CK elevation required for a diagnosis of rhabdomyolysis, but all agree that CK levels rising from normal to >10,000 U/L would meet that criterion. Interestingly, CK levels must rise to 50,000–75,000 U/L before clinical pigmenturia occurs (though myoglobin may be detected in the urine at lower levels than this). After a single episode of exertional rhabdomyolysis, the risk of recurrence is quite low, and further evaluation may not be warranted. However, after a second episode of rhabdomyolysis, evaluation may include serial CK levels, EMG, muscle biopsy and/or genetic testing. For patients with multiple, recurrent episodes of rhabdomyolysis, the most reasonable first step now, with the low cost of genetic testing, is to order a genetic testing panel covering 30–500 muscle genes (inclusive of the metabolic myopathy genes), exome sequencing, or genome sequencing. If genetic testing fails to return a definitive diagnosis, either negative testing or variant(s) of undetermined significance, then circling back to EMG and muscle biopsy with enzyme analysis will increase the diagnostic yield.

21. **Describe common genetic muscle diseases that may be confused with metabolic myopathies and childhood or adult polymyositis.**
   - **Dystrophinopathies:**
     - **Duchenne dystrophy:** X-linked disease due to a pathogenic variant in *DMD*, the gene for the protein, dystrophin, which connects the contractile proteins of muscle, the sarcomere, up to a protein complex at the muscle membrane, the sarcolemma. Onset of pelvic and shoulder girdle muscle weakness occurs by age 5. CK levels can be elevated to more than 50–150-fold normal at rest. Calf hypertrophy, scoliosis, loss of ambulation by age 13, and death from respiratory failure or cardiomyopathy in the third and fourth decades occurred in the past. Corticosteroids slow progression of skeletal and cardiac muscle dysfunction. Diagnosis is by genetic testing, and genetic therapies now are available to significantly slow the progression of the disease.
     - **Becker dystrophy:** X-linked disease also due to pathogenic variants in *DMD*, but that results in a partially functional dystrophin protein. Although somewhat like Duchenne muscular dystrophy, Becker muscular dystrophy patients walk beyond 16 years of age. Onset ranges from the first through the seventh decades. The extent of skeletal muscle and cardiac muscle dysfunction may be quite discordant with some ambulatory Becker patients requiring cardiac transplantation.
     - **Female carriers:** 10–30% of females with a pathogenic variant in *DMD* on one X chromosome (often mothers, sisters, or daughters of males with a dystrophinopathy) can develop skeletal muscle weakness and myalgias. An equal percentage may manifest cardiac dysfunction, arrhythmias, or heart failure, clinically or on testing (heart monitors, echocardiograms, and MRIs). Whenever a woman with muscle disease has symptoms that do not fit into a typical diagnosis, thought should be given to a genetic muscle disease.
   - **Facioscapulohumeral dystrophy.** Autosomal dominant disease due to a partial deletion located on chromosome 4. Variable disease expression with disease onset between adolescence

to middle-adult years. Facial muscle weakness (inability to whistle or asymmetric smile) often occurs first. Scapulohumeral weakness leading to winged scapulae is a prominent feature. Lower extremities are less involved. CK is elevated up to five times normal, and inflammation can be seen on muscle biopsy.

- **Limb-girdle muscular dystrophies (LGMD):** There are now more than 250 genetic muscle diseases that present with proximal weakness in the hip and shoulder girdle muscles. Fortunately, with large genetic testing panels encompassing 30–500 genes, many of these genetic muscle diseases can be cost-effectively diagnosed early in the evaluation. The most common limb-girdle muscular dystrophy confused with polymyositis include:
  - **LGMD2B – dysferlinopathy.** Autosomal recessive disease. LGMD2B stems from pathogenic variants in *DYSF*, the gene coding for dysferlin, a protein important in muscle repair. Patients present with progressive lower extremity followed by upper extremity proximal muscle weakness beginning in the second to fourth decades. Facial muscles and heart are spared and winged scapulae are not seen. The disease slowly progresses leading to 50% of patients requiring wheelchair use in 10–30 years. This dystrophy is the one most readily confused with adult polymyositis because CK is elevated, and inflammatory infiltrates may be seen on muscle biopsy. A diagnostic clue is that most patients have difficulty standing on their toes within the first 1–2 years of symptom onset due to early, concomitant calf muscle weakness. A trial of corticosteroids in dysferlinopathies failed to demonstrate any benefit.
  - **LGMD2C, 2D, 2E & 2F – the sarcoglycanopathies:** Autosomal recessive disorders due to pathogenic variants in the genes for the sarcoglycans, structural proteins along the sarcolemma. The sarcoglycans are a family of transmembrane proteins (α, β, γ, δ) involved in the protein complex responsible for connecting the muscle fiber cytoskeleton to the extracellular matrix, preventing damage to the muscle fiber sarcolemma through shearing forces. Patients present with a limb-girdle and Duchenne/Becker-like phenotypes. Most present by age 6–8 years old. Progression of weakness can be rapid. Cardiomyopathy occurs in 30%. Serum CK levels are high. Muscle biopsies may have inflammation, especially eosinophilic myositis. The sarcoglycanopathies do not respond to corticosteroids.
  - **LGMD2I – Fukutin-related protein (FKRP):** Autosomal recessive disorders due to pathogenic variants in a gene involved in glycosylation of alpha-dystroglycan. Alpha-dystroglycan forms pivotal, carbohydrate links from the sarcolemma up to the extracellular matrix. Onset of proximal weakness is in infancy, childhood, or early adulthood and may have associated brain and eye involvement. Cardiac and respiratory compromise may occur. CK levels are 5–25 times the upper limit of normal. Interestingly, associated with a febrile illness in early childhood, around one-quarter of alpha-dystroglycanopathy patients have an abrupt onset of weakness (often lose ambulation) along with respiratory compromise. Recovery ensues over 1–3 weeks. This acute illness-associated weakness occurs prior to onset of muscular dystrophy in half the cases.
- **Myotonic dystrophies.** Autosomal dominant diseases.
  - **Type 1** has temporalis muscle atrophy, sternocleidomastoid muscle wasting, ptosis, distal limb weakness, and systemic features (male pattern baldness, cataracts, cardiorespiratory, and gastrointestinal involvement). Characteristic physical finding is delayed relaxation and muscle stiffness (myotonia). Inability to relax handgrip when shaking hands and myotonic contraction of thumb when thenar eminence musculature is percussed by a reflex hammer are commonly observed. EMG shows excessive insertional activity and a "dive bomber" sound with contraction of muscle. Ringed myofibers may be seen in 70% of muscle biopsies as well as prominent atrophy of type I fibers.
  - **Type 2** has proximal muscle weakness, muscle pain, cataracts, infrequent clinical myotonia, tremors, cardiac disturbances (heart block), and hypogonadism. Neck flexors, hip flexors, and triceps are affected most. CK is elevated up to 4 times normal.
- **Lipin-1.** Autosomal recessive disease due to pathogenic variants in *LPIN1*, the gene for lipin-1. A common cause of rhabdomyolysis in children under 6 years of age. Baseline muscle strength and CK levels are often normal, but rhabdomyolysis may be severe with CK levels 10,000–1,000,000 U/L and up to a 30% mortality rate. Attacks are most often triggered by febrile episodes but are also associated with exercise, fasting, and anesthesia. Intravenous high-concentration glucose solutions during attacks and increased caloric intake during situations

of elevated energy demand (e.g., fever or exercise) resulted in decreased frequency and severity of episodes of rhabdomyolysis.

- **RYR1-associated myopathies.** Autosomal dominant disorder. Mutations in *RYR1*, the gene for the ryanodine receptor, may account for up to 30% of rhabdomyolysis episodes in otherwise healthy persons. Common triggers for episodes of rhabdomyolysis include exercise, heat, and viral infections. It is important to recognize and diagnose these patients since there can be concomitant malignant hyperthermia susceptibility with certain inhalational anesthetics. Modification of lifestyle through avoidance of overheating and modification of exercise programs can help reduce the frequency and severity of rhabdomyolysis episodes.

BIBLIOGRAPHY

Nagappa M, Narayanappa G. Approach to the diagnosis of metabolic myopathies. *Indian J Pathol Microbiol.* 2022;65:S277–S290.

Tarnopolsky M. Metabolic myopathies. *Continuum.* 2022;28(6):1752–1777.

Urtizberea J, Severa G, Malfatti E. Metabolic myopathies in the era of next-generation sequencing. *Genes.* 2023;14:954.

WEBSITES

www.mda.org.

www.neuro.wustl.edu/neuromuscular/index.html.

Amyloidosis

Tara Skorupa, MD

1. What is amyloidosis?

Amyloidosis is a disorder of protein folding in which normally soluble proteins are deposited as an insoluble proteinaceous material in the extracellular matrix of tissue. At least 36 human precursor proteins can form amyloid. The deposits may be localized to one organ or may be systemic. Amyloid deposition may be subclinical or may produce a diverse array of clinical manifestations.

2. Why is it called amyloid? How does its deposition result in clinical disease?

In 1854, Rudolph Virchow coined the term *amyloid* (starch-like) owing to the reaction of the material in a manner similar to cellulose when exposed to iodine and sulfuric acid. This designation has been retained despite the recognition of the proteinaceous nature of amyloid. Amyloid deposits encroach on parenchymal tissues, compromising their function. Organ compromise is related to the location, quantity, and rate of deposition, which varies within and between the types of amyloid.

3. Describe the structure of amyloid.

All amyloids share a unique ultrastructure as seen by electron microscopy. Thin, nonbranching protein fibrils constitute approximately 90% of amyloid deposits. Fibrils tend to aggregate laterally to form fibers. X-ray diffraction studies show that the polypeptide chains are oriented perpendicularly to the long axis of the fibril, forming a cross β-**pleated sheet conformation.** Serum amyloid P component (SAP), a protein composed of two pentagonal subunits forming a doughnut-like structure, makes up 5%. SAP is 50% homologous to C-reactive protein but is not an acute-phase reactant. The remainder of amyloid is composed of small amounts of certain glycosaminoglycans (GAGs) including heparan sulfate and dermatan sulfate as well as specific apolipoproteins (E and J).

4. Describe the light microscopic appearance of amyloid.

Without staining, amyloid appears as a homogeneous, amorphous, hyaline extracellular material. It is eosinophilic when stained with hematoxylin–eosin and metachromatic with crystal violet. Amyloid stains homogeneously with **Congo red (congophilic)** as a result of its β-pleated sheet configuration. Viewing of Congo red-stained tissue under polarized microscopy yields the pathognomonic **apple-green birefringence.**

5. Where do the amyloid proteins come from and why does amyloid deposition occur?

Fibrillar amyloid proteins are derived from either an intact protein or a fragment of a larger precursor molecule. Circulating forms of the relevant proteins that deposit and form amyloid fibrils are responsible for systemic forms of amyloidosis, whereas local production of protein subunits that are precursors to amyloid fibril formation are responsible for localized or organ-specific amyloidosis. There are four circumstances that predispose to amyloid deposition:

- Sustained high concentrations of normal proteins (i.e., serum amyloid A [SAA] in chronic inflammation and β2-microglobulin in renal failure)
- Exposure to normal concentrations of a weakly amyloidogenic protein over a prolonged period (i.e., amyloid β-protein in Alzheimer's disease)
- Acquired protein with an amyloidogenic structure (i.e., monoclonal immunoglobulin light chains in AL amyloid)
- Inherited variant protein with an amyloidogenic structure (i.e., TTR, others).

The pathogenesis of why certain proteins are capable of forming amyloid fibrils is unclear. Genetic factors are important in that mutations in certain proteins that circulate normally in plasma can result in structural changes that predispose them to the formation of an antiparallel beta-pleated sheet configuration when the protein deposits in the tissue. Indeed, certain protein variants are known to be "amyloidogenic" and may be more susceptible to the processing that leads to amyloidosis. For example, in systemic AL amyloidosis, the immunoglobulin light chain λ VI is highly associated with amyloidosis, whereas the more common κ light chains are not. In systemic AA amyloid, certain phenotypes of SAA are more likely to form amyloid. In hereditary systemic amyloidosis, single amino acid variants of TTR are most commonly found. Finally, in addition to these amyloidogenic precursor proteins undergoing misfolding, SAP and certain GAGs may contribute to the seeding, aggregation, and deposition of amyloid in tissues. Notably, little tissue reaction occurs around amyloid, and once deposited, amyloid resists proteolysis and phagocytosis. Features of the precursor proteins and/or host factors could result in abnormal processing by mononuclear phagocytic cells or ineffective degradation.

6. How are the amyloidoses classified?

By the major protein component of the fibril. This has also become the basis for defining the clinical syndromes with certainty. However, routine stains do not identify the major fibril protein, and specific immunohistochemical stains, or alternatively mass spectrometry proteomic-based analysis, are needed for identification (Table 72.1).

7. What is systemic AL amyloidosis?

Systemic AL amyloidosis, formerly called primary amyloidosis, is due to protein deposition derived from immunoglobulin light-chain fragments. AL amyloid appears to represent a spectrum of disease. At one end, the source of light chains is a malignant clone of plasma cells (myeloma-associated). At the other extreme, light chains are derived from a small, nonproliferative plasma cell population (immunocyte dyscrasia).

8. Describe the epidemiology of systemic AL amyloidosis.

Systemic AL amyloidosis occurs in 3–4% of individuals with monoclonal B-cell dyscrasias. Over 80% of cases are associated with "benign" monoclonal gammopathies with the remainder having multiple myeloma or, less often, Waldenstrom disease or non-Hodgkin lymphoma. Prevalence

TABLE 72.1 Classification of Amyloidoses

CLINICAL CATEGORIES	MAJOR PROTEIN TYPES	RELATIVE FREQUENCIES (%)
Systemic AL amyloidosis	AL	50–80
Systemic AA amyloidosis	AA	3–10
Age-related (senile) systemic amyloidosis	AATR	8–10
Organ-specific (localized) amyloidosis	AL, ALECT2, and others[a]	3
Dialysis-related amyloidosis	$A\beta_2M$	<2%
Heritable amyloidosis	ATTR and others[b]	5–10

[a]ALECT2, leukocyte chemotactic factor 2 (hepatic amyloid); Aβ, amyloid β protein (Alzheimer's disease, Down syndrome); AIAPP, islet amyloid polypeptide (type 2 diabetes, insulinoma); ACal, calcitonin (medullary thyroid cancer); AANF, atrial natriuretic factor (atrial amyloid); AMed, lactadherin (aortic media); ALac, lactoferrin (cornea, others)

[b]AApoA, apolipoprotein AI and AII; AGel, gelsolin; AFib, fibrinogen A alpha; ALys, lysozyme; ACys, cystatin C.

is slightly higher in men than in women. The median age at diagnosis is 63 years, and 90% of patients are aged >50 years.

9. What are the most common initial symptoms in patients with systemic AL amyloidosis?

- Fatigue and weight loss are most common
- Other early symptoms: pain, purpura, bleeding diathesis
  Diagnosis is often delayed as a result of the nonspecific nature of symptoms, with one-third of patients diagnosed >1 year after symptom onset. Weight loss can be striking, exceeding 40 lbs in some patients and prompting a search for occult malignancy. Pain is more common in those with myeloma (40%) than those without (8%). In those without myeloma, pain is frequently attributable to peripheral neuropathy (10%) and/or carpal tunnel syndrome (CTS; 20%). Other symptoms are often present in patients with specific organ involvement including edema secondary to nephrotic syndrome; dyspnea on exertion and edema due to a restrictive cardiomyopathy; abdominal discomfort from hepatosplenomegaly; seronegative arthropathy resembling RA; painful paresthesias with peripheral neuropathy; orthostasis, syncope, impotence, and gut dysmotility resulting from autonomic neuropathy.

10. What physical findings are common in patients with systemic AL amyloidosis?

- Edema (most common).
- Palpable liver (33%).
- Macroglossia (10%; pathognomonic when present).
- Purpura (15%).
- CTS (10–20%): can cause *claw hand* due to clumping of tendons together.
- Painful sensory polyneuropathy (15–20%).
  Edema may occur as a result of nephrotic syndrome, congestive heart failure, and, rarely, protein-losing enteropathy. Hepatomegaly is usually of only a modest degree. Macroglossia and purpura should particularly raise suspicion of systemic AL amyloidosis; both may be a source of patient complaints and are easily overlooked. Increased firmness of the tongue and dental indentations are helpful in determining the presence of macroglossia. Cutaneous purpura is generally localized to the upper chest, neck, and face. Purpura of the eyelids is a clue that may only be appreciated when the patient is asked to close their eyes. Gentle pinching of the eyelids may cause bruising (pinch purpura) due to vascular fragility caused by amyloid deposition in the blood vessels. Purpura around the eyes is called the "raccoon eyes" sign. Other findings include arthropathy ("shoulder pad" sign), CTS, nail dystrophy, adenopathy, and submandibular enlargement.

11. Because symptoms are nonspecific and physical findings insensitive, what clinical syndromes should suggest the presence of systemic AL amyloidosis?

Nephrotic syndrome	Autonomic neuropathy (orthostatic hypotension, gastric atony)
Congestive heart failure	CTS (especially if claw hand)
Peripheral neuropathy	Hepatic disease

The most common initial clinical manifestation is nephrotic syndrome. A distinguishing feature that allows it to be separated from many other causes of nephrosis is the finding of a monoclonal protein in the serum or urine (electrophoresis and immunofixation should be done). Although overt congestive heart failure can occur in up to one-third of patients, amyloid deposits in the heart are eventually seen on imaging in 90%. Peripheral neuropathy clinically resembles the neuropathy seen in diabetes, including the chronic course. Autonomic neuropathy may be superimposed on peripheral neuropathy or occur alone. A history of CTS is a very important clue to the presence of amyloidosis. It is typically bilateral, and surgical release may not provide complete relief.

12. What clues should alert you to the presence of hepatic amyloidosis?

- Proteinuria—high association with co-occurring renal involvement.
- Howell–Jolly bodies in the peripheral blood smear resulting from splenic infiltration and subsequent hyposplenism.

- Hepatomegaly (>15 cm) is out of proportion to liver function tests (one-third with hepatomegaly will have normal LFTs).
- Elevated alkaline phosphatase >1.5 times greater than the upper limit of normal.

13. Describe some of the characteristic findings in amyloid cardiomyopathy.

- Amyloid deposits cause diastolic dysfunction, leading to restrictive cardiomyopathy and heart failure with preserved ejection fraction (HFpEF). Involvement of the conduction system causes atrial fibrillation in up to 70%.
- Normal levels of N-terminal pro-brain natriuretic peptide (NT-proBNP) exclude cardiac amyloid. Elevated levels of NT-proBNP and cardiac troponin T are predictors of poor survival, especially if they do not decrease with therapy.
- Electrocardiogram shows reduced voltage as a result of replacement of myocardium by amyloid. A pseudo-infarct Q wave may be seen. Prolonged QTc interval is a poor prognostic indicator.
- Transthoracic echocardiogram has high sensitivity for detecting amyloid deposits. Symmetric thickening of the left ventricular (LV) wall (>12 mm) or thickening of the interventricular septum may lead to an erroneous diagnosis of concentric LV hypertrophy or asymmetric septal hypertrophy. Hypokinesis may suggest prior "silent" infarction. The combination of increased myocardial "sparkling" echogenicity and increased septal thickness (>6 mm) is 60% sensitive and 100% specific for the diagnosis of amyloidosis. Another characteristic finding is reduced global longitudinal strain with apical sparing (a "cherry on top" pattern).
- Cardiac magnetic resonance imaging shows diffuse late subendocardial gadolinium enhancement.

14. Name three presentations of amyloidosis that mimic other rheumatic diseases.

- Vascular involvement by amyloid can lead to claudication of the extremities and jaw as seen in temporal arteritis.
- Amyloid arthropathy can mimic seronegative RA or polymyalgia rheumatica. Clues are the lack of inflammation and frequent hip and shoulder involvement with periarticular amyloid infiltration, which leads to enlargement of the pelvic or shoulder girdle (shoulder pad sign). Synovial fluid analysis can be helpful in detecting amyloid deposits.
- Infiltration of amyloid into muscle may lead to weakness or pain, simulating polymyositis. Enlargement of involved muscles (pseudohypertrophy) can be striking and may not be associated with other symptoms.

15. Why does amyloid cause bruising and bleeding?

Amyloid deposition in blood vessels can lead to weakening of the vessel wall and easy bruising. A rare manifestation (8%) of AL amyloid is a bleeding diathesis as a result of an acquired factor X deficiency caused by factor X binding to widely deposited amyloid fibrils.

16. Do most patients with systemic AL amyloidosis display only one syndrome?

No. Most patients have widespread disease and more than one syndrome. CTS is seen more often in those with peripheral neuropathy and cardiomyopathy than in those with other syndromes.

17. What is systemic AA amyloidosis?

Systemic AA amyloidosis, formerly called secondary or reactive amyloidosis, is attributable to deposition of fragments of SAA that form amyloid fibrils. It can complicate any chronic inflammatory disorder, whether infectious, neoplastic, rheumatic, or heritable periodic fever syndromes. Notably, up to 6% of patients with AA amyloidosis have no clinically obvious chronic inflammatory disease. Some of these may have undiagnosed autoinflammatory syndrome (see Chapter 79: Familial Autoinflammatory Syndromes) or Castleman disease. The clinical feature most common in AA amyloidosis is renal involvement (with proteinuria in >90% and nephrotic syndrome in 50% at diagnosis) followed by hepatosplenomegaly. Cardiac and autonomic nerve involvement are less common than in AL amyloidosis. Patients with AA amyloidosis attributable to a chronic inflammatory disease tend to have a slow progression, whereas AA amyloid attributable to an untreated chronic infection can be rapidly progressive.

18. **Name the infectious and neoplastic disorders most commonly associated with systemic AA amyloidosis.**

Infections	*Neoplasms*
Tuberculosis	Hodgkin disease
Leprosy	Non-Hodgkin lymphoma
Chronic pyelonephritis	Renal cell carcinoma
Whipple disease	Melanoma
Osteomyelitis	Cancers of GI & genitourinary tract, lung
Chronic cutaneous ulcers	Sarcoma
Subacute bacterial endocarditis	

Conditions predisposing to chronic infection:
- Cystic fibrosis
- Bronchiectasis
- Injection drug use
- Sickle cell anemia
- Paraplegia

19. **What three rheumatic diseases are most commonly complicated by systemic AA amyloidosis, and how has the incidence of this complication changed over time?**

    Older studies reported a 5–15% overall incidence of amyloidosis in RA, juvenile idiopathic arthritis (JIA), and ankylosing spondylitis (AS). With newer and more effective therapies available for these diseases, the frequency of systemic AA amyloidosis is much lower today, and the median age of onset is later (ages 60–80, compared to 45–55 historically).

20. **Other than systemic AL amyloidosis, name two amyloidoses that occur more commonly in the elderly.**
    - **Age-related (senile) amyloidosis:** deposits of normal transthyretin amyloid (**ATTRwt**) are common in patients over the age of 70. Males are more commonly affected. Cardiac involvement is seen in almost all symptomatic patients, often presenting with a restrictive cardiomyopathy. Some patients have CTS. Other organs are rarely involved clinically.
    - **Aβ protein amyloidosis:** deposits of β-protein in Alzheimer's plaques. It can also be deposited in cerebral blood vessels (cerebral amyloid angiopathy) leading to strokes and hemorrhage, which can mimic central nervous system vasculitis.

21. **What is localized AL amyloidosis and how does it present?**

    Amyloid may occur in localized deposits, resembling tumors. The lung, skin, larynx, eye, and bladder are common sites. The deposits are attributable to a focal infiltrate of monoclonal B cells that produce amyloidogenic light chains. If the amyloid deposits are interfering with organ function or causing bleeding, surgical or laser excision can be done. Progression of this form of localized amyloid to systemic disease or myeloma is exceedingly rare.

22. **Name the forms of amyloid localized to endocrine tissue.**

    Acal (calcitonin)—medullary carcinoma of the thyroid.
    AANF (atrial natriuretic factor)—isolated atrial amyloid.
    AIAPP (islet amyloid polypeptide)—type 2 diabetes mellitus, insulinoma.
    Apro (prolactin)—local amyloid in prolactinomas.

23. **Describe the features of dialysis-related amyloidosis (DRA).**

    DRA is caused by β_2-**microglobulin amyloid** deposits. β_2-microglobulin is the invariant chain of the major histocompatibility complex class I molecule. β_2-microglobulin is renally cleared, so levels may be elevated 50-fold in patients on long-term dialysis. However, high levels alone do not predict the development of amyloid. Generally, patients with amyloidosis will have been on hemodialysis for at least 5 years. Up to 80% of patients who undergo dialysis for >15 years will have evidence of amyloidosis. Modern dialysis techniques with high flux, biocompatible membranes, are more effective at reducing β_2-microglobulin, yet osteoarticular complaints (the primary disease manifestation in DRA) are still reported. CTS is the first and most common clinical presentation. Chronic arthralgias, especially of the shoulders, may also occur. Patients can have the shoulder pad sign with inability to raise arms over their head. Persistent noninflammatory joint effusions in large joints can occur in up to 50% of patients. β_2-microglobulin amyloid deposits can be found in the synovial fluid with Congo red staining. A spondyloarthritis-like presentation with intervertebral disc destruction (mimics infection) and paravertebral erosions from amyloid deposits has been described. Cystic bone changes (carpal and other bones) can occur due to advanced glycation end products stimulating osteoclasts and leading to cyst formation. Rarely, other areas (skin, gastrointestinal tract, heart) are involved. The most effective treatment is renal transplantation.

24. Studies of hereditary amyloidosis have shown many cases are attributable to single amino acid variants of TTR (ATTR). What is their pattern of inheritance? How is it treated?

Hereditary transthyretin amyloidosis (variant transthyretin amyloidosis, or ATTRv) is an autosomal dominant disease. A family history of amyloidosis should be sought, but may or may not be present as spontaneous ATTR mutations can occur. Clinical features, age of onset, and rate of progression can vary among gene variants and among individuals. Most commonly, patients develop progressive peripheral and autonomic neuropathy and/or involvement of the heart and conduction system. The most definitive treatment is liver transplantation, which removes the source of the variant TTR production and replaces it with normal TTR. Death occurs within 2 to 12 years without liver transplantation. Patisiran, vutrisiran, inotersen, and eplontersen are novel RNA-targeted therapies that interfere with hepatic TTR synthesis and can reduce blood TTR levels by 70–90%. Trials have shown stabilization of peripheral neuropathy with these agents. Another medication, tafamidis, has been shown to bind to and stabilize TTR tetramers, preventing fibril formation and amyloid deposition. Randomized trials have shown slowing of neuropathy progression, as well as reduced all-cause mortality and cardiovascular-related hospitalization in cardiomyopathy patients. Interestingly, diflunisal, a nonsteroidal anti-inflammatory drug, also stabilizes TTR tetramers and has shown beneficial results in trials.

25. What other forms of hereditary systemic amyloidoses have been reported?

In addition to the >100 variant forms of TTR that have been reported to cause amyloidosis, other variant proteins that can cause amyloid deposits and symptoms include mutations in genes for cystatin C (cerebral amyloid angiopathy with hemorrhage in Icelandic patients) and gelsolin (cranial neuropathies). Mutations of lysozyme, fibrinogen A α-chain, apolipoprotein AI and AII, and apolipoprotein CII and CIII can cause visceral amyloid usually causing nephropathy. These autosomal dominant forms of amyloidosis have a worse prognosis than familial amyloidotic polyneuropathy (TTR mutations).

26. How is the diagnosis of amyloidosis established?

The diagnosis of amyloidosis is confirmed by tissue biopsy. The amyloid deposits appear as hyaline material on light microscopy. Congo-red stained tissue shows the characteristic apple-green birefringence under polarized light. Thioflavine T staining yields an intense yellow-green fluorescence. Immunohistochemical staining of tissue can characterize the amyloid fibril protein subunit type, especially amyloid AA and ATTR. The gold standard for amyloid subunit typing is mass spectrometry proteomic-based analysis, but this method is expensive and still not widely available.

27. Which tissue should be biopsied?

A screening biopsy should be performed first because the sensitivity is good and complications are few. Screening sites and their yields are:

Abdominal fat pad	70–80%
Bone marrow	56–70%
Rectal mucosa	50–84%
Gingiva/labial salivary gland	60–80%
Skin	50%

Of note, the use of rectal biopsy has declined in recent years, as evidence suggests diagnostic yield is low in the setting of a negative abdominal fat pat aspiration. Abdominal fat pad aspiration is performed by injecting saline into the abdominal wall fat about 10 cm laterally to the umbilicus using a 16-gauge needle attached to a 20-mL syringe and sucking back. Fat obtained is processed for Congo red staining. It is positive in 80% to 90% of patients with AL or ATTR amyloidosis, and in 60% to 70% of patients with AA amyloidosis (unfortunately, it is not typically helpful in diagnosing DRA). Note that 15% of patients with systemic AL amyloidosis will have both a negative abdominal fat pad and bone marrow biopsy.

28. If the screening biopsies for amyloid are negative, what should be done?

If biopsy screens are negative, biopsy of a clinically involved site may be undertaken, realizing that the risk of bleeding may be substantial. Therefore, do not biopsy a liver that is grossly enlarged. Yields for clinically involved sites are:

Kidney	90–99%
Carpal ligament	90–95%
Liver	92–97%
Sural nerve	100%
Skin	45–83%
Heart (endomyocardial biopsy)	92–100%

29. What additional laboratory and imaging studies should be performed?

- All patients with systemic amyloidosis should be evaluated for evidence of an associated plasma cell dyscrasia by ordering serum and urine protein electrophoresis and immunoelectrophoresis and free light chains. If all of these tests are negative, then it is unlikely that the amyloidosis is attributable to a plasma cell dyscrasia.
- In patients with symptoms consistent with hereditary systemic amyloidosis, DNA analysis to identify the amyloidogenic variant protein should be performed.
- MRI or ultrasound of involved joints (especially shoulders): ultrasound showing rotator cuff thickening (>8 mm) with echogenic deposits; joint space widening, likely due to amyloid deposition causing synovial hypertrophy; cysts at the site of synovial insertion. Erosive changes are rare (5%).
- Radiolabeled (I^{123}) SAP scintigraphy: if available, radioiodine-labeled SAP can be used for establishing the extent of disease and monitoring response to therapy. Sensitivity is 90% for detecting AL and AA amyloid but only 48% for ATTR.

30. How is systemic AL amyloidosis treated?

The control of light-chain production by proliferating plasma cells has been the rationale for the use of cytotoxic agents. In select lower-risk patients without severe organ involvement, induction chemotherapy followed by autologous peripheral blood stem cell transplantation can result in improvement of the patient's clinical condition, but treatment-related toxicity can be high. Thus, most patients with newly diagnosed AL amyloidosis who do not meet criteria for transplantation (~75%) receive conventional chemotherapy. Melphalan and dexamethasone are well-established agents in treatment of AL amyloidosis. However, more recently, regimens containing bortezomib (a proteasome inhibitor) and dartumumab (anti-CD38, targeting clonal B cells) have been used to induce deeper hematologic remission, leading to improved organ response and overall survival compared to prior regimens. Lenalidomide has also shown benefit but is associated with higher toxicity compared to other agents. These therapies need to decrease the serum/urine levels of free light chains by over 50% to effectively increase survival. Digitalis, calcium channel blockers, and β blockers should be avoided in patients with cardiac involvement due to the consequent adverse cardiac events. Other therapies under investigation include venetoclax, a B-cell lymphoma 2 gene inhibitor that impairs anti-apoptosis mechanisms to facilitate preferential killing of affected plasma cells; and birtamimab, an anti-amyloid fibril monoclonal antibody.

31. What factors are prognostic in systemic AL amyloidosis?

Median survival varies based on the degree of organ involvement and staging at time of diagnosis. Several staging systems utilize levels of NT-pro-BNP and troponin T (surrogates for severity of cardiac involvement) and free light chain levels (a marker of plasma cell clonality) to risk stratify patients. According to the Mayo 2012 staging system, median survival can range from 94 months in stage I disease, to 6 months in stage IV. As these staging criteria suggest, the most common cause of death is attributable to cardiac involvement. The best prognosis is in patients with peripheral neuropathy when it occurs as the sole manifestation. 24-hour urine protein excretion does not affect survival, but an elevated serum creatinine and failure of serum/urine-free light chains to decrease with therapy are poor prognostic signs.

32. Describe the treatment and prognosis of systemic AA amyloidosis.

Mobilization and clearance of amyloid deposits is possible and has been demonstrated in patients with AA. A basic tenet is to control the underlying inflammatory disease.

- Potent biologic agents are available to control the inflammatory arthritides (RA, JIA, and AS) and the autoinflammatory syndromes.
- Prophylactic colchicine (1.2–1.8 mg/day) is effective in suppressing the inflammatory episodes, as well as the subsequent amyloidosis, seen in familial Mediterranean fever.
- Surgical treatment of osteomyelitis with amputation, and aggressive surgical therapy for Crohn disease, have been reported to reverse or resolve nephrotic syndrome secondary to amyloidosis in these conditions.
- Measurement of SAA levels may be helpful in monitoring the success of therapy.
- Median survival in patients whose underlying inflammatory disease is not controlled is 6 to 9 years; older age and the presence of end-stage renal disease are associated with an increased risk of mortality.
- Other therapies being investigated include anti-amyloid immunotherapy as well as eprodisate, a molecule which competitively binds to the GAG-binding sites on SAA and inhibits fibril polymerization and amyloid deposition in tissues such as the kidneys.

ACKNOWLEDGMENT

The author would like to thank Dr. Sterling G. West for his contributions to this chapter in the previous edition.

BIBLIOGRAPHY

Benson MD, Buxbaum JN, Eisenberg DS, et al. Amyloid nomenclature 2020: update and recommendations by the International Society of Amyloidosis (ISA) nomenclature committee. *Amyloid.* 2020;27(4):217–222.

Bloom MW, Gorevic PD. Cardiac amyloidosis. *Ann Intern Med.* 2023;176(3):ITC33–ITC48.

Bomsztyk J, Khwaja J, Wechalekar AD. Recent guidelines for high-dose chemotherapy and autologous stem cell transplant for systemic AL amyloidosis: a practitioner's perspective. *Expert Rev Hematol.* 2022;15(9):781–788.

D'Aguanno V, Ralli M, Artico M, et al. Systemic amyloidosis: a contemporary overview. *Clin Rev Allergy Immunol.* 2020;59(3):304–322.

Gertz MA, Dispenzieri A. Systemic amyloidosis recognition, prognosis, and therapy: a systematic review. *JAMA.* 2020;324(1):79–89.

Gertz, M.A. Immunoglobulin light chain amyloidosis diagnosis and treatment algorithm 2018. Blood Cancer J **8**, 44 (2018).

Hoffman JE, Dempsey NG, Sanchorawala V. Systemic amyloidosis caused by monoclonal immunoglobulins: soft tissue and vascular involvement. *Hematol Oncol Clin North Am.* 2020;34(6):1099–1113.

Lachmann HJ, Goodman HJB, Gilbertson JA, et al. Natural history and outcome in systemic AA amyloidosis. *N Engl J Med.* 2007;356:2361–2371.

Lu R, Richards TA. AL Amyloidosis: unfolding a complex disease. *J Adv Pract Oncol.* 2019;10(8):813–825.

Muchtar E, Dispenzieri A, Lacy MQ, et al. Overuse of organ biopsies in immunoglobulin light chain amyloidosis (AL): the consequence of failure of early recognition. *Ann Med.* 2017;49(7):545–551.

Muchtar E, Dispenzieri A, Magen H, et al. Systemic amyloidosis from A (AA) to T (ATTR): a review. *J Intern Med.* 2021;289(3):268–292.

Papa R, Lachmann HJ. Secondary, AA, Amyloidosis. *Rheum Dis Clin North Am.* 2018;44(4):585–603.

Portales-Castillo I, Yee J, Tanaka H, et al. Beta-2 microglobulin amyloidosis: past, present, and future. *Kidney360.* 2020;1(12):1447–1455.

Riefolo M, Conti M, Longhi S, et al. Amyloidosis: what does pathology offer? The evolving field of tissue biopsy. *Front Cardiovasc Med.* 2022;9:1081098.

Sonthalia N, Jain S, Pawar S, et al. Primary hepatic amyloidosis: a case report and review of literature. *World J Hepatol.* 2016;8(6):340–344.

Taylor MS, Sidiqi H, Hare J, et al. Current approaches to the diagnosis and management of amyloidosis. *Intern Med J.* 2022;52(12):2046–2067.

Wechalekar AD, Cibeira MT, Gibbs SD, et al. Guidelines for non-transplant chemotherapy for treatment of systemic AL amyloidosis: EHA-ISA Working Group. *Amyloid.* 2023;30(1):3–17.

Wisniowski B, Wechalekar A. Confirming the diagnosis of amyloidosis. *Acta Haematol.* 2020;143(4):312–321.

FURTHER READING

www.amyloidosis.org.

CHAPTER 73

Raynaud's Phenomenon

Laura K. Hummers, MD, ScM

Symptoms then are in reality nothing but the cry from suffering organs.

—Jean-Martin Charcot (1825–1893)

> ### KEY POINTS
>
> 1. Vasospasm of the digital arteries and cutaneous arterioles causes Raynaud phenomenon (RP).
> 2. Color changes characteristic of Raynaud phenomenon are either blue or white in response to cold with subsequent erythema upon rewarming (many patients will not have all three color changes)
> 3. Nailfold capillary microscopy (NCM) and specific autoantibodies predict which patients with RP are likely to develop a rheumatic disorder.
> 4. Calcium channel blockers (CCBs) are often efficacious and well-tolerated in patients who require therapy and are considered first-line therapy.

1. What is RP?

In 1862, Maurice Raynaud described RP, which is a vasospastic disorder characterized by episodic attacks of well-demarcated color changes with numbness and pain of the digits on exposure to cold. It may be primary (idiopathic) or secondary to an underlying condition. Primary RP is also called Raynaud disease.

2. How common is primary RP? Who gets it?

The prevalence of primary RP is estimated to be 3% to 5% in most studies. Estimates based on patient questionnaires rather than medical provider diagnosis or fulfillment of strict criteria are higher at 10%. Prevalence is higher in colder climates and among women, younger age groups, and in patients with a family history of the phenomenon. RP commonly develops at a young age. New-onset disease after the age of 60 years is uncommon (prevalence, 0.1–1%). The female-to-male ratio ranges from 4:1 to 9:1. Estradiol increases the expression of alpha$_{2c}$ adrenoreceptors on smooth muscle cells leading to increased cutaneous vasoconstriction (see Question 5 for additional details). This has implications outside of RP as baseline digital blood flow in young females (but not postmenopausal females) is lower than that in males in the general population.

3. Which conditions are associated with secondary RP?

Conditions associated with secondary RP (or mimics of RP) may be grouped into seven broad categories: (1) systemic, (2) traumatic injury, (3) drugs or chemicals, (4) occlusive arterial disease, (5) hyperviscosity syndromes, (6) endocrine disorders, and (7) miscellaneous causes (Table 73.1).

4. Discuss the relevant pathophysiology of RP.

In the normal physiologic state, cutaneous blood flow to acral sites such as the fingers, toes, and tips of the nose and ears serves as an important part of the body's mechanism of thermoregulation. Cutaneous blood flow can exceed 6 L/minute in periods of hyperthermia when the body attempts to "vent" heat through such sites; in contrast, cold environments can drop cutaneous blood flow to nearly undetectable levels. RP represents an exaggerated vascular response to cold and stress, most commonly at acral sites responsible for thermoregulation.

Neural signals, circulating hormones, and mediators from immunomodulatory and endothelial cells all may affect blood vessel reactivity. Neural signals that modulate vascular reactivity include epinephrine, norepinephrine, vasopressin, bradykinin, histamine, and leukotrienes among others. Additional mediators from circulating cells include serotonin and ATP/ADP. Mediators from endothelial cells include both vasodilators and constrictors such as prostacyclin, nitric oxide, and endothelin. Patients with RP therefore suffer from diminished cutaneous blood flow due to

TABLE 73.1 Causes of Secondary Raynaud Phenomenon or Mimics of Raynaud Phenomenon

CATEGORY	CONDITION
Systemic rheumatic disorder	SSc, MCTD, UCTD, SLE, idiopathic inflammatory myopathies, SjD, RA, thromboangiitis obliterans, systemic vasculitis
Traumatic	Vibration injury: Rock drillers, lumberjacks, grinders, riveters, and pneumatic hammer operators. Frostbite. Carpal tunnel syndrome. Pressure injury (crutches or hypothenar hammer syndrome)
Drugs or chemicals	Beta-blockers[a], bleomycin[b], cisplatin[b], vinblastine[b], 5-fluorouracil, ergots, methysergide, bromocriptine, clonidine, cocaine, amphetamines, central nervous system stimulants (methylphenidate, dextroamphetamine), interferon-alpha, vinyl chloride, CGRP inhibitors
Occlusive arterial disease	Embolic/thrombotic arterial occlusion, thoracic outlet syndrome
Hyperviscosity/abnormal circulating proteins	Polycythemia, cryoglobulinemia, paraproteinemia, cold agglutinins, cryofibrinogens
Endocrine disorders	Carcinoid, pheochromocytoma, hypothyroidism
Miscellaneous	Infections (bacterial endocarditis, viral hepatitis), CRPS. peripheral arteriovenous fistula, malignancy/paraneoplastic (ovarian, angiocentric lymphoma), acrocyanosis, chilblains, Achenbach syndrome

CGRP, calcitonin gene-related peptide inhibitors (used to treat migraines); CRPS, complex regional pain syndrome; MCTD, mixed connective tissue disease; RA, rheumatoid arthritis; SSc, systemic sclerosis; SLE, systemic lupus erythematosus; SjD, Sjogren's disease; UCTD, undifferentiated connective tissue disease
[a]7% estimated prevalence of Raynaud phenomenon as a consequence of medication use.
[b]Commonly implicated chemotherapeutic medications; 20% to 30% estimated prevalence of Raynaud phenomenon.

alterations in the neural input (primary and secondary RP) as well as mediators from endothelial and immunomodulatory cells (secondary RP).

5. Compare the pathophysiology of primary RP with secondary RP.

Primary RP: individuals without RP exposed to cold experience increased sympathetic adrenergic input (vasoconstriction) to the cutaneous vasculature as well as increased alpha$_{2c}$ adrenoreceptor sensitivity. Activation of these receptors on vascular smooth muscle cells results in decreased blood flow through the digital arteries and arteriovenous anastomoses; this helps to divert blood flow and guard against excessive cutaneous heat loss. Nutritional blood flow to the skin supplied by capillary loops distal to the arteriovenous anastomoses, however, is not affected. In primary RP, there is **increased basal sympathetic adrenergic tone** as well as **increased alpha$_{2c}$ adrenoreceptor activity,** even at neutral temperatures. In cold environments, this adrenergic input is heightened and affects not only the arteriovenous anastomoses most prominently but also the digital arteries and veins, and less prominently, the nutritional blood flow through the distal capillary loops. Nutritional blood flow in primary RP is diminished but preserved due to intact endothelial function and structurally normal vessels.

Secondary RP: in patients with secondary RP, underlying vascular disease may disrupt the normal mechanisms responsible for the control of vessel reactivity. Examples include impaired endothelial vasodilatory function, diminished nitric oxide release, and increased generation of factors, such as endothelin. Furthermore, patients with systemic sclerosis (SSc) may have evidence of intimal proliferation and abnormal platelet adhesion to the endothelium, resulting in reduced vessel lumen size. Consequently, blood flow through the distal capillary loops may be severely decreased in secondary RP, and therefore could result in tissue injury.

PEARL: Primary RP will never cause digital ulcerations *(preserved nutritional blood flow to the skin)*. The presence of digital ulcerations and/or infarcts should prompt further evaluation for secondary causes of RP.

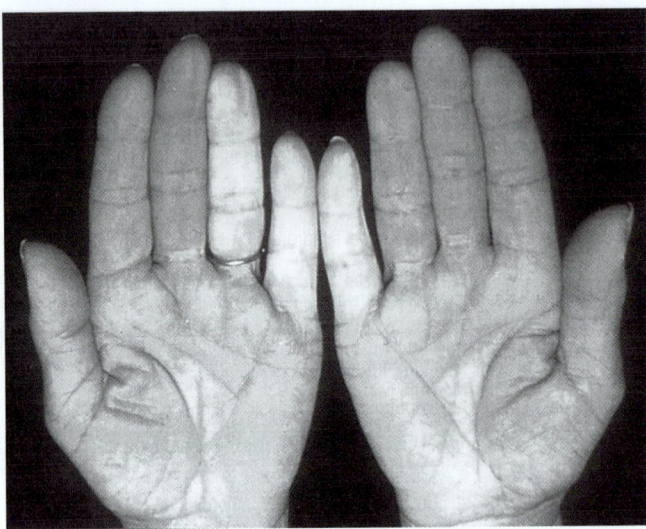

Fig. 73.1 The pallor (blanching) stage of Raynaud phenomenon.

6. Describe the triphasic color response of RP and briefly explain the pathophysiology of each phase.

The sequential color changes of RP classically are described as white to blue to red. Initial digital artery vasospasm causes a **pallor** (blanching) of the digit (Fig. 73.1), which gives way to **cyanosis** as static venous blood deoxygenates. With rewarming, the ischemic phase may be followed by reactive hyperemia, which causes the final stage, **rubor.** The classic triad in the classic order may not be seen in all patients. Either pallor or cyanosis, in response to cold exposure, is typically felt to be sufficient to make a diagnosis of Raynaud phenomenon.

7. Contrast the clinical presentations of primary and secondary RP.

The onset of primary RP usually occurs in women aged 15 to 30 years. The fingers are most commonly affected, but 40% of patients have attacks in the toes as well. Ears, nose, tongue, lips, and nipples may also be involved. The thumbs are frequently spared. The well-demarcated color changes involve part or all of one or more digits (never the "whole hand") typically with sharp demarcation on exposure to cold. The color changes may be accompanied by discomfort and numbness during the ischemic phase and by a throbbing pain during the reactive hyperemic phase. The frequency, duration, and severity of attacks vary widely, with some patients having several attacks per day and others having two or three per winter. *Primary RP patients never develop ischemic complications* such as digital ulceration, pitting, fissuring, or gangrene. NCM examination and serologies are normal/negative.

The onset of secondary RP is usually in the third and fourth decades and may be seen in either men or women depending on the underlying condition. The symptoms of digital vasospasm are the same as those of primary RP; however, secondary RP patients are more prone to complications. For example, up to 50% of patients with systemic sclerosis will develop digital ulcerations. Signs and symptoms related to an underlying condition may be discovered by a careful history and physical examination. NCM examination and serologies often will discriminate risk for CTD-associated Raynaud phenomenon from those with primary RP.

8. Is cold the only precipitant of RP?

Cold exposure is by far the most common precipitating cause of RP, especially when accompanied by pressure. Typical examples would be the gripping of a cold steering wheel, holding a cold soft drink can, or grasping items in the frozen food section of a grocery store. An attack of RP can also occur after stimulation of the sympathetic nervous system such as with pain and emotional distress. Other potential stimuli include trauma, medication exposure (decongestants, stimulants, beta-blockers), and certain chemicals such as those found in cigarette smoke. Additional "causes" such as vibration injury are more correctly attributed to the associated conditions of secondary RP.

9. In the evaluation of a patient with RP, what abnormalities may be noted on physical examination?

Patients may occasionally present to the clinic with an ongoing attack of RP, thereby allowing a definitive diagnosis. Induction of an attack in the physician's office by exposure to cold water is frequently unsuccessful, seldom necessary, and sometimes dangerous and therefore should be avoided. Patients should be instructed to take a picture of their fingers when having an attack for confirmation of typical findings.

The physical examination in primary RP is normal. A careful search for evidence of an underlying rheumatologic disease or other possible causes of RP is required. Abnormal peripheral pulses or asymmetric involvement may suggest macro-vascular disease, thromboembolic disease, or thoracic outlet syndrome (consider performing an Adson test; see Chapter 63: Entrapment Neuropathies). Puffy hands, tendon friction rubs, sclerodactyly, and telangiectasia suggest SSc. Rashes (particularly photosensitive rashes), arthritis or muscle weakness may suggest a myopathy or SLE. NCM is a useful technique in the evaluation of rheumatologic disease and should be performed.

10. Describe the technique, clinical findings, and prognostic value of NCM.

Along with the retina, the nailfold represents one of the only sites in the body where direct visualization of the vasculature is possible. NCM involves visualization of the capillaries through a magnifying device (an ophthalmoscope set at 40 diopters, dermatoscope, stereomicroscope, or digital video capillaroscopy) just proximal to the cuticle of the fingers (best to examine fingers 2–5). For some devices, visualization is enhanced by the use of microscope oil or surgical lubricant.

The normal nailbed demonstrates a confluent distribution of fine hairpin-shaped capillary loops (Fig. 73.2 photo A). **Dilated capillary loops and areas of avascularity ("dropout")** are often demonstrated in patients with underlying rheumatologic diseases such as SSc, dermatomyositis, and mixed connective tissue disease (Fig. 74.2 photo B, C, D). However, mild dilation of a few capillary loops, microhemorrhages, and abnormal shapes of capillaries may be seen in the normal population.

Some studies suggest that approximately 10% of patients initially diagnosed with primary RP will transition to a connective tissue disease (commonly limited SSc) during follow up. A large prospective cohort study demonstrated that only 2% of patients with a normal NCM and negative SSc-antibodies (Scl70, CENP, RNA pol III, or Th/To) developed subsequent SSc. In contrast, 80% of those with an abnormal NCM (vessel dropout and dilation) and a positive SSc-antibody went on to develop SSc. These patients may be diagnosed with mild or early systemic sclerosis and should be followed as such (i.e. evaluation for the presence of internal organ disease with pulmonary function testing etc.). The presence of either an abnormal NCM or SSc-antibody was associated with progression to SSc in 30% of patients and careful follow up in such patients is critical.

11. List the "red flags" that would be worrisome for the potential presence or later development of a disease associated with secondary RP.

- Onset of digital vasospasm after the age of 35 years
- Male sex
- Asymmetric attacks
- Trophic changes in the digits (ulcers, pits, gangrene)
- Ischemic signs/symptoms proximal to fingers or toes
- Color changes unrelated to ambient temperature
- Abnormal NCM
- Sclerodactyly, rashes, or other obvious evidence of an underlying condition
- Serologic presence of autoantibodies, especially anti-centromere antibodies or antibodies against a specific nuclear antigen (SCL-70, RNA polymerase 3, Th/To, RNP, Sm, SS-A, SS-B)

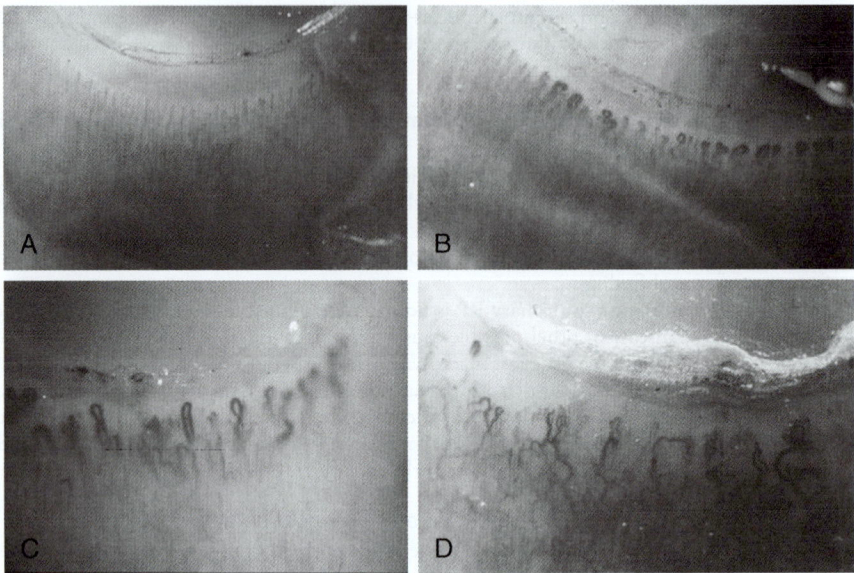

Fig. 73.2 Nailfold capillary microscopy. (A) Normal pattern. (B) Dilated capillary loops in systemic sclerosis. (C) Dilated loops and avascularity in adult dermatomyositis. (D) Childhood dermatomyositis.

12. Which laboratory studies are worthwhile in the evaluation of a patient with RP?

In cases of suspected primary RP (typical age of onset, normal examination and NCM, lack of "red flags" listed in Question 11), laboratory studies are typically unnecessary. In primary RP, laboratory tests will often be normal or negative, although up to one-third of patients will exhibit low titer of antinuclear antibodies in their serum, which means you are much more likely to find a false-positive antibody in this situation. In patients with clinical evidence suggestive of a secondary cause of RP, appropriate studies for the presence of a hypercoagulable state, cryoglobulins, hypothyroidism, and SSc-specific antibodies should be considered.

13. Describe the usefulness of vascular or other studies in the diagnosis of RP.

Patients with primary RP rarely, if ever, require noninvasive or invasive vascular studies. In patients with SSc or other secondary causes of RP, vascular studies may be helpful in a subset of patients when macrovascular disease is suspected. *Clinical scenarios in which vascular studies may be helpful include* asymmetric finger or hand involvement, high clinical suspicion of secondary causes of RP such as thromboembolism, thromboangiitis obliterans, an abnormal Allen's test suggestive of proximal artery disease, or severe disease resistant to initial vasodilator therapy.

Noninvasive studies include brachial-finger index measurement (gradients over 20 mmHg suggest a proximal fixed obstruction), Doppler ultrasound studies, and finger photoplethysmography (which can generate pulse-volume recordings). Significant vascular disease in SSc is typically confined to the level of the palmar arch and digital arteries ("vascular pruning"), but more proximal involvement (most commonly in the ulnar artery) can occur and may be suggested by an abnormal Allen's test and confirmed with vascular studies (see Question 20). Invasive angiography or magnetic resonance angiography may reveal an embolic source or proximal vessel disease such as with vascular thoracic outlet syndrome (vTOS), but these studies are often unnecessary in the initial evaluation of secondary RP. In patients with suspected vTOS, chest radiography may demonstrate a cervical rib as well.

14. Which general measures are important in the treatment of patients with RP?

The majority of RP patients often respond to simple prevention measures. Careful planning of one's activities of daily living minimizes unnecessary exposure to cold. Because reductions in core temperature as well as peripheral temperature may induce digital vasospasm, it is important to promote total body heat conservation. Layered clothing, warm socks, hats, and scarves should be worn in addition to gloves or mittens. Tobacco, sympathomimetic drugs (decongestants, amphetamines, diet pills), and beta-blockers must be avoided. Stress reduction techniques may be beneficial in those patients who identify emotional stress as a trigger for their symptoms.

15. **When is pharmacologic intervention indicated in the management of RP?**

Most patients with primary RP will not require pharmacologic therapy. Those with secondary RP more often require (but less often respond to) medication. Therapy for secondary RP should address the underlying disorder when possible and also treat the reversible component of vasospasm. Pharmacologic intervention is indicated in patients who suffer from frequent, prolonged, and/or severe episodes of RP in the setting of adequate preventative measures or with minimal provocation. Patients who manifest evidence of ischemic injury (digital pitting, etc.) should also be considered for medical management. Many patients who require medication may only need it during the colder months of the year. Other patients have year-round symptoms either due to more fixed vascular disease or changes in environmental temperature such as with air conditioning. Beta-blockers and smoking should be discontinued, if possible. Any evidence of digital infection should be treated with antibiotics. Analgesics may be necessary to reduce pain which can contribute to vasospasm.

16. **Which medications have been useful in the management of RP?**

All available therapies work better in primary RP than in secondary RP due to the lack of fixed vascular disease in primary RP. However, medications beyond CCB are not commonly required for primary RP.

PEARL: RP resistant to CCB therapy should prompt consideration of a workup for secondary disease.

Medications in the Management of RP

Medication Class	Specific drug/dosing	Possible side effects/monitoring
CCBs	Nifedipine 30–90 mg (extended release) daily	Lightheadedness/hypotension
	Amlodipine 2.5–10 mg daily	Headache
	Felodipine 2.5–10 mg daily	Lower extremity edema
	Diltiazem less effective	Worsening of GERD
	Verapamil and nicardipine are not effective	Constipation
PDE5 inhibitors	Sildenafil 20 mg two to three times daily	Lower extremity edema
	Tadalafil 5–20 mg daily	Lightheadedness/hypotension
		Avoid concurrent use of nitrates
Endothelin-1 antagonists	Bosentan 62.5–125 mg twice daily	Monthly LFT monitoring required (REMS program)
	Reduced new ulcer formation in clinical trials	Headache
		Lower extremity edema
Prostacyclin analogues	Epoprostenol, iloprost, treprostinil	Lightheadedness/hypotension
		Flushing
	Commonly administered intravenously in patients with refractory disease/ischemic crisis (i.e. threatened digital loss)	Diarrhea
		Jaw pain
		Short-term use for digital ischemia must be avoided in patients with possible pulmonary hypertension (screening for PAH is required prior to use)
Statins	Atorvastatin shown to decrease frequency of RP and reduce ulcer formation	Muscle pain
		LFT abnormalities
	Mechanism of action: potential vascular effects through inhibition of the rho-kinase pathway that regulates alpha$_{2c}$ adrenoreceptor expression	

Medications in the Management of RP

SSRIs	Fluoxetine 10–40 mg daily	Mood/sleep changes
	Other SSRIs also likely effective (class effect), but not trialed	Appetite/weight changes
ARBs	Losartan 25–100 mg daily	Lightheadedness/hypotension
Sympatholytic agents (e.g. prazosin)	Typically short-term use (loses effectiveness over time)	Lightheadedness/hypotension
Topical nitrates (2% nitroglyc-erin)	¼ to ½ inch ointment applied two to three times daily	Headache
		Hypotension
	A rest from nitrates for 12 hours is necessary to prevent development of a refractory state	Avoid concurrent use of PDE5 inhibitors
		Caution in patients with some cardio-vascular disease
Platelet-directed/ other therapy	ASA 81 mg daily	Bleeding
	Clopidagrel 75 mg twice daily	
	Pentoxyphylline 400 mg three times daily	
	Limited data, but commonly recommended in secondary RP with a history of digital infarcts or other signs of vascular insuf-ficiency, or those with concomitant macro-vascular disease	
Anticoagulation	Consider if evidence of embolization or new thrombosis	Bleeding
		INR monitoring
	Consider short-term use (heparin) in periods of critical ischemia (Question 18)	
	Consider long-term use (Coumadin) in resistant disease if antiphospholipid antibodies present	

ARBs, Angiotensin receptor blocker; *GERD,* gastroesophageal reflux disease; *LFT,* liver function test; *PDE5,* phosphodiesterase type 5 inhibitor; *PH,* pulmonary hypertension; *SSRIs,* selective serotonin reuptake inhibitors.

17. Describe an approach to treatment of patients with RP.

Step 1: Make sure to institute general measures such as heat conservation and cold protection. Counsel regarding the need for tobacco cessation. Consider stopping potential offending medications (e.g., beta-blockers) if medically feasible. If general measures are not effective, use medications. Try to use it only during cold months.

Step 2: Start low-dose dihydropyridine calcium channel blocker (nifedipine, amlodipine, felo-dipine). If no response in 1 week, increase the dose and continue to titrate subsequently every 2 weeks until maximum dose or side effects develop.

Step 3: If the patient has refractory RP that is significantly symptomatic or there is ongoing or re-current digital ischemic changes, consider adding other agents such as PDE5 inhibitors, ARB, ERA. In patients with baseline low blood pressure, consider changing to SSRI.

18. What are the characteristic features of an ischemic digital ulceration in systemic sclerosis?

By definition, an ischemic ulceration includes at least the loss of the epithelial layer but may involve deeper tissue as well. Lesions that are ischemic typically present with significant pain. Most ischemic ulcers occur distal to the DIP joint and are more common on the palmar surface of the digit. Digital ulcers are frequent in systemic sclerosis over the dorsal surface of the joints (particularly PIP and MCP), but lesions in these locations are considered to be multi-factorial with contractures and trauma playing a large role. Calcinosis in the digital pulp may also sponta-neously extrude from the skin and lead to ulcerations and often get confused with ischemic ulcers or infection.

19. What can be done medically in patients presenting with acute ischemic crisis that is digit threatening?

Step 1. Consider hospitalization to facilitate evaluation, control pain, titrate vasodilator therapy and possibly to consult surgery.

Step 2. Look for evidence of a secondary or exacerbating factor (OTC cold medication use, smoking, macro-vascular disease).

Step 3: Control pain. Pain control often requires opioid analgesics for severe ischemic pain. Consider short-term treatment such as a digital block with lidocaine.

Step 4. Escalate oral vasodilators as above in Question 17.

Step 5. Consider the need for intravenous prostaglandin/prostacyclin analogs in the appropriate setting (SSc and MCTD patients need to be screened for the presence of pulmonary hypertension prior to therapy initiation)

Step 6: Consider short-term anti-platelet therapy or anticoagulation in an ischemic crisis.

20. What surgical options can be performed for patients who are refractory to standard therapy?

Chemical sympathectomy via a **digital lidocaine block** can be performed promptly in the office for patients with acute episodes of ischemia and pain; this may provide lasting benefits beyond the temporary relief of the anesthetic. Chemical sympathectomy with botulinum toxin A has been described as well, but data on efficacy are conflicting.

Surgical sympathectomy may be considered in patients in whom more conservative measures have failed and who are at high risk for digital necrosis and other ischemic complications. It is commonly performed at either the superficial palmar arch, the common digital arteries, or the radial and ulnar arteries. Sympathectomy may not provide long-lasting benefits, so it should not be considered a definitive therapy.

The majority of patients with secondary RP due to SSc have vascular disease that is prominent at the level of the palmar arch and distal digital arteries. However, a small subset may have proximal vessel compromise that is discovered by an abnormal Allen's test. In this setting, angiography to identify occult disease at the ulnar artery (or less commonly the radial artery) should be performed to determine if the patient would benefit from surgical revascularization.

In patients presenting with dry gangrene of a digit, it is preferable to avoid surgery if possible and allow the necrotic area to clearly demarcate from viable tissue proximally. Allowing the digit to *autoamputate* preserves the greatest length possible of the involved finger and avoids surgery at a site with compromised blood flow. Surgical resection may be required in some patients with concern for infection and/or intractable pain.

21. What is the prognosis for patients with RP?

The prognosis for patients with primary RP is excellent. The vast majority of patients with primary RP never develop an underlying condition such as those associated with secondary RP. This is especially true if NCM and autoantibody testing are negative (<2% progression to SSc).

The prognosis for patients with secondary RP is generally dependent on the underlying condition. Intrinsic vascular disease is often present. Complications arising from vasospasm, such as digital ulcerations, are common.

ACKNOWLEDGMENT

The author would like to thank Drs. Marc Cohen & Jason Kolfenbach for their contributions to this chapter in prior editions.

BIBLIOGRAPHY

Flavahan NA. A vascular mechanistic approach to understanding Raynaud's phenomenon. *Nat Rev Rheumatol.* 2015;11:146–158.

Herrick AL. Raynaud's phenomenon and digital ulcers: advances in evaluation and management. *Curr Opin Rheumatol.* 2021;33(6):453–462 1.

Hirschl M, Hirschl K, Lenz M, et al. Transition from primary Raynaud's phenomenon to secondary Raynaud's phenomenon identified by diagnosis of an associated disease: results of ten years of prospective surveillance. *Arthritis Rheum.* 2006;54:1974.

Koenig M, Joyal F, Fritzler MJ, et al. Autoantibodies and microvascular damage are independent predictive factors for progression of Raynaud's phenomenon to systemic sclerosis: a twenty-year prospective study of 586 patients, with validation of proposed criteria for early systemic sclerosis. *Arthritis Rheum.* 2008;58:3902.

Lawson O, Sisti A, Konofaos P. The use of botulinum toxin in Raynaud phenomenon: a comprehensive literature review. *Ann Plast Surg.* 2023;91(1):159–186.

Satteson ES, Chung MP, Chung LS, et al. Microvascular hand surgery for digital ischemia in scleroderma. *J Scleroderma Relat Disord*. 2020;5(2):130–136.

Smith V, Herrick AL, Ingegnoli F, et al. Standardisation of nailfold capillaroscopy for the assessment of patients with Raynaud's phenomenon and systemic sclerosis. *Autoimmun Rev*. 2020;19(3):102458.

Taylor MH, McFadden JA, Bolster MB, Silver RM. Ulnar artery involvement in systemic sclerosis (scleroderma). *J Rheumatol*. 2002;29(1):102.

Wigley FM, Flavahan NA. Raynaud's phenomenon. *N Engl J Med*. 2016;375(6):556–565.

Wigley FM. Treatment of the Raynaud's Phenomenon Resistant to Initial Therapy. *UpToDate*. 2024. Waltham, MA.

Zahn C, Puga C, Malik A, et al. Painful Raynaud's mimics. *Best Pract Res Clin Rheumatol*. 2024;38(1):101948.

CHAPTER 74

Autoimmune Eye and Ear Disorders

Jason R. Kolfenbach, MD, Amit K. Reddy, MD, and Alan G. Palestine, MD

> **KEY SECRETS**
>
> 1. Ophthalmologic manifestations are common in patients with rheumatologic disease and should be considered in any such patient presenting with a red eye or other ocular symptoms.
> 2. Infectious causes are in the differential diagnosis of many common ophthalmologic conditions, and they are particularly important to keep in mind given the immune dysregulation and immunosuppression that is characteristic of patients with concurrent rheumatic illness.
> 3. The various causes of eye inflammation in a patient with rheumatologic disease can be difficult to distinguish, and prompt referral to an ophthalmologist is necessary for appropriate evaluation and assistance with management.

1. Why is a general understanding of the structures of the eye important to the field of rheumatology?

Systemic rheumatologic disease can affect ocular structures through inflammatory mechanisms (e.g., rheumatoid arthritis [RA], granulomatosis with polyangiitis [GPA], giant cell arteritis [GCA], and sarcoidosis among others), thrombotic disease (antiphospholipid antibody syndrome [APS]), and dryness (Sjögren disease [SjD]; see Chapter 21: Sjogren Disease). In some patients, the onset of inflammatory ocular disease (e.g., uveitis, scleritis) may represent the first manifestation of a systemic illness, requiring a rheumatologist to set forth a rational, targeted evaluation. Finally, some cases of idiopathic autoimmune eye disease require disease-modifying antirheumatic drugs or biologic therapy, which a rheumatologist may be called on to help manage.

A rheumatologist who is knowledgeable about ocular anatomy and inflammatory conditions affecting the various structures of the eye will be better equipped to recognize disease, perform appropriate evaluations, and communicate with partners in ophthalmology. In this chapter, we will describe the relationship between various ocular structures and rheumatic disease. See Fig. 74.1.

EPISCLERITIS/SCLERITIS

2. How is conjunctivitis separated clinically from episcleritis and scleritis?

Conjunctivitis is the most common cause of a red eye presenting to clinicians. Common etiologies include allergies, viral and bacterial infections, and local irritation (e.g., severe dryness), although it can also occur secondary to inflammatory disease (e.g., reactive arthritis). Conjunctivitis stemming from common etiologies is often bilateral and involves the palpebral and bulbar surfaces. In contrast, **episcleritis** and **scleritis** are commonly limited to the globe/bulbar surface and are often sectoral in location. Conjunctival vessels lie loosely on the superficial bulbar surface and can be moved across the underlying scleral surface by a cotton swab, helping the clinician distinguish redness originating from one of these sites.

3. List the basic exam elements that can be carried out by a non-ophthalmologist in a patient presenting with a red eye.

Important information can be elicited from a focused ocular exam even without tools such as a slit lamp or indirect ophthalmoscope. The following are basic clinical evaluations that can inform treatment and facilitate discussion with an ophthalmology consultant:

- Visual acuity testing (reading small print at 12 inches).
- Evaluation of external structures such as the lids and lashes (evaluating for lid swelling, blepharitis, entropion/extropion, overt proptosis, lacrimal gland enlargement).

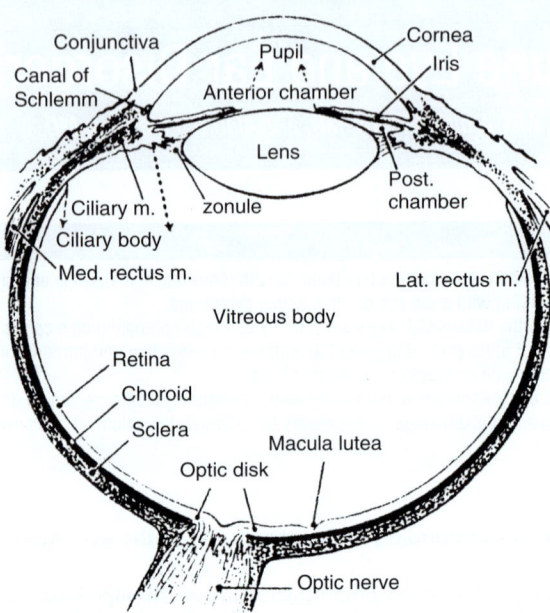

Fig. 74.1 Diagram of a human eye. (From Stedman T. *Stedman's Medical Dictionary*. 23rd ed. Baltimore, MD: Williams & Wilkins; 1976. with permission.)

- Evaluation of palpebral and bulbar conjunctiva.
- Evaluation for **ciliary flush** (erythema at the limbus area where the corneal dome meets the sclera).
- Evaluation of pupillary size, shape, and response to light.
- Gross examination of the cornea for signs of corneal opacity.
- Fundoscopic exam looking for obvious signs of retinal ischemia and/or retinal vessel abnormalities (exam may be limited due to pain or photophobia).

In a patient presenting with a red eye, certain findings by history and exam warrant immediate consultation with an ophthalmologist including extreme difficulty opening the eye (suggestive of corneal injury or keratitis), abnormal pupils (such as fixed, dilated pupils or synechiae), corneal opacities, or ciliary flush. Ciliary flush may represent significant pathology such as uveitis, keratitis, and/or acute angle closure glaucoma.

4. What is the clinical classification of episcleritis and scleritis?

Episcleritis (30–40% of cases).
    Simple ~75%
    Nodular ~25%
Scleritis (60–70% of cases).
    Anterior 98%.
        Diffuse 40%.
        Nodular 44%.
        Necrotizing 14%.
            With inflammation at 10%.
            Without inflammation 4%
            (scleromalacia perforans).
    Posterior 2%.

5. What are the typical features of episcleritis?

Episcleritis commonly presents as an acute onset of localized erythema and discomfort without significant pain. It affects women in two-thirds of cases. It is bilateral at some point over the course of disease in roughly half of patients, and is associated with a systemic autoimmune disorder in 30%. Tends to have a good prognosis, typically resolving in 2 to 3 weeks without complications, but may recur in most patients at 1- to 3-month intervals for several years. Rarely progresses to scleritis (~5%).

6. What are the typical features of scleritis?

Patients typically present with severe, boring, and persistent pain (except with scleromalacia perforans), with associated erythema, photophobia, and tearing. Less commonly, there can be a reduction in visual acuity. It affects women in two-thirds of cases. Bilateral disease develops in half of cases, with recurrence rates of up to 70%. Most patients (~95%) maintain the same clinical subtype. It is associated with a systemic disease in 50–60% of patients, with frequency depending on the subtype. Scleritis does not fully blanch with topical phenylephrine. Complications include keratitis, uveitis, glaucoma, cystoid macular edema, and exudative retinal detachment.

Subtypes of Scleritis

Diffuse	Most benign form, with ocular complications occurring in 50%, but only ~20% experiencing a decrease in visual acuity. 60% of patients have an associated systemic disease, with RA being the most common.
Nodular	Characterized by local inflammation with a tender immobile nodule. Nodules may have a dark red or violaceous hue. Ocular complications occur in 50%, with <10% experiencing decreased visual acuity. 45% have an associated systemic disorder such as RA.
Necrotizing	Most destructive form and can progress rapidly to scleral necrosis; ocular complications common. *Up to 95% have an associated systemic disorder.* Its presence may indicate increased activity of systemic vasculitis. **Scleromalacia perforans** is a subtype of necrotizing scleritis where the sclera becomes necrotic and thin **without pain or redness**. As a result, the disease presents with an insidious onset and poses a major challenge when attempting to gauge response to therapy.
Posterior	May be difficult to diagnose because redness may be absent (unless anterior involvement is also present) and pain and visual disturbance may be minimal. A clue on history and exam may be pain with eye accommodation. Orbital ultrasonography may demonstrate scleral thickening and magnetic resonance imaging (MRI) and computed tomography (CT) scans can also be helpful. Ocular complications occur in 85%, with retinal pathology (cystoid macular edema, exudative retinal detachment) being the most common. Associated with systemic disease in less than one-third when posterior involvement is isolated.

7. How are episcleritis and scleritis differentiated?

The significant **pain** associated with scleritis is the primary distinguishing feature. A blue/purple hue, rather than bright red discoloration, may be seen with scleritis. The presence of avascular areas within the regions of vascular engorgement is highly suggestive of necrotizing scleritis or scleromalacia perforans. In contrast, episcleritis is characterized by superficial inflammation of the loose vascular connective tissue overlying the sclera; it is typically brighter red in color, tender rather than overtly painful, and application of **phenylephrine** results in rapid resolution of erythema. Episcleritis and scleritis can coexist, which must be remembered when interpreting these results. Prompt evaluation by an ophthalmologist is necessary for an accurate diagnosis.

8. What systemic autoimmune/autoinflammatory diseases are associated with episcleritis?

Association in ~30% of cases: RA (11%), inflammatory bowel disease (IBD; 8%), vasculitis (5%), systemic lupus erythematosus (SLE; 3%), and other rheumatologic diseases (3%).

9. **What systemic autoimmune/autoinflammatory diseases are associated with scleritis?**

   Association in up to 60% of patients (see the following table). RA is the most common systemic condition, usually occurring in the setting of severely disabling and well-established disease. Joint inflammation may be "burnt out" and patients often have other extraarticular manifestations. When associated with peripheral ulcerative keratitis, RA, GPA, relapsing polychondritis, and SLE are most common. Necrotizing scleritis without inflammation (scleromalacia perforans) is seen almost exclusively in RA.

   SYSTEMIC DISEASES ASSOCIATED WITH SCLERITIS

Associated Condition	Cases of Scleritis (%)
RA	10-15
GPA	5-10
Relapsing polychondritis	<5
SLE	<5
IBD	<5
Seronegative spondyloarthropathies	1–2
Other[a]	≤1%

   [a]Other: Behçet, Takayasu, GCA, hypocomplementemic urticarial vasculitis, cutaneous vasculitis, hepatitis C virus-associated vasculitis, polymyalgia rheumatica, pyoderma gangrenosum, sarcoidosis, and Cogan syndrome.

10. **What nonrheumatologic diseases should be considered in a patient presenting with episcleritis or scleritis?**

    Infections such as herpes zoster (particularly in the setting of ipsilateral shingles in the V1 distribution), herpes simplex, aspergillus, tuberculosis (TB), syphilis, Lyme, pseudomonas, and other bacterial infections account for ~5% of episcleritis and 5% to 10% of scleritis cases. A high index of suspicion must be maintained for infectious causes in the setting of chronic immunosuppression typical of rheumatology patients. Scleritis in the setting of recent ocular surgery should also raise concern for an infectious etiology.

    Oral and intravenous (IV) **bisphosphonates, trauma,** and **malignancies** (penetration by ocular adnexal lymphoproliferative lesions and intraocular tumors) **are rare causes.**

11. **What workup is indicated for a patient presenting with episcleritis or scleritis?**

    A history, medication history, physical examination, chest x-ray, and routine laboratory exam (complete blood count [CBC], comprehensive metabolic panel, urinalysis [UA], erythrocyte sedimentation rate [ESR], and C-reactive protein [CRP]) evaluating for associated diseases are necessary. Routine testing for antineutrophil cytoplasmic antibody (ANCA) should be performed in all patients with scleritis, as positivity may be seen when other manifestations of ANCA-associated vasculitis are absent and positive results tend to indicate more aggressive disease. Further workup (e.g., antinuclear antibody [ANA], rheumatoid factor [RF], anticyclic citrullinated peptide, imaging, and microbiology studies) should be considered based on clinical suspicion following a thorough history and exam.

12. **How is episcleritis treated?**

    Initial symptomatic treatment includes cold compresses and topical lubricants. If frequent or prolonged use of topical lubricants is required, preservative-free formulations should be used to prevent irritation. If these measures fail, topical nonsteroidal anti-inflammatory drugs (NSAIDs) may be tried, but data suggest that they are no more effective than lubricants alone. **Topical corticosteroids** are extremely effective and should be considered the next line of therapy. Oral NSAIDs may be used if there is no response to local therapies. Systemic corticosteroids are rarely required.

13. **How is scleritis treated?**

    Systemic therapy is required for scleritis whether it is isolated or in the setting of systemic disease, and pain is often the best indicator of inflammation control. The selection of therapy is based on the subtype of disease and presence of associated systemic features. Oral NSAIDs are generally used as first-line therapy for non-necrotizing anterior scleritis and may be occasionally effective for idiopathic posterior scleritis. If inflammation is not controlled, or in necrotizing scleritis and most cases of posterior scleritis, systemic corticosteroids should be used. Subconjunctival corticosteroid injections may be useful for non-necrotizing scleritis but should be considered with caution due to the risk of scleral thinning and globe perforation; as such, corticosteroid injections should likely be avoided in necrotizing forms of disease.

In cases unresponsive to oral corticosteroids, or when the dose cannot be tapered to an acceptable level, steroid-sparing immunosuppressive agents such as methotrexate, azathioprine, mycophenolate mofetil, or cyclophosphamide may be required. In one study, such agents were required in 23% of diffuse anterior, 7% of nodular anterior, 70% of necrotizing, and 17% of posterior scleritis cases. Antitumor necrosis factor (TNF) therapies and rituximab have been used successfully in this setting as well. In cases associated with an underlying systemic disease, the choice of immunosuppression is commonly tailored to agents known to be effective for the systemic illness.

UVEITIS

14. What is uveitis and how is it anatomically classified?

Uveitis refers to inflammation of the uvea (the iris, ciliary body, and choroid). The term is broadly used to encompass inflammation within the eye and, therefore, includes adjacent anatomic locations and structures such as the aqueous, vitreous humor, and retina. Knowledge of this condition is important to rheumatologists as some cases (up to 40% in tertiary referral centers) are associated with systemic disease. Anatomic classification and additional clinical features (see Question 15) can be important clues to forming the differential diagnosis and guiding a rationale, targeted workup.

- **Anterior uveitis:** iris and ciliary body are the primary sites of inflammation; iritis (confined to iris) and iridocyclitis (iris + ciliary body) are examples (see Question 18).
- **Posterior uveitis:** choroid and/or retina are the primary sites of inflammation (see Question 24).
- **Intermediate uveitis:** vitreous is the primary site of inflammation; pars planitis and posterior cyclitis are examples (see Question 23).
- **Panuveitis:** when there is no predominant site and all intraocular locations are affected.

15. List the primary parameters used to characterize subsets of uveitis.

1. Anatomic location of inflammation: anterior, intermediate, posterior, or panuveitis.
2. Laterality: unilateral (can be asynchronous) or bilateral (occurring in both eyes simultaneously).
3. Onset: sudden or insidious.
4. Duration: limited (≤3 months) or persistent (>3 months).
5. Course: acute (sudden onset and limited duration), chronic (persistent disease with relapse within 3 months of discontinuation of therapy), recurrent (repeat episodes separated by ≥3 months).

16. How do the typical presenting symptoms differ among anterior, intermediate, and posterior uveitis?

Anatomic Classification	Patient-Reported Symptoms	Exam Findings
Anterior	Pain, redness, photophobia (chronic anterior uveitis may lack these) Variable degree of visual disturbance	*Ciliary flush* with acute onset. Chronic findings: cataract, synechiae, keratic precipitates, and band keratopathy
Intermediate	Blurry vision, floaters, distortion of central vision No pain or photophobia typically	Vitritis, with minimal involvement of anterior chamber May symptomatically present unilaterally, but evidence of bilateral disease in 80% on exam
Posterior	Blurred vision, floaters, scotomata No pain or photophobia typically	Evidence suggestive of inflammatory disease at choroid, retina, and/or retinal vessels by indirect ophthalmoscopy or fluorescein angiography
Panuveitis	Any combination of above	Any combination of above

17. List some common causes of uveitis based on the pattern of disease.

Pattern of Uveitis	Common Diseases Associated With Pattern[a]
Anterior	
Acute, recurrent unilateral	SpA (HLA-B27+), idiopathic (HLA-B27 and non-HLA-B27-associated), herpes viruses (HSV, VZV, CMV)
Acute, nonrecurrent unilateral	Idiopathic (HLA-B27 and non-HLA-B27 associated), SpA, herpes viruses
Acute bilateral	Idiopathic non-HLA-B27-associated, TINU, Behçet disease, SjD
Chronic	Idiopathic non-HLA-B27-associated, JIA, SjD, sarcoidosis, SpA, Lyme, syphilis, TB
Intermediate	Pars planitis, sarcoidosis, multiple sclerosis, Behçet disease, Lyme
Posterior	Toxoplasmosis, VKH, Behçet disease, sarcoidosis, herpes viruses, TB, Lyme, SpA (PsA, IBD)
Panuveitis	Toxoplasmosis, VKH, Behçet disease, sarcoidosis, IBD, herpes viruses, TB, bacterial, fungal

[a]*Behçet disease, sarcoidosis, Lyme, syphilis, and herpes viruses can present with any form of uveitis.* Various ophthalmologic syndromes (e.g., Fuchs' heterochromic cyclitis, birdshot retinochoroidopathy) are also common causes of uveitis. No etiology is identified in ~30%.

HLA, Human leukocyte antigen; *HSV,* herpes simplex virus; *JIA,* juvenile idiopathic arthritis; *PSA,* psoriatic arthritis; *SjD,* Sjogren's disease; *SpA,* spondyloarthritis; *TINU,* tubulointerstitial nephritis and uveitis syndrome; *VKH,* Vogt-Koyanagi-Harada syndrome; *VZV,* varicella zoster virus.

18. Define anterior uveitis and list the differential diagnosis associated with this finding.

Anterior uveitis is defined as inflammation occurring predominantly anterior to the lens of the eye. Iritis and iridocyclitis are examples of anterior uveitis. Anterior uveitis accounts for 50% to 80% of all cases of uveitis. Most cases are **idiopathic,** followed by **HLA-B27-associated** anterior uveitis. Other causes include sarcoidosis, Behçet disease, infectious etiologies (HSV, VZV, cytomegalovirus [CMV], Epstein–Barr virus, TB, syphilis, and Lyme), multiple sclerosis, Posner-Schlossman syndrome, drugs (e.g., bisphosphonates, rifabutin, cidofovir, sulfonamides, MEK and BRAF inhibitors, cancer immunotherapy agents), and trauma.

   JIA, TINU, and **Kawasaki disease** are the most common associations in the pediatric population.

   Fuchs heterochromic iridocyclitis is a common cause of chronic, unilateral anterior uveitis characterized by iris heterochromia.

19. How is HLA-B27 associated with anterior uveitis?

In Western populations, acute anterior uveitis (AAU) is associated with H0LA-B27 in 50% of patients. This group can be further subdivided into isolated HLA-B27-associated anterior uveitis (20–50%) and those associated with an underlying spondyloarthritis (50–80%; higher estimates of 80% identified in studies utilizing the Assessment of Spondyloarthritis International Society criteria for spondyloarthritis). Patients with HLA-B27-positive AAU are more likely to be White, younger, male sex, have an acute course, experience recurrences, develop hypopyon (the most common cause of hypopyon-complicated uveitis in North America), and have an associated systemic disease than patients with HLA-B27-negative AAU.

HLA-B27-Associated Disease	% of SpA Patients Developing AAU*	% of all AAU Patients Developing SpA	% of HLA-B27+ AAU Patients Developing SpA
Ankylosing spondylitis	20–40	15–40	55–80
Reactive arthritis	10–20	5–10	10–20
PsA	7–10	<5	<5
Enteropathic arthropathy	2–9	<5	<5

*The prevalence of uveitis among patients with spondyloarthritis (SpA) documented in this table is based on historical classifications of disease. Newer classification criteria for axial and peripheral SpA have resulted in patient populations with milder axial radiographic disease, increased prevalence of females, and decreased prevalence of HLA-B27. The decrease in HLA-B27 will likely change the prevalence of uveitis in future cohorts.

20. How does uveitis present differently depending on the associated SpA?

Ankylosing spondylitis and reactive arthritis: Historically, ~90% of patients are HLA-B27-positive. Typical presentation is sudden onset of anterior uveitis that is unilateral but alternating, has a recurrent course, and usually resolves completely within several months.

PsA and enteropathic: patients who are HLA-B27-positive (45–60%) may present with classic AAU. However, patients who are HLA-B27-negative may present with the insidious onset of bilateral, chronic uveitis that may be anterior, intermediate, or posterior in location.

As noted above (Question 19), the prevalence of HLA-B27 among cohorts fulfilling newer classification criteria for axial and peripheral SpA is lower than the historical prevalence in AS. This change in population characteristics will likely alter the prevalence, and presentation, of uveitis in this more diverse patient population.

21. How is the uveitis of JIA unique?

Unlike patients with almost all other causes of anterior uveitis, JIA patients with anterior uveitis (15% of all JIA patients) are usually **asymptomatic** and can have a normal-appearing eye. Consequently, complications of uveitis may develop before the inflammation is detected. As such, patients with JIA should undergo regular screening eye exams. Risk factors include young age (<7 years), female sex, ANA positivity, and pauciarticular disease.

22. Describe some ocular features that may be useful for distinguishing HSV and VZV from other causes of uveitis.

Uveitis caused by HSV and VZV may not be associated with other characteristic ocular, cutaneous, or systemic manifestations, making the diagnosis difficult to establish. An accurate and timely diagnosis is critical so appropriate treatment can be instituted. Suggestive findings include unilateral involvement, marked anterior chamber inflammation, elevated intraocular pressure, iris atrophy or nodules, iris transillumination, and corneal hypoesthesia. Polymerase chain reaction of the aqueous humor may be required for definitive diagnosis.

23. Define intermediate uveitis and pars planitis, and list the differential diagnosis associated with these findings.

Intermediate uveitis refers to ocular inflammation primarily affecting the anterior vitreous, pars plana (the area immediately posterior to the ciliary body where white blood cells may accumulate), and peripheral retina. It typically affects children and young adults, is bilateral in 80% of cases, and tends to be chronic with periods of exacerbation and remission. The hallmark finding is vitritis that can be associated with aggregates of exudates referred to as "snowballs" or "snowbanks" in the pars plana region. When anterior segment inflammation is present, it is typically only mild to moderate. Peripheral retinal vasculitis and cystoid macular edema resulting in visual loss may occur.

When the condition is **idiopathic** and pars plana exudation ("snowballs" or "snowbank") occurs, it is referred to as **pars planitis,** which accounts for >50% of intermediate uveitis cases and most commonly presents in children and adolescents.

The differential diagnosis also includes sarcoidosis, multiple sclerosis, infectious etiologies (Lyme disease, syphilis, herpes-family viruses, TB, Whipple's disease, rickettsiosis, human T-cell lymphotropic virus type 1, and toxocariasis), and Behçet disease.

24. Define posterior uveitis, and list the differential diagnosis associated with this finding.

Posterior uveitis describes inflammation of the choroid or retina, often associated with an overlying vitritis. **Toxoplasmosis** retinitis is the most common identifiable cause, and is particularly common in Central and South America. Other causes include Behçet disease, sarcoidosis, VKH disease, autoimmune retinopathy, cancer-associated retinopathy, retinal vasculitis, sympathetic ophthalmia, presumed ocular histoplasmosis syndrome, herpes-family viruses (HSV, VZV, and CMV), TB, and syphilis. TORCH organisms, Blau syndrome, and toxocariasis may be causes in the pediatric population.

There is also a group of posterior uveitides referred to as the "white dot syndromes". This group of inflammatory chorioretinopathies is characterized by the common presence of discrete, white lesions at the deeper retina and choroid. These conditions are typically idiopathic and include punctate inner choroiditis, multifocal choroiditis, serpiginous choroiditis, acute posterior multifocal placoid pigment epitheliopathy (APMPPE), and birdshot retinochoroidopathy. Birdshot retinochoroidopathy is characterized by multiple, discrete, cream-colored spots throughout the retina and choroid (primarily distributed around the optic nerve). It is highly associated with HLA-A29.

25. List the differential diagnosis of patients presenting with panuveitis.

Toxoplasmosis, VKH disease, Behçet disease, sarcoidosis, IBD, and infectious etiologies (herpes-family viruses, TB, bacterial and fungal infections). It is important to note that among rheumatologic conditions, Behçet disease and sarcoidosis can be associated with inflammation of any segment of the uveal tract.

26. Describe the typical features of VKH disease.

It is an idiopathic, bilateral, chronic panuveitis more commonly occurring in Asian, Hispanic, and Native American populations that progresses over phases (prodromal, uveitic, convalescent, and chronic/recurrent). It is thought to result from an inflammatory reaction against melanocytes. The prodromal phase may include an aseptic meningitis-like presentation (lymphocytic pleocytosis on lumbar puncture) and other neurologic deficits including auditory symptoms. The acute uveitic phase results in an exudative retinal detachment in over 80% of cases. The uveitic phase is followed by a convalescent period in which the fundus may demonstrate a characteristic "sunset glow" appearance resulting from choroid depigmentation. Skin changes (vitiligo, poliosis, and alopecia) do not typically appear until this convalescent phase; thus cutaneous findings cannot be relied on to make an early diagnosis. VKH must be distinguished from sympathetic ophthalmia, which is a bilateral, autoimmune uveitis resulting from trauma to one eye. The ocular findings can be very similar to VKH, but patients with sympathetic ophthalmia will not have the associated systemic signs and symptoms.

27. What masquerade syndromes mimic uveitis? How can they be distinguished clinically?

Masquerade syndromes present with ocular findings suspicious for immune-mediated uveitis, but are subsequently found to be related to hereditary, neoplastic, or mechanical mechanisms resulting in ocular irritation/inflammation. The most common is **ocular or central nervous system (CNS) B-cell lymphoma**. Others include retinitis pigmentosa, leukemia, melanoma, retinoblastoma, retained intraocular foreign body, and malpositioned postoperative intraocular lens. The diagnosis of a masquerade syndrome may be suggested by the appearance of the eye, age of the patient (e.g., malignancy in a patient aged >45 years, retinoblastoma in children), presence of neurologic signs or symptoms, or a lack of response (especially clinical worsening) to standard uveitis therapy.

28. Summarize the rheumatic diseases most likely to be associated with uveitis. Compare their typical onset, laterality, and location.

Rheumatologic Disease	Onset	Laterality	Location
HLA-B27 + SpA	Sudden	Unilateral	Anterior
PsA, enteropathic (non-B27+)	Insidious	Bilateral	Any segment
JIA	Insidious	Bilateral	Any segment
Sarcoidosis	Sudden	Bilateral	Anterior
Behçet disease	Sudden	Bilateral	Panuveitis

29. Which causes of uveitis have been associated with specific HLA types?

Axial SpA	HLA-B27.
Behçet disease	HLA-B51.
Birdshot retinochoroidopathy	HLA-A29.
Pars planitis	HLA-DR2, DR15.
VKH	HLA-DRB1, DR4, DQA1.
TINU	HLA DRB1, DQB1, DQA1.

30. What diagnostic workup is of value for a patient with unclassified uveitis?

History and physical examination should be used to guide further workup in all cases of uveitis. **Anterior uveitis is commonly idiopathic;** *therefore extensive evaluation is often unnecessary in a patient presenting with a single episode of uveitis without signs or symptoms of a systemic disease.* Patients with recurrent or chronic anterior uveitis, uveitis affecting the intermediate or posterior segments, panuveitis, or with an abnormal history or physical exam warrant additional testing. Routine labs including CBC, comprehensive metabolic panel, UA, ESR, and CRP should be considered in this setting. The need for further workup (e.g., infectious disease studies, imaging, autoantibodies) will depend on the results of initial testing as well as the history and exam.

Medication history (all patients): certain medications like bisphosphonates, moxifloxacin, sulfonamides, MEK and BRAF inhibitors, and cancer immunotherapy agents can cause uveitis.

Chest x-ray (all patients): sarcoidosis is part of the differential diagnosis of all patterns of uveitis. A chest x-ray is also a useful screen for TB.

Syphilis testing (all patients): like sarcoidosis, syphilis can cause any type of uveitis in the absence of characteristic systemic manifestations.

Purified protein derivative (PPD)/Quantiferon (select patients): positive results do not indicate active disease and can be misleading; therefore TB testing should be reserved for cases where there is suspicion of infection (exposure history, chest x-ray findings, and specific findings on ocular exam such as serpiginous choroiditis or focal choroidal nodules).

ANA (select patients): indicated only in the evaluation of pediatric patients with pauciarticular onset JIA and uveitis, as it has prognostic implications in these patients. It is not indicated for routine screening of adult patients with unclassified uveitis because it has an extremely low diagnostic and prognostic value unless other features of SLE, SjD, anti-C1q disease, or another ANA-associated disease are present. Note that many patients with SLE who develop uveitis frequently have anti-C1q antibodies.

HLA-B27 (select patients): appropriate for patients presenting with AAU, even in the absence of a demonstrable SpA given its prognostic implications.

The following are not recommended as part of the initial evaluation:

Angiotensin-converting enzyme level: elevations are nonspecific and may be seen in sarcoidosis, liver disease, granulomatous infections (TB, leprosy), Gaucher disease, hyperthyroidism, Hodgkin disease, and various causes of lung disease.

ANCA: ANCA-associated vasculitis is an extremely rare cause of uveitis. Routine testing is not recommended in the absence of retinal vasculitis.

31. Describe general treatment principles of uveitis.

- Infectious causes should be treated accordingly.
- Anterior uveitis:
  - Mydriatic and cycloplegic agents are commonly used to alleviate pain and prevent synechiae.
  - Topical corticosteroids are the hallmark of therapy (limited/no efficacy in posterior disease).
  - Oral corticosteroids are uncommonly required for isolated anterior uveitis.
- Uveitis in any segment:
  - Periocular or intravitreal corticosteroids may be useful for more severe cases or when posterior disease is prominent.
  - Oral corticosteroids are commonly effective; in severe cases, doses of 1 mg/kg may be required.
  - When systemic corticosteroids lead to an inadequate response, intolerance, or inability to taper, steroid-sparing immunosuppressive therapy may be required.
  - Immunosuppressive agents that have demonstrated efficacy in uveitis include methotrexate, azathioprine, mycophenolate mofetil, leflunomide, calcineurin inhibitors, cyclophosphamide, anti-TNF therapy (monoclonals > etanercept), and rituximab.
    - The FAST trial found that methotrexate was noninferior to mycophenolate mofetil in the treatment of noninfectious intermediate, posterior, and panuveitis (NIPPU).
- Adalimumab has demonstrated efficacy in NIPPU in several randomized controlled trials and is approved by the Food and Drug Administration for this indication.

- Disease-specific considerations:
  - Methotrexate plus adalimumab has been shown to be more effective than methotrexate alone for JIA-associated uveitis.
  - Anti-TNF therapy (monoclonal antibodies, not etanercept) has been found particularly beneficial in patients with uveitis due to Behçet disease, sarcoidosis, and HLA-B27-associated AAU.
  - Rituximab is increasingly utilized as an alternative to cyclophosphamide in ANCA-associated vasculitis with uveitis and other forms of ocular inflammation.

There is a balance between the use of systemic and local corticosteroids. All forms of corticosteroids (when used chronically) will lead to cataract, and some patients will develop corticosteroid-induced intraocular pressure rise. However, it is important to note that uncontrolled uveitis can cause cataract and elevated intraocular pressure (uveitic glaucoma) as well. The choice of local versus systemic corticosteroids is based on patient tolerance, risk factors, and the potential for side effects.

RETINAL VASCULITIS

32. Define retinal vasculitis.

Retinal vasculitis is defined as inflammation of the retinal vessel walls or perivascular spaces affecting veins more commonly than arterioles (except in polyarteritis nodosa, ANCA-associated vasculitis, SLE, and Susac syndrome). It occurs bilaterally in almost all cases. It can be complicated by occlusive retinal vascular disease secondary to obliterative or thrombotic processes. Can be primary or seen in conjunction with other forms of uveitis (e.g., posterior uveitis). Can be associated with systemic rheumatic disease, such as Behçet disease and sarcoidosis, but does not necessarily correlate well with systemic vasculitis.

33. What are the symptoms of retinal vasculitis?

Painless blurred vision, scotomata, and floaters are most common. Less frequently, dyschromatopsia (difficulty perceiving colors) and metamorphopsia (distorted vision where straight lines appear wavy) may be present. Pain and redness are uncommon if vasculitis is not associated with other ocular inflammatory conditions. Can be asymptomatic if only the peripheral vasculature is affected.

34. What ocular findings are seen in patients with retinal vasculitis?

Ophthalmoscopic examination and **fluorescein angiography** are required for the diagnosis. **Vascular sheathing** is the most characteristic feature and correlates with a perivascular infiltrate of inflammatory cells seen on pathologic specimens. Other findings may include cotton-wool spots, retinal hemorrhages, retinal or optic disc edema, vitritis, vascular leakage, and capillary dropout. Vessel occlusion *(occlusive vasculopathy)* can result from inflammatory and noninflammatory etiologies of retinal vasculitis (see Question 35) and may lead to subsequent retinal ischemia, an environment favoring neovascularization.

35. What is the differential diagnosis of retinal vasculitis?

May be inflammatory (vasculitis) or noninflammatory (vasculopathy), with atherosclerosis being the most common cause of abnormal retinal vessels. Inflammatory causes are generally grouped into three categories:

1. Systemic diseases: **Behçet disease, sarcoidosis,** and **multiple sclerosis** are the most common. SLE can be associated with retinal vasculitis, but it is more commonly associated with choroiditis. Retinal vasculitis is less frequently associated with other rheumatic diseases including ANCA-associated vasculitis, large- and medium-vessel vasculitis (e.g., GCA, Takayasu), Susac syndrome, and APS. Primary CNS lymphoma, acute leukemia, paraproteinemias, and cancer-associated retinopathy are other rare causes.
2. Infectious: toxoplasmosis, TB, Lyme disease, syphilis, cat scratch disease, herpes simplex, and varicella zoster are the most common. Less frequent associations include CMV, human immunodeficiency virus (HIV), Whipple disease, HTLV-1, brucellosis, and leptospirosis.

3. Primary ocular syndromes: idiopathic retinal vasculitis, pars planitis, birdshot retinocho-roidopathy, frosted branch angiitis, Eales' disease, and IRVAN syndrome.

36. What laboratory evaluation is indicated in the evaluation of retinal vasculitis?

Initial evaluation should include a CBC, comprehensive metabolic panel, UA, ESR, CRP, HIV screening, syphilis serology, chest radiograph, and TB screening (PPD or interferon-gamma release assay). Further evaluation is determined by the results of the history, physical examination, and initial screening studies and is guided by the suspected diagnosis based on the ocular exam.

Patients presenting with occlusive vasculopathy warrant additional discussion, given that non-inflammatory etiologies such as atherosclerosis represent a substantial proportion of cases. Inflammatory rheumatic disease is a less common cause of branch or central retinal vein occlusions as well as retinal artery occlusions. As such, routine evaluations for inflammatory disease should be reserved for patients with extraocular signs and symptoms suggestive of a rheumatic condition. APS may be an exception, however, especially in patients presenting with ischemic injury in other sites (e.g., stroke), as the diagnosis may lead to a change in therapy (anticoagulation).

37. Describe the treatment of retinal vasculitis.

The treatment of retinal vasculitis depends on the underlying diagnosis, the severity of the disease, and whether the process is unilateral or bilateral. If its cause is infectious, appropriate antimicrobial therapy should be initiated. Corticosteroids are needed in almost all cases, including those secondary to infection. Periocular or intraocular steroids may be used in patients with moderate to severe disease or in those with unilateral involvement. Systemic steroids are needed when bilateral involvement is present and in cases of moderate to severe inflammation with a marked decrease in visual acuity.

Steroid-sparing agents may be needed if there is an inadequate response to steroids or they cannot be tapered, and selection should be based on the underlying disease. Methotrexate, azathioprine, mycophenolate mofetil, anti-TNF therapies, and rituximab may be effective. Laser photocoagulation, antivascular endothelial growth factor agents (e.g., bevacizumab), and vitreoretinal procedures may also have a role in treating retinal neovascularization.

38. Briefly describe the defining features of Susac syndrome.

Susac syndrome is a microangiopathy of unclear etiology causing **encephalopathy** (corpus callosum involvement is prominent), **branch retinal artery occlusions (BRAOs)**, and **sensori-neural hearing loss** (SNHL). Headache can be a prominent feature (seen in >75% of patients). The disease commonly affects young women (80%) aged 15 to 40 years, with no racial or ethnic predilection. Diagnosis is based on characteristic clinical features and MRI findings and is made challenging by the fact that <20% of patients present with simultaneous involvement of the classic triad of clinical features.

The treatment regimen in the acute setting includes high-dose corticosteroids (3-day pulse therapy of solumedrol 500–1000 mg/day followed by prednisone 1 mg/kg for 2 to 4 weeks with subsequent taper) and consideration of intravenous immunoglobulin therapy. Corticosteroid-sparing immunosuppressive therapies that have been used include mycophenolate mofetil, rituximab, cyclophosphamide, azathioprine, and cyclosporine. Plasmapheresis has been described in the acute setting as well. Some experts recommend the addition of aspirin to reduce the risk of small-vessel thrombosis. Unfortunately, hearing and visual field loss suffered at the time of diagnosis is irreversible, and treatment is instituted to prevent further loss.

ORBITAL INFLAMMATORY DISEASE

39. What is orbital inflammatory disease (OID), and what rheumatic conditions are associated with it?

OID is a term that encompasses inflammation involving various structures in the orbital space outside of the globe, including the extraocular muscles, lacrimal gland, and orbital adipose tissue. Symptoms vary based on disease severity and the specific ocular structures involved but may include pain, orbital swelling, diplopia, chemosis, and proptosis. Severe forms of the disease may lead to optic nerve compression, and in some patients, proptosis may alter the shape of the eye and increase risk of exposure keratopathy. **GPA, sarcoidosis, and IgG4-related disease (IgG4-RD)** are among the most common rheumatologic conditions associated with OID, and an evaluation for those conditions should be considered in patients presenting with OID. Less common rheumatologic causes of OID include SjD (typically presenting with mild dacryoadenitis), IBD, Behçet disease, RA, SLE, adult-onset Still's disease, amyloidosis, and histiocytic disorders.

40. What nonrheumatologic conditions are associated with OID?

Thyroid eye disease is the most common cause of OID overall, representing half of cases. Other diseases associated with OID include ocular lymphoma/lymphoproliferative disease, metastatic disease affecting the orbit, and Tolosa–Hunt syndrome. Idiopathic disease (also referred to as **nonspecific orbital inflammation**) can be a common cause of OID and is a diagnosis of exclusion.

41. Describe an initial evaluation of a patient presenting with OID.

The history and examination should guide further testing. Initial laboratory studies may include a CBC, comprehensive metabolic panel, UA, ESR, CRP, thyroid studies (thyroid-stimulating hormone, T4, antithyroid antibodies including thyroperoxidase, thyroglobulin, and thyroid-stimulating antibodies), serum IgG4, and ANCAs. MRI of the orbits is commonly obtained to delineate the anatomic structures involved and may allow for discrimination between thyroid eye disease and other causes of OID. A chest radiograph or CT should be considered to rule out concurrent pulmonary involvement from sarcoidosis or GPA. Biopsy is required to rule out infectious and neoplastic etiologies in patients in whom the initial evaluation has not identified a clear etiology. In addition to histologic examination, staining should be performed for fungal and mycobacterial organisms as well as IgG4-specific staining to rule out IgG4-RD.

42. Describe the treatment of OID.

The treatment of OID depends on the etiology of the underlying condition. Patients with rheumatologic conditions such as GPA-causing OID are commonly treated with similar medications used for extraocular organ involvement (such as high-dose steroids, methotrexate, azathioprine, rituximab, or cyclophosphamide in the case of ANCA-associated vasculitis). Patients with sarcoidosis may have concurrent OID that is relatively mild in nature and warrants observation alone. More significant involvement may be treated with corticosteroids, methotrexate, azathioprine, or infliximab. Patients with IgG4-RD and OID may be treated with corticosteroids, with rituximab reserved for resistant disease, those failing steroid therapy, or patients with significant extraocular disease involvement.

The treatment of thyroid-associated ocular disease is beyond the scope of this chapter, but commonly includes reversal of hyperthyroidism if present (through oral medications and/or consideration of thyroidectomy), corticosteroids (including high-dose pulse intravenous therapy at onset), and complete cessation of tobacco use by the patient if applicable. In patients with sight-threatening disease, orbital decompression may be considered. Orbital radiation can be used in steroid-resistant cases, but its use may be limited by toxicity (risk of retinal and optic nerve damage). Steroid-sparing immunosuppression with rituximab and mycophenolate mofetil have mixed results in the literature. Teprotumumab is a newer monoclonal antibody directed against insulin-like growth factor-1 and is now FDA-approved for the treatment of thyroid eye disease.

IMMUNE-MEDIATED INNER EAR DISEASE

43. Define immune-mediated inner ear disease (IMIED; also known as autoimmune inner ear disease).

IMIED is a syndrome characterized by *rapidly progressive, bilateral SNHL* that can be responsive to immunosuppressive therapy. It is often accompanied by vertigo (50%), tinnitus, and a sense of aural fullness. It may exist as a primary illness or be associated with a systemic autoimmune disease (30% of cases). Although believed to be autoimmune, definitive evidence of an autoimmune etiology is lacking.

Caution should be taken to distinguish IMIED from idiopathic sudden SNHL, a very common cause of acute SNHL that is *unilateral,* rapidly progresses over 72 hours, *usually not associated with vestibular symptoms,* and commonly improves within 2 weeks (65% of cases) irrespective of treatment (although corticosteroids are frequently used). It is estimated that 85% of such cases are idiopathic (with up to 5% developing Ménière disease years later). All patients with sudden SNHL should be evaluated for secondary causes (15% of cases) including infection (HSV, VZV), vascular insult (vasculitis, APS, hypercoagulable diseases, atherosclerotic disease), medications, neoplasm (including those causing localized retrocochlear disease), and immune-mediated diseases. Patients with unilateral SNHL have diminished ability to hear a tuning fork and localize the sound during a Weber test (tuning fork on forehead) to the good ear. When they hum, the sound localizes to the good ear as well.

44. What is the differential diagnosis of IMIED?

Ménière disease, infection (syphilis, Lyme, viral, TB, fungal or bacterial labrynthitis), acoustic or barotrauma, perilymph fistula, hereditary hearing loss, drugs (e.g., aminoglycosides, hydroxychloroquine, NSAIDs, loop diuretics), mass effect from a tumor (acoustic neuroma, metastatic disease, lymphoma) or an abscess, presbycusis, ischemia, multiple sclerosis, basilar migraine, endocrine disease (diabetes mellitus, hypothyroid), sarcoidosis.

45. What characteristics help distinguish IMIED from other causes of inner ear dysfunction?

- **Relatively rapid time course,** with progression to severe irreversible damage within weeks to months of onset.
- **Bilateral disease** that may be asymmetric and asynchronous.
- **Fluctuating course**.
- *Vestibular symptoms* may be prominent (50%).

46. How is Ménière disease distinguished from IMIED?

Time course. Hearing loss typically occurs over several years in Ménière disease rather than weeks or months in IMIED. These two disease entities may be impossible to differentiate early in the disease course. Some data suggest that a subset of Ménière may be autoimmune in nature and possibly part of a spectrum of diseases including IMIED.

47. What systemic autoimmune diseases[*] are associated with SNHL?

Cogan syndrome, ANCA-associated vasculitides[**], relapsing polychondritis, polyarteritis nodosa and other vasculitides, SLE, SjD, RA, Susac syndrome, APS, Behçet disease, and sarcoidosis.

*When these systemic diseases are associated with sudden onset, bilateral SNHL, and other manifestations of IMIED, it is considered secondary IMIED.

**GPA is more commonly associated with conductive and mixed conductive-SNHL.

48. What diagnostic workup is indicated in a patient suspected of having IMIED?

Immediate referral to an otolaryngologist is necessary. Routine history, physical exam, and diagnostic tests including a CBC, comprehensive metabolic panel, ESR, CRP, testing for syphilis, and MRI to exclude a retrocochlear lesion should be performed to evaluate for other causes of SNHL or an associated systemic process. Disease severity should be measured at baseline and followed serially with audiograms.

The role of testing for ANCA, ANA, RF, complement levels, and APS studies in patients with no other evidence of a systemic autoimmune illness is unclear. ANA, RF, low-moderate titer antiphospholipid antibodies, and antithyroid antibodies are frequently detected in patients with IMIED who lack features of systemic disease and the antibodies do not have clear prognostic value in this setting.

49. Are there any specific diagnostic tests for IMIED?

Antibodies to a 68-kDa inner ear antigen, which is a heat shock protein (HSP-70), may be seen in up to 70% of patients with IMIED. Due to relatively low sensitivity, this test is unreliable to exclude a diagnosis of IMIED. Patients with Cogan syndrome and other autoimmune diseases associated with SNHL can also have these antibodies (<50%), although the specificity compared with normal control populations may be as high as 90%. Some studies suggest that their presence may have a prognostic role, in predicting both a more aggressive course and a more favorable response to steroids. Data on antibody specificity and association with steroid response are controversial, however, with conflicting data in the literature.

50. What is the treatment for IMIED?

Corticosteroids should be started at a dose of 1 mg/kg per day and continued for 2 to 4 weeks. If there is no response, they should be tapered off quickly over a period of 2 weeks. If a response in hearing is documented by repeat audiology testing after a 2- to 4-week trial of therapy, steroid tapering should be performed at a slower rate over an additional 2 to 3 months. There is no consensus regarding whether corticosteroid-sparing therapy should be given concurrently at the time of diagnosis or which agents to consider in patients who relapse during steroid taper, as data from clinical trials are limited. Methotrexate, azathioprine, mycophenolate mofetil, anti-TNF therapy (systemic and intratympanic), rituximab, cyclophosphamide, and intratympanic steroids have also been used with variable success (although a placebo-controlled trial of methotrexate failed to show benefit). Interpretation of the efficacy of these agents is limited given the lack of systematic studies. Given the toxicities of these therapies, cochlear implants should be considered as an alternative in severe cases.

COGAN'S SYNDROME

51. What is Cogan syndrome?

Cogan syndrome is often classified among the systemic vasculitides and is characterized by ocular inflammation (classically **interstitial keratitis**), **sensorineural hearing loss and vestibular symptoms**, and variable involvement with **systemic vasculitis**. Typical features include:
- Ocular involvement: classic lesion is nonsyphilitic interstitial keratitis
- Audiovestibular symptoms
- Constitutional symptoms (50%): fever, weight loss, adenopathy, hepatosplenomegaly, arthritis
- Systemic vasculitis (10–20%): Usually affects the large- and medium-sized vessels. Involvement of the aorta and its major branches is well described and typically manifests in a Takayasu-like manner, with risk for aortitis with aortic insufficiency/aneurysm (10%), coronary vasculitis, and aortic/mitral valvulitis.
- Other manifestations (most often seen with systemic involvement including vasculitis): gastrointestinal (pain, bleeding, hepatomegaly), cardiac (pericarditis), pulmonary (pleuritis), neurologic (headache, peripheral neuropathy, mononeuritis multiplex, meningitis), dermatologic (nodules, rash, purpura, digital gangrene), and lymphatic (lymphadenopathy, splenomegaly).
- Laboratory abnormalities: anemia, leukocytosis, thrombocytosis, elevated ESR and CRP. Rarely anti-myeloperoxidase (perinuclear antineutrophil cytoplasmic antibodies) and anti-Hsp-70 antibodies.

52. What is the epidemiology of Cogan syndrome?

Since its original description in 1945, approximately 250–300 cases have been reported. Mean age of onset is 30 years, although cases in children and the elderly have been reported. Distribution is equal between males and females, and there are no racial or ethnic differences. An upper respiratory syndrome precedes the onset in many cases, but no definite infectious etiology has been identified.

53. What are the specific ocular and auricular manifestations of Cogan syndrome?

Nonsyphilitic interstitial keratitis (IK) is the classic ocular manifestation and typically presents as the acute onset of unilateral or bilateral redness, pain, photophobia, and increased lacrimation. Other forms of ocular inflammation including uveitis, scleritis, choroiditis, and retinal artery occlusion can occur with or without concomitant keratitis.

Vestibuloauditory dysfunction is usually acute in onset and presents in a Ménière-like manner, with episodes of tinnitus, vertigo, and SNHL. Hearing loss is fluctuating but progressive, leading to deafness in >50% of cases. Unilateral involvement is typical, but bilateral disease can occur. Vestibular dysfunction may be prominent, manifesting as vertigo, ataxia, and nausea.

Eye and ear involvement usually occurs within 1 to 6 months of each other, but can be separated by years.

Atypical Cogan syndrome is defined as non-IK inflammatory ocular manifestations, typical or atypical ocular manifestations with audiovestibular symptoms different from Ménière-like episodes, or >2 years between the onset of eye and ear manifestations.

54. What is the differential diagnosis of Cogan syndrome?

Infection (syphilis, chlamydia, TB, viral infection, Whipple's disease), rheumatologic diseases (systemic vasculitides, relapsing polychondritis, Behçet, sarcoidosis), toxins, Ménière disease, and VKH syndrome.

55. How is the diagnosis of Cogan syndrome established?

It is a clinical diagnosis and should be suspected when IK or other ocular manifestations are accompanied by audiovestibular disease in the absence of another underlying disorder (see differential diagnosis earlier). The presence of either ocular or ear manifestations in isolation can make the diagnosis extremely challenging. Slit-lamp examination and audiovestibular testing are necessary. Laboratory evidence of systemic inflammation may be present. There is no role for checking autoantibodies unless clinical suspicion exists for a particular associated disorder. Microbiologic testing and MRI of the brain to evaluate for a tumor-causing inner ear disease can be considered.

56. How is Cogan syndrome treated? What is the prognosis?

Keratitis almost always responds to topical corticosteroid therapy. Topical cyclosporine is sometimes required, but the need for systemic steroids is rare (unless other ocular manifestations are present and dictate therapy). Note that keratitis resolves quickly on systemic corticosteroids. Therefore, an immediate eye exam is needed to document keratitis if the patient has another manifestation requiring high-dose corticosteroids. Otherwise, keratitis will be missed.

Vestibuloauditory dysfunction is less responsive to therapy in general. Oral prednisone is required and should be started at a dose of 1 mg/kg per day for 2 to 4 weeks. The usual tapering schedule is 10 mg every 2 to 4 weeks thereafter, with a total duration of 3 to 6 months (if positive treatment response). Audiovestibular testing should be repeated 2 to 4 weeks after the initiation of treatment, and prednisone should be tapered quickly if no response is noted. A response to additional immunosuppression is unlikely if prednisone has failed. If an initial response is noted but relapse occurs as prednisone is tapered, a steroid-sparing agent should be initiated (methotrexate, azathioprine, mycophenolate mofetil).

Systemic manifestations such as vasculitis should be treated by standard immunosuppressants (e.g., cytotoxic or biologic agents, azathioprine, methotrexate; cyclophosphamide is most commonly described in the literature for large and medium vessel vasculitis).

Some patients recover after a single episode. However, most patients have exacerbations with over 50% sustaining permanent hearing loss. Cochlear implants can be beneficial for these patients. Vascular surgery may be necessary for aortic valve replacement or aneurysm repair.

BIBLIOGRAPHY

Bañares A, Jover J, Fernández-Gutiérrez B, et al. Patterns of uveitis as a guide in making rheumatologic and immunologic diagnoses. *Arthritis Rheum.* 1997;40:358–370.

Broughton SS. Immune-mediated inner ear disease: 10-year experience. *Semin Arthritis Rheum.* 2004;34(2):544–548.

Ciorba A, Corazzi V, Bianchini C, et al. Autoimmune inner ear disease (AIED): a diagnostic challenge. *Int J Immunopathol Pharmacol.* 2018. doi:10.1177/2058738418808680.

Foster CS. The ocular immunology and uveitis foundation preferred practice patterns of uveitis management. *Surv Ophthalmol.* 2016;61(1):1–17.

Goodall AF. Current understanding of the pathogenesis of autoimmune inner ear disease: a review. *Clin Otolaryngol.* 2015;40:412–419.

Jabs DA, Mudun A, Dunn JP, Marsh MJ. Episcleritis and scleritis: clinical features and treatment results. *Am J Ophthalmol.* 2000;130(4):469–476.

Jabs DA. Immunosuppression for the uveitides. *Ophthalmology.* 2018;125(2):193–202.

Jabs DA. Interobserver agreement among uveitis experts on uveitic diagnoses: the standardization of uveitis nomenclature experience. *Am J Ophthalmol.* 2018;186:19–24.

Jakob E, Reuland MS, Mackensen F, et al. Uveitis subtypes in a German interdisciplinary uveitis center—analysis of 1916 patents. *J Rheumatol.* 2009;36:127–136.

Lutt JR, Rosenbaum JT. Orbital inflammatory disease. *Semin Arthritis Rheum.* 2008;37(4):207–222.

Mazlumzadeh M, Matteson EL. Cogan's syndrome: an audiovestibular, ocular, and systemic autoimmune disease. *Rheum Dis Clin N Am.* 2007;33:855–874.

Rathinam SR, Gonzales JA, Thundikandy R, et al. Effect of corticosteroid-sparing treatment with mycophenolate mofetil vs methotrexate on inflammation in patients with uveitis: a randomized clinical trial. *JAMA*. 2019;322(10):936–945.

Rauch SD. Idiopathic sudden sensorineural hearing loss. *N Engl J Med*. 2008;359:833–840.

Smith JR, Mackensen F, Rosenbaum JT. Therapy insight: scleritis and its relationship to systemic autoimmune disease. *Nat Clin Pract Rheumatol*. 2007;3:219–226.

Stacher RJ, Chandrasekhar SS, Archer SM, et al. Clinical practice guideline: sudden hearing loss. *Otolaryngol Head Neck Surg*. 2012;146(suppl):S1–S35.

Stone JH, Francis HW. Immune-mediated inner ear disease. *Curr Opin Rheumatol*. 2000;12:32–40.

Suslu N. Utility of anti-HSP 70, TNF-alpha, ESR, ANA, and antiphospholipid antibodies in the diagnosis and treatment of sudden sensorineural hearing loss. *Laryngoscope*. 2009;119:341–346.

Vodopivec I. Clinical features, diagnostic findings, and treatment of Susac syndrome: a case series. *J Neurol Sci*. 2015;357:50–57.

Zamecki KJ, Jabs DA. HLA typing in uveitis: use and misuse. *Am J Ophthalmol*. 2010;149:189–193.

WEBSITES

Learning the Lingo (a list of nomenclature commonly used in ophthalmology clinical notes, from the American Academy of Ophthalmology): https://www.aao.org/young-ophthalmologists/yo-info/article/learning-lingo-ophthalmic-abbreviations.

Uveitis Foundation: http://www.uveitis.org/default.html.

CHAPTER 75

Rheumatic Syndromes Associated With Sarcoidosis

Patompong Ungprasert, MD and Manuel L. Ribeiro Neto, MD

1. What is sarcoidosis?

The first description of sarcoidosis in the medical literature was in 1877 by Dr. Jonathan Hutchinson at King's College Hospital, London. It is a systemic inflammatory disorder characterized by **noncaseating granulomas** that classically involve the lung, but can affect virtually any organ. The classic sarcoidosis granuloma consists of a central area of epithelioid cells (activated macrophages which at times merge to form multinucleated giant cells), as well as tightly packed CD4-positive T lymphocytes, in the absence of necrosis. The central core is surrounded by CD4 and CD8 positive T lymphocytes, B lymphocytes, monocytes, mast cells and fibroblasts. The granuloma is often surrounded by fibrosis, especially in more established disease. Since there is no specific test for sarcoidosis, the diagnosis is established when the following criteria are met:

- A consistent clinical and radiographic presentation.
- Histologic evidence of noncaseating epithelioid granulomas in at least one organ.
- Exclusion of other granulomatous diseases caused by mycobacterial or fungal infection, berylliosis, medications, or local tissue reactions to adjacent malignancy.

While the diagnosis typically relies on tissue biopsy, there are certain situations in which a presumptive diagnosis can be made based on clinical and radiographic findings, such as the presence of asymptomatic bilateral hilar adenopathy, Lofgren syndrome, or Heerfordt syndrome (see Fig. 75.1).

2. Who is affected by sarcoidosis?

The highest incidence is among African Americans (20–35 cases per 100,000 person-years) and Whites (5–10 per 100,000 person-years). In the United States, the incidence is three-fold higher among African Americans than Whites, and the average age of onset is 10 years younger among African Americans. Sarcoidosis is less common among Asians and Hispanics (1–3 per 100,000 person-years). There appears to be a slight female predominance. The median age at diagnosis is between 35 and 45 years (70% of patients are diagnosed between 20 and 40 years of age). There is a higher prevalence of disease in first-generation relatives. Obesity is associated with an increased risk of sarcoidosis. Conversely, smoking is associated with a lower risk.

3. What are the immunopathologic features of sarcoidosis?

The etiology of sarcoidosis remains unknown, but it is believed to be caused by an abnormal immune response to environmental exposures in genetically susceptible individuals. Because the lungs are involved in 95% of those affected, it is likely that initial exposure to an inciting environmental or infectious agent is via the pulmonary route. The presence of foreign antigen(s) is thought to be the first step to stimulate monocytes to differentiate into macrophages or dendritic

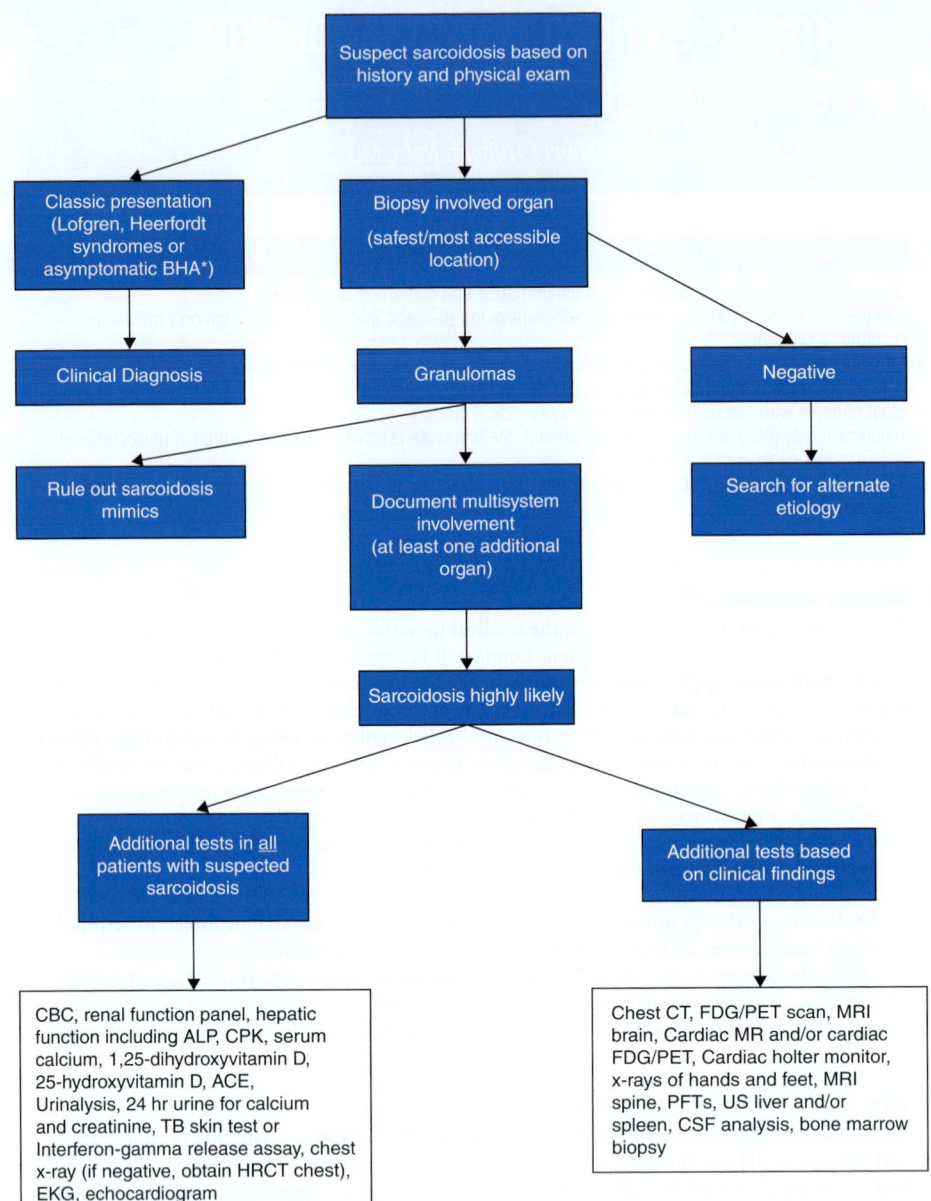

Fig 75.1 The Approach to Diagnosis of Sarcoidosis.

cells, which then present antigen(s) to CD4 positive T lymphocytes, resulting in increased secretion of cytokines including interferon (IFN)-gamma, interleukin-2 and tumor necrosis factor (TNF)-alpha. The release of IFN gamma and TNF alpha promotes macrophage activation and aggregation, resulting in the formation of noncaseating granulomas.

The abundance of CD4 positive T cells in the granuloma has diagnostic implications as well. Bronchoalveolar lavage (BAL) fluid typically reveals a lymphocytosis (>15%) and a marked increase in CD4/CD8 T-lymphocyte ratio (>3.5), especially in early and active disease.

TABLE 75.1 Frequency of Organ Involvement in Sarcoidosis

ORGAN	FREQUENCY
Pulmonary	95–98%
Hilar and mediastinal lymph nodes	80–90%
Lung parenchyma	40–50%
Skin	20–30%
Eye	10–25%
Joint	10–20%
Liver	5–20%
Hypercalcemia	5–10%
Nervous system	3–10%
Heart	1–3%
Kidney	1–3%
Bone	1–3%
Parotid gland	1%
Muscle	1%

Additionally, there is an influx of T-helper cells and an elevated ratio of CD4/CD8 T-cell subsets in other affected organs, hyperactivity of B cells, and circulation of immune complexes. Typical clinical observations related to these immunologic events include peripheral lymphopenia (due to sequestration at the site of inflammation), a low CD4/CD8 T-cell ratio in peripheral blood, cutaneous anergy, polyclonal gammopathy (30–80%), and autoantibody production (low titer rheumatoid factor and/or antinuclear antibody in approximately one-third of patients).

4. What organs are affected by sarcoidosis?

Virtually any organ can be affected by sarcoidosis. However, intrathoracic disease (either mediastinal/hilar adenopathy and/or pulmonary infiltration) is by far the most common organ involvement, seen in more than 95% of patients. Therefore, you should think twice before diagnosing someone with sarcoidosis without intrathoracic involvement. Multiple large series report that 50% of patients have extrathoracic involvement, and only 2% have isolated extrathoracic sarcoidosis. The frequency of organ involvement in sarcoidosis is summarized in Table 75.1. Notably, there are significant differences in clinical findings, incidence of organ involvement, and mortality between groups on the basis of race and ethnicity, sex, and age. Furthermore, because sarcoidosis is often asymptomatic, the reported prevalence of the disease and organ involvement is likely underestimated.

5. Describe the manifestations of pulmonary sarcoidosis.

Even though pulmonary involvement is extremely common in patients with sarcoidosis, only half of the patients have respiratory symptoms, including dry cough (30%) and dyspnea (30%). Crackles on exam are uncommon, even in the presence of lung parenchymal disease. As such, thoracic imaging is required if there is clinical suspicion for sarcoidosis, regardless of respiratory symptoms or exam findings. Pleural effusion is rare (<5%). Pulmonary hypertension has been increasingly recognized (up to 20%). The prognosis of pulmonary sarcoidosis is good, as spontaneous resolution is common, especially in early-stage disease. Chronic respiratory failure is seen in less than 10% over long-term follow-up.

6. Describe the imaging findings in pulmonary sarcoidosis.

Mediastinal/hilar lymphadenopathy and/or pulmonary infiltrates are the characteristic findings on chest X-ray. Radiographic classification is usually separated into four stages (**the Scadding staging system**), as described in Table 75.2. The different 'stages' are perhaps more aptly described as radiographic patterns, as they are not chronologic, do not indicate disease chronicity, and do not

TABLE 75.2 Radiographic Findings, Frequency, and Spontaneous Remission Rate

STAGE	CHEST RADIOGRAPHIC FINDINGS	FREQUENCY AT DIAGNOSIS (%)	SPONTANEOUS REMISSION RATE (%)
0	Normal	5	–
1	Hilar adenopathy (usually bilateral)	40–50	70–90
2	Hilar adenopathy (usually bilateral) *with pulmonary infiltrates*	30–40	50–60
3	Pulmonary infiltrates with lung insufficiency (no hilar adenopathy)	15–20	10–20
4	End-stage pulmonary fibrosis with volume loss	2–5	0

correlate with pulmonary function testing. Plain radiography is relatively insensitive for some of these imaging findings; therefore, high-resolution computed tomography (HRCT) of the chest should be performed if the initial chest X-ray is negative and clinical suspicion remains high. HRCT is often able to detect more subtle lymphadenopathy and parenchymal disease, including the characteristic finding of small (2–5 mm) nodules in a perilymphatic distribution (bronchovascular bundles, interlobular septa, interlobar fissures, and subpleural regions) with upper-middle lobe predominance. Importantly, imaging at presentation can be used to predict the probability of future spontaneous remission, which can help guide therapy.

7. **What are the cutaneous and ocular manifestations of sarcoidosis?**

The two most common extrathoracic manifestations of sarcoidosis are cutaneous and ocular involvement.

Cutaneous sarcoidosis (30% of patients) can be categorized into sarcoidosis-specific skin lesions (skin lesions with noncaseating granuloma on histopathology) and non-specific skin lesions commonly associated with sarcoidosis (such as erythema nodosum). Erythema nodosum (EN) more commonly occurs in acute-onset sarcoidosis, while subcutaneous nodules, papules, plaques, tattoo/scar sarcoidosis, and lupus pernio typically occur in chronic-onset disease.
- EN typically presents as painful, erythematous nodules on the anterior surface of the lower extremities. Histopathology reveals a **septal panniculitis without granuloma**, indistinguishable from idiopathic EN and other secondary forms.
- Papules, plaques, and subcutaneous nodules are the most common sarcoidosis-specific skin lesions.
- Cutaneous papules and plaques may be various colors on exam (skin-colored, yellow-brown, erythematous, violaceous, hyper/hypopigmented), including variation among patients of color; hence, a high index of suspicion should be maintained. These lesions are most commonly found on the extremities as well as the head and neck area.
- Erythematous and violaceous papules and plaques can also occur on the nose, cheeks, and ears; this form of cutaneous involvement is called **lupus pernio** due to the similar pattern of distribution as the malar rash in systemic lupus erythematosus (SLE). This term is sometimes considered a misnomer, as the lesion neither reflects SLE nor pernio (chilblains).
- Subcutaneous nodules represent granulomatous inflammation within the adipose tissue. These lesions are usually painless, with normal overlying skin, and are commonly found on the lower extremities.

Ocular involvement has been reported in up to **25% of patients**, with uveitis the most common form of involvement. Acute anterior uveitis is the most common subtype among White populations, while posterior uveitis (painless visual loss with floaters) and panuveitis are more prevalent among African Americans. Consultation with an ophthalmologist may provide useful clues to the diagnosis, as characteristic (but not pathognomonic) features such as granulomatous uveitis, 'mutton-fat' keratic precipitates, iris and/or trabecular meshwork nodules, and 'string of pearl' vitreous opacities, may be identified. Additional forms of ocular involvement include conjunctivitis/conjunctival nodules, scleritis, episcleritis, lacrimal gland involvement, choroidal nodules, optic neuritis, and orbital inflammatory disease.

TABLE 75.3 Comparison of Acute and Chronic Sarcoid Arthritis

FEATURES	ACUTE	CHRONIC
Initial clinical manifestation	Common	Not seen
Joint involvement	Symmetrical; ankles, knees, wrists, elbows, proximal interphalangeal joint	Same as acute, dactylitis
Hilar adenopathy	Common, no pulmonary infiltrates	May be seen with pulmonary involvement
Synovial fluid	Usually not obtainable	Mildly inflammatory; <5000 cells/mm^3
Synovial biopsy	Synovial hyperplasia, non-specific inflammation	Sarcoid granuloma
Destructive bony lesions	Absent	Present
Clinical course	Benign, self-limited	Chronic

Modified from Mathur A, Kremer JM. Immunology, rheumatic features, and therapy of sarcoidosis. *Curr Opin Rheumatol.* 1992;4:76–80.

8. Describe sarcoid arthropathy.

Arthralgias are present in the majority of patients, but **inflammatory arthritis is reported in** 10% to 20% and is classified as acute or chronic arthritis. The acute form is more common, and often occurs in the setting of Lofgren syndrome. The classic presentation is acute oligoarthritis with involvement of the medium to large joints, especially the ankles (in over 90% of cases). The joint swelling may be due to a periarthritis rather than true synovitis. Polyarthritis with involvement of the small joints of hands is seen very infrequently, and other diagnoses, such as rheumatoid arthritis, should be ruled out first. Resolution of inflammatory arthritis usually occurs within 6 weeks in most patients, and within 2 years in almost all patients. **As such, chronic inflammatory arthritis is extremely uncommon.** Tenosynovitis (especially Achilles tendinitis) has been reported in 5% to 10% of patients.

Synovial biopsy is typically not required, but if performed, may reveal non-specific inflammation in acute sarcoid arthritis and noncaseating granuloma in chronic arthritis. Table 75.3 lists additional distinguishing features of acute and chronic sarcoid arthritis.

9. Describe other musculoskeletal manifestations of sarcoidosis.

Osseous sarcoidosis is seen in up to 3% of patients. Over half of the cases are asymptomatic and found incidentally on imaging (Fig. 75.2). The phalanges of the hands and feet are classic locations, but any skeletal site can be involved. Bony lesions are associated with chronic overlying cutaneous lesions and multi-organ sarcoidosis. Typical radiographic findings include osteolysis, causing multiple cyst-like radiolucent areas within the trabecular bone (sometimes referred to as a 'lacy pattern') and punched-out cortical lesions that may be difficult to differentiate from malignancy. Bone scans, magnetic resonance imaging (MRI), and fluorodeoxyglucose-positron emission tomography (PET) scans are able to detect additional asymptomatic lesions, and have identified additional sites of skeletal involvement, including the axial spine.

Symptomatic **sarcoid myopathy** is rare (less than 1% of patients) and typically occurs in patients with multi-organ involvement. There are three clinical patterns in symptomatic disease: nodular myopathy, acute myositis, and chronic myopathy.
- Chronic myopathy is the most common pattern. Its clinical presentation includes the insidious onset of painless, progressive, symmetric, proximal muscle weakness. Muscle enzymes are usually normal or only mildly elevated, and atrophy can occur.
- The acute myositis form typically presents with the abrupt onset of painful, bilateral, proximal muscle weakness with elevated muscle enzymes. It is usually accompanied by constitutional symptoms (fever, fatigue, arthralgia, and erythema nodosum) and is more commonly seen in younger, female patients, especially African-American women.
- Nodular myopathy is the least common type, presenting as single or multiple painful nodules at the musculotendinous junction. It is not associated with muscle weakness or elevated

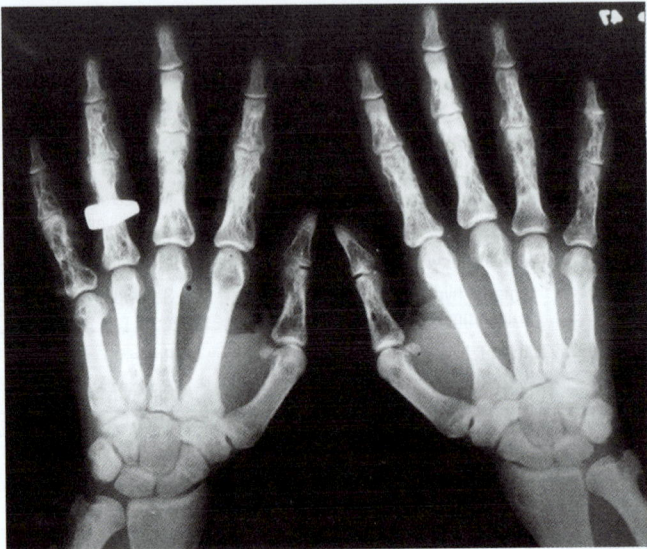

Fig 75.2 Osseous sarcoidosis involving the hands. The phalanges demonstrate a coarsened, reticulated, lacelike trabecular pattern.

muscle enzymes. It produces a distinguishing finding on muscle MRI: a star-shaped central structure of decreased signal intensity (the "dark star" sign), within the nodule.
- Muscle biopsy usually reveals noncaseating granulomas with a high CD4/CD8 T-lymphocyte ratio in all three patterns, which is helpful to differentiate from idiopathic inflammatory myositis.
- Asymptomatic patients with any of these patterns of myopathy do not typically require treatment.
- Corticosteroid injections have been attempted in patients with nodular myopathy, but systemic GCs may be required, given the relative inaccessibility of the lesions.
- Systemic GCs are typically utilized in acute myositis, and may be used in patients with chronic myopathy who have signs of ongoing inflammation (elevated CK, evidence of inflammation on muscle biopsy or MRI)

10. What is Lofgren syndrome? What is Heerfordt syndrome?

Lofgren syndrome is a triad of acute arthritis/periarthritis, erythema nodosum, and bilateral hilar adenopathy in a patient with sarcoidosis. This can be associated with fever and uveitis (6%). Joint involvement most commonly presents as an arthritis and/or periarthritis of the ankles. Nonsteroidal antiinflammatory drugs are recommended initially, but low-dose GCs may be clinically necessary to manage if severe symptoms exist. The ACE level is elevated in less than half of the cases. However, those with an elevated ACE level are more likely to have recurrence or persistence of the arthritis. Overall, these patients have a >90% remission rate. Acute histoplasmosis may simulate Lofgren syndrome and must be excluded by serologies, urine antigen, and cultures.

    Heerfordt syndrome (uveoparotid fever) is a combination of fever, parotid enlargement, uveitis, arthritis, and facial nerve palsy. It occurs most commonly in males and usually has a poor prognosis. Moderate-dose GCs and chronic immunosuppressive therapy are typically necessary to manage clinical manifestations.

11. What are some other extrathoracic manifestations of sarcoidosis?

Hepatic involvement (5–20%)
- Most patients are asymptomatic and diagnosed incidentally by abnormal liver chemistry tests and/or imaging studies. The most common laboratory pattern is elevated alkaline phosphatase and GGT, with normal or mildly elevated ALT and AST enzymes.
- Imaging studies may reveal hypodense nodules and/or hepatosplenomegaly.

Hypercalcemia (5–10%)
- Caused by overproduction of 1,25-dihydroxyvitamin D by activated macrophages, due to increased activity of the 1-α-hydroxylase enzyme in granulomas.
- This results in increased intestinal calcium absorption and resultant hypercalcemia and hypercalciuria. Calcium imbalance can be associated with nephrolithiasis and renal failure.

Nervous System (3–10%)
- May be the presenting manifestation of sarcoidosis (this is the case in 50–70% of patients with central nervous system [CNS] involvement)
- In patients with CNS sarcoidosis: cranial nerve involvement (optic and facial nerve most prominently) is most common (50–70% of cases), followed by meningeal disease (10–15%), parenchymal brain lesions, stroke-like presentations, and myelopathy.
- Patients with leptomeningeal involvement usually present with subacute to chronic onset of headache and constitutional symptoms. Cerebrospinal fluid (CSF) analysis usually reveals a monocytic pleocytosis with high protein and a normal glucose level. Elevated CSF CD4/CD8 ratio and IL-6 levels may help distinguish from other conditions such as multiple sclerosis and neuromyelitis optica (NMO).
- Intraparenchymal granulomatous lesions are less common. They present as a solitary mass or multiple nodules, and may cause focal neurologic deficit, seizure, or increased intra-cranial pressure. Sellar lesions can occur and may classically present as diabetes insipidus.
- Peripheral and small fiber-neuropathy can occur as well (see Question 18).

Cardiovascular (1–3%)
- Granulomatous inflammation of the myocardium and/or the conduction system can occur.
- Patients may present with dysrhythmia (most commonly atrioventricular block), conduction abnormalities, or cardiomyopathy.
- Many patients with such involvement (especially early in disease) may be asymptomatic. As such, most experts recommend a screening EKG and echocardiogram in patients diagnosed with sarcoidosis.
- Autopsy studies show that up to 25% of patients have evidence of granulomas on cardiac biopsy.

Hematologic
- Anemia and leukopenia can be seen. Anemia of chronic disease is most common, but bone marrow involvement may be found in up to 27% of anemic patients. Leukopenia may be due to sequestration of lymphocytes to sites of inflammation or hypersplenism.

Parotid gland enlargement
- Seen in approximately 1% of patients and can be associated with xerostomia and Heerfordt syndrome

  Kidney and **gastrointestinal** organs are rarely affected.

  Vasculitis of any size vessel has been described.

12. Describe a diagnostic approach to a patient with suspected sarcoidosis (Fig. 75.1).

The diagnosis of sarcoidosis is centered on the presence of noncaseating granuloma on histopathology, compatible clinical presentation, and exclusion of other causes of granulomatous inflammation. Tissue biopsy is not required for every affected organ, as presence of noncaseating granuloma in at least one site is generally considered sufficient for diagnosis. In this scenario, involvement of the other organs is generally assumed from a compatible clinical presentation and non-invasive studies. This is particularly important for hard-to-access organs, including the heart, central nervous system, and eyes.

Histopathologic confirmation is not typically pursued in patients with asymptomatic, isolated stage I pulmonary sarcoidosis. In these patients, the presence of bilateral hilar adenopathy alone is generally considered sufficient for diagnosis after exclusion of other possible etiologies, especially in light of the high rate of spontaneous resolution. Similarly, characteristic presentations such as Lofgren and Heerfordt syndromes are thought to be highly associated with sarcoidosis; hence, biopsy confirmation is not typically pursued. A proposed diagnostic algorithm is outlined in Fig. 75.1, including suggested baseline testing in patients with suspected sarcoidosis.

13. Which anatomic sites should be biopsied?

The skin, ocular conjunctiva, superficial lymph nodes, and lacrimal glands are all preferential sites for biopsy based on accessibility and safety of the procedure. The sensitivity of detecting noncaseating granuloma among the aforementioned sites is as high as 80–90%. Intra-thoracic sites (lymph nodes, airway lesions, and/or lung parenchyma) often are amenable to biopsy as well, as they are typically accessible with flexible bronchoscopy (for transbronchial needle aspirations, endobronchial and/or transbronchial biopsies).

14. Are serum biomarkers useful for the diagnosis of sarcoidosis?

Serum biomarkers have only a limited role in the diagnosis of sarcoidosis. Angiotensin-converting enzyme (ACE) is an enzyme produced by epithelioid cells and alveolar macrophages at the periphery of granulomas in response to an ACE-inducing factor released by T cells. The sensitivity of an elevated ACE level for the diagnosis of sarcoidosis is 40–60%, with a specificity of 80–90%, with resultant low positive and negative predictive values for diagnosis. Other diseases in which ACE levels can be elevated include tuberculosis, coccidioidomycosis, Gaucher disease, hypersensitivity pneumonitis, silicosis, asbestosis, leprosy, hyperthyroidism, lung cancer, and diabetes mellitus. Additionally, there are genetic causes of abnormal ACE levels due to ACE gene polymorphisms. Therefore, an elevated ACE level may be supportive (especially if >2 × upper limit of normal), but not diagnostic, of sarcoidosis. Of note, ACE inhibitors can suppress the serum ACE level.

Soluble interleukin-2 receptor (sIL-2R), which is produced by activated T cells, is a newer biomarker with slightly improved sensitivity (70–90%) and similar specificity compared to ACE levels. An elevated level is again supportive, but not diagnostic, of sarcoidosis. The rise and fall of both markers may reflect disease activity, but additional research is needed to define their use in the management of sarcoidosis.

15. Summarize the rheumatic manifestations of sarcoidosis and distinguish them from other autoimmune conditions (Table 75.4).

TABLE 75.4 Rheumatic Manifestations of Sarcoidosis

MANIFESTATION	FREQUENCY IN SARCOIDOSIS (% OF PATIENTS)	DIFFERENTIAL DIAGNOSIS
Arthritis	20	Rheumatoid arthritis, gonococcal arthritis, rheumatic fever, SLE, gout, spondyloarthritis
Parotid gland enlargement	1	Sjögren disease, IgG4-RD[a]
Upper airway disease (sinusitis, laryngeal inflammation, saddle nose deformity)	5–10	Granulomatosis polyangiitis
Uveitis Anterior Posterior	15–25[b]	Spondyloarthritis Behçet disease
Keratoconjunctivitis[c]	15–30	Sjögren disease
Proptosis	Rare	Granulomatosis polyangiitis, IgG4-RD
Myositis	≤1	Polymyositis
Mononeuritis multiplex	≤1	Systemic vasculitis
Facial nerve palsy	≤2	Lyme disease

[a]IgG4-RD = IgG4-Related Disease
[b]Sarcoid uveitis: 70–80% with anterior uveitis, 20–30% with posterior uveitis.
[c]Patients with keratoconjunctivitis may have lacrimal gland enlargement.

16. How is sarcoidosis usually treated?

Most patients with sarcoidosis do not require therapy. In patients with critical organ involvement, multi-organ disease, or symptoms that significantly affect quality of life, GCs remain first-line treatment.

In patients with isolated pulmonary sarcoidosis, only one-third of patients require medication, as the disease often undergoes spontaneous remission. Treatment for pulmonary involvement is indicated in patients with symptomatic disease, progressive pulmonary infiltrates, or progressive decline of lung function. Moderate dose GC (prednisone 0.5 mg/kg/day) is often used with a slow subsequent taper. Addition of steroid-sparing therapy is usually recommended in patients who experience relapse during GC taper. Steroid-sparing therapy can also be considered during initial treatment to minimize GC exposure. Methotrexate (MTX) is the most commonly used and well-studied steroid-sparing agent. The usual dose is between 15 and 25 mg weekly. Additional agents include azathioprine (AZA), leflunomide, mycophenolate (MMF), and hydroxychloroquine (HCQ). Biologic agents are considered third-line therapy for patients who do not respond to or cannot tolerate GC and the immunosuppressive agents outlined above. The most commonly used biologic agents are tumor necrosis factor (TNF)-alpha inhibitors. Infliximab has the most robust data in pulmonary sarcoidosis (including a randomized controlled trial). Adalimumab use may be considered as an alternative.

Extra-pulmonary sarcoidosis does not often undergo spontaneous remission, and usually requires treatment with GC and consideration of steroid-sparing therapy. In addition, inflammation and damage in some vital organs, such as the central nervous system, eyes, and heart, can lead to permanent disability. Therefore, treatment with GCs is more frequently required along with upfront use of a steroid-sparing agent/biologic agent. Oral GCs (up to 1 mg/kg per day) are used as first-line treatment for malignant hypercalcemia as well as severe ocular, neurologic, and cardiac involvement. The GC dose is typically tapered to 5–10 mg/day by 6 months, with the goal of coming off completely to avoid toxicity. If the patient continues to have progressive disease, or cannot taper prednisone to <10 mg daily, additional immunosuppressive therapy is indicated. Patients with severe cardiac or neurologic involvement typically benefit from additional immunosuppressive medication when corticosteroids are started initially. MTX at doses of 15–25 mg weekly is the most commonly used steroid-sparing agent for both pulmonary and extrapulmonary involvement. AZA (2 mg/kg per day), leflunomide (10–20 mg/day) and MMF (1000–15000 mg twice a day) have also been reported as effective. Failure to respond to at least one immunosuppressive/disease-modifying antirheumatic drug plus prednisone is an indication for treatment with anti-TNF-α agents. Not all anti-TNF-α agents are equally effective in sarcoidosis. Infliximab (5 mg/kg every 4–6 weeks) or adalimumab (40 mg subcutaneous weekly) is recommended. Etanercept appears to have limited benefit. Cyclophosphamide (oral and intravenous) has shown benefit in patients with cardiac or neurosarcoidosis, and is an option for treatment-resistant disease. Case reports have also described the use of rituximab, tocilizumab, and JAK inhibitors in treatment-resistant cases of sarcoidosis.

Isolated cutaneous involvement may respond to lower doses of oral GCs, topical therapy, and/or steroid-sparing agents such as HCQ, MTX, or MMF.

Acute manifestations such as Lofgren syndrome (Question #10) are short-lived and typically do not require chronic therapy.

Implantable pacemakers should be considered in patients with cardiac involvement and arrhythmias or heart block. Solid organ transplantation can be life-saving in patients who have failed all medical therapies.

Patients must be monitored for side effects, and prophylactic measures should be instituted to prevent toxicities. Patients on high-dose GCs should receive prophylaxis against *Pneumocystis jirovecii*. Osteopenia and osteoporosis due to dysregulated calcium metabolism and medications used in therapy can occur in up to two-thirds of patients (see Question 17). Vaccinations should be kept up to date.

17. What makes the treatment of osteopenia/osteoporosis unique in patients with sarcoidosis?

Hypercalcemia and hypercalciuria can occur in patients with sarcoidosis (Question 11).

This can lead to nephrocalcinosis and renal dysfunction, which can impact the selection of agents used for the treatment of osteoporosis. In addition, patients with sarcoidosis may have a high calcitriol (1,25-dihydroxyvitamin D) level despite a low 25-hydroxyvitamin D. Osteopenia and osteoporosis are well known adverse effects of GCs, and sarcoidosis can also cause direct bone lesions with subsequent bone loss. All sarcoidosis patients on GCs or who are postmenopausal should have bone density measurements. Appropriate therapy (anti-resorptive or anabolic agents) can be started in those at risk for fractures. However, calcium and vitamin D supplementation should be used with caution and monitored closely since sarcoid patients are prone to develop hypercalcemia and hypercalciuria.

18. What is parasarcoidosis syndrome?

The term *parasarcoidosis syndrome* is used to describe subjective symptoms experienced by patients with sarcoidosis that are not thought to be directly caused by granulomatous inflammation. These symptoms include fatigue (present in >50% of patients, and often disabling), myalgia/arthralgia, headache, depression (50–60% of patients), memory loss, and cognitive decline. Treatment of parasarcoidosis syndrome is mainly symptomatic. This syndrome is analogous to the concept of type 2 manifestations in SLE, which similarly have less evidence of being immunologically driven, and hence treatment approaches focus on non-immunosuppressive modalities.

Small fiber neuropathy (SFN) has been increasingly recognized as a parasarcoidosis manifestation (prevalence up to 10%). Patients usually present with pain, burning, numbness and tingling. These symptoms can be migratory and intermittent. It is often accompanied by autonomic neuropathy, causing orthostasis, palpitation, hyper/hypohidrosis, gastrointestinal dysmotility, or bowel/bladder disturbance. The diagnosis of SFN typically includes a characteristic skin biopsy showing decreased intraepidermal nerve fiber density (with no granuloma), or quantitative sudomotor axonal reflex testing showing reduced sweat output. The initial treatment of SFN in the setting of sarcoidosis includes symptomatic therapy with agents such as gabapentin, pregabalin, or amitriptyline. The use of intravenous immunoglobulin (IVIG) in this setting (similar to SFN described in Sjogren's) has been described for resistant disease.

19. Discuss the prognostic factors in sarcoidosis.

The extent of organ involvement in most cases is defined at presentation, with <25% of patients developing new organ involvement within 2 years of follow-up. Most patients (60%) undergo spontaneous remission, with an additional 10–20% resolving with GC therapy. However, in 10–30%, the course is chronic. In general, the more severe the involvement and the more organ systems (>3) involved at the time of diagnosis, the worse the prognosis. African–American heritage, disease onset after age 40, symptoms lasting over 6 months, advanced radiographic stage pulmonary disease (stages III & IV), pulmonary hypertension, and extrathoracic involvement (cardiac, neurologic, lupus pernio, panuveitis, hypercalcemia, and bone lesions) are poor prognostic signs. Overall mortality is 5%, with half dying of progressive pulmonary disease and half dying of cardiac or neurologic involvement.

ACKNOWLEDGMENT

The authors would like to thank Drs. Erica Hill and Daniel Battafarano for their contributions to this chapter in the previous edition.

BIBLIOGRAPHY

Baughman RP, Culver DA, Judson MA. A concise review of pulmonary sarcoidosis. *Am J Respir Crit Care Med.* 2011;183:573–581.

Birnie DH, Nery PB, Ha AC, et al. Cardiac sarcoidosis. *J Am Coll Cardiol.* 2016;68:411–421.

Chen ES, Moller DR. Etiology of sarcoidosis pathobiology. *Clin Chest Med.* 2008:365–377.

Tavee JO, Karwa K, Ahmed Z, et al. Sarcoidosis-associated small fiber neuropathy in a large cohort: clinical aspects and response to IVIG and anti-TNF alpha treatment. *Respir Med.* 2017;126:135–138.

Ungprasert P, Carmona EM, Crowson CS, et al. Diagnostic utility of angiotensin-converting enzyme in sarcoidosis: a population-based study. *Lung.* 2016;194:91–95.

Ungprasert P, Crowson CS, Matteson EL, et al. Clinical characteristics of sarcoid arthropathy: a population-based study. *Arthritis Care Res (Hoboken).* 2016;68:695–699.

Ungprasert P, Crowson CS, Matteson EL, et al. Epidemiology of sarcoidosis 1946–2013: a population-based study. *Mayo Clin Proc.* 2016;91:183–188.

Zhou Y, Lower EE, Li H, et al. Clinical characteristics of patients with bone sarcoidosis. *Semin Arthritis Rheum.* 2017;47:143–148.

FURTHER READING

http://www.stopsarcoidosis.org.

IgG4-Related Disease

John H. Stone, MD, MPH

1. What is IgG4-related disease (IgG4-RD)?

IgG4-RD is an immune-mediated fibroinflammatory condition that can affect multiple organ systems. Many aspects of the pathophysiology suggest that the condition may have an autoimmune basis, but this has not been established definitively. No single autoantibody has been identified to occur in all or even most patients. Tissue pathology is often characterized by a dense lymphoplasmacytic infiltrate enriched with IgG4-positive plasma cells, and associated fibrosis. Common sites of involvement include the retroperitoneum (especially peri-aortic distribution), pancreas, biliary tree, salivary glands, and orbit, among others (see Question #4).

2. When was IgG4-RD recognized?

IgG4-RD was recognized as a unique disease state in 2003, when a group of Japanese investigators discovered that similar pathology findings were evident in varied clinical syndromes across an array of different organs. This recognition was preceded 2 years earlier by research that demonstrated elevated levels of serum IgG4 in patients with "sclerosing pancreatitis", now known as IgG4-related autoimmune pancreatitis (IgG4-related AIP; also known as Type 1 AIP).

3. Which conditions previously known by other names are now considered to be part of IgG4-RD?

Mikulicz disease, the combination of enlarged lacrimal, parotid, and submandibular glands, was first described in the 1890s and was regarded as a variant of Sjögren disease (SjD) for decades. Küttner's tumors were the name given to isolated enlargement of the submandibular glands in the 1890s. Riedel's thyroiditis, a third diagnosis identified in the 1890s, is in fact IgG4-RD of the thyroid gland. Ormond's disease was the name originally given to retroperitoneal fibrosis in 1948. IgG4-RD is thought responsible for most cases of retroperitoneal fibrosis, and nearly all of those with inflammation centered around the abdominal aorta. Table 76.1 lists additional clinical syndromes now considered part of the spectrum of IgG4-RD.

4. Which organs are most commonly involved by IgG4-RD?

IgG4-RD can affect essentially any organ system, but there are several that are regarded as typical sites of involvement. These are outlined in the 2019 American College of Rheumatology/European Alliance of Associations for Rheumatology (ACR/EULAR) Classification Criteria (Table 76.2).

TABLE 76.1 Clinical Syndromes Now Considered Part of the IgG4-RD Spectrum		
Mikulicz disease	Type 1 AIP	Multifocal fibrosclerosis
Küttner's tumors	Hypertrophic pachymeningitis	Fibrosing mediastinitis
Riedel's thyroiditis	Inflammatory pseudotumor	Sclerosing mesenteritis
Retroperitoneal fibrosis	Inflammatory aortic aneurysm	

TABLE 76.2 Typical Sites of IgG4-RD Organ Involvement		
Pancreas	Kidneys	Retroperitoneum
Bile Ducts	Meninges	Lymph nodes
Lungs	Aorta	Glands[a]

[a]Most commonly includes submandibular, parotid, lacrimal, thyroid, and pituitary glands.

SPECIFIC ORGAN FEATURES

5. How does IgG4-related autoimmune pancreatitis (AIP) present?

While some cases of IgG4-related AIP present with significant abdominal pain, the majority of patients are diagnosed in the setting of longer-standing pancreatic injury (sometimes irreversible), with few or no symptoms. Due to its insidious nature, IgG4-related AIP is often recognized only long after the pancreas has been irreparably injured. Telltale signs of previously active AIP leading to subsequent damage include:

- Substantial weight loss caused by the development of exocrine pancreatic insufficiency
- New-onset diabetes
- A shrunken, fibrotic pancreas on imaging, despite the absence of a clinical history to suggest pancreatic inflammation or dysfunction.

Computed tomography (CT) imaging of the abdomen can be supportive in the diagnosis of IgG4-related AIP, often demonstrating diffuse or focal pancreatic enlargement. The diffuse form is often described as a 'sausage-like' enlargement of the pancreas, with loss of the organ's usual lobular shape. IgG4-related AIP can also manifest as a focal pancreatic enlargement, with CT scan revealing a well-defined focal mass that may compress adjacent pancreatic or common bile ducts, and mimic focal pancreatic cancer. Notably, pancreatic pseudocysts and/or retroperitoneal fluid collections are not common in IgG4-related AIP, which may help distinguish it from acute or chronic pancreatitis.

6. Name the sections of the eye commonly impacted by IgG4-RD.

Many unbiopsied cases of "idiopathic" orbital inflammation (IOI) may be secondary to IgG4-RD. Patients labelled as having IOI have often been treated empirically without biopsy, and thus the precise diagnosis is missed. Inflammation may occur in various structures within the orbit, as outlined below:

- **Extra-ocular muscle** involvement is usually a painless condition that is associated with enlargement of the muscles. Several muscles are typically involved (e.g., the lateral and superior rectus muscles) simultaneously. Proptosis and diplopia can occur.
- Inflammatory tissue invading the **retro-bulbar region** can be particularly concerning for severe (and potentially permanent) vision loss given the risk for optic nerve compression.
- The **cavernous sinus and Meckel's cave** are two additional sites where inflammatory tissue may invade, potentially leading to serious neurologic injury due to cranial nerve damage and/or vascular compromise.
- **Dacryoadenitis** (inflammation of the lacrimal gland) can occur in isolation or with other features of Mikulicz's disease (lacrimal, parotid, and submandibular enlargement).

Ocular involvement outside of the orbit is less common in IgG4-RD. Uveitis (including granulomatous pan-uveitis) and scleritis have both been described.

7. What is retroperitoneal fibrosis (RPF)?

In 1948, Ormond published the histopathologic findings of idiopathic **RPF.** Idiopathic RPF is thought to be a subset of **idiopathic multifocal fibrosclerosis**. IgG4-RD likely represents a subgroup of both conditions (see Question #8). Idiopathic RPF is rare and affects men more than women (3:1). It has been reported in all ethnicities and occurs at an average age of 40–60 years. Patients present with pain in the lower back, abdomen, flank, and/or scrotum. Some patients have systemic symptoms including fever, anorexia, and malaise. Physical exam is usually unremarkable, although lower extremity edema and phlebitis can be seen. Laboratory findings are nonspecific including elevated ESR/CRP (75–90%) and azotemia (50%). Medial deviation of the mid part of the ureter and hydronephrosis are common (60–75%). Open, laparoscopic, or CT-guided biopsy shows sclerosis and infiltration of mononuclear cells. Biopsy is helpful in ruling out malignant disease (lymphoma, sarcoma), histiocytic conditions (Erdheim–Chester disease), infections, and to identify features characteristic of IgG4-RD. Treatment for idiopathic RPF (not IgG4-related RPF) is high-dose prednisone (40–60 mg/d) for 2 to 4 weeks, with subsequent taper over the following 6 months. Low-dose maintenance prednisone (5–10 mg daily) may be continued for 1–3 years. Steroid sparing therapy may be used in treatment-resistant or relapsing disease, or alternatively, at treatment initiation to allow for lower dosing of glucocorticoids (rituximab, methotrexate, azathioprine, mycophenolate mofetil). Recurrence may occur in 30% of patients.

8. What is the relationship between IgG4-RD and retroperitoneal fibrosis?

Retroperitoneal fibrosis represents approximately 25–33% of all IgG4-RD cases. As outlined above, IgG4-RD is one of several conditions that can cause retroperitoneal fibrosis: Erdheim-Chester disease, sarcoidosis, ANCA-associated vasculitis, sarcomas, lymphomas, and infections such as tuberculosis may all be associated with RPF.

The pattern and distribution of involvement of IgG4-related RPF can be helpful in distinguishing it from other conditions, however. The retroperitoneal lesion in IgG4-RD typically extends from below the renal arteries caudally, encircling the aorta (an associated aortitis within the vessel wall may also be seen). The inflammation in IgG4-RD characteristically extends inferiorly beyond the aortic bifurcation into the iliac arteries.

9. What anatomic features of IgG4-related RPF elevate the risk for hydronephrosis?

The tendency of IgG4-RD to cause peri-aortitis in the infrarenal region increases the likelihood of ureter involvement and subsequent hydronephrosis. This occurs because the ureters cross the iliac arteries just inferior to the aortic bifurcation as they course from the renal pelvis to the bladder. The peri-aortitis in IgG4-related RPF often extends sufficiently inferior to involve the iliac arteries. In some cases, the inflammation may be more prominent around the iliac arteries than the aorta per se. Inflammation around the iliac arteries tends to entrap the ureters, leading to constriction and hydronephrosis.

10. Is IgG4-related RPF treatable?

Absolutely, and in many cases excellent results can be achieved. The earlier the disease is recognized and treatment started, the better the outcome. There appears to be an "inflammatory" (as opposed to "fibrotic") stage in IgG4-related RPF during which the process responds exceptionally well to glucocorticoids within days to weeks of high-dose (e.g., prednisone 40 mg/day) treatment. The challenge is that it is often difficult (if not impossible) to know precisely how long RPF has been present before the time of diagnosis. Given that the disease is clinically silent for long periods of time in the retroperitoneum, instances of such early recognition are the exception. It is more common to diagnose the condition at advanced stages of involvement—for example, when hydronephrosis necessitates the insertion of ureteral stents. Even in advanced cases, however, good therapeutic outcomes are possible. B-cell depletion appears to be more likely to lead to good outcomes (and fewer side effects) compared to glucocorticoid monotherapy. In some scenarios, it may be beneficial to use prednisone and rituximab together at treatment onset—for example, prednisone 40 mg/day tapered over 2 months combined with a typical remission induction course of rituximab (two 1-gram infusions separated by 2 weeks). Rituximab can also often achieve excellent results without concomitant glucocorticoid treatment in some patients.

Success in this condition is defined by improvement in patient symptoms and relief of urinary obstruction (including the ability to remove ureteral stents or nephrostomy tubes). This can often be achieved even when substantial residual fibrosis remains on imaging.

11. What are the neurologic complications of IgG4-RD?

- **Pachymeningitis:** One of the most common causes of hypertrophic pachymeningitis is IgG4-RD. Other potential causes include: ANCA-associated vasculitis, giant cell arteritis, sarcoidosis, Erdheim–Chester disease, and lymphoma, among others. Symptoms include headaches and neurologic dysfunction due to entrapment of cranial nerves. IgG4-related pachymeningitis usually responds very well to systemic treatment. Unusual cases have required intrathecal therapy.
- **Pituitary gland:** IgG4-RD can affect this gland just as it affects other glandular targets (submandibular, lacrimal, parotid, pancreas, and thyroid). In such cases, magnetic resonance imaging (MRI) may reveal dramatic pituitary enlargement. Partial or complete failure of the gland can result. Many patients will have radiographic improvement (decreased pituitary size) with immunosuppressive therapy, but the long-term prognosis for pituitary function is uncertain, with some patients experiencing recurrent loss of pituitary function after steroid cessation.
- Parenchymal brain involvement is very rare in IgG4-RD, albeit cases have been reported.

12. How does IgG4-RD affect the kidney?

- **Tubulo-interstitial nephritis (TIN)** is the principal lesion in the kidney. CT imaging appearance of IgG4-related TIN can be striking, with hypodense lesions concentrated in the renal cortex. Enlargement of the kidneys can be observed in cases of advanced disease. Renal biopsy of the lesion is expected to show the classic histopathologic and immunostaining characteristics of IgG4-RD (see Question #22). Slow onset of renal dysfunction can occur in this setting, occasionally culminating in end-stage renal disease if the diagnosis is not recognized until late. The urinalysis ranges from largely unimpressive to utterly unremarkable, posing a challenge to disease recognition. Low C3 and C4 levels may be seen in this setting, but hypocomplementemia is reported in one-third of patients with IgG4-RD overall and is not specific to patients with renal involvement.
- **Membranous nephropathy** (10% or less of IgG4-related kidney involvement): can lead to nephrotic syndrome. In some patients, both TIN and membranous GN occur simultaneously.
- **Ureteropelvic junction obstruction:** IgG4-RD can cause masses at the junction where the ureter attaches to the kidney. These are sometimes mistaken for renal cell carcinomas or other malignancies, leading unfortunately to nephrectomy.

13. List some of the common imaging findings in IgG4-RD in the lungs (Table 76.3).

TABLE 76.3 Common Pulmonary Imaging Findings in IgG4-RD[a]	
Pulmonary nodules or mass	Pleural thickening
Ground glass opacities	Interstitial lung disease
Peribronchovascular and septal thickening, similar to sarcoidosis	Paravertebral thoracic mass: typically confined to one side of column (more often right) and extending over several vertebral segments (T8-11 region). Rarely cause complications.

[a]Extensive pulmonary lesions can occur with surprisingly few symptoms in many cases.

EPIDEMIOLOGY

14. What do we know about the basic epidemiology of IgG4-RD?

The true incidence and prevalence of IgG4-RD is unknown. This lack of knowledge stems from the fact that the disease was unrecognized until the first few years of this century, and did not even have an ICD-10 code until 2023. Existing data suggest the disease has a male predominance, with a male:female ratio of approximately 2:1. Additional epidemiologic studies have suggested possible gender differences in disease presentation and course:

- Men with IgG4-RD tend to be at higher risk for multi-organ involvement
- Women with IgG4-RD tend to be at lower risk of internal organ involvement (pancreato-biliary tree, kidneys, and lungs); conversely, women may be more likely to have major salivary gland involvement
- Women may be more likely to experience disease flares than men.

15. Does IgG4-RD occur in children?

Yes. While the disease has a predilection for affecting adults (the classic patient is a middle-aged to elderly male), it has been well described in children also. Orbital disease appears to be particularly common among pediatric patients.

SERUM IGG4 CHARACTERISTICS

16. Do all patients with IgG4-RD have increased levels of serum IgG4?

No. Most patients with multi-organ disease have elevated serum IgG4 concentrations, but there is a subset of patients with classic organ involvement and characteristic histopathologic features with normal serum IgG4 concentrations. The prozone phenomenon may be responsible for some spuriously low serum IgG4 measurements, and this problem can be addressed by the laboratory by diluting the sample and repeating the assay. Nevertheless, some patients with IgG4-RD do not have elevated serum concentrations of this antibody (~30%). Of note, patients with the "fibrotic" as opposed to "proliferative" subset of IgG4-RD (retroperitoneal fibrosis, sclerosing mesenteritis, fibrosing mediastinitis) are more likely to have normal serum IgG4 concentrations (Zhang, 2019).

17. Do serum concentrations of IgG4 reflect disease activity?

Yes. Serum IgG4 concentrations can serve as good biomarkers in patients with elevated levels at baseline. They decline steadily following treatment and begin to rise when the disease is becoming active again, usually in advance of overt clinical manifestations of disease. As with most biomarkers, changes in the serum IgG4 level should be interpreted in the context of the patient history, physical exam findings, and other data.

18. Does the serum level of IgG4 normalize after treatment?

Usually not—*at least not quickly*. This is because there are long-lived plasma cells that have learned to make IgG4 during their sojourn as developing B cells. These cells continue to make IgG4 for long periods of time. Serum IgG4 concentrations do typically decline with treatment, and this is a reflection of reduced production by pre-plasma cell components of the B lymphocyte lineage. The overall serum concentration of IgG4 is unlikely to normalize for many months, particularly if levels were extremely high at treatment initiation. Given the characteristic slow rise and fall in serum antibody concentration, *the trend in IgG4 values* (whether the concentration is increasing or decreasing between measurements) may be more important than the total concentration at any single point in time.

19. Are there biomarkers other than IgG4 that are useful in IgG4-RD?

Serum IgE, IgG1, C3, and C4 can be useful biomarkers in some patients. Longitudinal management of patients may reveal that one or more of these biomarkers is helpful in gauging disease activity, and occasionally information from one of these other biomarkers is more useful than IgG4 for a particular patient. In most cases, however, the information provided by these other markers adds little to what can be gleaned from serum IgG4 values. Hypocomplementemia specifically is reported in one-third of patients with IgG4-RD overall, and is more prevalent in patients with multi-organ involvement (less common in patients with fibrotic manifestations and lacrimal gland involvement).

PATHOPHYSIOLOGY

20. Does IgG4 cause IgG4-RD?

No. Even though we call the condition IgG4-related disease, it is clear that it is not caused by IgG4. The IgG4 elevation in the peripheral blood is oligoclonal, and no specific autoantibody has been identified consistently. By its very nature, particularly the fact that IgG4 tends to undergo the process of Fab exchange (becoming unhinged and recombining with an unidentical half from another antibody), IgG4 antibody does not appear to activate complement efficiently in most circumstances and has long been viewed as an anti-inflammatory antibody. The role of IgG4 in the context of disease pathophysiology is currently conceived of as one that is counter-regulatory in nature—i.e., performing an anti-inflammatory function aimed at dampening the primary immune response.

21. What do we understand about the pathophysiology of IgG4-RD?

The chronic nature of IgG4-RD and its responsiveness to immunosuppression are both consistent with an immune-mediated pathophysiology. Although links established between IgG4-RD and several autoantigens are compatible with the concept that autoimmunity plays a role IgG4-RD, the specific details surrounding immunologic triggers, crucial disease pathways, and disease propagation remain poorly understood. IgG4-RD is associated with a symphony of inflammation, with contributions from multiple B- and T-cell subsets as well as macrophages, fibroblasts, and possibly complement components. IgG4-RD has been linked with expansions of a number of circulating and tissue-based cells, including B-cell subsets, cytotoxic T cells (both CD4+ and CD8+), T follicular helper cells, and T follicular regulatory cells (Perugino, 2020).

The lymphocytic infiltrates in IgG4-RD consist of $CD4^+$ cytotoxic T lymphocytes (CTLs) as well as B cells. It is believed that a central element of the pathophysiology of IgG4-RD is the presentation of antigens by B cells to CTLs. Interactions between B cells and other CD4+ T lymphocytes, such as T follicular helper cells, promote class switching to IgG4 and may play other important roles in disease development and propagation (Kubo, 2018).

PATHOLOGY

22. What are the key findings on pathology in IgG4-RD?

The pathology of IgG4-RD is characterized by several elements. First, there is a **dense lympho-plasmacytic infiltrate**. This infiltrate is comprised of B cells, plasma cells, and T cells, usually accompanied by a **mild eosinophilic infiltrate**. A disproportionate percentage of the plasma cells are IgG4+, with **IgG4 to IgG ratios of >40%** on tissue staining. Extra-nodal germinal centers are often observed at sites of disease. Some degree of **fibrosis** is present, even in the earliest stages of IgG4-RD, and the pattern of fibrosis observed typically has a **"storiform" pattern**. Finally, **phlebitis** is also seen in at least 50% of biopsies obtained from involved organs. This phlebitis may or may not be associated with the partial or complete obliteration of the vessel lumen. These pathology features, along with additional clinical, serologic, and radiographic findings can be used to classify a patient as having IgG4-RD according to the 2019 ACR/EULAR classification criteria.

23. Are the pathology findings of IgG4-RD diagnostic of this condition?

No. Although the pathology findings in IgG4-RD are distinctive and can be highly suggestive of this diagnosis, without having appropriate clinical context pathologists cannot render this diagnosis with certainty on the basis of the histopathologic and immunostaining findings alone. The diagnosis of IgG4-RD is made by synthesizing information related to the clinical presentation, serologic findings, radiographic data, and—when available—tissue biopsy.

24. If histopathology is not definitive, why do we perform biopsies?

Biopsies often provide critical information, even if they are not diagnostic. Biopsies can offer the missing piece of evidence that, in the context of other information, clinches the diagnosis of IgG4-RD. On the other hand, biopsies are often essential to excluding IgG4-RD and ruling in diseases for which the treatment and prognosis may be substantially different: adenocarcinoma, lymphoma, granulomatosis with polyangiitis, SjD, histiocytoses such as Rosai-Dorfman, and so on.

25. Are there pathology findings that exclude the diagnosis of IgG4-RD?

Absolutely. IgG4-RD is NOT associated with: fibrinoid necrosis, granulomatous inflammation, multinucleated giant cells, significant neutrophilic infiltrates, sheets of histiocytes, monoclonal cell populations, and emperiopolesis. The finding of any of these as a principal component of the pathology means that the diagnosis is something other than IgG4-RD.

DIFFERENTIAL DIAGNOSIS

26. **Outline the most common disease mimickers that should be considered in the evaluation of a patient with suspected IgG4-RD (Table 76.4).**

TABLE 76.4 Disease Mimickers Not to be Missed and Distinguishing Features From IgG4-RD

MIMICKER	WHAT'S DIFFERENT FROM IgG4-RD
Granulomatosis with polyangiitis (GPA)	• ANCA positivity in the great majority of cases • More rapid disease progression is typical, particularly in the setting of renal disease. • Alveolar hemorrhage does not occur in IgG4-RD • Cavitary pulmonary nodules do not occur in IgG4-RD • C-reactive protein is typically high during active GPA • Pathology features such as necrosis, neutrophilic abscesses, granulomatous inflammation, and multinucleated giant cells help exclude IgG4-RD
SjD	• Anti-Ro antibody positivity occurs in most cases of SjD • Isolated submandibular gland enlargement is not typical of SjD • Dryness of the eyes and mouth is usually more severe among patients with SjD
Rosai-Dorfman disease	• Lymphadenopathy is often out of proportion to extranodal features • Emperipolesis (histiocytic ingestion of whole lymphocytes, plasma cells, or other cell lines) is essentially unique to Rosai-Dorfman and not observed in the pathology of IgG4-RD
Lupus nephritis	• More likely to occur in a young woman than a middle-aged to elderly man (the classic IgG4-RD patient) • Mucocutaneous disease is unusual in IgG4-RD and photosensitivity highly atypical • Strong autoantibody findings such as antibodies to double-stranded DNA are not typical of IgG4-RD
Sarcoidosis	• Non-caseating granulomas on biopsy argue strongly for sarcoidosis
Lymphoma	• Evidence of a monoclonal lymphocyte population in biopsies
Adenocarcinoma	• Not anticipated to have a significant response to glucocorticoid treatment

TREATMENT

27. **What is the cornerstone of treatment for IgG4-RD across the world?**

Glucocorticoids are the principal treatment for IgG4-RD in most settings across the world. Even multi-organ IgG4-RD typically responds to doses of glucocorticoids on the order of prednisone 40 mg daily. The challenges to using glucocorticoids as the cornerstone of treatment for IgG4-RD, however, are obvious. IgG4-RD is a condition that preferentially effects middle-aged to elderly individuals and damages the pancreas in a high percentage of patients. Moreover, glucocorticoids do not cure the disease or even provide reliable remissions of any substantial length once the treatment is discontinued. This sets up scenarios of either repeated glucocorticoid treatments or ongoing maintenance therapy, both of which are associated with substantial adverse effects.

28. **What treatments other than glucocorticoids are useful for the treatment of IgG4-RD?**

Conventional synthetic disease-modifying anti-rheumatic drugs (csDMARDs) such as mycophenolate mofetil and leflunomide have proven useful in maintaining glucocorticoid-free remissions. B-cell depletion (traditionally with rituximab) is widely viewed, however, as being the most effective treatment strategy at the current time. Multiple prospective cohort studies have demonstrated successful response with rituximab in 90% of patients. Disease relapse, however, may occur in 25–40% of patients, including those with initial rituximab induction therapy. The MITIGATE trial, a randomized, double-blind, placebo-controlled trial of inebilizumab (targeted depletion of CD19+ B cells), reported its topline results in the summer of 2024. The study showed a reduced risk of flares and increased likelihood of complete remission at 1 year in treated patients. Of interest, CD19 is expressed across a wider range in the B-cell lineage, including plasmablasts and plasma cells, unlike the more restricted expression of CD20.

29. Are there nondrug interventions that are useful for the management of some IgG4-RD manifestations?

Temporary stent placements are frequently required in the biliary tree and ureters for complications associated with pancreatobiliary disease (IgG4-related sclerosing cholangitis and AIP) and retroperitoneal fibrosis. The goals of therapy include successful stent removal as soon as possible.

BIBLIOGRAPHY

AbdelRazek MA, Venna N, Stone JH. IgG4-related disease of the central and peripheral nervous systems. *Lancet Neurol.* 2018;17(2):183–192.

Carruthers MN, Topazian MD, Khosroshahi A, et al. Rituximab for IgG4-related disease: a prospective, open-label trial. *Ann Rheum Dis.* 2015;74(6):1171–1177.

Dahlgren M, Khosroshahi A, Nielsen GP, et al. Riedel's thyroiditis and multifocal fibrosclerosis are part of the IgG4-related systemic disease spectrum. *Arthritis Care Res (Hoboken).* 2010;62(9):1312–1318.

Inoue D, Yoshida K, Yoneda N, et al. IgG4-related disease: dataset of 235 consecutive patients. *Medicine (Baltimore).* 2015;94(15):e680.

Jha I, McMahon GA, Perugino CA, et al. Sex as a predictor of clinical phenotype and determinant of immune response in IgG4-related disease: a retrospective study of patients fulfilling the American College of Rheumatology–European League Against Rheumatism classification criteria. *Lancet Rheumatol.* 2024;6(7):e460–e468.

Kamisawa T, Funata N, Hayashi Y, et al. A new clinicopathological entity of IgG4-related autoimmune disease. *J Gastroenterol.* 2003;38(10):982–984.

Karim F, Loeffen J, Bramer W, et al. IgG4-related disease: a systematic review of this unrecognized disease in pediatrics. *Pediatr Rheumatol Online J.* 2016;14(1):18.

Khosroshahi A, Stone JH. IgG4-related sclerosing disease: the age of discovery. *Curr Opin Rheumatol.* 2011;23(1):72–73.

Khosroshahi A, Carruthers MN, Stone JH, et al. Rethinking Ormond's disease: "idiopathic" retroperitoneal fibrosis in the era of IgG4-related disease. *Medicine (Baltimore).* 2013;92(2):82–91.

Kubo S, Nakayamada S, Zhao J, et al. Correlation of T follicular helper cells and plasmablasts with the development of organ involvement in patients with IgG4-related disease. *Rheumatology (Oxford).* 2018;57(3):514–524.

Liu Y, Zhu L, Wang Z, et al. Clinical features of IgG4-related retroperitoneal fibrosis among 407 patients with IgG4-related disease: a retrospective study. *Rheumatology (Oxford).* 2021;60(2):767–772.

Masaki Y, Matsui S, Saeki T, et al. A multicenter phase II prospective clinical trial of glucocorticoid for patients with untreated IgG4-related disease. *Mod Rheumatol.* 2017;27(5):849–854.

Perugino CA, Stone JH. IgG4-related disease: an update on pathophysiology and implications for clinical care. *Nat Rev Rheumatol.* 2020;16(12):702–714.

Stone JH, Khosroshahi A, Zhang W, et al. Inebilizumab for treatment of IgG4-related disease. *N Engl J Med.* 2025;392(12):1168–1177.

Wallace ZS, Perugino C, Matza M, et al. Immunoglobulin G4-related disease. *Clin Chest Med.* 2019;40(3):583–597.

Wallace ZS, Naden RP, Chari S, et al. The 2019 American College of Rheumatology/European League against rheumatism classification criteria for IgG4-related disease. *Ann Rheum Dis.* 2020;79(1):77–87.

Yamamoto M, Takahashi H, Ohara M, et al. A new conceptualization for Mikulicz's disease as an IgG4-related plasmacytic disease. *Mod Rheumatol.* 2006;16(6):335–340.

Zhang W, Stone JH. Management of IgG4-related disease. *Lancet Rheumatol.* 2019;1(1):e55–e65.

CHAPTER 77

Rheumatic Disorders in Patients on Dialysis

Sterling G. West, MD

1. What are the rheumatologic complications that can occur in patients with end-stage renal disease (ESRD)?

Rheumatologic complications occur in up to 70% of patients with ESRD. There is a temporal relationship between the frequency of these disorders and the length of kidney disease. Some of the musculoskeletal disorders that develop in chronic renal failure and dialysis can be recalled with the mnemonic **VITAMINS ABCDE:**

V—Vascular calcification.
I—Infections (osteomyelitis, septic arthritis, septic discitis).
T—Tumoral calcifications, tendonitis, and tendon ruptures.
A—Amyloid arthropathy (β2-microglobulin).
M—Metabolic bone disease (osteomalacia, osteoporosis, adynamic bone dz), muscle cramps, myopathy.
I—Infarction (osteonecrosis).
N—Nodules (tophi).
S—Secondary hyperparathyroidism.
A—Aluminum toxicity.
B—Bursitis (olecranon).
C—Crystal arthropathy (gout, calcium pyrophosphate deposition disease [CPDD], hydroxyapatite, calcium oxalate).
D—Digital clubbing.
E—Erosive spondyloarthropathy, enthesitis.

2. What is renal osteodystrophy? What is chronic kidney disease-metabolic bone disease?

The term **renal osteodystrophy,** which was introduced by Liu and Chu in 1943, refers to the full spectrum of musculoskeletal disorders associated with renal failure. It is now called **chronic kidney disease-metabolic bone disease (CKD-MBD)**. Because the kidney plays a critical role in the overall regulation of mineral homeostasis, the development of renal failure has widespread consequences for the skeleton. The four principal types of renal osteodystrophy are:

- **Osteitis fibrosa:** bony lesions caused by accelerated bone turnover because of significant secondary hyperparathyroidism (PTH typically > 9x upper limit of normal). Hallmark lesion on bone biopsy is peritrabecular fibrosis in the setting of accelerated bone resorption and formation.
- **Osteomalacia:** reduced rate of bone turnover with increased osteoid volume and defective mineralization often associated with aluminum toxicity.
- **Adynamic bone disease:** bone turnover is markedly decreased because of excessive suppression of PTH (<100 pg/mL). Unlike osteomalacia, there is no increase in osteoid volume.
- **Mixed disease:** combined osteitis fibrosa and osteomalacia with marrow fibrosis.

The only way to separate these and definitively establish a diagnosis is by a tetracycline dual-labeled bone biopsy.

3. Why does secondary hyperparathyroidism develop in chronic renal failure? How does this lead to bone disease?

Secondary hyperparathyroidism starts relatively early, when the glomerular filtration rate (GFR) drops below 60 mL/minute, as evidenced by increased levels of PTH and histological changes in bone. As renal function deteriorates, these changes become more dramatic. Several factors in patients with chronic renal failure contribute to the sustained increases in PTH secretion and, ultimately, to parathyroid gland hyperplasia.

- Relative hyperphosphatemia resulting from impaired renal excretion occurs early and becomes overt as GFR drops to <20 mL/minute.
- Impaired renal hydroxylation of 25-hydroxyvitamin D to 1,25-dihydroxyvitamin D (calcitriol) attributable to reduced 1-α hydroxylase activity occurs early even before hyperphosphatemia develops because of the diseased kidney parenchyma. This enzyme is further inhibited by hyperphosphatemia and by increased fibroblast growth factor-23 (FGF-23) levels caused by reduced GFR. Notably, 1,25-dihydroxyvitamin D normally inhibits both parathyroid gland growth and PTH secretion; therefore, low levels cause secondary hyperparathyroidism.
- Decreased free calcium owing to poor gastrointestinal (GI) absorption resulting from reduced 1,25-dihydroxyvitamin D levels, skeletal resistance to PTH, and calcium deposition into vasculature, soft tissues, and viscera because of high calcium–phosphate product caused by hyperphosphatemia.
- Insensitivity of the parathyroid gland to the suppressive effects of calcium on PTH secretion. The end result of each of these defects (high phosphate, reduced calcitriol, and decreased free calcium) is stimulation of the parathyroid chief cell causing a sustained increase in PTH release. This increase in PTH (and FGF-23) is attempting to decrease phosphorous levels by reducing the renal reabsorption of phosphate as well as trying to stimulate 1-α hydroxylase activity. However, as kidney disease worsens and GFR decreases, this becomes ineffective and the resulting high PTH levels stimulate osteoclast activation and rapid bone resorption leading to osteitis fibrosa. This is usually asymptomatic but can be associated with bone pain/tenderness and proximal muscle weakness.

4. List the characteristic radiographic features of osteitis fibrosa attributable to secondary hyperparathyroidism.

Early: subperiosteal resorption in the hands, wrists, feet, and medial tibia, particularly on the radial side of the middle phalanx of the index and middle fingers (see Chapter 47: Endocrine-Associated Arthropathies); osteoporosis.

Intermediate: subchondral resorption of sternoclavicular, acromioclavicular, discovertebral, and sacroiliac joints and symphysis pubis; loss of the lamina dura around teeth; acroosteolysis of the phalangeal tufts; chondrocalcinosis of knees, wrists, and symphysis pubis (see Chapter 45: Calcium Pyrophosphate Deposition Disease); periarticular and soft tissue calcification; osteosclerosis.

Late: bone cysts (single or multiple; Fig. 77.1).

Brown tumor: osteoclastomas with dried blood (brown); typically occur at the medial end of clavicles or skull, long bones, sternum, and spine.

Subligamentous bone resorption: of trochanters, ischial tuberosities, humeral tuberosities, and calcanei.

5. What is a "salt and pepper" skull? What is "rugger-jersey spine"?

Trabecular bone resorption in hyperparathyroidism creates a characteristic mottling of the cranial vault with alternating areas of lucency and sclerosis, producing the **salt and pepper** radiographic appearance (see Fig. 77.1). **Rugger-jersey spine** refers to the band-like osteosclerosis of the superior and inferior margins of the vertebral bodies that are only seen in patients with secondary (not primary) hyperparathyroidism (Fig. 77.2).

6. Outline the prevention and treatment of secondary hyperparathyroidism.

- Dietary phosphate restriction (800–1000 mg/day). Avoid colas.

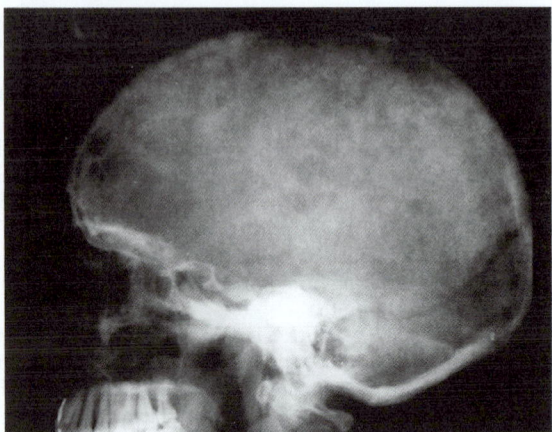

Fig. 77.1 Skull radiograph of a patient with renal failure and secondary hyperparathyroidism. Note the bone cysts ("brown tumors") superimposed on a "salt and pepper" skull.

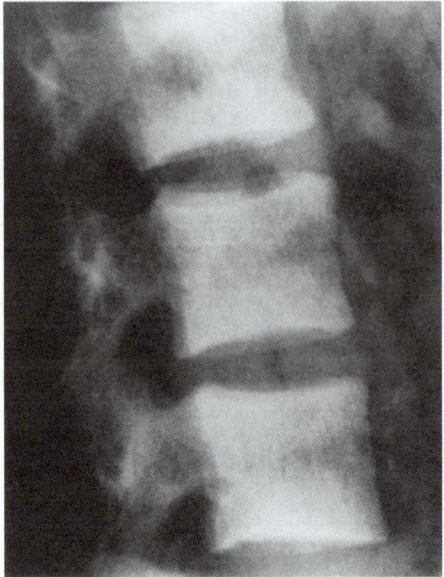

Fig. 77.2 Rugger-jersey spine.

- Calcium-based phosphate binders (calcium carbonate or calcium acetate limited to <1.5 g/day) or a noncalcium-based phosphate-binding resin (sevelamer, lanthanum) before meals if dietary restriction alone is unable to maintain serum phosphorous between 3.5 and 5.5 mg/dL (if on dialysis). If corrected total calcium is >9.5 mg/dL or vascular calcifications are present, a noncalcium-based phosphate-binding resin is preferred.
- Vitamin D derivatives (paricalcitol, doxercalciferol, calcitriol, others): if corrected total calcium is <9.5 mg/dL and PTH levels are still >300 pg/mL. There is a need to monitor for hypercalcemia causing a high calcium–phosphate product, which ideally should be <55 to prevent vascular calcifications.
- Calcimimetics (cinacalcet, etelcalcitide): if vitamin D derivatives are ineffective, corrected total calcium >8.4 mg/dL, and PTH >300 pg/mL. Use before vitamin D derivatives if calcium–phosphate product above 55.

- Once hyperparathyroidism has advanced, it may be refractory to these interventions, at which time subtotal parathyroidectomy is indicated to correct symptomatic hyperparathyroidism. Subtotal parathyroidectomy is also indicated in patients who develop **tertiary hyperparathyroidism,** which have symptoms such as high PTH levels (>800 pg/mL) and hypercalcemia in spite of being off all calcium and vitamin D therapies.

7. How does osteomalacia present? What role does aluminum play in this type of renal osteodystrophy?

In renal failure or hemodialysis, dietary aluminum is not adequately cleared and deposits in the osteoid lamellae of newly formed bone, inhibiting mineralization, which leads to osteomalacia. Therefore, in patients with ESRD, osteomalacia may be related to aluminum toxicity, although it can occur without aluminum toxicity. Therefore, other common causes of osteomalacia, such as vitamin D deficiency, need to be considered, although this is now uncommon with the routine supplementation of vitamin D in patients on dialysis. Chronic hypophosphatemia and metabolic acidosis can also cause osteomalacia in some patients.

Clinically, aluminum-induced osteomalacia presents as diffuse bone pain and predisposes to insufficiency fractures. Aluminum levels, PTH, and bone-specific alkaline phosphatase (BSAP) levels are increased. Radiographic findings are osteopenia and Looser's zones. Bone biopsy with aluminum staining is diagnostic and should be done for confirmation. Other manifestations of aluminum toxicity include an acute or chronic encephalopathy. Deferoxamine chelation therapy may be beneficial. This type of renal bone disease is becoming less common because aluminum-containing phosphate binders and antacids (including sucralfate) are now avoided, and aluminum levels are monitored in patients on dialysis.

8. What is adynamic bone disease?

Adynamic bone disease is the most common type of renal osteodystrophy and can lead to fragility fractures. Patients with ESRD who are older, diabetic, and on peritoneal dialysis are most at risk. The pathogenesis is unclear, but excessive suppression of PTH (<100 pg/mL) plays a major role. There is no diagnostic biochemical profile that can establish the diagnosis of adynamic bone disease. A low BSAP level <7 ng/mL with a PTH <100 pg/mL is highly suggestive of this disease. Alternatively, a PTH > 500 pg/mL or a BSAP >20 ng/mL with a PTH level >200 pg/mL makes adynamic bone disease unlikely. However, although often not done, a bone biopsy is necessary to establish a definitive diagnosis and will show a markedly reduced bone turnover resulting from lack of osteoblast and osteoclast activity. The suppressed PTH is often a result of excessive use of calcium-based phosphate binders, active vitamin D analogs, high calcium dialysate, or calcimimetics. Patients can be asymptomatic or have symptoms such as hypercalcemia and fractures. Treatment is aimed at eliminating PTH suppression to allow the PTH to rise to the recommended level of 150 to 300 pg/mL for patients on dialysis. Bisphosphonates should never be used to treat osteoporosis or fragility fractures in a patient with ESRD without first having a bone biopsy to rule out adynamic bone disease. Notably, teriparatide or abaloparatide have been used in some patients with success.

9. What is amyloid arthropathy of renal failure?

β2-**microglobulin** is an endogenous structural protein (molecular weight = 11.8 kDa) that is poorly cleared by standard dialysis membranes and accumulates to extremely high levels in patients on long-term hemodialysis. Owing to its high affinity for collagen, β2-microglobulin is deposited in bones, joints, and synovium. These deposits can lead to chronic arthralgias and carpal tunnel syndrome. This chronic arthropathy most commonly involves the shoulder, hip, wrist and finger tendon sheaths, and rarely the spine (especially cervical). Rotator cuff and subacromial bursae deposition lead to impingement syndrome.

Synovial fluid is noninflammatory but may be hemorrhagic because of anticoagulation use during dialysis. Synovial fluid or biopsy will identify amyloid fibrils when stained with Congo red. Radiographs are notable for erosions and large subchondral bony cysts that tend to occur at the ends of long bones (humerus, femur, tibia, and carpals). The use of more permeable, high-flux membranes may delay the onset of disease but does not prevent disease development. Kidney transplantation is the most effective therapy (see Chapter 72: Amyloidosis).

10. Which spondyloarthropathy is unique to dialysis patients?

A **destructive spondyloarthropathy** (DSA) is found only in long-term patients on dialysis and is defined by its radiologic picture. It can mimic infectious discitis. There is multilevel disc space narrowing with erosions and cysts of adjacent vertebral endplates without significant osteophytosis or sclerosis. Calcification of the surrounding vertebral discs is common. The cervical and lumbar spines are most frequently involved. The erosions progress radiographically over a few weeks or more, followed by reactive endplate sclerosis. Diffuse spinal involvement is unusual, although multi-segmented involvement has been described. Enthesitis can also occur.

This entity has been reported occasionally in patients who are uremic before dialysis but has not been reported following renal transplantation. Most patients are asymptomatic, which accounts for the rarity of its description. Neck pain or cervical radiculopathy is the most common complaint in symptomatic patients. Despite the severe radiologic picture, medullary compression is rare. Biopsies reveal calcium crystals (CPDD or hydroxyapatite) and/or β2-microglobulin. Hyperparathyroidism is usually also present and appears to play a role in the pathogenesis of DSA. Control of hyperparathyroidism, including subtotal parathyroidectomy, helps to slow down the progression of DSA.

11. What types of crystal deposition diseases occur in patients with renal disease?

- **Monosodium urate arthritis (gouty arthritis)** occurs occasionally, although less frequently than one would expect considering how common hyperuricemia is in patients with chronic renal failure. There is increased GI excretion of uric acid when patients are in renal failure. Uric acid is extensively removed during hemodialysis.
- **CPDD** is seen occasionally in secondary hyperparathyroidism (although less common than in primary hyperparathyroidism). CPDD is manifested by chondrocalcinosis (knee, wrist, and symphysis pubis), acute pseudogout, and/or degenerative arthritis.
- **Hydroxyapatite arthropathy** can present as acute episodes of joint pain or as a chronic periarthropathy resulting from calcium hydroxyapatite deposits. This arthropathy is strongly correlated with a high calcium–phosphate product. Periarticular and subcutaneous deposits may become quite large (tumoral calcinosis), particularly around the hips, knees, shoulders, and wrists, where they may cause pain, reduce range of motion, and predispose to infection. Enthesitis can also occur.
- **Secondary oxalosis** rarely develops in long-standing renal failure. It is marked by oxalate deposition in visceral organs, blood vessels, bones, and articular cartilage where it may contribute to chronic polyarthralgias. Oxalate is produced from ascorbic acid and is cleared very poorly in chronic renal failure (GFR <20 mL/minute) and dialysis. Most cases of oxalosis can be prevented by limiting ascorbic acid (vitamin C) and oxalate intake (tea, spinach, okra, sweet potatoes, nuts, and soy products). Treatment of established calcium oxalate arthropathy with nonsteroidal anti-inflammatory drugs (NSAIDs), colchicine, intraarticular corticosteroids, or increased dialysis has produced only slight improvement.

12. Where do soft tissue calcifications occur in renal osteodystrophy?

Soft tissue calcification is common in renal osteodystrophy. Sites of soft tissue deposition are multiple, including the cornea and conjunctiva, viscera, vasculature, and subcutaneous and periarticular tissues. Calcification consistently occurs in chronic renal failure when the concentration (mg/dL) product of plasma calcium and phosphorus exceeds 70. It can also occur at lesser levels. Of particular concern is the high incidence of coronary artery calcification in patients on hemodialysis, which can predispose them to coronary events. Additionally, vascular calcification may compromise blood flow leading to ischemic necrosis of skin and muscle, which is called **calciphylaxis**. The chemical composition of the calcium depends on the site of deposition. In subcutaneous, vascular, and periarticular sites, hydroxyapatite is observed, whereas in viscera, a magnesium whitlockite-like material is found.

13. A patient who is 3 months post renal transplant develops acute knee arthritis. Current medications include cyclosporine, mycophenolate mofetil, and prednisone. What is the most likely etiology for this patient's knee pain?

This is a common presentation of **acute gouty arthritis** associated with **cyclosporine** use. Cyclosporine blocks renal uric acid clearance, leading to marked hyperuricemia and gout. Polarized microscopy of the synovial fluid may identify numerous intracellular, negatively birefringent, needle-shaped crystals, confirming the diagnosis of gout (see Chapter 44: Gout). Positively birefringent rhomboid crystals of pseudogout also may be seen because of the association of secondary hyperparathyroidism and CPDD disease. Septic arthritis needs to be considered in the differential diagnosis because of the potent immunosuppressive therapy used in this post-transplant patient. Therefore, joint fluid should be sent for Gram stain and cultures to include bacteria, fungi, and mycobacteria. Note, when determining acute and long-term therapy, colchicine should not be used in patients taking cyclosporine owing to the risk of myotoxicity.

14. **What other musculoskeletal problems are increased in patients on dialysis?**
    - Erosive osteoarthritis.
    - Muscle cramps
    - Uremic myopathy (50%): due to vitamin D deficiency and/or hyperparathyroidism
    - Tendinitis and tendon ruptures (quadriceps, patellar, Achilles, triceps, finger extensors): attributable to secondary hyperparathyroidism.
    - Olecranon bursitis (dialysis elbow): occurs on same side as AV fistula used for dialysis. Due to mechanical irritation from elbow resting on hard surface. Infection needs to be excluded.
    - Osteonecrosis (avascular necrosis): does not improve with core decompression (see Chapter 53: Osteonecrosis).
    - Osteopenia: especially after renal transplantation (see Chapter 51: Metabolic Bone Disease). Note that FRAX risk calculation is <u>doubled</u> if patient's GFR is <30 mL/minute. Bone turnover markers (CTX, NTX) in the blood cannot be followed as they are cleared by the kidney and will be falsely elevated.
    - Nephrogenic systemic fibrosis (see Chapter 18: Scleroderma Mimics).

15. **What dose adjustments are needed for antirheumatic drugs in patients with renal insufficiency?**
    Serum creatinine may be an inaccurate measurement of renal function because as renal function declines, less creatinine is excreted by glomerular filtration and more is excreted by tubular secretion. The use of cimetidine (400 mg four times a day for 2 days) blocks the tubular secretion of creatinine and may improve accuracy of creatinine clearance measurements. Serum cystatin C may be a more accurate measure of estimated GFR since it is not affected by diet or muscle mass. After determining the correct GFR, the following guidelines can be used (also see chapters on medications):
    - Anakinra—GFR <30 mL/minute, decrease frequency from daily to 100 mg subcutaneously every other day.
    - Antimalarials—40% to 50% excreted by kidneys. Reduce dose 25% if GFR < 60 mL/min and reduce by 50% or do not use at all in severe renal insufficiency GFR <30 mL/minute. Neuromyopathy, cardiomyopathy, and retinal toxicity increase with renal insufficiency. Cannot be hemodialyzed. Follow hydroxychloroquine whole blood levels.
    - Allopurinol—GFR 30 mL/minute, use max 100 mg (start at 50 mg qod); GFR 60 mL/minute, use max 200 mg (start at 100 mg alternate with 50 mg qd); GFR 90 mL/minute, use max 300 mg daily (start with 100 mg qd). In patients on hemodialysis, give 100 mg daily after dialysis if needed. Dialysis usually lowers uric acid without the need for allopurinol.
    - Apremilast—GFR <60 mL/minute, max dose is 30 mg/day.
    - Azathioprine—GFR 15 to 30 mL/minute, reduce dose by 25%. GFR <15 mL/minute, reduce dose by 50%. Give after hemodialysis.
    - Baricitinib— GFR <60 mL/minute, max dose 2 mg/day or do not use; GFR <30 mL/minute, do not use. Can cause reversible increase in creatinine.
    - Biologics (monoclonal antibodies, decoy receptors, receptor antagonists)—most not tested but probably do not need dose adjustment. Chronic kidney disease is a risk factor for increased infections on biologic therapy.
    - Bisphosphonates—avoid in ESRD. Use half-oral dose or not at all in severe renal insufficiency (<30 mL/minute). Risedronate may be safer than alendronate. Intravenous (IV) bisphosphonates need to be administered more slowly with IV ibandronate safer than IV zoledronic acid in patients with moderate renal insufficiency (<50 mL/minute). Denosumab may be a better alternative but can cause hypocalcemia.

- Colchicine—avoid prolonged use in patients with GFR <50 mL/minute if possible. Use 0.6 mg daily for GFR <50 mL/minute and 0.3 mg daily for GFR <30 mL/minute. Do not use if GFR <10 mL/minute or on hemodialysis unless no other alternative. Watch for cytopenias and neuromyopathy. Cannot be hemodialyzed.
- Corticosteroids—no change in dose.
- Cyclophosphamide— GFR 15–30 mL/minute, reduce dose to 75% of usual dose. GFR <15 mL/minute, reduce dose to 50% usual dose if the patient has ESRD, give the dose after hemodialysis. Look at chapter 85 for IV dosing guidelines.
- Cyclosporine—no dose adjustment for renal insufficiency. However, using cyclosporine can worsen renal insufficiency. If creatinine rises, the cyclosporine dose needs to be lowered. Cannot be hemodialyzed. Monitor blood levels.
- Dapsone—GFR <50 mL/minute, give every other day.
- Deucravacitinib —no change in dose.
- Febuxostat—GFR <30 mL/minute, maximum dose is 40 mg/day.
- Leflunomide—insufficient data. The drug (40–50%) is eliminated by the kidneys although the active metabolite is not increased in renal insufficiency as a result of increased enterohepatic excretion. Cannot be hemodialyzed. Do not use if GFR < 15 mL/minute.
- Methotrexate—reduce dose 50% with renal insufficiency (GFR < 60 mL/min). Should not be used or used with extreme caution owing to hematologic toxicity when GFR <30–50 mL/minute (max dose 5 mg weekly). Cannot be hemodialyzed.
- Mycophenolate mofetil—hepatic metabolism with 90% renally excreted. Enterohepatic circulation can be safety valve with renal insufficiency. Do not exceed 1 g twice daily for GFR <30 mL/minute or on peritoneal dialysis. Do not exceed 500 mg twice daily if on hemodialysis.
- Narcotics—GFR 10 to 50 mL/minute, use 75% usual dose; GFR <10 mL/minute, cut dose 50%. Avoid meperidine. Fentanyl is safest.
- NSAIDs—most are metabolized by liver except for diflunisal. All NSAIDs except salsalate can make renal insufficiency worse. No need for dose adjustment for NSAIDs in ESRD, except for diflunisal (decrease dose 50%). Avoid sulindac, owing to renal stone formation in patients with low urine output. Also avoid ketoprofen, because it will be metabolized back to active drug if it cannot be renally excreted.
- Pegloticase—no change in dose. However, often given with methotrexate.
- Probenecid—does not work if GFR <30–50 mL/minute. No dosage changes for mild renal insufficiency. Same for lesinurad.
- Romosozumab—no dose change in renal insufficiency.
- Sulfasalazine—no change in dose but start with lower dose.
- Tacrolimus— Use with caution. Do not use if GFR<30 mL/min.
- Teriparatide—no change in dose. Teriparatide effective for osteoporosis in patients with GFR as low as 30 mL/minute even if PTH mildly elevated (up to 150 pg/mL) as long as vitamin D is repleted. Same for abaloparatide.
- Tofacitinib—GFR <50 to 60 mL/minute, max dose is 5 mg/day. Use with caution or not at all in patients on dialysis. Can cause reversible increase in creatinine.
- Tramadol—give dose (50 to 100 mg) every 12 hours instead of every 6 hours if GFR <30 mL/minute or on hemodialysis. Give after dialysis.
- Upadacitinib: no change in dose up to 15mg/d.

16. Which antirheumatic drugs are removed by hemodialysis?

- Allopurinol—removes 50%.
- Azathioprine.
- Methylprednisolone.
- Cyclophosphamide—removes 50%.
- Dapsone
- Tramadol—removes 70% (high permeability membrane).

These drugs should be given after hemodialysis. Other antirheumatic drugs are either not removed by hemodialysis (NSAIDs, narcotics, cyclosporine, methotrexate, leflunomide, colchicine, antimalarials, tacrolimus, bDMARDs, JAK inhibitors) or it is unknown if they are.

BIBLIOGRAPHY

Bardin T, Richette P. Rheumatic manifestations of renal disease. *Curr Opin Rheumatol.* 2009;21:55–61.

Golightly LK, Teitelbaum I, Simendinger BA, et al., eds. *Renal Pharmacotherapy. Dosage Adjustments of Medications Eliminated by the Kidneys.* New York: Springer Cham; 2021.

Hage S, Hage V, el-Khoury N, et al. Musculoskeletal disorders in hemodialysis patients: different disease clustering according to age and dialysis vintage. *Clin Rheumatol.* 2020;39:533–539.

Harty T, O'Shaughnessy MO, Harney S. Therapeutics in rheumatology and the kidney. *Rheumatology.* 2023;62:1009–1020.

Hu L, Napoletano A, Provenzano M, et al. Mineral bone disorders in kidney disease patients: the ever-current topic. *Int J Mol Sci.* 2022;23:12223.

Kidney Disease: Improving Global Outcomes (KDIGO) CKD-MBD Work Group: KDIGO clinical practice guidelines for the diagnosis, evaluation, prevention, and treatment of chronic kidney disease-mineral and bone disorder (CKD-MBD). *Kidney Int.* 2017(suppl 7):1–59.

Mehdi S, Prete P, Hashimzadeh M, et al. A study of musculoskeletal disease in two chronic hemodialysis populations and its impact on quality of life. *J Clin Rheumatol.* 2009;15:405–407.

Miller PD. Bone disease in CKD: a focus on osteoporosis diagnosis and management. *Am J Kid Dis.* 2014;64:290–304.

Moe S, Drueke T, Cunningham J, et al. Definition, evaluation, and classification of renal osteodystrophy: a position statement from Kidney disease: Improving Global Outcomes (KDIGO). *Kidney Int.* 2006;69:1945–1953.

Portales-Castillo I, Yee J, Tanaka H, Fenves AZ. Beta-2 microglobulin amyloidosis: past, present, future. *Kidney360.* 2020;1:1447–1455.

Portillo MR, ME Rodríguez-Ortiz. Secondary hyperparathyroidism: pathogenesis, diagnosis, preventive and therapeutic strategies. *Rev Endocr Metab Disord.* 2017;18:79–95.

Rafto SE, Dalinka MK, Schieber ML, et al. Spondyloarthropathy of the cervical spine in long-term hemodialysis. *Radiology.* 1988;166:201–204.

Sharma S, Gupta A. Adynamic bone disease: revisited. *Nefrologia.* 2022;42:8–14.

Vervloet MG, Massy ZA, Brandenburg VM, et al. Bone: a new endocrine organ at the heart of chronic kidney disease and mineral and bone disorders. *Lancet Diabetes Endocrinol.* 2014;2:427–436.

FURTHER READING

http://www.kidney.org.
http://www.kdigo.org.

CHAPTER 78

Rheumatic Disease and the Pregnant Patient

Kristen Demoruelle, MD, PhD, Daniele Marcy, MD, and JoAnn Zell, MD

> ## ≫ KEY POINTS
>
> 1. Maternal and fetal outcomes for pregnant patients with inflammatory rheumatic disease are best when the disease is well controlled prior to conception.
> 2. Patients who have anti-Ro (SS-A) or anti-La (SS-B) antibodies are at increased risk for having infants who develop neonatal lupus syndrome.
> 3. Hydroxychloroquine offers more benefit than risk when used in a pregnant patient with SLE.
> 4. Up to 50% to 75% of patients with rheumatoid arthritis (RA) improve during pregnancy.

1. List some of the physiologic changes that occur during pregnancy and their possible effects on patients with rheumatic diseases. See Table 78.1.

Additional notable changes during pregnancy include:

- The TH2 cytokine profile is dominant during pregnancy; this may explain why patients with SLE can flare during pregnancy while RA can improve.
- IgG can cross the placenta starting at 13 to 16 weeks of gestation.
- The risk of thrombosis increases during pregnancy due to increased hepatic protein synthesis. This can be exacerbated by the presence of antiphospholipid antibodies (aPLAs).
- Risk of osteoporosis increases during pregnancy and lactation as calcium is pulled from the bones; this calcium loss is reversible after pregnancy and lactation are completed.
- Edema of pregnancy can cause or worsen peripheral nerve compression, such as carpal tunnel syndrome, which can sometimes be misinterpreted as a disease flare.

2. What preconception counseling should I provide to my patients with rheumatologic disease?

- Consider routinely using the "one key question" that asks, "Would you like to become pregnant in the next year?" This provides a patient-centered framework to discuss a patient's desires and goals for pregnancy. If a patient answers "yes, unsure, or OK either way", counsel on potential pregnancy risk and medication safety. If a patient answers "no", counsel on contraception.
- High disease activity at conception has been associated with poor pregnancy outcomes in most autoimmune conditions. Therefore, the recommended timing of a planned pregnancy is when the rheumatologic disease is well controlled.
- Patients on immunomodulation or immunosuppression should be counseled regularly on potential risks of fetal exposure. For women planning pregnancy, prior to conception, medications should be optimized to avoid teratogenesis and maintain disease control. See Table 78.2.

3. Discuss key considerations regarding contraception in patients with rheumatic disease.

- Contraception is the key to ensuring optimized timing and safety of pregnancy.
- Long-acting reversible contraceptives (implants and intrauterine devices (IUDs) have the highest efficacy.
- Progesterone only oral contraceptives, progesterone-containing implants, and IUDs are considered safe in women with high clotting risk. Of note progesterone only oral contraceptives are only effective when taken within the same two-hour window each day.
- Estrogen-containing contraceptives should be avoided in women with a positive aPLA test, even with no history of clot or other clotting risk factors.
- Women with stable SLE, no aPLAs, no thrombotic risk factors, and no history of thrombosis may use estrogen-containing oral contraceptives if they have low to moderate disease activity.
- Contraceptive decisions should include the patient, gynecology, and rheumatology.

TABLE 78.1 Physiologic Changes During Pregnancy

ORGAN SYSTEM	CHANGES DURING PREGNANCY	EFFECTS ON A PATIENT WITH AUTOIMMUNE DISEASE
Cardiovascular	Increased plasma volume Increased heart rate Increased stroke volume Vasodilation	Can place strain on the heart if affected by CTD, and can potentially exacerbate heart failure Raynaud phenomenon can improve
Pulmonary	Increased minute ventilation Respiratory alkalosis	Can stress patients with underlying pulmonary disease such as PHTN or ILD
Renal	Increased glomerular filtration rate (renal blood flow increases by 50%) Increased urinary excretion of protein	Baseline proteinuria increases: can be difficult to differentiate from a flare of glomerular disease Possible increased excretion of renally cleared medication
Laboratory values	Acute-phase reactants can rise during pregnancy including ESR and alkaline phosphatase (secreted by the placenta)	Can make it difficult to distinguish a disease flare from normal physiologic pregnancy changes
Hepatic	Increased hepatic protein synthesis, complement, fibrinogen	Elevated ESR and complement May be hard to follow ESR
Hematologic	Leukocytosis Hemodilution	Can be confused with infection Anemia Thrombocytopenia
Muscle/MSK	Relaxation of skeletal muscle Relaxation of ligaments and tendons	Worsening GERD Predisposed to sprains/other injuries that may mimic disease activity
Dermatologic	Hyper-vascular changes Melasma	Can mimic a lupus rash

CTD, Connective tissue disease; *ILD*, interstitial lung disease; *PHTN*, pulmonary hypertension; *GERD*, gastroesophageal reflux disease; *ESR*, erythrocyte sedimentation rate.

4. How do I counsel my patients about medication safety during pregnancy and breastfeeding and effects on female and male fertility? See Table 78.2.

5. A young normotensive patient with a history of SLE is currently being treated with 5 mg of prednisone and hydroxychloroquine with good disease control. She would like to become pregnant. What labs should your order now? What are her risks for an adverse pregnancy outcome? What medications should be started or continued?

Labs in lupus pregnancy:
- aPL and anti-SSA/SSB antibodies should be tested in all SLE patients prior to conception or in early pregnancy as these labs may affect surveillance. Consider repeating these studies before conception even if they have been negative previously.

Risks for poor outcome in lupus pregnancy:
- Patients with SLE have an increased risk of preeclampsia, intrauterine growth restriction, and hypertension during pregnancy. The PROMISSE study prospectively studied pregnancies in patients with SLE and identified adverse pregnancy outcomes in 19% of SLE patients with mild to moderate activity. The five major predictors of adverse pregnancy outcomes in SLE were:
  1. Lupus anticoagulant positive.
  2. Hypertensive medication use.
  3. Physician global assessment >1 (i.e., greater disease activity).
  4. Non-Caucasian (notably, this predictor may be more reflective of other risk factors for poor pregnancy outcomes such as access to care and insurance status).
  5. Thrombocytopenia (per 50K decrease).

TABLE 78.2 Medication Considerations During Pregnancy, Breastfeeding, and in Men

	PREGNANCY	BREASTFEEDING	MEN	OTHER CONSIDERATIONS
Prednisone	Compatible; optimally <20 mg/day; potential increased risk of oral cleft, preterm birth, and low birth weight at higher doses	Compatible; optimally <20 mg/day and wait 2 hours after dose to breastfeed. If >20 mg/day, wait 4 hours after dose to breastfeed.	Long-term use can be associated with decreased testosterone levels	Difficult to determine if risks during pregnancy are independent of maternal disease activity
Methotrexate	Contraindicated; teratogenic	Not recommended; insufficient data	No evidence of teratogenicity in men taking MTX, but may be associated with reduced fertility	Before planned pregnancy, discontinue at least 1 month and preferably 3 months in women
Leflunomide	Contraindicated; teratogenic; if planning pregnancy, check blood level prior to ensure undetectable; if taking and unplanned pregnancy, administer cholestyramine	Not recommended; insufficient data	Insufficient data	Before planned pregnancy in women or men, discontinue 3.5 months to 2 years prior or consider cholestyramine
Sulfasalazine	Compatible; folate supplementation needed	Compatible	Reversible azoospermia that resolves 2–3 months after discontinuation	
Hydroxychloroquine	Compatible; reduces risk of SLE flare in pregnancy; may improve pregnancy outcomes in SLE	Compatible	No known risk	No known risk of teratogenicity with commonly used doses of ≤ 400mg/day.
Azathioprine	Compatible; crosses placenta but fetal liver lacks the enzyme to convert to the active metabolite	Compatible	Limited data, but no known risk	
Mycophenolate mofetil	Contraindicated; teratogenic; increased risk of first-trimester pregnancy loss	Not recommended; insufficient data	Limited data, but no known risk	Before planned pregnancy, discontinue at least 6 weeks, preferably 3 months, in women
Anti-tumor necrosis factor α agents	Compatible; if pregnant and taking, consider discontinuation during third trimester when placental transfer occurs	Compatible	Limited data but no known risk	Certolizumab has no active placental transfer, so can consider switching to certolizumab in pregnant women
Cyclophosphamide	Contraindicated; teratogenic; dose- and age-dependent infertility including premature ovarian failure	Contraindicated	Dose-dependent infertility including irreversible azoospermia	In men and women, stop at least 3 months before planned pregnancy

Cyclosporine and tacrolimus	Compatible; potential risk of preterm birth and low birth weight reported, but difficult to determine if risk is independent of other maternal factors. Monitor BP.	Limited data, low transfer into breast milk	Limited data, but no known risk	Tacrolimus dose may need to be increased during pregnancy. While voclosporin is also a calcineurin inhibitor, it should be avoided in pregnancy and lactation because its formulation contains alcohol
JAK inhibitors, apremilast	Insufficient data but can likely transfer across placenta and not recommended	Insufficient data but can likely transfer into breastmilk and not recommended	Insufficient data	
Abatacept, anti-IL-1, belimumab, anti-IL6, anti-IL17, anti-IL-23, anifrolumab	Insufficient data but not recommended; discontinue at conception	Insufficient data, minimal transfer, destroyed in baby's GI tract, and probably safe	Insufficient data	Most IgG molecules cross placenta in the second trimester and can therefore reach fetal circulation at that time
Rituximab	Can continue up to the time of conception	Compatible	Limited data, but no known risk	Can cross placenta starting in second trimester, but use can be considered in severe disease
Colchicine	Compatible	Compatible	Limited data, but no known risk	No need to hold in pregnant women with familial Mediterranean fever
Nonsteroidal anti-inflammatory drugs	First trimester: risk of miscarriage. Second trimester: risk of oligohydraminos Third trimester: premature closure of the fetal ductus arteriosus	Compatible, ibuprofen preferred.	Safe to use, but daily use, particularly for aspirin, could potentially reduce fertility	Could inhibit ovulation, consider avoiding days 8–20 of the menstrual cycle for planned pregnancy
ACEi/ARB	Contraindicated in second and third trimesters due to fetal renal effects	No known risk with enalapril and captopril; insufficient data for other ACEi/ARBs	No known risk	
Coumadin	Contraindicated; teratogenic	Compatible	Insufficient data	

ACEi, Angiotensin-converting enzyme inhibitor; *ARB,* angiotensin-receptor blocker; *IL,* interleukin; *JAK,* Janus kinase; *SLE,* systemic lupus erythematosus.
Compatible = low risk with no clear evidence of harm to fetus or infant.
Any medication not clinically indicated or needed should be avoided in pregnancy, with the exception of hydroxychloroquine, which should be continued during pregnancy in lupus to reduce the risk of flare.
Must always consider fetal risk of the medication versus fetal risk if disease flares.
Although most medications in the chart have been detected in small amounts in breast milk, those listed as compatible have been used historically without safety concerns.
Letter-based categories (i.e., A, B, C, D, and X) for medication risks in pregnancy and lactation are often confusing and not always clinically helpful. In June 2015, the Food and Drug Administration implemented a new Pregnancy and Lactation Labeling Rule to replace the letter-based categories.

SLE patients without these risk factors had poor pregnancy outcomes at rates similar to controls. Since this patient has none of the five risk factors, she has a lower chance of a poor pregnancy outcome.

Considerations for medications in lupus pregnancy:

- Low-dose prednisone (<20 mg/day) is considered safe in pregnancy, but for this patient, you could consider a prednisone taper prior to conception to minimize any immunosuppression. However, you must ensure any change in immunosuppression does not precipitate a flare of disease as pregnancy outcomes are worse when disease is active at conception.
- Hydroxychloroquine at doses of 400 mg or less per day is considered safe in pregnancy. Withdrawal of hydroxychloroquine when needed may result in poor outcomes. The 2020 ACR Reproductive Health Guidelines conditionally recommend starting HCQ in a lupus pregnancy if the mother is not already taking the medication.
- Low-dose aspirin (ASA) (75–100 mg/d) is recommended in all SLE patients for prevention of preeclampsia. Recommended to start at 12–28 weeks' gestation, preferably by 16 weeks, and continue until delivery.

6. What are the risks for a SLE patient with active lupus nephritis (LN) who would like to become pregnant?

The PROMISSE study excluded patients with severe renal disease (creatinine >1.2 mg/dL and >1 gram of proteinuria per day). However, sub-analysis of these patients showed that those with a history of complete or partial remission from renal disease and a low C4 all correlated with poorer obstetric outcomes.

Other studies indicate that active disease (including nephritis) portends a poor prognosis in SLE pregnancy. A history of LN or current LN correlates with poor fetal and maternal outcomes including an odds ratio (OR) of 9.0 for renal flare during/after pregnancy, OR of 7.3 for fetal loss, and OR of 18.9 for preterm delivery. Maternal hypertension and aPLAs may increase these risks as well as the risk of preeclampsia.

7. What should be considered when a patient with SLE nephritis desires pregnancy?

- **Stop renin–angiotensin blockade**: These medications are associated with oligohydramnios in fetuses exposed in the second and third trimesters of pregnancies. They should be stopped prior to or at conception and transitioned to pregnancy-compatible medications if needed for blood pressure control, such as labetalol.
- Patients should be in remission for at least 6 months prior to conception. The longer the remission, the better.
- Expect baseline proteinuria to increase with increased glomerular filtration rate during pregnancy.
- Hydroxychloroquine may help prevent intrauterine growth restriction and is generally considered safe in doses of 400 mg or less during pregnancy.
- Low-dose ASA started after 12 weeks gestation may lessen the chance of preeclampsia.
- Anti-dsDNA levels are not affected by pregnancy and can be followed as a sign of disease flare in some individuals with increasing proteinuria.
- The risk of renal biopsy is likely not increased for patients in the first and second trimesters (if aPLA-negative and not on anticoagulation), but best done prior to pregnancy if there is a concern for active nephritis.

PEARL: Complements are elevated during pregnancy, so even normal levels that are dropping may indicate an SLE flare.

8. How can you distinguish active SLE nephritis from preeclampsia?

Preeclampsia (formerly known as toxemia) typically occurs in late pregnancy (after 20 weeks of gestation) of primigravida. LN can occur at any time during pregnancy and is associated with active urine sediment. Since patients with SLE have an increased risk of preeclampsia, these conditions can be difficult to separate in a clinical scenario and can sometimes coexist. See Table 78.3 for distinguishing clinical findings.

TABLE 78.3 Clinical Findings Distinguishing Preeclampsia From a Lupus Flare

ABNORMALITY	PREECLAMPSIA	SLE
Blood pressure	High	Normal or high
Platelets	Low or normal	Low or normal
Complement	Variable[a]	Low or in normal range but down-trending
Uric acid	High	High or normal
Proteinuria	Present	Present
Active urine sediment	No	Yes
Anti-DNA antibody	Normal or stable	Rising or high
Other SLE symptoms	Absent	Can be present
sFlt-1/PlGF	>38	≤38

SLE, Systemic lupus erythematosus; *sFlt-1,* soluble fms-like tyrosine kinase; *PlGF,* placental growth factor.
[a]Patients with preeclampsia and eclampsia can develop low complement levels.

Interestingly, in the PROMISSE study the measurement of angiogenic factors such as placental growth factor (PGF) and soluble fms-like tyrosine kinase 1 (sFlt1) measured early in pregnancy (12–19 weeks) predicted preeclampsia (low PGF and high sFlt1). Other studies have shown that measuring these mediators can also help distinguish preeclampsia from active lupus nephritis later in pregnancy.

9. **Which lupus-related autoantibodies can cause problems for a fetus during pregnancy?**

Antibodies to Ro/SSA, especially when high titer, have been associated with neonatal lupus syndrome in patients with SLE or Sjogren disease (SjD). This can also occur in any woman who makes these antibodies regardless of whether she has an autoimmune disease or not. Antibodies to **La/SSB, especially in isolation,** have rarely been associated with this syndrome. Women with anti-Ro/SSA and/or anti-La/SSB antibodies should be monitored by high-risk OB/GYN for signs of neonatal heart block (see below) during 16–26 weeks of gestation.

aPLAs have been associated with an increased risk of recurrent first-trimester spontaneous abortion and stillbirths, preeclampsia, intrauterine growth restriction, and preterm birth. One hypothesis for this complication is that complement activation leading to influx of inflammatory cells results in thrombosis and placental insufficiency. Anticoagulation with unfractionated or low-molecular-weight heparin (in combination with low-dose aspirin) can dramatically improve obstetric outcomes (80% live birth rates) possibly due to their effect on the complement cascade. Rarely, neonatal antiphospholipid syndrome (APS) due to transplacental passage of aPLs may occur. There may be an increased risk of neurocognitive delay in children born to mothers with APS, perhaps due to microvascular insult on developing neural tissue.

Antiplatelet antibodies can occasionally cause autoimmune thrombocytopenia in the fetus with associated hemorrhage, especially at the time of delivery. The management of this complication can be challenging.

10. **Describe the typical clinical presentation of infants with neonatal lupus erythematosus (NLE) and speculate on pathogenesis. Are there treatments that can prevent NLE?**

Organ	*Manifestation*
Skin	Subacute SLE rash[a]
Liver	Elevation of liver function tests/hepatosplenomegaly
Hematologic	Cytopenias
Cardiac	Heart block/endocardial fibroelastosis

[a]Some patients with NLE and skin rash have ribonucleoprotein (anti U1 RNP) antibodies only.

Most noncardiac manifestations clear in approximately 6 months as this is when the maternal antibodies degrade. Congenital heart block (CHB) is the most common cardiac manifestation of NLE, and the accompanying myocarditis accounts for the majority of morbidity and mortality. The conduction defect is due to maternal IgG anti-Ro (SS-A) more than anti-La (SS-B) antibodies that cross the placenta and bind to fetal cardiocytes and heart conducting cells, eliciting an inflammatory injury during the second trimester of pregnancy. Any clinical manifestation of NLE occurs in approximately 5% to 20% of offspring of mothers with high circulating levels of these antibodies. The risk specifically of CHB is 2% in the offspring of seropositive mothers.

After a patient has one child with CHB, the risk of recurrent heart block in the fetus during another pregnancy is 15% to 20%. Hydroxychloroquine use is associated with a decreased rate of **recurrent** CHB in subsequent pregnancies. In the PATCH study, 400 mg of hydroxychloroquine started at 10 weeks gestation in women with a previous history of CHB reduced the rate of CHB to approximately 7.5% (secondary prevention). Studies are needed to determine if hydroxychloroquine can be used for primary prevention (i.e., preventing the initial development of CHB in seropositive mothers who have not had a previous child with CHB). However, the 2020 ACR Reproductive Health Guidelines do conditionally recommend the addition of HCQ in SSA/Ro positive pregnant women regardless of prior history of CHB. Monitoring of anti-SSA positive patients during pregnancy is outlined in Figure 78.1.

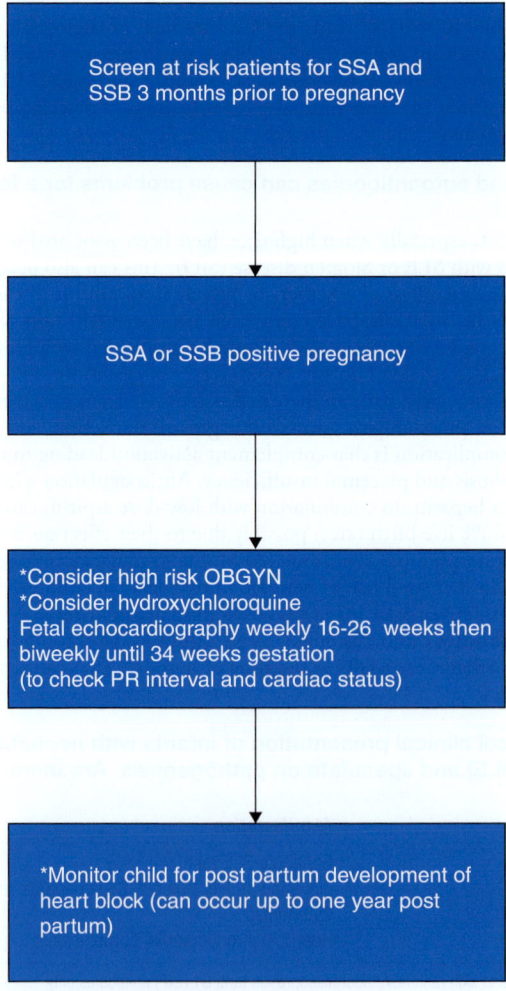

Fig 78.1 Monitoring of at-risk patients for complete heart block.

TABLE 78.4 Suggested Approach for the Treatment of Cardiac Neonatal Lupus Erythematosus

MANIFESTATION OF CARDIAC NEONATAL LUPUS ERYTHEMATOSUS	FEATURES	TREATMENT
First degree	Prolonged PR interval May revert back to sinus rhythm	Close monitoring Consider treatment with fluorinated steroids if persistent such as dexamethasone or betamethasone[a]; data limited
Second degree	Likely to progress to third-degree atrioventricular block but can revert to sinus rhythm without treatment	Consider fluorinated steroids, IVIG
Third degree	Irreversible Associated with fetal demise in up to 9–25% of cases	Possible neonatal or post-natal pacemaker No treatment has been clearly shown to correct this for rhythm disturbance If endocardial inflammation is present, see below
Cardiomyopathy/endocardial fibroelastosis/hydrops	Global disease can accompany heart block	Fluorinated steroids and/or IVIG may be considered for inflammatory cardiac disease ± heart block; data limited

IVIG, Intravenous immunoglobulin.
[a]dexamethasone and betamethasone are fluorinated glucocorticoids and are not inactivated by the placental 11 beta hydrogenase. Infants born to mothers with anti-SSA and/or SSB antibodies should have an EKG at birth even if monitoring was normal during pregnancy. Any evidence of heart block indicates a risk of progression during the first year of life.

11. Is there a treatment for CHB in neonatal lupus syndrome?

Consider treatment (see table 78.4) if a fetus develops (1) heart block or (2) signs of myocardial inflammation. Notably, data on the treatment of CHB yield conflicting results and much of it is anecdotal. Currently, there does not appear to be an effective treatment option for third-degree heart block.

12. What are the obstetric complications that can be associated with APS?

See Chapter 22: Antiphospholipid Syndrome for details regarding the classification and diagnosis of APS. The following adverse pregnancy outcomes are included in the Obstetric domain of the 2023 ACR/EULAR APS Classification Criteria:

- Pre-fetal death – otherwise unexplained pregnancy loss before 10 weeks gestation
- Fetal death – otherwise unexplained pregnancy loss between 10 and 34 weeks' gestation.
- Pre-eclampsia with severe features. Severe features can include severe blood pressure elevation (systolic ≥160 or diastolic ≥110 on 2 occasions), CNS dysfunction (new headache unresponsive to medication), visual disturbances, pulmonary edema, impaired liver function, renal dysfunction, thrombocytopenia.
- Placental insufficiency (i.e. intrauterine fetal growth restriction (IUGR)) with severe features. Severe features can include abnormal fetal surveillance tests, severe IUGR <3rd percentile, oligohydramnios, maternal vascular malperfusion on placental histology.

Notably, the 2023 ACR/EULAR APS Classification Criteria includes an additive weighted points system in which only 1 point is given for ≥3 consecutive pre-fetal pregnancy losses (<10 weeks gestation) and/or 3 early fetal deaths (10–16 weeks gestation), or ≥1 fetal death (16–34 weeks gestations). This deemphasis on obstetric features of APS compared to prior APS guidelines results in the potential that a woman with only obstetric features of APS may not meet the 2023 classification criteria for APS.

TABLE 78.5 Suggested Treatment During Pregnancy for Women With aPLAs or APS

CLINICAL SCENARIO	REGIMEN SUGGESTED
Repeatedly positive aPLAs, but no history of pregnancy morbidity	Consider low-dose aspirin Consider prophylactic dose heparin for 6 weeks postpartum in patients with LAC and/or high titer aPLAs due to risk of thrombosis
High-risk repeatedly positive aPLAs (triple positive or LAC positive) and less than three consecutive pregnancy losses.	Consider prophylactic dose heparin and aspirin[a]
All SLE patients during pregnancy +/− aPLAs Patients with a history of preterm birth due to preeclampsia and positive aPLAs	Low-dose aspirin
Women with SLE +/− APS with pregnancy failure despite treatment with low-dose aspirin Patients with severe preeclampsia and positive aPLAs	Aspirin plus prophylactic dose heparin or LMWH
Patients with positive aPLAs and a prior thrombotic event (meets criteria for APS prior to pregnancy) Pregnancy loss with positive aPLAs despite prophylactic dose heparin and aspirin[a]	Full dose LMWH and aspirin
Obstetric APS	Combined low-dose aspirin and prophylactic dose LMWH Consider addition of hydroxychloroquine Consider treating with prophylactic heparin or LMWH for 6–12 weeks postpartum
Thrombotic APS	Combined low-dose aspirin and therapeutic dose LMWH throughout pregnancy and postpartum period Consider addition of hydroxychloroquine

aPLAs, Antiphospholipid antibodies; *LAC,* lupus anticoagulant; *LMWH,* low-molecular-weight heparin; *SLE,* systemic lupus erythematosus.
[a]Controversial.

13. How does APS affect pregnancy outcomes? How it is best treated?

- Patients with APS with or without SLE are at risk for poor pregnancy outcomes (OR 9.2) including IUGR (OR 4.7), preeclampsia (OR 2.3), thrombosis (OR 12.1), and early and late fetal loss.
- Lupus anticoagulant conveys the greatest risk for adverse pregnancy outcomes (RR 12.2).
- A systematic review found that for recurrent early miscarriage associated with APS, the addition of heparin plus ASA provided an estimated 54% reduced risk of pregnancy loss. No universally accepted guidelines exist for prophylaxis in pregnancy with persistently positive aPL antibodies. Most determine treatment based on prior obstetric complications. It is recommended to start ASA 4 weeks prior to conception if possible. See Table 78.5 for additional details regarding treatment during pregnancy in patients with aPLAs or APS.

14. How does pregnancy affect rheumatoid arthritis (RA)?

- Two-thirds of patients with RA have improvement in RA symptoms during pregnancy, but <20% achieve drug-free remission.
- Symptom improvement is highest during the third trimester.
- Two-thirds of RA patients have a flare of RA symptoms in the first 6 months postpartum.
- Erythrocyte sedimentation rate increases during pregnancy and should not be used in the measurements of disease activity.

15. A patient with RA is currently being treated with adalimumab with good disease control. They would like to become pregnant. What labs should you order now?

What are the risks for an adverse pregnancy outcome? Should adalimumab be continued? Does taking adalimumab affect the vaccination schedule for the baby?

- Five percent of RA patients are anti-SSA positive. Screening for anti-SSA in RA women who are pregnant or planning pregnancy can inform risk of neonatal CHB.
- Women with RA are at increased risk of preterm birth (OR 1.9), small for gestational age (SGA) babies (OR 1.9), and pre-eclampsia.
- Moderate or high disease activity at conception and during pregnancy is associated with preterm birth and SGA. Risk is lowered (OR 1) if RA is in low disease activity or remission prior to and during pregnancy.
- TNF inhibitors are compatible with pregnancy and can be continued after conception. TNF inhibitors other than certolizumab can cross the placenta and it is recommended to discontinue them during the third trimester to minimize immunosuppression of the baby. Certolizumab does not contain an Fc fragment resulting in minimal to no placental transfer; as such, it can be continued throughout pregnancy.
- Babies exposed to TNF inhibitors in utero should avoid live vaccines until 6 months of age. One exception is rotavirus vaccination, which is conditionally recommended by the American College of Rheumatology to be given on schedule (within the first 6 months) for babies exposed to TNF inhibitors. Nonlive vaccines can be given on schedule.

16. What effect does pregnancy have on the spondyloarthropathies and *vice versa?*

- The course of ankylosing spondylitis varies during pregnancy (33% improve, 33% worsen) and up to 60% worsen postpartum (mostly low back pain).
- Up to 50% of patients with PsA may improve during pregnancy.
- Hip involvement can increase the incidence of cesarean section. Notably, hip arthroplasty and SI joint fusion are not contraindications for vaginal delivery. Patients with severe back and/or hip disease should be assessed for their capability to deliver vaginally.
- Both elevated disease activity and anti-TNF discontinuation in early pregnancy are associated with increased risk of disease flare later in pregnancy.
- Incidence of preterm birth and IUGR is increased in women with SpA and PsA.
- Pre-eclampsia risk may be higher in women with PsA.

17. How does systemic sclerosis (SSc) affect pregnancy?

- Pregnancy is not recommended in women with underlying pulmonary hypertension (PHTN). If a woman with PHTN does desire pregnancy, very close follow-up with high-risk OB and pulmonology is necessary.
- Women with early disease should delay pregnancy until disease stabilization.
- Patients with SSc have an increased risk of: (1) preterm delivery, (2) intrauterine growth restriction, and (3) low birth weight.
- Risk factors for worse outcomes include: (1) early disease, (2) diffuse cutaneous SSc, (3) anti-Scl-70 ab, and (4) anti-RNA polymerase III ab.
- Pregnancy does not cause progressive visceral involvement or an increased risk of scleroderma renal crisis.
- Raynaud symptoms often improve and gastrointestinal reflux and arthralgias often worsen during pregnancy.
- Anti-SSA positivity is present in 15–30% of patients with SSc. Screening for anti-SSA in women with scleroderma who are pregnant or planning pregnancy can inform risk of neonatal CHB.

18. How does CTD-ILD affect pregnancy?

- Women with CTD-ILD have increased rates of adverse pregnancy outcomes (56% had either preeclampsia, preterm delivery, small for gestational age baby, fetal death or neonatal death).
- Rates of adverse pregnancy outcomes were higher in women with more severe ILD.

19. How does inflammatory myositis affect pregnancy?

Like other rheumatic diseases, active myositis during pregnancy correlates with poorer obstetric outcomes such as increased rate of fetal death, preterm birth, and IUGR. Hypertension during pregnancy appears to be relatively common and could be related to medication use. Some data suggest that myositis may improve during pregnancy as has been reported in some other rheumatic conditions. Postpartum flare can occur. For treatment of myositis during pregnancy, IVIG appears to be relatively safe (watch for risk of thrombosis) as do other medications commonly used including corticosteroids, azathioprine, and calcineurin inhibitors.

20. How do pregnancy outcomes vary among different types of vasculitis?

- **Anti-neutrophil cytoplasmic antibody-associated vasculitis:** increased risk of preterm delivery (18%) and IUGR (20%). Poor outcomes occur when pregnancy occurs in the setting of high disease activity, but even if conception occurs with controlled disease, up to 40% of patients will flare during pregnancy. Disease activity during pregnancy is associated with preterm delivery and miscarriage as well as more serious outcomes.
- **Polyarteritis nodosa (PAN):** conception during remission results in good outcomes with rare flares. Onset of disease during pregnancy has a high maternal mortality.
- **Takayasu arteritis:** pregnancies are more likely to be complicated by hypertension (40%) and preeclampsia (20%). Limited case series show 3–25% of patients can experience a flare during pregnancy. Most adverse pregnancy outcomes are not due to disease flares but due to vascular sequelae from previously active disease.
- **Behçet disease:** pregnancy outcomes are similar to the general population, but preterm delivery may be more common. Up to 30% have an increase in disease activity during pregnancy. Patients with prior thrombosis should be considered for intrapartum anticoagulation.

21. Is male fertility affected by rheumatic disease?

- **Vasculitis:** decreased fertility if testicular involvement in PAN; patients with Behçet disease have normal fertility. Data are lacking for other forms of vasculitis.
- **Ankylosing spondylitis:** higher rates of varicocele which can affect sperm production.
- **Psoriatic arthritis:** conflicting data if inflammatory arthritis affects sperm quality and decreases fertility.
- **RA:** active RA is associated with hypogonadism as well as decreased sperm production and function.
- **SLE:** decreased libido, erectile dysfunction, and failure to ejaculate, though it is difficult to sort out medication effect.
- **Medications:** see Table 78.2.
- Common comorbidities also affect fertility and libido including NSAID use, obesity, chronic kidney disease, and depression.

22. What are some helpful resources for working with patients with rheumatic disease who have questions about pregnancy or contraception?

- **Organization of Teratology Information Specialists.** This organization runs MotherToBaby (https://mothertobaby.org), which is an excellent source of information for patients and healthcare professionals that includes up-to-date information regarding the effects of medications and rheumatologic disease in pregnancy. They can be reached by calling 1-866-626-6847.
- 2020 ACR Reproductive Health Guidelines. This resource includes a summary of data and consensus agreement as well as easily visualized figures covering a range of topics that include contraception and pregnancy in women with rheumatic disease.
- Lactmed is a database that can be used to query medication safety in breastfeeding.
- www.lupuspregnancy.org. Includes multiple resources to facilitate conversations with lupus patients regarding contraception and pregnancy.
- www.reprorheum.duke.edu. Includes multiple resources to facilitate conversations related to contraception and pregnancy in women with a range of autoimmune diseases.

ACKNOWLEDGMENT

The authors would like to thank Dr. Jennifer Stichman, Dr. Sterling West, and Dr. Mark Jarek for their contributions to this chapter in earlier editions.

BIBLIOGRAPHY

Andreoli L, Bertsias GK, Agmon-Levin N, et al. EULAR recommendations for women's health and the management of family planning, assisted reproduction, pregnancy and menopause in patients with systemic lupus erythematosus and/or antiphospholipid syndrome. *Ann Rheum Dis.* 2017;76:476–485.

Barbhaiya M, Zuily S, Naden R, et al. The 2023 ACR/EULAR Antiphospholipid syndrome classification criteria. *Arthritis Rheumatol.* 2023;75:1687–1702.

Branch DW, Lim MY. How I diagnose and treat antiphospholipid syndrome in pregnancy. *Blood.* 2024;143:757–768.

Buyon JP, Kim MY, Guerra MM, et al. Predictors of pregnancy outcomes in patients with lupus: a cohort study. *Ann Int Med.* 2015;163:153–163.

Clowse M, Addae-Konadu K, Federspiel J, et al. The utility of the sFlt1:PlGF ratio to rule out and predict preeclampsia in women with lupus [abstract 0809]. *Arthritis Rheumatol.* 2024;76(suppl 9).

de Jesus GR, Lacerda MI, Rodrigues BC, et al. Soluble Flt-1, placental growth factor, and vascular endothelial growth factor serum levels to differentiate between active lupus nephritis during pregnancy and preeclampsia. *Arthritis Care Res (Hoboken).* 2021;73:717–721.

Empson M, Lassere M, Craig JC, Scott JR. Recurrent pregnancy loss with antiphospholipid antibody: a systematic review of therapeutic trials. *Obstet Gynecol.* 2002;99:135–144.

Garcia D, Erkan D. Diagnosis and management of the antiphospholipid syndrome. *N Engl J Med.* 2018;378:2010–2021.

Hellgren K, Secher AE, Glintborg B, et al. Pregnancy outcomes in relation to disease activity and anti-rheumatic treatment strategies in women with rheumatoid arthritis: a matched cohort study from Sweden and Denmark. *Rheumatology (Oxford).* 2022;61:3711–3722.

Izmirly PA, Kim M, Friedman DM, et al. Hydroxychloroquine to prevent recurrent congenital heart block in fetuses of anti-SSA/Ro-positive mother. *J Am Coll Cardiol.* 2020;76:292–302 21.

Jakobsson GL, Stephansson O, Askling J, Jacobsson LTH. Pregnancy outcomes in patients with ankylosing spondylitis: a nationwide register study. *Ann Rheum Dis.* 2016;75:1838–1842.

Lightstone L, Hladunewich MA. Lupus nephritis and pregnancy: concerns and management. *Semin Nephrol.* 2017;37:347–353.

Lockshin MD, Kim M, Laskin CA, et al. Prediction of adverse pregnancy outcome by the presence of lupus anticoagulant, but not anticardiolipin antibody, in patients with antiphospholipid antibodies. *Arthritis Rheum.* 2012;64:2311–2318.

Machen L, Clowse ME. Vasculitis and pregnancy. *Rheum Dis Clin North Am.* 2017;43:239–247.

Maguire S, Molto A. Pregnancy & neonatal outcomes in spondyloarthritis. *Best Pract Res Clin Rheumatol.* 2023;37:101868.

Marder W, Littlejohn EA, Somers EC. Pregnancy and autoimmune connective tissue diseases. *Best Pract Res Clin Rheumatol.* 2016;30:63–80.

Noviani M, Wasserman S, Clowse ME. Breastfeeding in mothers with systemic lupus erythematosus. *Lupus.* 2016;41:476–481.

Partalidou S, Mamopoulos A, Dimopoulou D, et al. Pregnancy outcomes in ANCA-associated vasculitis patients: a systematic review and meta-analysis. *Joint Bone Spine.* 2023;90:105609.

Perez-Garcia LF, Roder E, Goekoop RJ, et al. Impaired fertility in men diagnosed with inflammatory arthritis: results of a large multicentre study (iFAME-Fertility). *Ann Rheum Dis.* 2021;80:1545–1552.

Polachek A, Li S, Polachek IS, Chandran V, Gladman D. Psoriatic arthritis disease activity during pregnancy and the first-year postpartum. *Semin Arthritis Rheum.* 2017;46:740–745.

Sammaritano LR. Contraception in patients with rheumatic disease. *Rheum Dis Clin North Am.* 2017;43:173–188.

Sammaritano LR, Bermas BL, Chakravarty EE, et al. 2020 American College of Rheumatology guideline for the management of reproductive health in rheumatic and musculoskeletal diseases. *Arthritis Rheumatol.* 2020;72:529–556.

Scriffignano S, Perrotta FM, Lubrano E. male fertility in spondyloarthritis: from clinical issues to cytokines milieu. A narrative review. *Curr Rheumatol Rep.* 2024;26:321–331.

Sims C, Clowse MEB. A comprehensive guide for managing the reproductive health of patients with vasculitis. *Nat Rev Rheumatol.* 2022;18:711–723.

Tang K, Zhou J, Lan Y, et al. Pregnancy in adult-onset dermatomyositis/polymyositis: a systematic review. *Am J Reprod Immunol.* 2022;88:e13603.

van den Brandt S, Zbinden A, Baeten D, Villiger PM, Østensen M, Forger F. Risk factors for flare and treatment of disease flares during pregnancy in rheumatoid arthritis and axial spondyloarthritis patients. *Arthritis Res Ther.* 2017;19:64.

Young A, Khanna D. Systemic sclerosis: commonly asked questions by rheumatologists. *J Clin Rheumatol.* 2015;21:149–155.

CHAPTER 79

Autoinflammatory Syndromes

Katharine F. Moore, MD and Robert C. Fuhlbrigge, MD, PhD

> ## KEY POINTS
>
> 1. Autoinflammatory syndromes are disorders of the innate immune system, and typically present as recurring episodes of inflammation without evidence of infection, autoantibodies, or antigen-specific T cells.
> 2. Autoinflammatory syndromes are often characterized by episodes of fever, rash, arthritis, peritonitis, eye inflammation, and elevated acute-phase reactants in various combinations that normalize between flares; there is a great deal of symptom overlap among different autoinflammatory syndromes.
> 3. Many autoinflammatory syndromes are monogenetic diseases with mutations altering the function of the inflammatory cascade.
> 4. Autoinflammatory syndromes most commonly present in infancy or childhood, but some patients are diagnosed in adulthood.
> 5. AA Amyloidosis is a rare and late complication of some autoinflammatory syndromes and can lead to renal failure, especially in untreated patients or those with inadequately controlled disease.
> 6. Autoinflammatory syndromes can be categorized according to the primary immune regulatory pathway affected, including inflammasomopathies, interferonopathies, disorders of NF-κB and/or aberrant TNF activity, or miscellaneous mechanisms.

1. What characterizes an autoinflammatory syndrome?

- Abnormal and excessive inflammation driven by aberrant activation of the innate immune system.
- Recurrent (not necessarily periodic) bouts of antigen-independent systemic or localized hyper-inflammation, occurring spontaneously or with minimal trigger.
- Absence of infection or autoimmunity (no autoantibodies).
- Autoinflammatory syndromes are a subset of the broad category of immune dysregulation disorders (which includes autoimmunity and immune deficiency).
- Periodic fever syndromes represent a subset of autoinflammatory syndromes.
- Although fever is a common feature, not all autoinflammatory conditions are periodic or associated with fever.
- Autoinflammatory syndromes can be monogenic or polygenic and can arise from germline or somatic mutations.

2. What are the characteristic clinical features of autoinflammatory syndromes?

- Episodes of fever, elevated inflammatory markers (e.g., erythrocyte sedimentation rate [ESR], C-reactive protein [CRP], white blood cells [WBC]), and multi-organ manifestations involving joints, internal organs, skin and mucosa, and/or eyes.
- Some syndromes manifest nearly continuous symptoms, some by irregular flares, and some by regularly occurring discrete acute attacks that resolve spontaneously.
- Outside of the most severe/persistent syndromes, patients are usually asymptomatic between episodes with normal laboratory values.
- Although infectious illnesses and routine vaccinations may provoke flares, flares often occur spontaneously and without features of common infectious disorders.
- Due to genetic founder effects, some autoinflammatory syndromes are seen more often in particular ethnic groups from defined geographical areas and in populations with significant consanguinity.

See Table 79.1 for specific details regarding the most common autoinflammatory syndromes.

3. What conditions need to be ruled out in patients with recurrent fevers?

1. Infectious disorders:
   - Recurrent or persistent infection (frequent exposures such as in daycare, chronic sinusitis, etc.; if severe, consider host defense defect/primary immunodeficiency)

TABLE 79.1 Comparison of the Most Common Monogenetic Autoinflammatory Syndromes

MECHANISM	SYNDROME	GENE	CLINICAL FEATURES	THERAPY
Inflammasomopathies				
Pyrin activation	FMF	MEFV	Erysipelas-like rash, sterile peritonitis, monoarthritis, pleuritis	Colch., IL-1i
	HIDS	MVK	Maculopapular rash, abdominal pain, polyarthritis, splenomegaly, cervical adenopathy, aphthous ulcers	IL-1i
	PAPA	PSTPIP1	Pyoderma gangrenosum, arthritis	IL-1i, TNFi
Cryopyrin activation	FCAS	NLRP3	Cold-induced urticaria, arthralgia, conjunctivitis	IL-1i
	MWS	NLRP3	Urticarial rash, arthralgia/arthritis, conjunctivitis/episcleritis, sensorineural hearing loss	IL-1i
	NOMID	NLRP3	Urticaria, epiphyseal overgrowth, arthritis, conjunctivitis, vision loss, hearing loss, chronic aseptic meningitis, hepatosplenomegaly	IL-1i
NLRC4 activation	AIFEC	NLRC4	Enterocolitis, rash, arthritis, fever, MAS	IL-1i, IL-18i
Receptor antagonist deficiency	DIRA	IL1RN	Pustulosis, sterile osteomyelitis, periosteitis, fever	IL-1i
	DITRA	IL36RN	Pustular psoriasis, fever, arthralgia, glossitis, nail dystrophy	TNFi IL-17i? IL-12/23?
Interferonopathies				
Nucleicacid processing	Aicardi-Goutières	TREX1, IFIH1, others	Fever, encephalopathy, basal ganglia lesions, chilblains/pernio, autoantibodies	JAK
	Monogenic lupus	DNASE1/2/1L3, complements	Autoantibodies, cytopenias, glomerulonephritis, rash, arthritis, oral ulcers	JAK ?
Nucleic acid sensing	SAVI	TMEM137	Chilblains/pernio, small-vessel vasculitis, arthritis, ILD	JAK
Proteasome	CANDLE	PSMB8 and others	Fever, annular rash, lipodystrophy, lip swelling, aseptic meningitis, developmental delay, conjunctivitis, cardiomyopathy, diarrhea, hepatomegaly, arthropathy	JAK
NF-κB and/or Aberrant TNF Activity				
Dysregulation of NF-κB	HA20	TNFRAIP3	Behcet's-like syndrome with oral and genital ulcerations, intestinal inflammation/ulceration, arthritis, fevers	TNFi, IL-1i JAK ?
Dysregulation of TNF	TRAPS	TNFRSF1A	Myalgias with overlying rash, conjunctivitis or periorbital edema, peritonitis, large joint arthritis	IL-1i, etan.
	Blau	NOD2	Polyarthritis, tenosynovitis, anterior or panuveitis, granulomatous dermatitis	TNFi
	DADA2	ADA2	Fever, livedo reticularis, early-onset vasculopathy (stroke and/or polyarteritis nodosa presentation), mild immunodeficiency	TNFi

Continued

TABLE 79.1 Comparison of the Most Common Monogenetic Autoinflammatory Syndromes—cont'd

MECHANISM	SYNDROME	GENE	CLINICAL FEATURES	THERAPY
Miscellaneous / Other Mechanisms				
Golgi-ER transport	COPA	COPA	ILD, alveolar hemorrhage, autoantibodies, arthritis	
Proteosome	VEXAS	UBA1	Multi-system inflammation having clinical overlap with: relapsing polychondritis, vasculitis, inflammatory lung disease, Sweet Syndrome	
Lyn kinase activity	LAVLI	LYN	Skin vasculitis, fever, hepatosplenomegaly, periorbital edema/conjunctivitis, arthralgia, liver fibrosis, leukocytosis	Src kinase inhibitor

Adapted from Nigrovic PA, Lee PY, Hoffman HM. Monogenic autoinflammatory disorders: conceptual overview, phenotype, and clinical approach. *J Allergy Clin Immunol.* 2020;146(5):925–937.
AEFIC, Autoinflammation with infantile enterocolitis; CANDLE, Chronic atypical neutrophilic dermatosis with lipodystrophy and elevated temperature; Colch, colchicine; COPA, COPI coat complex subunit alpha; DADA2, deficiency of adenosine deaminase 2; DIRA, deficiency of IL-1 receptor antagonist; DITRA, deficiency of IL-36 receptor antagonist; Etan, etanercept; FCAS, familial cold autoinflammatory syndrome; FMF, familial Mediterranean fever; HA20, haploinsufficiency of A20; HIDS, hyperimmunoglobulin-D syndrome; ILD, interstitial lung disease; MWS, Muckle Wells syndrome; NOMID, neonatal onset multisystem inflammatory disease; PAPA, pyogenic sterile arthritis, pyoderma gangrenosum, and acne syndrome; SAVI, STING-associated vasculopathy with onset in infancy; TRAPS, TNF-receptor-associated periodic syndrome; VEXAS, vacuoles in myeloid progenitors, E1 ubiquitin ligase, X-linked, autoinflammatory, somatic syndrome;

- Specific infections with recurrent features (Borrelia or other relapsing fever, malaria, Whipple disease)
2. Noninfectious inflammatory disorders:
    - Systemic juvenile idiopathic arthritis, adult-onset Still's disease
    - Relapsing/remitting manifestations of systemic rheumatic illness: Behcet's disease, relapsing polychondritis, sarcoidosis, systemic lupus erythematosus, systemic vasculitis
    - Inflammatory bowel disease (particularly Crohn's disease).
    - Sweet syndrome
    - Schnitzler syndrome (IgM gammopathy, fever, urticarial rash, dermatographism, bone pain, splenomegaly, systemic symptoms; hematologic malignancy may be seen in 20% to 30%; reports of success with IL-1 inhibition)
3. Cyclic neutropenia (ELANE mutation)
4. Malignancy: hematologic or solid tumors; paraneoplastic syndromes

4. How do you diagnose autoinflammatory syndromes?
- Pattern recognition, symptom diary, exclusion of other causes, and response to empiric medication trials all are helpful.
- Ultimately, genetic testing may provide a definitive diagnosis, but not all classically symptomatic patients will be found to have a known pathogenic mutation.

5. What is the most common autoinflammatory syndrome in pediatric patients, and how does it present?
- **Periodic Fever with Aphthous Stomatitis, Pharyngitis, and Adenitis (PFAPA)** affects approximately 2–20 per 100,000 children worldwide.
- There are no known genetic mutations or ethnic factors associated with PFAPA, and it remains a clinical diagnosis.
- PFAPA is characterized by recurrent episodes lasting ~5 days that occur predictably ~every 28 days. Children are well in between episodes and will be growing and developing normally.
- Typical onset is under age five, and most cases resolve by adolescence.
- Diagnosis of PFAPA is based on pattern recognition and confirmed by response to appropriate treatment and is thus largely a diagnosis of exclusion.
- Because manifestations of PFAPA overlap with many monogenetic autoinflammatory illnesses, genetic testing may be considered, especially if there are atypical features or lack of response to standard treatments.

- PFAPA has excellent outcomes, although there is a large impact on quality of life associated with flares (missed school, medical workup prior to diagnosis, unnecessary diagnostic or therapeutic procedures, missed work for caregivers, etc.).

6. How is PFAPA treated?
Treatment selection depends on severity, and may include:
- Nonsteroidal antiinflammatory drugs (NSAIDs)/acetaminophen during flares.
- Prednisone 1 - 2 mg/kg × 1 dose at fever onset (or before fever if patient has a characteristic prodrome). The dose can be repeated once if still febrile after >12 hours; Prednisone is a highly effective abortive therapy for most patients but is often associated with a shorter period between flares.
- Cimetidine and colchicine can be used for prophylaxis.
- Tonsillectomy can be curative, though not necessary for many as the disorder characteristically self-resolves over time.
- Case reports and series of successful treatments for refractory disease with anti-IL1 therapies (e.g., anakinra or canakinumab).

7. What are the primary categories of genetic autoinflammatory syndromes?
1. Inflammasomopathies
2. Type 1 Interferonopathies
3. NF-κB and/or aberrant TNF activity
4. Miscellaneous / other mechanisms

INFLAMMASOMOPATHIES

8. What is an inflammasome, and what is its function?
- Inflammasomes are protein complexes that assemble in the cytosol following stress- or infection-related triggers, resulting in the activation of caspases, which mediate cleavage of inactive cytokine precursors (e.g., pro- IL-1β and pro-IL-18) and ultimately the release of activated pro-inflammatory cytokines (See Fig 79.1)
- Each inflammasome complex mediates the innate immune response to a unique subset of pathogen-associated or danger-associated molecular patterns (PAMPs and DAMPs).
- IL-1β and IL-18 are powerful activators of macrophages and neutrophils. Inflammasomopathies resulting in IL-1 and IL-18 overproduction are characterized by rapid and intense inflammatory responses.

9. How does IL-1β contribute to the regulation of inflammasome activation?
- After active IL-1β is produced from inflammasome assembly and cleavage of the precursor protein, it will self-propagate through a positive feedback loop in which binding to the cell's IL-1 receptor (IL-1R1) induces further inflammasome activity.
- This self-propagation is down-regulated by endogenous IL-1 receptor antagonist (IL-1ra), which inhibits IL-1β from binding to and activating IL-1R1 (See Fig. 79.1).

10. What is the genetic basis for inflammasomopathies?
- Inflammasomopathies are caused by mutations in the genes encoding inflammasome proteins or their regulators that result in a pathologic excess of IL-1β and related cytokines.
- Overproduction of inflammatory cytokines can result from either gain-of-function (GOF) mutations that cause overactivity of the inflammasome (resulting in increased production of activated IL-1β), or from loss-of-function (LOF) mutations that decrease the ability of IL-1ra to down-regulate inflammasome activation.

11. What are some examples of specific inflammasomes, and associated clinical syndromes?
- **NLRP1** - Mediates response to bacterial toxins (e.g., *B. anthracis* toxin) and muramyl dipeptide. Mutations associated with arthritis and dyskeratosis, Crohn's disease, Familial Keratosis Lichenoides Chronica (FKLC).

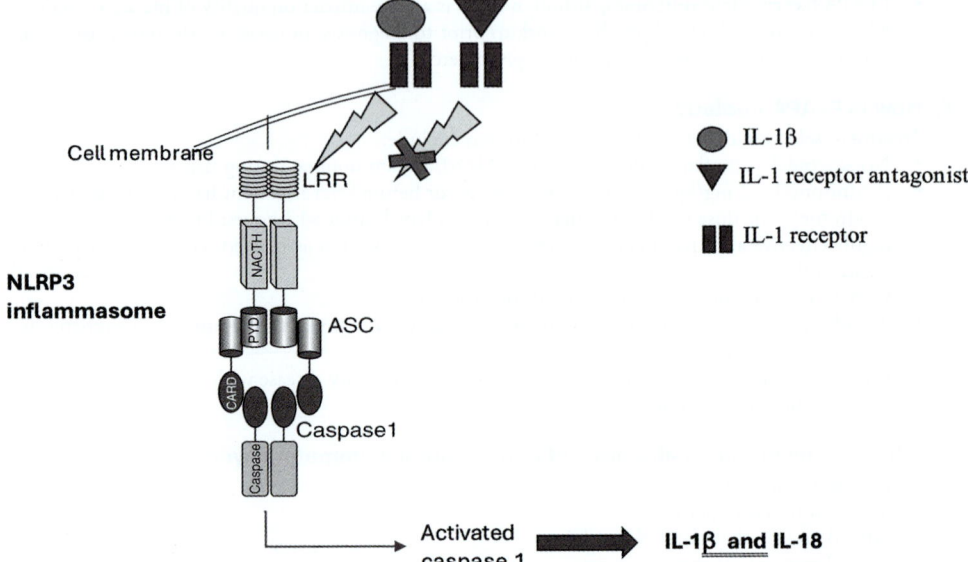

Fig. 79.1 NLRP3 as an example of the role of an inflammasome and IL-1β in the pathogenesis of inflammasomopathies. In CAPS, mutated NLRP3 is constitutively activated, leading to caspase-1 activation and increased cleavage of pro- IL-1β to active IL-1β. IL-1β can also act in an autocrine fashion to further activate the inflammasome, leading to a positive amplification loop. IL-1 receptor antagonist (IL-1ra) is an endogenous inhibitor of the IL-1 receptor, and deficiency of IL-1ra (e.g. in DIRA) can result in unrestricted inflammasome activation. Of note, IL-18 is the primary proinflammatory produced by the NLRC4 inflammasome. Figure adapted from both: Petty RE, Laxer RM, Lindsley CB, Mellins ED, Fullbrigge RC, 2021. *Textbook of Pediatric Rheumatology.* 8th ed. Philadelphia, PA: Elsevier and de Jesus AA, Canna SW, Liu Y, Goldbach-Mansky R. Molecular mechanisms in genetically defined autoinflammatory diseases: disorders of amplified danger signaling. *Annu Rev Immunol.* 2015;33:823–874.

- **NLRP3 (cryopyrin)** - Mediates response to pore-forming toxins (e.g., *Nigericin*) as well as crystalline (e.g., gout and pseudogout) and particulate (e.g., silica, alum, amyloid-β) irritants. Mutations associated with the Cryopyrin-Associated Periodic Syndromes (CAPS): Familial Cold Autoinflammatory Syndrome (FACS), Muckle-Wells Syndrome (MWS), and Neonatal-Onset Multisystem Inflammatory Syndrome (NOMID).
- **NLRC4** - Mediates response to flagellin (e.g., *S. typhimurium*) and Type III secretion system components (e.g., *E. coli*). Mutations associated with Autoinflammation with Infantile Enterocolitis (AIFEC) and macrophage activation syndrome (MAS).
- **AIM2** - Mediates response to cytosolic double-stranded DNA (e.g., herpes and papilloma viruses, *M. tuberculosis*). Mutations associated with defects in the DNA mismatch repair system (Lynch Syndrome) and development of colorectal cancer.
- **Pyrin (MEFV gene)** - Mediates response to a variety of bacterial toxins (e.g., *B. pertussis, B. cenocepacia, C. botulinum, Y. pestis,* etc.). Mutations in MEFV are associated with Familial Mediterranean Fever (FMF) and Pyrin-Associated Autoinflammation with Neutrophilic Dermatosis (PAAND). Mutations in proteins that bind or regulate the pyrin inflammasome are associated with Mevalonate Kinase Deficiency/ Hyper-IgD Syndrome (MVK/HIDS- mutations in the MVK gene), Pyogenic Arthritis/ Pyoderma gangrenosum/ Acne syndrome (PAPA-mutations in PSTPIP1).

SPECIFIC INFLAMMASOMOPATHIES

12. What is Familial Mediterranean Fever (FMF)?

- FMF is the most common monogenetic autoinflammatory syndrome. It is caused by gain-of-function mutations in the MEFV locus on chromosome 16p, which encodes the pyrin protein. These mutations lead to activation of the pyrin inflammasome, resulting in increased production of activated IL-1β (see Fig. 79.1).

- The most common inheritance pattern of FMF is autosomal recessive, but there are cases of autosomal dominant inheritance with incomplete penetrance.
- Over 80 mutations of MEFV have been described. However, 10% to 20% of patients with a classic FMF phenotype do not carry MEFV mutations.
- FMF is most often seen among populations originating from the Mediterranean basin (e.g., Turks, Armenians, Jews, and Arabs) due to an increased prevalence of MEFV mutations. This is postulated to reflect a historical evolutionary advantage in which people with a single copy of a mutated MEFV gene, which results in an enhanced pyrin-mediated inflammatory response without the episodic flares seen in patients with two mutated copies of MEFV, experienced enhanced survival during cycles of plague (infection with *Y. pestis*), which was a significant danger in that region during much of human history.

13. What are the symptoms of FMF?

The majority (~90%) of patients have onset within the first or second decade of life. FMF causes acute and self-limited flares characterized by:

- Fever
- Serositis: generalized peritonitis (80–90%), pleuritis (25–50%). Abdominal pain is often severe, presenting as an acute abdomen.
- Arthritis: large joint oligoarticular arthritis (50–75%), most commonly of the hip, knee, ankle, or wrist. Pain out of proportion to swelling. Poor response to prednisone.
- Rash: erysipelas-like rash (30%).
- Less common manifestations include polyarthritis, prolonged arthritis, aseptic meningitis, pericarditis, scrotal swelling, and lymphadenopathy.
- Flares typically last 1-3 days and recur every 2 to 4 weeks.
- Systemic amyloidosis (AA) can develop as a sequel of chronic inflammation and can lead to renal failure. A subset of patients presents with AA as their initial manifestation, without a history of recognized inflammatory episodes.
- Prevalence of AA increases with age and is not associated with the severity or frequency of acute attacks (but is associated with untreated disease).
- End-stage renal disease as a result of AA is treated with renal transplantation and continuation of colchicine therapy.

14. How is FMF treated?

- For most patients, colchicine is highly effective in preventing flares of FMF and reducing the incidence of secondary amyloidosis. Gastrointestinal (GI) side effects are often a dose-limiting barrier; gradually increasing to the goal dose can help minimize GI symptoms. Colchicine is typically given indefinitely, presuming normal renal and liver function.
- For patients with nephrotic syndrome from AA, colchicine reduces proteinuria and the risk of further progression. Higher doses of colchicine have been found to be more effective (1.8 mg/day). However, dosing may be limited by renal disease and patients with significant renal insufficiency (creatinine ≥1.5 mg/dL) may not experience an improvement in proteinuria with colchicine.
- The IL-1β inhibitors anakinra and canakinumab are also effective in refractory FMF. However, data regarding their effectiveness for the prevention of secondary amyloidosis are limited, and most experts suggest using these agents in addition to colchicine if possible.

15. What is Mevalonate Kinase Deficiency/ Hyper-Immunoglobulin-D Syndrome (MVK/ HIDS) and what causes it?

- HIDS is an autosomal recessive inflammasomopathy caused by LOF mutations in the MVK gene on chromosome 12 (MVK encodes mevalonate kinase, an enzyme involved in the cholesterol synthesis pathway). Reduced enzyme levels lead to dysregulation of RhoAGTPase, which leads to activation of the pyrin inflammasome. HIDS is at the less-severe end of the spectrum of MVK deficiency; complete enzyme deficiency results in mevalonic aciduria, with developmental delay, dysmorphism, organomegaly, and sometimes periodic inflammatory crises.

16. What are the clinical features of HIDS?

- Onset in infancy. 90% of cases have onset at <1 year of age.

- Recurrent episodes of fever/chills, abdominal pain, nausea/vomiting, erythematous fixed rash (typically macular, can be papular or morbilliform), arthritis, headache, adenopathy, orogenital ulcers, splenomegaly.
- Duration of attacks is variable, but on average last 3–7 days with recurrence every 4–6 weeks.
- Can be associated with palpable purpura or erythema elevatum diutinum.
- Amyloidosis is rare.
- IgD levels are elevated in 80% of patients; as such, elevation of IgD is not necessary for the diagnosis of HIDS and may represent an epiphenomenon.
- In patients with elevated IgD levels, the levels remain elevated between disease flares.

17. How do you treat HIDS?
- Canakinumab is the only FDA-approved therapy.
- Anakinra and rilonacept, which also target IL-1, can be effective.
- Successful use of etanercept and simvastatin has been reported.
- NSAIDs may be a helpful adjunctive treatment.
- Steroids, intravenous immunoglobulin, colchicine, and cyclosporine have variable efficacy.

18. What are Cryopyrin-Associated Periodic Syndromes (CAPS)?
CAPS is a continuum of autoinflammatory syndromes related to dysfunction of the cryopyrin inflammasome. In order of increasing severity, these include familial cold autoinflammatory syndrome (FCAS), Muckle-Wells syndrome (MWS), and neonatal-onset multisystem inflammatory disease (NOMID). CAPS results from autosomal dominant, GOF mutations in the gene encoding cryopyrin (NLRP3; formerly denoted CIAS1), leading to variable activation of the cryopyrin inflammasome (see Fig. 79.1). Specific mutations are associated with the different clinical phenotypes. Cases of somatic mosaicism can lead to a CAPS phenotype without easily identifiable NLRP3 mutations.

19. What are the clinical characteristics of the three major phenotypes of CAPS?
Neonatal onset multisystem inflammatory disease (NOMID):
- Most severe; mortality rate ~20% in childhood.
- Symptoms begin at birth or early infancy; classic triad of rash (commonly urticaria), arthropathy, and chronic aseptic meningitis; Sensorineural hearing loss, daily fever, and other multisystem abnormalities are common.
- Growth restriction and abnormal facies with frontal bossing, "saddle-shaped" nose, and protruding eyes may occur.
- Focal epiphyseal overgrowth may be substantial in some patients.
- Renal AA amyloidosis can occur.
  Muckle Wells syndrome (MWS):
- Intermediate in severity among CAPS presentations.
- Episodic fever, headache, urticarial rash, limb pain, conjunctivitis, arthralgias > arthritis. Sensorineural hearing loss may wax and wane but is progressive over time.
- Symptoms commonly develop in adolescence.
- Renal AA amyloidosis can occur.
- Variable duration/frequency of flares: attacks on average last 2–3 days, but frequency can be irregular or even seem continuous in some patients.
  Familial cold autoinflammatory syndrome (FCAS):
- Mildest form of CAPS.
- Self-limited episodes of urticarial rash, fever, arthralgia, conjunctivitis, headache, malaise, and diaphoresis following cold exposure (or even a relative drop in temperature).
- Begins in infancy (95% of patients); can decrease in severity over time.
- Average time to symptom onset following exposure ~6 hours.
- Flare duration: hours to 2–3 days (commonly <24 hours).
- Urticarial rash is ubiquitous during flares; erythematous macules and petechiae have been described; often begins on extremities.
- Renal amyloidosis is rare.

- Ice cube test (immediate appearance of skin changes after contact) is typically negative. This helps distinguish FCAS from acquired cold urticaria, which is a nongenetic condition that does not present in infancy and lacks systemic features.
- *Absence* of deafness, periorbital edema, lymphadenopathy, and serositis.

20. How do you treat CAPS?

- Three IL-1β inhibitors are approved: anakinra, canakinumab, and rilonacept.
- NSAIDs, antihistamines, and prednisone may provide temporary symptom relief, but are not effective long-term treatments.
- No benefit from colchicine.

21. What is pyogenic sterile arthritis, pyoderma gangrenosum and acne syndrome (PAPA)?

- PAPA is an autosomal dominant episodic disorder caused by a mutation of PSTPIP1, which leads to hyperphosphorylation and a stronger interaction between PSTPIP1 and pyrin, which leads in turn to enhanced activation of the pyrin inflammasome.
- Onset of arthritis is typically in the first decade of life and affects one joint at a time. Fever is not prominent. Skin manifestations typically start around puberty.
- Treatment options include glucocorticoids, IL-1 antagonists, or TNF inhibitors.

22. Describe the genetic basis and clinical features of NLRC4 inflammasomopathy.

Autoinflammation with infantile enterocolitis (AIFEC) results from GOF mutations causing activation of the NLRC4 inflammasome. These patients can present with CAPS-like features, but colitis is a prominent feature due to the abundance of NLRC4 in the gut lining. Other symptoms include rash, hepatosplenomegaly, and severe systemic inflammation with features of macrophage activation syndrome including hyperferritinemia, cytopenias, and hepatobiliary dysfunction. Treatment with IL-1 inhibitors can be beneficial, but growing data support IL-18 playing a central role. There are no anti-IL-18 drugs available yet, but there are agents in development.

23. What are Deficiency of the IL-1 Receptor Antagonist (DIRA) and Deficiency of IL-36 Receptor Antagonist (DITRA) syndromes?

DIRA results from a mutation leading to loss of IL-1ra production and unchecked IL-1β signaling. DITRA results from a mutation leading to unchecked IL-36 signaling (which has effects very similar to IL-1). See Table 79.1

INTERFERONOPATHIES

24. What are the 3 types of interferon (IFN), and how do they relate to interferonopathies?

IFNs are a family of immune defense cytokines:

- **Type 1:** IFNα, IFNβ; Regulation of antiviral defense responses. Receptor signaling is through Janus kinase (JAK) 1 and tyrosine kinase (TYK) 2.
- **Type 2:** IFN-γ; involved in multiple facets of innate and adaptive immunity. Receptor signaling is through JAK1 and JAK2.
- **Type 3:** IFN-λ, less understood; similar kinases as Type1 IFN.

Currently recognized interferonopathies involve abnormal activation of Type 1 IFN pathways. (See Table 79.1 for list and comparison of interferonopathies). Type I IFNs are potent pyrogens, and fever is a prominent feature of these interferonopathies. Other manifestations include rashes, cutaneous vasculitis/vasculopathy, and sometimes basal ganglia lesions. Interestingly, some interferonopathies are associated with autoantibodies, underscoring the intersection of innate and adaptive immune responses and the blurred distinction between the concepts of autoimmunity and autoinflammation.

SPECIFIC INTERFERONOPATHIES

25. What is the Chronic Atypical Neutrophilic Dermatosis with Lipodystrophy and Elevated temperature (CANDLE) syndrome?

Patients with CANDLE syndrome have recurrent (almost daily) fever in infancy in addition to skin rash (erythematous annular plaques) and unique facial features including facial lipodystrophy. CANDLE is associated with mutations in the *PSMB8* gene, which encodes components of cellular proteasomes, resulting in an increased Type 1 IFN signaling. Treatment is with JAKinibs such as baricitinib or ruxolitinib, and corticosteroids or methotrexate also may be helpful.

DISORDERS OF NF-κB AND/OR ABERRANT TNF ACTIVITY

26. What is NF-κB and how does it relate to autoinflammatory syndromes?

NF-κB is a complex of intracellular transcription factors that mediates response to multiple danger signals outside and within the cell to prompt the expression of pro-inflammatory genes. Defects in positive or negative regulators of NF-κB can lead to dysregulation of this pathway. Receptors in the TNF family are upstream regulators of NF-κB, and NF-κB activation leads to increased TNF secretion, resulting in positive feedback amplification. Autoinflammatory syndromes caused by aberrant NF-κB activity often present with fevers, systemic inflammation, and granuloma formation. Many of the NF-κB inflammatory syndromes show at least partial response to TNF inhibitors.

SPECIFIC DISORDERS OF NF-κB AND/OR ABERRANT TNF ACTIVITY

27. What is Tumor necrosis factor Receptor-Associated Periodic Syndrome (TRAPS)?

- TRAPS is an autoinflammatory syndrome caused by autosomal dominant mutations in the TNFRSF1A gene on chromosome 12p13. Reduced penetrance and *de novo* mutations are also observed, so a family history of similar symptoms may be lacking.
- The mechanism of disease is unclear but suspected to be related to ligand-independent activation of TNF receptor 1 (receptor signaling in the absence of TNF binding) that leads to downstream enhancement of inflammasome activity.

28. What are the clinical features of TRAPS?

- Recurrent episodes of fever, painful erysipelas-like rash, myalgia, serositis (peritonitis in 90%), and conjunctivitis. Periorbital swelling is common and is a distinguishing characteristic.
- Onset is generally in the first and second decades of life but can vary up to middle age.
- Rash is more common on the distal extremities and face (centrifugal pattern) and may be migratory.
- Arthralgias > arthritis (arthritis is typically monoarticular, if present).
- Myalgia commonly involves the thighs; may migrate to additional areas.
- Average duration of episodes is 2–4 weeks, with a recurrence of 2–6 episodes per year.
- Amyloidosis occurs in ~10% of patients (less than what is seen in untreated FMF). Monitor with urinalysis to identify proteinuria, as well as serum creatinine.

29. What is the treatment for TRAPS?

- Prednisone during flares (tapering course over duration of flare); alternatively, consider NSAIDs if mild symptoms.
- Both anakinra and canakinumab are effective (only canakinumab is FDA-approved) and considered standard of care.
- Etanercept (soluble TNF receptor 1) is effective for many patients, although efficacy is often lost.
- Infliximab often worsens disease (mechanism unknown)
- Colchicine is not effective.

30. What is the basis of Blau syndrome and how does it present?

- Associated with GOF mutations in the NOD2/CARD15 gene on chromosome 16. Of note, although polymorphisms in NOD2/CARD15 are associated with susceptibility to Crohn's disease, there is no bowel inflammation in Blau syndrome.
- Characterized by recurrent granulomatous inflammation of the joints (boggy polyarthritis or tenosynovitis), eyes (anterior uveitis or panuveitis), and skin (dermal granulomas), with onset before the age of 5 years. The severity of arthritis may lead to joint contractures.
- Other less common manifestations include CNS inflammation, cranial neuropathy, and vasculitis.

- TNF inhibitors and corticosteroids are typically the most beneficial. Response to IL-1 blockade is variable.

31. What are the clinical features of Deficiency of Adenosine Deaminase 2 (DADA2)?

- DADA2 is monogenic autoinflammatory disease caused by biallelic pathogenic mutations in the ADA2 gene (AKA CERC1) on chromosome 22q11.
- The clinical spectrum of DADA2 is broad and can be quite severe, including systemic vasculitis, early-onset stroke, bone marrow failure, and/ or immunodeficiency.
- The vasculitis of DADA2 is a medium vessel vasculitis that clinically resembles polyarteritis nodosa, often with prominent livedo racemosa.
- Some patients experience cytopenias and immunodeficiency.
- TNF inhibitors are the mainstay of treatment of the vasculitis/ vasculopathy phenotype and are very effective in treating symptoms and preventing stroke. Hematopoietic stem cell transplant has been used for patients with severe bone marrow failure.

32. What is haploinsufficiency of A20 (HA20), and what are the clinical manifestations?

- HA20 is a monogenic autoinflammatory disease caused by loss-of-function mutations in the TNFAIP3 gene which encodes the protein A20. As A20 is a negative regulator of NF-κB, insufficiency of A20 results in upregulation of inflammatory genes regulated by this immune response pathway.
- Patients with HA20 present with a juvenile-onset Behcet's-like phenotype, including recurrent orogenital ulcerations and relapsing/remitting systemic inflammatory symptoms. Some reported patients were initially diagnosed with related disorders, including PFAPA, systemic-onset JIA, FMF, Crohn's disease, and autoimmune lymphoproliferative syndrome.
- HA20 is characterized by overproduction of TNF, IL-1β, IL-6, and IFN-γ and biologics targeting these cytokines can be effective at controlling the symptoms. An elevated type I IFN signature may predict response to JAK inhibitors in patients refractory to anti-cytokine therapies.

MISCELLANEOUS / OTHER MECHANISMS

33. What causes COPA Syndrome and what are its primary manifestations?

- COPA syndrome is an autosomal dominant immune dysregulation disorder caused by mutations in the COPA gene encoding the coatamer complex-I alpha protein (COPα) protein. These mutations result in aberrant intracellular trafficking that leads to aberrant cellular autophagy/ endoplasmic reticulum stress and causes a shift in effector T cells to a TH17 phenotype. This in turn is associated with increased pro-inflammatory cytokine expression including IL-17, IL-1β, and IL-6.
- COPA Syndrome presents in childhood with autoimmunity (often with multiple high-titer autoantibodies), inflammatory arthritis, nephritis, and interstitial lung disease with diffuse alveolar hemorrhage.

34. What is the pathophysiology that leads to Vacuoles, E1 Enzyme, X-Linked, Autoinflammatory Somatic (VEXAS) Syndrome?

- VEXAS is an immune dysregulation disorder caused by somatic loss-of-function mutations of the UBA1 gene located on the X chromosome. Loss of UBA1 function results in decreased ubiquitination and altered proteosome function (i.e., dysregulation of intracellular protein processing).
- Defective proteosome function (i.e., proteosome-opathy) in myeloid cells activates the unfolded protein response and type I interferon production which results in activation of innate immune pathways including increased production of TNF, IL-6, and IFNγ. The development of VEXAS reflects the expression of mutant UBA1 in myeloid precursor cells and the severity of symptoms reflect the proportion of circulating myeloid cells involved. Typical enlarged vacuoles are observed in hematopoietic precursor cells on bone marrow biopsy.
- VEXAS is an adult-onset inflammatory syndrome, typically presenting in the 5th to 7th decade of life. As the gene is on the X chromosome, the disorder is primarily observed in

males, though cases have been described in females with inherited or acquired X-monosomy or chromosomal defects.
- VEXAS syndrome manifests as treatment-refractory fevers, arthritis, chondritis, vasculitis, cytopenias, and neutrophilic skin and pulmonary inflammation.

35. When should VEXAS be considered?
VEXAS should be a consideration in patients with adult-onset multi-system inflammatory disease who show progressive anemia or other evidence of myelodysplasia. VEXAS can mimic and over-lap with other inflammatory conditions, including relapsing polychondritis, inflammatory lung disease, polyarteritis nodosa, and Sweet's syndrome. First described in 2020, the true incidence and spectrum of VEXAS syndrome are still being delineated but may explain the historic association of increased risk of malignancy and myelodysplastic syndrome reported in patients with these diagnoses.

36. What causes LAVLI Syndrome and what are its primary manifestations?
- Lyn kinase-associated vasculopathy and liver fibrosis (LAVLI) is an autosomal dominant disorder caused by de novo gain of function mutations in the Src-family tyrosine kinase gene, *LYN*, resulting in constitutive activation of Lyn kinase. This causes increased expression of ICAM-1 on endothelial cells and β2-integrins on neutrophils causing increased neutrophil adhesion and vascular transendothelial cell migration.
- LAVLI Syndrome was previously called systemic autoinflammatory disease with vasculitis (SAIDV). It manifests soon after birth with neutrophilic cutaneous small vessel vasculitis, fever, hepatosplenomegaly, periorbital edema/conjunctivitis, and arthralgias. Laboratory studies show leukocytosis, elevated C-reactive protein, and autoantibodies. A subset of patients develops liver fibrosis. Treatment includes Src kinase inhibitor or TNF inhibitor.

AUTOINFLAMMATORY BONE DISEASE

37. What is chronic nonbacterial osteomyelitis (CNO)?
CNO, which is the preferred label for the condition previously termed chronic recurrent multifocal osteomyelitis (CRMO), is a noninfectious autoinflammatory lytic bone disorder.

No specific gene mutation has been identified, but there is a susceptibility locus on chromosome 18. Mutations in LPIN2 on chromosome 18 are associated with Majeed syndrome, an autosomal recessive disorder in which CNO develops in conjunction with fever, rash, and congenital dyserythropoietic anemia.

38. What are the clinical features of CNO?
- The peak age of onset at 7–12 years, but variable and can have onset in adulthood. Of those with childhood onset, most will have spontaneous resolution by adolescence.
- Biologic females are two to four times more affected than males.
- Wide variability of bone lesions: unifocal or multifocal, monophasic, recurrent, or persistent.
- Bone pain (often insidious onset) is the primary symptom. It is often worse at night and can present with or without fever.
- The most commonly affected areas include the metaphyses of long bones, vertebrae, clavicle, and pelvis; involvement is symmetric in 25–40%; Spinal involvement is associated with a high risk of vertebral collapse.
- There is an association with inflammatory bowel disease, psoriasis, and pyoderma gangrenosum. CNO is also seen as a part of the SAPHO syndrome (Synovitis, Acne, Pustulosis, Hyperostosis, Osteitis) See Fig. 79.2

39. How do you diagnose CNO?
- X-rays: mixed osteolytic and sclerotic lesions, although may be normal initially
- As asymptomatic lesions are possible, non-contrast whole-body magnetic resonance imaging (MRI) with STIR imaging is preferred; otherwise, MRI of symptomatic sites is used to characterize the presence and extent of lesions. Technetium bone scan was used historically but is no longer recommended.

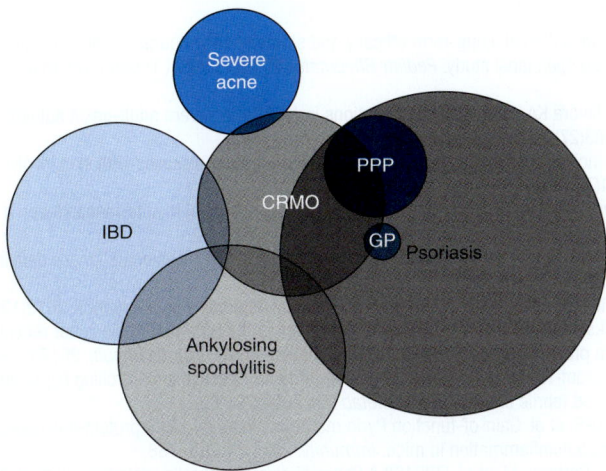

Fig. 79.2 Overlap of chronicrecurrent multifocal osteomyelitis (CRMO) and other inflammatory illnesses. *GP,* Generalized pustulosis; *IBD,* inflammatory bowel disease; *PPP,* palmoplantar pustulosis. From Petty RE, Laxer RM, Lindsley CB, Wedderburn L, 2015. *Textbook of Pediatric Rheumatology,* 7th ed. Philadelphia, PA: Elsevier 629.

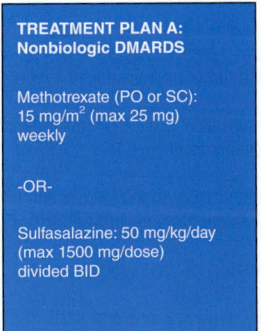

TREATMENT PLAN A:
Nonbiologic DMARDS

Methotrexate (PO or SC):
15 mg/m^2 (max 25 mg)
weekly

-OR-

Sulfasalazine: 50 mg/kg/day
(max 1500 mg/dose)
divided BID

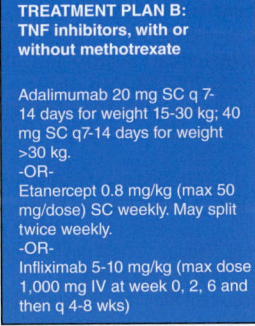

TREATMENT PLAN B:
TNF inhibitors, with or
without methotrexate

Adalimumab 20 mg SC q 7-
14 days for weight 15-30 kg; 40
mg SC q7-14 days for weight
>30 kg.
-OR-
Etanercept 0.8 mg/kg (max 50
mg/dose) SC weekly. May split
twice weekly.
-OR-
Infliximab 5-10 mg/kg (max dose
1,000 mg IV at week 0, 2, 6 and
then q 4-8 wks)

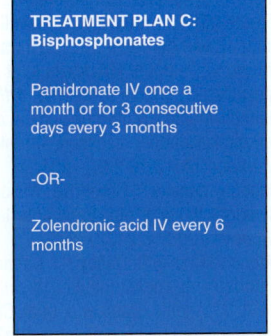

TREATMENT PLAN C:
Bisphosphonates

Pamidronate IV once a
month or for 3 consecutive
days every 3 months

-OR-

Zolendronic acid IV every 6
months

Fig. 79.3 Childhood Arthritis and Rheumatology Research Alliance Consensus treatment plans for the first 6 to 12 months in patients with chronic noninfectious osteomyelitis refractory to nonsteroidal anti-inflammatory drugs (NSAIDs) or with active spinal lesions (all plans allow concurrent use of NSAIDs and/or prednisone). *BID,* Twice a day; *DMARDs,* disease-modifying antirheumatic drugs; *IV,* intravenous; *PO,* orally; *SC,* subcutaneously; *TNF,* tumor necrosis factor.

- Many, but not all, patients have elevations in acute phase reactants such as ESR, CRP, and/or leukocyte count.
- Bone biopsy is often performed to confirm inflammatory changes and exclude infection and malignancy.

40. How do you treat CNO?

- If no active spinal lesions: NSAIDs initially, which for many patients is sufficient for disease control.
- If refractory or intolerant of NSAIDs: nonbiologic disease-modifying antirheumatic drugs (methotrexate or sulfasalazine), TNF-inhibitors, and/or bisphosphonates have been shown to be effective (Fig 79.3).
- For patients with vertebral involvement, treatment with TNF inhibitors or bisphosphonates is indicated.

BIBLIOGRAPHY

Arostegui JI, Anton J, Yague J, et al. Long-term efficacy and safety of canakinumab in active Hyper-IgD syndrome (HIDS): results from an open label study. *Pediatr Rheumatol.* 2015;13(suppl 1):058 Erratum in: *Arthritis Rheum.* 2009; 60:1851–1861.

Beck DB, Ferrada MA, Sikora KA, et al. Somatic mutations in *UBA1* and severe adult-onset autoinflammatory disease. *N Engl J Med.* 2020;383(27):2628–2638.

Beer HD, Contassot French LE. The inflammasomes in autoinflammatory diseases with skin involvement. *J Invest Dermatol.* 2014;134(7):1805–1810.

Ben-Zvi I, Kukuy O, Livneh A, et al. Anakinra for colchicine-resistant familial Mediterranean fever: a randomized, double-blind, placebo-controlled trial. *Arthritis Rheumatol.* 2017;69(4):854–862.

Bodar EJ, Kuijk LM, Drenth JPH, et al. On demand anakinra is effective in mevalonate kinase deficiency. *Ann Rheum Dis.* 2011;70:2155–2158.

Borzutzky A, Stern S, Reiff A, et al. Pediatric chronic nonbacterial osteomyelitis. *Pediatrics.* 2012;130(5):e1190–e1197.

Bulua AC, Mogul DB, Aksentijevich I, et al. Efficacy of etanercept in the tumor necrosis factor receptor–associated periodic syndrome: a prospective, open-label, dose-escalation study. *Arthritis Rheum.* 2012;64:908–913.

Cailliez M, Garaix F, Rousset-Rouvière C, et al. Anakinra is safe and effective in controlling hyperimmunoglobulinaemia D syndrome-associated febrile crisis. *J Inherit Metab Dis.* 2006;29:763.

Chae JJ, Cho Y-H, Lee G-S, et al. Gain-of-function Pyrin mutations induce NLRP3 protein-independent interleukin-1β activation and severe autoinflammation in mice. *Immunity.* 2011;34:755–768.

De Benedetti F, Anton J, Gattorno M, et al. FRI0488 A Phase Iii pivotal umbrella trial of canakinumab in patients with autoinflammatory periodic fever syndromes (Colchicine Resistant FMF, HIDS/MKD and TRAPS). *Ann Rheum Dis.* 2016;75:615–616.

de Jesus AA, Canna SW, Liu Y, Goldbach-Mansky R. Molecular mechanisms in genetically defined autoinflammatory diseases: disorders of amplified danger signaling. *Annu Rev Immunol.* 2015;33:823–874.

de Jesus AA, Chen G, Yang D, et al. Constitutively active Lyn kinase causes a cutaneous small vessel vasculitis and liver fibrosis syndrome. *Nat Commun.* 2023;14:1502. doi:10.1038/s41467-023-36941-y.

de Zoete MR, Palm NW, Zhu S, Flavell RA. Inflammasomes. *Cold Spring Harb Perspect Biol.* 2014;6(12):a016287.

Drenth JP, van der Meer JW. The inflammasome—linebacker of innate defense. *N Engl J Med.* 2006;355:730–732.

Gattorno M, Pelagatti MA, Meini A, et al. Persistent efficacy of anakinra in patients with tumor necrosis factor receptor–associated periodic syndrome. *Arthritis Rheum.* 2008;58:1516–1520.

Goldbach-Mansky R. Immunology in clinic review series; focus on autoinflammatory diseases: update on monogenic autoinflammatory diseases: the role of interleukin (IL)-1 and an emerging role of cytokines beyond IL-1. *Clin Exp Immunol.* 2012;167:391–404.

Goldbach-Mansky R, Shroff SD, Wilson M, et al. A pilot study to evaluate the safety and efficacy of the long-acting inter-leukin-1 inhibitor rilonacept (interleukin-1 Trap) in patients with familial cold autoinflammatory syndrome. *Arthritis Rheum.* 2008;58:2432–2442.

Goldbach-Mansky R, Dailey NJ, Canna SW, et al. Neonatal-onset multisystem inflammatory disease responsive to interleuking-1beta inhibition. *N Engl J Med.* 2006;355:581–592.

Golla A, Jansson A, Ramser J, et al. Chronic recurrent multifocal osteomyelitis (CRMO): evidence for a susceptibility gene located on chromosome 18q21.3–18q22. *Eur J Hum Genet.* 2002;10(3):217–221.

Hoffman HM. Therapy of autoinflammatory syndromes. *J Allergy Clin Immunol.* 2009;124:1129–1138.

Hoffman HM, Throne ML, Amar NJ, et al. Efficacy and safety of rilonacept (interleukin-1 Trap) in patients with cryopyrin-associated periodic syndromes: results from two sequential placebo-controlled studies. *Arthritis Rheum.* 2008;58(8):2443–2452.

Jansson A, Renner ED, Ramser J, et al. Classification of non-bacterial osteitis: retrospective study of clinical, immuno-logical and genetic aspects in 89 patients. *Rheumatology (Oxford).* 2007;46(1):154–160.

Lachmann HJ, Kone-Paut I, Kuemmerle-Deschner JB, et al. Use of canakinumab in the cryopyrin-associated periodic syndrome. *N Engl J Med.* 2006;360:2416–2425.

Mankan AK, Kubarenko A, Hornung V. Immunology in clinic review series; focus on autoinflammatory diseases: update on monogenic autoinflammatory diseases: inflammasomes: mechanisms of activation. *Clin Exp Immunol.* 2012;167:369–381.

Masters SL, Simon A, Aksentijevich I, Kastner DL. Horror autoinflammaticus: the molecular pathophysiology of autoin-flammatory disease. *Annu Rev Immunol.* 2009;27:621–668.

Nigrovic PA, Lee PY, Hoffman HM. Monogenic autoinflammatory disorders: conceptual overview, phenotype and clinical approach. *J Allergy Clin Immunol.* 2020;146:925–937.

Ozen S, Bilginer Y, Ayaz NA, Calguneri M. Anti-interleukin 1 treatment for patients with familial Mediterranean fever resistant to colchicine. *J Rheumatol.* 2011;38:516–518.

Ozkurede VU, Franchi L. Immunology in clinic review series; focus on autoinflammatory diseases: update on mono-genic autoinflammatory diseases: role of inflammasomes in autoinflammatory syndromes. *Clin Exp Immunol.* 2012;167:382–390.

Petty RE, Laxer RM, Lindsley CB, Wedderburn L, Fuhlbrigge RC, Mellins ED. *Textbook of Pediatric Rheumatology.* 8th ed. Philadelphia, PA: Elsevier; 2020.

Shohat M, Halpern GJ. Familial Mediterranean fever—a review. *Genet Med.* 2011;13:487–498.

Simon A, Drewe E, van der Meer JW, et al. Simvastatin treatment for inflammatory attacks of the hyperimmunoglobu-linemia D and periodic fever syndrome. *Clin Pharmacol Ther.* 2004;75:476–483.

Simon A, Park H, Maddipati R, et al. Concerted action of wild-type and mutant TNF receptors enhances inflammation in TNF receptor 1-associated periodic fever syndrome. *Proc Nat Acad Sci USA.* 2010;107:9801–9806.

Soriano A, Soriano M, Espinosa G, et al. Current therapeutic options for the main monogenic autoinflammatory diseases and PFAPA syndrome: evidence-based approach and proposal of a practical guide. *Front Immunol.* 2020;11:865.

Van der Hilst JC, Bodar EJ, Barron KS, et al. Long-term follow up, clinical features, and quality of life in a series of 103 patients with hyperimmunoglobulinemia D syndrome. *Medicine (Baltimore).* 2008;87:301–310.

Zhao Y, Wu E, Furguson P, et al. Consensus treatment plans for chronic nonbacterial osteomyelitis refractory to nonste-roidal antiinflammatory drugs and/or with active spinal lesions. *Arthritis Care Res.* 2018;70(8):1228–1237.

FURTHER READING

https://infevers.umai-montpellier.fr.

www.autoinflammatory.org.

Odds and Ends

Sterling G. West, MD

PERIODIC ARTHRITIS SYNDROMES

1. Name the nonhereditary periodic arthritis syndromes. Why are they grouped together?

- Intermittent hydrarthrosis.
- Palindromic rheumatism.
- Eosinophilic synovitis.
- Remitting seronegative symmetrical synovitis with pitting edema (RS3PE) syndrome (see Chapter 14: Rheumatoid Arthritis).

These syndromes are grouped together because they share four features: (1) intermittent arthritis followed by periods of remission; (2) complete resolution between attacks; (3) rare development of joint damage; and (4) unknown cause. These disorders should not be confused with periodic fever syndromes.

2. Are all disorders with intermittent arthritis encompassed by the periodic arthritis syndromes?

No. Many other disorders may include intermittent joint swelling and other characteristics of the periodic syndromes. Among these are mechanical and inflammatory disorders. Thus, a broad differential should be kept in mind in patients with intermittent arthritis.

Periodic syndromes

- Intermittent hydrarthrosis
- Palindromic rheumatism
- Eosinophilic synovitis
- Familial autoinflammatory syndromes

Crystalline arthropathies

- Gout
- Calcium pyrophosphate dihydrate (pseudogout)
- Hydroxyapatite

RS3PE

Spondyloarthropathies

- Reactive arthritis
- Enteropathic arthritis

Sarcoidosis

Infections

- Lyme disease
- Whipple's disease

Mechanical

- Loose bodies
- Meniscal tears

3. Describe the typical clinical features of intermittent hydrarthrosis.

Intermittent hydrarthrosis is characterized by recurrent joint effusions occurring at regular intervals. Men and women are equally affected. The episode may parallel menses in women and resolve after menopause. The knee or another large joint (elbow, ankle) develops an effusion over 12 to 24 hours with no or minimal discomfort or signs of inflammation. Attacks last for 3 to 5 days and can recur in cycles of usually 7–11 days. There are no systemic symptoms. The recurrent episodes may occur lifelong. No treatment is proven to prevent or abort attacks, although low-dose colchicine has been used with success in some patients.

4. **What do laboratory studies and joint radiographs show in intermittent hydrarthrosis?**

Laboratory tests, including the erythrocyte sedimentation rate (ESR), are normal even during an attack. Synovial fluid is normal or mildly inflammatory (white blood cells [WBCs], 5000/mm^3) with a slight increase in polymorphonuclear leukocytes. An effusion may be seen on radiographs, but no other abnormalities are seen even after years of attacks. Recently, some patients have been found to be heterozygous for MEFV gene mutations without other features of familial Mediterranean fever (FMF). TRAPS-related genes have also been reported in some patients. This suggests that some patients with intermittent hydrarthrosis may have a mild autoinflammatory syndrome that can be colchicine-responsive.

5. **What is palindromic rheumatism? What does it mean?**

Palindromic rheumatism is a recurrent syndrome of acute arthritis and periarthritis. Palindromic means "recurring" and is derived from a Greek word that literally means "to run back." The term *palindromic* was introduced by Hench and Rosenberg in 1944 as descriptive of the syndrome. They preferred rheumatism to arthritis because of the frequent involvement of periarticular structures and occasional presence of subcutaneous nodules.

6. **How do the clinical features of palindromic rheumatism differ from those of intermittent hydrarthrosis?**

Palindromic rheumatism, similar to intermittent hydrarthrosis, affects both men and women, often begins in the third to fifth decade, frequently affects the knees, and is rarely associated with constitutional symptoms. However, unlike intermittent hydrarthrosis, palindromic rheumatism attacks occur irregularly and may involve more than one joint (usually two to five joints). Arthritic attacks may last hours to several days. The pattern of attacks tends to be characteristic in an individual patient. Symptoms may begin in one joint while waning in another. Attacks are sudden and pain may be intense, often reaching a peak within a few hours. Signs of joint inflammation (swelling, warmth, redness) can be noted soon after pain begins. Small joints of the hands, wrist, and feet may be affected, and occasionally the temporomandibular joints. Also, unlike intermittent hydrarthrosis, periarticular attacks (occurring in one-third of cases) and transient subcutaneous nodules may be seen.

7. **What do laboratory studies and joint radiographs show in palindromic rheumatism?**

The ESR and other acute-phase reactants may be elevated during attacks but are normal between them. Rheumatoid factor (RF) and anticyclic citrullinated peptide (anti-CCP) are positive in 30% to 50% of cases and identify patients who are most likely to develop RA. Antinuclear antibodies (ANAs) are typically negative and serum complement levels are normal. There have been few studies of synovial fluid in palindromic rheumatism. Leukocytes may vary from a few hundred to several thousand, with the magnitude poorly correlated with symptom severity. Radiographs show only soft tissue swelling. Ultrasound can show synovitis and/or periarticular inflammation. Similar to intermittent hydrarthrosis, some patients (10%) have been found to be heterozygous for mutations of the MEFV gene similar to those reported in FMF. These patients tend to have more constitutional symptoms (e.g. fever) and serositis associated with their arthritic attacks. Whipple's disease should always be considered in patients presenting with palindromic rheumatism.

8. **How is palindromic rheumatism treated?**

Nonsteroidal anti-inflammatory drugs (NSAIDs) may provide some relief from joint symptoms but do not reliably prevent attacks. A variety of other agents have been used including colchicine, antimalarial agents, sulfasalazine, methotrexate, and leflunomide.

9. **Describe the course of palindromic rheumatism**

Although the course is variable, <10% of patients experience a spontaneous complete remission. Some patients continue to have the disease for many years. However, 30% to 50% of cases evolve into a chronic inflammatory polyarthritis, usually RA. Less commonly, a diagnosis of systemic lupus erythematosus (SLE) or other connective tissue disease (CTDs) is eventually made especially in patients with a positive ANA. Antimalarials, methotrexate, and leflunomide have been reported to reduce the risk of subsequent development of RA or other CTD.

10. What features are predictive of a patient with palindromic rheumatism later developing RA?

Female sex, proximal interphalangeal (PIP) and wrist involvement, positive RF and/or anti-CCP, synovitis on ultrasound, and HLA-DR4 positivity increase the likelihood of evolution to RA.

FOREIGN BODY SYNOVITIS

11. Define foreign body synovitis.

Foreign body synovitis is an inflammatory reaction of the synovium (from joint, bursa, or tendon sheath) attributable to the introduction of a foreign material. Most commonly, it results from a traumatic event, but it may also follow surgical introduction of foreign material.

12. Name the foreign bodies most commonly associated with foreign body synovitis.

Foreign bodies can be organic or inorganic materials. Plant thorns, wood splinters, seashell fragments, and sea urchin spines are the most common. Other recognized materials include fish bones, chitin fragments, stones, gravel, brick fragments, lead, glass, fiberglass, plastic, and rubber. Surgically implanted materials include metallic fragments, cement (methylmethacrylate), and silicone (silicone synovitis).

13. Name five activities that are risk factors for foreign body synovitis.

Professional fishing, professional diving, marine recreational activities, farming, and gardening.

14. Describe the clinical, laboratory, and radiographic features of foreign body synovitis.

The joints of the hands and knees are most commonly affected. There is sudden onset of pain at the site of injury, which may be forgotten by the patient or overlooked by the physician. The patient may be seen with acute synovitis several days after the injury, ranging from months to years later, with chronic synovitis (particularly of the knee). The inflammatory synovitis may be episodic. The ESR is usually normal, and synovial fluid is inflammatory with a predominance of neutrophils. Radiographs may show soft tissue swelling only and can be useful to detect radiodense particles (metal, fish bones, and sea urchin spines) but not wood, plastic, or plant thorns. Chronic changes of periarticular osteoporosis, osteolysis, osteosclerosis, and periosteal new bone formation can mimic osteomyelitis or bone tumors. Synovial biopsies show a nonspecific granulomatous synovitis that may be confused with sarcoidosis.

15. How is foreign body synovitis diagnosed and treated?

In approximately two-thirds of patients with foreign body synovitis attributable to exogenous particles who develop a chronic or relapsing course, diagnosis and treatment usually necessitate excisional biopsy with synovectomy. Because of its resolution, ultrasound is better than computed tomography (CT) scanning and magnetic resonance imaging (MRI) in detecting particles that are too small or radiolucent to be seen with conventional radiography. Bacteriologic studies (including fungal and mycobacterial studies) and histopathologic examination of tissue are essential. Polarized microscopy is useful in detecting birefringent fragments of plant origin, sea urchin spines, and polymethylmethacrylate.

16. What is silicone synovitis?

Silicone-containing joint implants have been used to replace the metacarpophalangeal (MCP), PIP, first metatarsophalangeal, and wrist joints. Wear particles from fracturing of the prosthesis can be ingested by macrophages generating an inflammatory response, leading to a destructive synovitis. This occurs most commonly with wrist implants. Patients who develop this condition receive NSAIDs for symptom control but frequently require removal of the prosthesis and synovectomy.

RARE ARTHRITIC SYNDROMES

17. What is multicentric reticulohistiocytosis (MRH)?

MRH is a rare disease with prominent skin and joint manifestations that is classified among the non-Langerhans cell histiocytoses. It affects women more than men (3:1), most commonly in the fourth decade. Most patients have symmetric polyarthritis. The cutaneous manifestations occur after a mean of 3 years (66%), although in one-third of patients, the skin lesions will occur before or simultaneously with the arthritis. Systemic manifestations including fever, weight loss, and fatigue commonly occur. Pulmonary, cardiac, laryngeal, and myopathy symptoms can occur.

18. How does the arthritis of MRH resemble that of RA? How does it differ?

Similar to RA, the arthritis of MRH is inflammatory, usually chronic, symmetric, and polyarticular; it characteristically affects the interphalangeal joints of the hands and is destructive. Large joints, the feet, and occasionally C1 to C2 can also be involved. However, unlike RA, DIP synovitis and destruction may be prominent (75%), and severely deforming arthritis mutilans occurs in 50% of patients. Fever and weight loss can occur. Glucocorticoid therapy has little, if any, effect on the arthritis. Also, in contrast to RA, radiographs in MRH feature well-circumscribed erosions, widened joint spaces, and absent or disproportionately mild periarticular osteopenia for the degree of erosive change. Serologies are negative, and 50% have a moderately elevated ESR. Synovial fluid can range from mildly to significantly inflammatory.

19. Describe the cutaneous manifestations of MRH.

Firm papulonodules, reddish-brown or yellow, occur most commonly on the face, hands, ears, arms, scalp, neck, and chest. A classic finding is "coral beads" around the nailbeds. These nodules may wax and wane and even disappear completely. They can be induced by sun exposure and may be pruritic. The nodules may coalesce on the face leading to a "leonine facies." Lesions are less common on the legs.

20. Several disorders have been associated with MRH. Name them.

- Tuberculin skin test positivity is seen in 12% to 50% of patients, but only two patients have been reported to have active tuberculosis.
- Xanthelasma occurs in one-third of patients. Up to 60% have hyperlipidemia.
- Malignant disease of various types has been reported in approximately 15–30% of patients. Breast, heme, and gastric malignancies are most common. The cancer may precede, be concurrent with, or follow the development of MRH. Treatment of the malignancy can lead to improvement of the MRH.
- Autoimmune diseases occur in 5% to 20% of patients. Multiple different autoimmune diseases have been reported.

21. What are the typical histologic findings of MRH on biopsy of skin or synovium?

The characteristic findings are aggregates of multinucleated giant cells and histiocytes (i.e., tissue macrophages) having a granular, ground-glass appearance. This ground-glass cytoplasm contains a periodic acid–Schiff-reactive material thought to be attributable to a mucoprotein or glycoprotein. This cellular tissue reaction has prompted the idea that MRH represents a histiocytic granulomatous reaction to an unidentified stimulus. Fat stains, such as Sudan black, are also positive. Cell markers indicate a monocyte/macrophage lineage (CD68+) of the histiocytes and multinucleated giant cells. Some have osteoclast markers.

22. How is MRH treated?

No treatment has consistently shown benefit. In patients with mild disease, symptomatic therapy with NSAIDs or nonnarcotic analgesics should be tried. Unfortunately, the arthritis in 40% to 50% of patients progresses to arthritis mutilans. Glucocorticoids, methotrexate, leflunomide, and antitumor necrosis factor (anti-TNF) agents have been effective for severe cases. Cyclophosphamide has also been reported to achieve partial and complete remissions. As a result of some of the cells exhibiting osteoclastic markers, intravenous (IV) bisphosphonates have shown efficacy in some patients. Most cases of MRH will resolve within 10 years leaving behind joint deformities.

23. What is fibroblastic rheumatism?

Fibroblastic rheumatism can resemble MRH. It is a rare fibroblastic (not histiocytic) disease with at least 33% of cases occurring in children. Patients develop the rapid onset of symmetric polyarthritis, mainly of the upper extremities. DIP joints can be involved. Palmar thickening and inability to extend fingers is seen in 80% of cases, leading to functional disability. Sclerodactyly and skin thickening of the arms and trunk can be seen. Raynaud's phenomenon occurs in 50%

of cases. Cutaneous manifestations start as maculopapular lesions that develop into flesh-colored nodules over the extensor surfaces of the MCP joints and fingers. They usually develop after the arthritis. There is no association with malignancy or autoimmune disease. Serologies are unremarkable. Radiographs can show joint destruction resembling MRH. Nodule and synovial biopsies show "spindle-shaped" fibroblastic cells that are myofibroblasts which stain for α-smooth muscle actin. Elastic fibers are reduced. Treatment with prednisone, methotrexate, and TNF antagonists has had variable results. Fibroblastic rheumatism may remit spontaneously but usually recurs.

24. What are the clinical characteristics of idiopathic eosinophilic synovitis?

- Many have a history of atopy; some have dermatographism.
- Both sexes, age of onset 20 to 50 years. Can occur in childhood.
- Minor trauma causes acute onset (within 12–24 hours) of painless monoarthritis (usually knee) without warmth or erythema. Trauma may activate mast cells which attract eosinophils.
- Synovial fluid shows mildly inflammatory fluid with up to 50% eosinophils. Charcot–Leyden crystals (bipyramidal, hexagonal-shaped crystal made of products of intracellular lipases in eosinophils) may be seen.
- Peripheral blood WBC count normal. Peripheral blood eosinophilia in only 10%. Most have a normal ESR.
- Attacks last 1 to 2 weeks. Can have recurrences. Therapy includes NSAIDs.

RARE SYSTEMIC DISEASES

25. What is the differential diagnosis of a patient with fever and generalized lymphadenopathy?

- Infections: toxoplasmosis, Epstein–Barr virus (EBV), cytomegalovirus, human immunodeficiency virus (HIV), Whipple's disease, secondary syphilis, bartonella, brucellosis, tularemia, Yersinia pestis, mycobacterial, fungal.
- Malignancies: lymphoma, acute leukemia.
- Multicentric Castleman's disease.
- Systemic inflammatory disease: SLE, adult-onset/juvenile Still's disease, sarcoidosis.
- Medications: allopurinol, phenytoin, carbamazepine, sulfa antibiotics, others.
- Autoimmune lymphoproliferative syndrome (Canale–Smith syndrome).

26. What is the Canale–Smith syndrome?

Canale–Smith syndrome (autoimmune lymphoproliferative syndrome [ALPS]): a rare autosomal dominant disorder typically presenting in childhood and characterized by generalized lymphadenopathy, hepatosplenomegaly, and autoimmune hemolytic anemia and thrombocytopenia. Other organs (neurologic, lung, kidney, skin, etc.) can also be involved. Rarely patients with mutations causing a milder phenotype may not have symptoms until adulthood. Patients are diagnosed by increased numbers (≥5% of all T cells) of circulating double-negative T cells (CD3$^+$, CD4$^-$, CD8$^-$) which comprise >1.5% of all circulating lymphocytes. Approximately 66% of patients have an identifiable genetic defect. Most of these are germline mutations in the *Fas* gene (*TNFRSF6*), leading to abnormalities in the intracellular "death domain" of the receptor Fas (APO-1, CD95). This leads to the inability of the T cell to be signaled to undergo programmed cell death (apoptosis). Consequently, autoreactive T cells will downregulate CD4 and CD8 molecules but cannot be disposed of by Fas-mediated apoptosis (similar to *lpr* mice), leading to autoimmune disease. Patients without *Fas* gene mutations have been found to have mutations in the *Fas ligand* gene (similar to *gld* mice) or enzymes involved in apoptosis (caspase 10). Corticosteroid therapy has variable effects. Mycophenolate mofetil and sirolimus have been effective steroid-sparing medications. Notably, up to 10% of patients can develop neoplasms (lymphoma). Hematopoietic cell transplantation can be curative.

27. What is Erdheim–Chester disease (polyostotic sclerosing histiocytosis)?

Similar to MRH, **Erdheim–Chester disease** is classified among the non-Langerhans cell histiocytoses. It is a malignancy of myeloid progenitor cells. Patients usually have symptoms of bilateral, symmetric long bone pain which occurs in middle age. More than 50% of cases can

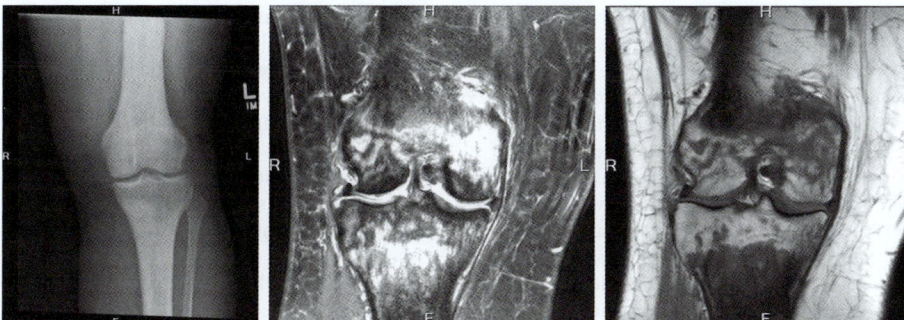

Fig. 80.1 Erdheim–Chester disease. Plain radiograph showing sclerosis of diaphysis and metaphysis. Magnetic resonance imaging (T1 and T2) showing heterogenous signal intensity due to replacement of normal bone marrow fat.

have extraskeletal involvement including painless exophthalmos (can precede other manifestations), brain (pituitary and cerebellum), kidney, lung, heart (recurrent pericardial effusions), or skin involvement (xanthomas). Retroperitoneal fibrosis can occur. Radiographs of involved areas show osteosclerosis. Long bone (diaphysis > metaphysis) and facial bones are commonly affected (Fig. 80.1). Bone biopsy shows xanthogranulomatous infiltration with foamy histiocytes surrounded by fibrosis. Approximately 50% of patients have a point mutation of the *BRAF* gene. These patients respond to vemurafenib (BRAF inhibitor) therapy. Other gene mutations have been reported. Patients with gene mutations in other components of the MAPK signaling pathway are treated with cobimetinib (MEK inhibitor) or interferon-alpha. Overall, prognosis is variable depending on the extent of disease with 5YS of 70% in some series.

28. What is Kikuchi disease?

Kikuchi–Fujimoto disease is a histiocytic, necrotizing lymphadenitis. Most patients are aged <30 years (range 2–75 years) and previously well. The most common presentation is fever (30–70%) and cervical lymphadenopathy (80–100%). Fever is low grade and lasts 1 to 4 weeks. Cervical adenopathy is usually unilateral and affects the posterior more than the anterior lymph nodes. Up to 20% can have other nodal involvement. Nodes are usually <2 cm, firm, discrete, and mobile. Some patients (up to 50%) have a flu-like prodrome with extranodal involvement including night sweats, joint pain (7%), variable rashes (5–30%), weight loss (10%), gastrointestinal (GI) symptoms, neurologic involvement (ataxia, aseptic meningitis), hepatosplenomegaly (5%), as well as others. Laboratory evaluation can show an elevated ESR (40–70%), leukopenia (25%), atypical lymphocytes (25%), and elevated liver function tests (especially lactate dehydrogenase). ANA and RF are negative and if positive suggest an associated rheumatic disease with SLE being most common. Lymph node biopsy will establish the diagnosis and exclude lymphoma, infections (tuberculosis, others), sarcoidosis, and unicentric Castleman's disease that can present with cervical adenopathy. The biopsy classically shows <u>necrosis</u> without a neutrophilic infiltrate. Histiocytes and $CD8^+$ T cells predominate. The etiology is unknown but suspected to be an immune response to an infectious agent or autoimmune in nature. Most patients (90%) improve in 1 to 6 months without treatment. Others will have relapses (3%) or persistent symptoms which can be treated with hydroxychloroquine, corticosteroids, or IV immunoglobulin.

29. What is Castleman's disease (angiofollicular lymph node hyperplasia)?

Castleman's disease is a heterogeneous group of lymphoproliferative disorders that share histopathologic features including germinal-center formation and marked capillary proliferation. The etiology is unknown but appears to be a result of impaired immunoregulation that causes abundant proliferation of B lymphocytes and plasma cells in lymphoid organs. There are three subtypes:
- **Unicentric:** involves one or more lymph nodes in one region of the body. Histopathology can vary between hyaline vascular subtype (90%) and plasma cell subtype (10%). Patients usually do not have systemic features. Treatment is surgical removal.

- **Multicentric:** presents with lymphadenopathy in multiple regions of the body. Histopathology can vary between hyaline vascular subtype and plasma cell subtype. Half the patients with multicentric disease will have a human herpes virus (HHV)-8 infection and be immunocompromised (usually HIV infected), and half of the patients will have no evidence of HHV-8 or HIV infection. Some of these patients without evidence of a viral infection will have an associated POEMS syndrome.
  - Patients who have the plasma cell subtype of multicentric Castleman's disease frequently have systemic symptoms which can mimic autoimmune diseases including fever, night sweats, hepatosplenomegaly, cytopenias, elevated ESR, autoantibodies (Coombs, ANA), and a polyclonal gammopathy.
  - Patients with symptomatic multicentric Castleman's disease who are not infected with HHV-8 can be treated with anti-IL6 therapy (siltuximab or tocilizumab). Rituximab is used as first-line therapy in those infected with HHV-8. Patients with HHV-8 infections or POEMS receive additional directed therapy (e.g., antivirals or plasma cell-directed therapy).

30. What is POEMS syndrome?

POEMS syndrome is a paraneoplastic syndrome that stands for:
- **P**olyneuropathy: a demyelinating sensorimotor peripheral neuropathy is seen in 100% of patients. At least 50% of patients develop severe muscle weakness.
- **O**rganomegaly: hepatomegaly, splenomegaly, or lymphadenopathy develops in 45–85%.
- **E**ndocrinopathy: 67–89% have or develop at least one endocrine abnormality. The most common is hypogonadism (55–89%). Abnormalities of the adrenal and pituitary gland can occur. DM and hypothyroidism also can be present but do not count as criteria due to their frequency in the general population.
- **M**onoclonal proteins: 100% have a monoclonal protein in the serum and/or urine. It is almost always associated with a lambda light chain.
- **S**kin changes: occur in 67–93% of patients. Hyperpigmentation and hemangiomas are most common (40–93%). Hypertrichosis is also common. Scleroderma-like changes with Raynaud's or acrocyanosis can also be seen (20–30%).
- There are numerous other manifestations such as extravascular volume overload (edema, ascites, etc.) (29–89%), hematologic abnormalities, papilledema (29–64%), clubbing, as well as others.

Diagnostic criteria have been developed. POEMS syndrome occurs in middle-aged patients with a slight male predominance. It is commonly associated with osteosclerotic bone lesions (27–97%) and has been called osteosclerotic myeloma. Multicentric Castleman's disease is seen in 15% to 20% of patients who have POEMS syndrome. This is notable because proinflammatory cytokines (IL-1, TNF, and IL-6) are elevated in both diseases. However, patients with POEMS also have significantly (more than three to four times the upper limit of normal) elevated levels of vascular endothelial growth factor (VEGF) (60–70%) that is produced by platelets and plasma cells. This may contribute to some of the clinical manifestations. Patients with disseminated disease are treated similar to patients with multiple myeloma.

ABNORMAL CALCIFICATIONS

31. Discuss the differences between the various types of soft tissue calcifications.

- **Calcinosis cutis:** calcium deposits form in the skin (see Question 32).
- **Calciphylaxis:** calcification occurs in the intima of blood vessels and subcutaneous tissue. This is primarily seen in patients with chronic renal failure, uremia, and a high-calcium/phosphorous product (>70). This frequently presents with ischemia and skin ulceration. Treatment is to control the hyperphosphatemia (<5.5 mg/dL) and uremia. Calcimimetic agents are used to treat secondary hyperparathyroidism. In severe cases, IV sodium thiosulfate has been used.
- **Tumoral calcinosis:** large calcific nodules in juxtaarticular locations causing pain and limited range of motion. There are three types: primary hyperphosphatemic, primary normophosphatemic, and secondary tumoral calcinosis. The primary hyperphosphatemic subtype is autosomal recessive and tends to affect adolescents and young adults. The basic defect is

thought to be in the proximal renal tubular cell with an elevated renal phosphate reabsorption threshold and increased production of 1,25-dihydroxyvitamin D. Mutations of the *GALNT3, KLOTHO,* and *FGF23* genes have been described. Notably, fibroblast growth factor (FGF) 23 is an important phosphaturic hormone. Mutations that cause inactivation of FGF 23 cause hyperphosphatemia. Treatment is inadequate and includes low-phosphate diet, phosphate-binding antacids, acetazolamide, and surgical excision. Tumoral calcinosis tends to recur after surgical removal. The primary normophosphatemic subtype may be due to mutations of the *SAMD9* gene that is important in cellular apoptosis. It is unclear how this causes tumoral calcinosis. Secondary tumoral calcinosis is usually due to chronic renal failure with secondary or tertiary hyperparathyroidism and is treated by subtotal parathyroidectomy or renal transplantation.

- **Heterotopic ossification:** abnormal formation of lamellar bone within soft tissues such as tendons, ligaments, or muscles. It commonly occurs in patients with traumatic brain injuries or spinal cord injuries. Patients with these neurologic problems as well as patients with diffuse idiopathic skeletal hyperostosis (DISH) or ankylosing spondylitis are at risk for developing this following total joint arthroplasty. Patients have pain and a limited range of motion. Patients at high risk should receive indomethacin, IV bisphosphonates, or local radiation therapy before arthroplasty to prevent this complication. Recurrence is common after surgical removal.

32. What is dystrophic calcification? What CTDs are associated with it?

When calcification occurs in cutaneous tissues, it is called **calcinosis cutis** and can be divided into four categories: dystrophic, metastatic (high-calcium × phosphorous product >70–75), idiopathic (e.g., tumoral calcinosis), and iatrogenic. **Dystrophic calcification** is the most common type (95%) and is secondary to nonmetabolic diseases such as CTDs or due to deposition of calcium salts in the damaged tissue. Calcium is deposited either as numerous large masses (calcinosis universalis) or a few small, localized masses (calcinosis circumscripta). Dystrophic calcifications are most commonly associated with systemic sclerosis, dermatomyositis, SLE, MCTD, pseudoxanthoma elasticum, panniculitis, and trauma. Tests for serum calcium and phosphorus should be normal. Medical therapy is poor. Small lesions may be improved with intralesional corticosteroids, low-dose (1 mg/day) warfarin, minocycline (50–100 mg/day), ceftriaxone (2 g/day IV for 20 days binds calcium salts), carbon dioxide laser, or surgical excision. Larger lesions may be improved by high-dose diltiazem (3 mg/kg per day), probenecid (1.5 g/day), IV bisphosphonates (zoledronic acid 4 mg IV every 3–4 months for a year inhibits calcium apposition onto hydroxyapatite), topical sodium thiosulfate 25%, or surgical excision.

33. What benign synovial tumor can cause synovial calcifications?

Primary synovial osteochondromatosis is a benign condition occurring most commonly in patients aged 30 to 50 years where an inflamed synovium undergoes metaplasia resulting in cartilage nodules that can undergo calcification and ossification. The calcifications can break free as loose bodies into the joint space leading to locking and articular cartilage damage causing osteoarthritis. It most commonly occurs in the knee, hip, or shoulder, but any joint can be involved. Radiographs demonstrate multiple calcific densities looking like "popcorn". The etiology is unknown. Malignant transformation to chondrosarcoma is rare. Treatment is symptomatic but often requires surgical removal of the loose bodies and synovectomy. Incomplete synovectomy can result in disease recurrence.

34. What is diffuse idiopathic skeletal hyperostosis (DISH)?

DISH has also been called **Forestier's disease** and ankylosing hyperostosis. It is a bone-forming condition in which ossification occurs at skeletal sites subjected to stress. It occurs most frequently in the thoracic spine, leading to stiffness or decreased motion. Pain is usually not a significant symptom; if severe, the patient should be evaluated for other causes of pain. Involvement of the cervical spine can cause dysphagia. DISH occurs in approximately 12% of the elderly population and may coexist with other disorders, particularly type 2 diabetes mellitus.

Radiographically, normal bone mineralization is seen in addition to "flowing" ossification of the anterior longitudinal ligament connecting at least four contiguous vertebral bodies. The calcification of the anterior longitudinal ligament is seen as a radiodense band separated from the

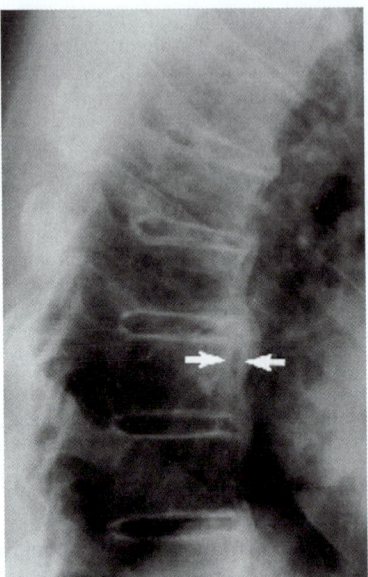

Fig. 80.2 Lateral radiograph of the thoracic spine showing calcification of the anterior longitudinal ligament connecting four vertebrae. Note the space between the calcified ligament and the anterior border of the vertebral bodies *(arrows)*.

anterior aspect of the vertebral bodies by a thin radiolucent line, similar to flowing candle wax (Fig. 80.2). Ossification of multiple tendinous or ligamentous sites in the appendicular skeleton may also be seen. Disc spaces, apophyseal joints, and sacroiliac joints are typically normal on radiographs, helping differentiate DISH from OA and ankylosing spondylitis.

SKIN MANIFESTATIONS OF DISEASE

35. What is erythromelalgia?

Erythromelalgia is a neurovascular peripheral pain disorder in which blood vessels are episodically blocked and then become hyperemic and inflamed. The attacks are episodic and characterized by red, warm, swollen, and painful (burning) extremities. Feet are affected more than hands. Attacks are triggered by exertion, heat, pressure, caffeine, and alcohol. Symptoms are bilateral but not necessarily symmetric. Rarely symptoms may progress to gangrene. Other diseases such as Fabry disease, peripheral neuropathy, complex regional pain syndrome, and vasculitis can mimic erythromelalgia and need to be excluded. Erythromelalgia is categorized as primary or secondary.

- **Primary erythromelalgia:** may be genetic or idiopathic in origin. Early-onset erythromelalgia is usually familial with an autosomal dominant inheritance. It is associated with a gain-of-function mutation of the voltage-gated sodium channel α subunit gene *(SCN9A, SCN10A, or SCN11A)*. The mutation causes hyperexcitability of dorsal root ganglion of the sympathetic ganglion neurons leading to symptoms similar to chronic regional pain syndrome. The severity of the mutation determines if the clinical symptoms start at puberty or later in adulthood. Elevation and cold exposure including emersion of feet in ice water give relief. There is no consistently effective therapy. Triggers (heat, exercise, standing) should be avoided. Topical therapy (lidocaine, others) can be effective. It does not respond to aspirin therapy. Medications affecting voltage-gated sodium channels (mexiletine, lidocaine, carbamazepine) may be helpful. Prostacyclin, venlafaxine, and gabapentin/pregabalin have also been used. Most of the patients presenting with adult-onset erythromelalgia do not have an identifiable genetic mutation or an associated disease and are considered to have primary idiopathic erythromelalgia.
- **Secondary erythromelalgia:** is similar to primary erythromelalgia clinically, has its onset during adulthood, and is associated with various diseases or medications. Treatment of the underlying disease or withdrawal of the offending medication is helpful. There are two types of secondary erythromelalgia: aspirin sensitive and aspirin insensitive.

- Aspirin-sensitive erythromelalgia is associated with polycythemia vera, essential thrombocytosis, and other chronic myeloproliferative disorders. In 85% of patients, the cutaneous symptoms precede the myelodysplastic syndrome by months to years (median 2.5 years). Erythromelalgia is diagnosed on the basis of platelet counts exceeding 400,000/mm^3, relief of symptoms lasting for days with low-dose aspirin (81–640 mg/d), and histopathologic evidence of arterioles with fibromuscular proliferation. The response to aspirin suggests that platelet-derived prostaglandins cause the symptoms.
- Aspirin-insensitive erythromelalgia is typically attributable to a medication (calcium channel blockers, bromocriptine, others) or another disease (small fiber neuropathy, autoimmune disease, mushroom poisoning). Treatment is similar to primary erythromelalgia if stopping possible precipitating medications is ineffective.

36. Describe the histologic classification of the panniculitides and the most common CTDs associated with each.

- **Septal panniculitis:**
  - With vasculitis: cutaneous PAN, Behcet disease
  - Without vasculitis: erythema nodosum (R/O sarcoidosis), α1-antitrypsin deficiency
- **Lobular panniculitis:**
  - With vasculitis: erythema induratum/nodular vasculitis.
  - Without vasculitis: Weber–Christian syndrome (relapsing febrile nodular nonsuppurative panniculitis), enzymatic panniculitis attributable to pancreatic enzymes, and connective tissue panniculitis.
- Mixed panniculitis: lupus profundus.

37. Describe the histologic classification and clinical associations with pyoderma gangrenosum.

- **Ulcerative pyoderma gangrenosum:** ulceration, purulent. Associated with poorly controlled RA and inflammatory bowel disease (IBD).
- **Pustular pyoderma gangrenosum:** discrete pustules. Associated with IBD.
- **Bullous pyoderma gangrenosum:** superficial bullae that develop ulcerations. Associated with myeloproliferative diseases.
- **Vegetative pyoderma gangrenosum:** erosions, superficial ulcers.

  Juvenile-onset pyoderma gangrenosum may be associated with other clinical manifestations and should suggest an autoinflammatory syndrome (PAPA, PASH, PAPASH, others) which are caused by gene mutations leading to dysfunction of inflammasomes (Chapter 79).

38. Differentiate the following skin manifestations that can mimic vasculitis: livedo reticularis, livedo racemosa, livedoid vasculopathy, and malignant atrophic papulosis.

- **Livedo reticularis:** macular, violaceous, netlike, patterned erythema of the skin. The livid rings are due to reduced blood flow and low oxygen tension at the periphery. Skin biopsy is unrevealing. There are four types:
  - Physiologic (also called cutis mamorata): mainly occurs on legs of young women. Typically, worse in cold and resolves with warming.
  - Primary: has fluctuant course but does not resolve with warming.
  - Idiopathic: persistent and unresolving livedo. May be early form of livedo racemosa.
  - Amantadine-induced: occurs in 2% to 28% of patients on amantadine. Vascular reaction due to catecholamine depletion.
- **Livedo racemosa:** resembles livedo reticularis but is persistent and more widespread. The pattern is irregular, broken circles. Associated with a secondary cause including Sneddon syndrome, antiphospholipid antibody syndrome (APS), SLE, essential thrombocythemia, thromboangiitis obliterans, polycythemia vera, and polyarteritis nodosa. Skin biopsy shows thrombi and/or vessel inflammation. Strong association with cerebral and ocular ischemic arterial events, valve disease, and seizures in patients with APS (Sneddon syndrome).
- **Livedoid vasculopathy (atrophie blanche):** is included as a cause of livedo racemosa. It is a vascular disease characterized by thrombosis and skin ulcerations on bilateral lower extremities. It occurs predominantly in middle-aged women and is not associated with another

disease. Some patients are hypercoagulable (Factor V Leiden, APS, etc). Skin biopsy shows segmental hyalinization of dermal vessels and thrombi, but no vasculitis. There is no internal organ manifestation unless associated with another disease. Skin lesions respond poorly to therapy and heal with characteristic stellate ivory scars.

- **Malignant atrophic papulosis (Kohlmeier-Degos disease):** a rare thrombo-occlusive vasculopathy that presents with erythematous papular skin lesions with a porcelain-white depressed center. There is an average of 30 lesions scattered on trunk and extremities. Up to 33% develop systemic manifestations due to involvement of small- and medium-sized arteries of the GI tract, central nervous system (CNS), pericardium, and bladder. Laboratory tests are nonspecific. Diagnosis is made by skin biopsy showing endothelial proliferation, thrombosis, and infarction. Vasculitis is not present. Treatment is poor and many patients die of sepsis from GI perforation. Immunosuppressives are ineffective, although eculizumab and teprostinil have been reported to be beneficial.

OTHER DISEASES WITH RHEUMATIC MANIFESTATIONS

39. Stiff-person syndrome (SPS): a disorder characterized by muscle rigidity and episodic muscle spasms, primarily involving the trunk. Episodes can be prolonged, painful, and precipitated by loud noises. There are three types:

- The most common (60–80%) type is associated with **antibodies against glutamic acid decarboxylase** (GAD65) and frequently with autoimmune diseases (e.g., type I DM, Graves' disease, hypothyroidism, pernicious anemia, vitiligo) because of its high association with HLA DQ-0201. Electromyography demonstrates involuntary motor unit firing. It is postulated that the anti-GAD antibodies inhibit the enzymes in the CNS responsible for production of gamma-aminobutyric acid (GABA), which is an inhibitory neurotransmitter. In addition, many of these patients also have antibodies that inhibit GABA-associated receptor protein, which prevents GABA from binding to its receptor. Consequently, neural transmission is unopposed and can lead to muscle rigidity. This type of SPS is treated with diazepam, baclofen, plasmapheresis, immunosuppressives including rituximab, and/or IV gammaglobulin.
- The other two types of SPS are not associated with anti-GAD antibodies or a certain HLA phenotype. One type (5% of cases) is a **paraneoplastic** manifestation of cancers (lymphoma, breast, lung, colon, thyroid), whereas the other type (15–35% of cases) is **idiopathic.** Paraneoplastic SPS tends to involve the neck and arms, has a rapid onset, and is very painful. Patients with paraneoplastic SPS have been found to have **anti-amphiphysin** (128-kd protein on the surface of synaptic vesicles) or less commonly anti-gephyrin antibodies. These two SPS types do not respond to immune-modulating therapies and are treated with high doses of muscle relaxants such as diazepam or baclofen that are GABA agonists.
- Variants of SPS: (1) stiff-limb syndrome has stiffness limited to one limb, usually the leg. This can resemble dystonia. Up to 25% will develop other manifestations of classical SPS over time; (2) progressive encephalomyelitis with rigidity and myoclonus (PERM) has brainstem, cerebellar, and spinal cord involvement with autonomic dysfunction, anti-glycine receptor antibodies; and (3) jerking man syndrome begins as classical SPS, but patient develops limb myoclonic jerks over time.

40. How does Tietze syndrome differ from costochondritis?

Tietze syndrome is a syndrome of pain, tenderness, and non-suppurative swelling of joints of the chest wall, typically the costochondral joints (second or third most commonly). In comparison, costochondritis is a much more common syndrome characterized by costochondral joint pain and tenderness without objective signs of swelling or inflammation. Tietze syndrome occurs in both men and women age usually <40 years. It usually (80%) involves a single joint and is rarely bilateral. Polyarticular disease can affect neighboring articulations on the same side of the sternum. Unlike costochondritis, radiographs and ultrasound show soft tissue swelling of the involved articulation(s). The etiology is unknown, but an attack may be precipitated by trauma, coughing, vomiting, or a viral syndrome. In older patients, it is seen more frequently in those with costal cartilage calcification, suggesting that hydroxyapatite may play an etiologic role. Attacks usually resolve within 2 weeks. NSAIDs, toradol, glucocorticoid injections, and local therapy with heat or ice may help symptoms. Other causes of costochondral joint swelling such as infection, spondyloarthropathies, SAPHO, and relapsing polychondritis must be excluded before diagnosing a patient with Tietze syndrome.

41. Discuss the musculoskeletal complications of cystic fibrosis.

Cystic fibrosis is an autosomal recessive disease characterized by decreased mucous production leading to obstructive lung disease and malabsorption. Other organs, including sinuses, pancreas, liver, sweat glands, and reproductive tract can be affected. It is attributable to a defect in the *CFTR* gene on chromosome 7, which encodes for a membrane glycoprotein (CFTR) that is a chloride ion channel. In cystic fibrosis, one of the chloride ion channels present on the apical membrane of the epithelial cell is either absent or defective. This leads to increased sodium absorption and decreased chloride secretion, resulting in decreased extracellular water content. Patients have obstruction with infections in the lung and malabsorption from the gut. Consequently, patients are susceptible to osteoporosis (up to 75% of adults) attributable to poor calcium and vitamin D absorption. Kyphoscoliosis and muscle weakness are also increased. Additionally, 2% to 9% of patients have episodic nondestructive oligoarthritis most commonly involving the fingers and lower extremity large joints. The arthritis is felt to be a result of immune complexes attributable to chronic lung infection. Attacks last for a few days (median 7 days) and may be associated with fever and painful nodular skin lesions and purpura. Rarely, hypertrophic osteoarthropathy (5%) and small vessel vasculitis can occur. Musculoskeletal symptoms are more common the longer the disease duration (adults > adolescence > children), the more severe the disease, and in patients infected with *Pseudomonas aeruginosa*.

MEDICATION-INDUCED RHEUMATIC MANIFESTATIONS AND ASIA SYNDROME

42. What rheumatic and autoimmune syndromes have been associated with the following medications?
- Fluoroquinolones: Achilles tendinitis and rupture.
- Minocycline: drug-induced lupus, autoimmune hepatitis, perinuclear ANCA positivity and vasculitis.
- Statins: myopathy, myositis (anti-HMG-CoA reductase antibodies), subacute cutaneous lupus erythematosus (SCLE) rash.
- Rifabutin: drug-induced lupus.
- Hydralazine: ANCA vasculitis, drug-induced lupus.
- Zafirlukast: Churg–Strauss syndrome.
- Antithyroid medications (propylthiouracil): ANCA vasculitis.
- Anti-TNF agents: drug-induced lupus, vasculitis, sarcoidosis, SCLE rash.
- Interferon-α: thyroiditis, drug-induced lupus, sarcoidosis.
- Protease inhibitors (HIV): osteonecrosis, adhesive capsulitis.
- Cancer chemotherapy: isolated case reports of several rheumatic diseases caused by various chemotherapies (e.g., hydroxyurea causing dermatomyositis-like rash).
- Immune checkpoint inhibitors (anti-CTLA-4, anti-PD-1, anti-PD-L1): multiple immune-related adverse events (arthritis, sicca, colitis, pneumonitis, others).
- Myopathies: corticosteroids, antimalarials, colchicine, zidovudine, antifungals (triazoles, imidazoles), oncologic drugs, succinylcholine, others.
- Drug-induced antiphospholipid antibodies: procainamide, quinidine, antipsychotics, phenytoin, interferon-α, hydralazine, TNF-α antagonists.
- Drug-induced SCLE: (frequently with anti-SSA): calcium channel blockers, angiotensin-converting enzyme inhibitors, diclofenac, proton pump inhibitors, TNF antagonists, terbinafine, buproprion, statins, and antiepileptics.
- Bisphosphonates: uveitis, atypical femoral fractures.
- Retinoids: extraspinal hyperostosis (DISH-like).
- Voriconazole: nodular hypertrophic osteoarthropathy.
- See individual chapters on other medications causing drug-induced lupus, gout, vasculitis, myopathies, etc.

43. What is the ASIA syndrome?

ASIA stands for **A**utoimmune/inflammatory **S**yndrome **I**nduced by **A**djuvants. This is a controversial concept suggesting that certain environmental exposures (infections, vaccines, adjuvants, silicone, and drugs) can act as an adjuvant stimulating the innate immune system, resulting in symptoms and/or subsequent stimulation of the adaptive immune system leading to autoantibodies and/or an autoimmune disease. In patients who already have a defined autoimmune disease, these adjuvants may exacerbate their disease. Because this only occurs in a small fraction of patients exposed to these adjuvants, causality is difficult to prove.

The proposed diagnostic criteria are: (1) development of symptoms (muscle, joint, fatigue, demyelination, cognitive impairment, pyrexia) or (2) development of an undifferentiated CTD and/or autoantibodies within proximity to exposure to an adjuvant. Some examples are:

- **Immunizations:** associated with causing demyelinating syndromes, reactive arthritis, and small vessel vasculitis. Recombinant hepatitis B vaccination has been associated with a higher-than-expected number of rheumatic disorders including vasculitis (especially central retinal vein occlusion), RA, SLE, reactive arthritis, as well as various demyelination syndromes. These rheumatic disorders occur within 1 to 2 months of the first, second, or third vaccination. Unlike other typical side effects of an immunization, these rheumatic disorders may not resolve. Other vaccines (influenza, HPV, COVID-19) have also been associated with ASIA syndrome.
- **Silicone:** breast implants (especially those that ruptured) and oil injections for cosmetic purposes have been reported to cause scleroderma-like diseases. Very controversial.
- **Alum adjuvant:** aluminum in vaccines has been associated with causing the macrophage myofasciitis syndrome.
- **Gulf War syndrome:** soldiers exposed to multiple vaccinations and other environmental hazards in a short period of time developed fibromyalgia-like symptoms and cognitive dysfunction. Many patients had antisqualene antibodies due to the anthrax vaccine they received although the significance of this is debated.
- **Sick building syndrome:** SBS is a complex spectrum of ill health symptoms, such as mucous membrane irritation, asthma, neurotoxic effects, gastrointestinal disturbance, skin dryness, sensitivity to odors that may appear among occupants in office and public buildings, schools and hospitals. Environmental exposures are postulated to trigger these symptoms by causing a chronic inflammatory response. Autoantibodies to various neuronal antigens have been reported.
- Case reports of parvovirus infection with arthritis evolving into RA, EBV infection evolving into SLE, COVID infection causing a variety of autoimmune syndromes, and procainamide exposure triggering SLE that does not resolve with drug withdrawal.

BIBLIOGRAPHY

Burg MR, Mitschang C, George T, Schneider SW. Livedoid vasculopathy—a diagnostic and therapeutic challenge. *Front Med*. 2022;9:1–15.

Cavalli G, Guglielmi B, Berti A, et al. The multifaceted clinical presentations of Erdheim-Chester disease: comprehensive review of the literature and of 10 new cases. *Ann Rheum Dis*. 2013;72:1691–1695.

Corradini D, Di Matteo A, Emery P, Mankia K. How should we treat palindromic rheumatism? A systemic literature review. *Seminars Arth Rheum*. 2021;51:266–277.

Dispenzieri A. POEMS syndrome: 2021 update on diagnosis, risk-stratification, and management. *Am J Hematol*. 2021;96:872–888.

Fathi I, Sakr M. Review of tumoral calcinosis: a rare clinicopathological entity. *World J Clin Cases*. 2014;2:409–414.

Guo H, Liang Q, Dong C, Zhang Q, Gu ZF. Systemic review of fibroblastic rheumatism: a case report. *World J Clin Cases*. 2023;11:5136–5146.

Hench PS, Rosenberg EF. Palindromic rheumatism. *Arch Intern Med*. 1944;73:293–321.

Khouri J, Nakashima M, Wong S. Update on the diagnosis and treatment of POEMS (polyneuropathy, organomegaly, endocrinopathy, monoclonal gammopathy, and skin changes) syndrome: a review. *JAMA Oncol*. 2021;7:1383–1391.

Lambrechts M. Musculoskeletal abnormalities caused by cystic fibrosis. *Advances in Skeletal Muscle Health and Disease. IntechOpen*; 2023. doi:10.5772/intechopen.104591.

Mader R, Verlaan JJ, Buskila D. Diffuse idiopathic skeletal hyperostosis: clinical features and pathogenic mechanisms. *Nat Rev Rheumatol*. 2013;9:741–750.

Mann N, King T, Murphy R. Review of primary and secondary erythromelalgia. *Clin Exp Dermatol*. 2019;44:477–482.

Martinez-Lopez J, Marquez A, Pegoraro F, et al. Brief report: Genome-wide association study identifies the first germline genetic variant associated with Erdheim-Chester disease. *Arthritis Rheumatol*. 2024;76:141–145.

Masab M, Farooq H. Kikuchi disease. *Clin Rheumatol*. 2017;27:1073–1075.

Mor A, Pillinger MH, Wortmann RL, Mitnick HJ. Drug-induced arthritic and connective tissue disorders. *Semin Arthritis Rheum*. 2008;38:249–264.

Newsome SD, Johnson T. Stiff person syndrome spectrum disorders; more than meets the eye. *J Neuroimmunol*. 2022;369:577915.

Parker LK, Ponte C, Howell KJ, Ong VH, Denton CP, Schreiber BE. Clinical features and management of erythromelalgia: long term follow-up of 46 cases. *Clin Exp Rheumatol*. 2017;35:80–84.

Rieux-Laucat F, Magérus-Chatinet A, Neven B. The autoimmune lymphoproliferative syndrome with defective FAS or FAS-ligand functions. *J Clin Immunol*. 2018;38:558–568.

Roehmel JF, Kallinich T, Staab D, Schwarz C. Clinical manifestations and risk factors of arthropathy in cystic fibrosis. *Respir Med*. 2019;147:66–71.

Sanmarti R, Haro I, Canete JD. Palindromic rheumatism: a unique and enigmatic entity with a complex relationship with rheumatoid arthritis [review]. *Expert Rev Clin Immunol*. 2021;17:375–384.

Saternus R, Schwingel J, Müller CSL, Vogt T, Reichrath J. Ancient friends, revisited: Systematic review and case report of pyoderma gangrenosum-associated autoinflammatory syndromes. *J Transl Autoimmun*. 2020;3:1–9.

Schoenfeld Y, Agmon-Levin N. ASIA"– autoimmune/inflammatory syndrome induced by adjuvants. *J Autoimmun*. 2011;36:4–8.

Seida I, Seida R, Elsalti A, Mahroum N. Vaccines and autoimmunity—from side effects to ASIA syndrome. *Medicina*. 2023;59:364.

Van der Linden PD, van Puijenbroek EP, Feenstra J, et al. Tendon disorders attributed to fluoroquinolones: a study on 42 spontaneous reports in the period 1988–1998. *Arthritis Care Res*. 2001;45:235–239.

Xu X-L, Liang X-H, Liu J, et al. Multicentric reticulohistiocytosis with prominent skin lesions and arthritis: a case report. *World J Clin Cases*. 2022;10:7913–7923.

Yu L, Tu M, Cortes J, et al. Clinical and pathological characteristics of HIV- and HHV-8 negative Castleman disease. *Blood*. 2017;129:1658–1668.

FURTHER READING

https://raredisease.

CHAPTER 81

Nonsteroidal Anti-Inflammatory Drugs

Trevor McKown, MD

"No drug is as good as the day it is first thought of."

-Sir William Osler

> **KEY POINTS**
>
> 1. NSAIDs' beneficial and adverse effects arise from blocking prostaglandin synthesis by inhibiting cyclooxygenase.
> 2. The risk of gastrointestinal bleeding from NSAIDs can be reduced through appropriate selection of NSAID and use of proton pump inhibitors.
> 3. Chronic use of NSAIDs increases the risk of coronary thrombosis.
> 4. Patients with advanced chronic kidney disease are at greatest risk of renal toxicity from NSAIDs.

1. What are nonsteroidal anti-inflammatory drugs (NSAIDs) and how were they named?

NSAIDs are a class of medications that interfere with the production of prostaglandins, which are important mediators of pain and inflammation. NSAIDs are among the most widely used classes of medications in the United States. In the National Health And Nutrition Examination Survey (NHANES) from 1999 to 2004, 11.6% of adults reported regular use of non-aspirin NSAIDs. The term *NSAIDs* was coined in the 1970s, when the only other major class of anti-inflammatory drug used at the time were glucocorticoids. There are now many other medications that interfere with various inflammatory pathways that are neither steroids nor NSAIDs, but the name has stuck.

2. What are prostaglandins?

Prostaglandins are a class of lipid molecules that act locally (via autocrine or paracrine signaling) to regulate physiologic processes and act as mediators of inflammation. Prostaglandins are derived from arachidonic acid, a 20-carbon polyunsaturated fatty acid that is a dietary essential fatty acid. Arachidonic acid is stored in phospholipid within the plasma membrane until released by phospholipases in response to cellular stimuli. Various enzymes act on free arachidonic acid and its derivatives to produce a variety of lipophilic signaling molecules, called eicosanoids (from the Greek *eikosi-*, meaning "twenty"); important eicosanoids include the prostaglandins (which also include prostacyclin and thromboxane) and the leukotrienes.

3. How are prostaglandins produced from arachidonic acid?

The prostaglandins are formed through the action of cyclooxygenase, a class of enzyme that peroxidizes and reduces arachidonic acid. A constitutively expressed form of cyclooxygenase, called **COX-1**, is present in many different tissues, including the endothelium, platelets, and gastric mucosa. An inducible form of cyclooxygenase, called **COX-2**, is produced by certain cells in response to tissue injury, inflammatory signals, or other stimuli; it also is constitutively produced in some areas of the body. Both COX-1 and COX-2 act to convert arachidonic acid into prostaglandin H_2 (PGH_2). Prostaglandins D_2, E_2, F_2, prostacyclin (PGI_2), and thromboxane A_2, among others, are produced from PGH_2 by enzymes that are differentially expressed in the body according to tissue type (anatomic location) and physiologic state (normal versus inflamed tissue).

4. What are the biological functions of prostaglandins?

Prostaglandins exert their physiologic effects primarily through binding to prostaglandin receptors on target cells. The same type of prostaglandin can regulate different physiologic processes in different tissues. For example, PGE_2 produced by myeloid cells at sites of inflammation causes sensitization of nerve endings in pain-signaling neurons, thereby increasing pain sensitization in inflamed tissue. Meanwhile, circulating fever-producing signals such as interleukin-1β trigger endothelial cells in the hypothalamus to produce PGE_2 using COX-2; PGE_2 then acts on hypothalamic neurons to cause fever. Finally, PGE_2 sustains and protects the gastric mucosa by enhancing mucus production and increasing submucosal blood flow in the stomach, demonstrating the widespread biological effects of PGE_2.

Some representative functions of the major prostaglandins include:

- Prostaglandin D_2: eosinophil activation, migration; smooth muscle proliferation (airway smooth muscle)
- Prostaglandin E_2: fever (hypothalamic neurons); pain response (sensory nerve endings), oocyte maturation (ovarian follicle); bone resorption (osteoclasts); mucus, bicarbonate secretion (gastric mucosa)
- Prostaglandin F_2: smooth muscle contraction (uterus)
- Prostacyclin (prostaglandin I_2): vasodilation, platelet declumping
- Thromboxane A_2: vasoconstriction, platelet aggregation

5. Describe the mechanism of action of NSAIDs.

NSAIDs reversibly inhibit cyclooxygenase (COX-1, COX-2, or both), preventing production of prostaglandins and their downstream physiologic effects. Most NSAIDs inhibit both COX-1 and COX-2 to varying degrees. The therapeutic effects of NSAIDs largely arise from inhibition of COX-2-derived prostaglandins in inflamed tissues. The disruption of normal physiologic actions of prostaglandins by COX-1 inhibition is responsible for some adverse effects of NSAIDs. However, experience with COX-2-selective agents has shown that several important adverse effects of NSAIDs arise from specific COX-2 inhibition as well.

6. Name some NSAIDs and describe how they can be classified according to chemical structure (Table 81.1).

7. How do NSAIDs differ in potency and efficacy?

There are significant differences in the relative potency of the NSAIDs. For instance, meloxicam is approximately 200 times more potent than ibuprofen: 15 mg of meloxicam daily has roughly the same therapeutic effects as 3000 mg of ibuprofen daily. However, the comparative clinical efficacy of NSAIDs generally does not differ if they are adequately dosed. An individual patient may experience better efficacy or more adverse effects from a particular NSAID, which may be due to differences in how the drug is absorbed and metabolized; for example, polymorphisms in the CYP2C9 gene alter the clearance of celecoxib, ibuprofen, and meloxicam.

8. What routes are available for administration of NSAIDs?

The majority of NSAIDs are administered by mouth, with several available in liquid form. Ketorolac can be given intravenously or intramuscularly for treatment of severe acute pain. Topical formulations of salicylates and diclofenac can be used to treat musculoskeletal pain. Systemic absorption of topical diclofenac is significantly lower compared to oral (between 5- and 15-fold, depending on the dose applied), meaning that some patients with relative contraindications to systemic NSAIDs can safely use topical diclofenac. Several NSAIDs also come as rectal suppositories.

9. Describe the indications for NSAIDs.

The vast majority of NSAIDs, either as prescription or over-the-counter drugs, are used for pain. In rheumatology, NSAIDs are used to treat pain from inflammatory arthritis, including rheumatoid arthritis and spondyloarthritis. NSAIDs are effective for the treatment of acute gout as well as for anti-inflammatory prophylaxis to prevent gout flares. NSAIDs are also effective for treating pain from noninflammatory conditions including osteoarthritis, soft tissue injuries, headaches, and dysmenorrhea. NSAIDs are also widely used as a fever reducer (antipyretic).

There are also several specialized indications for NSAIDs. PGE_2 supports patency of the ductus arteriosus in the fetus, so NSAIDs can be used in newborns with patent ductus arteriosus to

TABLE 81.1 Non-steroidal anti-inflammatory drug classes

CLASS	DRUG	TYPICAL DOSE (MG)	FREQUENCY	MAXIMUM DAILY DOSE (MG)
Salicylic acid derivatives	Aspirin[a,b]	650–975	q4–6h[d]	3900
	Salsalate	1000–1500	q8–12h	3000
	Diflunisal	500	q8h	1500
Propionic acid derivatives	Ibuprofen[b]	400–800	q4–6h	3200
	Naproxen[b]	220–500	q12h[d]	1500
	Ketoprofen	50–75	q6–8H[d]	300
Acetic acid derivatives	Diclofenac[c]	50–75	q6–8h[d]	200
	Ketorolac	10–20 PO 30–60 IV or IM	q4–6h PO q6h IV or IM	40 PO 60 IV-IM
	Etodolac	200–400	q6–8[d]	1000
	Indomethacin	25–50	q6–8h	150
	Sulindac	150–200	q12h	400
	Tolmetin	600	q8H	1800
	Nabumetone	1000–1500	q12–24h	2000
Enolic acid derivatives	Meloxicam	7.5–15	q12–q24h	15
	Piroxicam	10–20	q12–q24h	20
Fenamic acid dervatives	Mefenamic acid	250–500	q8h	1500
Selective COX-2 inhibitors	Celecoxib	100–200	q12h	400

[a]Sometimes considered a non-NSAID; see below.
[b]Available over the counter in the United States.
[c]Topical only available over the counter the United States.
[d]Extended-release form available.

promote closure. Chronic NSAID use decreases the risk of colorectal cancer (via a decreased risk of adenomatous polyps) and has been recommended as prophylaxis for certain patients at high risk of cancer. Rectal administration of indomethacin decreases the risk of pancreatitis following endoscopic retrograde cholangiopancreatography (ERCP) in higher-risk patients.

10. What is the guiding principle of NSAID dosing?

Use the lowest dose and shortest duration of an NSAID that produces the desired therapeutic effect. As-needed use is preferable to continuous use for most indications. Many of the adverse effects of NSAIDs are dose and duration dependent, so this principle helps maximize the ratio of therapeutic benefits to risk of adverse effects.

11. Is aspirin an NSAID?

Aspirin (acetylsalicylic acid) is often separated from other NSAIDS due to an important difference in its mechanism of action. Aspirin acetylates and thereby **irreversibly inactivates COX**, unlike the reversible COX inhibition by NSAIDs. Thus, while aspirin's half-life is only 15–20 minutes, its effects can be longer-lasting. Aspirin is an efficient COX-1 inhibitor, and low doses (81–100 mg/day) have potent antiplatelet effects by inhibiting platelet COX-1. Aspirin is less effective as a COX-2 inhibitor, and higher doses of aspirin are required to exert analgesic and anti-inflammatory effects.

12. Describe how aspirin and NSAIDs differ in their effects on platelet function.

In platelets, COX-1 inhibition prevents production of thromboxane A_2, an important mediator of platelet activation and vasoconstriction. NSAIDs inhibit platelet COX-1 to a degree proportional to their COX-1 selectivity; since NSAIDs bind reversibly, any effects on platelet function are temporary. In contrast, aspirin irreversibly inhibits platelet COX-1. Platelets cannot synthesize new proteins and so aspirin's effects last for the lifetime of the platelet (8-10 days).

13. What is a selective COX-2 inhibitor? How do its effects differ from conventional NSAIDs?

Selective COX-2 inhibitors preferentially inhibit COX-2 compared to COX-1, with the intent of inhibiting inflammation-related prostaglandin production without affecting the "housekeeping" functions of COX-1-derived prostagladins. Drugs designed to be selective COX-2 inhibitors include celecoxib, rofecoxib, and valdecoxib. However, the relative selectivity of COX-1 versus COX-2 inhibition varies between different NSAIDs, and the COX-2-selectivity of certain traditional NSAIDs, such as diclofenac, approaches that of celecoxib (see below).

Chronic use of selective COX-2 inhibitors is associated with a lower gastrointestinal bleeding risk compared to traditional NSAIDs. However, post-marketing studies identified an increased risk of cardiovascular events, leading to the removal of rofecoxib and valdecoxib from the US market. There remains uncertainty about the relative importance of COX-2-selectivity on determining increased risk of cardiovascular disease in chronic NSAID users (see Question #18). Selective COX-2 inhibitors have a similar risk of renal adverse effects as traditional NSAIDs. The adverse effect profile of selective COX-2 inhibitors has led to a reappraisal of the older paradigm that all "housekeeping" functions of prostaglandins are carried out through COX-1; constitutively expressed COX-2 is now known to play a role in the normal physiology of several organs.

Nomenclature	NSAIDs in This Classification
COX-1 selective	Low-dose ASA
COX nonselective	Ibuprofen, naproxen, meclomen, indomethacin
COX-2 selective	Etodolac, diclofenac, nabumetone, meloxicam
COX-2 highly selective	Celecoxib

14. Is acetaminophen an NSAID?

No. Acetaminophen has occasionally been categorized as an NSAID; however, it has long been recognized that beyond analgesia and fever reduction, acetaminophen causes almost none of the other characteristic physiologic effects of NSAIDs. More recent evidence suggests that metabolites of acetaminophen cause analgesia via action on ion channels in the central nervous system.

ADVERSE EFFECTS

15. How do NSAIDs cause gastrointestinal (GI) bleeding?

Chronic NSAID use is a major risk factor for peptic ulcer disease (PUD) and complications such as perforation. PGE_2 produced via COX-1 is important for maintaining GI mucosal integrity via stimulation of mucus and bicarbonate production, epithelial cell proliferation, and increased mucosal blood flow. Blockade of PGE_2 production allows initiation and progression of mucosal ulceration by gastric acid and enzymes, although non-COX-mediated mechanisms of NSAIDs may also contribute. NSAID-related enteropathy can manifest as GI bleeding from the small bowel or colon as well.

16. Describe how to stratify and manage the risk of upper gastrointestinal bleeding from NSAIDs.

The risk of NSAID-related PUD is higher in patients who are over 60, who have a history of PUD, and who are concomitantly using certain medications, including other NSAIDs, steroids, antiplatelet medications, and anticoagulants. SSRIs have also been implicated, although evidence is more mixed. Heavy alcohol use may also be a risk factor. Use of selective COX-2 inhibitors is associated with a lower risk compared to traditional NSAIDs. Addition of gastroprotective agents such as proton pump inhibitors (PPIs) significantly decreases the risk of GI bleeding. H2 blockers have been shown to prevent GI bleeding from aspirin, but there is no strong data for efficacy for non-aspirin NSAIDs. Thus, in patients at high risk for NSAID-related PUD for whom there are no good alternatives to NSAIDs, a selective COX-2 inhibitor combined with a PPI may offer the lowest risk.

17. Describe the effects of NSAIDs on the kidneys.

Several prostaglandins regulate renal blood flow and have effects on the renin-angiotensin-aldosterone system (RAAS). As such, prostaglandin inhibition can have major effects on renal physiology. NSAIDs can lead to AKI via acute tubular necrosis, especially in states such as hypovolemia in which renal blood flow is already compromised. NSAIDs can also cause fluid retention, alterations in blood electrolytes, and decreased efficacy of antihypertensives that act via the kidneys (such as ACE inhibitors and diuretics) via these same mechanisms. These risks are greater in patients with preexisting chronic kidney disease. Short-term use (i.e., <5 days) of NSAIDs in patients with mild to moderate CKD (i.e., stage 2 or 3) is generally thought to be safe in the absence of other predisposing factors (such as dehydration or RAAS inhibitor use). The renal effects of COX-2-selective inhibitors do not differ from those of traditional NSAIDs. Chronic high-dose NSAID use increases the risk of progression of CKD, although in prospective studies the effect size is small (hazard ratio 1.2).

18. What are the cardiovascular risks of NSAIDs?

There is robust evidence that chronic NSAID use increases the risk of atherosclerotic cardiovascular disease, primarily coronary artery thrombosis. In a major 2013 meta-analysis of placebo-controlled NSAID trials, use of ibuprofen, diclofenac, or selective COX-2 inhibitors increased the frequency of major coronary events by 80% (rate ratio 1.8). The number of excess cardiovascular events caused by NSAID use varied with baseline risk: an extra 9–12 cardiac events are anticipated among NSAID users per 1000 person-years assuming a 2% annual risk of a major cardiovascular event, compared to 2 additional events if a baseline annual risk of 0.5% is used.

There remains disagreement about whether this effect is related primarily to COX-2 inhibition or if the cardiovascular risk is similar across NSAIDs. In the metanalysis mentioned above, naproxen (a less COX-2-selective agent) was not associated with a higher risk of cardiovascular disease. However, a safety advantage for naproxen over celecoxib or ibuprofen was not seen in an industry-funded 2016 trial mandated by the US Food and Drug Administration (FDA). Based on this result, the FDA requires a label warning about cardiovascular risk for all NSAIDs. The risk of cardiovascular events may increase even after short-term NSAID use, although this is less well understood. NSAID use also increases risks of hospitalization for heart failure, likely through adverse effects on blood pressure and fluid retention.

19. Which other major adverse effects of NSAIDs are common to the entire class?

- **Bleeding**. NSAIDs reversibly interfere with platelet function, so are typically held prior to elective surgery.
- **Reproductive**. Prostaglandins are involved in maintenance of early pregnancy; some but not all studies show higher risk of miscarriage with first-trimester NSAID use. Use in pregnancy after 20 weeks gestation is contraindicated due to risk of oligohydramnios (via effects on the fetal kidney) and premature closure of the ductus arteriosus.
- **NSAID-exacerbated respiratory disease (N-ERD)**. NSAIDs may trigger flares of sinopulmonary disease in patients with N-ERD, formerly known as aspirin-exacerbated respiratory disease (A-ERD). Patients with N-ERD present with adult-onset chronic rhinosinusitis followed by nasal polyps, and frequently asthma. When exposed to NSAIDs or aspirin, patients experience a flare-up of upper and/or lower respiratory symptoms. The combination of nasal polyposis, asthma, and exacerbation with aspirin is known as **Samter's triad** and historically was used to define A-ERD; it is now known that some patients will not experience asthma, and any COX-1 inhibitor may lead to a flare. Patients with N-ERD will have basal symptoms even without NSAID exposure. Acutely, aspirin and NSAID exposure worsens the disease, but cautious exposure to low doses of aspirin can lead to desensitization, and chronic aspirin use actually improves asthma control in patients with N-ERD. Use of other COX-1-targeting NSAIDs for desensitization is less well studied, and selective COX-2 inhibitors appear not to provoke N-ERD flares. Patients with N-ERD have chronic overproduction of leukotrienes and certain prostaglandins, but the pathophysiology of N-ERD and its interactions with COX-1 inhibitors is incompletely understood.

20. Name some idiopathic adverse effects of NSAIDs.

There are myriad adverse effects of NSAIDs that are idiopathic (not mediated by COX inhibition). Some of these may be specific to individual NSAIDs or chemical classes and might not occur when challenged with an NSAID from a different chemical class. However, cross-reactivity between NSAID classes can occur, and the benefits of NSAID use in patients with a prior serious adverse effect should be weighed against the risk of recurrent toxicity.

- Neurologic: aseptic meningitis
- Allergic/cutaneous: urticaria/angioedema; anaphylaxis; drug reaction with eosinophilia and systemic symptoms (DRESS) syndrome; fixed drug eruption; Stevens-Johnson syndrome/toxic epidermal necrolysis; acute generalized exanthematous pustulosis (AGEP)
- Pulmonary: acute eosinophilic pneumonia
- Hepatic: drug-induced liver injury; Reye's syndrome (hepatic failure and encephalopathy in children after taking aspirin during viral illness); transaminase elevation (up to 15% of regular users)
- Gastrointestinal: GI ulcers and bleeding (as outlined above); dyspepsia, GERD; diarrhea
- Renal: acute interstitial nephritis, renal papillary necrosis
- Hematologic: thrombocytopenia, hemolytic anemia

21. Do NSAIDs interact with methotrexate?

Yes, but not at doses used for rheumatic diseases. Certain NSAIDs increase the total exposure to high-dose methotrexate used for cancer treatment, potentially causing fatal methotrexate toxicity. In contrast, low-dose methotrexate for rheumatologic indications does not have clinically meaningful interactions with NSAIDs, either by pharmacokinetic studies or in clinical trials. The distinction between high- and low-dose methotrexate is frequently not recognized by automated medication interaction checking, so this is a frequent "pain point" for methotrexate prescribers.

22. How do NSAIDs interact with aspirin?

At least some NSAIDs (ibuprofen, naproxen, indomethacin) have been shown to interfere with platelet inactivation by low-dose aspirin; the mechanism is thought to be due to competition with aspirin for binding sites on COX-1. Dosing aspirin at least 2 hours before a *single* dose of ibuprofen preserves the antiplatelet activity of aspirin, but importantly, aspirin has reduced antiplatelet efficacy when ibuprofen is taken chronically, regardless of the timing of the aspirin dose. Diclofenac, sulindac, and celecoxib do not appear to interfere with aspirin's antiplatelet activity.

23. List other drugs with important interactions with NSAIDs.

- Anticoagulants: Increased gastrointestinal bleeding risk
- ACEI/ARBs: Reduced antihypertensive efficacy; increased risk of AKI
- Diuretics: Reduced natriuretic and antihypertensive efficacy; increased risk of AKI
- CCBs, beta-blockers: More modest reduction of antihypertensive efficacy
- Lithium: Increases serum lithium levels by about 20% (via decreased renal clearance of lithium)

BIBLIOGRAPHY

Baker M, Perazella MA. NSAIDs in CKD: are they safe? *Am J Kidney Dis.* 2020;76(4):546–557. doi:10.1053/j.ajkd.2020.03.023.

Bhala N, Emberson J, et al. Coxib and traditional NSAID Trialists' (CNT) Collaboration. Vascular and upper gastrointestinal effects of non-steroidal anti-inflammatory drugs: meta-analyses of individual participant data from randomised trials. *Lancet.* 2013;382(9894):769–779. doi:10.1016/S0140-6736(13)60900-9.

Bonnesen K, Schmidt M. Recategorization of non-aspirin nonsteroidal anti-inflammatory drugs according to clinical relevance: abandoning the traditional NSAID terminology. *Can J Cardiol.* 2021;37(11):1705–1707. doi:10.1016/j.cjca.2021.06.014.

Funk CD. Prostaglandins and leukotrienes: advances in eicosanoid biology. *Science.* 2001;294(5548):1871–1875. doi:10.1126/science.294.5548.1871.

Kowalski ML, Asero R, Bavbek S, et al. Classification and practical approach to the diagnosis and management of hypersensitivity to nonsteroidal anti-inflammatory drugs. *Allergy.* 2013;68(10):1219–1232. doi:10.1111/all.12260.

Mackenzie IS, Coughtrie MW, MacDonald TM, Wei L. Antiplatelet drug interactions. *J Intern Med.* 2010;268(6):516–529. doi:10.1111/j.1365-2796.2010.02299.x.

Masclee GM, Valkhoff VE, Coloma PM, et al. Risk of upper gastrointestinal bleeding from different drug combinations. *Gastroenterology.* 2014;147(4):784. e14. doi:10.1053/j.gastro.2014.06.007.

Nissen SE, Yeomans ND, Solomon DH, et al. Cardiovascular safety of celecoxib, naproxen, or ibuprofen for arthritis. *N Engl J Med.* 2016;375(26):2519–2529. doi:10.1056/NEJMoa1611593.

Vane JR, Botting RM. Anti-inflammatory drugs and their mechanism of action. *Inflamm Res.* 1998;47(Suppl 2):S78–S87. doi:10.1007/s000110050284.

CHAPTER 82

Glucocorticoids—Systemic and Injectable

Sarah L. Dill, MD

1. List some general indications for implementation of GC therapy in rheumatology.

GCs are potent medications discovered in 1949 (Drs. Hench and Kendall won the Nobel Prize in 1950) and have been used since then for various medical indications. In the management of rheumatic disorders, there are two primary indications for their use:
- Suppression of the inflammatory cascade.
- Modification of the immune response.

2. How are the anti-inflammatory effects of GCs mediated?

GCs have anti-inflammatory effects through both genomic and nongenomic mechanisms. GCs influence the expression of 20% of all genes including both immune and nonimmune cells such as chondrocytes and fibroblasts. Their action is variable between different cell types, stage of differentiation, and even disease state resulting in a myriad of changes in cell function, survival, and protein expression.

Genomic effects:

Glucocorticoid receptors (GRs) can either be cytosolic or membrane bound, with two main subtypes of GRs (GRα and GRβ). GRα can actively bind glucocorticoids while GRβ cannot. The unbound cytosolic GR is typically complexed with multiple other proteins. GCs are lipophilic and freely diffuse across cell membranes and interact with cytoplasmic GRα homodimers, activating them and releasing the receptor from some of the proteins in the complex. The ligand-bound receptor then translocates to the nucleus where it may recruit coactivators or tether to other transcription factors. The GR then binds to glucocorticoid response elements (GREs), altering their expression, typically through transactivation of anti-inflammatory GREs and transrepression of proinflammatory GREs.

GRβ antagonizes the action of GRα through both direct binding and blockage of GREs and via formation of GRα-GRβ heterodimers which have reduced ability to bind GCs, GREs, and other transcription factors. The balance of these actions results in both increasing anti-inflammatory proteins (IL-10, annexin A1, IκB) and regulator proteins (tyrosine aminotransferase, serine dehydrogenase, phosophoenolpyruvate) while decreasing transcription of proinflammatory cytokines (IL-1, IL-2, IL-6, IL-8, TNFα, and IFNγ) and signaling pathways.

GCs saturate 90% of the cytosolic GRs at prednisone doses of 30 mg/day. Higher doses have fewer genomic effects. GCs take >30 minutes to exert their genomic effects and hours to days for these effects to cause changes at a cellular or tissue level.

Nongenomic effects

Nongenomic effects occur quickly, particularly when glucocorticoids are given in higher doses.
- GCs (≤ 30 mg/d): when the cytosolic GR binds GCs, the other proteins it is bound to (heat shock proteins, Src, p23 and multiple kinases) are released and have downstream effects on metabolism and inflammation. This occurs within minutes of GC exposure. The GC bound GR may also translocate to the mitochondria, triggering apoptosis in certain cell types.

- GCs (≥ 30 mg/d): moderate dose GCs can bind to membrane bound GR which are present on some cell types (lymphocytes and T cells) and may be upregulated by systemic inflammation. This binding to the membrane GR results in altered cell signaling and cytokine production.
- GCs (≥ 100 mg/d): high doses of GC can intercalate into cell membranes and change calcium and sodium cell cycling across the plasma and mitochondrial membranes, altering immune function, and reducing ATP production.

3. What are the effects of GCs on the innate and adaptive immune systems?

Innate
- Decreased Toll like receptor (TLR) signaling in macrophages, mast cells, eosinophils, and basophils.
- Mast cells decrease degranulation (may affect allergy testing).
- Basophils and eosinophils increase apoptosis and migration to bone marrow and lymphatic tissue (leading to eosinopenia).
- GCs upregulate enzymes that degrade bradykinin. This results in vasoconstriction which leads to less swelling. There is also ↓pain.
- GCs suppress production of prostaglandins by inducing synthesis of lipocortin-1 (annexin-1), which inhibits phospholipase A2-mediated liberation of arachidonic acid from cell membranes.
- GCs inhibit NF-κB which suppresses COX-2 synthesis. Does not affect COX-1 so platelet function preserved.
- GCs interfere with phagocytosis and cytokine production by macrophages and neutrophils.
- Neutrophilia results from a combination of increased neutrophil production and decreased tissue extravasation related to downregulation of adhesion molecules on endothelial cells.
- Inhibition of multiple inflammatory cytokines including multiple interleukins, TNFα, GM-CSF, and interferon-γ.

Adaptive
- Increased rates of apoptosis of dendritic cells. Decreased antigen presentation.
- Decreased differentiation of TH1, TH17 cells and increased differentiation of TH2 cells.
- Decreased cytokine production by TH1, TH17, cytotoxic T cells, dendritic cells. This causes anergy to tuberculosis and other skin testing.
- Decreased rates of TLR and B cell receptor signaling.
- B cells are less affected by GCs than T cells. Immunoglobulin production preserved unless prolonged (>1 yr) use at nonphysiologic doses (prednisone >12.5 mg/d).
- T cells and monocytes redistribute to tissues (leading to lymphopenia and monocytopenia).
- Natural killer cell cytolytic activity decreased.

4. How is prednisone metabolized?

Prednisone is metabolized in the liver to the active form, prednisolone. This conversion is impaired in patients with significant liver disease and impaired synthetic function, which is present if the patient has an elevated international normalized ratio (INR) that cannot be normalized with supplemental vitamin K. In those patients, prednisolone or methylprednisolone should be given rather than prednisone.

The half-life for prednisolone is 2.1 to 3.5 hours, so there is a waning effect after 10–18 hours (five half-lives). This means that splitting the dose of high-dose prednisone to twice a day when treating severe disease manifestations will assure that therapeutic effects last for 24 hours.

Glucocorticoid receptors are fully saturated at prednisone equivalent doses of >30 mg, so a single dose of 30 mg once a day is more immunosuppressive than a split-dose regimen of 10 to 15 mg twice daily. At the tissue level, GCs are inactivated by 11-β hydroxysteroid dehydrogenase type 2 isoenzyme. This isoenzyme has various polymorphisms that determine how sensitive a person is to GCs and may help explain why some patients get more side effects than others.

5. Outline a general clinical baseline that should be established to prevent potential complications before instituting GC therapy.

- **Chronic infection screening** – necessary to exclude quiescent or latent infections which may become reactivated by instituting GC therapy.

- Latent tuberculosis: Interferon gamma release assay or tuberculin skin testing and chest Xray. Interferon gamma release assays may be indeterminate if checked after starting moderate or high dose glucocorticoids.
- Viral hepatitis: hepatitis C antibody, hepatitis B core total antibody, hepatitis B surface antibody and antigen.

- **Glucose intolerance** – Glucocorticoids may cause or exacerbate insulin resistance. Use fasting glucose or hemoglobin A1c to identify patients at risk for glucocorticoid induced diabetes. Use fasting glucose of >126 mg/dL or hemoglobin A1c of >6.5 mg/dL to identify patients who may require treatment. Hemoglobin A1c may be inaccurate in patients with increased erythrocyte turnover/blood loss. Patients receiving high or moderate doses of glucocorticoids should be intermittently monitored either with random glucose or hemoglobin A1c. Random glucose (2 hours postprandial) of ≥200 mg/dL warrants further evaluation.
- **Bone health** – bone mineral densitometry prior to or early in course of therapy, (particularly if prolonged therapy is anticipated), significant bone loss occurs in first 3 months of therapy. Screen for vitamin D deficiency (25-OH vitamin D level) and correct deficiency. Keep 25-OH vitamin D level > 30 ng/mL.
- **Gastrointestinal erosive disease** – screen for history of gastrointestinal bleeding, check complete blood count with MCV prior to therapy and intermittently monitor CBC to identify progressive anemia or microcytosis suggestive of gastrointestinal losses. Additional evaluation should be pursued in patients with concerning history or findings.
- **Cardiovascular disease and hypertension** – may be aggravated by GC use. Baseline blood pressure and exam for peripheral edema with periodic reevaluation. Listen for carotid bruits.
- **Cognitive and psychiatric effects** – consider cognitive evaluation or mini mental status exam, particularly in patients with baseline issues. Screen for mood disorders and psychiatric comorbidity.
- **Ocular effects** – Encourage baseline eye exam, particularly in older patients, to evaluate for pre-existing glaucoma or cataracts which may be exacerbated by GC use.

6. To minimize the risk of hypothalamic–pituitary–adrenal (HPA) axis suppression, when should patients take their daily dose of GC medication?

The body makes 10 to 12 mg/day of cortisol (equivalent to 2.5–3 mg/day prednisone). Because natural cortisol secretion in humans has a circadian rhythm with the peak level in the morning, taking the GC at that time will have less of a suppressive effect on the release of cortisol-releasing factor and consequently less suppression of the HPA axis. Additionally, the effect of GC is greater if taken in the morning because its clearance is 25% less. However, when taking GCs long term, this probably is less important.

7. What is considered low, medium, high, and pulse dosing of steroids, and how does dosing affect GR saturation and physiologic action?

See Table 82.1.

8. Compare the potency, duration of action and mineralocorticoid activity of common glucocorticoids.

GCs may be divided into three main groups according to their duration of biologic activity. These categories and their pharmacologic properties are presented in Table 82.2.

PEARL: Cortisol (Solu-Cortef) 20 mg = prednisone 5 mg = prednisolone 5 mg = methylprednisolone (Solu-Medrol) 4 mg = dexamethasone (Decadron) 0.75 mg.

---

9. What factors may affect GC dose efficacy?

- Age
  Children aged <12 years clear GCs 33% faster.
- Comorbid diseases
  Severe liver disease - may not convert prednisone to prednisolone (active form). Failure to normalize the INR with vitamin K indicates severe liver disease.
  Hyperthyroidism, nephrotic syndrome, and hemodialysis all increase GC clearance.
- Medications
  - Aluminum/magnesium antacids reduce absorption by 40%.

TABLE 82.1 Dosing Classification of Glucocorticoids and General Indications

CLASSIFICATION	PREDNISONE EQUIVALENTS	GR[a] SATURATION	INDICATION
Low dose	≤7.5 mg/day	40–50%	Chronic adjunctive therapy
Medium dose	7.5–30 mg/day	50–90%	Initial therapy or treatment of flares in chronic rheumatic diseases
High dose	30–100 mg/day	Near complete	Serious, organ-threatening disease or exacerbations of disease
Very high dose	>100 mg/day	Complete	Life-threatening disease
Pulse dose	>250 mg/day for 1–5 days	Complete	Induction therapy in organ/life threatening-disease

[a]GR=glucocorticoid receptor.

TABLE 82.2 Physiologic Duration, Potency, and Mineralocorticoid Activity of Common Glucocorticoid Medications*

SHORT ACTING (HALF-LIFE 12 HOURS)	GLUCOCORTICOID POTENCY	EQUIVALENT DOSE	MINERALOCORTICOID POTENCY
Hydrocortisone	1	20 mg	1
Cortisone	0.8	25 mg	0.8
Intermediate acting (half-life 12–36 hours)			
Prednisone	4	5 mg	0.8
Prednisolone	4	5 mg	0.8
Methylprednisolone	5	4 mg	Minimal
Triamcinolone	5	4 mg	0
Long acting (half-life 48 hours)			
Dexamethasone	30–40	0.75 mg	Minimal
Betamethasone	25	0.6 mg	Minimal

*Glucocorticoid and mineralocorticoid potency is determined with cortisol as a reference value of 1.

- Most anticonvulsants and rifampin enhance GC metabolism by upregulating the CYP3A4 hepatic enzyme. On these medications, the GC dose will need to be increased (often doubled) to achieve the same immunosuppressive effects.
- Ritonavir, saquinavir, clarithromycin, erythromycin, and ketoconazole all decrease GC metabolism (increase steroid exposure, need to decrease dose).

10. What are some of the adverse consequences of GC therapy? At what dose (prednisone) does risk increase the most?
- CUSHINGOID Mnemonic summarizes major effects (Table 82.3).
- Weight gain (>5 mg/day). Up to 25% of patients appear Cushingoid on >7.5 mg/day.
- Glucose intolerance and increased triglycerides attributable to insulin resistance (doses >10 mg/day).
- Hypertension (doses >10 mg/day).
- Abnormal menstruation (decreased follicle-stimulating hormone and luteinizing hormone) and depressed hormone levels (thyroid-stimulating hormone, testosterone).
- Growth suppression in children (less if dose kept ≤0.5 mg/kg).
- Osteoporosis (≥5 to 7.5 mg/day for 3 months).
- Osteonecrosis (risk at dose >20 mg/day for 1 month).

TABLE 82.3	CUSHINGOID Mnemonic
C	Cataracts
U	Ulcers
S	Striae & skin thinning
H	Hypertension and hirsutism (female)
I	Immunosuppression and infections
N	Necrosis of femoral heads
G	Glucose elevation
O	Osteoporosis & obesity
I	Impaired wound healing
D	Depression & mood changes

- Ophthalmologic: Posterior subcapsular cataract formation (risk even at 5 mg/day), glaucoma (>10 mg/day), central serous choroidopathy—accumulation of subretinal fluid resulting in central blurry vision, thought to be precipitated or exacerbated by corticosteroid use (any dose).
- Skin disorders (thinning, bruising, striae, delayed wound repair, hirsutism).
- Muscle weakness and wasting (>10–20 mg/day): worse with fluorinated GCs, recovery may take months to a year.
- Peptic ulcer disease (doses >10 mg/day, combination with nonsteroidal anti-inflammatory drugs [NSAIDs] increases risk 3 ×).
- Infection (doses >20–25 mg/day [≥0.3 mg/kg] cause significant risk). Dose-dependent increased risk starts at >6 to 10 mg/day. Staph Aureus most common.
- *Pneumocystis jiroveci* infection increased risk >15 to 20 mg/day for >3 to 4 weeks.
  - Prophylaxis options: trimethoprim/sulfamethoxazole 1 single strength tab daily or double strength thrice a week. If have a sulfa allergy, options include: dapsone (100 mg daily, check G6PD level prior), atovaquone 1500 mg daily, or monthly inhaled pentamidine (300 mg) (less effective, particularly in patients with underlying lung pathology).
  - Prophylaxis should be started sooner and continued longer (even at doses <15 mg daily) if have two or more risk factors: age >60 years, lung involvement from underlying disease (e.g., granulomatosis with polyangiitis, dermato/polymyositis, etc.), additional immunosuppressive use (e.g., cyclophosphamide, rituximab, antitumor necrosis factor), low CD4 count (<200 cells/μL), lymphopenia (<1000 lymphs/μL).
  - Without multiple risk factors, prophylaxis can be stopped at <15 mg/day.
- Mycobacterial (especially *Mycobacterium tuberculosis*) risk increases at >10 to 15 mg/day for a month.
- Anergy can occur within 2 to 4 weeks on prednisone 30 mg/day.
- Fungal infections, particularly Candida.
- Viral infections, especially herpes (cytomegalovirus, herpes zoster) (>5 mg/day).
- Increased risk for perioperative infection if given within 30 days of surgery.
- Vaccinations: if necessary, live-attenuated vaccines can be given if on <20 mg/day for adults or <2 mg/kg per day if child weighs <10 kg. Ideally holding prednisone for 4 weeks before and after a live-attenuated vaccine is recommended if disease activity permits.
- Response to inactivated and other non-live vaccines: decreased response if on ≥20 mg/day of prednisone. Other than influenza vaccine, prednisone dose should be tapered to less than 20 mg a day for at least a month before vaccine given.
- Mental disturbance (≥20–30 mg/day): may include depression, anxiety, psychosis. Mental disturbances rarely occur in children.
- Allergy skin test results can be affected by 15–20 mg/day for 2 to 4 weeks.
- Hypercoagulability with long-term use.

PEARL: Even with short-term use of prednisone (<30 days), up to 20% of patients will experience an adverse event particularly with higher doses or split doses of GCs.

11. Which group of corticosteroid medications results in the least amount of sodium retention?

Sodium retention is dependent upon the mineralocorticoid effect of the preparation. This is an important consideration in patients with comorbid cardiac systolic dysfunction or fluid balance issues to avoid causing or exacerbating volume overload. Mineralocorticoid activity is insignificant with typical doses of methylprednisolone, triamcinolone, betamethasone, and dexamethasone (Table 82.2).

12. How common is adrenal atrophy in patients taking GCs?

Exogenous administration of GCs is the most common cause of adrenal insufficiency, resulting from suppression of adrenocorticotropic hormone (ACTH). Any patient who is Cushingoid in appearance, has received >20 mg of daily prednisone for >3 weeks, has been on ≥5 mg/day for >1 year, or has a fasting morning plasma cortisol <5 to 10 μg/dL should be considered to have a potentially suppressed HPA axis. In some patients, 10 to 15 mg/day of prednisone for as little as 4 to 6 weeks can cause adrenal suppression that cannot respond to physiologic stress. When patients with adrenocortical functional impairment are stressed by infection, trauma, or surgery, they may not be able to respond optimally (the body's normal cortisol output when under stress is up to 200–300 mg/day) resulting in fluid unresponsive hypotension. Proper management during periods of physiologic stress aims to mimic the normal cortisol response. Full recovery of the HPA axis may take 6 to 9 months after stopping GC therapy. The responsiveness of the adrenal gland to stress can be tested with a short ACTH (Cortrosyn) stimulation test (250 μg [40 IU] intramuscularly [IM], measure baseline and 60-minute plasma cortisol levels). A normal response is doubling of baseline cortisol and a 60-minute level >18 μg/dL. In patients at risk for adrenal insufficiency who are undergoing surgery or experiencing a severe infection, "stress dose steroids" may be needed to prevent hemodynamic instability (for a recommended regimen, see Chapter 13: Perioperative Management of Patients with Rheumatic Diseases). Patients who become hypotensive during a period of "stress" and do not respond to intravenous fluids should immediately receive 100 mg of Solu-Cortef intravenously.

13. List eight basic measures that should be performed routinely for patients receiving GCs to reduce the chance of an adverse reaction.

- Document patient education concerning the adverse effects of therapy, particularly risk of osteonecrosis.
- Prescribe corticosteroids at the lowest possible dose and taper the dose as soon as the disease activity permits.
- Encourage physical activities and avoid immobilization (helps prevent myopathy and deconditioning).
- Implement fall prevention program to reduce risk of fractures.
- Prescribe dietary and supplemental calcium to achieve intake of 1000 to 1200 mg/day.
- Prescribe vitamin D at a minimum of 1000 IU/day and correct underlying deficiency.
- Consider bisphosphonate therapy implementation (if >7.5 mg/day for >3 months) particularly if the patient is post-menopausal or has underlying osteopenia (see Chapter 51: Metabolic Bone Disease).
- Vaccination: Patients should receive appropriate inactivated and other non-live vaccines (e.g. influenza, pneumococcal, COVID, zoster, others). Notably, the vaccination response will be decreased if the patient's prednisone dose is ≥20 mg/day. Furthermore, patients on prednisone ≥20 mg/day should **not** receive live-attenuated vaccines. In addition, they should avoid contact with children recently vaccinated with oral polio vaccine, smallpox, or rotavirus because the virus is shed in their stool. They should also avoid contact with patients who received the live influenza virus intranasally and those who develop a rash following the live herpes zoster vaccine. After a patient has tapered to less than 20 mg/day of prednisone for at least a month, they can receive a live-attenuated vaccine.

14. Outline a tapering regimen for glucocorticoids.

Glucocorticoid (GC) dosing and tapering are complex and depend on several factors including the underlying disease process, severity of illness, concurrent DMARD therapy, and patient comorbidities. With life and organ-threatening diseases like systemic lupus with nephritis or vasculitis, patients often require prolonged courses, although recent studies do suggest that GCs can be tapered more quickly than was previously thought, particularly when they are combined with targeted immunosuppressive therapies.

In life- or organ-threatening conditions, an initial pulse of steroids is often administered (methylprednisolone 500–1000 mg daily for 3 days), typically followed prednisone 0.5–1 mg/kg of body weight, with a maximum oral daily dose of 60–80 mg. In cases where patients are receiving concurrent targeted biologic therapy or DMARDs, steroids can often be tapered by 10–20% per week, often with a goal of reducing their dose to ≤5 mg daily by 16 weeks. The patient's symptoms and disease-specific laboratory monitoring may affect tapering speed. An example tapering scheme is listed below:

- Prednisone 60 mg (30 mg twice daily) for 2–4 weeks
- 50 mg (25 mg twice daily) for 1 week
- 40 mg and under—reduce by 5 mg every week
- 20 mg and under—reduce by 2.5–5 mg every 2 weeks
- 10 mg and under—reduce by 1–2.5 mg every 2 weeks
- 5 mg and under—taper by 1 mg every 4 weeks (some patients may need to remain on doses of up to 5 mg chronically)

Some patients may develop steroid withdrawal syndrome (Slocumb's syndrome) with rapid tapering causing arthralgias and myalgias. These symptoms should be controllable with acetaminophen and resolve within 3 to 4 days after the dose has been lowered. If symptoms do not resolve, consider a disease flare may be causing the symptoms.

15. What is Acthar gel? What is it used for?

Acthar gel (repository corticotropin) is a purified preparation of ACTH extracted from slaughtered pigs' pituitary glands. It is in a gel form designed to provide extended release of ACTH following injection. ACTH stimulates the adrenal cortex gland to secrete cortisol, corticosterone, and aldosterone. In addition, it is postulated to have other substances (e.g., melanocortins) from the pig's pituitary that have additional immunomodulatory effects above that of just ACTH alone. However, the substances responsible for these additional effects are unclear. Acthar gel is Food and Drug Administration (FDA)-approved for the treatment of various diseases (19 current indications including dermatomyositis/polymyositis, SLE, nephrotic syndrome, multiple sclerosis, sarcoidosis, inflammatory eye disease, Stevens–Johnson syndrome) as well as for infantile spasms. These FDA indications date back to the 1950s, which is prior to the 1962 Kefauver Harris Amendment, which necessitated rigorous evidence of efficacy from randomized controlled trials for drug approval. The manufacturer of Acthar gel has funded more recent research, and the FDA has upheld the drug's current indications in more recent years. However, the use of Acthar gel remains somewhat controversial with recent reviews calling the drug's efficacy into question, arguing that there is limited evidence for efficacy over much cheaper corticosteroids. Acthar gel is very expensive (current list price is approximately $40,000 per vial), currently costing Medicare hundreds of millions of dollars a year. The high price is related to its orphan drug status for infantile spasms, although the manufacturer has also cited the costs of process improvement, modernization, and research as contributing factors. Acthar gel is supplied in 5 mL multidose vials (80 USP units/mL). The dose varies depending on the disease being treated (80 units IM daily to 80 units IM twice a week).

15. What is Rayos?

Rayos is the brand name of delayed-release prednisone tablets (1, 2, and 5 mg). Compared with immediate-release prednisone, it has a formulation that results in a 4-hour lag time for its release. Otherwise, its mode of action and pharmacokinetics are identical to immediate-release prednisone. Rayos is administered at 10:00 p.m. and prednisone is released during the night when cytokine release is increased. The delayed release is purported to mimic endogenous cortisol effect, decreasing side effects, and allowing for improved symptoms in the morning. It is primarily for use in patients with rheumatoid arthritis, polymyalgia rheumatica, asthma, and chronic obstructive pulmonary disease. The average retail cost for brand name is $3300/month (#30, 5-mg tablets with copay assistance available to commercially insured patients). The recently approved

TABLE 82.4 Glucocorticoid Preparations Suitable for Joint or Other Injection

PREPARATION	STRENGTHS (MG/ML)	PREDNISONE EQUIVALENT (MG)[a]
Short-acting, soluble		
Dexamethasone sodium phosphate (Decadron, Hexadrol)	4	40
Hydrocortisone acetate (Hydrocortone)	25, 50	5, 10
Long-acting, less soluble		
Prednisolone tebutate (Hydeltra-TBA)	20	20
Methylprednisolone acetate (Depo-Medrol)	20, 40, 80	25, 50, 100
Dexamethasone acetate (Decadron-LA)	8	80
Longest-acting, least soluble		
Triamcinolone acetonide (Kenalog, Aristocort, Zilretta)	10, 40	12.5, 50
Triamcinolone hexacetonide (Aristospan)	20	25
Combination		
Betamethasone sodium phosphate/acetate[b] (Celestone Soluspan)	6	50

[a]Of 1 mL of injected steroid preparation.
[b]Has longest-acting and short-acting steroid combined.

generic form costs $10 to $30/month which is comparable to immediate-release prednisone (#30, 5-mg tablets).

16. List some of the general indications for GC injection therapy in rheumatic conditions.

- Monoarthritis or disproportionate joint inflammation (after joint infection is ruled out).
- Recurrent joint effusion.
- Tendon sheath inflammation.
- Bursitis or tendinitis refractory to NSAIDs and/or physical therapy.

Note that the effectiveness of a single GC injection ranges from 50% to 100% and lasts for days to months.

17. Construct a summary table of GC preparations available for injection into a joint, bursa, or tendon sheath.

GC preparations suitable for joint or other injections are presented in Table 82.4.

18. What characteristics of GC preparations are important to consider when determining which to use for injection therapy?

Solubility of the GC preparation is an important factor when considering injection therapy. Reducing the solubility of a compound increases the duration of the local effect because diffusion of the medication will be slower. Thus, less soluble (i.e., fluorinated) preparations have greater potency but are also more likely to result in adverse consequences (soft tissue atrophy, tendon rupture, etc.).

19. How often can a joint or tendon sheath be injected with GC medications?

The main concern with frequent injections is accelerated deterioration of the joint attributable to cartilage breakdown or weakening of the tendon. A single GC injection into a tendon sheath can weaken the tendon up to 40% for 3 to 12 weeks. Thus, the longer the interval between injections, the better it is. A minimum of 4 to 6 weeks between injections is recommended with a risk of tendon rupture between 3% and 8%. Weight-bearing joints should not be injected more frequently than every 6 to 12 weeks. If patients do not experience relief or if relief lasts only a few days, repeat injection may not be worth the potential risks. A good general rule is not to inject the same joint or tendon sheath more than three times yearly. However, cumulative steroid exposure (oral steroids, epidural injections, other injections) should also be considered, with many experts recommending limiting total glucocorticoid exposure (prednisone equivalent) in patients over the age of 50 to 200 mg per year and 400 mg per 3 years.

20. Are there any contraindications to joint injection or areas that should not be injected?

Intraarticular steroids should not be administered if there is concern for active infection.

Achilles tendon sheath and insertion are not typically injected due to risk of tendon rupture. Repeat bursa or tendon sheath insertions should also raise concern for underlying pathology or injury that may be masked or exacerbated by repeat glucocorticoid injection.

Glucocorticoid injections should be avoided if the patient plans to undergo joint replacement surgery in the subsequent 3–6 months, as there are data showing increased risk of prosthetic joint infection in patients who have received intraarticular steroids in the 3–6-month perioperative period.

21. Can GC preparations for injection be combined with an anesthetic to minimize the number of needle sticks to the patient?

Yes, anesthetic preparations can be safely mixed with GC preparations. If the GC preparation contains a paraben compound as a preservative, flocculation of the suspension is likely to occur. Immediately before injecting, shake the syringe vigorously to minimize joint precipitation. There is experimental data that anesthetics like lidocaine and bupivacaine can be toxic to chondrocytes, so limiting the number of injections of GC with these anesthetics is prudent. Ropivacaine at low concentrations (0.5% or less) may be less toxic than other anesthetics.

22. Is there an optimal amount of GC that should be injected into a joint, bursa, or tendon sheath?

It is generally recommended that short-acting (soluble) or long-acting GCs (less soluble) be injected into tendon sheaths because they are more soluble and cause less soft tissue atrophy or chance of tendon rupture (see Table 82.2). The longest-acting, least-soluble GC preparations are typically injected into inflamed joints because they tend to be more effective. There is an extended-release triamcinolone acetonide (Zilretta, 32 mg/5 mL) which is specifically approved for joint injections. It costs $730 compared with $18 to $34 for triamcinolone acetonide (Kenalog, 40 mg/mL).

The dose and volume of GCs that can be safely injected depends on the size of the joint (Table 82.5) and the degree of inflammation present. The provider must be aware of the volume to be injected and attempts should be made to avoid overdistention of the joint capsule, often by using a higher or lower concentration to achieve the desired volume. This is especially important for small joints (e.g., metacarpals) that should receive <0.5 mL with an injection.

23. List some concerning problems and sequelae that may occur from GC injections, including any systemic effects.

- Infection (1 in 50,000 injections).
- Skin hypopigmentation (1–2%).

TABLE 82.5 Dosing Guidelines for Intraarticular Glucocorticoid Injections

SITE	PREDNISONE DOSE EQUIVALENT (MG)	METHYLPREDNISOLONE ACETATE OR TRIAMCINOLONE ACETONIDE DOSE (MG)
Bursa (hip, shoulder, knee)	25–50	20–40
Tendon sheath	12.5–25	10–20
Small joints of hands and feet	6–12.5	5–10
Medium-sized joints (wrist, elbow)	12.5–50	10–40
Large joints (knee, shoulder, ankle)	25–100	20–80

The dose for injection into a child's knee is 1 mg/kg.

- Subcutaneous tissue atrophy (1–2%).
- Steroid crystal-induced synovitis (postinjection flare; 2%, typically lasting 2–3 days).
- Tendon rupture (<1%, never inject Achilles tendon area).
- Osteonecrosis (rare, typically affecting femoral head).
- Erythroderma (particularly in patients with psoriasis).
- Vasovagal response (1–20%).
- Transient hyperglycemia in diabetic patients (monitor glucose for 1 week post injection, particularly in patients with elevated hemoglobin A1c or poor baseline glycemic control).
- Iatrogenic adrenal insufficiency (2 weeks post injection).
- Iatrogenic Cushing's syndrome (particularly with multiple injections).
- Short-term hypogonadism.

24. How might a postinjection flare be distinguished from infection after a GC injection?

Post-injection flares occur in 1% to 2% of patients receiving GC injections and are most likely to occur with use of least soluble (i.e., longest-acting) GC preparations. Injections of the lateral epicondyle of the elbow are particularly prone to this complication. The flare occurs within 6 to 18 hours after an injection. In contrast, an infection usually becomes apparent 2 to 4 days after an injection. If need be, the joint can be aspirated and will show intracellular steroid crystals in a post-injection flare (look like calcium pyrophosphate dihydrate crystals but polarize with first-order red compensation like gout crystals). Treat with ice, NSAIDs, and pain medications. A post-injection flare should resolve within 24 hours, whereas an infection will not.

ACKNOWLEDGMENT

The author would like to thank Dr. Sterling West for his contributions to this chapter in the previous edition.

BIBLIOGRAPHY

Bass AR, Chakravarty E, Akl EA, et al. 2022 American College of Rheumatology guideline for vaccinations in patients with rheumatic and musculoskeletal diseases. *Arthritis Care Res.* 2023;75:449–464.

Cain D, Cidlowski J. Immune regulation by glucocorticoids. *Nat Rev Immunol.* 2017;17:233–247.

Curtis JR, Westfall AO, Allison J, et al. Population-based assessment of adverse events associated with long-term glucocorticoid use. *Arthritis Rheum.* 2006;55:420–426.

Duarte-Monteiro AM, Dourado E, Fonseca JE, Saraiva F. Safety of intra-articular glucocorticoid injections—state of the art. *ARP Rheum.* 2023;2:64–73.

Hardy RS, Raza K, Cooper MS. Therapeutic glucocorticoids: mechanisms of actions in rheumatic diseases. *Nat Rev Rheumatol.* 2020;16:133–144.

Hench PS, Kendall EC, Slocumb CH, et al. The effects of the adrenal cortex (17 hydroxy-11-dehydrocorticosterone: compound E) and of pituitary adrenocorticotropic hormone on rheumatoid arthritis: preliminary report. *Proc Staff Meet Mayo Clin.* 1949;24:181–197.

Jayaram P, Kennedy DJ, Yeh P, Dragoo J. Chondrotoxic effects of local anesthetics on human knee articular cartilage: a systematic review. *PMR.* 2019;11:379–400.

Liu D, Ahmet A, Ward L, et al. A practical guide to the monitoring and management of the complications of systemic corticosteroid therapy. *Allergy Asthma Clin Immun.* 2013;9:30.

Saag KG, Buttgereit F. Systemic glucocorticoid therapy in rheumatology. In: Hochberg MC, Gravallese EM, Smolen JF, et al. (Eds). *Rheumatology.* 8th ed. Philadelphia, PA: Elsevier; 2023:490–500.

Stout A, Friedly J, Standaert CJ. Systemic Absorption and Side Effects of Locally Injected Glucocorticoids. *PMR.* 2019;11:409–419.

Tran KA, Harrod C, Bourdette DN, Cohen DM, Deodhar AA, Hartung DM. Characterization of the clinical evidence supporting repository corticotropin injection for FDA-approved indications: a scoping review. *JAMA Intern Med.* 2022;182:206–217.

Waljee AK, Rogers MA, Lin P, et al. Short-term use of oral corticosteroids and related harms among adults in the United States: population based cohort study. *BMJ.* 2017;357:j1415.

Winthrop KL, Baddley JW. Pneumocystis and glucocorticoid use: to prophylax or not to prophylax (and when?); that is the question. *Ann Rheum Dis.* 2018;77:631–633.

Yang X, Li L, Ren X, Nie L. Do preoperative intra-articular injections of corticosteroids or hyaluronic acid increase the risk of infection after total knee arthroplasty? A meta-analysis. *Bone Joint Res.* 2022;11:171–179.

CHAPTER 83

DMARDs: csDMARDs and tsDMARDs

Marcus H. Snow, MD and Amy C. Cannella, MD

If many drugs are used for disease, all are insufficient.
—Sir William Osler

> ## ⟫ KEY POINTS
>
> 1. Choice of disease-modifying antirheumatic drug (DMARD) therapy is based on disease severity, comorbidities, and fertility plans.
> 2. Hydroxychloroquine (HCQ) or sulfasalazine (SSZ) monotherapy is best used for mild rheumatoid arthritis (RA).
> 3. Methotrexate (MTX) is the most common initial treatment choice for patients with RA and is the anchor drug for most combination therapies for RA.
> 4. Janus tyrosine kinase inhibitors (JAKi) are a newer oral class of medication that has shown significant benefit in treating many types of inflammatory disease.

1. What is meant by a DMARD?

Without a cure for most rheumatic diseases, such as RA or systemic lupus erythematosus (SLE), the goal is to utilize drugs that can modulate the immune system to induce remission, and these are known as DMARDs. To be designated a DMARD, a drug must change the course of the disease for at least 1 year as evidenced by one of the following: sustained improvement in physical function, decreased inflammatory synovitis, slowing or prevention of structural joint damage. There are three general classes of DMARDs used in rheumatology:

- Conventional synthetic DMARDs (csDMARDs): see Chapters 83 and 85.
- Targeted synthetic DMARDs (tsDMARDs): apremilast, JAK inhibitors, avacopan: Chapters 83 and 85.
- Biologic DMARDs (bDMARDs): see Chapter 84.

csDMARDs

2. How quickly can traditional csDMARDs be expected to work?

Most csDMARDs take 3 to 6 months to achieve a full response. It is important to educate patients about this timeline, so they are not discouraged when immediate results are not seen.

3. How are antimalarials used in the treatment of rheumatic diseases such as RA or SLE?

Antimalarials are the **least toxic** of all DMARDs and can be safely combined with other DMARDs. They are particularly effective in early treatment or add-on therapy for mild to moderate RA. They are almost universally employed in SLE. Due to a more favorable toxicity profile, HCQ is most commonly used.

Dosage:

Hydroxychloroquine (HCQ; Plaquenil), 200 to 400 mg/day (<5 mg/kg actual body weight). Maximum daily dose 400 mg/day even if obese. Also available as a functionally scored 300-mg tablet (Sovuna®).

Chloroquine (CQ; Aralen), 250 mg/day (≤3.0 mg/kg ideal body weight or ≤2.3 mg/kg actual body weight).

Quinacrine (Atabrine), 100 to 200 mg/day. Quinacrine is supplied by a compounding pharmacy and can be used in a dose of 50 to 100 mg/day as adjunctive therapy with either HCQ or CQ without increasing retinal toxicity.

Food does not affect absorption of antimalarials. About 50% is excreted in urine. Patients with renal insufficiency (<30–60 mL/min) should receive a reduced dose and a close evaluation for side effects (ocular, myopathy, cardiomyopathy). HCQ whole blood levels can be monitored but are not routinely used in clinical practice. Antimalarials are not effectively dialyzable.

Side effects (HCQ):

- Nausea and vomiting (5%): this is less likely to occur by dose titration (start at ½ dose) over 2 to 4 weeks and split dose (i.e., BID instead of qd). Coating the pill with butter before ingestion to delay pill dissolution can also help. If this fails, prescribe brand name Plaquenil, which is coated and dissolves more slowly.
- Retinal toxicity: The risk is proportional to the dose and length of exposure for HCQ. Enhanced screening can detect early toxicity and this risk is increased with renal insufficiency and concomitant use of tamoxifen.
- Central nervous system effects (2%): these can include headache, dizziness, and tinnitus.
- Myopathy and neuropathy: a neuromyopathy can rarely occur usually after prolonged use or in patients with renal insufficiency. Creatine phosphokinase (CK) can be normal or slightly elevated. Muscle pathology shows a vacuolar myopathy with the classic findings of curvilinear and/or myeloid bodies. A cardiomyopathy with similar histologic features presenting as congestive heart failure can also occur in this setting. Use antimalarials with caution or not at all in patients with a prolonged QT interval or in those taking medications known to prolong the QT interval. A baseline and follow-up ECG may be warranted in those patients.
- Aplastic anemia (quinacrine): this may be heralded by a lichen planus rash.
- Hemolysis: this is rare unless the patient has a glucose-6-phosphate dehydrogenase (G6PD) deficiency.
- Rash: rarely, an acute erythroderma-like reaction can occur, and may be more common in patients with psoriasis or dermatomyositis. Hyperpigmentation of the skin (gray-black with HCQ and CQ; yellow with quinacrine) is common with long-term use. Bleaching of hair has been described.

Monitoring: a baseline retinal examination including automated visual fields plus spectral-domain optical coherence tomography (SDOCT) is recommended. Low-risk patients may have follow-up retinal screening at year 5 and then yearly. However, some experts recommend yearly examinations regardless of risk (see Question 7).

PEARL: HCQ comes in 200-mg tablets. Patients on 300 mg a day do not need to cut pills in half. (The cut pills taste terrible.) Due to HCQ long half-life, a patient can alternate 400 mg with 200 mg daily. HCQ 300-mg tablet is now available.

---

4. What is the mechanism of action (MOA) of antimalarials?

The precise MOA is unknown. Antimalarials are weak bases and accumulate in acidic vesicles such as lysosomes. Alteration of lysosomal pH prevents functional transformation and activation of Toll-like receptors (TLRs) and alters antigen processing and presentation by disrupting the normal assimilation of peptides with the class II major histocompatibility complex. Antimalarials also physically block TLR binding of nucleic acids, especially TLR7 and TLR9. The actions of antimalarials decrease cellular production of interleukin-1 (IL-1), IL-6, interferons, and prostaglandins.

Antimalarials have other beneficial cellular effects, including increased lipoprotein (low-density lipoprotein) receptors, thus helping lower lipid levels. They also decrease insulin degradation, lessening glucose intolerance, and they can inhibit platelet aggregation and adhesion, helping prevent thrombosis.

5. In which rheumatic conditions has treatment with antimalarials been effective?

- RA.
- Juvenile idiopathic arthritis (JIA).
- SLE.
- Discoid lupus, skin rash of dermatomyositis.
- Antiphospholipid antibody syndrome.
- Palindromic rheumatism.
- Psoriatic arthritis (controversial)—use with caution as antimalarials may exacerbate psoriatic skin lesions.
- Sarcoidosis
- Use in Sjögren's syndrome and erosive OA is controversial.

6. Discuss the use of antimalarial therapy in SLE.

Antimalarial therapy is very useful in treating patients with SLE. Skin manifestations, serositis, fatigue, and joint disease are especially responsive to treatment. Additionally, antimalarials are useful in **maintaining remissions** and **preventing flares** of disease. Women with lupus and/or anti-Ro/SSA positivity are less likely to have a child with neonatal lupus and/or congenital heart block if they remain on antimalarials during pregnancy. Due to their effects on platelet inhibition, antimalarials may decrease the risk of thrombosis, especially in patients with antiphospholipid antibodies. Unless contraindicated, patients with SLE and pregnant patients who are anti-Ro/SSA positive should be on HCQ.

Some experts recommend monitoring whole blood (not serum or plasma) HCQ levels after 3–6 months of use. These levels can assure compliance, account for individual variations in absorption and metabolism, and have been correlated with response to therapy and toxicity. The ideal therapeutic HCQ whole blood level is reportedly 1000–1500 ng/mL. Levels <500 ng/mL are subtherapeutic and associated with more SLE flares. Levels ≥750 ng/mL are associated with better control of skin disease, and patients with levels ≥1000 ng/mL have fewer venous and arterial thrombotic events. Mean levels over 1200 ng/mL may have a higher risk of retinal toxicity. SLE patients with renal insufficiency should have HCQ blood levels monitored.

7. How common is antimalarial retinopathy and what steps can be used to decrease this toxicity?

Antimalarial distribution in the body is highest in melanin-containing cells, such as the skin and retina, making retinal toxicity a particular concern. CQ binds more avidly to corneal and retinal pigmented epithelium than HCQ and causes more corneal deposits and retinopathy. Corneal deposits are not an indication to stop antimalarials, but retinopathy is an absolute indication to stop therapy.

The overall risk of HCQ retinopathy has been estimated from 1% to 7.5% of patients and is strongly tied to the overall dose and duration of HCQ. Historically, dosing was 6.5 mg/kg of ideal body weight, but newer guidelines have recommended dosing HCQ at ≤5 mg/kg of actual body weight with a maximum daily dose of 400 mg/day to reduce the risk of retinal toxicity. The dose must be decreased further if there is renal dysfunction (≤60 mL/min), liver dysfunction, or concomitant tamoxifen use. At a daily dose of ≤5 mg/kg/day of actual body weight, the risk of retinal toxicity is less than 1% at 5 years of use and less than 2% in the first 10 years of use. With regular screening, the risk remains low even after 20 years of use with less than 5% developing retinopathy in the year after a normal screening examination.

For chloroquine, patients <1.57 m (62 inches) in height should receive <250 mg of chloroquine a day. Notably, owing to a different chemical composition, quinacrine does not cause retinopathy. Consequently, quinacrine can be combined with chloroquine or HCQ without added retinal toxicity.

A baseline ophthalmologic examination should be done on all patients during the first year of therapy. Revised recommendations state that annual screening using Humphrey automated visual fields 10-2 perimetry as well as newer objective tests (SDOCT, electroretinography, fluorescein angiography) should begin at 5 years of usage. Patients who are at higher risk for toxicity should be examined more frequently (i.e., every year after baseline examination). These high-risk patients include those who are on higher than recommended doses, have a coexistent eye disease, are over age 60 years, are taking tamoxifen (has its own risk of retinal toxicity that is adversely synergistic with HCQ), have renal or liver dysfunction, or on chloroquine instead of HCQ. Some experts advise yearly retinal screening, even in low-risk individuals.

The first evidence of toxicity is loss of red-light perception. If this is detected, the antimalarial can be stopped and there will be no loss of vision. However, if toxicity progresses to a decrease in visual acuity and/or macular retinal pigment epithelium changes ("bulls eye"), the patient may lose further vision despite discontinuation of the antimalarial.

8. What can interfere with antimalarial effectiveness? What drug interactions can occur?

Smoking can induce hepatic cytochrome P450 enzymes resulting in accelerated metabolism of antimalarials, causing them to be less effective. Cimetidine can decrease the clearance of antimalarials. Antimalarials can increase digoxin levels and conversely antagonize the effects of anticonvulsants and amiodarone. Due to the effect on insulin degradation, they may also potentiate the glucose-lowering effects of hypoglycemic agents, and diabetic patients are advised to closely monitor blood sugars with initiation of treatment.

9. **Discuss the use of SSZ in RA.**

   SSZ (Azulfidine, Azulfidine EN-tabs, others) is often used in early and mild RA. Its potential for toxicity is low, and it is often combined with other DMARDs.

   Dosage: 1 to 3 g/day in divided doses. To reduce gastrointestinal (GI) toxicity, start at 500 mg/day and increase by 500 mg each week.

   Side effects:
   - Nausea and vomiting: less likely to occur with slow dose titration, the use of enteric coated tablets, and if taken with meals.
   - Rash: occurs in approximately 1% to 5%, usually within first 3 months.
   - Headache and dizziness.
   - Azoospermia: reversible within 3 months upon cessation of therapy.
   - Agranulocytosis: occurs in <3% of patients and usually within the first 3 months of therapy. Prescribers should be vigilant in monitoring for this potentially fatal toxicity.
   - Hemolysis: can occur if the patient has G6PD deficiency.
   - Pulmonary infiltrates with eosinophilia.
   - Hypersensitivity reactions: can include hepatic enzyme elevation with or without fever, adenopathy, and rash.

   Monitoring: complete blood count (CBC), creatinine, and liver transaminases every 2 to 4 weeks for the first 3 months, then every 8 to 12 weeks for the next 3 to 6 months, then every 12 weeks.

   Precautions: dose should be decreased by 50% if creatinine clearance (CrCl) <50 mL/min with close monitoring.

10. **What are the metabolism and MOA of SSZ?**

    SSZ was designed as a two-component drug including sulfapyridine, which is antimicrobial, and 5-aminosalicylic acid (5-ASA), which is anti-inflammatory. Only 10% to 30% of SSZ is ultimately absorbed in the small intestine. The azo-bond of SSZ is reduced by colonic bacteria, resulting in liberation of the sulfapyridine and 5-ASA components. Sulfapyridine is absorbed (90%) and 5-ASA remains in the bowel. With differential absorption of the components of SSZ, it is difficult to know exactly which component is most responsible for its multiple anti-inflammatory effects, including upregulation of adenosine similar to MTX. SSZ concentrations are highest in the gut's mucosa-associated lymphoid tissue (MALT), and this may be an important site of action for the drug's immunomodulatory properties.

11. **In what rheumatic diseases is SSZ used?**
    - RA.
    - JIA.
    - Reactive arthritis (Reiter's syndrome).
    - Psoriatic arthritis.
    - Ankylosing spondylitis (peripheral arthritis).
    - Enteropathic arthritis.

12. **Discuss the role of MTX in RA.**

    MTX (Rheumatrex, Trexall, Otrexup, Rasuvo) is considered the most effective csDMARD for RA. Approximately 30% of patients will achieve low disease activity on MTX monotherapy. MTX acts relatively quickly after initiation, often within several weeks, but significant clinical improvement may take over 3 months. In addition to its clinical efficacy, MTX decreases new erosions. Using other drugs (HCQ and SSZ) in combination with MTX ("triple therapy") has resulted in improved efficacy over MTX alone without an additive increase in side effects.

13. **What dose of MTX is used to treat RA and what toxicities are associated with its use?**

    The usual dose is 7.5 to 25 mg orally, subcutaneously, or intramuscularly **weekly**. The absorption of oral and parenteral MTX is equivalent at doses <15 mg per week. At doses >15 mg per week, absorption is diminished and parenteral MTX gives serum levels 30% higher. At oral doses above 15 mg week, absorption is improved <u>if the oral dose is split</u> within a 24-hour period.

    Dosage:
    - Generic oral MTX is available in 2.5 mg tablets, *Rheumatrex* comes in dose packs (5 to 20 mg) containing 2.5-mg tablets, and *Trexall* is available in 5-, 7.5-, 10-, and 15-mg tablets. Most rheumatologists only use 2.5-mg tablets to reduce the risk of dose confusion.

- Subcutaneous MTX (generic) is supplied as a solution of 25 mg/mL (supplied in 2-mL and 10-mL vials). The patient must draw up the correct dose (2.5 mg/0.1 mL). MTX solution can be with or without preservatives. At the doses used in rheumatology, patients can take either type. Preservative-free solution can be used if there are injection site reactions.
- Fixed-dose individual syringes *(Otrexup, Rasuvo, RediTrex)* for subcutaneous injection are supplied as single-dose autoinjectors (0.4 mL) with prefilled doses of 10, 15, 20, or 25 mg. Folic acid 1 mg/day reduces some of MTX's toxicity and should be given with MTX. The dose can be increased to 2 to 5 mg per day to mitigate toxicity without reducing efficacy. Folinic acid (leucovorin) 5 mg given as one dose 24 hours after a weekly dose of MTX can sometimes help mouth sores even if folic acid fails.

Side effects:
- Oral ulcers: this may be prevented with the use of folic acid.
- Photosensitivity.
- Hepatic toxicity: folic acid and subcutaneous dosing may reduce this side effect. Concern has lessened with further experience, and routine liver biopsy is not currently recommended. Alcohol use as well as obesity and diabetes mellitus which increases fat in the liver all increase the chance of MTX hepatotoxicity.
- Hematologic toxicity: this includes leukopenia, thrombocytopenia, pancytopenia, and megaloblastic anemia. **This is most likely to occur in patients with renal insufficiency**.
- Pneumonitis: pulmonary toxicity from MTX can be myriad. In true pneumonitis, it is critical to eliminate infectious causes such as *Pneumocystis jiroveci* pneumonia, and if MTX is felt to be the causative agent, it should be discontinued indefinitely. The mortality rate upon rechallenge is up to 50%.
- Flu-like symptoms: these include nausea, fatigue, fever, chills, myalgias, and are called "MTX flu."
- Worsening nodulosis (5%) and leukocytoclastic vasculitis.
- Lymphoma: if a patient on MTX is diagnosed with Epstein–Barr virus–positive lymphoma, discontinuation of MTX may be the only needed treatment for the lymphoma.
- Skin cancer: 2x increased risk. Need sun protection and skin exams.
- Teratogenicity: MTX is an abortifacient and should not be used in pregnancy
- Neurotoxicity: headache, dizziness, cognitive dysfunction, mood alterations

PEARL: Patients who have neurotoxicity may prevent these symptoms if they take two Mucinex-DM (dextromethorphan) tablets or drink 8–10-ounce cup of coffee (90–135 mg caffeine) on days they take MTX. Dextromethorphan or caffeine blocks the NMDA receptor activation by homocysteine.

14. Discuss the precautions and monitoring required for patients taking MTX.

Monitoring: before starting MTX, a CBC with platelets, hepatitis B and C serologies, aspartate aminotransferase (AST), alanine aminotransferase (ALT), albumin, and creatinine (Cr) should be obtained. A chest x-ray may be considered if the patient has not had one in the past year. Monitor CBC, creatinine, and liver transaminases every 2 to 4 weeks for the first 3 months, then every 8 to 12 weeks for the next 3 to 6 months, and then every 12 weeks.

Precautions: MTX should not be used in patients on dialysis or who have a CrCl <30 mL/minute. The dose should be reduced by 25% and 50% for CrCl <80 mL/minute and <50 mL/minute, respectively. Patients should also avoid or limit alcohol (hepatoxicity) and trimethoprim–sulfamethoxazole (decreases excretion).

MTX is contraindicated in pregnancy due to teratogenic and abortive properties, and female patients of child-bearing age should use a reliable form of contraception. MTX should be stopped for 3 months in both males and females before attempting to get pregnant, since the normal life cycle from oocyte to mature egg is 90 days (though this is more based on expert opinion in males). In a patient with a pleural effusion, MTX should be used with caution, since it can accumulate in the pleural effusion and be reabsorbed causing neutropenia. MTX should not be used without consultation with a hepatologist in patients with hepatitis B or C virus infections.

15. When should a liver biopsy be performed on patients receiving MTX?

Routine baseline or periodic liver biopsies in patients receiving MTX are not recommended. Patients with underlying fatty liver disease and/or those that consume alcohol are most at risk for MTX hepatotoxicity. When liver function tests (LFTs) are persistently or significantly elevated in patients on MTX, the dose is reduced, and reevaluation is performed. If the LFTs continue to be significantly elevated, MTX is usually stopped in favor of non-hepatotoxic therapies. In patients who need to remain on MTX, consultation with a hepatologist will guide biopsy decision making.

16. What is the MOA for the immunologic effects of MTX at the doses currently used?

MTX enters the cell via the reduced folate carrier (RFC) and leaves the cell via members of the ATP-binding cassette (ABC) protein family. Intracellular MTX undergoes polyglutamation by the enzyme folylpolyglutamate synthase (FPGS). Polyglutamation of MTX prevents intracellular MTX from being transported out of the cell, resulting in its immune-modulating effects and long duration of action. It takes 4 to 6 weeks after starting MTX for the effect to be seen clinically. Polymorphisms of RFC, ABC proteins, and FPGS account for variations in the efficacy and toxicity of MTX among patients.

MTX has multiple effects on the immune system, including inhibition of 5-aminoimidazole-4-carboxamide ribonucleotide (AICAR) transformylase, thymidylate synthetase, and dihydrofolate reductase, with resultant anti-inflammatory and antiproliferative effects. At the doses used in rheumatology, the effects of MTX are more likely via its anti-inflammatory properties. MTX inhibition of AICAR transformylase leads to increases in the intracellular concentration of its substrate AICAR, which stimulates the release of adenosine. Adenosine is a tissue protective retaliatory metabolite with potent anti-inflammatory properties, including counter-regulation of neutrophils and dendritic cells, downregulation of macrophages, cytokine modulation, and inhibition of collagenase synthesis. In addition, adenosine has multiple effects on the cardiovascular system. It is a potent vasodilator, has negative inotropic and chronotropic effects, and downregulates vascular smooth muscle cell proliferation. It is likely via these cardioprotective mechanisms that MTX has been shown to have a preferential effect on cardiovascular mortality when compared with other DMARDs in RA.

17. In what rheumatologic conditions is MTX used?

- RA.
- JIA.
- Psoriatic arthritis.
- Reactive arthritis (Reiter's syndrome).
- Ankylosing spondylitis (peripheral arthritis).
- Polymyositis/dermatomyositis.
- Antineutrophil cytoplasmic antibody (ANCA) associated vasculitis.
- Adult-onset Still's disease.
- SLE.
- Polymyalgia rheumatica and giant cell arteritis.
- Sarcoidosis.
- Uveitis.

18. Discuss the role of leflunomide in RA.

Leflunomide (Arava) is a csDMARD engineered and approved for the treatment of active RA. Studies support leflunomide's comparable efficacy to low-dose MTX and to SSZ. Additionally, leflunomide has been shown to slow radiographic progression in RA. Leflunomide may be used when MTX is contraindicated or not tolerated. It can also be added at a reduced dose (10 mg per day) to MTX in patients who have received benefit from MTX, but still have active disease, although the potential of liver toxicity is increased.

19. Discuss the dosing and side effects of leflunomide.

Dosage: 10 to 20 mg daily. It is primarily metabolized by the liver. Leflunomide 20 mg every other day may be more cost effective. While approved with a loading dose (100 mg daily × 3 days), it is rarely given due to significant GI toxicity.

Side effects:
- Nausea, vomiting, diarrhea: diarrhea is the most common (17%) and may be abrogated by dose reduction.
- Skin rash (8%): most commonly occurs during the second and fifth months.

- Reversible alopecia
- Cytopenias: neutropenia occurs more commonly than thrombocytopenia and usually in patients who already have a hematologic disorder.
- Hepatotoxicity: usually occurs when used with other hepatotoxic agents, but fatal hepatotoxicity can occur, and prudent monitoring is required.
- Cardiovascular: hypertension and hyperlipidemia can occur.
- Weight loss: can occur in absence of any other factor.
- Teratogenicity: contraindicated in pregnancy based on embryo lethality in mice
- Pneumonitis: seen less commonly than with MTX.
- Neuropathy: peripheral neuropathy can occur.

20. What is the MOA of leflunomide?

Leflunomide is metabolized by the liver to its active metabolite, teriflunomide (A77 1726), which inhibits dihydroorotate dehydrogenase and decreases *de novo* synthesis of uridine and subsequently pyrimidines. Activated but not resting lymphocytes (B cells > T cells) have low pools of pyrimidine nucleotides, making them sensitive to this drug. When uridine is lowered below a critical level, the tumor suppressor p53 is activated, arresting lymphocyte cell division in the G1 stage of the cell cycle.

21. Is leflunomide used in diseases other than RA?

Yes. Although not Food and Drug Administration (FDA) approved, leflunomide has been used in most diseases where MTX is used with similar results.

22. What precautions and monitoring are required in patients taking leflunomide?

Before starting leflunomide, a CBC with platelets, hepatitis B and C serologies, AST, ALT, albumin, and creatinine (Cr) should be obtained. Monitor with a CBC, creatinine, and liver transaminases every 2 to 4 weeks for the first 3 months, then every 8 to 12 weeks for the next 3 to 6 months, and then every 12 weeks.

Leflunomide should not be used in patients with hepatic impairment or positive viral hepatitis serology and is also contraindicated in pregnancy and lactation. Caution should be used in patients with renal impairment because there is currently no clinical data available in this group of patients. However, leflunomide has been used successfully in patients on hemodialysis without need for dose adjustment.

Leflunomide has an extremely long half-life (15.5 days) due to enterohepatic recirculation; in some cases, it may take up to 2 years to reach undetectable plasma concentrations. Because of this, an enhanced drug elimination procedure has been developed in cases of overdose, toxicity, or desire for pregnancy. Cholestyramine 8 g three times daily for 11 days (does not have to be consecutive days) will rapidly reduce plasma concentrations in these situations. In patients desiring to become pregnant, the A77 1726 level must be <0.02 µg/mL on two occasions at least 14 days apart.

Rifampin increases the serum level of leflunomide, which can increase toxicity. Warfarin therapy may be potentiated by leflunomide.

23. Discuss the management of hepatotoxicity attributable to leflunomide

Severe hepatotoxicity, liver failure, and death attributable to leflunomide have been reported. Most occurred within the first several months of therapy. Most patients were taking concomitant hepatotoxic medications (such as MTX) or had coexistent hepatitis B that was reactivated. Appropriate precautions can decrease the chance of this toxicity:

- Limit the use of other drugs with potential for additive liver toxicity.
- Do not use leflunomide in patients with hepatitis B or C.
- Monitor CBC, creatinine, and liver transaminases every 2–4 weeks for the first 3 months, then every 8–12 weeks for the next 3–6 months, and then every 12 weeks.
  The following are recommendations should LFTs become elevated:
- Minor sporadic LFT elevations (1–2 times the upper limit of normal [ULN])—follow with repeat testing.
- LFTs >2× ULN or persistent minor elevations—dose reduction
- LFTs >3× ULN—stop leflunomide and consider abbreviated (cholestyramine 4 g three times daily for 5 days) or full drug elimination protocol.

24. How is minocycline used for RA?

Minocycline (Minocin, others**)** is a tetracycline antibiotic that has been shown to reduce disease activity in seropositive RA. In clinical practice, it is used more commonly in mild disease and in patients who have significant comorbidities and risk with immunosuppression that limit other more toxic DMARD choices. It does not require laboratory monitoring. It is dosed at 100 mg twice daily, and side effects include hyperpigmentation (with long-term use, blue-black in arms and legs), dizziness, and photosensitivity. Doxycycline at 100 mg twice daily can be substituted for minocycline if hyperpigmentation is a concern.

25. Can combinations of two or more DMARDs be used in the treatment of RA?

Yes. The role of combination DMARD therapy in the treatment of RA has been well established, and there are multiple combinations that can be employed. Most clinical trials of combination therapy with DMARDs have included MTX. Several studies have shown that combination therapy with MTX, whether step-up or as initial therapy, is more beneficial than MTX alone. The following are some combinations that have been studied:
- MTX and HCQ
- MTX, HCQ, and SSZ (triple therapy)
- MTX and leflunomide (typically MTX plus 10 mg of leflunomide)
- MTX and azathioprine
- MTX and tsDMARDs
- MTX and bDMARDs

26. How is dapsone used in the treatment of rheumatic diseases?

Dapsone is a sulfone. It is poorly water-soluble, poorly absorbed through the GI tract, and metabolized by the liver. It is used as an antimicrobial agent for leprosy treatment. However, it also has anti-inflammatory effects and is particularly useful in dermatoses involving polymorpho-nuclear leukocytes. It is a free oxygen radical scavenger and impairs the myeloperoxidase system. In rheumatic diseases, it is particularly useful for skin vasculitis (leukocytoclastic, urticarial, cutaneous polyarteritis nodosa), skin lesions of Behçet's disease, SLE rashes (particularly bullous disease and panniculitis), relapsing polychondritis, dermatitis herpetiformis, and pyoderma gangrenosum. Doses range from 50 to 200 mg with an average of 100 mg/day. The major drug interaction is probenecid, which slows its renal excretion. Dapsone is also used as *P. jiroveci* prophylaxis in patients allergic to sulfa antibiotics.

27. What are the major toxicities of dapsone?

All patients treated with dapsone will have some degree of hemolysis and methemoglobinemia and should be thus supplemented with 1 mg of folate daily. Patients with G6PD deficiency will have severe hemolysis, so all patients should be screened. The hemolysis is attributable to a metabolite of dapsone causing oxidation of glutathione, which is essential for erythrocyte membrane integrity. G6PD is necessary to produce nicotinamide adenine dinucleotide phosphate, also called NADPH, which is a cofactor for glutathione reductase, which reduces the oxidized glutathione back to an active form.

Other side effects can include leukopenia, hypersensitivity syndrome, liver toxicity, nausea, and peripheral neuropathy (high doses). Monitoring should include CBC and reticulocyte count every month for 3 months, then every 3 months with renal and liver tests.

tsDMARDs

27. What is apremilast (Otezla), how is it supplied, and how is it used in the treatment of rheumatic diseases?

Apremilast is an immune modulator rather than an immunosuppressant. It is an inhibitor of phosphodiesterase 4 (PDE4) which results in an elevation of intracellular cAMP in multiple cell types (T cells, mononuclear cells, and others). A downstream effect is a decrease in the production of several proinflammatory mediators (TNF-α, IL-12, IL-23, IFNγ), and inducible nitric oxide synthase) and an increase in the production of anti-inflammatory cytokines (IL-10).
FDA-approved indications: psoriasis, psoriatic arthritis, and oral ulcers in Behcet disease.
Available formulation: starter therapy pack (10-, 20-, 30-mg tabs); 30-mg tablets

Dosage: use a starter pack to start with 10 mg qd and escalate up to 30 mg BID over 1–2 weeks. Decrease dose by 50% if severe renal insufficiency (CrCl <30 mL/min).

Monitoring: no specific blood tests required.

Adverse effects: most common side effects are diarrhea (15–20%), weight loss, and headache.

Precautions: monitor for depression. Dexamethasone and rifampin decrease effectiveness of apremilast by increasing its metabolism. Ketoconazole/fluconazole decreases its metabolism.

28. What are the Janus tyrosine kinase (JAK) inhibitors (JAKi)?

The Janus tyrosine kinases (JAKs) are intracellular proteins that associate with and transduce signals from multiple cytokine and growth factor receptors. There are four JAKs (JAK1, JAK2, JAK3, and TYK2) that form various homo- and heterodimers, and different pairings are associated with different cell surface receptors. When a specific cytokine or growth factor binds to its cognate receptor, a conformational change occurs which results in the recruitment of transcription factors. The JAK dimers associated with a specific receptor phosphorylate the recruited transcription factors (e.g. STAT family). These phosphorylated transcription factors dimerize and translocate to the nucleus where they initiate gene transcription resulting in the production of a variety of inflammatory mediators. The following are the JAKs associated with specific cytokine receptors.

JAK1
- IL-2, IL-4, IL-7, IL-9, IL-15
- IL-6, IL-10, IL-21, IL-27, IFNα/β, IFNγ

JAK2
- EPO, TPO, prolactin, growth hormone, GM-CSF
- IFNγ, IL-6, IL-12, IL-27

JAK3 (primarily on hematopoietic cells)
- IL-2, IL-4, IL-7, IL-9, IL-15, IL-21

TYK2
- IL-6, IL-10, IL-12, IL-23, IL-27, IFNα/β

Several small molecules have been developed or are in development that can inhibit one or more of these JAKs. The inhibition of these JAKs will abrogate the effect of specific cytokines/growth factors depending on which JAK is inhibited, and may result in differences in clinical and adverse effects (e.g., inhibition of interferons results in herpes infections). The nomenclature assigned to class of JAKi includes " –itinib" indicating tyrosine inhibition. The following are some of the JAKi that are currently used in rheumatology:

FDA approved

Tofacitinib: JAK3>JAK1>JAK2

Baricitinib: JAK1= JAK2

Upadacitinib: JAK1 highly selective

It is important to note that all the JAKi inhibit all the JAK kinases to some degree even if listed as inhibiting a specific JAK significantly. Although there are differences in immunologic effects in vitro among the various JAKi, none of them inhibit a cytokine for a full 24 hours due to their short half-life (2–6 hours). At therapeutic doses, they all seem to have similar effects and adverse effects.

29. What is tofacitinib (Xeljanz, Xeljanz XR)?

Tofacitinib acts on JAK1/JAK2 (important for IL-6 and IFN signaling), JAK1/JAK3 (important for T- and B-cell signaling), and JAK2/JAK2 (growth factor signaling) dimer pairs. With JAK3 inhibition, there is decreased production of IL-2, IL-4, IL-7, IL-9, IL-15, and IL-21, which are important in T- and B-cell activation and function. Additionally, with JAK1 inhibition, IL-6 and IFN-γ production are attenuated. Finally, IL-2-dependent differentiation of Th2 and Th17 cells is decreased. Tofacitinib is metabolized and eliminated primarily by the liver (70%), with the remainder excreted by the kidneys (30%). The half-life is 3 hours for the 5-mg tablet and 6 hours for the extended-release tablet.

FDA-approved indications: Patients with RA, PsA, ulcerative colitis, axial spondyloarthritis (axSp), and polyarticular juvenile idiopathic arthritis (pcJIA) who have failed tumor necrosis factor inhibition (TNFi.).

Available formulation: 5-mg tablet, 11-mg extended-release (XR) tablet. There is a 10 mg tablet for use in ulcerative colitis.

Dosage (RA,PsA, axSp): 5-mg tablet twice a day or 11-mg XR tablet daily. Dosing for pcJIA ranges from 3.2 mg bid (10–20 kg) to 4 mg bid (20–40 kg) to 5 mg bid (for those over 40 kg). Not affected by food. Dose should be decreased to 5 mg daily if severe liver or renal disease. Can be used alone or in combination with MTX. Avoid use with azathioprine, cyclosporine, or bDMARDs.

Follow-up: CBC (with differential), creatinine, and hepatic enzymes monthly for 3 months, then every 3 months. Maximum effect on lipids (below) occurs by 6 to 8 weeks, thus lipid panel should be done by 12 weeks.

Adverse reactions: common symptoms (4–5%) include nasopharyngitis, diarrhea, and headache.

Serious adverse event risk: In 2021, the FDA placed a Boxed Warning on tofacitinib, baricitinib and upadacitinib due to data demonstrating increased risk of patients on tofacitinib of major adverse cardiovascular event (MACE), malignancy, thrombotic events and mortality when tofacitinib was compared to TNFi in long term surveillance data. With the placement of the Boxed Warning, the FDA amended its approval of these three JAKi after a TNF failure/intolerance.

Infections: any (20%), serious (2.7 events/100 patient years), opportunistic (0.3 events/100 patient years). Herpes zoster may be increased more than with other cs- and bDMARDs.

Hematologic: lymphopenia <500/mm^3 (0.3%), ANC <1000/mm^3 (0.07%), or hemoglobin drop >2 g/dL. Stop tofacitinib until counts recover, then restart at lower dose. Lymphopenia is associated with a higher infection rate.

Hepatic enzyme elevations: >3 × ULN (1.3%), stop tofacitinib until enzymes improve, restart at lower dose.

Lipid abnormalities: LDL increases 15% and HDL increases 10%.

Creatinine: increase >50% of baseline (2% of patients): etiology unknown. Usually reversible if tofacitinib is stopped.

Malignancy: solid tumors (0.6 events/100 patient years) and lymphoma reported in tofacitinib group but not placebo-treated group.

Gastrointestinal perforations: have been reported.

Immunizations: decreases response to inactivated vaccines.

Precautions: do not use in patients with active infection. Patients with hepatitis B and hepatitis C viral infections were excluded from trials. Drug interactions include decreased effectiveness if used with rifampin. The tofacitinib dose needs to be decreased by half if the patient is put on ketoconazole/fluconazole. Do not use during pregnancy or breast feeding.

30. What is baricitinib (Olumiant) and how is it different from tofacitinib?

Baricitinib blocks both JAK1 and JAK2 with expected inhibition of cytokines and growth factors which depend on JAK1 and JAK2. It is eliminated primarily by the kidney (75%) and thus dose adjustments should be made in patients with significant renal insufficiency (2 mg/d max if CrCl <60 mL/min or patient on probenecid). Do not use in patients with CrCl <30 mL/min. Half-life is 12.5 hours.

FDA-approved indication: RA after failure of MTX and TNFi. It also is FDA approved for COVID-19 and for alopecia areata. Outside of the US it is approved for RA without need to fail an anti-TNF.

Available formulations: 2-mg tablet. Ex-US there is also a 4-mg tablet.

Dosage: 2 mg daily. For COVID-19 infection, 4 mg daily. Ex-US can also use 4 mg daily. Not affected by food. Can be used alone or in combination with MTX.

Follow-up: same as tofacitinib

Adverse reactions, laboratory abnormalities, and precautions: similar to tofacitinib. Notable differences were:

- Venous thromboembolism was numerically more common in patients receiving the 4-mg daily dose. For this reason, the FDA approved only the 2-mg daily dose for use in the United States. Baricitinib (and all JAK inhibitors) should be used with caution in patients with a prior history of DVT/PE or multiple risk factors.
- Creatine kinase (CK) elevations: CK elevations >5x upper limit of normal (1.5% of pts on 4 mg/d; 0.8% of pts on 2 mg daily). No evidence of muscle weakness or rhabdomyolysis. Etiology unclear. CK usually improves without interruption of therapy.
- Creatinine elevations have not been observed but need to be monitored due to renal excretion.

31. What is upadacitinib (Rinvoq)?

Upadacitinib is a JAKi that blocks primarily JAK1. It reaches steady state within 4 days and is a strong CYP3A4 inhibitor. There are no dosing changes for renal disease or mild to moderate hepatic impairment. It is not recommended for pregnant women and conception is not recommended for four weeks after cessation of upadacitinib.

FDA-approved indication: RA, PsA, axSpA, nonradiographic axial spondyloarthropathy, atopic dermatitis, Crohn's disease, and ulcerative colitis. In the US, all JAKi approved for rheumatologic use are recommended after TNF failure (black box warning).

Available formulations: 15-mg tablet, 30-mg tablet (Crohn's and ulcerative colitis only), 45-mg tablet (Crohn's and ulcerative colitis induction dosing).

Follow-up: same as tofacitinib

Adverse events: similar to other JAK inhibitors.

32. Should patients on csDMARDs and tsDMARDs be vaccinated?

All patients on csDMARDs, tsDMARDs, glucocorticoids, immunosuppressives, and bDMARDs should receive appropriate vaccinations. However, there are special considerations based on DMARD used and dosing regimen. It is also important to know if the vaccine is live or inactivated/nonlive. Without other contraindications, patients on csDMARDs, JAKi, or apremilast can receive any of the inactivated and other nonlive vaccines. Immunosuppressive medications may blunt the immune response to vaccines, but this effect may be diminished by timing of the vaccination.

Patients on JAKi should **not** receive live-attenuated virus vaccines. Furthermore, they should avoid contact with children recently vaccinated with oral polio vaccine, smallpox, or rotavirus because the virus is shed in their stool. They should avoid contact with patients who received the live influenza virus intranasally and those who develop a rash following the live herpes zoster vaccine.

Inactivated and other nonlive vaccines:
- Studies support that patients on MTX have a better protective response to influenza and pneumococcal vaccination if they skip two weekly doses immediately after they receive the vaccine. Although data is limited, this same protocol is also used for other inactivated and nonlive vaccinations in patients on MTX. Holding MTX for two weeks after vaccination in a patient with active disease is a clinical decision and may not be possible. Other csDMARDs and tsDMARDs detailed in this chapter do not need to be held after vaccination with inactivated and other non-live vaccines.
- Influenza A/B/H1N1 vaccine: give yearly.
- COVID vaccination: follow current CDC guidelines. Recommended to hold all csDMARDs and tsDMARDs for one week after each COVID vaccination.
- Pneumococcal vaccine: PCV 20 is considered a complete vaccination.
- Hepatitis B vaccine: at-risk patients on MTX or leflunomide.
- Age-appropriate vaccinations: tetanus diphtheria/acellular pertussis, meningococcal, *Haemophilus influenzae* B, RSV.
- Other inactivated/non-live vaccines as appropriate: inactivated polio, rabies, hepatitis A, hepatitis B, human papilloma virus, typhoid polysaccharide.
- Zoster Vaccine Recombinant, Adjuvanted (Shingrix): Recommended for those over 50 or those >18 years of age on immunosuppression.

Live-attenuated vaccines.
- Live-attenuated vaccines currently available: mumps/measles/rubella, live attenuated influenza (nasal), varicella zoster (Zostavax), yellow fever, oral typhoid, Bacillus Calmette–Guérin, rotavirus, oral adenovirus, smallpox.
- At the doses used in rheumatology, patients on csDMARDs or apremilast can receive live-attenuated vaccines. It is recommended patients hold MTX and leflunomide for 4 weeks before and 4 weeks after receiving a live-attenuated vaccine.
- Patients on JAKi should be off the agent for at 1 week before receiving a live-attenuated vaccine and not restart the agent until 1 month after administration of the vaccine.

33. What are the monthly costs for csDMARDs and tsDMARDs?

The monthly costs for these medications are outlined in Table 83.1.

TABLE 83.1 Approximate Monthly Costs (Dollars) of csDMARDs and tsDMARDs

GENERIC MEDICATION AND DOSE	COST WITHOUT INSURANCE/MONTH[a]
Methotrexate 2.5-mg tablets 25 mg/week orally, (#40)	$25
Generic Methotrexate solution for injection 25 mg weekly, 25 mg/mL (4 mL)	$10
Brand name autoinjector ("fixed dose") Methotrexate (Otrexup, Rasuvo, RediTrex)	$500
Hydroxychloroquine 200-mg tablet 1 twice daily (#60)	$20
Sulfasalazine 500-mg delayed-release tablet 1000 mg twice daily (#120)	$15
Leflunomide 20-mg tablet 1 daily (#30)	$25
Minocycline 100-mg capsule 1 twice daily (#60)	$30
Dapsone 25-mg tablets 100 mg daily (#120)	$130
Tofacitinib 5-mg tablet 5 mg twice daily (#60)	$2800
Upadacitinib 15-mg tablet 1 daily (#30)	$6200
Barcitinib 4-mg tablet[b]	$5400
Apremilast 30-mg tablet 1 twice a day (#60)	$4500

[a]All cost is from online search through http://goodrx.com in early 2024.
[b]Cost of the 2-mg tablet is unavailable through goodrx.com in early 2024.

BIBLIOGRAPHY

Bass AR, Chakravarty E, Akl EA, et al. 2022 American College of Rheumatology guideline for vaccinations in patients with rheumatic and musculoskeletal diseases. *Arthritis Care Res.* 2023;75:333–338.
Bird P, Griffiths H, Tymms K, et al. The SMILE study—safety of methotrexate in combination with leflunomide in rheumatoid arthritis. *J Rheumatol.* 2013;40:228–235.
Braun J, Kastner P, Flaxenberg P. Comparison of the clinical efficacy and safety of subcutaneous versus oral administration of methotrexate in patients with active rheumatoid arthritis. *Arthritis Rheum.* 2008;58:73–81.
Cannella AC, O'Dell JR. Traditional DMARDs: methotrexate, leflunomide, sulfasalazine, hydroxychloroquine, and combination therapies. In: Firestein GS, Budd RC, Gabriel SE, et al. (Eds.). *Firestein & Kelley's Textbook of Rheumatology.* 11th ed. Philadelphia, PA: Elsevier; 2021:1007–1030.
Fraenkel L, Bathon JM, England BR, et al. 2021 American College of Rheumatology guideline for the treatment of rheumatoid arthritis. *Arthritis Care Res (Hoboken).* 2021;73:924–939.
Hoekstra M, Haagsma C, Neef C, et al. Splitting high-dose oral methotrexate improves the bioavailability: a pharmacokinetic study in patients with rheumatoid arthritis. *J Rheumatol.* 2006;33:481–485.
Izmirly PM, Costedoat-Chalumeau N, Bunyon JP, et al. Maternal use of hydroxychloroquine is associated with a reduced risk of recurrent anti-SSA/Ro-antibody–associated cardiac manifestations of neonatal lupus. *Circulation.* 2012;126:76–82.
Katz SJ, Russell AS. Re-evaluation of antimalarials in treating rheumatic diseases: re-appreciation and insights into new mechanisms of action. *Curr Opin Rheumatol.* 2011;23:278–281.
Kremer J. Toward a better understanding of methotrexate. *Arthritis Rheum.* 2004;50:1370–1382.
Moreland LW, O'Dell JR, Paulus HE, et al. A randomized comparative effectiveness study of oral triple therapy versus etanercept plus methotrexate in early aggressive rheumatoid arthritis: the treatment of early aggressive rheumatoid arthritis trial. *Arthritis Rheum.* 2012;64:2824–2835.
O'Dell JR, Haire C, Erikson N, et al. Treatment of rheumatoid arthritis with methotrexate, sulfasalazine, and hydroxychloroquine, or a combination of these medications. *N Engl J Med.* 1996;334:1287–1291.
O'Dell JR, Haire CE, Moore GF, et al. Treatment of early rheumatoid arthritis with minocycline or placebo. *Arthritis Rheum.* 1997;40:842–848.

Plosker G, Croom K. Sulfasalazine: a review of its use in the management of rheumatoid arthritis. *Drugs.* 2005;65:1825–1849.

Rosenbaum JT, Costenbader KH, Desmarais J, et al. ACR, AAD, RDS and AAO 2020 joint statement on hydroxychloroquine use with respect to retinal toxicity. *Arthritis Rheumatol.* 2021;73:908–911.

Schwartz DM, Kanno Y, Villarino A, et al. JAK inhibition as a strategy for immune and inflammatory diseases. *Nature Rev Drug Discovery.* 2017;16:843–862.

Shawky AM, Almalki FA, Abdalla AN, Abdelazeem AH, Gouda AM. A comprehensive overview of globally approved JAK inhibitors. *Pharmaceutics.* 2022;14:1001.

Smolen JS, Landewé RBM, Bergstra SA, et al. EULAR recommendations for the management of rheumatoid arthritis with synthetic and biological disease-modifying antirheumatic drugs: 2022 update. *Ann Rheum Dis.* 2023;82:3–18.

Ytterberg SR, Bhatt DL, Mikuls TR, et al. Cardiovascular and cancer risk with tofacitinib in rheumatoid arthritis. *N Engl J Med.* 2022;386:316–326.

CHAPTER 84

Disease Modifying Anti-Rheumatic Drugs: Biologic Agents

Sterling G. West, MD

A cynic is someone who knows the cost of everything but the value of nothing.
—Anonymous

> ## KEY POINTS
>
> 1. Biologic agents differ in their effectiveness for controlling specific rheumatic diseases depending on what immunologic process and/or cytokines are driving the patient's inflammation.
> 2. Tumor necrosis factor (TNF) inhibitors are more effective when combined with methotrexate (MTX).
> 3. Interleukin-1 inhibitors are most effective for Still's disease, the cryopyrinopathies, recurrent pericarditis, and treatment-resistant gout.
> 4. Interleukin (IL) 6 receptor inhibitor is effective for rheumatoid arthritis (RA), giant cell arteritis (GCA), polymyalgia rheumatica (PMR), polyarticular JIA, and systemic sclerosis-ILD.
> 5. Risk of hepatitis B reactivation, mycobacterial, and opportunistic infections is increased in patients on biologics.
> 6. Live vaccines when clinically necessary should not be given to patients on biologic agents without appropriate precautions.

1. What biologic agents (biologic disease-modifying antirheumatic drugs [bDMARDs]) are currently available for use in the treatment of inflammatory rheumatic diseases?

With our increased understanding of the pathogenesis of autoimmune rheumatic diseases, several bDMARDs have been developed for treatment, especially for RA, ankylosing spondylitis (AS), psoriatic arthritis (PsA), juvenile idiopathic arthritis (JIA), cryopyrinopathies/cryopyrin-associated autoinflammatory syndromes (CAPS), systemic lupus erythematosus (SLE), and primary vasculitides. The bDMARDs used in the treatment of rheumatic diseases can be classified as follows:

Cytokine-targeted therapies:
- TNF-α inhibitors: etanercept (ETN), infliximab (INF), adalimumab (ADA), golimumab (GOL), certolizumab.
- TNF-α inhibitor biosimilars: ETN-szzs, ETN-ykro; INF-dyyb, INF-abda, INF-axxq, INF-qbtx; ADA-atto, ADA-abdm, ADA-adaz, ADA-aacf, ADA-aaty, ADA-afzb, ADA-aqvh, ADA-bwwd, ADA-fkjp, ADA-ryvk.
- IL-1 inhibitors: anakinra, rilonacept, canakinumab.
- Anti-IL-5: mepolizumab. Anti-IL-5 alpha receptor: benralizumab.
- Anti-IL-6 receptor: tocilizumab (TCZ), sarilumab. Anti-IL-6 receptor biosimilars: TCZ-bavi, TCZ-aazg.
- Anti-IL-12/IL-23: ustekinumab (UST). Anti-IL-12/IL-23 biosimilars: UST-auub, UST-aekn, USK-ttwe, UST-aauz, UST-srlf.
- Anti-IL-17A: secukinumab, ixekizumab. Anti-IL-17A/F: bimekizumab
- Anti-IL-23: guselkumab, risankizumab.
- Anti-interferon alpha receptor: anifrolumab
B-cell-targeted therapies:
- Anti-CD19: inebilizumab
- Anti-CD20: rituximab (RTX)
- Anti-CD20 biosimilars: RTX-abbs, RTX-arrx, RTX-pvvr
- B-cell growth factor inhibitors: belimumab (anti-Blys)
T-cell-targeted therapies:
- Costimulatory molecule inhibitors: abatacept (anti-CD80/86).
Complement-targeted therapies:
- Anti-C1q: sutimlimab
- Anti-C5: eculizumab (ECZ), ravulizumab. Anti-C5 biosimilars: ECZ-aagh, ECZ-aeeb

2. What nomenclature is used in naming the biologic agents?

- **cept:** receptor drug which prevents a ligand from binding to its receptor (e.g., ETN, abatacept, rilonacept).
- **ximab:** chimeric monoclonal antibody (e.g., INF, RTX).
- **zumab:** humanized monoclonal antibody (e.g., certolizumab, tocilizumab, ixekizumab, eculizumab).
- **umab:** fully human monoclonal antibody (e.g., ADA, golimumab, belimumab, ustekinumab).
- **ra:** receptor antagonist (e.g., anakinra).

3. List the precautions that should be taken before starting any biologic agents.

- Establish and record disease activity.
- Screen for comorbidities: skin examination for malignancy, infection risk, human immune deficiency virus (HIV) risk factors, hepatitis B/C risk factors, history of malignancy (lymphoma, melanoma, others), history of demyelinating disease, history of tuberculosis (TB) or other mycobacterial infections, history of fungal exposure, hyperlipidemia, liver disease, congestive heart failure, pregnancy, medications.
- Vaccination status: patients should receive inactivated influenza vaccine (seasonal), SARS-CoV-2 (COVID-19), respiratory syncytial virus (RSV), human papilloma virus (age 11–45), pneumococcal (all ages), and herpes zoster vaccines (age >18). Hepatitis B virus vaccination for at-risk patients.
- Tests before use: complete blood count (CBC), creatinine, hepatic enzymes, lipids, C-reactive protein, hepatitis B and C serologies, purified protein derivative (PPD) (or interferon [IFN]-γ release assay [IGRA]), chest x-ray, HIV (if risk factors). Chest radiograph if not done within last year.

4. What is the rationale behind the use of biologics to inhibit cytokines in various inflammatory diseases?

- **TNF-α** is initially expressed as a transmembrane molecule primarily on the surface of monocytes and macrophages. The extracellular portion is cleaved by TNF-α-converting enzyme to form a soluble molecule that circulates as a homotrimer. TNF-α (and TNF-β from T cells) binds to two receptors, TNF-RI (p55) and TNF-RII (p75), both of which are found on the surface of most cells. Binding of TNF-α to its receptor triggers a variety of intracellular signaling events, inducing production of prostaglandins and proinflammatory cytokines/chemokines, endothelial cell expression of adhesion molecules that help recruit neutrophils and monocytes into the synovium, and synoviocyte/chondrocyte production of matrix metalloproteinases (e.g., collagenase) and upregulation of RANK-L with osteoclast activation which can destroy cartilage and bone.
- **IL-1** is a proinflammatory cytokine that exists in two forms, IL-1α and IL-1β, which are transcribed from closely related but distinct genes. IL-1α is in the cytosol and is membrane-bound. IL-1β is secreted into the extracellular space after cleavage of pro-IL-1β by IL-1β-converting enzyme (caspase 1). Thus, IL-1β is the predominant form that binds to the IL-1 receptor triggering intracellular signaling leading to a proinflammatory response, (which is synergistic to that induced by TNF-α), B-cell activation and rheumatoid factor production, cartilage degradation by induction of synoviocyte/chondrocyte production of enzymes resulting in proteoglycan loss, and stimulation of osteoclasts causing bone resorption. Notably, cells producing IL-1 also produce IL-1Ra. However, in patients with inflammatory synovitis such as RA, the amount of IL-1Ra in the synovium is produced in insufficient amounts to neutralize the amount of locally produced IL-1.
- **IL-5** is produced by Th2 cells and mast cells. It binds to its receptor, IL-5R, and stimulates B-cell growth, immunoglobulin production, and eosinophil activation and survival.
- **IL-6** is critical for inflammatory and immune responses. It binds to its receptor, IL-6R, which is constitutively associated with glycoprotein 130 (gp130) on the cell membranes of hepatocytes and some leukocytes. Notably, binding of IL-6 to this cell membrane-bound IL-6R on hepatocytes and leukocytes has an antiapoptotic/antiinflammatory effect. Additionally, there is a soluble form of IL-6R which can bind IL-6, and this complex can interact with gp130 on a wide variety of cells that are usually not affected by IL-6. This soluble IL-6/IL-6R complex is proinflammatory. IL-6 stimulates the development of T helper 17 (Th17) cells which produce

IL-17, have a role in the activation of B cells and osteoclasts, help recruit neutrophils, and act synergistically with other cytokines to cause pannus formation.

- **IL-17** has six subtypes (A–F) of which IL-17A and IL-17F are most important in inflammation. IL-17 is produced by multiple cells with IL-17A produced mainly by Th17 cells. Th17 cells are derived from CD4+ T cells that have been stimulated with IL-6 or IL-1β and transforming growth factor β. IL-17 dimers bind to the IL-17 receptor on multiple cells resulting in IL-6, IL-8, and granulocyte-macrophage colony-stimulating factor production by epithelial cells, endothelial cells, and fibroblasts, TNF-α production by monocytes, matrix metalloproteinase production, and osteoclastogenesis.
- **IL-23** is produced mainly by macrophages and dendritic cells (DCs). It binds to its receptor on multiple cells resulting in enhanced survival of Th17 cells, induction of memory T cells, and stimulation of antigen presentation by DCs.
- **Interferon-alpha** proteins (13 subtypes) are type 1 interferons. They are produced mainly by plasmacytoid dendritic cells and have a variety of immunoregulatory functions including proliferation of B cells, enhanced expression of MHC molecules, and antiviral activity. All type I interferons (IFNα, IFNβ, IFNε, IFNκ, IFNω) bind to the interferon alpha receptor on cell surfaces.

5. What biologic agents are currently available to inhibit TNF-α?

ETN (Enbrel): a bioengineered molecule derived from Chinese hamster ovary cells, which consists of a fusion protein created by linking the extracellular binding regions from two TNF-RII (p75) receptors to the Fc portion of human immunoglobulin G1 (IgG1). This molecule is a dimeric soluble TNF receptor that binds soluble TNF-α and lymphotoxin (TNF-β). Its half-life is 3 to 5 days.

INF (Remicade): chimeric mouse–human monoclonal antibody composed of the constant regions of human IgG1 heavy and partial kappa light-chain domains coupled to the variable region of a mouse light chain with high affinity for human TNF-α. INF binds both soluble and cell-bound TNF-α and thus can induce apoptosis of cells with TNF-α bound to its surface. It does not bind lymphotoxin (TNF-β). Its half-life is 8 to 9 days. Concomitant use of MTX increases the amount of INF exposure by 30%.

ADA (Humira): fully human IgG1κ monoclonal antibody that binds soluble and transmembrane forms of TNF-α. Its half-life is 10 to 13 days. Simultaneous use of MTX increases a patient's exposure to ADA by 30%.

GOL (Simponi): fully human IgG1κ monoclonal antibody that binds soluble and transmembrane forms of TNF-α. Median half-life is 14 days. Concomitant MTX use increases trough concentrations of golimumab by 30%.

Certolizumab pegol (Cimzia): Fab fragment of a recombinant, humanized anti-TNF monoclonal antibody that has been fused to a polyethylene glycol moiety. Cannot bind to Fc receptors, fix complement, or cross placenta due to not having a functional Fc fragment. Its half-life is 14 days. The PEGylation delays clearance and may help localize the molecule to acidic, inflammatory sites.

6. How are TNF inhibitors supplied and used for their Food and Drug Administration (FDA)-approved indications in rheumatic diseases?

ETN (Enbrel).

- Available formulations: single-use 25-mg and 50-mg prefilled syringes; single-use 50-mg Sure-Click autoinjector; single-use 50-mg prefilled cartridge (Enbrel Mini) for use with reusable AutoTouch autoinjector; single-use vial with 25 mg of lyophilized powder for reconstitution. Should be refrigerated but can be stable for up to 2 weeks at room temperature.
- Adult dosage: RA, PsA, AS: 25 mg subcutaneously (SC) twice a week or 50 mg SC once a week.
- Pediatric dosage: JIA (>138 lbs) 50 mg SC once a week; JIA (<138 lbs, age >2 years) 0.8 mg/kg SC once a week.
- In RA, typically used in conjunction with MTX or another conventional synthetic disease-modifying antirheumatic drug (csDMARD). Not effective for uveitis in spondyloarthropathies. Should not be used if a patient with AS has uveitis or inflammatory bowel disease (IBD).

INF (Remicade).
- Available formulations: single-use vials with 100 mg of lyophilized powder for reconstitution.
- RA dose: loading dose 3 mg/kg intravenous (IV) at weeks 0, 2, and 6, and then every 8 weeks. Dose can be increased as high as 5–10 mg/kg every 4 to 8 weeks.
- PsA, AS dose: loading dose 5 mg/kg IV at weeks 0, 2, and 6; then every 8 weeks for PsA and every 6 weeks for AS. Dose can be increased as high as 5 to 10 mg/kg every 4 weeks.
- Initial infusion takes 2 hours. If tolerated, subsequent infusions can be shortened.
- In RA, typically used in conjunction with MTX or other conventional synthetic DMARD (csDMARD) to decrease development of human anti-chimeric antibodies (HACAs), which can neutralize/increase clearance of INF and/or cause infusion reactions. Concomitant csDMARD (MTX) use is less important for spondyloarthropathies because HACAs are less likely to occur.

PEARL: If a patient is not responding initially, increasing the frequency of infliximab infusions is more efficacious than increasing the dose. Try not to increase dose higher than 5 mg/kg every 4 weeks because of infection and malignancy concerns.

ADA (Humira).
Available formulations: single use 10, 20, 40, and 80-mg prefilled syringe; single use 40 and 80-mg autoinjector pen. There is a citrate-free option for the prefilled syringe and autoinjector pen. Citrate-free formulations sting less when injected.
Adult dosage: RA, PsA, AS: 40 mg SC every other week.
Adult dosage: uveitis: initial dose 80 mg, then 40 mg every other week starting 1 week after initial dose.
Pediatric dosage: JIA and uveitis (≥66 lbs) 40 mg SC every other week; (33 to <66 lbs) 20 mg every other week; (22 to <33 lbs) 10mg every other week.
Although approved for use as monotherapy, ADA works better in association with MTX in RA. Some patients who do not respond to every other week dosing may respond to weekly dosing, although this is unusual and expensive.

GOL (Simponi and Simponi Aria).
Available formulation: 50-mg and 100-mg single-use prefilled syringes or SmartJect autoinjectors; single-use vials (50 mg/4 mL) for IV use.
Dosage: Simponi: RA, PsA, AS: 50 mg SC once a month. Simponi Aria: RA, PsA, AS:2 mg/kg infused IV over 30 minutes at 0, 4, and then every 8 weeks. Simponi Aria for polyarticular JIA: 80 mg/m^2 IV at 0, 4 and then every 8 weeks.
Although SC formulation is prescribed as a once-a-month dose, some patients do not get a full month of benefit.

Certolizumab pegol (Cimzia).
Available formulation: single use 200-mg prefilled syringe with specially designed grip. There is also a 200 mg/vial lyophilized formulation that can be reconstituted and administered in physician's office by a healthcare professional (this makes it eligible for Medicare part B insurance coverage).
Dosage: RA, PsA, AS, nonradiographic axial spondyloarthritis (nr-axSpA): loading dose 400 mg (two syringes) SC at weeks 0, 2, and 4; then 200 mg every 2 weeks (or 400 mg every 4 weeks).
Owing to lack of functional Fc fragment, may be less injection site reactions and safer during pregnancy (does not cross placenta).

Other diseases anti-TNF-α inhibitors used in:
FDA-approved indications: psoriasis (ETN, INF, ADA, certolizumab), Crohn's disease (INF, ADA, certolizumab), ulcerative colitis (INF, ADA, golimumab), hidradenitis suppurativa (ADA).
Off-label use: sarcoidosis, Takayasu's arteritis, Behćet's disease, pyoderma gangrenosum, reactive arthritis, adult-onset Still's disease, Dada2 PAN, others.

7. What are some of the side effects observed with anti-TNF-α biologic agents? How can these toxicities be limited?

1. Injection site and infusion reactions.
   - All injectable TNF inhibitors: injection site reaction (up to 40% of patients) lasting 3 to 5 days. Some cause "bee sting" pain due to the preservative in the liquid. Treat with topical steroid or antihistamine. Rotate the injection sites. Usually, reactions stop after 3 months

of continued use. Citrate-free formulations cause less injection site pain. If problems persist, lyophilized ETN or certolizumab pegol can be used, which seem to have fewer injection site reactions.

- INF: moderate infusion reactions occur in <6% of patients. Common complaints include headache (20%), nausea (15%), flushing, and dyspnea. Treat by stopping the infusion and restarting at a slower rate. If the patient has more than three drug allergies or has an infusion reaction, premedicate with Allegra (180 mg) 45 minutes before infusion; may also premedicate with aspirin (better than acetaminophen) and, if necessary, Solu-Cortef (100–125 mg IV).
- GOL: infusion reactions can occur (1.1%) but are less common than with INF because GOL is fully human and not a chimeric monoclonal antibody.

2. Infections.
   - **Serious bacterial infections:** the overall prevalence of serious infections is 3% to 4% and overall relative risk is 1.5 to 2 times compared with csDMARDs alone. However, when disease severity, comorbidities, and corticosteroid use are controlled for, the risk of serious infections may not be much higher than with other csDMARDs. Infections tend to be pneumonias which occur more commonly within the first 6 months of use. TNF inhibitors should be stopped in all patients who develop a febrile infection, except for the "common cold." Patients with an open skin wound are most prone to develop cellulitis, so stopping the TNF inhibitor until the wound is healed is prudent. TNF inhibitors should be avoided in patients with chronic ongoing infections such as osteomyelitis and bronchiectasis with recurrent pneumonias.
   - **Opportunistic infection (TB):** TNF is important for granuloma formation and integrity. Therefore, all TNF inhibitors can cause reactivation of latent TB (risk increased 2.4 to 8.7 ×). Owing to long half-life and blood levels, INF may cause more of these infections than subcutaneous formulations. Anti-TNF monoclonal antibodies are more likely (3–4 ×) than ETN to reactivate latent TB. Patients who reactivate their TB typically do so within 6 to 9 months of starting a TNF inhibitor. In >50% of cases, the reactivation is at a site other than the lung (lymph nodes commonly). Therefore, all patients should be screened for risk factors for TB exposure and should be screened with an *ex vivo* interferon-gamma release assay (IGRA) or PPD for TB and chest radiograph before starting a TNF inhibitor. IGRA is recommended over PPD. This should be repeated yearly in patients at risk for further TB exposure. Because patients are on immunosuppressants, a PPD ≥5 mm is considered positive even in patients who have received a bacillus Calmette–Guérin (BCG) vaccine previously. The *ex vivo* IGRA (QuantiFERON-TB Gold and T-SPOT.TB) may be a better screening test for TB than PPD, since the skin test is only 70% sensitive. The IGRA test is particularly useful in patients with a history of previous BCG vaccination, which can cause a false-positive PPD, and in patients on immunosuppressive medications, which have a high false-negative rate for PPD skin testing. However, an indeterminant and/or false-negative IGRA can also occur in patients on moderate doses of corticosteroids. Note that the T-SPOT.TB test is more sensitive than the QuantiFERON-TB test in patients on immunosuppressives. If one IGRA test is indeterminate, the other test should be performed. If either test is positive, the patient should be considered to have latent TB. Patients who have a positive TB screening test need treatment with a Centers for Disease Control and Prevention-recommended anti-TB prophylaxis regimen. After 4 weeks of therapy, the TNF inhibitor can be started. In patients with active TB, patients should complete anti-TB therapy before starting a TNF inhibitor; however, in some cases it could be started sooner if necessary.
   - **Opportunistic infections (hepatitis B/C):** all TNF inhibitors increase the risk of hepatitis B reactivation. Patients with resolved hepatitis (HBsAg–, HBcAb⁺, undetectable viral load) have <2% risk of reactivation. As a result of this low rate, these patients can receive TNF inhibitors and have their symptoms, hepatic enzyme tests, and viral DNA loads checked periodically. Alternatively, patients with chronic and inactive hepatitis B (HBsAg⁺) should either not receive TNF inhibitors or must receive concomitant antiviral prophylaxis (lamivudine, other) starting 2 to 4 weeks before and continuing while on TNF inhibitors. Patients with hepatitis C can receive TNF agents without antiviral therapy but need hepatic enzyme and viral RNA load monitoring.

- **Opportunistic infections (other):** TNF inhibitors increase risk of nontuberculous mycobacterial infections, *Pneumocystis jirovecii*, *Listeria monocytogenes*, *Legionella*, herpes zoster, cytomegalovirus, and fungal infections. Patients with previous or current exposure to endemic fungi (*Histoplasmosis*, *Coccidioidomycosis*, others) need to be evaluated for these infections if they develop a febrile illness. INF may be associated with increased risk of fungal infections compared with SC-administered TNF inhibitors.

3. Malignancy.

   TNF is important for inducing apoptosis in tumor cells. However, it is unclear if TNF inhibitors increase the risk of malignancy, particularly lymphoma. Studies vary and state that the relative risk may or may not be increased for lymphoma. However, most large studies report that it is not increased over the increased baseline risk (2–3 ×) of lymphoma associated with the underlying autoimmune disease being treated. Solid tumors are not increased. Melanoma and other skin cancers may be increased (relative risk 1.79 × and 1.45 ×, respectively). Patients who develop cancer (other than melanoma) while receiving a TNF inhibitor do not have worse histology, more widespread disease, or worse prognosis. Whether or not patients with active cancer or recently treated cancer can safely receive a TNF inhibitor is controversial, although it should not be used in patients with melanoma or lymphoma. Some experts recommend not starting these agents until a patient is cancer-free for 5 years, while others will use TNF inhibitors in any patient with a previously treated solid organ malignancy.

4. Demyelinating syndromes.

   Brain demyelination (multiple sclerosis-like), optic neuritis, Guillain–Barré syndrome, myelitis, polyradiculopathy, and peripheral demyelinating neuropathy have been reported rarely. Most are reversible when the TNF inhibitor is stopped. Therefore, TNF inhibitors should not be given to patients with a history of multiple sclerosis, optic neuritis, or other demyelinating disorders. Some experts recommend brain magnetic resonance imaging in patients with a strong family history of demyelinating disease to look for occult lesions. If silent lesions are present, do not give TNF inhibitors to the patient.

5. Autoimmune phenomenon.

   Between 10% and 50% of patients on TNF inhibitors will develop a positive antinuclear antibody, 5% to 10% of patients develop anti-dsDNA antibodies (usually IgM isotype), and a small number (0.2–0.4%) develop drug-induced lupus (DIL; aka TNF-α inhibitor-induced lupus-like syndrome). A few patients have developed antiphospholipid antibodies and antineutrophil cytoplasmic antibodies (ANCAs) that are rarely clinically significant. Patients who develop DIL have mild symptoms of arthritis, cytopenias, and serositis that resolve with TNF inhibitor discontinuation. Small-vessel leukocytoclastic vasculitis has rarely been reported. Concomitant use of MTX does not lessen the frequency of these manifestations. Pretreatment and/or routine monitoring of autoantibody levels is not indicated in the absence of symptoms.

   Antidrug antibodies: over 30% of patients treated with anti-TNF monoclonal antibodies (INF or ADA) but only 5% to 10% treated with TNF receptor fusion antibody (ETN) will develop HACAs. Patients who develop HACAs may lose their response to the TNF inhibitor (i.e., neutralizing antibodies) and/or experience more severe infusion reactions. Concomitant MTX therapy in RA patients (not spondyloarthropathy patients) is recommended to decrease the risk of developing HACAs. Fewer patients receiving SC formulations of TNF inhibitors develop antidrug antibodies. The risk of developing HACAs is decreased with concomitant MTX use. These antibodies can be neutralizing but more often bind to and increase drug clearance, making the TNF inhibitor less effective. Drug levels/activity and antidrug antibodies can be measured in patients on INF or ADA. Note that chimeric (-ximab) and humanized (-zumab) monoclonal antibodies cause more antidrug antibodies than fully human (-umab) monoclonals or receptor fusion (-cept) antibody proteins. This applies to all bDMARDs.

6. Others.

   - **Congestive heart failure (CHF):** avoid TNF inhibitors (especially INF) in patients with class III or IV CHF.
   - **Hematologic:** neutropenia, thrombocytopenia, and pancytopenia have rarely been reported. Monitoring with periodic CBC (every 3–6 months) is recommended.

- **Palmoplantar psoriasis:** less than 5% of patients develop worsening psoriasis on palms and soles. Not prevented by using MTX. Etiology unknown but may be attributable to increased IFN-α production. Patients with SAPHO (acronym for synovitis, acne, pustulosis, hyperostosis, and osteitis) or pustular psoriasis are more likely to get this with INF or ADA.
- **Additional toxicities:** sarcoidosis, subacute cutaneous lupus-like rash, seizures, colonic perforations, increased liver enzymes > three-fold elevation (2–4%), severe hepatotoxicity (rare but most common with INF), and noninfectious pulmonary infiltrates have been reported.
- **Nonresponse:** although technically not a side effect, failure to respond adequately to a bDMARD therapy is costly. The blood test, PrismRA, is approved to predict if a patient with RA will respond to TNF inhibitor therapy. Cost of test: $750.

8. **Can more than one TNF inhibitor be tried in a patient? Any guidelines for switching?**

Most physicians and patients feel that at least a 50% overall clinical response is necessary to justify the cost and risk of using a TNF inhibitor. At least 50% of patients with RA, AS, or PsA may not achieve this response or will develop an intolerance to the first TNF inhibitor they are put on. Although controversial, many physicians will try a second TNF inhibitor. The effectiveness of switching TNF inhibitors and the "rules" for switching can be summarized as follows:

- Patients who fail to respond to the first TNF inhibitor (primary failures) are less likely to get a good response to a second TNF inhibitor compared with patients who initially responded to a TNF inhibitor and then lose that response (secondary failures) or who had to stop the TNF inhibitor because of an adverse event (intolerance). Only 4% to 5% of primary failures will get a good response to a second TNF inhibitor compared with 27% to 30% of patients who had secondary failure/intolerance.
- Patients who had an adverse event to their first TNF inhibitor are more likely (2–3 ×) to develop an adverse event to a second TNF inhibitor.
- To increase the chance of a response in a primary failure patient, choose a second TNF inhibitor which is a different molecule. For example, if the patient fails ADA (monoclonal antibody), put them on ETN (soluble receptor) and *vice versa*. Usually this is not successful and switching from a TNF inhibitor to a bDMARD with a different mechanism of action is usually the best approach in patients who are primary TNF inhibitor failures.
- Patients who are secondary failures or have developed adverse events to a TNF inhibitor (especially INF) may have developed neutralizing antibodies, and switching to a second TNF inhibitor of any type can be beneficial.
- Patients who have failed two TNF inhibitors should probably not be tried on a third.

9. **What biologic agents are currently available to inhibit IL-1?**

Anakinra (Kineret): a recombinant, non-glycosylated form of the human IL-1 receptor antagonist (IL-1Ra). It blocks the biologic activity of IL-1 by competitively inhibiting IL-1 binding to the IL-1 type I receptor. The half-life is 4–6 hours.

Rilonacept (Arcalyst): dimeric fusion protein that incorporates in a single molecule the extracellular domains of both IL-1 receptor (IL-1R) and IL-1 receptor accessory protein (IL-1RAcP) fused to the Fc portion of an IgG1 molecule. Targets both IL-1α and IL-1β. Also known as IL-1 TRAP. The half-life is 128 to 214 hours (average 8.6 days).

Canakinumab (Ilaris): fully human IgG1κ monoclonal antibody that specifically targets IL-1β. The half-life is 624 hours (26 days).

10. **How are IL-1 inhibitors supplied and used? What are their indications and toxicities?**

- **Anakinra (Kineret).**
  Available formulation: single-use vial of 100 mg.
  Dosage: adults 100 mg SC daily; children 1 to 2 mg/kg (up to 8 mg/kg) daily.
  Follow-up: CBC monthly for 3 months, then every 3 months.
  Adverse reactions: serious infections (2%), neutropenia (3%).
  Injection site reactions (70%): less likely if ice is placed on skin before injection. Treat with topical steroids.

Precautions: do not use in patients with active infection. Do not combine with other
biologics.

FDA-approved indication: RA, neonatal-onset multisystem inflammatory disease (NOMID),
deficiency of interleukin-1 receptor antagonist (DIRA).

- **Rilonacept (Arcalyst).**

  Available formulation: single-use, glass vial containing 220 mg of lyophilized powder for
  reconstitution.

  Pediatric dose. Ages 12 to 17 dose: load with one dose 4.4 mg/kg (maximum 320 mg) followed by 2.2 mg/kg (maximum 160 mg) SC weekly.

  Adult dose: load with one dose 320 mg followed by 160 mg SC weekly.

  Follow-up: CBC periodically. Get lipid profile at 3 months.

  Adverse reactions: injection site reaction (48%), infections (25%), serious infections (rare),
  other common symptoms.

  Precautions: do not use in patients with active infection; warfarin interaction.

  FDA-approved indication: CAPS (familial cold autoinflammatory syndrome [FCAS],
  Muckle–Wells syndrome [MWS]), DIRA, recurrent pericarditis.

- **Canakinumab (Ilaris).**

  Available formulation: glass vial containing 150 mg of lyophilized powder for reconstitution;
  150 mg/mL solution in single-dose vials.

  Adult and pediatric dose:

  Patient weight ≥40 kg: 150 mg SC (max 300 mg) every 8 weeks.

  Patient weight 7.5 to 40 kg: 2 mg/kg (max 4 mg/kg) every 8 weeks.

  Can be increased to every 4-week dosing if inadequate response.

  Follow-up: CBC and hepatic enzymes periodically.

  Adverse reactions: nasopharyngitis, diarrhea, vertigo (10%), headache, injection site reactions
  (ISR) (9%), other common symptoms.

  Precautions: do not use in patients with active infection; warfarin interaction.

  FDA-approved indication: CAPS (FCAS, MWS), adult-onset and systemic JIA (Still's disease), HIDS/MKD, FMF, TRAPS, treatment-resistant gout.

  Other diseases IL-1 inhibitors used with success: gout, pseudogout, Behćet's, PAPA
  syndrome, Sweet syndrome, Schnitzler syndrome, pyoderma gangrenosum, hidradenitis
  suppurativa, and others.

11. What biologic agent can inhibit IL-5? What are its uses and toxicities?

Mepolizumab (Nucala) is a humanized IgG1κ monoclonal antibody that binds to IL-5. This
antibody inhibits IL-5 which profoundly affects the activation and survival of eosinophils. Half-
life with subcutaneous administration is 16 to 22 days.

- Available formulations: 100 mg of lyophilized powder in a single-dose vial for reconstitution.
- FDA indications: eosinophilic granulomatosis with polyangiitis (EGPA), eosinophilic asthma.
- Dose (EGPA): 300 mg (3 × 100-mg vials) SC once every 4 weeks.
- Monitoring: no specific tests.
- Adverse reactions: headache, pharyngitis, hypersensitivity reactions, and potentially helmin-
  thic infections. Herpes zoster reported.

  Benralizumab (Fasenra) is a humanized IgG1κ cytolytic monoclonal antibody directed
  against the IL-5 receptor alpha expressed on eosinophils. Half-life with subcutaneous administration is approximately 15 days.

- Available formulations: 30 mg/mL solution in a single-dose prefilled syringe and autoinjector.
- FDA indications: EGPA, eosinophilic asthma.
- Dose (EGPA): 30mg SC once every 4 weeks.
- Monitoring: no specific tests.
- Adverse reactions: similar to mepolizumab.

12. What biologic agent can inhibit IL-6? What are its uses and toxicities?

Tocilizumab (Actemra) is a humanized IgG1κ monoclonal antibody that binds to the soluble
and membrane-bound forms of the IL-6 receptor (IL-6R). This antibody inhibits IL-6 signaling
of cells that constitutively express IL-6R as well as cells that bind the soluble form of IL-6R that
interacts with gp130 on a wide variety of cells. Half-life is 8 to 14 days depending on dose. MTX

does not help increase the exposure to tocilizumab. It is controversial whether or not tocilizumab is more effective when used in combination with MTX.

- Available formulation: 80-mg, 200-mg, 400-mg single-use vials for IV administration; 162-mg prefilled (1 mL) ready-to-use, single-use syringe for SC administration or 162 mg prefilled single-dose autoinjector (ACTpen). FDA-approved for diseases and doses listed below.
- Adult RA IV dose: 4 mg/kg IV once every 4 weeks as a 60-minute infusion. Can increase to 8 mg/kg IV (not to exceed 800 mg) monthly if needed.
- Adult RA SC dose: if ≥100 kg body weight 162 mg SC weekly; if <100 kg body weight, 162 mg SC every other week. If not effective, the dose can be increased to weekly.
- Adult giant cell arteritis (GCA) SC dose: 162 mg SC weekly. IV dose: 6 mg/kg every 4 weeks but not yet FDA-approved for IV dosing.
- Systemic JIA (Still's disease; aged >2 years) and cytokine release syndrome from chimeric antigen receptor T-cell therapy: patient weight <30 kg: use 12 mg/kg IV every 2 weeks; ≥30 kg: use 8 mg/kg IV every 2 weeks.
- Polyarticular JIA (age >2 years) IV dose: patient weight <30 kg: use 10 mg/kg IV every 4 weeks; ≥30 kg: use 8 mg/kg IV every 4 weeks.
- Polyarticular JIA (age >2 years) SC dose: patient weight <30 kg: use 162 mg every 3 weeks; ≥30 kg: use 162 mg every 2 weeks.
- Systemic sclerosis-ILD: 162 mg SC weekly
- Tocilizumab can be used with or without MTX or another csDMARD.
- Monitoring: CBC (with differential) and hepatic enzymes monthly until stable dose, then every 1 to 2 months. Lipid panel every 1 to 2 months until stable dose, then every 3 to 6 months.
- Adverse reactions: all adverse events more common on 8 mg/kg than on 4 mg/kg dose.
- Infusion reactions (8%): headaches, hypertension. Premedication usually not necessary. Serious reactions rare.
- Infections: upper respiratory (8%), serious infections (3–5 events/100 patient years), Herpes zoster, opportunistic (rare).
- Elevated hepatic enzymes: attributable to binding IL-6R on liver cells, which blocks antiapoptotic effects of IL-6 on liver cells.
  Enzymes between 1 and 3 times upper limit of normal (ULN; 35–50% of patients): reduce tocilizumab dose and/or modify DMARD (MTX) dose.
  Enzymes more than three to five times ULN (5%): stop tocilizumab until enzymes less than three times ULN, then restart at lower dose and/or modify DMARD dose.
  Enzymes more than five times ULN (0.5–1.5%): discontinue tocilizumab.
- Neutropenia (29%): as a result of binding IL-6R on neutrophils.
  Absolute neutrophil count (ANC) >1000/mm³: continue tocilizumab.
  ANC 500 to 1000/mm³ (2–4% of patients): stop tocilizumab until ANC >1000/mm³, then restart at lower dose.
  ANC <500/mm³ (0.4%): discontinue tocilizumab.
- Thrombocytopenia (8%): discontinue if <50,000/mm³ (0.8%).
- Lipid elevations: mean increase low-density lipoprotein was 10 to 20 mg/dL and mean high-density lipoprotein increase was 3 to 5 mg/dL.
- Gastrointestinal perforations (0.26 events/100 patient years): IL-6 important for fibrotic healing and repair of gastrointestinal inflammation. More common in patients on nonsteroidal antiinflammatory drugs, corticosteroids, and who have previous history of diverticulitis.
- Macrophage activation syndrome: seen in 3% of systemic JIA patients treated with tocilizumab.
- No increase in malignancy, CHF, or demyelinating disease noted. Patients with hepatitis B were excluded from trials, and thus reactivation risk is unknown.
- HACAs can develop in up to 20% of treated patients.
- Precautions: do not use in patients with active infection, hepatic enzymes >1.5 × upper limit, platelet count <100,000/mm³, history of diverticulitis or other IBD. Drug interactions include affecting blood levels of warfarin, cyclosporine, and theophylline. Lowers blood levels of omeprazole, atorvastatin, simvastatin, and birth control pills. Advise patients about birth control.

- Other diseases that it has been used with success: Castleman disease, Takayasu's arteritis, Behćet's disease, relapsing polychondritis, adult-onset Still's disease, polymyalgia rheumatica (PMR) and SLE. Does not work for spondyloarthropathies.
  Sarilumab (Kevzara) is a fully human anti-IL-6Rα monoclonal antibody that binds the soluble and membrane-bound human IL-6Rα.
- Available formulation: 150-mg and 200-mg solution in a single-dose prefilled syringe and pen. FDA-approved for RA and PMR.
- Adult RA dose: 200 mg SC every 2 weeks. If toxicity develops, can decrease to 150-mg dose. Can be combined with other csDMARDs (e.g., MTX).
- PMR dose: 200 mg SC every 2 weeks.
- Toxicity profile and monitoring schedule similar to tocilizumab.

13. What is ustekinumab and why is it effective in PsA?

Ustekinumab (Stelara) is a human IgG1κmonoclonal antibody that binds to the p40 subunit of both IL-12 and IL-23 preventing their binding to their shared cell surface receptor chain, IL-12β. The inhibition of IL-12 signaling abrogates Th1 response with reduction in TNF-α, IFN-γ, and IL-2 production. The inhibition of IL-23 signaling abrogates Th17 response with reduction in IL-6, IL-17, IL-21, IL-22, and TNF-α production. Th17 cells and IL-23 production by DCs and keratinocytes are important in the pathogenesis of psoriasis. Half-life is 15 to 45 days.

- Available formulation: single-use 45-mg and 90-mg prefilled syringes. A 45-mg single-dose vial for SC administration and a 130-mg single-dose vial for IV administration (Crohn's disease) are also available.
- FDA-approved indications: psoriasis (age >12 years), PsA (> age 12 yrs), Crohn's disease (adults), ulcerative colitis (adults). Although not FDA-approved, it has been used with some success in patients with AS.
- Adult psoriasis and PsA dosage: patient ≤100 kg: 45 mg SC initially, followed by 45 mg in 4 weeks, then 45 mg every 12 weeks. Dosage for >100 kg: 90 mg SC initially, followed by 90 mg in 4 weeks, then 90 mg every 12 weeks. Can be combined with a csDMARD (e.g., MTX).
- Pediatric (age >12 years) psoriasis and PsA dosage: weight < 60 kg: 0.75 mg/kg SC initially and 4 weeks later, then every 12 weeks. Weight >60 kg use adult dosing.
- Monitoring: routine monitoring for other csDMARDs (MTX).
- Adverse reactions: nasopharyngitis (10%), nonmelanoma skin cancers.
- Serious infections (2%–3%): IL-12/IL-23 are important for resistance against mycobacterial and salmonella infections. IL-17 is important for resistance against fungal infections.
- Precautions: do not use in patients with active infection.

14. What bDMARDs are available to inhibit IL-17 in rheumatic diseases?

Secukinumab (Cosentyx) is a human IgG1κmonoclonal antibody which blocks IL-17A. It is FDA-approved to treat psoriasis (age >6 yrs), PsA (age >2 yrs), adult AS, nr-axSpA, enthesitis-related JIA (age >4 yrs), hidradenitis suppurativa. Not effective for RA.

- Available formulations: 300 mg/2 mL solution in a single-use UnoReady pen or prefilled syringe, 150 mg/mL solution in a single-use Sensoready pen or prefilled syringe, and 75 mg/0.5 mLsingle dose prefilled syringe. All pens and syringes are self-administered. IV formulation comes as 125 mg/5 mL solution in a single-dose vial.
- Adult PsA, AS, and nr-axSpA dosage: 150 mg SC weekly × 4 (loading dose), then 150 mg SC every 4 weeks. IV dosing is 6 mg/kg x 1 (loading dose), then 1.75 mg/kg (max 300 mg) every 4 weeks. Can be combined with a csDMARD (e.g., MTX).
- Pediatric PsA and enthesitis-related JIA dosage: weight 15–50 kg the dose is 75mg SC weekly × 4, then 75 mg SC every 4 wks. Weight >50 kg, dosing is same as adults.
- Monitoring: routine monitoring for other csDMARDs (e.g., MTX).
- Adverse reactions: ISR, nasopharyngitis, and acne are most common. IL-17 is important for resistance to fungal infections. Opportunistic infections, especially *Candida,* have been reported. Development and/or exacerbation of Crohn's disease have been reported.
- Precautions: do not use in patients with active infection. Use with caution or not at all in patients with inflammatory bowel disease. Do not combine with other bDMARDs.
  Ixekizumab (Taltz) is a humanized IgG4 monoclonal antibody to IL-17A, which is FDA-approved to treat psoriasis, PsA, AS, and nr-axSpA.

- Available formulations: 80-mg/mL solution in a single-dose prefilled autoinjector or syringe.
- Adult dosage for all indications: 160-mg SC loading dose, then 80-mg SC every 4 weeks. Can be combined with a csDMARD (e.g., MTX).
- Adverse reactions, monitoring, and precautions similar to secukinumab.

Bimekizumab (Bimzelx) is a humanized IgG1 monoclonal antibody that selectively inhibits both Il-17A and IL-17F. It is FDA-approved to treat psoriasis, PsA, AS, and nr-axSpA.

- Available formulations:160 mg/mL solution in single-dose prefilled autoinjector or syringe.
- Dosage: 160 mg SC q 4 wk. Patients with severe skin psoriasis may use higher doses.
- Adverse reactions, monitoring, and precautions similar to secukinumab

15. What bDMARDs are available to inhibit IL-23 in the rheumatic diseases?

Guselkumab (Tremfya) is a human IgG1 λ monoclonal antibody that selectively blocks IL-23 by targeting the p19 subunit. It is FDA-approved to treat skin psoriasis and PsA. Effective but not yet approved for inflammatory bowel disease. The IL-23 inhibitors are less effective for treating the axial manifestations of PsA.

- Available formulations: 100 mg/mL solution in single-dose prefilled autoinjector (One-Press) or syringe.
- Dosage: 100 mg SC at weeks 0 and 4 then every 8 weeks thereafter. Can be combined with other csDMARDs (e.g. MTX)
- Monitoring: Routine monitoring if combined with csDMARDs (e.g. MTX).
- Adverse reactions: URTI/bronchitis, ISR, headaches, tinea.
- Precautions: do not use in patients with active infection. Do not combine with other bDMARDs, however, IL-23 inhibitors are probably the safest to combine if absolutely necessary.

Risankizumab (Skyrizi) is a humanized IgG1 monoclonal antibody that selectively blocks IL-23A by targeting the p19 subunit. It is FDA-approved to treat psoriasis, PsA, ulcerative colitis, and Crohn's disease.

- Available formulations: 75 mg, 90 mg, and 150 mg prefilled syringes. 150 mg/mL in prefilled pen. Other doses and IV formulation are available to treat Crohn's disease and ulcerative colitis.
- Dosage: 150 mg SC at weeks 0 and 4 then every 12 weeks thereafter. Can be combined with csDMARDs (e.g., MTX).
- Monitoring, adverse reactions, and precautions similar to guselkumab.

16. What bDMARD can inhibit interferon alpha?

Anifrolumab (Saphnelo) is a human IgG1 κ monoclonal antibody that blocks type I interferon (IFN) signalling by binding to the type I IFN receptor subunit 1. It is FDA-approved to treat SLE. It is most effective in patients with a high interferon α gene signature.

- Available formulation: 300 mg/2 mL solution in single dose vial.
- Dosage: 300 mg IV over 30 minutes every 4 weeks. Can be combined with csDMARDs.
- Monitoring: routine monitoring if combined with other immunosuppressive meds.
- Adverse effects: URTI, headache, and herpes zoster (6%) were most common. Serious infections and hypersensitivity reactions are possible.
- Precautions: do not use in patients with active infection. Do not combine with other bDMARDs. All patients should get shingles vaccine prior to starting.

17. What are B-cell-targeted therapies?

RTX (Rituxan): chimeric mouse–human IgG1κ type I monoclonal antibody directed against extracellular domain of CD20 antigen on B cells. B cells are eliminated by complement-mediated lysis, antibody-dependent cell-mediated cytotoxicity, or apoptosis. All peripheral B cells are eliminated within days. Patients who fail to deplete their B cells respond less well. Notably, Ig levels are preserved due to preservation of plasma cells which lack the CD20 antigen on their cell membranes. However, repeated infusions can cause decreased Ig levels (IgM > IgG > IgA). Half-life is 18 to 21 days.

Belimumab (Benlysta): fully human IgG1λ monoclonal antibody directed against B lymphocyte stimulator protein (BLyS)/B-cell activating factor (BAFF). BLyS is the same as BAFF and promotes B-cell survival, growth, and maturation by binding to three different B-cell receptors.

Inhibition of BLyS causes peripheral B-cell counts to decrease by 40% to 50%. Ig levels are usually not affected. Half-life is 11 to 14 days.

Other B cell-targeted therapies: several other therapies have been tested in autoimmune rheumatic diseases but are not yet FDA-approved. These include anti-CD20 monoclonal antibodies (obinutuzumab, ocrelizumab, ofatumumab), recombinant TACI-Fc fusion protein inhibitor of BlyS/APRIL signaling molecules (telitacicept), and CAR T cells targeting CD19.

18. What are the indications and toxicities of RTX (Rituxan)?

- FDA-approved rheumatologic indications: RA after MTX and anti-TNF failure; ANCA-associated vasculitis (granulomatosis with polyangiitis [GPA], microscopic polyangiitis [MPA]), pemphigus.
- Available formulation: single-use vial of 100 mg and 500 mg.
- Dosage. RA: 1000-mg IV infusion repeated once 2 weeks later. Some physicians feel 500-mg dose is as effective as 1000 mg particularly on subsequent infusions. Can be used with concomitant csDMARDs (e.g., MTX).
- ANCA-associated vasculitis: 375 mg/m^2 IV infusion once weekly for 4 weeks. Can also use RA dosage (1 g on days 1 and 15). Maintenance dose: 500 mg IV every 6 months.
- First infusion lasts 3 to 5 hours, subsequent infusions 1.5 to 3 hours. Patients are typically premedicated 30 to 60 minutes before each infusion with acetaminophen 1000 mg and an antihistamine to decrease the chance of infusion reaction. Some physicians also premedicate with an IV glucocorticoid particularly with the first infusion or in patients with three or more drug allergies.
- Follow-up: CBC every 2 to 4 months to monitor for late-onset neutropenia. Get IgG level prior to RTX infusions to make sure patient is not hypogammaglobulinemic.
- Adverse reactions:
  - Infusion reaction (10–35%): usually not severe if use premedication. Respond to stopping infusion until symptoms gone, then restart at slower rate. Stop infusion if patients start clearing their throat due to a scratchy feeling. Serious reactions (1%). Risk does not increase with subsequent infusions. May not need premedication with subsequent infusion if tolerated well. If an anaphylactic reaction develops, stop drug, treat with epinephrine, H1/H2 blockers, fluids, oxygen, and observe for 24 hours for late-onset reactions. Do not use RTX again.
  - Infection: any (35% or 78 events/100 patient years); serious (2% or 3 events/100 patient years); opportunistic (0.05/100 patient years, very low rate).
  - Viral infections: reactivation of resolved hepatitis B (HBsAg–, HBcAb$^+$) occurs in 5% to 10%. Patients with chronic and inactive hepatitis B (HBsAg$^+$) should either not receive RTX or must receive concomitant antiviral prophylaxis (lamivudine, other) starting 2 to 4 weeks before and continuing while on RTX and for 1 month after stopping. Patients with hepatitis C can receive RTX without antiviral therapy but need hepatic enzymes and viral RNA load monitoring. The risk of JC virus infection resulting in progressive multifocal leukoencephalopathy (PML) may vary by disease being treated and previous immunosuppressive medications (1:25,000 RA patients, 1:4000 SLE patients compared with 1:200,000 in the general population). Owing to frequency of JC virus exposure (60–70%) and low rate of PML in RA patients treated with RTX, it is not recommended to screen patients with antibody testing for previous JC virus exposure. Herpes zoster appears increased.
  - Hypogammaglobulinemia: only occurs in patients after multiple courses of RTX therapy. IgG becomes low in 3.5% to 12% of patients, IgM low in 22% to 26%. Patients who develop low IgG (<600 mg/dL) are more likely (2–4 ×) to get a serious infection. Treating hypogammaglobulinemia with IVIG can prevent infection.
  - Late-onset neutropenia: occurs in 3% of patients with RA and up to 20% of SLE or ANCA-associated vasculitis patients treated. Occurs an average of 3 to 4 months post-therapy and is associated with increased infection risk (16%). Neutropenia can last several weeks. Etiology is unclear. Tends to recur with subsequent doses.
  - HACAs can develop in up to 50% of patients.
  - Immunizations: response to T-cell-independent antigen vaccines (influenza, pneumococcal) is severely decreased if given after RTX. Give vaccines 2 (nonlive) to 4 (live vaccines) weeks before or 6 months post-RTX infusion. Tetanus vaccination is not impaired.

- Other: severe mucocutaneous reactions, hypertension/arrhythmias/myocardial infarction during infusions. Note that CHF, demyelinating disease, malignancy (except skin cancer), and mycobacterial infections were not increased over placebo. RTX may be used ahead of TNF inhibitors in patients with one of these conditions that make TNF inhibitors contraindicated.
- Precautions: do not use in patients with active infection. However, many physicians regard RTX as the safest therapy in RA patients with ongoing chronic infections (e.g., osteomyelitis), recently treated cancer, or history of lymphoma. Use *P. jirovecii* prophylaxis for patients with ANCA-associated vasculitis and lung disease. Consider prophylaxis in any patient with an autoimmune rheumatic disease treated with RTX who are > age 60, on prednisone (≥20 mg/d for over 4 wks) or other immunosuppressive medication, or has underlying lung disease.
- Other diseases that RTX has been used for: SLE, antiphospholipid antibody syndrome, extraglandular Sjögren's syndrome, IgG4 disease, neuromyelitis optica spectrum disorder (NMOSD), idiopathic thrombocytopenic purpura, autoimmune hemolytic anemia, Castleman's disease, cryoglobulinemia, inflammatory myopathies, others. Does not work in spondyloarthropathies.

19. When can/should RTX be repeated? Can other immunosuppressive medications be used with it?

Among RA patients, the response is variable. Patients who are seropositive (rheumatoid factor and/or anticyclic citrullinated peptide) and have hypergammaglobulinemia are more likely to respond. Most RA patients deplete their B cells after RTX. Those who deplete their plasmablasts (CD27$^+$CD38$^+$) get the best response. B-cell repopulation occurs at a mean of 8 months post-therapy. Patients who respond tend to by 4 to 6 months. The duration of response varies (median 30 weeks) and patients tend to relapse with reappearance of memory B cells (CD19$^+$CD27$^+$CD38$^-$) and not naïve B cells (CD19$^+$CD27$^-$CD38$^-$). Retreatment is done when clinical symptoms recur and are not based on B-cell counts; however, retreatment is usually not done sooner than 4 months after previous therapy unless patients fail to deplete their B cells. Recently, some physicians are giving one infusion of 500 to 1000 mg of RTX every 6 months to maintain remission in responders to prevent relapse. Primary nonresponders usually do not respond to additional RTX courses. RA patients who fail to respond to RTX can be started on another biologic agent at 6 months after the initial course of two RTX infusions even if B cells are still depleted without a significant increase in infection risk.

Among ANCA-associated vasculitis patients, RTX is noninferior to cyclophosphamide. Patients can be treated with an RA dose schedule or lymphoma (4 weekly doses) schedule. All patients deplete their B cells. Patients relapse with recurrence of B cells at an average of 12 months. Patients can relapse before the reappearance of ANCA. Many physicians advocate giving 500 mg every 6 months to maintain remission and avoid relapse. In patients that relapse, a second course of RTX is as effective as the first course. RTX is reportedly effective in GPA and MPA patients who are ANCA negative.

20. What are the indications, efficacy, and toxicities of belimumab (Benlysta)?

- FDA-approved indication: adult and pediatric SLE. Does not work in RA.
- Available formulation: single-use vial containing 120 mg or 400 mg of lyophilized powder for reconstitution. A 200-mg/mL single-dose prefilled autoinjector or syringe is also available.
- IV dosage (adult and pediatric) for SLE and lupus nephritis: loading dose of 10 mg/kg IV at 0, 2, and 4 weeks; maintenance 10 mg/kg IV every 4 weeks. Does not need premedication. Infusion takes 1 hour.
- Subcutaneous dose (adult): SLE: 200 mg SC weekly. Lupus nephritis: 400 mg SC weekly for four doses then 200 mg SC weekly.
- Follow-up: routine monitoring for SLE.
- Efficacy: SLE patients who were not responding to standard therapy achieved primary endpoint in 43% to 61% of cases. It seems to be most effective in patients with active serologies (low C3/C4, elevated anti-dsDNA antibody) and high BLyS levels (not readily available for testing). Manifestations that respond best are fatigue, rash, and arthritis. Hematologic abnormalities do not respond well. Recently, belimumab plus standard immunosuppressive therapy

was found effective (43% of cases) for treatment of lupus nephritis as well as the prevention of renal flares.
- Adverse reactions: infections and infusion reactions/ISR can occur. Serious infections and malignancies were not increased over placebo rate. Two cases of PML reported.
- Depression and suicide mildly increased over placebo rate.
- Immunizations: response to killed/inactivated vaccines may be decreased.
- Precautions: do not use in patients with active infection. Can be given with background immunosuppressive therapy including csDMARDs and glucocorticoids.

21. What T-cell-targeted therapies are available and how are they used?

Abatacept (Orencia): a fully human fusion protein comprising the extracellular portion of CTLA4 and the Fc fragment of IgG1 (CTLA4Ig). Abatacept binds to CD80/CD86 on antigen-presenting cells (APCs) preventing these molecules from binding to their ligand, CD28, on T cells. This interferes with optimal T-cell activation resulting in decreased production of proinflammatory cytokines. Notably, T-cell activation is not completely inhibited because other interactions between APCs and T cells (ICAM-1: LFA-1; CD40:CD40L; LFA-3:CD-2) are not inhibited.
- FDA-approved indication: RA, adult and pediatric PsA, and polyarticular JIA (age >2 years) who are inadequate responders to DMARDs (MTX). Can use with csDMARDs (MTX).
- Available formulation: single-use vial containing 250 mg of lyophilized powder for reconstitution for IV infusion; also available are 50-, 87.5-, and 125-mg single-dose prefilled syringes and a 125-mg single-dose ClickJect autoinjector for SC administration.
- IV dose: weight based (adults with RA or PsA: 500 mg if <60 kg; 750 mg if 60 to 100 kg; 1000 mg if >100 kg); (child with JIA or PsA: 10 mg/kg if <75 kg; same as adult dose if >75 kg). Loading dose at 0, 2, and 4 weeks, then every 4 weeks. Does not need premedication. Infusion takes 30 minutes.
- SC dose: adult RA or PsA: 125 mg SC weekly with or without IV loading dose. Child with JIA or PsA: 10 to <25 kg: 50 mg weekly; 25 to 50 kg: 87.5 mg weekly; >50 kg: 125 mg weekly with or without IV loading dose.
- Follow-up: routine monitoring for csDMARDs.
- Adverse reactions:
  - Infusion reactions: rare. Routine premedication not necessary.
  - Infections: routine similar to placebo. Serious infections (3%). Pneumonias increased in patients with chronic obstructive pulmonary disease. Opportunistic infections rare (0.01–0.05 events/100 patient years). Abatacept may be the safest biologic to use in patients at risk for contacting TB.
  - Malignancy: standardized incidence rates for lung cancer, lymphoma, and other malignancies are not increased over background rates of patients with RA who are not on biologics.
  - Immunizations: response to killed/inactivated vaccines may be decreased.
  - Others: headache. No increased rate of demyelinating disease, autoimmune phenomenon, CHF, hematologic abnormalities.
- Precautions: do not use in patients with active infection. Do not use in patients with cancer being treated with immune checkpoint inhibitors.

22. What is eculizumab?

Eculizumab (Soliris) is a humanized IgG2/4κmonoclonal antibody that binds C5 to inhibit its cleavage to C5a and C5b preventing the generation of the terminal complement complex, C5b-9. **Ravulizumab (Ultomiris)** was bioengineered from eculizumab to have a four times longer half-life. They are approved for use to treat the complement-mediated thrombotic microangiopathy occurring in patients with atypical hemolytic uremic syndrome and to prevent the hemolysis that occurs in patients with paroxysmal nocturnal hemoglobinuria. It also is used to treat aquaporin-4 antibody-positive NMOSD and AchR antibody-positive generalized myasthenia gravis patients. Their most feared side effect is meningococcemia. Therefore, all patients should be immunized against meningococcemia and be on antibiotic prophylaxis during treatment. It costs $500,000 to $700,000 annually for therapy.

23. What factors can make a patient less likely to respond to bDMARD therapy? Can two biologic agents be used together?

Recent reports suggest that 5% to 10% of patients will fail three or more bDMARDs used to treat their underlying rheumatic disease. These patients are defined as being bDMARD-resistant.

The most important factor is to ensure the patient is compliant in taking the bDMARD. Other factors contributing to bDMARD resistance include obesity and smoking, which reduce the effectiveness of many bDMARDs. Younger age, female sex, and high disease activity scores are also factors predicting nonresponse. In patients with a partial response to bDMARDs, it may be tempting to combine two biologic agents. This should not be done due to an increased risk of serious infections although clinical trials are ongoing (e.g., anti-TNF and anti-IL23 for PsA).

24. What are the guidelines for giving vaccines to patients on biologics?

Nonlive attenuated vaccines can be given to rheumatic disease patients on bDMARDs. Several are recommended. Since immunogenicity can be affected by bDMARDs, the vaccinations should ideally be given at least 2 weeks prior to starting a bDMARD. In patients already on a bDMARD there are several timing recommendations to follow (see below). In addition, glucocorticoids (prednisone >20 mg/d) and immunosuppressive medications (e.g., MTX, MMF) that patients may be on concurrently can also affect the immunogenicity of vaccines.

- **Seasonal influenza:** high-dose quadrivalent vaccine should be given to all patients. Patients on RTX, abatacept, or high-dose glucocorticoids should not wait to get this vaccine if flu season is imminent even though immunogenicity will be less.
- **Pneumococcal:** all patients should receive PCV20 (Prevnar-20) vaccine if not previously immunized. If previously immunized, the patient should receive PCV20 if they received only one dose of either the PCV13 (Prevnar-13) or PPSV23 (Pneumovax-23) greater than one year previously or received both the PCV13 and PPSV23 vaccines more than 5 years previously.
- **Recombinant herpes zoster:** all patients 18 years or older should receive this vaccine. Of all the vaccines, this is the one most likely (24%) to cause a disease flare due to its adjuvant effect.
- **Human papilloma virus:** all patients 11 to 45 years old should be offered this vaccine. This is especially important for SLE patients.
- **SARS-CoV-2 (COVID-19) and Respiratory syncytial virus:** all patients should receive this vaccine according to CDC guidelines (https://www.cdc.gov/vaccines/hcp/imz-schedules.).
- **Timing of nonlive attenuated vaccination**: RTX, belimumab, and abatacept can affect immunogenicity of these vaccines.
  - RTX: for all vaccinations (including influenza if flu season is not imminent) the vaccine should be given at the end of one dosing interval for RTX (5–6 months) and RTX not given for 2 weeks after the vaccination.
  - Belimumab and abatacept: vaccines can be given 4 weeks after last IV infusion or one week after a subcutaneous injection. Belimumab and abatacept can be restarted 1 to 2 weeks after the vaccination.
  - Other cytokine inhibitors and prednisone (≤10 mg/d) do not affect immunogenicity of vaccines (except hepatitis B) and do not need to be held/adjusted for vaccinations.
  - MTX should be held for 2 weeks after influenza, pneumococcal, and COVID-19 vaccinations. Although data is not available, some recommend MTX be held for 1 to 2 weeks after all vaccinations.
  - MMF should be held for 1 to 2 weeks after COVID-19 (and possibly all) vaccinations as disease activity allows.
  - Vaccinations can be given to patients regardless of level of disease activity. The decision to hold bDMARDs, MTX, or MMF after vaccination depends on disease activity and shared decision making with the patient.

Live-attenuated vaccines should not be given to patients on bDMARDs unless clinically necessary. Commonly used live-attenuated vaccines include measles (MMR, Proquad), varicella (Varivax), oral rotavirus, Zostavax, and intranasal influenza (Flumist). Yellow fever, BCG, oral typhoid, and adenovirus (military personnel) are live vaccines given only to high-risk groups, whereas smallpox and oral polio are rarely given today. Patients who need to receive a live-attenuated vaccine should receive the vaccine at least 4 weeks before starting a biologic therapy. If already on a biologic agent, the patients are recommended to hold the bDMARD for at least one dosing interval prior to getting the vaccine and to not restart the bDMARD until 4 weeks after getting the live-attenuated virus vaccination.

25. What are the recommendations for holding bDMARDs for elective surgery?

Due to infection risk, recommendations for holding bDMARDs have been made for patients undergoing total hip and knee surgery. These have also been used as guidelines for other elective surgeries. The recommendation is to schedule the surgery for one dosing cycle plus one week after the prior dose. If a bDMARD has more than one dosing interval (e.g., 1 week vs. 2 weeks), the longest interval is selected. For example, a patient on adalimumab 40 mg SC every week would have their surgery scheduled for 3 weeks after their prior dose because the longest dosing interval for adalimumab is 2 weeks. The bDMARD is restarted 2 weeks after the surgery (usually after stitches removed) if the wound is healing well and without signs of infection.

26. Can biologic agents be given during pregnancy and breastfeeding?

TNF inhibitors and ustekinumab are FDA Pregnancy Classification B (old classification) medications. They can be used if clinically necessary for the mother's health. It should be noted that only 4% of the maternal blood level of ETN is detected in the fetal circulation. Immunoglobulins do not cross placenta before 13 to 16 weeks of gestation, thus TNF inhibitors that are monoclonal antibodies should not cross the placenta until then. Studies support that certolizumab pegol crosses the placenta much less than other monoclonal antibodies because it does not have a functional Fc fragment attributable to the pegylation and is, therefore, likely the safest anti-TNF agent that can be used throughout pregnancy, whereas the other TNF inhibitors should be stopped at the end of the second trimester. Animal and observational data support that the congenital malformation rate is not more than the 3% risk in the general population, and the incidence of serious or opportunistic infections in infants born to mothers with RA on biologics was similar to infants born to mothers with RA who did not receive biologics (4% vs. 2.6%). Importantly, infants born to mothers who have received a TNF inhibitor (not certolizumab) throughout pregnancy should not receive BCG which is a live vaccine until at least 6 months of age because of the TNF inhibitor crossing the placenta and remaining in the infant's circulation for a prolonged period. Rotavirus vaccine is also a live vaccine, but some (not all) experts conditionally recommend that it can be given within the first 6 months after birth to infants of mothers treated with TNF inhibitors during pregnancy. Finally, only 4% of ETN gets into breast milk, whereas very little of the monoclonal TNF inhibitors get into breast milk because IgG antibodies are not transferred from the maternal circulation to breast milk in high amounts. Any biologic that does get into the breast milk will be destroyed by the infant's digestive system and is unlikely to be harmful. Therefore, breastfeeding is allowed in patients on TNF inhibitors.

All other biologic agents are FDA Pregnancy Classification C (old classification) medications. They have not been studied sufficiently and are therefore not recommended or should be used with caution during pregnancy. RTX has been reported to cause transient B-cell depletion in the fetus and infant when given to the mother during pregnancy and thus it is recommended to not give live vaccines (rotavirus and BCG) to infants within the first 6 months after birth if the mother received RTX during the last two trimesters of pregnancy. The outcome of pregnancies of patients who receive any biologic agent during pregnancy should be reported to the Organization of Teratology Information Specialists registry at 1-866-626-6847. There is also limited data on safety of breastfeeding with these biologics. However, if any biologic does get into the breast milk, it is likely destroyed by the infant's digestive system.

27. What are the annual costs of bDMARDs?

The wholesale acquisition cost (WAC) for most biologic agents with patent protection used to treat rheumatic diseases range from $25,000/year to over $50,000/year depending on dose and route of administration. The retail price is usually 20% higher than the WAC. A few biologics (rilonacept, canakinumab, eculizumab) with specific indications for uncommon diseases cost considerably more. There is concern about the cost-effectiveness of using expensive bDMARDs compared with csDMARDs for the treatment of rheumatic diseases. It was hoped that competition between biologic agents and introduction of biosimilars would decrease these costs.

28. What are biosimilars?

A biosimilars is a copy of a biologic (bio-originator) made by a different manufacturer from the original innovator of the biologic agent that is no longer protected by patent. The manufacturer does not have access to the originator's molecular clone or the exact fermentation and purification process. The biosimilars have undergone rigorous assessment in comparison to its reference product and have been approved by a regulatory agency (e.g., FDA). It is estimated that the cost of biosimilars will be 80% of the original product and lead to cost savings. Direct comparison of the biosimilar with the bio-originator shows that efficacy and side effects are similar and switching does not cause problems with immunogenicity. Presently several biosimilars have been FDA-approved for the TNF inhibitors, tocilizumab, ustekinumab, and rituximab (see question #1). Other biosimilars for other biologics are in development.

BIBLIOGRAPHY

Ascef BDO, Almeida MO, Medeiros-Ribeiro ACD, et al. Therapeutic equivalence of biosimilar and reference biologic drugs in rheumatoid arthritis: a systematic review and meta-analysis. *JAMA Netw Open.* 2023;6:e2315872.

Bass AR, Chakravarty E, Akl EA, et al. 2022 American College of Rheumatology guideline for vaccinations in patients with rheumatic and musculoskeletal diseases. *Arthritis Care Res (Hoboken).* 2023;75:449–464.

Bitoun S, Hässler S, Ternant D, et al. Response to biologic drugs in patients with rheumatoid arthritis and antidrug antibodies. *JAMA Netw Open.* 2023;6(7):e2323098.

Bredemeir M, de Oliveira FK, Rocha CM. Low- versus high-dose rituximab for rheumatoid arthritis: a systemic review and meta-analysis. *Arthritis Care Res.* 2014;66:228–235.

Campbell L, Chen C, Bhagat SS, et al. Risk of adverse events including serious infections in rheumatoid arthritis patients treated with tocilizumab: a systematic literature review and meta-analysis of randomized controlled trials. *Rheumatology.* 2011;50:552–562.

Chen L, Flies DB. Molecular mechanisms of T cell co-stimulation and co-inhibition. *Nat Rev Immunol.* 2013;13:227–242.

Curtis JR, Johnson SR, Anthony DD, et al. American College of Rheumatology guidance for COVID-19 vaccination in patients with rheumatic and musculoskeletal diseases: version 4. *Arthritis Rheumatol.* 2022;74:e21–e36.

Dorner T, Kay J. Biosimilars in rheumatology: current perspectives and lessons learnt. *Nat Rev Rheumatol.* 2015;11:713–724.

Engel P, Gomez-Puerta JA, Ramos-Casals M, et al. Therapeutic targeting of B cells for rheumatic autoimmune diseases. *Pharmacol Rev.* 2011;6:127–156.

Flint J, Panchal S, Hurrell A, et al. BSR and BHPR guideline on prescribing drugs in pregnancy and breastfeeding—part I: standard and biologic disease modifying anti-rheumatic drugs and corticosteroids. *Rheumatology.* 2016;55:1693–1697.

Fragoulis GE, Nikiphorou E, Dey M, et al. 2022 EULAR recommendations for screening and prophylaxis of chronic and opportunistic infections in adults with autoimmune inflammatory rheumatic diseases. *Ann Rheum Dis.* 2023;82:742–753.

Goodman SM, Springer BD, Chen AF, et al. 2022 American College of Rheumatology/American Association of Hip and Knee Surgeons guideline for the perioperative management of antirheumatic medication in patients with rheumatic diseases undergoing elective total hip or total knee arthroplasty. *Arthritis Care Res (Hoboken).* 2022;74:1399–1408.

Gossec L, Baraliakos X, Kerschbaumer A, et al. EULAR recommendations for the management of psoriatic arthritis with pharmacological therapies: 2019 update. *Ann Rheum Dis.* 2020;79:700–712.

Hellmich B, Sanchez-Alamo B, Schirmer JH, et al. EULAR recommendations for the management of ANCA-associated vasculitis: 2022 update. *Ann Rheum Dis.* 2023. doi:10.1136/ard-2022-223764.

Joensuu JT, Huoponen S, Aaltonen KJ, et al. The cost-effectiveness of biologics for the treatment of rheumatoid arthritis: a systemic review. *PLoS One.* 2015;10:e0119683.

Kerschbaumer A, Sepriano A, Bergstra SA, et al. Efficacy of synthetic and biological DMARDs: a systematic literature review informing the 2022 update of the EULAR recommendations for the management of rheumatoid arthritis. *Ann Rheum Dis.* 2023;82:95–106.

Min HK, Kim SH, Kim HR, Lee SH. Therapeutic utility and adverse effects of biologic disease-modifying anti-rheumatic drugs in inflammatory arthritis. *Int J Mol Sci.* 2022;23:13913.

Muller F, Taubmann J, Bucci L, et al. CD19 CAR T-cell therapy in autoimmune disease—a case series with follow-up. *N Eng J Med.* 2024;390:687–700.

Pang M, Sun Z, Zhang H. Biologic DMARDs and targeted synthetic DMARDs and the risk of all-cause mortality in rheumatoid arthritis: a systematic review and meta-analysis. *Medicine (Baltimore).* 2022;101:e29838.

Ramos-Casals M, Brito-Zeron P, Munoz S, et al. A systematic review of the off-label use of biological therapies in systemic autoimmune diseases. *Medicine.* 2008;87:345–364.

Russell MD, Dey M, Flint J, et al. British Society for Rheumatology guideline on prescribing drugs in pregnancy and breastfeeding: immunomodulatory anti-rheumatic drugs and corticosteroids. *Rheumatology.* 2023;62(4):e48–e88.

Schett G, Dayer J-M, Manger B. Interleukin-1 function and role in rheumatic disease. *Nat Rev Rheumatol.* 2016;12:14–24.

Singh JA, Cameron C, Noorbaloochi S, et al. Risk of serious infection in biological treatment of patients with rheumatoid arthritis: a systemic review and meta-analysis. *Lancet.* 2015;386:258–265.

Smolen JS, Landewé RBM, Bergstra SA, et al. EULAR recommendations for the management of rheumatoid arthritis with synthetic and biological disease-modifying antirheumatic drugs: 2022 update. *Ann Rheum Dis.* 2023;82:3–18.

Solomon DH, Rassen JA, Kuriya B, et al. Heart failure risk among patients with rheumatoid arthritis starting a TNF antagonist. *Ann Rheum Dis.* 2013;72:1813–1818.

Stone JH, Merkel PA, Spiera R, et al. Rituximab versus cyclophosphamide for ANCA-associated vasculitis. *N Engl J Med.* 2010;363:221–232.

Stone JH, Tuckwell K, Dimonaco S, et al. Trial of tocilizumab in giant cell arteritis. *N Engl J Med.* 2017;377:317–328.

Tanaka T, Kishimoto T. The biology and medical implications of interleukin-6. *Cancer Immunol Res.* 2014;2:288.

Tarp S, Amarilyo G, Foeldvari I, et al. Efficacy and safety of biological agents for systemic juvenile idiopathic arthritis: a systemic review and meta-analysis of randomized trials. *Rheumatology.* 2016;55:669–679.

US Preventative Services Task Force. Screening for latent tuberculosis infection in adults. *JAMA.* 2023;329:1487–1494.

van Sleen Y, van der Geest KSM, Huckriede ALW, et al. Effect of DMARDs on the immunogenicity of vaccines. *Nat Rev Rheumatol.* 2023;19:560–575.

Wallace ZS, Putman M. Weighing the risks and benefits of *Pneumocystis jirovecii* pneumonia prophylaxis in rituximab users. *Arthritis Rheumatol.* 2023;75:1904–1906.

Webers C, Ortolan A, Sepriano A, et al. Efficacy and safety of biological DMARDs: a systematic literature review informing the 2022 update of the ASAS-EULAR recommendations for the management of axial spondyloarthritis. *Ann Rheum Dis.* 2023;82:130–141.

Winthrop KL, Baxter R, Liu L, et al. Mycobacterial diseases and antitumor necrosis factor therapy in USA. *Ann Rheum Dis.* 2013;72:37–42.

FURTHER READING

www.rheumatology.org.

CHAPTER 85

Immunosuppressive and Immunoregulatory Agents

Michael G. Feely, MD and Amy C. Cannella, MD

The physician without physiology and chemistry practices a sort of popgun pharmacy, hitting now the malady and again the patient, he himself not knowing which.

–Sir William Osler

 KEY POINTS

1. Cyclophosphamide is best used for remission induction in severe rheumatic diseases.
2. Azathioprine (AZA) is best used for remission maintenance of rheumatic diseases.
3. AZA-induced myelosuppression is increased in patients with low thiopurine methyltransferase (TPMT) enzyme activity.
4. Mycophenolate mofetil (MMF) can be used for remission induction and maintenance for lupus nephritis.
5. Calcineurin inhibitors may be effective as adjunctive therapy for rheumatic disorders including inflammatory autoimmune lung disease and lupus nephritis.
6. Avacopan is a complement C5 inhibitor that is effective as an adjunctive induction therapy which has a steroid sparing effect in ANCA-associated vasculitides

IMMUNOSUPPRESSIVE AGENTS

1. How is AZA (Imuran, Azasan) supplied and used?

- Available formulations: 50-mg tablets (Imuran), 75-mg tablets (Azasan), 100-mg/20-mL vial.
- Side effects: bone marrow depression, nausea, vomiting, skin rash, malignancy (some studies show lymphoma increased two times, non-melanoma skin cancer), hepatotoxicity (liver enzymes mildly increased in 33%, isolated hyperbilirubinemia, severe toxicity is rare), infections (herpes zoster, cytomegalovirus [CMV]), pancreatitis, hypersensitivity syndrome (rash, fever, hepatitis, renal failure within first 2 weeks of use).
- Dosage: 50 to 200 mg/day (1–2.5 mg/kg per day). Start 25 to 50 mg/day and increase by 25 to 50 mg every 1 to 2 weeks to the desired dose.
- Cost (150 mg/day): generic ($28/month; Imuran ($770/month). **TPMT testing:** genetic ($395) and phenotypic or functional enzyme ($220) testing for TPMT are commercially available. TPMT is the enzyme responsible for the metabolism of thiopurines, including AZA and 6-mercaptopurine (6-MP). Genetic polymorphisms can result in functional inactivation of the enzyme and lead to potentially fatal myelosuppression. The US Food and Drug Administration (FDA) recommends that "consideration be given to either genotype or phenotype patients for TPMT" prior to initiating therapy with AZA. Some practitioners routinely order the TPMT test prior to administration of AZA or 6-MP, but this has not been universally adopted. Ordering the phenotype/functional enzyme test provides more clinically useful information than the genetic test. However, with a lack of cost-effective data, other practitioners do not routinely do TPMT enzyme testing and elect for slow dose escalation with close monitoring of the blood counts. Even in the absence of TPMT genetic polymorphisms, close monitoring should occur for anyone taking AZA or 6-MP.
- Monitoring: a complete blood count (CBC) and platelet count and liver transaminases should be monitored every 1-2 weeks during dose escalation and every 8 to 12 weeks after dose stability. If leukopenia or thrombocytopenia occurs, the dose should be reduced by 50% or the drug discontinued. Patients developing macrocytosis require closer monitoring once alternative causes have been excluded.
- Precautions: AZA has been used in pregnancy and breastfeeding without demonstration of teratogenicity or serious harm to the fetus or infant. AZA is metabolized by xanthine oxidase (XO), and XO inhibitors can lead to fatal bone marrow suppression. Use of AZA or 6-MP with allopurinol or febuxostat requires a reduction of AZA/6-MP dose by 75%. Many would

advocate to avoid using this combination. Sulfasalazine and trimethoprim/sulfamethoxazole increase the risk of leukopenia. AZA may cause **warfarin resistance.** Patients more likely (3 ×) to get a rash if treated with ampicillin or amoxicillin. Risk of lymphoma and skin cancer increased.

> **PEARL:** Patients who cannot tolerate AZA due to nausea, vomiting, or rash may be able to tolerate 6-MP (Purinethol), which is the active product of AZA. However, 6-MP cannot be used in patients who develop pancreatitis or liver toxicity on AZA. The effective dose of 6-MP is half the dose of AZA (i.e., 50 mg 6-MP = 100 mg AZA).

2. Describe the mechanism of action (MOA) and metabolism of AZA.

AZA is a prodrug converted to 6-MP, which is then converted to thiopurine nucleotides (6-TGN), which decrease de novo synthesis of purine nucleotides with subsequent inhibition of DNA, RNA, and protein synthesis. This results in both cytotoxicity and decreased cellular proliferation. 6-TGN metabolite levels can be measured within 4 hours of taking AZA with 230 to 400 pmole/8 × 10^8 red blood cells being therapeutic (cost: $270).

XO and TPMT metabolize 6-MP into the inactive metabolites, 6-Methylthiouric acid and 6-Methylmercaptopurine, respectively. Inhibition of XO (by allopurinol, febuxostat) or TPMT (possibly by sulfasalazine) causes an accumulation of 6-MP resulting in toxicity. In addition, TPMT enzyme activity is affected by genetic polymorphisms with 90% having high activity, 10% intermediate activity, and 0.3% low activity. Black people have 17% less TPMT activity than white people. Patients with low TPMT activity are at risk for the sudden onset of severe myelosuppression occurring between 4 and 10 weeks after starting AZA. Patients with intermediate activity have more frequent adverse side effects, particularly gastrointestinal (GI). TPMT genotype and phenotype can be measured. Notably, the TPMT enzyme activity (i.e., phenotype) cannot always be predicted by the genotype. Whether or not this is necessary prior to starting AZA is controversial since over half of all cases of leukopenia are seen in patients with normal TPMT activity (Fig. 85.1).

3. What rheumatic diseases are commonly treated with AZA?
- Rheumatoid arthritis (RA; less effective than methotrexate [MTX] and slower onset).
- Systemic lupus erythematosus (SLE).
- Idiopathic inflammatory myopathies (polymyositis, dermatomyositis, necrotizing myopathies).
- Behçet's syndrome.
- Antineutrophil cytoplasmic antibody (ANCA)-associated vasculitis (remission maintenance).
- Many other rheumatic diseases (in an attempt to decrease glucocorticoid dosage).

> **PEARL:** AZA is more effective as a maintenance therapy than for induction of remission in rheumatic disease.

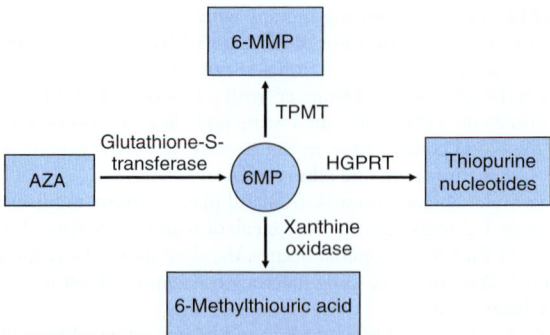

Fig. 85.1 Azathioprine metabolism. *AZA,* Azathioprine; *HGPRT,* hypoxanthine-guanine-phosphoribosyl-transferase; *6-MP,* 6-mercaptopurine; *6-MMP,* 6-methylmercaptopurine; *TPMT,* thiopurine methyltransferase. From Van Laar JM. Immunosuppressive Drugs in Kelley's Textbook of Rheumatology. 9th ed. Philadelphia: Elsevier; 2013.

4. How is MMF (Cellcept) supplied and used?

- Available formulations: 250-mg, 500-mg capsules; oral suspension (200 mg/mL), and intravenous (IV) form (500 mg/20 mL) available.
- Side effects: GI (especially diarrhea 25%), leukopenia, anemia, hepatotoxicity, infections (*Pneumocystis jirovecii*, progressive multifocal leukoencephalopathy, herpes zoster, and CMV); lymphoproliferative malignancies (Epstein–Barr virus [EBV]-associated).
- Dosage: 500 to 1500 mg two times a day (BID). Taking with food may decrease not only absorption but also GI side effects. Decrease maximum dose to 1000 mg BID if severe renal insufficiency (creatinine clearance [CrCl] <30 cc/minute) and in Asian people.
- Cost (1000 mg BID): generic ($50/month); Cellcept ($2080/month).
- Monitoring: baseline CBC with differential, hepatic function tests, creatinine, serologic testing for hepatitis B and C, and screening for latent tuberculosis. Follow CBC and liver enzymes weekly with dose change and then CBC every 6 to 8 weeks.
- Precautions: **do not use in pregnancy and lactation;** can reduce the efficacy of oral contraceptive pills; vaccinate appropriately. Cholestyramine and administration with food or antacids/**proton pump inhibitors** decrease bioavailability. Tacrolimus may potentiate the effects of MMF.

> **PEARL:** Good alternative to AZA in patients with gout who need allopurinol or febuxostat and in patients who need warfarin.

5. What is mycophenolic acid (MPA; Myfortic)?

MPA (Myfortic) is enteric-coated, delayed-release mycophenolate sodium. It comes in 180-mg and 360-mg delayed-release tablets. Dose conversion is 360 mg of Myfortic is equivalent to 500 mg of MMF. Some patients will tolerate Myfortic when they have experienced severe GI side effects with MMF. Cost of 720 mg BID is $60/month for generic; $1570/month for brand name.

6. What is the MOA of MMF?

MMF is an inactive prodrug that is hydrolyzed to active MPA. MPA is a reversible inhibitor of inosine-5'-monophosphate dehydrogenase (IMPDH), which is an enzyme necessary for the de novo synthesis of the purine, guanosine. Lymphocytes (T and B cells) depend on IMPDH to generate sufficient guanosine levels to initiate a proliferative response to antigen. Cytokine production is not affected. MPA also inhibits carbohydrate (fucose, mannose) transfer to glycoproteins, resulting in less production of adhesion molecules (VLA-4, ICAM-1). In summary, MPA inhibits lymphocyte proliferation and migration. It also has antifibrotic activity. Notably, neutrophils are less affected by MPA than lymphocytes. The enterohepatic recycling of glucuronide-conjugated MPA contributes to GI toxicity since GI mucosal cells are 50% dependent on de novo synthesis pathway of purines. Therapeutic trough level of MPA is 1.0–3.5 ug/mL on 2 gram of MMF and up to 5.0 ug/mL on 3 gram of MMF.

7. What rheumatic diseases have been treated successfully with MMF? Which diseases have not been treated successfully with MMF?

Use is similar to AZA. Good success has been seen in lupus nephritis (diffuse proliferative glomerulonephritis membranous) especially in Black and Hispanic patients. It has been used successfully for treating cutaneous lupus (discoid and subacute cutaneous lupus), systemic sclerosis, myositis, uveitis, and vasculitis. Patients with RA or psoriatic arthritis (PsA) usually do not respond to MMF. MMF is less effective than AZA in maintaining remission in patients with granulomatous polyangiitis and other ANCA-associated vasculitides. Due to its lymphocyte and antifibrotic effects, it has been effective in treating interstitial lung disease (ILD) associated with many rheumatic diseases.

8. Discuss the use of cyclophosphamide (Cytoxan) in rheumatic diseases.

- Available formulations: 25-and 50-mg tablets; 100-, 200-, 500-, and 1000-mg vials.
- Dosage: multiple dosing regimens including (1) daily oral, 50 to 200 mg (0.7–2 mg/kg per day); (2) monthly IV, 0.5 to 1 g/m² body surface area or 15 mg/kg; and (3) 500 mg IV every 2 weeks for 6 doses (Euro-Lupus Protocol).

> **PEARL:** Dose of cyclophosphamide is based on actual body weight even if patient is obese.

- Cost (150 mg/day): oral generic tablets $1100/month.
- Follow-up: daily dosing, CBC every 2 weeks until stable dose, then monthly; serum creatinine, blood urea nitrogen, and electrolytes every 2 to 4 weeks, liver transaminases every 4 weeks. Urinalysis monthly while on therapy; urinalysis with cytology every 12 months after cessation of therapy. For monthly IV dosing, CBC, urinalysis, and pregnancy test (women) before each dose, CBC 10 to 14 days after each dose to see nadir. If total white blood cell (WBC) count falls below $3500/mm^3$ or neutrophil count falls below $1500/mm^3$ at the nadir, the dose should be reduced by 20% to 25%. If the nadir total WBC count is above $4000/mm^3$, the dose may be increased if patient's disease is not controlled.
- Precautions: avoid in pregnancy and breastfeeding, avoid live vaccines, use lower doses in elderly (> age 60) due to less bone marrow reserve (cellularity = 100% − age). Cimetidine and allopurinol increase frequency of leukopenia. IV cyclophosphamide interferes with stable warfarin dosing.

9. Describe the MOA and metabolism of cyclophosphamide (CYC).

Cyclophosphamide is an inactive prodrug that is activated by hepatic cytochrome P-450 enzymes. Genetic polymorphisms of cytochrome P-450 enzymes can affect response to cyclophosphamide. The major active metabolite is phosphoramide mustard, which alkylates DNA and results in crosslinking of DNA, breaks in DNA, decreased DNA synthesis, and apoptosis. CYC synthesis has a marked effect on rapidly dividing cells and throughout the cell cycle, resulting in alterations in humoral and cellular immunity (B > T cells).

Liver disease does not increase the toxicity of CYC so dose does not have to be altered. However, with renal insufficiency the oral dose is decreased by 30% if CrCl <30 cc/minute and by 50% if CrCl <15cc/min. Intravenous CYC dose is reduced by 33% if creatinine >3.4 mg/dL and/or patient >60 years old. CYC is dialyzable and should be administered more than 12 hours before a dialysis or administered any time after dialysis.

Acrolein is a major metabolic product of cyclophosphamide metabolism. It is responsible for causing hemorrhagic cystitis and bladder cancer. Bladder lavage should be considered in patients with low urine output to reduce this toxicity.

10. In which rheumatic diseases is cyclophosphamide therapy indicated? How effective is it?

- Granulomatosis with polyangiitis (GPA) and other ANCA-associated vasculitides.
- SLE (particularly lupus nephritis, severe manifestations).
- ILD in systemic sclerosis patients.
- Other systemic vasculitis syndromes.
- Other rheumatic diseases refractory to conventional therapy.
  Cyclophosphamide is considered to be one of the most potent immunosuppressive drugs available. It has been used successfully in almost all rheumatic diseases, particularly when other less potent and usually less toxic forms of therapy have failed. Once remission is induced by cyclophosphamide (usually by 3–6 months), less toxic agents, such as AZA or MMF, are used for maintenance.

11. What are the major toxicities of cyclophosphamide? What can be done to prevent them?

- **Bone marrow suppression:** the WBC nadir after an IV dose is 8 to 14 days later. Start at 50 mg/day orally or 500 mg/m^2 IV, with slow escalation and close monitoring.
- **Infection (all types, especially herpes viruses):** screen for hepatitis B and C, human immunodeficiency virus, and tuberculosis prior to therapy. Keep WBC nadir >3000/mm^3 and preferably >4000/mm^3. Decrease prednisone dose to <20 to 25 mg/day as soon as possible. Prophylaxis for *P. jirovecci* pneumonia with TMP/SMX, dapsone, or inhaled pentamidine. Pneumococcal, recombinant VZV, and influenza vaccines should be given.

- **Hemorrhagic cystitis and bladder cancer:** hemorrhagic cystitis is more common in patients with BK virus. Non-glomerular hematuria occurs in up to 50% of patients with 5% developing bladder cancer (31-fold increased risk). The risk of bladder cancer is reduced by IV dosing and giving concomitant MESNA, which is a sulfhydryl compound that binds and inactivates acrolein in the urine. Cigarette smoking increases the risk of bladder toxicity. With daily oral therapy, cyclophosphamide should be dosed in the morning, and patients should be educated to maintain adequate hydration (>2 L/day) and empty their bladder frequently.
- **Malignancy:** risk increased two- to four-fold. Increased risk if given daily oral versus monthly IV; the higher the cumulative dose, the greater the risk (50% in patients receiving ≥80 g total dose develop a malignancy).
- **Infertility:** the risk for ovarian failure ranges from 30% to 70% and varies depending on the patients' age and cumulative dose. The risk may be less likely with monthly IV than with daily oral dosing. Female risk of premature ovarian failure is age dependent as follows: age <20 years, 13% risk, 20 to 30 years, 50% risk, and >30 years, 100% risk. Ovarian failure is unlikely if women receive less than 6 monthly doses and common if they receive over 15 monthly doses (50% with 8 g/m^2 and 90% with 12 g/m^2). It is rare in patients who receive the Euro-lupus protocol (500 mg IV every 2 weeks × 6 doses). Azoospermia is found in 50% to 90% of males. Various strategies have been tried to limit this toxicity. Banking ova and sperm can be done but may be costly. In females, using gonadotropin-releasing hormone analog (Lupron depot, 3.75 mg intramuscular [IM] monthly or 11.25 mg IM every 3 months plus estradiol 0.3 mg/day [or biweekly patch if patient hypercoagulable]) will reduce hot flashes and protect bone mineral density. In males, testosterone 100 mg IM every 15 days may be protective. Antimullerian hormone levels are a good marker of ovarian reserve and can be measured at any time during the cycle.
- **Pulmonary:** less than 1% of patients get pneumonitis or pulmonary fibrosis.
- **Others:** reversible alopecia, the syndrome of inappropriate antidiuretic hormone secretion, nausea (use antiemetics), teratogenicity, and reversible posterior leukoencephalopathy syndrome after IV administration.

12. What other alkylating agent has been used to treat rheumatic diseases?

Chlorambucil (Leukeran) has been used to treat several rheumatic diseases. The usual dose is 0.1 mg/kg per day (2–8 mg/day). It has been used primarily to treat the ocular and neuropsychiatric complications of Behçet's disease. It has also been used in cryoglobulinemia, refractory dermatomyositis, lupus nephritis, and amyloidosis secondary to chronic inflammatory arthritis (RA, juvenile idiopathic arthritis, ankylosing spondylitis). Major toxicities are myelosuppression, infection (herpes zoster), and induction of myeloid leukemia and other malignancies.

13. How is cyclosporine microemulsion (Gengraf, Neoral) used in the treatment of rheumatic diseases?

- Available formulations: 25- and 100-mg capsule; oral solution 100 mg/mL; IV solution 50 mg/mL.
- Dosage: 2.5 to 4 mg/kg ideal body weight for most rheumatic diseases. Start low in divided doses and increase 0.5 mg/kg per day every 4 to 8 weeks.
- Cost (200 mg/day): $450 to $500/month.
- Follow-up: monitor creatinine and blood pressure every 2 weeks for 3 months, then monthly; periodic CBC, liver function tests, magnesium, potassium, uric acid, and lipid levels. Therapeutic trough blood level is 100-300 ng/mL.
- Precautions: concurrent use of nonsteroidal anti-inflammatory drugs (NSAID), aminoglycosides, and angiotensin-converting enzyme (ACE) inhibitors may contribute to renal insufficiency. Erythromycin/clarithromycin, azole antifungals, diltiazem/verapamil, and other CYP3A4 inhibitors increase cyclosporine levels causing toxicity. Consider stopping cyclosporine if the creatinine increases 30% over baseline, even if still in normal range. Cyclosporine can increase toxicity of statins (myopathy), colchicine (neuromyopathy), digoxin, and potassium-sparing diuretics (hyperkalemia). **Do not use colchicine in patients on cyclosporine.**
Cyclosporine is a potent immunomodulating agent that works by inhibition of T-cell activation (primarily T helper cells). It does so by binding to a cytoplasmic protein (immunophilin) called cyclophilin, which in turn binds to calcineurin. This blocks the interaction of calcineurin with

calmodulin, which is necessary to dephosphorylate nuclear factor of activated T cells (NF-AT)—a transcription factor which activates genes for T-cell for stimulation, such as interleukin (IL)-2.

14. What affects cyclosporine absorption?

Cyclosporine is poorly absorbed from the gut with a bioavailability of 30%, though substantial individual variability exists. Absorption can be increased by a high-fat meal. Grapefruit juice and marmalade from Seville oranges contain dihydroxy-bergamottin, which inhibits the cytochrome P450 enzyme in the small intestine, resulting in increased absorption and decreased metabolism of cyclosporine, statins, and ACE inhibitors. St. John's Wort decreases cyclosporine levels by inducing cytochrome P450 3A4, duodenal P-glycoprotein, and MDR-1 gene.

15. What are tacrolimus (Prograf) and sirolimus (Rapamune)?

Tacrolimus is a macrolide produced by a fungus (actinomycete). It has immunosuppressive effects similar to cyclosporine but at a dose 10 to 100 times lower (0.1–0.25 mg/kg per day; usual dose 2–5 mg BID). Tacrolimus, like cyclosporine, is a potent inhibitor of T-cell activation and inhibits transcription of early T-cell activation genes, such as IL-2, by interfering with the binding of nuclear regulatory factor, NF-AT, to its target in the enhancer region of these inducible genes (see Question 13). Notably, tacrolimus causes less increase in uric acid than cyclosporine and it may be useful to switch from cyclosporine to tacrolimus in transplant patients with tophaceous gout. Tacrolimus has shown efficacy in treatment-refractory myositis with or without lung involvement. Therapeutic trough blood level is 5–15 ng/mL.

Sirolimus (rapamycin) and its derivative, everolimus (Afinitor), inhibit T-cell proliferation by binding to its cytoplasmic immunophilin (FK-binding protein, TOR, or FRAP), which inhibits IL-2 receptor transduction events after the receptor has bound IL-2. This blocks progression of the T-cell cycle from G1 to S phase. Sirolimus has not been used much in the treatment of rheumatic diseases.

16. What rheumatic syndromes have been treated with cyclosporine and tacrolimus?

- RA (especially when combined with MTX).
- Polymyositis/dermatomyositis (especially with ILD): tacrolimus may be a better option.
- PsA and psoriasis.
- SLE (especially membranous glomerulonephritis due to its effect on podocytes).
- Uveitis.
- Others: Behçet's, macrophage-activation syndrome (Still's disease, SLE), pyoderma gangrenosum, Sjogren's dry eyes (ophthalmic emulsion), sarcoidosis.

17. What are the major toxicities of cyclosporine and tacrolimus?

- Decreased renal function (usually reversible with discontinuation of drug).
- Hypertension (treat with nifedipine or labetalol).
- Anemia (note that they do not decrease WBC count).
- Malignancies (lymphomas and skin cancers): lymphoma (EBV related) may regress with stopping drug.
- Hyperuricemia and gout (switch to tacrolimus which causes less hyperuricemia).
- Bone pain (treat with calcium channel blockers and lower cyclosporine dose).
- Others: infections, headaches, tremors, hyperpigmentation, anorexia, hepatotoxicity (rare).

18. What is voclosporin (Lupkynis)?

- Voclosporin is a calcineurin inhibitor used in the management of lupus nephritis. It is particularly effective for proteinuria. Approved for use in combination with corticosteroids and/or mycophenolate mofetil.
- Available formulation: 7.9 mg capsule
- Dosage: 23.7 mg BID on empty stomach
  - Does not require monitoring of drug levels which gives it an advantage over cyclosporine and tacrolimus.
- Cost: $15,500/month
- Follow-up: monitor BP, eGFR, and potassium every 2 weeks for first month then monthly.
- Precautions: Avoid in CKD if eGFR <45 mL/min/1.73 m^2. If baseline eGFR <60 mL/min/1.73 m^2 and decreases by 20% from baseline decrease dose by 7.9 mg BID. If decreases

by 30% then discontinue voclosporin until eGFR improves to >80% of baseline, then restart at lower dose. In patients with liver disease decrease dose to 15.8 mg BID. Avoid in combination with strong CYP3A4 inhibitors (e.g., clarithromycin, azoles) and reduce dose for moderate inhibitors (e.g., diltiazem/verapamil). Multiple other potential drug interactions. Avoid use in pregnancy and breast-feeding.
- Common side effects (≥10%): headache, decreased GFR, HBP, diarrhea, cough, UTI

19. What is avacopan (Tavneos)?
- Avacopan is a complement C5a receptor inhibitor used as adjunctive therapy for induction treatment in the management of ANCA-associated vasculitides. It helps achieve remission with reduced reliance on corticosteroids.
- Available formulation: 10 mg capsule
- Dosage: 30 mg BID with food (high-fat)
- Cost: $16,200/month
- Follow-up: screen for Hepatitis B (HBsAg, anti-HBc) infection prior to treatment. Monitor liver function tests every 4 weeks for first 6 months and then periodically. Hold avacopan if AST/ALT >3x upper limit of normal (ULN) and stop if >5x ULN or total bilirubin >2x ULN. Monitor for angioedema.
- Precautions: avoid in untreated or active liver disease or in combination with strong CYP3A4 inhibitors. Reduce dose to 30mg daily if used with moderate CYP3A4 inhibitors. Multiple other potential drug interactions. No dose adjustment for renal insufficiency.
- Common side effects (10%): headache, nausea, diarrhea

20. What precautions should be observed when giving vaccinations to patients on immunosuppressive medications.
All patients on immunosuppressive medications covered in this chapter should get recommended vaccinations per CDC recommendations.
- Inactivated and other non-live vaccines (e.g., influenza, pneumococcal, recombinant VZV, HPV, others): immunosuppressive medications (excluding MTX) do not need to be stopped before or after these vaccinations. However, note that protective titers may be diminished. Also note that unlike other non-live vaccines, it is recommended to hold all immunosuppressives detailed in this chapter for one week following each COVID vaccination if disease activity permits.
- Live-attenuated vaccines (e.g. MMR, smallpox, yellow fever, others):immunosuppressive medications should be stopped 4 weeks prior to and 4 weeks after live vaccine is given.
- Note that in patients also on prednisone (especially ≥20mg/day) adjustments to prednisone dose should also be made for effectiveness and safety (see chapter 82).

OTHER IMMUNOREGULATORY THERAPIES

21. Why do physicians use "pulse" glucocorticoids (GCs)?
Many clinicians use IV pulse GCs as the initial treatment of severe life or organ-threatening manifestations of rheumatic diseases. Methylprednisolone is typically given in doses of 1 g per day for 3 to 5 consecutive days. Many physicians split the dose (500 mg IV every 12 hours or 250 mg IV every 6 hours) on inpatients to lessen potential side effects. This regimen of GC administration is considered to have more immunomodulating effects than high-dose daily oral GCs through rapid (within minutes) nongenomic mechanisms including cell membrane physiochemical effects (controversial). As the sole therapeutic intervention, pulse steroids probably have no role in long-term therapy. However, in combination therapy with a cytotoxic agent, pulse steroids may provide time for a second agent to achieve its therapeutic effect.

The effect of pulse steroids usually lasts 4 to 6 weeks with wide variation between patients. It has been used most often in the treatment of severe vasculitis, lupus nephritis, and neuropsychiatric lupus. Side effects include psychosis, arrhythmias (some from hypokalemia), glucose intolerance, hypertension, glaucoma, and, rarely, sudden death. The risk of these adverse effects may be lessened by using a slow rate of infusion and ensuring that the serum potassium level is normal.

22. How is IV gamma globulin (IVIG) used as an immunomodulator in rheumatic diseases?

- Available formulations: multiple suppliers; solution concentrations vary from 3% to 12% Immunoglobulin; cost is $100 to $300/g.
- Dosage: 1 to 2 g/kg administered over 1 to 5 days.
- Side effects: headache (2–20%), flushing, chest tightness, back pain/myalgias, fever, chills, nausea, diaphoresis, hypotension, aseptic meningitis, thrombosis, leukopenia, serum sickness.
- Follow-up: creatinine 24 hours after infusion if baseline renal insufficiency.
- Precautions: anaphylactic reaction in patients with hereditary IgA deficiency (1/700 patients); transmission of infectious agents (rare). IVIG can diminish effectiveness of live-attenuated vaccines depending on timing of administration and vaccination.

Some side effects of IVIG are avoided by premedicating patients with acetaminophen and diphenhydramine hydrochloride (Benadryl) or hydrocortisone sodium succinate (Solu-Cortef) and by slowing the rate of infusion. Infusion is started at 30 mL/hour and increased to a maximum of 250 mL/hour (sometimes higher). Patients who get migraine headaches may benefit from premedication with sumatriptan. Avoid sucrose containing IVIG (Carimune), which can cause acute renal failure. Avoid sugar containing IVIG in diabetics. Use iso-osmolar IVIG (240–300 mOsm/kg) to reduce the chance of thrombosis. Use IVIG preparations (PrIVIGen, Gammagard S/D) containing low IgA levels in IgA-deficient patients. In a patient who is not IgA-deficient, Gamunex-C (10%) may be best tolerated.

23. In which rheumatic diseases is IVIG indicated? How might it work in these diseases?

- Autoimmune thrombocytopenia: Fc portion of IVIG binds the Fc receptor on reticuloendothelial cells blocking the removal of antibody-coated cells.
- Kawasaki disease: IVIG reduces expression of adhesion molecules on endothelial cells, binds cytokines that cause inflammation, reduces number of activated T cells, and binds staphylococcal toxin superantigens.
- Dermatomyositis and polymyositis: the Fc portion of IVIG can bind to C3b and C4b, decreasing complement activation.
- Chronic inflammatory demyelinating polyneuropathy.
- Antiphospholipid antibody syndrome (off-label).
- Autoimmune hemolytic anemia and neutropenia (off-label).

Other proposed mechanisms that may explain IVIG effectiveness in autoimmune diseases include:

- Anti-idiotypic antibodies bind surface Ig on B cells, preventing binding to target autoantigen.
- Monomeric IgG in high dose IVIG causes blockade of activating FcgRs by saturating them on immune cells attenuating immune complex-mediated inflammation and autoimmunity.
- Saturation of neonatal Fc receptor resulting in accelerated degradation of pathogenic IgG.
- Sialylated fraction of IVIG (5% of total IVIG) binds to the protein, DC-SIGN, on dendritic cells resulting in enhanced expression of inhibitory FcγRs (FcγRIIb) on effector macrophages which can attenuate inflammation.
- Others: enhancement of Treg function, inhibition of dendritic cells, inhibition of macrophages/monocytes, others.

24. Why is plasma exchange (PLEX) used in the treatment of rheumatic diseases?

Theoretically, PLEX should remove immune complexes and autoantibodies that contribute to the pathogenesis of some of the rheumatic diseases. It is most effective when used acutely to gain a rapid response in life-threatening situations. PLEX is usually used in combination with GCs and/or cytotoxic therapy to decrease the risk of a rebound flare of the underlying immunologic disease once the pheresis is stopped.

Most PLEX protocols remove 2 to 4 L (40 mL/kg = 1 plasma volume) of plasma over a 2-hour period daily. Each exchange of 1 to 1.5 plasma volumes removes 60% to 70% of plasma constituents. Replacement fluid is generally albumin-saline or another protein-containing solution. To decrease the risk of infection and bleeding, 1 to 2 units of fresh frozen plasma (FFP) are included as part of the replacement solution. If not, monitoring of fibrinogen, coagulation studies, and immunoglobulin levels are important. If the patient develops a low fibrinogen level (<200 mg/dL) or elevated international normalized ratio/partial thromboplastin time, then FFP is given. If patient develops hypogammaglobulinemia, IVIG (0.4 g/kg × 1 dose) is given. Cost of PLEX: >$5000 per session.

25. In which rheumatic diseases has PLEX been beneficial?

- Thrombotic thrombocytopenia purpura (TTP) associated with rheumatic diseases.
- Catastrophic antiphospholipid syndrome.
- SLE: diffuse alveolar hemorrhage; neuropsychiatric lupus with coma; TTP.
- Neuromyelitis optica spectrum disorder.
- ANCA-associated vasculitis with diffuse alveolar hemorrhage and/or rapidly progressive crescentic glomerulonephritis (Cr >3.5; controversial).
- Hepatitis B-associated polyarteritis nodosa (combined with antiviral agent).
- Hepatitis C-associated cryoglobulinemia (combined with antiviral agent).
- Goodpasture syndrome with progressive renal failure and/or diffuse alveolar hemorrhage.
- PANDAS—pediatric autoimmune neuropsychiatric disorders associated with streptococcal infections.

26. Discuss the use of high-dose immunoablative therapy with autologous hematopoietic stem cell transplantation for the treatment of severe autoimmune disease.

Autologous (using patient's own stem cells) hematopoietic stem cell transplantation is a method of increasing the intensity of chemotherapy that can be given to a patient with a severe autoimmune disease who is failing standard therapy. By collecting stem cells (CD34+) prior to chemotherapy, higher doses of cyclophosphamide (200 mg/kg) can be given to ablate the immune system because the patient can be rescued from bone marrow failure by reinfusion of the patient's own stem cells. Some patients may also receive lymphoablative antibodies or total body irradiation to eradicate residual autoreactive cells. This stem cell transplantation strategy allows the patient to reconstitute their immune system without redeveloping their autoimmune disease or developing graft versus host disease. This procedure is most often used for treatment resistant SLE, systemic sclerosis, multiple sclerosis, and other autoimmune diseases. Success rates are variable, mortality rates are as high as 8%, and the procedure costs can exceed $100,000. Other immunoablative and/or transplantation strategies are also being investigated.

27. What is CD-19-targeting chimeric antigen receptor (CAR) T-cell therapy in autoimmune diseases?

CD-19-targeting CAR T cells are autologous cytotoxic T cells that have been genetically engineered to express chimeric antigen receptors directed against the CD-19 antigen expressed on all B cells and most but not all plasma cells. This therapy which is not FDA-approved for autoimmune diseases causes prolonged depletion of B cells and has been successfully used to treat presumably B-cell–mediated autoimmune diseases (SLE, antisynthetase syndrome, systemic sclerosis, NMOSD, myasthenia gravis, others) which have failed multiple other therapies. The process is complex and costly. The patient undergoes leukapheresis to obtain peripheral blood leukocytes. In a laboratory, T cells are isolated, genetically engineered to express a CD-19 CAR, and expanded in culture over 10–15 days to produce a large number of CAR T-cells. The patient then undergoes lymphocyte depleting chemotherapy (e.g., fludarabine and cyclophosphamide) followed by the infusion of CD-19 CAR T-cells into the patient. Potential immediate side effects include cytokine release syndrome and neurotoxicity. Potential long-term toxicities include cytopenias, hypogammaglobulinemia, infection, and development of T-cell lymphoma. Notably all these have been relatively rare. CAR T cells against BCMA antigen, CAR Treg cell therapy for immunosuppression, and CAAR T cells that target autoantibodies expressed on autoreactive B cells are also being investigated. Total cost $500,000–1,000,000.

BIBLIOGRAPHY

Hochberg MC, Gravallese EM, Smolen JS, et al. Immunosuppressive agents: cyclosporine, cyclophosphamide, azathioprine, mycophenolate mofetil, and tacrolimus. In: Hochberg MC et al, ed. *Rheumatology*. 8th ed. Philadelphia, PA: Elsevier; 2023:518–526.

Ballow M. The IgG molecule as a biological immune response modifier: mechanisms of action of intravenous immune serum globulin in autoimmune and inflammatory disorders. *J Allergy Clin Immunol*. 2011;127:315–323.

Bass AR, Chakravarty E, Akl EA, et al. 2022 American College of Rheumatology guideline for vaccinations in patients with rheumatic and musculoskeletal diseases. *Arthritis Rheumatol*. 2023;75:333–348.

Blumenfeld Z, Shapiro D, Shteinberg M, et al. Preservation of fertility and ovarian function and minimizing gonadotoxicity in young women with systemic lupus erythematosus treated by chemotherapy. *Lupus*. 2000;9:401–405.

Gerbino AJ, Goss CH, Molitor JA. Effect of mycophenolate mofetil on pulmonary function in scleroderma-associated interstitial lung disease. *Chest*. 2008;133:455–460.

Haubitz M, Bohnenstengel F, Brunkhorst R, et al. Cyclophosphamide pharmacokinetics and dose adjustments in patients with renal insufficiency. *Kidney Int*. 2002;61:1495–1501.

Jayne DRW, Merkel PA, Schall TJ, et al. Avacopan for the treatment of ANCA-associated vasculitis. *N Engl J Med*. 2021;384:599–609.

Majhail NS, Farnia SH, Carpenter PA, et al. Indications for autologous and allogeneic hematopoietic cell transplantation: guidelines from the American Society for Blood and Marrow Transplantation. *Biol Blood Marrow Transplant*. 2015;21:1863–1869.

Medication cost information. http://www.goodrx.com.

Monach PA, Arnold LM, Merkel PA. Incidence and prevention of bladder toxicity from cyclophosphamide in the treatment of rheumatic diseases. A data driven review. *Arthritis Rheum*. 2010;62:9–21.

Muller F, Taubmann J, Bucci L, et al. CD19 CAR T-cell therapy in autoimmune disease—a case series with follow-up. *N Eng J Med*. 2024;390:687–700.

Perez EE, Orange JS, Bonilla F, et al. Update on the use of immunoglobulin in human disease: a review of evidence. *J Allergy Clin Immunol*. 2017;139:S1–S46.

Schedel J, Godde A, Schutz E, et al. Impact of thiopurine methyltransferase activity and 6-thioguanine nucleotide concentrations in patients with chronic inflammatory diseases. *Ann NY Acad Sci*. 2006;1069:477–491.

Schwartz J, Padmanabhan A, Aqui N, et al. Guidelines on the use of therapeutic apheresis in clinical practice-evidence-based approach from the writing committee of the American Society for Apheresis: the seventh special issue. *J Clin Apher*. 2016;31:149–162.

Smolen JS, Landewé RBM, Bergstra SA, et al. EULAR recommendations for the management of rheumatoid arthritis with synthetic and biological disease-modifying antirheumatic drugs: 2022 update. *Ann Rheum Dis*. 2023;82:3–18.

Touma Z, Gladman DD, Urowitz MB, et al. Mycophenolate mofetil for induction treatment of lupus nephritis: a systemic review and metaanalysis. *J Rheumatol*. 2011;38:69–78.

Vazquez SR, Rondina MT, Pendleton RC. Azathioprine-induced warfarin resistance. *Ann Pharmacother*. 2008;42:1118–1123.

Witt LJ, Demchuk C, Curran JJ, et al. Benefit of adjunctive tacrolimus in connective tissue disease-interstitial lung disease. *Pulm Pharmacol Ther*. 2016;36:46–52.

FURTHER READING

www.rheumatology.org.

CHAPTER 86

Hypouricemic Agents and Colchicine

Jennifer Stichman, MD

Jennifer Stichman, MD

KEY POINTS

1. Treat to target with urate-lowering therapy (ULT)—aim for serum uric acid <6.0 mg/dL.
2. Continue ULT in patients having an acute flare of gouty arthritis.
3. Colchicine, allopurinol, and probenecid have many drug–drug interactions—use a drug interaction checker to avoid causing harm.
4. Start allopurinol at a low dose and titrate to reach the goal serum uric acid level.
5. Avoid pegloticase in patients with glucose-6-phosphate dehydrogenase (G6PD) deficiency.

1. Identify the goals in the treatment of gout.

The goal in treatment of acute gouty arthritis is to quickly alleviate pain and restore joint function. The long-term treatment goals and purpose of ULT are to prevent recurrent attacks and the development of destructive arthropathy, tophi formation, or renal complications.

2. What is colchicine?

Colchicine, an alkaloid derivative from the plant *Colchicum autumnale,* has been used in the treatment of acute gout for nearly two centuries and for joint pain since the 6th century. Clinical response to colchicine in the setting of acute arthritis is not diagnostic for gout as it also treats other inflammatory arthropathies including pseudogout and familial Mediterranean fever (FMF).

3. Discuss the mechanism of action and pharmacokinetics of colchicine.

- Irreversibly binds free tubulin dimers → disrupts microtubule polymerization → inhibition of neutrophil chemotaxis, phagocytosis, and cytokine secretion.
- Inhibits phospholipase A2, which leads to lower levels of inflammatory prostaglandins and leukotrienes (LTB4).
- May modulate pyrin expression.
- Colchicine is not bound to plasma proteins and is highly lipid soluble, readily passing into all tissues.
- Colchicine achieves much higher intraleukocyte concentrations than plasma concentration— can be detected in neutrophils up to 10 days after a single dose
- Hepatic metabolism, predominantly excreted in feces; 40% to 65% excreted unchanged in urine.

4. Name clinical scenarios where colchicine may be used.

Treatment of acute gout or pseudogout attacks	Prevention of recurrent pseudogout flares
Prophylaxis against recurrent gout flares	Prevention of cardiovascular disease
FMF	Pericarditis, initial and recurrent episodes
Periodic fever, aphthous stomatitis, pharyngitis and cervical adenitis syndrome (PFAPA)	Post-procedurally for atrial fibrillation ablations
Behćet disease	Sweet syndrome
Cutaneous vasculitis (e.g., LCV)	Recurrent aphthous stomatitis

5. How should colchicine be dosed in the treatment of gout?

Management of the Rheumatic Diseases: 1.2 mg followed by 0.6 mg in 1 hour.

Most effective if started in first few hours of gout attack. Similar efficacy to prior "high-dose" regimens used in the past, with fewer side effects. Some patients may benefit from a more prolonged course after Day 1 (0.6 mg once or twice daily for 7–10 days).

Gout prophylaxis: 0.6 mg once or twice daily (or renally dosed as appropriate).

Colchicine has no effect on serum urate concentration or on urate metabolism and is **inappropriate as monotherapy** if the patient has indication for ULT. Colchicine is available as 0.6-mg tablets in the United States and 0.5-mg tablets elsewhere in the world. In addition, a liquid formulation (Gloperba®; 0.6 mg/5 mL) is available and may allow for more precise dosing when <0.6 mg daily is desired.

6. When should colchicine be avoided?

- Concurrent use of cytochrome P450 3A4 (CYP3A4) and P-glycoprotein (P-gp) inhibitors (see Table 86.1) in the setting of renal or hepatic impairment.
- Patients with concurrent renal and hepatic disease.
- Patients with severe hepatic disease.

7. How should colchicine be managed in pregnancy?

Gout does not typically occur in premenopausal women outside the setting of advanced renal disease. Similarly, pseudogout would be uncommon in this age group as well. As such, the use of colchicine for crystalline arthritis in this population is expected to be rare. However, women who become pregnant may use colchicine for another indication (see Question #4). Colchicine was previously designated as pregnancy risk category C, based on suggestion of harm in animal but not human studies. The FDA eliminated such risk category reporting in 2015, and given lack of data demonstrating clear harm, the American College of Rheumatology 2020 Reproductive Guidelines list colchicine as an acceptable medication for use during pregnancy. In general, discussions regarding medication use during pregnancy should be tailored for each patient (taking in to account specific patient-related and disease-related factors).

8. In patients at high risk of toxicity, how can colchicine be adjusted to mitigate risk?

Avoidance is the safest route; no antidotes exist to treat overdose and **hemodialysis is ineffective.** In patients with refractory disease and limited options (i.e., NSAIDs and glucocorticoids are contraindicated), dose adjustments can be made as described in Table 86.1.

TABLE 86.1 Colchicine Dose Adjustments

	DOSE ADJUSTMENT FOR ACUTE GOUT FLARE	DOSE ADJUSTMENT FOR GOUT PROPHYLAXIS
Strong CYP3A4 inhibitors[a]	0.6 mg × 1 dose, 0.3 mg 1 hour later Do not repeat in <3 days	0.3 mg QOD, can increase to 0.3 mg QD with monitoring
Moderate CYP3A4 inhibitors[b]	1.2 mg × 1 dose Do not repeat in <3 days	0.3 mg QD, can increase to 0.6 mg QD with monitoring
Weak CYP3A4 inhibitor[c]	No dose adjustment required	No dose adjustment required
P-gp inhibitors[d]	0.6 mg × 1 dose Do not repeat in <3 days	0.3 mg QOD, can increase to 0.3 mg QD with monitoring
Severe renal impairment (CrCl <30 mL/minute)	1.2 mg × 1 dose, 0.6 mg 1 hour later Do not repeat more than once per 2 weeks	0.3 mg QD
Dialysis	0.6 mg × 1 dose Do not repeat more than once per 2 weeks	0.3 mg twice a week, monitor closely

[a]Clarithromycin, erythromycin, ketoconazole, ritonavir.
[b]Diltiazem, verapamil.
[c]Azithromycin.
[d]Cyclosporine, voclosporin, sunitinib, clarithromycin, erythromycin, tacrolimus (weaker P-gp inhibitor than cyclosporine), carvedilol.
Note:
Clarithromycin and erythromycin are inhibitors of both CYP3A4 and P-gp.
Cyclosporine use is especially problematic due to scheduled, chronic dosing and common use in patients with solid organ transplant (a population at risk for gout). Colchicine should be avoided if possible (elevated risk of neuromyopathy reported).
CrCl, Creatinine clearance; *QD,* every day; *QOD,* every other day.

9. **Describe manifestations of colchicine toxicity and identify patients most at risk.**

Risk factors for toxicity include: older age, renal impairment, hepatic impairment, chronic use, and concomitant interacting medications. Most adverse effects are **related to dose and duration.**

- Common: gastrointestinal (GI) effects (nausea, vomiting, especially diarrhea) can occur even at recommended doses.
- Acute toxicity: renal failure, circulatory collapse, marrow failure, rhabdomyolysis, and respiratory failure.
- Chronic toxicity: most common in elderly, renal insufficiency, and interacting medications. Marrow suppression, irreversible neuromyopathy (elevated creatinine kinase, proximal weakness, peripheral neuropathy, lysosomal vacuoles on biopsy).
- Rare (<1%): alopecia, azo- or oligospermia, amenorrhea, dysgeusia, central nervous system dysfunction, malabsorption syndrome (especially of vitamin B_{12}), hemorrhagic gastritis.

10. **What are the indications for initiating ULT in patients with gout?**

- Recurrent attacks (≥ 2 per year).
- Tophus or tophi (can take months to years to resorb).
- Gouty arthropathy and a history of nephrolithiasis.
- Gouty arthropathy and a serum uric acid >9 mg/dL.
- Renal insufficiency (chronic kidney disease [CKD] stage 3 or worse; creatinine clearance <60 mL/min).
- Asymptomatic hyperuricemia in the absence of clinical disease is **not** an indication for ULT. The decision to use ULT in this setting is a lifelong commitment, so it is essential that these agents be initiated only when the diagnosis is assured.

11. **In addition to gout, when else might xanthine oxidase inhibitors (XOIs) be used?**

- Hyperuricosuria (24-hour urine uric acid >1100 mg) due to risk of uric acid nephrolithiasis.
- Hypoxanthine phosphoribosyltransferase deficiency (Lesch–Nyhan syndrome).
- Hyperuricemia due to myeloproliferative disorders.
- Prophylaxis against tumor lysis syndrome.
- Hyperuricemia with nephrolithiasis of any type.

12. **How can you decrease the risk of precipitating gout flares when initiating ULT?**

Acute gout flare is the most common side effect of ULT initiation.

- Gradual dose increases. Start at 100 mg/day (50 mg if glomerular filtration rate [GFR] <30 mL/min) and increase by 100-mg (50 mg) increments, every 2 to 5 weeks.
- Use of prophylaxis with colchicine, nonsteroidal anti-inflammatory drugs (NSAIDs) or low-dose prednisone (see Chapter 44: Gout).

13. **When should ULT be initiated?**

Classic teaching is that initiation of ULT should be avoided in the presence of acute flares. American College of Rheumatology (ACR) Guidelines from 2012 give the option to start ULT during a flare as long as appropriate flare prophylaxis is initiated concomitantly.

14. **What types of urate-lowering agents are available?**

- **XOIs** inhibit uric acid synthesis by inhibiting xanthine oxidase, the final enzyme involved in the production of uric acid. XOIs, specifically allopurinol, are **first-line** in the absence of contraindications.
- **Uricosurics** reduce the serum urate concentration by enhancing the renal excretion of uric acid. Typically used as add-on therapy with XOIs.
- **Uricase** converts relatively insoluble uric acid into allantoin, which is 5 to 10 times more soluble.

15. **Outline an algorithm for instituting and optimizing ULT for a patient with gout (Fig. 86.1).**

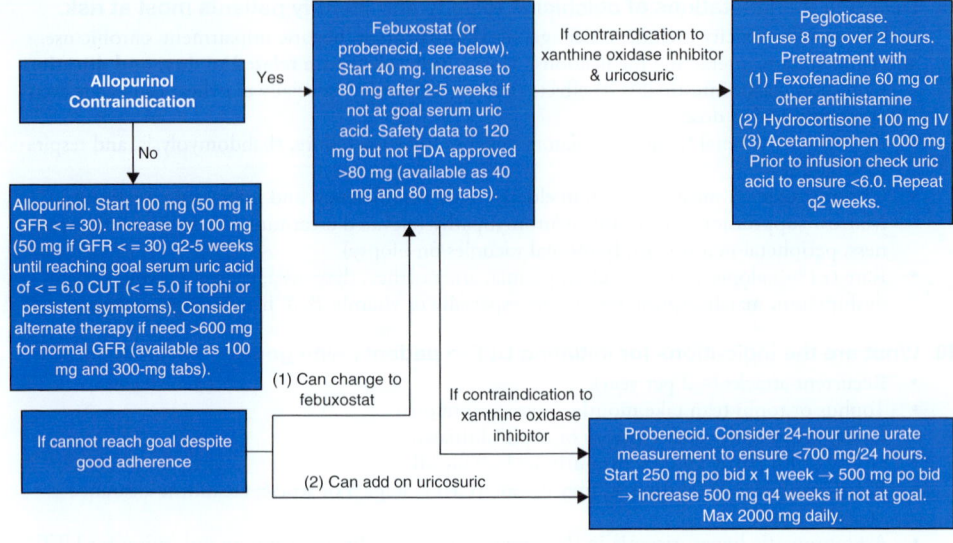

Fig. 86.1 See also Chapter 44: Gout.

16. Compare and contrast XOIs (Table 86.2).

Patients with gout have an increased baseline risk for cardiovascular (CV) events. In 2018, a large randomized controlled trial (CARES trial) was conducted in patients with gout and concurrent CV disease to determine if risk was heightened with the use of febuxostat compared to allopurinol. Feboxostat use was associated with increased all-cause and CV-specific mortality (secondary end-points). No differences were observed in the primary study end-point nor the secondary end-points of nonfatal myocardial infarction, nonfatal stroke, or need for urgent revascularization. Based on this study, the 2020 American College of Rheumatology Guideline for the Management of Gout conditionally recommended changing from feboxostat to an alternative agent in patients with gout and concurrent CV disease. CARES was followed later in 2020 by a second trial (FAST) which failed to show an increased risk for CV endpoints with the use of feboxostat compared to allopurinol. In FAST, all study participants had at least one CV risk factor, but only one-third of patients had concurrent CV disease. Given the conflicting data in the literature, a risk-benefit discussion should be carried out on a case-by-case basis with each patient, ensuring appropriate emphasis is placed on the fact that uncontrolled hyperuricemia itself is a risk factor for CV disease. See Table 86.2 for additional details on the differences between allopurinol and febuxostat.

17. What are the most common reasons for inadequate response of serum uric acid to allopurinol?

Poor adherence and under-dosing of allopurinol by physicians (failure to titrate dose to goal serum uric acid level) are the two most common causes. Adherence may be as low as 50%. Patients are asymptomatic in the intercritical period, and there may be a lack of understanding about the need for daily long-term medication. Adherence can be evaluated by checking serum oxipurinol levels in patients on allopurinol and evaluating pharmacy fill data. About half of patients do not achieve a serum uric acid goal of ≤ 6.0 at an allopurinol dose of 300 mg. Some patients do have "resistance" to allopurinol, but this is less common.

18. What is the allopurinol hypersensitivity syndrome (AHS)?

- AHS is a rare (0.1–0.4% of patients) complication of allopurinol use with high morbidity and mortality (25% in some studies).

TABLE 86.2 Comparison of Xanthine Oxidase Inhibitors

	ALLOPURINOL	FEBUXOSTAT
Mechanism of action	XOI Hypoxanthine analog	XOI (more potent than allopurinol) Not a hypoxanthine analog
Pharmacokinetics	80–90% bioavailability Half-life of 60 minutes Oxipurinol metabolite long-lived ($t_{1/2}$ 14–28 hours) Max antihyperuricemic effect seen after 7–10 days	~50% bioavailability Extensive hepatic metabolism Equal hepatic and renal excretion Max antihyperuricemic effect seen after 5–7 days
Adverse events	**Common** Acute gouty arthritis: use prophylaxis Maculopapular erythematous rash: 3% (risk 3x higher if on ampicillin/amoxicillin) Gastrointestinal symptoms (nausea, diarrhea): 5–10% Abnormal liver-associated enzymes: 6% Headache **Uncommon (<1%) but serious** Allopurinol hypersensitivity syndrome DRESS, SJS, TEN, vasculitis Oxipurinol xanthine nephrolithiasis Bone marrow suppression can occur early or late in treatment Hepatitis, peripheral neuropathy, interstitial nephritis, death Cataracts: dose and duration associated The overall incidence of side effects is around 20%, but only 5% of patients discontinue therapy as a result of drug toxicity	**Common** Acute gouty arthritis: use prophylaxis Nausea, rash, arthralgia: ~1% **Uncommon but serious** DRESS, SJS, TEN Abnormal AST or ALT (~5%)
Contraindications or cautions to use	Interacting medications, especially azathioprine and 6-MP Avoid if history of rash with allopurinol Dose adjust for renal insufficiency	CrCl 15–29: do not exceed 40 mg daily Not studied and thus consider avoiding in patients with dialysis dependence or severe hepatic disease (Child–Pugh class C)
Drug interactions	**AZA[a]:** decrease azathioprine dose 50–75%; safest to avoid concurrent use **6-MP[a]:** as per azathioprine Theophylline: metabolized by xanthine oxidase; increased concentration and marrow suppression Ampicillin/amoxicillin: increased risk of rash Thiazide diuretics: decreased allopurinol excretion Cyclophosphamide, warfarin, cyclosporine: levels all increased by allopurinol	**AZA[a]: avoid combination** **6-MP[a]: avoid combination** Theophylline: increased plasma concentration
Cost	$15/month (30 tablets of 300 mg)	$40/month (40-mg and 80-mg tablets cost approx the same)

[a]AZA and 6-MP are both metabolized by xanthine oxidase, and hence use of xanthine oxidase inhibitors increases drug levels of both medications leading to an increased risk of bone marrow toxicity.
6-MP, 6-Mercaptopurine; *AZA,* azathioprine; *CrCl,* creatinine clearance; *DRESS,* drug rash with eosinophilia and systemic symptoms; *SJS,* Stevens–Johnson syndrome; *TEN,* toxic epidermal necrolysis.

- AHS typically occurs 2 to 4 weeks after initiating therapy.
- Clinical manifestations include severe skin rash (e.g., Stevens–Johnson syndrome, toxic epidermal necrolysis), fever, eosinophilia, hepatic necrosis, leukocytosis, and renal failure.
- Treatment of AHS includes high-dose steroids and hemodialysis (to remove oxipurinol).

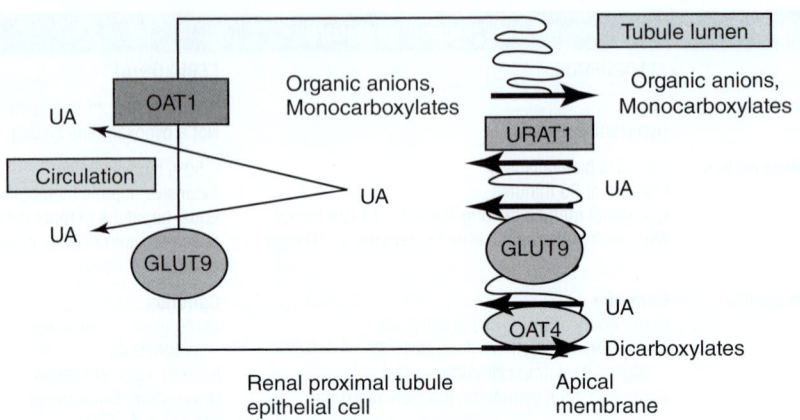

Fig. 86.2 Renal handling of uric acid.

19. Which patients are most at risk of developing AHS?

- Risk factors for developing AHS include: female sex, renal insufficiency, concomitant diuretic therapy, and older age. History of rash on allopurinol (5–10% of patients) is also a risk for AHS and patients should not be rechallenged if they have previously developed a rash on allopurinol.
- **HLA-B∗5801.** This test should be checked in populations with a high prevalence of the polymorphism: Korean descent with CKD stage ≥3, ethnic Han Chinese and Thai patients, and African Americans patients.

PEARL: Starting dose of allopurinol is associated with AHS. Start at 100 mg daily if GFR >30 mL/minute (50 mg daily for GFR ≤30 mL/minute) and titrate every 2 to 4 weeks by 100-mg increments (50 mg for GFR <30 mL/min). Start low and go slow.

PEARL: Ask patients about ethnic background regardless of the country of origin. Check HLA-B∗5801 in patients listed above and choose alternative ULT if HLA-B∗5801 is present.

20. Describe the renal handling of uric acid (see Fig. 86.2).

Uric acid is a weak organic acid. It is excreted primarily (66%) through the kidney. Up to a third is excreted through the GI tract. In cases of renal failure, GI excretion is increased.

There are four components of renal excretion of uric acid:

1. Glomerular filtration: near complete excretion of urate.
2. Proximal tubule reabsorption of urate in exchange for organic acids and monocarboxylates (lactate/pyruvate/acetoacetate/hydroxybutyrate): mediated by URAT1 and GLUT9 transporters.
3. Tubular secretion of urate more distal in the tubule, mediated by ABCG2 and MRP4 transporters.
4. Tubular reabsorption of urate a second time in exchange for dicarboxylates (oxalic acid/malonic acid/succinic acid): mediated by OAT4 and OAT 10 transporter.

21. Discuss the pharmacology of probenecid (Table 86.3).

22. What medications have uricosuric effect even if not prescribed for this reason?

Losartan: modest uricosuric effect, plateaus at 50 mg daily.
Fenofibrate: may induce ∼20% decrease in serum uric acid.
Atorvastatin (note the risk of myopathy with statins + fibrates).
High-dose (>4 g/day) salicylates.
Sodium-glucose cotransporter-2 (SGLT2) inhibitors

TABLE 86.3 Clinical Pharmacology of Probenecid	
	PROBENECID
Mechanism of action	Competitively inhibits URAT1 & GLUT9 → decreased tubular reabsorption of urate → increased uricosuria
Pharmacokinetics	Hepatic metabolism Half-life 6–12 hours → BID dosing Decreases serum uric acid by ~33%
Adverse events	**Preventable** Acute gouty attacks: use prophylaxis **Relatively common** Nausea, loss of appetite (10%) Dermatitis (5%) Headache, flushing **Rare but serious** Urate nephropathy Urate nephrolithiasis Cytopenias, aplastic anemia Stevens–Johnson syndrome Anaphylaxis Nephrotic syndrome
Contraindications or cautions to use	History of nephrolithiasis CrCl ≤ 50 mL/minute (lack of efficacy) G6PD deficiency (risk of hemolytic anemia) Avoid with salicylates On Beers list of medications to avoid in elderly No hepatic adjustment required
Drug interactions	Increases the half-life of many meds Probenecid increases serum concentration of many antibiotics, NSAIDs, dapsone, methotrexate, sulfonylureas, and heparin among others Aspirin diminishes effectiveness of probenecid
Cost	With drug discount cards: $60/month (1000 mg BID dosing)

BID, Twice a day; *CrCl,* creatinine clearance; *G6PD,* glucose-6-phosphate dehydrogenase; *NSAIDs,* nonsteroidal antiinflammatory drugs. NOTE: Probenecid is the only uricosuric medication available in the United States; sulfinpyrazone and benzbromarone are available outside the United States.

PEARL: Consider choosing medications with urate-lowering "side effect" for patients with gout and comorbid hypertension, diabetes mellitus, or dyslipidemia.

23. Discuss the use of uricosuric medications.

In the United States, probenecid is the only available uricosuric and in practice is used rarely. It can be effective as add-on therapy to XOI to achieve goal serum uric acid levels. Efficacy decreases in CKD and probenecid should not be used in CKD ≥3 (GFR <50 mL/min). Patients who use uricosurics should be instructed to consume adequate fluid intake. Evidence for alkalinization of the urine is limited and not recommended in current guidelines.

24. What is pegloticase and when should its use be considered?

In contrast with other mammals, *Homo sapiens* (and other higher primates) lack uricase, an enzyme which converts uric acid to the more soluble allantoin. Pegloticase is a recombinant mammalian uricase attached to polyethylene glycol (PEGylated). Due to high cost and risk of adverse events (including anaphylaxis), it is recommended for cases with severe disease burden (especially tophaceous burden) and either intolerance of usual ULT or refractory disease despite appropriate dosing of ULT.

25. What are the major risks of pegloticase?

- **Hemolytic anemia and methemoglobinemia in the setting of low G6PD** enzyme activity (deficiency). Screen patients for G6PD deficiency and do not use if deficiency is present.
- **Acute gout flares.** Pegloticase profoundly lowers the uric acid level in 24 hours; without prophylaxis, 80% of patients will suffer an acute gout flare. Start flare prophylaxis (NSAIDs, colchicine, or prednisone) 1 week prior to initial infusion.
- **Infusion reactions** occur in 25% of patients even if uric acid is <6 mg/dL. Incidence increases with longer gaps between infusions.

26. What steps can be taken to decrease the risk of infusion reaction with pegloticase?

- Check serum uric acid prior to each infusion after the initial dose. A serum uric acid level >6 mg/dL while on treatment reflects loss of efficacy due to antibody development— discontinue pegloticase.
- Pegloticase should **not** be used in conjunction with other ULT; it can confound interpretation of uric acid levels
- Pretreatment with each infusion (antihistamines, acetaminophen, and corticosteroids; see Question 14 for a typical pretreatment regimen).
- In the absence of contraindication, consider use of an immunosuppessive agent to decrease the risk of anti-pegloticase antibodies which are associated with infusion reactions including ana-phylaxis (7%). Start methotrexate (15 mg/wk) 4 weeks prior to initial infusion and continue through duration of pegloticase use. Alternative immunosuppressants (e.g., mycophenolate mofetil, azathioprine) may be considered.

BIBLIOGRAPHY

Botson JK, Saag K, Peterson J, et al. A randomized, double-blind, placebo-controlled multicenter efficacy and safety study of methotrexate to increase response rates in patients with uncontrolled gout receiving pegloticase: 12-month findings. *ACR Open Rheumatol.* 2023;5(8):407–418.

Choi H, Neogi T, Stamp L, et al. Implications of the cardiovascular safety of febuxostat and allopurinol in patients with gout and cardiovascular morbidities (CARES) trial and associated FDA public safety alert. *Arthritis Rheumatol.* 2018;70(11):1702–1709.

FitzGerald JD, Dalbeth N, Mikuls T, et al. 2020 American College of Rheumatology guideline for the management of gout. *Arthritis Rheumatol.* 2020;72(6):879–895 Erratum in: *Arthritis Rheumatol.* 2021;73(3):413.

Fralick M, Chen SK, Patorno E, et al. Assessing the risk for gout with sodium-glucose cotransporter-2 inhibitors in patients with type 2 diabetes: a population-based cohort study. *Ann Intern Med.* 2020;172(3):186–194.

Khanna D, Fitzgerald JD, Khanna PP, et al. American College of Rheumatology guidelines for management of gout. Part 1. Systematic nonpharmacologic and pharmacologic therapeutic approaches to hyperuricemia. *Arth Care Res.* 2012;64:1431–1446.

Khanna D, Khanna PP, Fitzgerald JD, et al. American College of Rheumatology guidelines for management of gout. Part 2: therapy and antiinflammatory prophylaxis of acute gouty arthritis. *Arthritis Care Res.* 2012;64:1447–1461.

Stamp LK, Merriman TR, Barclay ML, et al. Impaired response or insufficient dosage? Examining the potential causes of "inadequate response" to allopurinol in the treatment of gout. *Semin Arthritis Rheum.* 2014;44(2):170–174.

Terkeltaub RA, Furst DE, Digiacinto JL, et al. Novel evidence-based colchicine dose-reduction algorithm to predict and prevent colchicine toxicity in the presence of cytochrome P450 3A4/P-glycoprotein inhibitors. *Arthritis Rheum.* 2011;63:2226–2237.

CHAPTER 87

Bone Strengthening Agents

Michael T. McDermott, MD

Treatment without prevention is simply unsustainable.
—Bill Gates

KEY POINTS

1. Nonpharmacological measures that are effective for prevention and treatment of osteoporosis include adequate calcium and vitamin D nutrition, regular exercise, fall prevention, smoking cessation, and limitation of alcohol and caffeine intake.
2. Pharmacological therapy should be initiated in people who have had a fragility fracture, a BMD T-score ≤ −2.5, or a FRAX-derived 10-year risk of ≥3% for hip fractures or ≥20% for other major osteoporosis fractures.
3. There are two primary categories of effective medications for treating osteoporosis: anti-resorptive agents and anabolic agents.
4. Osteonecrosis of the jaw and atypical femoral fractures have been reported in some people using anti-resorptive medications but not anabolic medications.
5. BMD loss during osteoporosis therapy is most often due to therapy nonadherence but affected individuals should also be investigated for other causes of bone loss.
6. Bisphosphonates, teriparatide, and denosumab improve BMD and reduce fractures in people with glucocorticoid (GC)-induced osteoporosis.

1. What nonpharmacologic measures help prevent and treat osteoporosis?

Adequate calcium intake (diet plus supplements):*
    1000—1200 mg/day, premenopausal women and men
    1200—1500 mg/day, postmenopausal women and men ≥age 65 years
Adequate vitamin D intake: 800–1200 IU/day*,†
Regular exercise (30 min, 3–5 times/week): aerobic, strength, flexibility, balance
Limitation of alcohol consumption to ≤2 drinks/day
Limitation of caffeine consumption to ≤2 servings/day
Smoking cessation
Fall prevention, avoid high-impact/twisting motion, do not flop into a chair

2. How can dietary calcium intake be accurately assessed?

The major bioavailable sources are dairy products and calcium-fortified fruit drinks. The following approximate calcium contents should be assigned for dairy product intake:

Milk/Yogurt	300 mg/cup
Cheese	300 mg/oz
Fruit juice with calcium	300 mg/cup

In addition to calcium from dairy, add another 300 mg for the general nondairy diet for a reasonable estimate of total daily calcium intake.

3. How do you ensure adequate intake of calcium?

Low-fat dairy products are the *best* sources of calcium. Calcium supplements should be added when the desired goals cannot be reached with dietary sources. Calcium carbonate and calcium

---

*Taking more than the stated amounts of calcium and vitamin D is not recommended. Higher amounts may be associated with more kidney stones as well as more vascular calcifications, particularly in patients with renal insufficiency.

†Vitamin D3 (cholecalciferol) and vitamin D2 (ergocalciferol) are equivalent when taken on a chronic basis.

citrate are both well absorbed when taken with meals. Gastric acid is needed for normal calcium absorption; calcium carbonate absorption may be significantly reduced in patients who have achlorhydria or who use a proton pump inhibitor (PPI). Calcium citrate absorption is less likely to be affected by PPI use. Calcium citrate is also a better choice in patients with a history of kidney stones, since citric acid is often low in the urine of stone formers. Total calcium intake (dietary + supplements) should not exceed 2000 mg/day chronically.

Note: the addition of magnesium, boron, and vitamin K does not increase the effectiveness of calcium supplementation but does add to cost. Patients on warfarin should be warned to avoid calcium preparations that contain vitamin K (e.g., viactiv). Patients who experience constipation with calcium supplements may benefit from formulations that contain magnesium.

4. What are the best ways to achieve adequate vitamin D intake?

Vitamin D exists in two natural forms: cholecalciferol (D3) and ergocalciferol (D2). Fatty fish (salmon, tuna, mackerel; D3 = 400 IU/3.5 oz), fortified milk (400 IU/quart), and cereal products (50 IU/cup) are good dietary sources. Vitamin D2 and D3 supplements are available over the counter in multiple doses and 50,000 IU vitamin D2 supplements can be given by prescription. Ten minutes of midday summer sunlight exposure to a fair-skinned person in a tank top and shorts not wearing sunscreen produces 10,000 IU of vitamin D3. Dark-skinned individuals and the elderly get less production. However, many individuals wear sunscreen (SPF >8) which prevents vitamin D production by the skin. Therefore, oral vitamin D is necessary for most people. The optimal vitamin D intake is 800–1200 IU daily and should not exceed 4000 IU/day chronically.

5. How do you treat patients with vitamin D deficiency?

The goal serum 25 OH vitamin D level is 30–100 ng/mL. In general, 1000 units (U) daily of vitamin D will raise the serum level by 6–10 ng/mL. I recommend the following:

25 OH D Level	Management
20–30 ng/mL	2000 U D3 daily
10–20 ng/mL	50,000 U D2 weekly for 3 months, then 2000 U D3 daily
≤10 ng/mL	50,000 U D2 twice weekly for 3 months, then 2000 U D3 daily

People with malabsorption syndromes, bowel bypass surgery, severe liver disease, and those who take anti-epileptic drugs may require higher doses. Some may need to be treated with calcitriol. However, noncompliance is the most common reason for persistently low vitamin D levels.

6. Does calcium or vitamin D supplementation promote vascular calcification or coronary artery disease?

The suggestion that calcium and/or vitamin D supplementation promotes calcification of coronary arteries came from several early, small studies that gained significant attention from the lay press. However, subsequent large reviews and meta-analyses demonstrated clearly that the existing published evidence does not support the hypothesis that calcium and/or vitamin D supplementation, in the recommended doses, increases the risk of coronary artery disease (CAD) or CAD mortality. As stated above, however, excessive doses should be avoided especially in patients with renal insufficiency.

7. When should pharmacological therapy be initiated for osteoporosis?

Pharmacological therapy should be advised for high and very high fracture risk patients:
A *high fracture risk* patient is defined as having any *one* of the following:
- History of a fragility fracture (vertebral, hip, wrist, humerus)
- T-Score ≤ −2.5 (at any site)
- FRAX 10 Year Risk ≥3% for hip fracture or ≥20% for major osteoporosis fractures*
- *The FRAX tool (Search Engine: FRAX), developed by the World Health Organization (WHO), is recommended for making treatment decisions in drug-naïve patients over age 40 years with osteopenia on BMD testing.

A *very high fracture risk* patient is defined as having a fragility fracture *plus* a T score ≤ –2.5 (at any site).

Many experts recommend using teriparatide, abaloparatide, or romosozumab as the first therapy in these high/very high fracture risk patients followed by an anti-resorptive.

8. Describe bone remodeling.

Bone remodeling is the process that removes old bone and replaces it with new bone. Osteoclasts attach to bone surfaces and secrete acid and enzymes that dissolve away underlying bone. This resorptive phase takes 3–4 weeks. Osteoblasts then migrate into these resorption pits and secrete osteoid, which becomes mineralized with calcium phosphate crystals (hydroxyapatite). This formative and mineralization phase takes 3 months. Osteocytes serve as the mechanoreceptors that sense skeletal stress and send signals, such as sclerostin, to orchestrate the process of bone remodeling in areas of bone that need renewal (Fig. 87.1).

9. What are RANK, RANK-L, and osteoprotegerin?

RANK (receptor activator of nuclear factor κ) is a specific receptor on osteoclasts. RANK-L (RANK ligand) binds to RANK to stimulate osteoclastic bone resorption. Osteoprotegerin (OPG) is a soluble decoy receptor produced by osteoblasts and bone marrow stromal cells that binds to RANK-L, preventing it from binding to RANK. Bone resorption is driven by RANK-L and inhibited by OPG.

10. How do the pharmacological agents for osteoporosis work?

Osteoporosis medications are classified into two main categories: *anti-resorptive* agents and *anabolic* agents. Anti-resorptive medications include bisphosphonates, denosumab, estrogens, raloxifene, and calcitonin; they inhibit osteoclastic bone resorption. Teriparatide and abaloparatide are anabolic agents; they stimulate osteoblastic bone formation. Romosozumab has both anabolic and anti-resorptive actions.

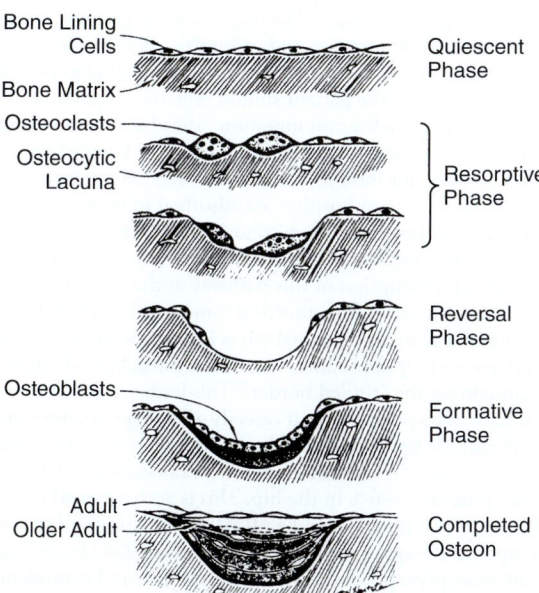

Fig. 87.1 Bone remodeling. Osteoclasts resorb old bone, leaving an empty resorption pit. Osteoblasts then fill the pit by secreting osteoid, which is subsequently mineralized by calcium and phosphate from the extracellular fluid, forming new bone. (From Peck WA, ed. *Bone and Mineral Research Annual 2.* New York: Elsevier. Used with permission.)

11. What pharmacological agents are FDA approved and how are they used?

Mechanism	Route	Dose	Frequency
Anti-Resorptive Agents			
Bisphosphonates			
Alendronate (Fosamax)*	Oral	10 mg	Daily
		70 mg	Weekly
Risedronate (Actonel)	Oral	5 mg	Daily
		35 mg	Weekly
		150 mg	Monthly
Risedronate SR (Atelvia)	Oral	35 mg	Weekly
Ibandronate (Boniva)	Oral	150 mg	Monthly
	IV+	3 mg	Q3 Months
Zoledronic Acid (Reclast)	IV+	5 mg	Yearly
Non-Bisphosphonates			
Denosumab (Prolia)	SQ	60 mg	Q6 Months
Raloxifene (Evista)	Oral	60 mg	Daily
Calcitonin (Miacalcin)	Nasal	200 U	Daily
	SQ	100 U	Daily
Estrogen Therapy (multiple preparations and regimens)			
Anabolic Agents			
Teriparatide (Forteo)	SQ	20 mcg	Daily (prolonged use approved)
Abaloparatide (Tymlos)	SQ	80 mcg	Daily (18–24 months)
Combination Agent			
Romosozumab (Evenity)	SQ	210 mg	Monthly (1 year)

*Note that there is a Fosamax plus D preparation containing 70 mg of alendronate and either 2800 IU or 5600 IU of vitamin D3.
+Infusion times: IV ibandronate 1–3 minutes; IV zoledronic acid 15–60 minutes.

12. Explain how bisphosphonates are taken and why they work for osteoporosis

The oral nitrogenous bisphosphonates are analogs of pyrophosphate that avidly bind to bone. They have very poor intestinal absorption (<1%) that is further inhibited by the presence of food or medications in the gastrointestinal tract. The major side effects are esophageal and gastrointestinal pain. To maximize intestinal absorption and minimize gastrointestinal toxicity, they should be taken first thing in the morning on an empty stomach with a full glass of water on the day they are scheduled to take the medication. The patient should remain upright and take nothing by mouth for at least 30–60 minutes after medication ingestion. The absorbed bisphosphonate goes through the bloodstream and binds to bone with a terminal half-life in bone of up to 10 years. Approximately 50–60% of a dose does not bind to bone and is excreted unchanged in the urine. There are no drug interactions. Some of the bisphosphonate adsorbed to bone is ingested by osteoclasts during bone remodeling. Within the osteoclast, bisphosphonates bind to and block the intracellular enzyme, farnesyl diphosphate synthase (FPPS), in the HMG CoA-reductase pathway (also known as the mevalonate pathway). Disruption of this pathway at the FPPS level prevents the formation of two metabolites that are essential for connecting some small proteins (Ras, Rho, Rac) to the cell membrane, a process known as prenylation, which is important for proper sub-cellular protein trafficking. This interferes with lipid modification of the osteoclast cell membrane/cytoskeleton that is needed for maintaining the "ruffled border." This leads to osteoclast apoptosis, causing significantly reduced bone resorption without directly affecting bone formation. As a result, bone formation temporarily exceeds resorption, and bone mass increases. After about 24 months, bone formation declines to the level of resorption and bone mass stabilizes. Over this time bone mass increases 4–8% in the spine and 3–6% in the hip. This is accompanied by a 33–68% relative risk reduction for incident vertebral fractures and a 40–50% reduction in hip fractures (not with ibandronate) depending upon the bisphosphonate that is studied. Zoledronic acid may be the most effective due to its anti-resorptive potency, IV administration, and compliance.

13. What precautions should be considered before prescribing bisphosphonates?

- Oral bisphosphonates are contraindicated in patients with esophageal problems [strictures, achalasia or severe dysmotility (scleroderma), varices], malabsorption, or inability to sit upright. These are indications for an IV formulation.

- Oral bisphosphonates are contraindicated in patients with an estimated glomerular filtration rate (eGFR) <30–35 cc/min and IV bisphosphonates are contraindicated if eGFR <35–40 cc/min due to renal excretion. Patients with severe stage 3 chronic kidney disease (eGFR 35–40 cc/min) who are receiving IV bisphosphonates should be taken off drugs affecting renal function, if possible (NSAIDs, diuretics), be well hydrated, and have slower infusion rates (ibandronate 15 minutes; zoledronic acid 60 minutes). IV ibandronate is probably safer than IV zoledronic acid due to less effect on renal tissue.
- All planned invasive dental work should be performed prior to starting a bisphosphonate, if possible, to lessen future risk for osteonecrosis of the jaw. It is recommended that providers do an oral examination before starting therapy with bisphosphonates.
- 25OH vitamin D should be >20 (preferably 30) ng/mL before starting bisphosphonate therapy.
- IV bisphosphonates can cause a flu-like illness and bone pain lasting up to 2–3 days in 10% (ibandronate) to 30% (zoledronic acid) of individuals. Premedication with acetaminophen will often prevent or lessen these symptoms.
- Compliance is important. Failure to take a bisphosphonate at least 70% of the time significantly decreases its fracture protection.
- Bone mineral density increase is less with low turnover and perimenopausal patients.
- Fracture protection has not been proven in osteopenic patients especially those aged less than 65. FRAX can help determine the need for therapy.
- Bisphosphonates are contraindicated in women who are pregnant or breastfeeding due to unknown effects on the developing skeleton. In the rare person who requires a bisphosphonate and may want to get pregnant in the future, risedronate may be the safest to use due to more rapid clearance from the blood after it is stopped. However, risedronate should be stopped 6 months prior to getting pregnant.
- Unusual side effects from bisphosphonates: ocular symptoms including uveitis, keratitis, optic neuritis, and orbital swelling have been reported.

14. What is denosumab and how does it work in osteoporosis?

Denosumab is a monoclonal antibody directed against RANK-L. It interferes with the ability of osteoblasts (and other cells with RANK-L on their surface) to bind to RANK and stimulate osteoclastic bone resorption. Denosumab is given in a clinic or an infusion center at a dose of 60 mg subcutaneously (SC) every 6 months. This medication is well tolerated although there is a potential concern that infections could be increased, since RANK-L is also on T helper cells and involved in dendritic cell activation. In trials, denosumab increased lumbar spine bone mass by 6.5% and hip mass by 3.5%. This was accompanied by a 68% reduction in vertebral and 40% reduction in hip fractures over 3 years. Denosumab is cleared by the reticuloendothelial system and can thus be used in osteoporotic patients with Class 4 CKD (eGFR 15–30 cc/min) although *there is an increased risk of hypocalcemia* for one week after administration in patients with significant renal insufficiency. As with bisphosphonates, any planned invasive dental work (extractions, implants) should be done prior to starting denosumab or a week prior to the next dose, if possible, to reduce the risk for osteonecrosis of the jaw. It also is recommended that providers do an oral examination before starting therapy with denosumab.

15. What happens when denosumab is stopped and what precautions are recommended?

Discontinuation of denosumab has been reported to result in rapid bone loss and, in some patients, the development of multiple vertebral fractures. For this reason, if denosumab therapy is stopped after at least 2 doses, it is recommended that bisphosphonate therapy be started; if an oral bisphosphonate is used, it should be started 6 months after the last denosumab injection, whereas if IV Zoledronic acid is chosen, it should be given 6–9 months after the last denosumab injection.

16. What is osteonecrosis of the jaw (ONJ) and which medications may cause it?

ONJ presents as persistently exposed nonhealing bone following an invasive dental procedure (extractions and implants); it does not occur after root canal procedures, fillings, and dental cleaning. It has been reported mainly in people on strong anti-resorptive medications (bisphosphonates or denosumab) and does not occur with anabolic bone agents. ONJ develops most often during high-dose, frequent administration of anti-resorptive agents for the treatment of multiple myeloma or bone metastases; however, it has also been reported, though much less often (0.01–0.15%/year), in people taking anti-resorptive agents for osteoporosis. Good oral hygiene and regular dental care are the best preventive measures. As discussed above, an oral exam should be done by the prescribing provider prior to starting an anti-resorptive medication. Temporarily stopping anti-resorptive therapy for invasive dental procedures (3 months prior) is a common and reasonable practice but has not been proven to prevent ONJ. Some oral surgeons require a serum C-telopeptide to be in the normal range before they will do surgery.

17. What about atypical femoral fractures with anti-resorptive medication use?

Atypical femoral fractures (AFF) have been reported in people being treated with anti-resorptive agents (1:1000 treated patients). Anabolic agents have not been implicated as causing AFF. AFF has very rarely occurred in patients treated with romosozumab which has both anabolic and anti-resorptive effects. The absolute risk of AFF increases with duration of bisphosphonate use being 2, 20, and 100/100,000 patient-years after 2, 5, and 10 years on therapy. The relative risk is increased 9x in patients who have received bisphosphonates for 3–5 years and 44x in patients on bisphosphonates over 8 years. Any such person with unexplained thigh pain should be evaluated with a radiograph looking for a "bird-beak" on the lateral aspect of the femoral shaft indicating a stress fracture (see Fig. 87.2). These fractures are frequently bilateral (30%) and require femoral rods to stabilize. The risk appears increased in physically active patients, females, Asians, those on glucocorticoids, and those with very low bone turnover markers. AFF have less commonly been reported in patients treated with denosumab. However, they can occur particularly in patients previously treated with long-term bisphosphonates before switching to denosumab.

Currently, no data exist regarding preventive measures. However, after 5 years of oral bisphosphonate or 3 years of IV zoledronic acid use, many providers recommend a 1–3-year drug holiday for people whose BMD has risen into the osteopenic range or a temporary switch to an anabolic for people with previous fragility fractures or very low BMD. A drug holiday decreases the risk for AFF by 70% per year. Drug holidays are not recommended for denosumab because of the rapid bone loss and vertebral fractures that have been reported after its discontinuation.

18. Briefly discuss the issues regarding hormone replacement therapy.

The Women's Health Initiative (WHI) report in 2002 confirmed the efficacy of estrogen replacement therapy (ERT) and hormone replacement therapy (HRT; estrogen plus progesterone) for prevention of fractures but also confirmed a previously reported increased risk of breast cancer and

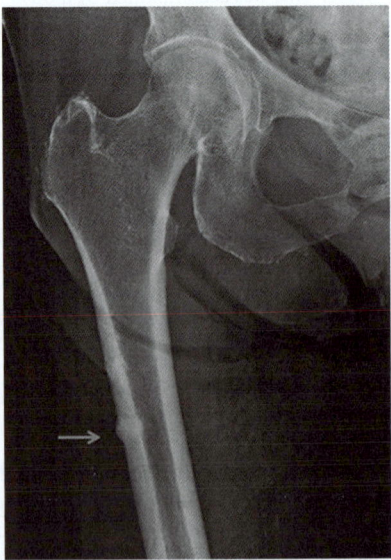

Fig. 87.2 Atypical femoral fracture (*arrow*) with bisphosphonate use.

cardiovascular events. After this report, the use of ERT and HRT significantly decreased. Subsequent studies have cast significant doubt on the risk of these adverse events with ERT and HRT, especially ERT. Currently, ERT (women without an intact uterus) and HRT (women with an intact uterus) are recommended mainly for limited use for up to 3 years to treat postmenopausal hot flashes.

19. Discuss selective estrogen receptor modulators (SERMS) for the management of osteoporosis.

Selective estrogen receptor modulators (SERMS) are agents that function as estrogen agonists in some tissues (bone) and estrogen antagonists in other tissues (breast). **Raloxifene (Evista)** is a SERM that has been shown to improve bone mass and to reduce spine fractures; it is FDA approved for the treatment of postmenopausal osteoporosis. Raloxifene has also been shown to reduce the risk (76%) of developing invasive breast cancer. The dose is 60 mg daily. Side effects include hot flashes, leg cramps, and an increased risk of thromboembolic disease (especially in smokers) similar to that seen with HRT. Raloxifene increases BMD by 2–3% in the spine and hip while reducing the relative risk of vertebral fractures by 31–49% without an effect on hip fracture reduction. An ideal person to receive raloxifene is an osteoporosis patient with a personal or family history of breast cancer. It can also be used in osteoporotic patients with CKD although little data are available to support its efficacy in this group.

20. How can PTH and PTHrP be anabolic agents for treating osteoporosis?

Persistently elevated serum parathyroid hormone (PTH) levels (hyperparathyroidism) or parathyroid hormone-related peptide (PTHrP) levels promote osteoclastic bone resorption, hypercalcemia and bone loss. In contrast, intermittent daily pulses of exogenous PTH or PTHrP, by promoting WNT signaling, actually stimulate osteoblast differentiation, proliferation, and survival, resulting in osteoid formation and increased bone mass. They also decrease the production of the bone_inhibiting protein, sclerostin, from osteocytes.

21. How effective are the currently available anabolic bone agents?

Teriparatide is a 34-amino acid fragment of intact PTH that retains the ability to bind to and activate PTH receptors on osteoblasts and osteoblast precursors. It is self-administered as a 20 mcg SC injection daily for 18–24 months. In trials, teriparatide increased lumbar spine BMD by 9–13% and hip BMD by 2.5–5% while decreasing the relative risk of new vertebral fractures by 65% and nonvertebral fractures by 50%. Side effects are similar to placebo and include headache, nausea, arthralgias, orthostasis, and flushing. Teriparatide must be refrigerated for the duration of its use; it becomes inactivated if left unrefrigerated for over 24 hours. Teriparatide was recently approved for prolonged use beyond 2 years during a patient's lifetime. This should be considered in:

- High fracture risk patients (see question #7) whose P1NP level remains above the upper limits after 2 years on teriparatide.
- High fracture risk patients with multiple vertebral compression fractures (VCF) at baseline but none while on teriparatide
- Patients with adynamic renal bone disease
- Severe COPD patients with VCF
- Very high fracture-risk patients unable to come off glucocorticoids

Abaloparatide is a 34 amino acid fragment of PTHrP that also activates osteoblast recruitment and activity. It is self-administered as an 80 mcg SC injection daily for 18–24 months. Spine BMD has been shown to increase by 10.4% and hip BMD by 4% compared to placebo. In a head-to-head trial against teriparatide, abaloparatide reduced new vertebral fractures by 86%, nonvertebral fractures by 43%, and major osteoporosis fractures by 70% (the reduction in major osteoporosis fractures was statistically significantly better than teriparatide). Side effects are similar to those reported with teriparatide. Abaloparatide does not require refrigeration. Abaloparatide is currently limited to 24 months of use but is likely to get a change to its label similar to teriparatide in the future.

22. What precautions should be considered prior to prescribing teriparatide or abaloparatide?

- Teriparatide and abaloparatide are contraindicated in people at increased risk for osteosarcomas: Paget's disease, unexplained alkaline phosphatase elevation, children and young adults with open epiphyses, prior external beam or implant radiation therapy involving the skeleton.

- In people without contraindications, teriparatide does not cause an increased risk of osteo-sarcomas compared to general population (1: 250,000). Data on osteosarcoma in adults on long-term abaloparatide therapy is not yet available.
- Use in patients with skeletal metastases and myeloma is contraindicated.
- May cause hypercalcemia (digoxin toxicity, kidney stones) and hyperuricemia (gout).
- Expensive. They are cost effective when used in patients at highest risk for osteoporotic fractures (T score < −2.5 to −3.0 with history of fragility fracture; T score ≤ −3.0) or in patients who develop a fragility fracture while on an oral bisphosphonate.
- Teriparatide and abaloparatide can promote healing of stress fractures (especially sacral, pelvic), nonunion fractures, ONJ and AFF. However, this is not an FDA-approved use for these agents.
- Teriparatide and abaloparatide should not be used concurrently with an anti-resorptive agent. Blunting of the anabolic response has been demonstrated in people who have previously received prolonged alendronate therapy prior to starting teriparatide. This blunting was not apparent when teriparatide was used concurrently with zoledronic acid or denosumab. However, fracture reduction efficacy has not yet been demonstrated with combination therapy.
- A PTH level should be checked prior to use of anabolic bone drugs. If elevated, secondary causes (vitamin D deficiency) should be corrected to normalize the PTH level. The benefit of teriparatide and abaloparatide in people with persistent mild PTH elevations is unclear but many experts feel it can still be effective. It can be used with severe kidney disease but the effectiveness in these people (who frequently have an elevated PTH) is unknown but felt to be useful if the PTH level is less than 150 pg/mL.
- After treatment with teriparatide or abaloparatide, an anti-resorptive agent should be started to preserve the gains in bone mass. Otherwise, bone mass declines significantly after these agents are stopped.

23. What is romosozumab and how does it work?

Romosozumab is a monoclonal antibody directed against sclerostin, an intrinsic inhibitor of the WNT pathway that stimulates bone formation. By inhibiting the inhibitor (sclerostin) of bone formation, romosozumab stimulates bone formation and therefore is an anabolic agent. Through other less clear mechanisms, it also inhibits bone resorption resulting in dual anabolic and anti-resorptive activity. Romosozumab is administered in an infusion center or office as a 210 mg SC total dose (two 105 mg injections) once every month for 1 year.

Compared to placebo, romosozumab increased BMD by 12.7% in the lumbar spine, 5.8% in the total hip, 5.2% in the femoral neck, and reduced vertebral fractures by 73%. The most common side effects in clinical trials were joint pain and headaches. Allergic reactions can occur. Serum calcium levels often decrease transiently after administration. Both ONJ and AFF have been reported with romosozumab. Serious adverse events in clinical trials included strokes, myocardial infarctions and cardiovascular deaths. As a result, it is recommended that romosozumab be avoided in people who have had a stroke or major cardiovascular event within the past year and in those at high risk of stroke or cardiovascular disease.

24. Discuss the role of testosterone for the treatment of osteoporosis.

Men with osteoporosis and symptoms of hypogonadism may benefit from testosterone replacement therapy (TRT), especially if the serum testosterone level is less than 150 ng/dL. Testosterone replacement increases bone mass in men with baseline low testosterone levels but there has been no fracture reduction data reported; for this reason, it is not an FDA-approved treatment for osteoporosis.

Testosterone cypionate or enanthate can be administered intramuscularly (IM) (100–400 mg every 1–4 weeks; lower doses at more frequent intervals are preferred), as a transdermal patch (AndroDerm) or gel (Testim, AndroGel, Fortesta, Axiron, Vogelxo), as a buccal patch (Striant), testosterone undecanoate (oral or IM) or testosterone pellets. We do not recommend injectable testosterone pellets because supraphysiological testosterone levels often result from this therapy. TRT has not been shown to cause prostate cancer but has clearly been shown to increase the risk of growth of existing prostate cancer. TRT can also precipitate or worsen sleep apnea. The TRAVERSE study, a large multi-center randomized controlled trial of TRT in hypogonadal men with pre-existing or a high risk of cardiovascular disease, reported in 2023 that physiologic testosterone doses do not promote the development of cardiovascular disease. Patients without improvement in hypogonadal symptoms should not continue testosterone as other therapies for osteoporosis are more beneficial.

25. Have all of these medications been shown to prevent fractures?

The FDA-approved medications have all been demonstrated in randomized controlled trials (RCTs) to significantly reduce vertebral fractures in women with postmenopausal osteoporosis. Hip fractures have also been reduced by alendronate, risedronate, zoledronic acid, and denosumab. Nonvertebral fracture reduction has been reported with alendronate, risedronate, zoledronic acid, denosumab, teriparatide, and abaloparatide. As discussed, there is no fracture prevention data for testosterone replacement therapy.

26. Should osteoporosis medications be used in combination?

No, not yet. Combining anti-resorptive medications should be avoided because of concerns about excessively suppressing bone remodeling. Combining anabolic and anti-resorptive medications is an appealing notion with emerging clinical trial data. The combination of teriparatide and alendronate had no synergy and resulted in inferior bone mass increases compared with teriparatide alone. In contrast, teriparatide combined with zoledronic acid or with denosumab did show synergy in regard to improvements in bone density. Despite these promising results, combination therapy is not currently recommended because there are no data showing superior fracture reduction compared to monotherapy. Furthermore, the cost of using combinations is certainly additive and may cause significant problems with insurance coverage. While combination therapy is not recommended, sequential therapy is clearly beneficial in many patients and is supported by a strong evidence base. Leaders in the field suggest that patients with severe osteoporosis may have maximal benefit by receiving anabolic therapy first, followed by an anti-resorptive agent.

27. Summarize the benefits and risks of pharmacological osteoporosis medications.

Benefits
　　Fracture Reduction (significant for all FDA-approved agents)
Risks
　　Common Side Effects
　　　　Upper GI Symptoms – oral bisphosphonates
　　　　Acute Phase Reactions – IV bisphosphonates (1st dose)
　　　　Transient decrease in serum calcium – zoledronic acid, denosumab, romosozumab
　　　　Transient increase in serum and urine calcium – teriparatide, abaloparatide
　　Uncommon / Rare Side Effects
　　　　Osteonecrosis of the Jaw – anti-resorptive agents
　　　　Atypical Femoral Fractures – anti-resorptive agents
　　　　Uveitis, Keratitis, Optic Neuritis, Orbital Swelling – bisphosphonates
　　　　Hypercalcemia – teriparatide, abaloparatide
　　　　Stroke, Myocardial Infarction – romosozumab

28. Describe a recommended risk stratification strategy for approaching osteoporosis therapy.

Low/Moderate-Risk Patients
　　Oral Bisphosphonates (alendronate, risedronate, ibandronate)
　　Zoledronic Acid
　　Denosumab
High-Risk Patients*
　　Zoledronic Acid
　　Denosumab
　　Teriparatide
　　Abaloparatide
　　Romosozumab

---

*High-risk Patients: old age, prior fracture, very low BMD, high fall risk, glucocorticoid use. In high-risk patients, use an anabolic agent before an anti-resorptive agent.

29. What is the optimum duration of treatment with osteoporosis medications?

Oral Bisphosphonates

    5 years (low/moderate risk patients)

    6–10 years (high-risk patients*)

Zoledronic Acid

    3 years (low/moderate risk patients)

    6 years (high-risk patients*)

Denosumab – stopping is not recommended without substituting another agent.

Teriparatide – approved for long-term use (>24 months lifetime). Best if used long term in high-risk fracture patients whose serum P1NP remains >ULN while on teriparatide. Stopping is not recommended without substituting another agent.

    Abaloparatide – 18–24 months. Stopping is not recommended without substituting another agent.

    Romosozumab – 12 months. Stopping is not recommended without substituting another agent.

30. Should patients on osteoporosis medications be given a drug holiday? If so, how long should the drug holiday last?

Bisphosphonates are the only osteoporosis medication class for which a drug holiday should be considered. Drug holidays are not recommended with denosumab, teriparatide, abaloparatide, or romosozumab for reasons stated above; if and when these medications are stopped, another agent should be substituted.

Bisphosphonate drug holidays may be considered after a person has had the optimum duration of treatment (see previous question). Bisphosphonate drug holidays should end under the following circumstances:

- Fragility fracture (spine, hip, wrist, humerus) occurs.
- Bone density decreases more than the least significant change (LSC) established for that specific instrument (see question #32).
- Bone turnover markers (urine n-telopeptide, serum c-telopeptide, serum bone-specific alkaline phosphatase) increase by ≥30% or rise into the upper 50% of the reference range.

31. How should bone mineral density (BMD) testing be used to monitor the response to osteoporosis therapy?

BMD testing to monitor osteoporosis therapy responses is most often repeated after 1–2 years of treatment. To accurately interpret serial changes, BMD should be measured on the same instrument and the least significant change (LSC) for that specific instrument must be known. The LSC is a precision estimate that informs the user about the minimum BMD change that should be considered significant. Standard procedures for performing the LSC assessment are available on the International Society for Clinical Densitometry website, www.iscd.org.

32. How do you interpret BMD changes in patients on osteoporosis medications?

BMD Change	Interpretation	Recommended Action
Increase ≥ LSC	Good Response	Continue Therapy
No Change or < LSC	Adequate Response	Continue Therapy
Decrease ≥ LSC	Treatment Failure	Evaluate; Consider Therapy Change

33. What markers are available to assess bone remodeling and how are they used?

Bone Formation	Bone Resorption
Serum Alkaline Phosphatase	Urine or Serum N-telopeptides NTX)
Serum Osteocalcin	Serum C-telopeptides (CTX)
Serum P1NP	

An increase in P1NP by 10 mcg/L after initiation of an anabolic agent predicts an increase in bone mass. A 30% reduction of bone resorption biomarkers after anti-resorptive therapy is initiated

---

*High-risk Patients: old age, prior fracture, very low BMD, high fall risk, glucocorticoid use. Due to risk of AFF with prolonged use, consider switching to an anabolic rather than continuing long-term bisphosphonate therapy.

verifies compliance and predicts an increase in bone mass. A serum CTX <312 ng/L indicates good control. However, marked variability in biomarker measurement limits the utility of this tool.

34. What constitutes a treatment failure to osteoporosis therapy?

This is controversial because no treatment completely eliminates the risk of fractures, since these people are already at high risk. **Falls are the major reason for fracture while on therapy**. Therefore, exercise and other measures to reduce the number of falls is as important as medications to treat osteoporosis. At best, pharmacologic therapy can reduce the risk of fracture following a fall by 50%.

Currently suggested criteria to define treatment failure are (any of these, while on treatment):
1. Development of two or more fragility fractures
2. Decrease in BMD by more than the LSC on the same DXA machine.
3. Increase in bone remodeling biomarkers by 30% or into the upper half of the reference range.

35. What do you do when BMD falls significantly during osteoporosis therapy?

The common causes of BMD loss on treatment and their management are listed below.

Cause	Management
Nonadherence →	Encourage Adherence
Calcium Deficiency →	Adequate Calcium Intake
Vitamin D Deficiency →	Adequate Vitamin D Intake
Secondary Bone Loss →	Treat the Cause
Treatment Failure →	Change Medication

36. Which medications are effective in preventing and treating glucocorticoid-induced osteoporosis (GIOP)?

Bisphosphonates (alendronate, risedronate, zoledronic acid), denosumab, and teriparatide have been shown in randomized controlled trials to significantly improve BMD and reduce fractures in glucocorticoid-treated people. They are instituted based on FRAX risk assessment score (high, medium, low), T score, history of fragility fracture, and age.

37. What are the costs for osteoporosis medications?

The table shows wholesale acquisition costs (WAC) from the two sources cited below and the nondiscounted retail costs for multiple pharmacies were obtained from GoodRx.

Drug	WAC $/Month	Retail $/Month
• Alendronate (generic)	21	11.97–48.07
• Alendronate (Fosamax)	129	165.00–191.00
• Fosamax plus D	173	185.78–228.33
• Alendronate effervescent (Bonisto)	300	309.62–339.55
• Risedronate (generic)	166	55.15–190.90
• Risedronate (Actonel)	369	434.00–478.00
• Risedronate DR (Atelvia)	267	192.00–227.00
• Ibandronate (generic)	10	24.49–104.54
• Ibandronate (Boniva)	115	226.00–281.33
• Zoledronic Acid (Reclast)	1,084/yr[a]	1,300–1,500/yr[a]
• Denosumab (Prolia)	2,558/yr[a]	3,249.08/yr[a]
• Raloxifene (generic)	60	13.85–67.33
• Raloxifene (Evista)	198	185.67–207.69
• Calcitonin (generic)	75	29.54–89.99
• Teriparatide (generic)	2,475	3,306.00–5,124.00
• Teriparatide (Forteo)	3,598	6,578.00
• Abaloparatide (Tymlos)	1,966	4,372.00
• Romosozumab (Evenity)	1,825	2,434.36[a]

[a]Additional administration costs for infusion center or office.

From Crandall C. Pharmacotherapy for postmenopausal osteoporosis. *JAMA.* 2021;325:1888–1889 and No Authors Listed. Drugs for postmenopausal osteopororis. *Med Lett Drugs Ther.* 2020;62(1602):105–112.

38. What new and emerging osteoporosis therapies are in development?

- Anti-resorptive drugs
  - New SERMs: lasofoxifene, bazedoxifene, arzoxifene
- Osteoanabolic drugs
  - Teriparatide: transdermal, intranasal
  - Abaloparatide: transdermal
  - Calcilytic (stimulates endogenous PTH release): ronacaleret
  - Tryptophan hydroxylase 1 (Tph 1) inhibitor: inhibit gut-derived serotonin

39. Develop an algorithm for the diagnosis and management of osteoporosis

See Fig. 87.3.

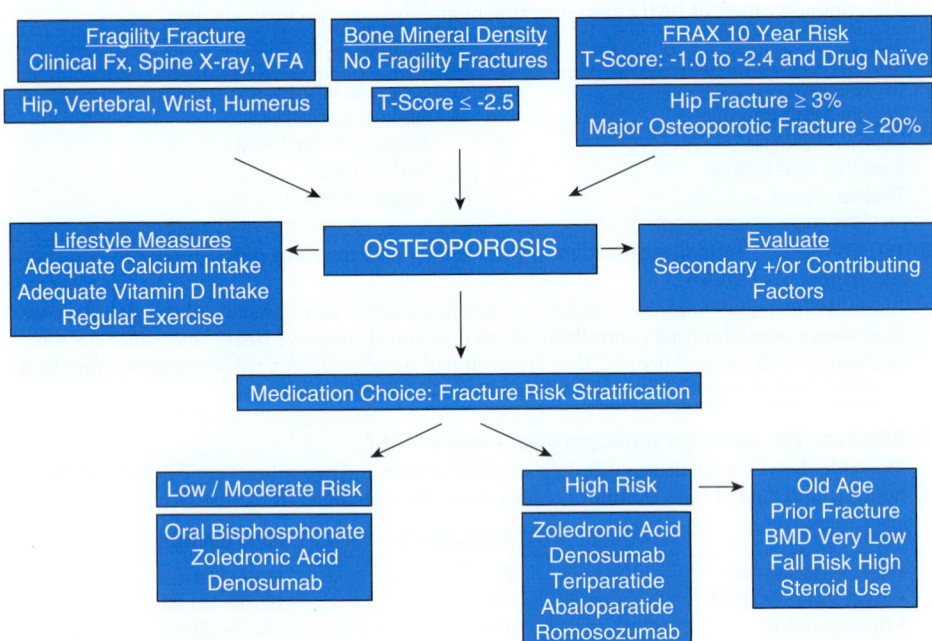

Fig. 87.3 Osteoporosis diagnosis and management. *High-Risk Patients: old age, prior fracture, very low BMD, high fall risk, glucocorticoid use. Use anabolic agent before anti-resorptive agent when possible.

BIBLIOGRAPHY

Adler RA, Fuleihan GE-H, Bauer DC, et al. Managing osteoporosis in patients on long-term bisphosphonate treatment: report of a task force of the American Society for Bone and Mineral Research. *J Bone Min Res.* 2016;31:16–35.

Adler RA. Management of endocrine disease: atypical femoral fractures: risks and benefits of long-term treatment of osteoporosis with anti-resorptive therapy. *Eur J Endocrinol.* 2018;178:R81–R87.

Albert SG, Wood E. Meta-analysis of clinical fracture risk reduction of antiosteoporosis drugs: direct and indirect comparisons and meta-regressions. *Endocr Pract.* 2021;27:1082–1092.

Anastasilakis AD, Polyzos SA, Makras P, et al. Clinical features of 24 patients with rebound-associated vertebral fractures after denosumab discontinuation: systematic review and additional cases. *J Bone Min Res.* 2017;32:1291–1296.

Axelsson KF, Nilsson AG, Wedel H, et al. Association between alendronate use and hip fracture risk in older patients using oral prednisolone. *JAMA.* 2017;318:146–155.

Ayers C, Kansagara D, Lazur B, et al. Effectiveness and safety of treatments to prevent fractures in people with low bone mass or primary osteoporosis: a living systematic review and network meta-analysis for the American College of Physicians. *Ann Intern Med.* 2023;176:182–195.

Bindon B, Adams W, Balasubramanian N, et al. Osteoporosis fractures during bisphosphonate drug holidays. *Endocr Pract*. 2018;24:163–169.

Black DM, Rosen CJ. Postmenopausal osteoporosis. *N Engl J Med*. 2016;374:254–262.

Bone HG, Wagman RB, Brandi ML, et al. 10 years of denosumab treatment in postmenopausal women with osteoporosis: results from the phase 3 randomized FREEDOM trial and open label extension. *Lancet Diabet Endocrinol*. 2017;5:513–523.

Bonnick S, Johnston CC, Kleerekoper M, et al. Importance of precision in bone density measurements. *J Clin Densitometry*. 2001;4:1–6.

Buckley L, Guyatt G, Fink HA, et al. 2017 American College of Rheumatology guideline for the prevention and treatment of glucocorticoid-induced osteoporosis. *Arthritis Rheumatol*. 2017;69:1521–1537.

Burckhardt P, Faouzi M, Buclin T, Lamy Othe Swiss Denosumab Study Group. Fractures after denosumab discontinuation: a retrospective study of 797 cases. *J Bone Min Res*. 2021;36:1717–1728.

Camacho PM, Petak SM, Binkley N, et al. American Association of Clinical Endocrinologists and American College of Endocrinology clinical practice guidelines for the diagnosis and treatment of postmenopausal osteoporosis—2016. *Endocr Pract*. 2016;22(suppl. 4):1–42.

Chapurlat R. Effects and management of denosumab discontinuation. *Joint Bone Spine*. 2018;85:515–517.

Chung M, Tang AM, Fu Z, Wang DD, Newberry SJ. Calcium intake and cardiovascular disease risk: an updated systematic review and meta-analysis. *Ann Intern Med*. 2016;165:856–866.

Cosman F, Crittenden DB, Adachi JD, et al. Romosozumab treatment in postmenopausal women with osteoporosis. *N Engl J Med*. 2016;375:1532–1543.

Cosman F, Miller PD, Williams CG, et al. Eighteen months of treatment with subcutaneous abaloparatide followed by 6 months of treatment with alendronate in postmenopausal women with osteoporosis: resultys of the ACTIVExtend trial. *Mayo Clin Proc*. 2017;92:200–210.

Cosman F, Nieves JW, Dempster DW. Treatment sequence matters: anabolic and antiresorptive therapy for osteoporosis. *J Bone Min Res*. 2017;32:198–202.

Cosman F, Crittenden DB, Adachi JD, et al. Romosozumab treatment of postmenopausal women with osteoporosis. *N Engl J Med*. 2016;375:1532–1543.

Cotts KG, Cifu AS. Treatment of osteoporosis. *JAMA*. 2018;319:1040–1041.

Crandall CJ, Newberry SJ, Diamant A, et al. Comparative effectiveness of pharmacologic treatments to prevent fractures: an updated systematic review. *Ann Intern Med*. 2014;161:711–723.

Crandall C. Pharmacotherapy for postmenopausal osteoporosis. *JAMA*. 2021;325:1888–1889.

Cummings SR, Cosman F, Lewiecki EM, et al. Goal-directed treatment for osteoporosis: a progress report from the ASBMR-NOF Working Group on Goal-Directed Treatment for Osteoporosis. *J Bone Min Res*. 2017;32:3–10.

Cummings SR, Ferrari S, Eastell R, et al. Vertebral fractures after discontinuation of denosumab: a post hoc analysis of the randomized placebo-controlled FREEDOM trial and its extension. *J Bone Min Res*. 2018;33:190–197.

Dawson-Hughes B, Bischoff-Ferrari HA. Therapy of osteoporosis with calcium and vitamin D. *J Bone Min Res*. 2007;22:V59–V63.

Eastell R, Szulc P. Use of bone turnover markers in postmenopausal osteoporosis. Osteoporosis treatment: recent developments and ongoing challenges. *Lancet Diabetes Endocrinol*. 2017;5:908–923.

Grassi G, Chiodini I, Palmieri S, et al. Bisphosphonates after denosumab withdrawal reduced the vertebral fractures incidence. *Eur J Endocrinol*. 2021;185:387–396.

Holick MF. Vitamin D deficiency. *N Engl J Med*. 2007;357:266–281.

Kendler DL, Marin F, Zerbini CAF, et al. Effects of teriparatide and risedronate on new fractures in post-menopausal women with severe osteoporosis (VERO): a multicentre, double-blind, double-dummy, randomised controlled trial. *Lancet*. 2018;391:230–240.

Khan AA, Morrison A, Hanley DA, et al. Diagnosis and management of osteonecrosis of the jaw: a systematic review and international consensus. *J Bone Min Res*. 2015;30:3–23.

Kosla S, Hofbauer L. Osteoporosis treatment: recent developments and ongoing challenges. *Lancet Diabetes Endocrinol*. 2017;5:898–907.

Langdahl BL, Libanati C, Crittenden DB, et al. Romosozumab (sclerostin monoclonal antibody) versus teriparatide in postmenopausal women with osteoporosis transitioning from oral bisphosphonate therapy: a randomised, open-label, phase 3 trial. *Lancet*. 2017;390:1585–1594.

Leboff MS, Greenspan SL, Insogna KL, et al. The clinician's guide to prevention and treatment of osteoporosis. *Osteoporos Int*. 2022;33:2049–2102.

Leder BZ, O'Dee LS, Zanchetta JR, et al. Effects of abaloparatide, a human parathyroid hormone-related peptide analog, on bone mineral density in postmenopausal women with osteoporosis. *J Clin Endocrinol Metab*. 2015;100:697–706.

Leder BZ, Tsai JN, Uihlein AV, et al. Two years of denosumab and teriparatide administration in postmenopausal women with osteoporosis (the DATA Extension Study): a randomized controlled trial. *J Clin Endocrinol Metab*. 2014;99:1694–1700.

Leder BZ, Tsai JN, Uihlein AV, et al. Denosumab and teriparatide transitions in postmenopausal osteoporosis (the DATA-Switch study): extension of a randomized controlled trial. *Lancet*. 2015;336:1147–1155.

Lewiecki EM. Nonresponders to osteoporosis therapy. *J Clin Densitometry*. 2003;6:307–314.

Lewiecki M, Cummings SR, Cosman F. Treat-to-target for osteoporosis: is now the time? *J Clin Endocrinol Metab*. 2013;98:946–953.

Lewis JR, Radavelli-Bagatini S, Rejnmark L, et al. The effects of calcium supplementation on verified coronary heart diseas hospitalization and death in postmenopausal women: a collaborative meta-analysis of randomized controlled trials. *J Bone Min Res.* 2015;30:165–175.

Lincoff AM, Bhasin S, Flevaris P, et al. Cardiovascular safety of testosterone replacement therapy. *N Engl J Med.* 2023;389:107–117.

Lloyd AA, Gludovatz B, Riedel C, et al. Atypical fracture with long-term bisphosphonate therapy is associated with altered cortical composition and reduced fracture resistance. *Proc Natl Acad Sci USA.* 2017;114:8722–8727.

Long F. Building stronger bones: molecular regulation of the osteoblast lineage. *Nat Rev Mol Cell Biol.* 2011;13:27–38.

Malouf-Sierra J, Tarantino U, García-Hernández PA, et al. Effect of teriparatide or risedronate in elderly patients with a recent per-trochanteric hip fracture: final results of a 78-week randomized clinical trial. *J Bone Miner Res.* 2017;32:1040–1051.

Marie PJ, Cohen-Solal M. The expanding life and functions of osteogenic cells: from simple bone-making cells to multifunctional cells and beyond. *J Bone Min Res.* 2018;33:199–210.

McClung MR, Lewiecki EM, Geller ML, et al. Effect of denosumab on bone mineral density and biochemical markers of bone turnover: 8 year results of a phase 2 clinical trial. *Osteoporos Int.* 2013;24:227–235.

McClung MR. Cancel the denosumab holiday. *Osteoporos Int.* 2016;27:1677–1682.

McClung MR, Wagman RB, Miller PD, Wang A, Lewiecki EM. Observations following discontinuation of long-term denosumab therapy. *Osteoporos Int.* 2017;28:1723–1732.

McClung MR. Clinical utility of anti-sclerostin antibodies. *Bone.* 2017;96:3–7.

McClung MR. Using osteoporosis therapies in combination. *Curr Osteoporos Rep.* 2017;15:343–352.

Miller PD, Pannacciulli N, Brown JP, et al. Denosumab or zoledronic acid in postmenopausal women with osteoporosis previously treated with oral bisphosphonates. *J Clin Endocrinol Metab.* 2016;101:3163–3170.

Miller PD, Hattersley G, Riis BJ, et al. Effect of abaloparatide vs placebo on new vertebral fractures in postmenopausal women with osteoporosis: a randomized clinical trial (ACTIVE trial). *JAMA.* 2016;316:722–733.

Miller PD, Lewiecki EM, Krohn K, Schwartz E. Teriparatide: label changes and identifying patients for long-term use. *Clev Clinic J Med.* 2021;88:489–493.

No Authors Listed. Drugs for postmenopausal osteopororis. *Med Lett Drugs Ther.* 2020;62(1602):105–112.

Olivier L, Gonzalez-Rodriguez E, Stoli D, Hans D, Aubry-Rozier B. Severe rebound-associated vertebral fractures after denosumab discontinuation: 9 clinical cases report. *J Clin Endocrinol Metab.* 2017;102:354–358.

Park-Wyllie L, Mamdani MM, Juurink DN, et al. Bisphosphonate use and the risk of subtrochanteric or femoral shaft fractures in older women. *JAMA.* 2011;305:783–789.

Qaseem A, Forciea MA, McLean RM, Denberg TD. Treatment of low bone density or osteoporosis to prevent fractures in men and women: a clinical practice guideline update from the American College of Physicians. *Ann Intern Med.* 2017;166:818–839.

Qasseem A, Hicks LA, Etxeandia-Ikobaltzeta I, et al. Pharmacologic treatment of primary osteoporosis or low bone mass to prevent fractures in adults: a living clinical guideline from the American College of Physicians. *Ann Inter Med.* 2023;176:224–238.

Rothman MS, Lewiecki EM, Miller PD. Bone density testing is the best way to monitor osteoporosis. *Am J Med.* 2017;130:1133–1134.

Ruggiero SL, Dodson TB, Fantasia L, et al. American Association of Oral and Maxillofacial Surgeons position paper on medication-related osteonecrosis of the jaw—2014 update. *J Oral Maxillofac Surg.* 2014;72:1938–1956.

Saag KG, Petersen J, Brandi ML. Romosozumab or alendronate for fracture prevention in women with osteoporosis (EVENITY). *N Engl J Med.* 2017;377:1417–1427.

Shane E, Burr D, Abrahamsen B, et al. Atypical subtrochanteric and diaphyseal femoral fractures: second report of a task force of the American Society for Bone and Mineral Research. *J Bone Min Res.* 2014;29:1–23.

Singh S, Dutta S, Khasbage S, et al. A systematic review and meta-analysis of efficacy and safety of romosozumab. *Osteoporos Int.* 2022;33:1–12.

Wu C-H, Li C-C, Hsu Y-U, et al. Comparisons between different anti-osteoporosis medications on postfracture mortality: a population based study. *J Clin Endocrinol Metab.* 2023;108:827–833.

CHAPTER 88

Rehabilitative Techniques

Kristina Barber, MD and Venu Akuthota, MD

 KEY POINTS

1. Maximizing function and quality of life are the goals of employing rehabilitative techniques.
2. Exercise should be promoted in patients with rheumatic disease. Start low and go slow to reach the goal of 150 minutes of moderate-intensity exercise per week.
3. Exercise should be reduced or modified if patients experience prolonged soreness or pain for more than 2 hours after exercise.
4. For joint protection, patients with arthritis should focus on stretching, proper biomechanics, and range-of-motion exercises. Splints or orthoses can assist with positioning.
5. Physical modalities are used as an adjunct to facilitate active therapy and to reduce inflammation and pain associated with the disease state.

REHABILITATION BASICS

1. **What are the goals of rehabilitation for a patient with rheumatic disease?**

   Rehabilitation has a critical role in the management of rheumatic disease. The overarching goal is to improve a patient's function allowing them successful personal, family, and community lives. Focus on patient-centered functional goals (e.g., gardening or playing with grandchildren) can enhance quality of life. Addressing range of motion and strength is critical. Stretching and bracing can prevent contractures and deformities. Strength and endurance training lead to increased activity tolerance and lessen fatigue. Lastly, many modalities can be utilized to reduce pain.

2. **How can function be assessed in a patient with rheumatologic disease (Table 88.1)?**

TABLE 88.1 Elements of a Functional Assessment

Physical history	• Review of medical diagnoses
	• Assessment of pain and fatigue
	• Review of durable medical equipment use (e.g., cane, walker, wheelchair)
	• Ability to perform activities of daily living (eating, toileting, personal hygiene)
	• Ability to participate in:
	  • Recreational (avocational) and leisure activities
	  • Occupational (vocational) activities (job, housework, schoolwork)
	  • Sexual activity

Psychological & cognitive history	• Affective function (depression, anxiety, mood) • Cognitive function • Coping skills • Sleep history

Social history	• Social supports and obligations
	  • Community
	  • Interpersonal relationships
	• Social ability and integration
	• Socioeconomic factors
	  • Finances
	  • Insurance
	  • Transportation, housing, food security
	• Health literacy

Physical Exam	• Strength assessment (manual muscle testing) • Joint range of motion (can use goniometer). • Transfers and ambulation.

3. Management of the Rheumatic Diseases.

Physical Therapists:
- Assess for deficiencies in joint range of motion, strength, balance, gait, and transfers.
- Improve imbalances, deficiencies, and pain with modalities (thermal agents, electrical stimulation, dry needling, cupping, myofascial release, manual manipulation), therapeutic exercise, and stretching.
- Determine optimal gait aid and lower extremity bracing. Educate on appropriate use.
- Improve fear avoidance and kinesiophobic behaviors.

Occupational therapists:
- Assess for ways to improve energy conservation and joint protection with activities of daily living.
- Determine optimal upper extremity splinting/orthoses and recommend adaptive equipment for activities of daily living (e.g., shower chair).
- Assist with sexual therapy.

Podiatrists and Orthotists:
- Evaluate and treat foot and ankle deformities and painful conditions.
- Recommend appropriate orthoses and custom shoes.

Psychologists:
- Assist the patient in coping with pain and loss of function.

Social workers:
- Assist in the management of social, economic, and psychological barriers to health, function, and quality of life.

Recreational therapists:
- Assist with reintegration into community and avocational activities.

Vocational rehabilitation counselors:
- Mobilize community resources to retrain and restore the patient to the workplace.

Arthritis Rehabilitation Nurses and Patient Educators:
- Educate about rheumatic disease and management.
- Provide emotional support to the patient and family.

EXERCISE AND ENERGY CONSERVATION

4. Describe different energy conservation techniques for a person with arthritis.

Patients with rheumatic disease should receive education on energy conservation techniques. During activity, a focus on paced breathing, body biomechanics, and joint protection is essential. Advanced planning for rest and activity prioritization can also maximize generalized function.

- **Joint protection:** is a self-management approach that aims to maintain the function and integrity of joints by reducing loading on vulnerable joints. Techniques include maintaining good posture and joint alignment, altering movement patterns, avoiding static positions, and maintaining proper body weight. Joint protection also includes environmental modification, utilization of assistive devices, and allowing for adequate rest periods throughout the day.
- Types of Rest:
  - **Local rest** of a specific joint utilizing splinting techniques can reduce pain, inflammation, or prevent contracture. However, excessive inactivity or rest must be avoided as a muscle's mass may decrease by 5% to 10% within 1 week if a joint is immobilized.
  - **Systemic rest** can be considered for up to 4 weeks if appropriate anti-inflammatory medication and outpatient rehabilitation management are ineffective in alleviating pain from systemic diseases such as rheumatoid arthritis (RA) or polymyositis. Generalized deconditioning and increased cardiometabolic side effects can ensue if prolonged.
  - **Short rest periods** can be utilized throughout the day as a preventative means of managing pain and fatigue. The patient interrupts daily activities of >30 continuous minutes to take short breaks, thereby allowing for energy conservation.

5. How does exercise benefit a patient with rheumatic disease?

Fatigue, weakness, and decreased endurance are common symptoms in patients with rheumatic disease. Disuse, inactivity, and excessive rest can lead to significant deconditioning and loss of strength. In addition, joint immobility can lead to loss of range or motion and contractures. Therapeutic exercise can prevent or improve these problems.

6. Which factors need to be considered in prescribing an exercise program for a patient with a rheumatic disease?

- Stage of disease.
- Extent of inflammation and deformity.
- Patient's general medical condition.
- Types of activities the patient enjoys. This can increase adherence.

7. What types of exercise can be used in a patient with arthritis (Table 88.2)?

TABLE 88.2 Types of Exercise Used in Patients With Arthritis

TYPE OF EXERCISE	DESCRIPTION	USE	EXAMPLES
Isometric	Static muscle contraction with no change in length which does not lead to any visible movement in the angle of the joint.	• Helps maintain or increase muscle bulk and strength without increasing joint inflammation in a patient with active arthritis.	• Wall squat • Straight leg quadricep activation and hold • Plank
Isotonic	Dynamic muscle contraction changing muscle length which leads to movement of a joint against a fixed resistance.	• Can exacerbate flares and should be used when inflammation is controlled.	• Bicep curl • Squat
Isokinetic	Muscle contraction is performed at a constant velocity, made possible with a preset rate-limiting device.	• Rarely used in arthritis rehabilitation. • Typically used for higher performance athletes.	• Stationary bike
Aerobic	Combination of cardiopulmonary endurance exercises with strengthening.	• Can reduce joint damage, risk of cardiovascular disease, relieve fatigue, improve muscular strength, improve quality of life.	• Walking, jogging, bicycling • Aquatic-based exercises can improve tolerance
Mobility	Joint-dependent exercises to improve flexibility or ability to move through the entire range of motion.	• Exercises are specific to joint. • 3–5 repetitions, 1–2 times per day, 3 times per week.	• Ankle dorsiflexion to stretch gastrocnemius-soleus complex

8. How does strength training differ from endurance training?

Strength is the amount of force a muscle can lift or move at one time whereas endurance is the number of times a muscle can perform the action without becoming exhausted. Strength can be increased with isometric and isotonic exercise. Strength improves as resistance increases with isotonic exercise, resulting in fewer repetitions. Endurance increases with aerobic exercise and isotonic exercises with low resistance, enabling multiple repetitions (3 sets of 10 repetitions).

9. Which aerobic activities should be recommended to patients with rheumatic disease to improve cardiovascular fitness and promote weight loss?

Swimming, walking, elliptical training, and treadmill walking are recommended to increase cardiovascular fitness. The intensity should be sufficient to elevate the heart rate to 75% of maximum (220 minus age in years) for 20 to 40 minutes. Walking at a brisk pace for 30 to 70 minutes/day for 6 days/week is recommended if weight loss is indicated.

10. How often should a patient with arthritis exercise?

Patients with arthritis who exercise have improved quality of life, fatigue, joint pain, and cardio-vascular fitness. Stretching and range of motion exercises can be performed daily to prevent joint contractures. Current recommendation is for 150 minutes of moderate-intensity aerobic exercise or 75 minutes of vigorous-intensity aerobic activity per week, similar to recommendations for the general population. Strengthening exercises are recommended two to three times per week.

For those with active joint inflammation or more severe functional limitations, the American College of Sports Medicine has issued a separate set of guidelines. These recommendations state that adults with a chronic condition and/or functional limitation should perform at least 30 min-utes of moderate-intensity activity on most days of the week or vigorous-intensity aerobic physical activity for a minimum of 20 minutes on 3 days each week. Starting slowly with low-intensity exercise, perhaps involving isometric exercises and aquatic therapy, can help to improve adherence to routine exercise.

11. What are the signs that a patient with arthritis has over-exercised?

- Excessive pain during the exercise session.
- Post-exercise soreness lasting >2 hours.
- Increased joint pain or swelling the day following exercise.

PHYSICAL MODALITIES

12. What physical modalities are available for management of musculoskeletal pain?

The purpose of physical modalities is to decrease pain, allowing the patient to participate in thera-peutic exercises. Many of the commonly used modalities are listed in Table 88.3, with a notable (but not exhaustive) list of contraindications.

13. What are different types and uses of cryotherapy?

Cryotherapy can be delivered locally or to a broad area. Local applications include vapocoolant sprays (Fluori-Methane), ice massage, and locally applied cold packs. General applications include ice water immersion (ice bath), thermal blankets, and contrast baths. Cryotherapy decreases the excitability of free nerve endings of peripheral nerve fibers and small nerve endings in the muscle spindle and Golgi tendons. This leads to decreased nerve conduction velocity leading to analgesic effect approximately 15 minutes after the onset of application, and also reduces muscle spasm. In rheumatic disease, local cryotherapy induces a decrease in intra-joint temperature that can down-regulate inflammatory mediators (cytokines, cartilage degrading enzymes, pro-angiogenic factors). The administration of cryotherapy is recommended for 20-minute increments, as it takes at least 15 minutes to achieve an analgesic effect.

14. What are the different types and uses of thermotherapy?

Thermotherapy can be either deep (diatheramy) or superficial. Deep heat warms tissues at 3–5 cm depth without affecting superficial tissue, whereas superficial heat addresses cutaneous tissue less than 1 cm from the surface. Superficial heat increases cutaneous blood flow initially and, if used for a long enough duration, triggers a hypothalamic-mediated reflex increase in blood flow to underlying tissues as well. Heat produces analgesia by stimulation of afferent c-fibers under the gate-control theory of pain. Heat also decreases the stimulus threshold of muscle spindles and decreases the gamma efferent firing rate, contributing to a negative biofeedback loop resulting in reduced muscle tension.

Superficial heat can be delivered by heating pads, paraffin baths, hot whirlpools, infrared, and hydrocollator packs. Paraffin wax baths have specifically been shown to improve objective hand function measures (ROM, pinch function, grip strength, pain, and stiffness) after 4 weeks of treatment.

Diatheramy is delivered by ultrasound, shortwave, or microwave with the intention of affect-ing deeper structures like ligament, tendon, muscle, and joint capsules. Ultrasound converts ultra-sound energy to thermal energy, whereas shortwave converts electromagnetic energy into thermal energy. Thermotherapy is typically applied for 15–20 minutes per treatment.

TABLE 88.3 Commonly Used Physical Modalities

CATEGORY	MODALITIES	IMPORTANT CONTRAINDICATIONS

Thermal agents	• Cryotherapy (cold)
	  • Local
	  • Generalized
	• Thermotherapy (heat)
	  • Superficial
	  • Deep (diathermy)
	• Ultrasound
	• Shortwave, microwave
		• General
		  • Local sensory deficits
		  • Impaired ability to communicate pain
		  • Underlying malignancy
		  • Impaired circulation
		  • Underlying infection
		  • Gravid uterus
		• Specific to ultrasound
		  • Near pacemaker or plastic implant
		• Specific to shortwave, microwave
		  • On metal implant or epiphysis

Electrotherapy & local drug delivery	• Transcutaneous electrical nerve stimulation (TENS)
	• Iontophoresis
	• Phonophoresis
		• General:
		  • Local sensory deficits
		  • Impaired ability to communicate pain
		  • Underlying implants including pacemaker
		• Specific to Iontophoresis/Phonophoresis:
		  • Allergy to medication used

Traction	• Continuous • Sustained • Intermittent	• Inflammatory arthritis • Bone disease (osteoporosis, fracture, tumor) • Spinal instability • Neurologic injury • Spinal infection • Pregnancy (lumbar) • Atlantoaxial subluxation (cervical) • Vertebrobasilar insufficiency (cervical)
Manipulation	• High Velocity, low amplitude	• Inflammatory arthritis • Bleeding disorders • Underlying bone disease (tumor, osteoporosis, infection) • Neurologic compromise
Myofascial	• Soft Tissue Mobilization • Myofascial release • Massage • Muscle Energy • Strain, Counterstain	• Underlying DVT • Cellulitis • Lymphangitis • Malignancy

15. What are the contraindications to treating with thermotherapy?

Thermal modalities should be avoided in patients with impaired circulation or sensation, infection, or altered mental status leading to inability to report adverse effects. Thermotherapy should generally be avoided on a gravid uterus, gonads, or with an acute musculoskeletal injury. Ultrasound, shortwave, and microwave diathermy are contraindicated if there are underlying plastic or metal components, or malignancy. These modalities should also be avoided around bony epiphyses.

16. What are electrotherapy and phonophoresis?

Electrotherapy includes, but is not limited to, transcutaneous electrical nerve stimulation (TENS) and iontophoresis. TENS has been described in the use of chronic pain syndromes and peripheral neuropathic pain, though evidence is lacking in effectiveness compared to sham procedures. The use of TENS is often patient directed after initial training, and may provide temporary pain relief after 10–15 minutes of use. Iontophoresis uses direct electrical current to induce topically applied medications to migrate into soft tissues and nerves up to 1 cm deep. Common topical medications applied with this modality include lidocaine gel, corticosteroid (usually dexamethasone) gel, and analgesics. This therapy has been used in tendonitis (especially Achilles), bursitis, and neuritis. Treatment time is typically 20–30 minutes.

Phonophoresis is similar to iontophoresis but uses ultrasonic waves to deliver medication more deeply (up to 5 cm below the skin). Treatment time is typically 10 minutes.

17. When is traction used for the management of cervical and lumbar spinal disorders?

Traction utilizes a pulling force to stretch soft tissue or separate joint surfaces. It is most often used on the cervical and lumbar spine to increase the intervertebral foraminal area, allowing more space for the exiting nerve root. It can stretch ligaments and muscles and may decrease muscle spasms and pressure on intervertebral discs. There is no consensus on the indications for traction, and the evidence for benefit is limited outside of cervical radicular pain.

Both cervical and lumbar traction work best if applied two or three times a day until pain relief occurs. Failure to improve within 2–4 weeks and/or exacerbation of pain during traction are indications to stop therapy. Contraindications to traction include spinal malignancy or infection, osteoporosis, fracture, ligamentous instability, neurologic injury, atlantoaxial subluxation with instability, pregnancy, aortic aneurysm, restrictive lung disease, and inflammatory arthritis.

18. What are some types of manual therapy?

There are many manual therapy techniques. Soft tissue mobilization can be used to relax muscles and fascia via lateral force to stretch the muscle, direct longitudinal stretching, or careful kneading. Direct myofascial release is also used to improve tissue restriction by loading the tissue via stretch, holding in position, and waiting for a release. Additional techniques include muscle energy and strain-counterstain. High-velocity manipulation, particularly of the cervical spine, is generally contraindicated for patients with rheumatic conditions. Massage techniques can be used to create tissue compression, shearing, or vibration to address lymphatic, muscular, fascial, and deep connective tissue-related pain. It is generally well tolerated, with few contraindications (such as underlying DVT, cellulitis, lymphangitis, and malignancy).

ORTHOSES AND ASSISTIVE DEVICES

19. Why are orthoses (splints and braces) used in arthritis patients?

Orthoses are used in the treatment of inflammatory and degenerative arthritis for a variety of reasons, with underlying principles including pain relief and joint stability. Splinting generally immobilizes range of motion, while bracing supports the range of motion. Both can create stability, modify range of motion, or support the joint in the position of maximal function. Orthoses can be purchased off-the-shelf or custom-molded for the individual patient. Often, if the need for intervention is less than 6 months and there are no notable contractures or abnormal anatomy, a prefabricated orthosis is appropriate. Evidence for efficacy in reducing pain and disability is perhaps best for the use of orthoses in thumb carpometacarpal joint osteoarthritis (OA). Splinting in this setting allows joint rest and opening of the first web space. Additionally, unloader (valgus) knee braces have level B evidence for improving pain related to medial joint space narrowing.

20. Name the major factors associated with patient adherence to the use of splints and orthoses.

The effectiveness of an orthosis is only as good as adherence to use. Disuse is commonly associated with patient dissatisfaction with one of the following: appearance, weight, usefulness, reliability, fitness, and comfort. Patients may dislike the appearance of the orthosis or be concerned with discrimination due to use, leading to decreased utilization. Pain and skin breakdown secondary to the orthosis itself can occur, but importantly, these represent modifiable factors. Inquiring about each of the aspects associated with patient dissatisfaction, and addressing them with an appropriate intervention, is likely to improve use. Finally, adherence is increased when the splints significantly improve pain or function and when family members or support groups reinforce the importance of regular use.

21. How can the use of assistive devices and mobility aids benefit a patient with arthritis?

Assistive devices that substitute for deficient function help a patient improve energy conservation and pain via reduced joint loading. The type of aid used depends on the severity of impairment. Adaptive devices that aid functionality in the kitchen, bathroom, and for self-care are readily available. A few examples of devices for patients with decreased hand function are built-up utensil handles, zipper pulls, and adaptive shoelaces.

For lower extremity deficits or generalized weakness, raised toilet seats and shower chairs are helpful. Mobility aids can assist a patient in maintaining their center of gravity safely over their support area. Examples include canes (quad, single point), crutches (axillary, forearm, triceps, platform), walkers (two wheel, four wheel), wheelchairs (manual, powered), and scooters. Ambulatory patients with diminished endurance can benefit from a seated walker.

22. How should patients be instructed to use a cane?

Canes are indicated in individuals who would benefit from mild to moderate reduction in weight bearing on an affected limb, and in those with mild to moderate balance impairments. There are multiple types of canes, but a single-point cane is typically used in arthritic conditions. If pain is resulting from hip level or above, the cane should be held by the contralateral hand. This creates a moment arm that counteracts the patient's weight and significantly reduces (by 25%) the amount of force applied to the hip joint. For painful joints below the hip, the cane should be held in the ipsilateral hand. Although the use of a cane can negatively impact gait speed, it helps offload the painful joint leading to improved gait mechanics.

23. How can you tell if a cane has been properly fitted to the patient?

When the patient is standing, the cane should reach the level of their greater trochanter. The arm using the cane should be flexed at the elbow to about 20 degrees for optimal positioning.

24. When should a walker be considered?

Walkers are utilized when a patient would benefit from moderate to high-level weight-bearing reduction on an affected limb, or to compensate for moderate to severe balance deficits. For patients with unilateral upper extremity impairment, a hemi-walker can be considered over a standard walker. For those with significant hand or wrist impairment, a platform walker facilitates weight bearing through the forearms rather than the hands. A fold-down seat can benefit patients with impaired endurance or walking-related symptoms that require intermittent rest. Use of a walker can lead to decreased gait speed, but can improve gait mechanics and pain.

25. When should a power mobility device (PMD; electric wheelchair, scooter) be considered?

Patients meet criteria for power mobility when they have limitations in mobility-related activities of daily living (ADL) (e.g., moving from room to room, dressing, grooming, toileting, feeding, bathing) that cannot safely or sufficiently be resolved with a fitted cane or walker (or if impaired upper extremity function). **CMS will only approve PMD when it facilitates movement around the home, but the use of power mobility can improve access in the community as well.**

26. What are the documentation requirements required by the Centers for Medicare and Medicaid Services to justify reimbursement for a PMD?

A provider must complete a face-to-face examination and document how the patient's medical conditions affect mobility and ADLs. Documentation should include all elements outlined in Table 88.4, and must be forwarded to the PMD supplier within 45 days of the encounter.

TABLE 88.4 Face-to-Face Documentation Elements

History of Present Condition(s) and Medical History	• Symptoms limiting ambulation • Timeline and trajectory of ambulation difficulty • Other diagnoses related to ambulatory difficulty • Current ambulatory ability (distance without stopping, pace) • Current assistive device and why no longer sufficient • Ability to stand from a seated position without assistance • Description of home set up and ADL abilities
Physical Exam	• Weight and height • Cardiopulmonary examination • Musculoskeletal examination (range of motion, contractures, etc) • Neurologic examination (weakness, hypertonia, gait impairment, etc)
Supporting Data	• Pertinent laboratory tests • Pertinent imaging • Other diagnostic tests related to mobility needs

27. **What are the seven elements that must be included in the written order for any PMD (Table 88.5)?**

TABLE 88.5 Seven Elements in Written Prescriptions for PMD

1. Patient's Name
2. Date of the face-to-face examination
3. Pertinent diagnoses/conditions that relate to the need for PMD (International Classification of Diseases-10 codes)
4. Description of the item ordered (power mobility device)
5. Length of need in months (99 = lifetime)
6. Treating/ordering provider's signature
7. Date of provider's signature

28. **Describe footwear considerations for patients with foot pain/arthritis.**

Footwear should be worn with the goal of maximizing foot function by accommodating for pain and structural deficiencies. Providers can use orthoses and recommend specific shoe types to assist patients. Foot orthoses can be soft, semirigid, or rigid depending on the level of support needed. They can be purchased prefabricated or custom molded. For patients with leg length discrepancy of more than half of an inch, heel (and if needed sole) lifts can be recommended. Metatarsal pads can assist with forefoot pain. Heel lifts can temporarily relieve pain associated with Achilles tendinopathy/enthesopathy.

Minimalist shoes do not assist with correction and are not recommended when there is lower extremity pathology. High heels and pointed-toe shoes should be avoided, as they put the foot and ankle in a biomechanically disadvantaged position for normal ambulation. A wide, deep toe box is recommended to allow sufficient space for the foot. Proper fit should be assessed by a trusted vendor. Tight fit may lead to the development of corns over bony prominences, while loose fit may lead to increased friction and callous formation. Custom-made shoes may be indicated if the foot deformity is severe. For patients with limited hand function, adaptive shoelaces or Velcro closures should be recommended.

DISEASE SPECIFIC REHABILITATION

29. **What kinds of exercise are available for a patient with OA?**

While patients may be concerned that exercise will worsen their pain or advance their arthritis, exercise should be promoted in this population as it helps promote general health and has evidence of alleviating the degenerative process. In mouse models, running and swimming have been shown at a cellular level to subdue the degradation of extracellular matrix (ECM), cell apoptosis, and inhibit intraarticular inflammatory response. Aerobic exercise, resistance exercise, and neuromuscular training have been shown to relieve pain and improve function and quality of life in patients with knee and hip OA. Adherence to the exercise program is the best predictor for improvement. Aquatic exercise should be considered for obese patients or individuals with more severe disease.

30. What is the best method for a patient with knee arthritis to walk up and down the stairs?

Patients with knee arthritis commonly have increased pain with ascending and descending stairs. To reduce force across the painful joint, they should lead with their unaffected leg going up the stairs, and lead with their affected leg going down the stairs. **This can be remembered by the phrase, "Up to heaven (good leg), down to hell (bad leg)."** If using a cane, the patient should advance the cane with the affected leg. Exercises focused on strengthening the knee extensors should improve knee pain and stair-climbing ability.

31. Can patients with inflammatory arthritis benefit from a regular exercise program?

Patients with inflammatory arthritis should be encouraged to follow the recommendation of at least 150 minutes of moderate-intensity activity per week, with strength training of all muscle groups at least twice per week (per EULAR guidelines). A gradual increase in activity to reach this goal may be required depending on the current activity level. Modifications may be required depending on disease activity and symptoms. Isometric exercises are preferred for joints with active inflammation. Patients can benefit from low-repetition, low-resistance isotonic exercises taken through shorter arcs. Resistance and repetitions can be gradually increased. Paraffin wax baths for the hands can be particularly helpful to warm joints before exercise. Using a behavioral change framework when counseling on physical activity may lead to improved adherence.

32. What rehabilitative techniques can be used for specific rheumatic diseases?

Ankylosing spondylitis: Focus on pain relief, improvement of posture, and maximizing mobility. Before aerobic exercise, thermotherapy to affected areas and a 10-minute warm up are recommended. Swimming may be the best aerobic exercise as it promotes spinal extension and shoulder range of motion. Stretching should include suboccipital muscles, pectoral muscles, hamstrings, hip flexors, and spinal rotators. Range of motion exercises should focus on spine, neck, shoulders, and hips.

    Inflammatory myositis: Focus on aerobic endurance training (walking, swimming, stationary bike). Strength training should be modified to avoid muscle damage by limiting muscle exhaustion. The intensity of resistance training should not lead to delayed onset muscle soreness (1–2 days after exercise) or post-workout weakness. Both aerobic and strength training are recommended in this patient population outside of periods of disease exacerbation. Daily ROM exercises are important to prevent contractures. Aquatic exercise is recommended to allow higher-intensity exercise with reduced delayed-onset muscle soreness.

    Steroid-induced myopathy: Aerobic and strength training is recommended. These modalities can attenuate muscle atrophy in this setting, but not prevent it entirely.

    Systemic sclerosis: Focus on improving hand range of motion and stretching exercises. Some studies suggest improvement with preceding paraffin wax baths but assess for the presence of digital ulcers prior to use. Additional focus on orofacial range of motion improves patient-reported quality of life.

    Fibromyalgia: Education on the importance of aerobic and strengthening exercises. Acupuncture, cognitive behavioral therapy, and mindfulness techniques may improve adherence to exercise regimens and reduce pain.

    Complex Regional Pain Syndrome (CRPS): Structured rehabilitation by a physical or occupational therapist is recommended. There is uncertainty on which specific exercises and modalities lead to the most benefit. Recommendations should include gradual increase in the range of motion and weight bearing of the affected limb. Graded motor imagery, mirror therapy, and modalities including massage, TENS, and contrast baths have been suggested. Intervention techniques, such as stellate ganglion blocks, lumbar sympathetic blocks, or spinal cord stimulators may be used to facilitate active exercise treatment.

    Systemic Lupus Erythematosus: Regular exercise has been shown to improve fatigue, stress, depression and quality of life. Patients benefit from explicit counseling on exercise. Aerobic exercise may improve systemic inflammation and cardiovascular health.

Rheumatoid Arthritis: During acute stages of the disease, isometric exercise at submaximal effort is recommended. Once disease activity is better controlled, isotonic exercise of gradual increasing repetition and resistance is recommended, in addition to endurance training and aerobic exercise.

ACKNOWLEDGMENT

The author would like to thank Dr. Alexandra Garnett for her contributions to this chapter in previous editions.

BIBLIOGRAPHY

Bearne LM. Physical activity in rheumatoid arthritis—is it time to push the pace of change? *Rheumatol Adv Pract*. 2023;7(1):rkac107. https://doi.org/10.1093/rap/rkac107.

Cameron MH. *Physical Agents in Rehabilitation: An Evidence Based Approach to Practice*. 5th ed. Philadelphia, PA: Elsevier Health Sciences; 2018.

Casaña J, Calatayud J, Silvestre A, et al. Knee extensor muscle strength is more important than postural balance for stair-climbing ability in elderly patients with severe knee osteoarthritis. *Int J Environ Res Public Health*. 2021;18(7):3637. https://doi.org/10.3390/ijerph18073637.

Cifu DX. *Braddom's Physical Medicine and Rehabilitation*. 5th ed. Philadelphia, PA: Elsevier, Inc.; 2016.

da Silva BISL, Dos Santos BRJ, Carneiro JA, Silva FMFE, de Souza JM. Physical exercise for dermatomyositis and polymyositis: a systematic review and meta-analysis. *Clin Rheumatol*. 2022;41(9):2635–2646. https://doi.org/10.1007/s10067-022-06281-1.

Frontera W. *Delisa's Physical Medicine and Rehabilitation: Principles and Practice*. 6th ed. Philadelphia, PA: Wolters Kluwer; 2020.

Kong H, Wang XQ, Zhang XA. Exercise for osteoarthritis: a literature review of pathology and mechanism. *Front Aging Neurosci*. 2022;14:854026. https://doi.org/10.3389/fnagi.2022.854026.

Medicare Learning Network. *Power Mobility Devices*. 2017. https://www.cms.gov/outreach-and-education/medicare-learning-network-mln/mlnproducts/downloads/pmd_doccvg_factsheet_icn905063-text-only.pdf.

Ye Hui, Weng H, Xu Y. Effectiveness and safety of aerobic exercise for rheumatoid arthritis: a systematic review and meta-analysis of randomized controlled trials. *BMC Sports Sci Med Rehabil*. 2022;14(17y). https://doi.org/10.1186/s13102-022-00408-2.

CHAPTER 89

Surgical Treatment and Rheumatic Diseases

Craig Hogan, MD, Bradley Reeves, MD and Jonathan T. Bravman, MD

Surgery is the cry of defeat in medicine.
  —Martin H. Fischer, MD (1879–1962)

 KEY POINTS

1. Inability to walk more than one block or stand longer than 20 to 30 minutes as a result of pain despite nonoperative measures are indications for total hip and knee replacement.
2. The most common cause of periprosthetic osteolysis resulting in implant loosening is a chronic proinflammatory biologic response to particulate debris.
3. Arthroscopic debridement is most beneficial in patients with osteoarthritis (OA) with mechanical symptoms such as locking, popping, and catching.
4. Lumbar spine surgery is most successful in addressing radicular symptoms confirmed by clinical examination, electromyography (EMG), and magnetic resonance imaging (MRI) in patients who responded favorably to transforaminal epidural corticosteroid injections.

1. What are the major indications for total joint replacement surgery in patients with arthritis?

Joint replacement is indicated when pain has failed to respond to nonoperative management and is limiting activities of daily living. Pain relief is the most attainable result of surgery. Deformity correction, restoration of motion and function are secondary goals of surgery and are less predictable.

2. What medical factors require preoperative attention in patients undergoing total joint replacement?

- All surgical candidates for orthopedic reconstructive procedures require a comprehensive history and physical examination to assess the overall general operative risks. Patients should be examined for carious teeth, skin ulcerations (especially around the feet), and symptoms of urinary tract infection or prostatism because these could increase the risk of postoperative infections.
- Routine preoperative urinalysis is not recommended to screen for asymptomatic urinary tract colonization, as treatment increases antibiotic utilization without an observed decrease in surgical site infections (SSI) or catheter-associated urinary tract infections (CAUTI).
- If patients are receiving nonsteroidal anti-inflammatory drugs (NSAIDs), these medications should be switched to a COX-2-specific NSAID or stopped several days (at least five half-lives) before surgery to prevent bleeding because of their antiplatelet effects. Aspirin should be held for 7–10 days preoperatively.
- Management of acute and chronic anticoagulation therapy in the perioperative time frame requires careful consideration and a multidisciplinary approach to balance bleeding and embolic risks. Patients should be stratified according to their risk for perioperative thromboembolism. Multiple national and international organizations (ie. American College of Cardiology (ACC), American Academy of Orthopaedic Surgeons (AAOS), etc.) have published guidelines for the management of perioperative anticoagulation therapy and venous thromboembolism prophylaxis. Generally, in the preoperative period therapeutic dosed DOACs are held for 4–5 half-lives, prophylactic dosed DOACs for 2–3 half-lives, and antiplatelet agents are held for 5–7 days. Typically, these therapies are resumed 24–72 hours postoperatively. DOACs are associated with spinal epidural hematoma from neuraxial anesthesia and

need to be stopped 72 hours prior to catheter insertion and cannot be restarted for at least 6 hours following catheter removal. Discontinuation of warfarin therapy and bridging with low-molecular-weight heparin are based on INR and specific guidelines should be referred to for details.

- Perioperative management of antirheumatic medications should be based on the guidelines published by the American College of Rheumatology and the American Association of Hip and Knee Surgeons.

3. What other factors must be addressed preoperatively in patients with rheumatoid arthritis (RA) (see Chapter 13: Perioperative Management of Patients With Rheumatic Diseases)?

- **Cervical spine**—an unstable cervical spine attributable to arthritic involvement places a patient at risk for catastrophic neurologic loss when the neck is manipulated during intubation. Preoperative lateral flexion and extension radiographs of the cervical spine are mandatory in patients with RA, especially if they have neck symptoms or long-standing disease with peripheral joint deformities. An increased anterior atlantodens interval >3 mm indicates disruption of the transverse ligament. When unstable, the interval usually increases with flexion and decreases in extension. An anterior atlantodens interval >7 mm or posterior atlantodens interval of ≤14 mm suggests cervical spine instability.
- **Blood transfusion**—Transfusion of packed red cells, platelets, or plasma can precipitate immune dysregulation and remain associated with transmissible infections, particularly in immunosuppressed recipients. Conservative transfusion strategies and preoperative autologous blood donation should be discussed.
- **Temporomandibular arthritis** (especially patients with juvenile idiopathic arthritis [JIA]) and **cricoarytenoid arthritis**—may make intubations more difficult.
- **Immune status**—infection rates are significantly higher in patients with RA, partly because of the disease process and partly because of the immunosuppressive drugs used to control it. Patients should be on the lowest glucocorticoid dosage possible, since even low doses increase the risk of infection. Conventional synthetic disease-modifying antirheumatic drugs (DMARDs) do not need to be stopped prior to surgery. At least one dose of a biologic DMARD should be held before surgery. Janus kinase (JAK) inhibitors should be stopped for 4 days prior to surgery.
- **Nutritional status**—patients with RA may be relatively malnourished, which predisposes them to infection. Patients with a total lymphocyte count >1500/mm^3, hemoglobin A1C ≤ 7.5%, albumin level >3.5 g/dL, hemoglobin >13.0 g/dL in men or >12.0 g/dL in women, and body mass index <40 kg/m^2 are less prone to infections.
- **Hypothalamic–pituitary–adrenal axis**—patients on chronic corticosteroid therapy may not be able to respond normally to surgical stress. Perioperative stress-dose corticosteroids may be needed in some patients undergoing moderate/major-risk surgery (see Chapter 13: Perioperative Management of Patients With Rheumatic Diseases).
- **Intraarticular corticosteroids**—patients who received intraarticular corticosteroids should not receive a total joint arthroplasty of that injected joint for at least 3 months.
- **Cardiovascular status**—patients with RA are at risk for premature atherosclerosis (relative risk 1.5 ×). Attention should be given to anginal chest pain and bruits.

4. Patients with RA frequently have multiple joints involved. What is the recommended sequence for reconstructive surgery?

- Lower extremity (LE) surgery is done before upper extremity (UE) surgery because crutch use postoperatively would place excessive demands on any UE reconstructive surgery.
- In the multiple involved LE, the hip is reconstructed before the knee to get the best possible alignment of the knee and relieve referred pain from the hip to the knee. However, in patients with normal knee alignment, foot and ankle surgery should be performed before hip and knee replacement to provide stability for LE rehabilitation. Ankle and hindfoot procedures are done before forefoot reconstruction.
- In the UE, the preferred order is controversial. Usually, proximal joints, nerve, and tendon problems are addressed before the hand and wrist. The wrist is done before the hand joints to help with alignment. For the shoulder and elbow, the most symptomatic joint is usually done first.

5. What additional intraoperative and postoperative medical procedures are done to prevent postoperative complications following total hip arthroplasty or total knee arthroplasty?

Intraoperative prophylactic antibiotics are given to decrease the chance of infection. There may be a potential benefit for mixing antibiotic powder with cement in arthroplasty, but currently there is no strong consensus. For LE total joint replacement (hip, knee), sequential compression devices, early ambulation, and anticoagulation are done to prevent postoperative deep venous thrombosis. Deep venous thrombosis occurs in 50% to 60% of patients, pulmonary embolus in over 10% of patients, and fatal pulmonary embolus in 0% to 3% of patients if postoperative anticoagulation (1–6 weeks) is not done.

6. What is Steel's rule of thirds?

At the level of the first cervical vertebra (C1), the anteroposterior diameter is divided into thirds, allowing one-third for the dens, one-third for the spinal cord, and one-third for free space. Because there is significant free space at this level, small degrees of C1 to C2 subluxation (3–7 mm) usually do not compromise the cord. However, when the anterior atlantodens interval (measured from the posterior part of the anterior arch of C1 to the anterior aspect of odontoid) measures >10 to 12 mm, significant disruption of the atlantoaxial ligamentous complex has occurred, and the space available for the spinal cord is usually compromised. Likewise, when the posterior atlantodens interval (measured from posterior aspect of the odontoid to the anterior aspect of the posterior arch of C1) is <14 mm, the spinal cord is usually compressed. (See also Chapter 13: Perioperative Management of Patients with Rheumatic Diseases.)

7. When should the cervical spine (C1 to C2) be fused in patients with RA?

- Overall, rates of cervical spine fusions for RA patients have declined in the setting of expanded disease-modifying drug therapies. Operative stabilization of the rheumatoid cervical spine is indicated in patients with the following structural abnormalities:
  - Have atlantoaxial subluxation with a posterior atlantodens interval of ≤14 mm.
  - Have atlantoaxial subluxation and at least 5 mm of basilar invagination.
  - Have subaxial subluxation and a sagittal diameter of the spinal canal of ≤14 mm.
- Indications for surgical stabilization based on the presence of neurologic symptoms can be prognostically classified as follows:
  - Ranawat Class I: no neurologic deficits. Neurologic deterioration rarely (10%) occurs. Conservative and surgical outcomes are similar, so patients should be treated conservatively with medical treatment of their RA. The 10-year survival rate is 75%.
  - Ranawat Class II: subjective weakness with hyperreflexia and/or dysesthesia. Neurologic deterioration will occur in 67% with conservative therapy. With surgery, 50% improve and 40% stabilize neurologically. The 10-year survival rate is 65%.
  - Ranawat Class IIIA: objective weakness and long tract signs but able to walk. Neurologic deterioration occurs in all with conservative therapy. With surgery, 55% improve and 35% stay the same. The 10-year survival rate is 50%.
  - Ranawat class IIIB: quadriparetic and unable to walk. Neurologic deterioration occurs in all with conservative therapy. With surgery, 60% improve. The 10-year survival rate is 30%.

8. What are the potential intraoperative and postoperative complication rates following cervical spine fusion in a patient with RA?

- Postoperative mortality: 0% to 10%. Has been as high as 33% for patients with severe neurologic compromise.
- Wound infections and dehiscence.
- Nonunion rates: 0% to 50%. Average is 20%.
- Late subaxial subluxation below previous fusion as a result of transfer of increased stresses.

9. What surgical procedures are available for patients with RA with shoulder involvement?

Surgical procedures of the shoulder are performed predominantly for pain control. An increase in range of motion (ROM) usually does not occur. Replacement arthroplasty can include the entire joint, termed **total shoulder arthroplasty,** or only the humeral head, termed **hemiarthro-plasty.** The principal factor in choosing between the two is the status of the glenoid. For maximal functional use and stability of a total shoulder arthroplasty, soft-tissue tension from an intact rotator cuff plays an integral role. If the rotator cuff is not intact and cannot be repaired, then a constrained arthroplasty, reverse total shoulder arthroplasty (ball on glenoid side), bipolar arthro-plasty, or an oversized hemiarthroplasty is chosen.

10. What are the surgical options for management of arthritis involving the elbow joint?

- In **inflammatory arthritis** not responsive to medical management, synovectomy will tem-porarily control the disease and reliably decrease pain, but it infrequently has any positive effect on joint motion. Open synovectomy may also include excision of the radial head if significantly involved. However, total elbow arthroplasty is preferred to radial head resection/synovectomy in most patients. Arthroscopy is used for diagnostic purposes, removal of loose bodies, and synovectomy for both biopsy and treatment purposes.
- **OA:** the ulnohumeral articulation is predominantly affected, usually by osteophytes that develop on the coronoid process or olecranon. Surgically, these osteophytes are removed arthroscopically or through an open incision. When the articular cartilage is lost, a soft tissue arthroplasty can be performed to resurface the joint with autologous tissue: fascia lata most commonly, or allograft.
- In **posttraumatic arthritis** involving the radiohumeral or proximal radioulnar joint, a radial head excision can be performed with predictably good results as long as the medial collateral ligament of the elbow is intact.

Total elbow arthroplasty is becoming the surgical option of choice for most arthritic condi-tions of the elbow. This is attributable to the increasing reliability of the current prostheses and the magnitude of functional improvement for a patient. Overall pain relief is 90% with long-term complications of 10%, most commonly loosening. Elbow arthrodesis should be a very last resort because this procedure makes it impossible to position the hand for functional use. It is reserved for an end-stage arthritic elbow from previous septic arthritis and in patients when total elbow replacement is not feasible.

11. How are the common problems of the wrist in RA managed surgically?

RA has a predilection for the small joints of the hand and wrist. The wrist is almost universally involved and usually presents predictable patterns of involvement and resultant deformities. The goal of medical management lies in control of the inflammatory synovitis to prevent destruction of bony and soft tissue structures. When this fails, surgery can be used to remove inflammatory synovium or correct deformity.

The dorsal wrist capsule and dorsal tendon sheath are commonly involved with synovitis and tenosynovitis that can lead to extensor tendon rupture. Prevention of tendon rupture is far better than tendon transfer and, therefore, if medical control is inadequate, early surgical synovectomy and tenosynovectomy are warranted. The term **Vaughn-Jackson syndrome** is applied when the extensor tendons of the ring and small finger have ruptured. Primary tendon repair is usually not possible, especially if the rupture occurred longer than a few days previously. Tendon transfer surgery is then required to restore function.

On the volar aspect of the wrist, tenosynovitis of the flexor tendons can cause compression of the median nerve in the carpal canal, leading to carpal tunnel syndrome. It can also lead to rupture of the flexor pollicis longus tendon, leading to inadequate thumb flexion and resting hyperextension at the interphalangeal joint. This is the **Mannerfelt syndrome** and requires ten-don transfer or arthrodesis of the interphalangeal joint of the thumb.

The distal radioulnar joint is commonly involved by synovitis, which leads to laxity of this joint, osseous destruction of the ulnar head, and pain with forearm rotation. The ulnar head becomes dorsally prominent and adds to stress on the ulnar extensor tendons. This constellation of findings is called the **caput ulna syndrome.** Its surgical management entails aggressive syno-vectomy, ulnar head excision, capsulorrhaphy, and lateral tenodesis using a portion of the extensor carpi ulnaris tendon.

When the radiocarpal joint is involved with advanced changes, total wrist arthroplasty (TWA) or wrist arthrodesis can be used to control pain and improve function in over 90% of patients. However, over 20% of patients receiving a TWA will need a revision within 10 years.

12. What are the surgical options for basilar thumb OA?

The carpometacarpal joint of the thumb, also known as the trapeziometacarpal or basilar thumb joint, is a saddle-shaped articulation with a high propensity for degenerative change. Surgical procedures include implant arthroplasty, tendon interposition arthroplasty, tendon suspension arthroplasty, and arthrodesis. Implants have a high rate of failure, and work continues on a better prosthetic design, most recently with pyrocarbon hemi and total joint components. Tendon interposition ("anchovy procedure") entails placing a wad of tendon into the cavity created by removal of some or all of the trapezium. Tendon suspension is similar, except after the trapezium is removed, a weave of tendon is created that supports the thumb metacarpal base like a sling. Both tendon procedures result in a 30% to 40% loss of pinch strength. Arthrodesis is probably the best procedure for longevity of the reconstruction, but it restricts metacarpal motion and requires very precise positioning, or function will not be optimal.

13. How is a mucous cyst and OA of the distal interphalangeal (DIP) joints managed?

Mucous cysts are commonly associated with OA of the DIP joints of the fingers. They present as a clear mucin-filled cystic mass, usually between the DIP joint and the proximal aspect of the nail. Mucous cysts result from chronic inflammation secondary to a dorsal osteophyte of the DIP joint. Therefore, appropriate evaluation includes an x-ray, and definitive management must be directed at removal of the osteophyte, not just the cyst alone. If the DIP joint is significantly painful or unstable, fusion of the DIP joint in mild flexion becomes the treatment of choice.

14. How are deformities of the proximal interphalangeal (PIP) joints managed surgically in patients with RA?

Boutonnière deformities result from synovitis within the PIP joints, causing extensor tendon elongation and rupture, and leading to progressive flexion contractures. During early stages, synovectomy may be helpful.

Swan-neck deformities progress through four stages of deformity. During the first three stages, splinting, synovectomy, and surgical release of intrinsic muscle tightness and tendon adhesions are used. In the last stage, when the PIP joint is destroyed, surgical options include joint replacement or fusion.

In patients with destroyed PIP joints, total joint replacement is preferred for PIPs involved in grasping (third, fourth, and fifth PIPs), whereas fusion is used more for PIPs involved in pinch (thumb IP, second PIP).

15. Describe the results of metacarpophalangeal (MCP) joint surgery in patients with RA.

Synovitis of the MCP joints ultimately leads to joint destruction, volar subluxation of the MCP joints, and ulnar drift of the fingers. There is little evidence that prophylactic synovectomy slows joint destruction, but it may postpone the need for joint replacement surgery when done early before x-ray changes. MCP arthroplasty is indicated when synovitis has resulted in cartilage destruction, decreased motion, pain, ulnar drift, deformity, and loss of function. MCP arthroplasties, irrespective of design, result in 50 degrees of motion which may decrease to 30 degrees over time. Ulnar deviation can be improved to <20 degrees. Postoperative splinting and hand rehabilitation are critical for optimal results. Arthrodesis is not done except for the thumb MCP joint. This is because the thumb needs strength for pinch, whereas motion is less important.

16. Name several symptoms that are indications for joint replacement surgery in a patient with arthritis of the hip or knee.

- Significant pain refractory to nonoperative interventions that interferes with activities of daily living.
- Inability to walk more than one block as a result of pain.
- Inability to stand in one place for >20 to 30 minutes as a result of pain.
- Inability to obtain restful sleep resulting from pain when rolling over in bed at night.
- Inability to climb stairs without a railing (fall risk).
- Difficulty putting on pants, socks, and shoes.

17. How do cemented, cementless, and hybrid prostheses differ?

The terms cemented and cementless refer to methods of fixation of total joint arthroplasty prostheses for the hip and knee. Most experience is with **cemented** prostheses where a self-curing acrylic cement, polymethylmethacrylate, is used to improve fixation between the prosthetic component and bone. Advances in cementing techniques and materials have led to improved longevity and fewer problems with aseptic loosening, particularly in patients with poor bone quality.

Cementless prostheses include press fit and porous ingrowth prostheses. Press fit relies on a snug fit between prosthesis and bone without the use of cement. Porous ingrowth prostheses contain pores or trabeculated metal located on the proximal portion of the femoral component and acetabulum that allow ingrowth or ongrowth of bone. Hydroxyapatite or growth factors may be incorporated into the porous coating to stimulate bone ingrowth and better fixation. Overall, there is bone ingrowth into approximately 10% of the porous-coated surface. Often, patients with press-fit components are able to progress with immediate unrestricted weight bearing.

Cemented stems and cementless acetabular components have demonstrated the best longevity. Consequently, many surgeons use a cementless acetabular component with a cemented femoral component. This is termed a **hybrid hip replacement.**

18. Who should get a cemented arthroplasty and who should get a cementless prosthesis?

In the **hip,** this is an area of controversy. Conventional wisdom in the United States suggests that younger, active patients with good bone quality in whom intimate apposition of prosthesis to bone can be achieved intraoperatively are the best candidates for cementless total hip arthroplasty (THA). This is usually a patient aged <50 to 60 years with OA of the hip. Cemented prostheses remain the "gold standard" and preferred in patients with RA with poor bone stock, in the elderly with low activity levels, and in hybrid hip implants. Regardless of the prosthesis, over 90% of THAs are pain-free and without complications 10 to 15 years postoperatively.

In the **knee,** cemented implants (posterior cruciate retaining, posterior stabilized condylar, and total condylar prosthesis) demonstrate 90% to 95% satisfactory results at 5 to 10 years for both patients with RA and OA. Cementless prostheses are gaining popularity with new 3-D printed trabeculated metal manufacturing techniques but are reserved for younger active patients with good bone quality. In a **hybrid knee replacement,** the cementless component is reserved for the femur, whereas tibia and patella components are cemented.

19. What are the differences between minimally invasive and traditional/standard techniques for THA?

The traditional/standard technique for THA is a posterior lateral, direct lateral, or anterior approach with an incision that is 6 to 12 inches long. This technique provides good visualization for component placement. The posterior lateral approach and direct lateral approach have a longer recovery time resulting from splitting and dissection of hip musculature (gluteus maximus/external rotators or hip abductors). The posterior approach results in more risk for postoperative hip dislocation (1% to 2%). The anterior approach gains exposure to the hip without detachment of surrounding muscles. Recently, some surgeons have been performing a minimally invasive (solely based on length of incision) incision technique where the incision is only 4 inches, but the approaches and postoperative complication rates are the same. Additionally, most studies suggest similar recovery times and outcomes between minimally invasive and standard techniques.

20. How commonly does aseptic loosening occur?

In cemented THA done using inferior techniques, the rate of aseptic loosening requiring revision was 10% to 15% at 10 to 15 years of follow-up (1%/year). Radiographic loosening of the femoral prosthetic component was as high as 30% to 40%. With contemporary cement techniques there is now <3% loosening at 10 years, 5% at 15 years, and 10% at 20 years. These rates are comparable to the frequency of loosening in the best porous-coated cementless prostheses. Patients who are young (<50 years) and/or heavy (>200 lb) have the highest incidence of loosening for both cemented and cementless methods.

21. **Why does aseptic loosening occur and what is periprosthetic osteolysis?**

Osteolysis around prosthetic joints causing loosening of the components is the most important long-term complication of total hip and knee surgery. It is reported that between 30% and 70% of prosthetic components (both cemented and cementless) have evidence of periprosthetic osteolysis at 10 years post arthroplasty as evidenced by a radiolucent line >2 to 3 mm in thickness around the prosthesis. It is caused by polyethylene particles or metal debris produced by wear at the articulating surfaces of the prosthesis. The particulate debris tracks down the side of the prosthesis where it is ingested by macrophages in the membrane lining the bone–cement or bone–implant interfaces. These macrophages produce prostaglandins and cytokines, such as interleukin-1 and tumor necrosis factor (TNF), which leads to osteoclast stimulation and endosteal bone resorption. Treatment has included bisphosphonates (downregulates macrophages and osteoclasts), indomethacin (decreases prostaglandin production), anti-TNF-α therapy, as well as revision surgery with bone grafting. However, with newer bearing surface materials over the last 20 years the above numbers are no longer commonly accepted. With current implants the survivorship for both hip and knees when solely looking at wear debris and osteolysis is >90% at 20 years.

22. **What is metallosis?**

Metallosis is a complication of metal-on-metal implants used predominantly for THAs. It occurs in 1% of patients by 5 years. The metal implants contain chromium and cobalt which can be released as wear particles during use. The metal debris (particularly cobalt) is highly reactive and attracts lymphocytes more than macrophages. This can cause a cytotoxic local tissue effect and/or a hypersensitivity reaction. This can lead to necrosis/fibrosis of periprosthetic tissue leading to muscle necrosis, osteolysis with loosening, effusions, solid soft tissue masses, and aseptic cysts. Metal ion blood levels (>7 ppb), skin patch testing, and lymphocyte transformation tests are used for diagnosis but give inconsistent results so infection should always be ruled out first.

In addition, metal ions can gain entry to the blood stream and cause heavy metal poisoning characterized by skin rashes, cardiomyopathy, hearing and vision problems, depression, cognitive difficulties, renal impairment, and thyroid dysfunction. These patients typically have high metal ion blood levels (>17–20 ppb) with this complication. Treatment of metallosis requires revision arthroplasty with removal of the metal-on-metal implant.

23. **What unique postoperative complication occurs in patients receiving cementless THA?**

Mild to moderate **thigh pain** occurs in approximately 20% of patients receiving a porous-coated THA. This pain is attributable to a bony stress reaction occurring at the tip of the femoral stem which can often be identified on radiographs. It usually does not require medication and resolves in 12 to 18 months. Additionally, modern implant design has dramatically reduced the incidence of this given more bone friendly ingrowth surfaces and geometry which produces more physiologic loading in the proximal femur.

24. **How is arthroscopy used in the management of knee OA?**

Arthroscopic debridement of the knee is indicated in patients with mechanical symptoms (e.g., locking) resulting from an internal derangement, such as a meniscal tear. Arthroscopic debridement and lavage may provide several months of lessened pain in some patients with more advanced degenerative arthritic changes. However, this remains controversial as blinded studies have shown no significant difference in outcomes between arthroscopic debridement and sham surgery.

25. **When should osteotomy about the knee be chosen over total knee replacement?**

Osteotomy is appropriate in the young, active patient with unicompartmental arthritis. The **high tibial osteotomy** is the most commonly performed realignment procedure for the knee with degenerative changes limited to either the medial or lateral compartment. Involvement of the patellofemoral compartment, inflammatory arthritis, marked loss of motion, and instability are contraindications. This procedure is usually intended to relieve pain, preserve functional status, and delay the need for a total knee replacement. The most common complications include under correction and peroneal nerve injury when correcting a valgus deformity.

26. What are the indications for unicompartmental arthroplasty of the knee?

This is an area of some controversy, and some surgeons are opposed to unicompartmental arthroplasty. It is indicated in a patient with at least 90 to 110 degrees of flexion arc and arthritic involvement of only one compartment of the knee. It is contraindicated in inflammatory arthritis, <90 to 110 degrees arc of motion, absence of the anterior or posterior cruciate ligaments, flexion contracture (>15 degrees), fixed angular deformity (varus >15 degrees or valgus >20 degrees), and/or involvement of the patellofemoral compartment. It is accomplished by resurfacing the femoral and tibial joint surface in the involved compartment. Revision to total knee replacement is possible, but this is technically more difficult and has higher complication and failure rates than primary arthroplasty.

27. Discuss the problems that can occur with a revision THA/total knee arthroplasty.

Revision arthroplasties are technically more challenging than primary arthroplasty, and the outcome (longevity) of the revision is significantly shorter and attendant complications higher. One of the significant problems encountered during revision is loss of bone stock, irrespective of mode of fixation. Another problem is soft tissue balance producing instability in the revised hip and altered mechanics in the revised knee.

28. How frequently does infection complicate total hip and total knee replacements?

Early postoperative infection rates are typically <0.5% with use of perioperative antibiotics. Late infections (>1 year postoperatively) occur in 1% to 3% of patients with RA and fewer patients with OA. Infection rate in revision arthroplasties can be as high as 4%. A patient with a painful prosthesis or loosening and an elevated C-reactive protein should be evaluated for an infected prosthesis regardless of the absence of systemic symptoms such as fever.

29. Should patients with total joint replacements receive prophylactic antibiotics before having dental work done?

Controversial. The American Academy of Orthopedic Surgeons (orthopedists) and the American Dental Association (dentists) issued a joint guideline stating there is insufficient evidence to recommend antibiotic prophylaxis for dental procedures in patients who have a history of total joint replacement. Some physicians disagree and use prophylactic antibiotics for at least the first 2 years postoperatively, especially in patients they consider immunosuppressed. The author uses amoxicillin, cephalexin, or cephadrine 2000 mg orally 1 hour before the procedure. If allergic to penicillin, a patient should get clindamycin 600 mg orally 1 hour before the procedure.

30. How is a prosthetic joint infection (PJI) managed?

Early infections (<2–4 weeks postoperatively; < 2–3 weeks acute hematogenous infection) with a well-fixed prosthesis and no sinus tract can be managed with open synovectomy, thorough debridement, antibiotics, and retention of the prosthesis, often with removal and replacement of the polyethylene insert in TKA (i.e., debridement, antibiotics, and implant retention [DAIR]). Additional surgical debridements may be necessary. Antibiotics duration consists of intravenous antibiotics for 4–6 weeks followed by oral antibiotics for a prolonged duration depending on pathogen and site of joint infection (total antibiotic duration 3–6 months). This is curative in up to 70% to 75% of patients. Some patients with an early PJI may be better managed with a one-stage revision arthroplasty.

　　Late infections usually present with only pain but can present with obvious sepsis of the involved joint. Initial workup involves obtaining a CBC with differential, sedimentation rate, and C-reactive protein. Arthrocentesis, preferably by the index surgeon, should be considered if clinical suspicion is high. If empiric antibiotics were initiated but the patient is clinically stable, a minimum 2-week antibiotic holiday is recommended prior to arthrocentesis to optimize culture yield. Alpha-defensin is a synovial biomarker that has recently demonstrated high sensitivity and specificity for prosthetic joint infections. Once the diagnosis is made, the gold standard for treatment is a 2-stage revision arthroplasty. The first stage is done after a 2-week antibiotic holiday and involves removal and culture of prosthetic components, thorough debridement, and antibiotic cement or polyethylene spacer placement. This is followed by intravenous antibiotics for 4–6 weeks. Typically, an antibiotic holiday (2 weeks) is then initiated and repeat testing for infection is performed. If this is negative, then the second stage of reimplantation and culture is performed generally about 2–3 months after the initial resection and antibiotic spacer placement surgery. This two-stage resection arthroplasty with reimplantation is curative in 80% to 90% of patients. Long-term oral antibiotic suppression therapy is necessary in patients whose cultures are positive from tissue specimens obtained during the second stage of reimplantation. Recently, comparison studies have shown that selected patients with a late PJI may be successfully treated with a one-stage revision arthroplasty.

31. Name the two most common etiologies of ankle arthritis. How are they managed surgically?

Posttraumatic arthritis and RA. The ankle joint very rarely develops OA compared with the hip and knee, but when it does, it is most commonly related to posttraumatic changes. Fractures that result in minimal amounts (1–2 mm) of lateral talar subluxation will produce degenerative changes in a relatively short time because of decreased surface area contact and increased joint reactive forces.

Regardless of the etiology, functional bracing (Arizona brace) should be pursued until a patient can no longer tolerate this form of management. Total ankle arthroplasty (TAA) and arthrodesis are the two definitive options for end-stage ankle arthritis. While arthroplasty aims to preserve motion and better facilitates ambulating on uneven surfaces, outcomes are not as reliable or long lasting as seen in hip and knee arthroplasty, with TAA 10-year survivorship ranging from 70–90%. Ankle arthrodesis currently remains the most reliable salvage procedure for an end-stage arthritic ankle but can lead to accelerated arthrosis in adjacent joints (e.g., subtalar and transtarsal joints).

32. Which joints are fused in a triple arthrodesis?

The subtalar, calcaneocuboid, and talonavicular joints. Both RA and JIA affect the subtalar and transtarsal joints. These joint involvements can be isolated or combined, and there has been a trend toward isolated arthrodesis of involved joints rather than triple arthrodesis when possible. Particularly common is isolated talonavicular joint destruction. If this occurs in an adult with RA, then isolated fusion is recommended. Conversely, if the involvement occurs at a young age secondary to JIA, then the entire transtarsal joint (talonavicular, calcaneocuboid) should be arthrodesed because this will provide a longer-term satisfactory result.

Isolated subtalar arthrodesis is commonly performed when the remaining articulations of the triple joint are uninvolved and supple. Triple arthrodesis requires similar precision in positioning to that of ankle arthrodesis to maximize walking biomechanics. In general, insensate feet (usually secondary to diabetes) are a contraindication to bony fusion because of the high likelihood of skin ulceration and subsequent infection.

33. What is hallux valgus and how is it evaluated for surgery?

Hallux valgus is the most common affliction of the normal adult foot. It is a condition where the large toe is deviated laterally with the first metatarsal head deviated medially causing bunion deformity. The hallux valgus angle is measured by a line drawn through the proximal phalanx of the large toe and through the first metatarsal. A normal angle is 0 to 15 degrees with moderate (>25 degrees) and severe (>35 degrees) deformities commonly occurring.

The cause of hallux valgus can be attributable to heredity, especially in combination with a short hallux relative to the second toe (Greek foot). Other congenital causes include pes planovalgus (flat feet) and metatarsus primus varus. The intermetatarsal angle between the first and second metatarsals is measured by a line drawn through the first and second metatarsals. The intermetatarsal angle is normally 0 to 10 degrees, whereas angles >16 degrees are moderate and >21 degrees are severely deformed. The need for surgical correction is considered if the painful deformity interferes with a patient's lifestyle or ability to wear shoes and there is a failure of conservative management (wider toe box shoes). There are over 100 different operations for correction of hallux valgus. The choice depends on the surgeon's skill and how the deformity needs correction (i.e., proximal metatarsal wedge osteotomy if intermetatarsal angle is too great, etc.). Implant arthroplasty does not provide reliable long-term results compared with arthrodesis (15 degrees valgus, 25 degrees dorsiflexion).

34. What is a Clayton-Hoffman procedure?

A commonly performed salvage procedure for advanced rheumatoid forefoot deformity. The rheumatoid forefoot pattern of involvement usually includes degeneration and instability at the first metatarsophalangeal (MTP) joint, leading to hallux valgus and bunion deformity. The lesser toes are also involved with synovitis, leading to subluxation and eventual dislocation at the remaining MTP joints. This results in prominent metatarsal heads on the plantar surface and the development of intractable plantar keratoses. This progressive deformation commonly involves all the MTP joints to some degree.

The **Clayton-Hoffman procedure** entails resection of all the metatarsal heads through either a plantar or dorsal approach. Rarely, only two metatarsal joints will be involved, and the procedure can be performed only on the involved joints. However, it is not recommended to remove only one or three involved metatarsal heads. Fusion of the first MTP joint is often done concurrently with the Clayton-Hoffman procedure.

35. Differentiate between hammer toe, claw toe, and mallet toe.

Differences among hammer toe, claw toe, and mallet toe are outlined in Table 89.1.

36. Discuss the indications for surgery in a patient with symptomatic disc herniation.

Overall, approximately 1% of patients with herniated discs eventually require surgery. Absolute indications include disc herniation causing cauda equina syndrome, progressive spinal stenosis, or marked muscular weakness and progressive neurologic deficit despite conservative management. Controversy arises over indications for surgery in patients with less severe symptoms and signs. Relative indications for laminectomy and disc removal include intolerable pain with sciatica symptoms unrelieved by nonsurgical treatment (including corticosteroid injections) and recurrent back pain and sciatica that fail to improve significantly so that a patient can participate in activities of daily living after 6 to 12 weeks of conservative nonsurgical therapy.

Overall, long-term relief of sciatica has been shown to be the same in operative versus nonoperative patients, although the operative patients achieve their degree of relief more rapidly. The best results from surgery are obtained in the emotionally stable patient who has unequivocal disc herniation documented by consistent symptoms, compatible physical examination and tension signs, abnormal EMG that confirms the physical examination, and an abnormal MRI of the spine or myelogram confirming the EMG. The most common cause for surgical failure is poor initial patient selection. Patients should be warned that surgery will help the radicular symptoms but may not help the back pain.

TABLE 89.1 Differences Among Hammer Toe, Claw Toe, and Mallet Toe

| FLEXIBLE TOE DEFORMITY | JOINT POSITION | | | SURGICAL MANAGEMENT |
	MTP	PIP	DIP	
Hammer toe	Uninvolved, neutral	Flexion	Uninvolved, neutral	Flexible—flexor to extensor transfer Fixed—hemiresection arthroplasty, excision of distal portion of proximal phalanx
Claw toe	Fixed, extension	Fixed, flexion	Uninvolved, neutral or flexion	Resection of both sides of the PIP joint; joint dorsal capsulotomy and extensor tenotomy, flexor to extensor transfer
Mallet toe	Uninvolved, neutral	Uninvolved, neutral	Fixed, flexion	Excision of middle phalanx and/or flexor tenotomy if flexible

DIP, Distal interphalangeal; *MTP*, metatarsophalangeal; *PIP*, proximal interphalangeal.

37. List and discuss some of the recent advances in lumbar spine surgery.

- Chronic (>1 year) low back pain with degenerative disc disease:

  Spinal fusion with bone graft: this is the most common surgery. Fusion can be done with or without instrumentation (plates, screws, cages) that serve as internal splints. Bone morphogenic proteins are frequently used to improve fusion. Unfortunately, there is little evidence that this improves pain more than conservative nonsurgical therapy.

  Lumbar artificial disc replacement: theoretic advantage over fusion is that the prosthetic disc will help preserve ROM and lessen the chance for progressive degeneration of discs above and below a fusion. There is little evidence that an artificial disc is any better than fusion. Patients who are candidates are aged <60 years, have disease limited to one disc space, and have no back deformities or neurologic deficits.

- Lumbar disc prolapse meeting criteria for surgery (see Question 36):

  Open discectomy: standard technique. Frequently involves a laminectomy.

  Microdiscectomy: most common procedure performed. Smaller incision. Involves a hemilaminectomy and removal of disc material.

  Minimally invasive techniques to remove the disc: tubular or trocar discectomy, percutaneous manual nucleotomy, endoscopic discectomy, coblation nucleoplasty, disc DeKompressor, others. Smaller incisions and quicker recovery times.

- Spinal stenosis:

  Decompressive laminectomy: most common surgery. Fusion with or without instrumentation is also done especially for multilevel laminectomy and for degenerative spondylolisthesis causing stenosis. Interbody cages are indicated when neuroforaminal stenosis exists in the cranial-caudal plane as restoration of disc height is necessary to restore the neuroforamen. Instrumentation and bone morphogenic proteins improve the chance of fusion but not clinical outcomes.

  Interspinous spacer implantation (X-STOP, Coflex, TOPS): titanium implant placed between two spinous processes. Patients who may be candidates for this procedure are aged over 50 years, have no or low-grade spondylolisthesis, suffer from intermittent claudication/leg pain exacerbated by back extension and relieved by sitting forward, and have only one or at most two lumbar levels involved. Certain deformities and severe osteoporosis are contraindications.

- Spondylolysis and isthmic spondylolisthesis:

  Spondylolysis, seen in 6% of the population, is a lytic defect of the pars interarticularis. Isthmic spondylolisthesis is much less common and is attributable to lytic defects in the pars interarticularis bilaterally with anterior subluxation occurring most commonly (90%) at L5 on S1. This differs from degenerative spondylolisthesis, which occurs most commonly with L4 disc degeneration leading to posterior subluxation of L4 vertebrae causing spinal stenosis. Posterolateral fusion is the procedure of choice for isthmic spondylolisthesis.

BIBLIOGRAPHY

Azar FM, Beaty JH, eds. *Campbell's Operative Orthopedics*. 14th ed. Philadelphia, PA: Elsevier; 2021.

Challoumas D, Murray E, Ng N, Putti A, Millar N. A meta-analysis of surgical interventions for base of thumb arthritis. *J Wrist Surg*. 2022;11:550–560.

Chou R, Baisden J, Carragee EJ, et al. Surgery for low back pain: a review of the evidence for an American Pain Society clinical practice guideline. *Spine (Phila, PA 1976)*. 2009;34:1094.

Chou R, Loeser JD, Owens DK, et al. Interventional therapies, surgery, and interdisciplinary rehabilitation for low back pain: an evidence-based clinical practice guideline from the American Pain Society. *Spine (Phila, PA 1976)*. 2007;32:2403.

Douketis JD, Spyropoulos AC, Murad MH, et al. Perioperative management of antithrombotic therapy. *Chest*. 2022;162:e207–e243.

Ekman P, Möller H, Hedlund R. The long-term effect of posterolateral fusion in adult isthmic spondylolisthesis: a randomized controlled study. *Spine J*. 2005;5:36–44.

Goodman SM, Springer BD, Chen AF, et al. 2022 American College of Rheumatology/American Association of hip and knee surgeons guideline for the perioperative management of antirheumatic medication in patients with rheumatic diseases undergoing elective total hip or total knee arthroplasty. *Arthritis Care Res (Hoboken)*. 2022;74:1399–1408.

Goodman SB, Gallo J. Periprosthetic osteolysis: mechanisms, prevention and treatment. *J Clin Med*. 2019;8:2091.

Goubran H, Ragab F, Seghatchian J, et al. Blood transfusion in autoimmune rhematic diseases. *Transfus Apher Sci*. 2022;61:103596.

Granchi D, Savarino LM, Ciapetti G, Baldini N. Biological effects of metal degradation in hip arthroplasties. *Crit Rev Toxicol.* 2018;48:170–193.

Hannon CP, Goodman SM, Austin MS, et al. 2023 American College of Rheumatology and American Association of hip and knee surgeons clinical practice guideline for the optimal timing of elective hip or knee arthroplasty for patients with symptomatic moderate-to-severe osteoarthritis or advanced symptomatic osteonecrosis with secondary arthritis for whom nonoperative therapy is ineffective. *Arthritis Care Res (Hoboken).* 2023;75:2227–2238.

Holelnbeck BL, Hoffman M, Fang CJ, et al. Elimination of routine urinalysis before elective orthopaedic surgery reduces antibiotic utilization without impacting catheter-associated urinary tract infection or surgical site infection rates. *Hip Pelvis.* 2021;33:225–230.

Jacobs WC, van der Gaag NA, Kruyt MC, et al. Total disc replacement for chronic discogenic low back pain: a Cochrane review. *Spine (Phila, PA 1976).* 2013;38:24.

Kirkley A, Birmingham TB, Litchfield RB, et al. A randomized trial of arthroscopic surgery for osteoarthritis of the knee. *N Engl J Med.* 2008;359:1097.

Liu C, Ferreira GE, Abdel Shaheed C, et al. Surgical versus non-surgical treatment for sciatica: systematic review and meta-analysis of randomized controlled trials. *BMJ.* 2023;381:e070730.

Longo UG, De Salvatore S, Bandini B, et al. Debridement, antibiotics, and implant retention (DAIR) for the early prosthetic joint infection of total knee and hip arthroplasties: a systematic review. *J ISAKOS.* 2024;9:62–70.

MacMahon A, Rao SS, Chaudhry YP, et al. Perioperative optimization in total joint arthroplasty—the paradigm shift from preoperative clearance: a narrative review. *HSS J.* 2022;18:418–427.

McKee L, Malhotra A. The rheumatoid hand: a review of current medical and surgical management. *Ortho Trauma.* 2023;37:118–124.

Mizra SK, Deyo RA. Systematic review of randomized trials comparing lumbar fusion surgery to nonoperative care for treatment of chronic back pain. *Spine (Phila, PA 1976).* 2007;32:816.

Ortega-Avila AB, Moreno-Velasco A, Cervera-Garvi P, et al. Surgical treatment for the ankle and foot in patients with rheumatoid arthritis: a systematic review. *J Clin Med.* 2019;9:42.

Pivec R, Johnson AJ, Mears SC, Mont MA. Hip arthroplasty. *Lancet.* 2012;380:1768–1777.

Ravi B, Escott B, Shah PS, et al. A systematic review and meta-analysis comparing complications following total joint arthroplasty for rheumatoid arthritis versus for osteoarthritis. *Arthritis Rheum.* 2012;64:3839.

Sahan I, Anagnostakos K. Metallosis after knee replacement: a review. *Arch Orthop Trauma Surg.* 2020;140:1791–1808.

Santana DC, Hadad MJ, Emara A, et al. Perioperative management of chronic antithrombotic agents in elective hip and knee arthroplasty. *Medicine.* 2021;57:188.

Shlobin NA, Dahdaleh NS. Cervical spine manifestations of rheumatoid arthritis: a review. *Neurosurg Rev.* 2021;44:1957–1965.

Sollecito TP, Abt E, Lockhart PB, et al. The use of prophylactic antibiotics prior to dental procedures in patients with prosthetic joints: Evidence-based clinical practice guideline for dental practitioners—a report of the American Dental Association Council on Scientific Affairs. *J Am Dent Assoc.* 2015;146:11–16.

Tosteson AN, Tosteson TD, Lurie JD, et al. Comparative effectiveness evidence from the spine patient outcomes research trial: surgical versus nonoperative care for spinal stenosis, degenerative spondylolisthesis, and intervertebral disc herniation. *Spine (Phila, PA 1976).* 2011;36:2061–2068.

Weinstein JN, Lurie JD, Tosteson TD, et al. Surgical versus nonoperative treatment for lumbar disc herniation: four-year results for the spine patient outcomes research trial (SPORT). *Spine (Phila, PA 1976).* 2008;33:2789.

Wolfs JFC, Klopenburg M, Fehlings MG, et al. Neurologic outcome of surgical and conservative treatment of rheumatoid cervical spine subluxation: a systemic review. *Arthritis Rheum.* 2009;61:1743.

Yan L, Ge L, Dong S, et al. Evaluation of comparative efficacy and safety of surgical approaches for total hip arthroplasty: a systematic review and network meta-analysis. *JAMA Netw Open.* 2023;6:e2253942.

Zhu XM, Perera E, Gohal C, Dennis B, Khan M, Alolabi B. A systematic review of outcomes of wrist arthrodesis and wrist arthroplasty in patients with rheumatoid arthritis. *J Hand Surg Eur.* 2021;46:297–303.

FURTHER READING

www.orthoinfo.aaos.org/main.cfm.

CHAPTER 90

Disability

Audrey Leung, MD and Namrata Singh, MD, MSCI

1. What options are available for an individual who can no longer perform his or her job satisfactorily because of a musculoskeletal problem?

- Adapt the workplace
  Obtain or modify special equipment or devices
  Modify work schedules
  Job restructuring
- Consider switching jobs or reassignment to another position
- Vocational rehabilitation
- Apply for disability benefits.

2. What is disability?

Disability can be defined generally as *not being able to do something because of an illness or injury.* Most often, disability refers to an **individual** economic loss (by not being able to work at a previously acceptable level) because of a physical or mental condition. In insurance policies, laws, and regulations, the word "disability" has a more specific definition and needs to be distinguished from two similar yet specific terms: **impairment** and **handicap**.

3. Give a specific definition of disability.

Disability is an alteration of an individual's capacity to meet personal, social, or occupational demands because of an impairment. It is the gap between what an individual can do and what the individual needs or wants to do. The degree of disability is affected by not only the individual's impairment but also the economic and social aspects of that person's life (i.e., age, education, training). People with the same impairment do not necessarily have the same disability. Disability is assessed by nonmedical means.

4. Define impairment.

Impairment is a physical or mental **limitation to normal function** resulting from a disease process. Impairment is determined by a physician. An impairment does not necessarily mean that a person is disabled.

5. What is a handicap?

Handicap refers to the **social consequences** that relate to an impairment or disability. A handicap is present if an individual has:
1. An impairment or disability that substantially limits one or more of life's activities or prevents the fulfillment of a role that is normal for that individual;
2. Medical record of such an impairment;
3. Barriers to accomplishing life's tasks that can be overcome only by compensating in some way for the effects of the impairment. Such compensation involves things like crutches, wheelchairs, prostheses, or even the amount of time necessary to complete a task.

6. Management of the Rheumatic Diseases.

Disease	Work
• Type of musculoskeletal disease	• Occupation
• Disease severity	• Job autonomy
• Impairment severity	• Work experience

Personal	Social
• Age	• Social support
• Gender	• Peer and social pressures for or against disability
• Education/training	
• Personality	

Most physicians concentrate on trying to alleviate the disease factors to decrease disability. The other factors may be just as important in determining whether a patient considers himself or herself disabled.

7. What state and federal programs are set up to deal with disability?

There are two major government programs that deal with a person's inability to work: **Social Security Disability** and **Worker's Compensation**. The Social Security Administration administers two programs that differ mainly in eligibility criteria: Social Security Disability Insurance (Title II) (SSDI, also called Disability Insurance Benefits) and Supplemental Security Income (Title XVI) (SSI). According to the annual statistical report on Social Security Disability in 2021, 9.2 million people received SSD benefits with payments totaling over $11.9 billion. The most common reason (34% of all claims) was for musculoskeletal and connective tissue conditions.

8. Who is eligible for Social Security disability (SSDI) payments?

Any employee 18–64 years of age with an appropriate work history
Dependent of a deceased person who was receiving SSDI (survivor SSDI benefits) includes:
• Unmarried son or daughter disabled before age 22
• Spouse who is caring for a child who is <16 years
• Spouse who is ≥age 60 years
• Disabled widow or widower ≥50 years of age whose disability started within 7 years of spouse's death
• Disabled, divorced widow or widower ≥ age 50. Must have been married at least 10 years.

9. Describe Social Security Disability Insurance (SSDI).

SSDI is a federally regulated program that was established in the 1950s. It is the largest disability insurance program in the world. In SSDI, employers and workers pay into a trust fund. Workers contribute through payroll taxes (FICA) and receive benefits (based on lifetime earnings) if they meet certain listed criteria:
• Age: over 18 and less than 65 years.
• If over age 31, need 40 work credits with at least 20 of them earned in the last 10 years prior to year of disability onset. As of 2023, a person can only get 4 work credits a year which is met if that person earns over $6560 for that year and has paid FICA on that amount. Disabled worker's less than age 31 have prorated criteria for work credit requirements.
• Unable "to engage in any substantial gainful activity (SGA)" by reason of any medically determinable physical or mental impairment which can be expected to result in death, or which has lasted or can be expected to last for a continuous period of not less than 12 months. SGA is defined as unable to earn over $1470/month for non-blind (in 2023).

A person can apply for SSDI immediately upon becoming disabled. The Social Security Administration tries to take into account individual variations in impairment, vocational, and educational backgrounds. SSDI considers only <u>global</u> disability, so there are no partial awards. Disability payments can start 5 months after the date of disability onset. Persons may also qualify for Medicare to help cover medical expenses after receiving SSDI benefits for 24 months. A disabled person who cannot afford medical expenses during this 24 month waiting period can receive Medicaid if they qualify.

10. **How much are the SSDI benefits and how long can they be received? What are auxillary benefits?**

The monthly benefit varies and is based on a complex formula that looks at the average covered earnings over a period of years that the patient has paid into the social security system. The average monthly benefit as of 2021 is $1358.30/month. A person on SSDI has a case review every 3–7 years to determine if they still qualify for disability. They can receive SSDI up to age 65 at which time they receive their monthly retirement benefit payment. The following dependents of a disabled worker can receive auxillary benefits which can be up to 50% of the monthly benefit that the disabled worker is receiving:

- Unmarried sons or daughters < 18 years old (can be 18 years of age if attending high school)
- Unmarried son or daughter disabled before age 22
- Spouse ≥ age 62 years
- Spouse who is caring for a child who is disabled
- Ex-spouse if previously married over 10 yrs, ≥ age 62 yrs, and unmarried

11. **What is Supplemental Security Income (SSI)?**

Individuals not qualifying for SSDI because of a lack of work experience may be covered by another program, SSI. SSI pays monthly sums to financially needy people who are either >65 years of age or qualified persons of any age with documented disabilities. SSI requires an evaluation of assets, sometimes called a "means" test. Usually, those who receive SSI are eligible to have some medical expenses covered by Medicaid and will be eligible for Supplemental Nutrition Assistance Program (SNAP; previously called food stamps). Disabled persons are eligible for SSI if they meet the following asset limits (means test):

- Individual has less than $2000 ($3000 if a couple) in liquid assets (bank account, stocks, bonds, etc).
- Gross wages are less than $1913/month for an individual or less than $2827/month for a couple. Wages used to pay for items or services that help the person work are not counted as part of the gross wages.
- Income from pensions or gifts is less than $834/month for an individual or less than $1391/month for a couple.
- Can have one vehicle for transportation.
- Can have a house that is the person's principal residence.
- Life insurance policies with combined face values less than or equal to $1500.
- Burial plots for oneself or one's family.
- Burial funds up to $1500 in a separate bank account.

12. **How much are SSI benefits?**

The monthly SSI payment is based on the federal benefit rate (FBR). In 2023, the FBR was $914/month for individuals and $1371/month for a couple who has one disabled person. In most states, there is a monthly state supplement ($10–200) added to the monthly SSI benefit payment. If a disabled person receives an SSDI benefit that is less than the FBR, then they can also receive SSI in an amount that brings the monthly benefit up to the FBR. If a disabled person earns any income, half of whatever they earn over $85 is subtracted from the SSI monthly payment.

13. **Describe the workers' compensation program.**

Workers' compensation is primarily a state-based system, although there is also a program for federal employees under the auspices of the U.S. Department of Labor. Any worker who incurs an illness or sustains an injury during and because of employment is entitled to protection against financial loss. It is a "no-fault" insurance system that provides benefits to all workers who are covered and who meet criteria. It removes the necessity to sue the employer. The program is designed to pay medical expenses and a portion of lost income during the period of disability arising out of gainful employment. Workers' compensation deals effectively with work-related traumatic accidents but has more difficulty with occupational illnesses. Determining if an illness is related to a person's employment may be difficult but only has to exceed a 50% probability that it is related.

Workers' compensation determines disability based on the "whole person concept". Unlike SSDI, it can award partial disability. The disability can be temporary or permanent and it can be partial or total. Disability payments can be a lump sum or structured payments over a period of time depending upon the state-based system.

14. What paperwork is necessary to apply for Social Security Disability?

Social Security number
Birth certificate or other proof of age
Names and addresses of doctors, hospitals, clinics, and institutions involved in medical care
W2 forms or tax return from previous year
Summary of work history for past 15 years
Date employee stopped working
Marital history (if spouse is applying)
Dates of military service

15. For those who meet the eligibility criteria and assemble the required application items, the Social Security Administration then evaluates four major factors. Name them.

- **Inability to perform substantial gainful activity** (work). Gainful activity is defined as earnings that average > $1470/month for non-blind individuals and $2460 for blind individuals (in 2023).
- **Work credits.** Workers > age 31 must have contributed to the Social Security fund for 20 of the preceding 40 quarters. For younger workers, fewer years are required.
- **Severity and extent of impairment**. Objective evidence of a physical or mental impairment is required. Symptoms alone are never sufficient for a determination of disability. There must be corroborating physical, laboratory, and/or radiographic findings. The impairment must interfere with basic work-related activities.
- **Does the impairment meet or exceed listed criteria for disability for that impairment**? The patient's individual physician does not determine if the person is disabled. The Social Security Administration has a list of defined impairments under each body system. If the patient's disease meets the listed measurements of disease severity, then the patient is assumed to have a disabling impairment. These listings make the system more objective and uniform. If the impairment is severe but does not meet the criteria for disability, the Social Security Administration will determine if the individual can perform the work they did previously. If not, the Social Security Administration will try to determine if other work could be done based on the medical condition(s), age, education, past work experience, and transferrable skills.

16. What is residual functional capacity? What is a functional capacity evaluation?

If an applicant's impairment fails to meet the listed criteria for automatic disability, a physician or vocational specialist employed by the Social Security Disability Determination Service must make a determination of the applicant's residual functional capacity (RFC). RFC is the degree to which the applicant has the capacity for sustained performance of the physical requirements of certain levels of work. RFC is determined by a functional capacity evaluation (FCE). The FCE can be performed by appropriately trained physicians or therapists. This is a physical ability test that is specifically related to the individual's occupational requirements. Specific abilities and endurances are measured such as standing, sitting, crawling, lifting, bending, strength, flexibility, pushing, pulling and climbing stairs. These abilities and endurances are quantified according to Department of Labor standards, according to weight and frequency of the activity for five categories of work.

17. Outline the physical requirements as defined by the Department of Labor for each of the five categories of work.

Sedentary work
- Sitting most of the time
- Occasional (up to one-third of an 8-hour day) lifting of ≤10 lbs
- Occasional walking or standing

Light work
- Lifting of ≤ 20 lbs
- Frequent (up to two-thirds of an 8-hour day) lifting or carrying of ≤10 lbs
- Walking or standing to a significant degree
- Sitting with push/pull arm or leg controls

Medium work
  - Occasional lifting of 20–50 lbs
  - Frequent lifting or carrying of 10–25 lbs
  - Physical demands in excess of those for light work

Heavy work
- Occasional lifting of 50–100 lbs
- Frequent lifting or carrying of 25–50 lbs
- Physical demands in excess of those for medium work

Very heavy work
- Occasional lifting of > 100 lbs
- Frequent lifting or carrying of > 50 lbs
- Physical demands in excess of those for heavy work
  Other factors taken into account when determining a person's RFC are fatigue; ability to see, hear, and speak; adequate mental capacity; ability for social interaction with coworkers; and skills to adapt to changes in work routine.

18. How does the Social Security Administration use the RFC in determining disability?

The disability examiner determines the physical demands of the work previously done by the applicant and judges whether the individual has the RFC to do such work. If not, the examiner considers whether the applicant's RFC, coupled with the individual's age, education, and previous work experience, makes it possible for the applicant to do any work. If not, the applicant can be declared disabled, even though his or her impairment did not meet listed disability criteria.

19. How is an application for disability benefits evaluated? Can a decision be appealed?

An application to the Social Security Administration for disability benefits is first evaluated by a physician panel without a personal appearance by the applicant. A decision is supposed to be made within 90 days of filing the disability application, however, due to backlogs this may take up to a year. Consequently, a person should file for disability as soon as they become disabled. Approximately one-third of applications are approved at this point. If denied, an individual has the option of appeal at many stages, while the Social Security Administration does not. After initially being denied, an individual may appeal within 60 days. They can have the application reviewed again by a separate physician panel. However, only about 10–15% of these appeals are granted benefits. A denial at this stage may be appealed to a third level, an administrative law judge, where a personal appearance may first take place. Approximately 50–60% of the cases appealed to administrative law judges are subsequently approved, making this application step very important. Applications denied by the administrative law judge can be appealed to the Social Security Appeals Council and ultimately to a U.S. District Court. Few of these cases (2%) are ultimately approved. Overall, approximately 40–50% of all applications to the Social Security Administration are ultimately approved.

20. If an individual who is receiving disability benefits returns to work, will their benefits be stopped?

Disability recipients continue to receive full disability benefits for up to 9 months after returning to work. This 9-month period is called a trial work period. The 9 months need not be continuous, and only months count in which the individual earns >$1050 (gross)/month or works >80 hours/month (in 2018). Disability benefits are reassessed after the trial work period. If it is decided that disability benefits are no longer needed, the individual receives three more monthly checks. Subsequently, benefits are paid for any month the individual is disabled and unable to perform substantial gainful activity (earn >$1470/month in 2023) for up to 36 months after the trial work period ends. If disability payments end but the individual continues with impairment, the Medicare benefit can be continued for up to 39 months, even though the person is no longer receiving disability payments. If after returning to work a person subsequently discovers they can't work at a level that earns the SGA minimum ($1180/month) due to their disability, they can then apply for expedited reinstatement of their disability benefits if filed within 5 years after benefits ceased due to returning to work.

21. What is vocational rehabilitation?

Vocational rehabilitation (VR) is a service provided for by the Federal Rehabilitation Act of 1973. Funded by both state and federal governments, VR agencies assist people with disabilities to find and keep employment. Every state is required to have a VR program, although the range of services varies among states. Private vocational rehabilitation agencies also provide a wide array of services to disabled and injured individuals.

Any person applying for disability is referred to and considered for vocational rehabilitation. The participating agencies provide counseling, interest/skills evaluation, basic living expenses, education expenses, transportation costs, purchase of special equipment, job training, and placement. These agencies may also acquire services from other public programs. Not all VR services are provided free of charge, but in some cases VR does pay for all expenses when an individual has very limited resources. Disability benefits may be continued while an individual receives VR services. Notably, refusal of VR services may stop disability benefits. If a person recovers while participating in VR services, disability benefits continue if the VR services are likely to enable the person to return to work.

22. What is the primary physician's role while the patient is applying for disability?

The primary physician may be asked to fulfill several roles:
- Information source for the patient
- Details of the disability insurance system
- Options to be pursued if the request is denied
- Information source for the agency by documenting the impairment
- Prior health status
- Objective evidence of impairment (physical findings, radiographs, laboratory abnormalities)
- Progression of symptoms
- Impact the impairment has on the patient's activities of daily living
- Response to therapy
- Patient advocate, supporting the patient during the process of application
- Monitor of ongoing therapy
- Independent validator of an impairment
- Expert witness for litigation

Difficulties arise for both the physician and patient when these roles become contradictory. A physician who tries to be an effective patient advocate and an impartial adjudicator at the same time may be risking a strain of the physician–patient relationship.

23. What are "activities of daily living"?

Usual activities that need to be assessed and documented when evaluating or documenting impairments. Over 60% of patients with chronic musculoskeletal disorders report some limitation with one or more of these activities of daily living.

ACTIVITIES OF DAILY LIVING

CATEGORIES	SPECIFIC ACTIVITIES
Self-care and personal hygiene	Bathing, dressing, brushing teeth, combing hair, eating, toileting
Communication	Writing, speaking, hearing
Ambulation, travel, and posture	Walking, climbing stairs, driving, riding, flying, sitting, standing, lying down
Movement	Lifting, grasping, tactile discrimination
Sleep, social activities, and sexual function	—

24. Does the Americans with Disabilities Act of 1990 apply to musculoskeletal conditions?

Yes. This Act makes it unlawful to discriminate in employment against a qualified individual with a disability. It also outlaws discrimination against individuals with disabilities in state and local government services, public accommodations, transportation, and telecommunications. To be protected, one must have a "substantial" impairment (one that significantly limits or restricts a major life activity) and must be otherwise qualified to perform the essential functions or duties of a job with or without reasonable accommodation. Reasonable accommodations include modifying work schedules, equipment, or environment. An employer may deny providing reasonable accommodations for either financial hardship or business necessity.

BIBLIOGRAPHY

Association American Medical. *Guides to the Evaluation of Permanent Impairment*. 6th ed. Chicago, IL: AMA; 2007.
Carey TS, Hadler NM. The role of the primary care physician in disability determination for Social Security Insurance and Worker's compensation. *Ann Intern Med*. 1986;104:706.
Katz RT, Rondinelli RD. Impairment and disability rating in low back pain. *Occup Med*. 1998;13:213–230.
King PM, Tuckwell N, Barrett TE. A critical review of functional capacity evalutions. *Phys Therapy*. 1998;78:852–866.
Michalopoulos C, Wittenburg D, Israel DA, Warren A. The effects of health care benefits on health care use and health: a randomized trial for disability insurance beneficiaries. *Med Care*. 2012;50:764.
Minnigerode LK. Social Security and the physician. *Missouri Med*. 2000;97:156–158.
Stewart AL, Painter PL. Issues in measuring physical functioning and disability in arthritis patients. *Arthritis Care Res*. 1997;10:395–405.
US Government Printing Office. *Social Security Administration Disability Evaluation Under Social Security*. Washington, DC; 2006.

WEBSITES FOR ADDITIONAL READING

Department of Labor: http://www.dol.gov.
Office of Administrative Law Judges: http://www.oalj.dol.gov.
Social Security Administration: www.ssa.gov.
Qualifications for Disability: https://www.ssa.gov/benefits/disability/qualify.html#anchor0.

CHAPTER 91 Complementary and Alternative Medicine

Amrita Bath, MBBS and Alan R. Erickson, MD

"I didn't say it was good for you," the king replied, "I said there was nothing like it."
–Lewis Carroll (1832–1898) Through the Looking Glass

KEY POINTS

1. Most rheumatology patients are considering, have tried, or are presently using complementary and alternative medicine (CAM) therapies.
2. Some CAM therapies have proven but limited benefits for patients with certain rheumatic diseases.
3. Some CAM therapies can be harmful to patients undergoing surgery or taking particular medications.
4. Physicians should ask patients about CAM therapies, discuss their benefits and risks, and record them in their medical record.

1. What is the definition of CAM?

The term *CAM* describes therapies that have not been scientifically proven to be beneficial. The World Health Organization defines CAM as "A broad set of healthcare practices that are not part of the country's own tradition and are not integrated into the dominant healthcare system." This is not to be confused with quackery or fraud, which is a false claim made deliberately to promote a product or treatment.

2. Justify how widely used are CAM remedies?

Over 130 unconventional modalities and >500 remedies to treat patients have been described. Previous studies indicated that 60% to 90% of patients with rheumatic diseases have used some form of CAM. Rheumatologic conditions are among the most common disease conditions encountered by CAM practitioners. According to the 2007 National Health Institute Survey, 83 million US adults spent $33.9 billion out-of-pocket on visits to CAM practitioners and on purchases of CAM products, classes, and materials. In total, there were approximately 354 million visits to CAM practitioners and approximately 835 million purchases.

3. Why do rheumatology patients choose CAM therapies?

Rheumatic diseases are associated with reduced productivity, increased risk of disability, and lowered quality of life. Conventional therapies for rheumatic diseases like nonsteroidal anti-inflammatory drugs (NSAIDs), disease-modifying antirheumatic drugs, and biologics have potential and realized side effects. Consequently, some patients decline these conventional therapies, opting for other forms of treatments such as CAM, with the belief that these therapies are effective and safer.

4. Does the ACR support CAM therapies?

The ACR developed a position statement concerning complementary and alternative medicine (CAM) for rheumatic diseases for the American College of Rheumatology (ACR) in 1998 that has subsequently been updated several times, including in 2020. It states:

"The American College of Rheumatology (ACR) recognizes the interest in complementary and alternative medicine (CAM) by persons with arthritis. The ACR believes health care providers should be informed about more common CAM modalities such as mind-body interventions, herbal therapy, and nutritional therapy, and should be willing and able to discuss them openly with patients. The ACR supports rigorous scientific evaluation of all modalities that can improve outcomes for patients with rheumatic diseases and recommends continued support of

the National Center for Complementary and Integrative Health. The ACR understands that certain characteristics of some CAM modalities make it difficult or impossible to conduct standard randomized controlled trials. For these modalities, innovative methods of evaluation are needed, as are measures and standards for the generation and interpretation of evidence. The ACR supports the integration of those modalities proven to be safe and effective by scientifically rigorous clinical trials into clinical practice. The ACR advises caution in the use of modalities not studied scientifically. In the absence of rigorous clinical trials, the ACR recommends advising patients that potential harm can occur from unproven therapies. The ACR recommends practitioners be proactive in inquiring about patients' interest and use of CAM."

In 2024, the ACR updated their position statement by making the distinction that some CAM therapies have been shown to be safe and effective in treating rheumatic disease patients. Consequently, these therapies are not alternative to conventional therapy but can be integrated into the patient's care. These therapies are labeled in the position statement as complimentary and integrative medicine for the rheumatic diseases.

5. List the various categories of CAM remedies, procedures, and tests.

Alternative Medical Systems

Holistic medicine	Homeopathy
Naturopathy	Indian traditional medicine (Ayurveda, Siddha)
Chinese traditional medicine	Anthroposophical medicine

Biologically based therapies
Diet therapies

Low-fat diet	Macrobiotic diet
Unpasteurized milk	Vegetarian
Elimination diet	

Nutraceuticals

Glucosamine/Chondroitin	Antioxidants
Cod liver oil	Amino acids
Fish oil (omega-3 fatty acids [FAs])	Green-lipped mussel
Propolis, royal jelly, bee pollen	Cartilage (shark, bovine, chicken)
Megavitamins and supplements	S-adenosylmethionine (SAM-e)

Herbal and natural remedies

Devil's claw	Ginger, nettle, turmeric, wild yam, bromelain
Alfalfa	Chinese herbs (corydalis, genetian, paeonia, scutellaria,
Garlic	*Tripterygium wilfordii* Hook F, and Ma-Huang)
Willow bark	Kelp, sarsaparilla, boswellia, meadowsweet
Herbs rich in γ-linoleic acid (evening primrose oil, borage oil, blackcurrant seed oil)	Marijuana (cannabis) and cannabinoids

Body-based and manipulative therapies

Chiropractic	Rolfing
Massage	Reflexology
Osteopathy	Movement (Feldenkrais method, Alexander technique)

Mind-body interventions and spiritual medicine

Biofeedback	Meditation
Relaxation techniques	Guided imagery
Hypnotherapy	Prayer
Yoga, Tai Chi, Qi Gong	

Energy therapies

Magnets	Pulsed electric field
Reiki	Therapeutic (healing) touch
External qi gong	

Procedures

Acupuncture	Chelation
Colon cleansing	Hydrotherapy
Mineral baths	

Diagnostic tests

Cytotoxic testing
Iridology

Hair analysis
Kinesiology

Miscellaneous

Copper bracelets
Snake oil
Antimicrobials
Leech therapy

Dimethyl sulfoxide (DMSO)
Venoms
Exercise

---

6. Define holistic medicine, homeopathy, and naturopathy.

Holistic medicine holds that people should try to maintain a balance between their physical and emotional processes while seeking harmony with the environment. Disease occurs when this balance is disrupted. **Ayurveda** is an ancient Hindu variation of holistic medicine that uses meditation, breathing exercises, reciting mantras, yoga, and herbal medicines to restore balance of the three basic energy types called doshas within the body and with nature. Some Ayurveda herbs have been found to contain heavy metals (mercury, lead, arsenic) that may cause health problems.

Homeopathy principles were set forth in the 1800s by German physician Samuel Hahnemann. They use dilute preparations of substances that cause the same symptoms the patient is experiencing to stimulate the body's natural defenses to fight disease.

Naturopathy claims that disease is an imbalance in the body that results from the accumulation of waste products. Natural therapies are said to remove the body's "poisons."

7. Is there any evidence that diet affects arthritis?

The subject of diet has attracted many claims of cures for patients with arthritis. This interest stems from various known facts. Historically, autoimmune disease is a relatively recent phenomenon and may correlate with our changing diet. In the late paleolithic period, the human diet was rich in protein as opposed to our current diet, which is rich in fat. This increase in dietary fat can affect the composition of cellular membrane fatty acids (FAs). These membrane FAs are the source of arachidonic acid-derived prostaglandins (PGs) and leukotrienes (LTs), which contribute to inflammation. It has been noted that some patients with inflammatory arthritis may be deficient in zinc, selenium, and vitamins A and C, which are involved in the scavenging or inactivation of oxygen free radicals. Though no convincing scientific evidence indicates that diet causes or cures arthritis, there are observations that diet may modulate the immune system. Innovative research has noted the importance of the gastrointestinal (GI) tract along with our intestinal and mucosal microbiomes in autoimmunity.

8. What is an anti-inflammatory diet?

Many patients with rheumatoid arthritis (RA) report symptom relief from eliminating certain foods (e.g dairy, gluten) and/or including certain other foods in their diet. Some studies modelled on the Mediterranean-style diet (with or without exercise) have indicated positive effects of an anti-inflammatory diet on disease activity in RA patients. The Mediterranean-style diet has been shown to have a greater effect on pain scores than vegetarian or vegan diets. However, special consideration should be given when recommending a Mediterranean diet to RA patients as gluten sensitivity is more common in patients with rheumatic diseases than the general population. In addition, due to a possible link between intestinal dysbiosis and the immune response, a few studies have given RA patients different strains of probiotics to ameliorate symptoms with conflicting results.

9. Can FA ingestion alter our inflammatory response to rheumatic disease?

Yes. FAs are essential to the human diet, with omega-3 and omega-6 FAs being the two major groups. FAs are responsible for the composition of the phospholipids in cellular membranes, and thus these membranes can be altered by dietary intake of omega-3 or omega-6 FA. Additionally, FAs are the precursors for LTs and PGs, the agents (among many) responsible for our inflammatory response. Omega-3 FAs are the precursors of PGE3 and LTB5, which are less inflammatory than PGE2 and LTB4 that come from omega-6 FA. Long-chain omega-3 FAs (Krill oil, fish [salmon] oil) are more effective than short-chain omega-3 FAs (plant oil, e.g., flaxseed). The recommended dose for dietary supplements containing long-chain omega-3 FA is 2000 mg/day (eicosapentaenoic acid [EPA] and docosahexaenoic acid combined) for a safe anti-inflammatory effect.

10. How do fish oils and evening primrose oil affect rheumatic diseases?

It is known that ethnic cultures with diets rich in fish oils (10 g/day), which are primarily long-chain omega-3 FAs, tend to have less autoimmune disease. Omega-3 FA diets can reduce arachidonic acid levels by 33% and increase EPA levels in cellular membranes by 20 times. This results in production of PGE3 and LTB5, which have less inflammatory potential than those agents made from omega-6 FAs.

Evening primrose oil (also **borage seed oil** and **blackcurrant seed oil**) is rich in gamma-linolenic acid (GLA), which is an omega-6 FA. In experimental animal models, excess dietary GLA results in more PGE1 compounds and less LT production, leading to less inflammation. Some studies support that this therapy reduces inflammation in rheumatoid arthritis (RA).

11. What is the theory behind the use of antioxidants?

Antioxidants interfere with the production of free radicals, compounds with an unpaired free electron that takes electrons from others, potentially affecting the immune system or cell membranes. One well-known free radical is superoxide, which is formed using NADPH. Superoxide is both a reducing and oxidizing agent and can spontaneously undergo a reaction to form hydrogen peroxide and oxygen. Hydrogen peroxide can also react with superoxide to produce a hydroxyl radical (the most reactive of the oxygen products) or chloride ions to form hypochlorous acid (the active ingredient in chlorine bleach).

A variety of antioxidants exist including vitamins A, C, D, and E and the trace elements copper, zinc, iron, and selenium, which scavenge free radicals and may protect cells against oxidation. To date, there is little evidence to support that this therapy is helpful in patients with arthritis.

12. Many patients with RA wear copper bracelets. Why?

Copper bracelets were used by the ancient Greeks for their healing powers. Copper salts have been used for the treatment of RA, achieving generally favorable responses, unfortunately along with significant side effects. Copper in bracelets is absorbed through the skin (turning the skin green) and is said to improve arthritis symptoms in some patients, perhaps by binding oxygen free radicals. Interestingly, d-penicillamine, a proven therapy for RA, binds copper, which would suggest that copper is not a useful therapy.

13. Are herbal remedies used by patients with osteoarthritis (OA) and RA?

Yes. Herbal products have been referred to as the most commonly used and abused form of alternative therapies. Herbs are claimed to treat arthritis and other diseases, but is there truth to that claim? Yes. Data does point toward a potential for Phyto antiinflammation, likely through effects on eicosanoid metabolism.

OA: randomized controlled trials (RCTs) have shown that **devil's claw** (*Harpagophytum procumbens*), **bromelain** (a pineapple extract), and **willow bark extract** are effective in reducing pain in patients with OA. **Phytodolor** (golden rod, aspen leaf/bark, and ash bark) has been shown in RCTs to be as effective as NSAIDs in treating OA pain. **Nettle** (*Urtica dioica*) inhibits cyclooxygenase and lipoxygenase pathways as well as suppresses cytokine release. **Ginger** (*Zingibar officinale*) contains gingerol and shogaol that inhibits PG and LT production. It inhibits neutrophil hyperactivity and NETosis. Uncontrolled studies have shown benefit. Note that ginger can interact with antiplatelet and anticoagulant medications, which may cause excess bleeding during surgery. **Avocado soybean unsaponifiables** (ASU) are reported to slow progression of hip and knee OA. ASU contain plant sterols that are chondroprotective by their anti-inflammatory and proanabolic effects on articular chondrocytes. **Green-lipped mussels** (*Perna canaliculus*) contain omega-3 FAs, which are converted into less inflammatory mediators (PGE3, LTB5).

RA: an herb used in China is extract of **thunder god vine** (*Tripterygium wilfordii* Hook F). Its active compounds are celastrol and triptolide, which inhibit nuclear factor κβ and T-cell proliferation as well as production of proinflammatory cytokines to include interleukin (IL)-2 and gamma-interferon. A RCT showed that it was superior to sulfasalazine in the treatment of RA.

Side effects, however, were significant. **Cat's claw** (*Uncaria tomentosa*) and **turmeric** (*Curcuma longa*) contain immunomodulatory and anti-inflammatory ingredients and have been shown in small RCTs to be moderately effective in RA. Turmeric is also used to treat OA pain by depleting substance P from nerve root endings similar to capsaicin. **Cinnamon** (*Cinnamomum burmannii*) contains trans-cinnamaldehyde which has been shown to down-regulate multiple cytokines in mouse models and in a small randomized controlled trial (RCT) was beneficial in RA. Dose should be less than 3 grams/day to avoid potential liver toxicity. **Tibetan five-nectar formula** medicated bath therapy is derived from five types of plants that are considered anti-inflammatory. Studies in RA demonstrating benefit are of poor quality and cannot be critically evaluated.

14. **What are some other herbs and dietary supplements do Rheumatology patients commonly use to control symptoms?**
   - **Black cohosh**
     Uses: treats hot flashes and moodiness at menopause.
   - **Cayenne**
     Uses: contains the chemical capsaicin that gives hot cayenne peppers their heat. When applied as a skin cream, it can deplete substance P from nerve endings, thus decreasing pain. Used for postherpetic neuralgia and rubbed on single joint with arthritis.
   - **Coenzyme Q-10**
     Uses: relieves chronic fatigue, immune stimulant, heart failure. Contains ubiquinone, which is a cofactor for metabolic pathways that generate ATP. Also, a free radical scavenger and can act as an antioxidant.
     Drug interactions: can decrease warfarin's effect.
   - **Echinacea**
     Uses: stimulates immune system, upper respiratory infections.
     Disease precautions: liver disease, myositis, autoimmune skin diseases.
     Drug interactions: chemotherapy drugs for cancer treatment, HIV drugs, anticoagulants, immunosuppressive drugs, drugs that may be toxic to liver.
   - **Garlic**
     Uses: lowers low-density lipoprotein cholesterol, platelet inhibition.
     Disease precautions: surgery.
     Drug interactions: anticoagulants, antiplatelet medications.
   - **Ginkgo biloba**
     Uses: treatment of dementia, vertigo, ringing in ears. Can inhibit platelets and increase blood flow.
     Disease precautions: intracranial bleeding, GI bleeding, seizures, surgery, peripheral vascular disease. Ginkgo has anticoagulant effects and decreases platelet aggregation. Can cause GI upset.
     Drug interactions: anticoagulants, antiplatelet medications, thiazide diuretics, tricyclic antidepressants, monoamine oxidase (MAO) inhibitors.
   - **Glucosamine & chondroitin: see** chapter 50.
   - **Ginseng**
     Uses: to fight fatigue, improve performance, reduce stress. Can inhibit platelets.
     Disease precautions: heart disease, diabetes, pregnancy/nursing, surgery.
     Drug interactions: caffeine (using both may cause high blood pressure [BP]), antiplatelet medications, insulin (ginseng may lower blood sugar), anticoagulants, MAO inhibitors, loop diuretics.
   - **Indian frankincense (*Boswellia serrata*)**
     Uses: anti-inflammatory by inhibiting LTs.
     Disease precautions: none.
     Drug interactions: none.
   - **St. John's wort (*Hypericum perforatum*) (Nature's Prozac)**
     Uses: treatment of mild depression.
     Disease precautions: can cause photosensitivity.
     Drug precautions (induces P450 3A4 and 2C9 isoforms): MAO inhibitors (Nardil, Parnate), SSRIs (Prozac, Zoloft, Paxil) (mild serotonin syndrome), digoxin (decreases blood concentration), tramadol, oral contraceptives (decreased efficacy), photosensitizers (tetracycline,

quinolones, Feldene), Dyazide, Bactrim, Septra, theophylline (decreased levels of theophylline), HIV protease inhibitors (decreased levels of Indinavir), cyclosporine (decreases levels of cyclosporine), warfarin (decreased efficacy).
- **Zinaxin**—Ginger root extract called hydroxy-methoxy-phenyl-33 (see Ginger).
- **Other herbs to ask patients about:** feverfew, goldenseal, green tea, grape seed extract, kava kava, Ma-Huang (very dangerous herb), milk thistle, pycnogenol, saw palmetto (herbal catheter), valerian root (Nature's ambien), wild yam, yucca (Adam's needle), others.

> **PEARL:** There is no standardization of herbal medicine in the United States. Consequently, a patient has little idea of how much active herb they are getting in what they buy over the counter. The daily cost of most herbs ranges between $0.30 and 1.50 a day. In addition, herbal medications from some sources have been found to be adulterated with undeclared ingredients such as NSAIDs and corticosteroids.

15. What is the evidence that medical cannabis and cannabinoids are effective for the treatment of pain due to rheumatic diseases?

Marijuana is the dried leaves/flowers of the plant, *Cannabis sativa.* It contains over 500 different compounds of which more than 125 are classified as phytocannabinoids. Two of these phytocannabinoids, 9-tetrahydrocannabinol (THC) and cannabidiol (CBD), are most relevant to medicine. THC is the most psychoactive compound and has pain-relieving effects, whereas CBD has effects on immunologic function and can counteract some of the psychoactive effects of THC. CB1 and CB2 are the main receptors that both these cannabinoids bind to and exert their effects to varying degrees. Other receptors (TRPV1, GPR55) may also be important. CB1 is primarily found in the brain and responsible for the psychoactive effects. CB1 is also found in a few tissues/organs outside the brain. CB2 is found primarily on immune cells and thought to modulate pain and inflammation. CB2 is also found in a few other tissues including brain microglial cells and peripheral nerve terminals where they are anti-inflammatory and antinociceptive. The scientific basis to support medical cannabis/cannabinoids is based on the evidence that endocannabinoids are endogenous ligands derived locally from the breakdown of phospholipids during inflammation and tissue injury that bind to CB2 to dampen inflammation. However, to date there is little evidence (<200 patients total randomized to trials) that medical cannabis/cannabinoids significantly modulate pain and inflammation in any of the rheumatic diseases.

16. What information should a rheumatologist give if their patient wants to try using medical marijuana to treat their rheumatic disease?

- Cannabinoid absorption is dependent on the route of administration. Inhaled/vaporized (10–35% absorption) has rapid onset of effects (minutes) compared with oral (6% absorption, 2–6 hours to peak concentration). Transmucosal preparations have better absorption (15%) than oral ingestion. Most of an orally or transmucosally ingested cannabinoid is metabolized to an inactive form by its first pass through the liver. This is why oral formulations are not very effective in rheumatic diseases.
- In spite of better absorption and rapid onset, smoking marijuana (cannabis) daily cannot be recommended due to multiple harmful compounds in marijuana smoke that can cause health issues including bronchitis, cardiovascular, and mental health issues. THC can have psychoactive effects, which impairs alertness and reaction time. Patients who smoke marijuana should not drive for up to 24 hours after consuming herbal cannabis.
- Cannabinoids, especially if smoking marijuana, can have multiple drug interactions. Some dangerous interactions include anticoagulants/warfarin, anti-platelet drugs, sedatives, anti-anxiety meds, antidepressants, pain meds, anticonvulsants, others.
- Medical cannabis should not be used in children, adolescents, adults < age 25), pregnant and breast-feeding women, or patients with previous abuse of psychoactive or pain medications.
- If the patient plans on trying medical cannabis and has been certified to need it in a state that has legalized medical cannabis, the following guidance could be helpful:
  - Chronic pain-management options other than medical cannabis are available with better evidence for safety and effectiveness. Most physicians agree that medical cannabis/

cannabinoids should only be considered after all other measures for chronic pain control (except opioids) have been tried.

- Recommend oral preparations (sublingual oil, capsule) over inhaled formulations. However, the caveat remains that there is little standardization or regulation assuring product formulations and degree of bioavailability. Get medical cannabis from a licensed provider or dispensary.
- Start with low-dose CBD (little or no THC), up to 2.5 mg qd. Increase by 2.5 mg every 2–3 days to 5 mg bid. If an inadequate clinical response the CBD dose can be increased by an additional 10 mg (i.e. 5 mg bid) every 2–3 days to max dose of 20 mg bid.
- If the patient's response to CBD is inadequate, THC can be added. Start with dosing at bedtime. The initial dose (1-2.5 mg) of THC should start with CBD:THC ratio of 20:1 (i.e. 20 mg bid CBD: 1mg bid THC). The THC can be increased by a total dose of 1-2.5 mg per day every 7 days to max of 10–20 mg bid if necessary to control pain.
- A THC dose titrated up to 5 mg is relatively well tolerated with few side effects. Higher doses can cause cannabis-related disorders and toxic effects.
- Cannabis users may require more anesthesia during surgery and require more opioids postoperatively for pain control than nonusers. Patients should not consume cannabis on day of surgery and be monitored for withdrawal symptoms postoperatively.

17. **In the digitization era of health care, patients have easy access to information about diet and health care. Physicians are often asked about what patients should eat and what they should avoid. Name three common dietary items that rheumatology patients ask about during routine visits.**

A. Is turmeric good for me?

The use of **curcumin,** the principal active component in turmeric, dates back >4000 years in cuisine and religious ceremonies in India; it was later adopted in Ayurvedic medicine. The mechanisms by which it has been shown to attenuate the immune system are mainly via antioxidative and anti-inflammatory actions. Turmeric is used to treat OA pain by depleting substance P from nerve root endings like capsaicin. A review of RCTs in inflammatory diseases found turmeric and/or the more potent curcumin or nanocurcumin may be beneficial in RA, psoriatic arthritis, axial spondyloarthritis, and Behcet's disease. Another small trial has shown improvement in lupus nephritis. However, the efficacy of turmeric has been questioned due to its low bioavailability and unstable, reactive nature. Curcumin has better bioavailability. To improve the bioavailability, turmeric has been formulated with black pepper or piperine. Unfortunately, piperine can cause liver injury. Therefore, turmeric is safe to consume at recommended doses (recommended therapeutic dose is 400–600 mg three times a day) if it is not adulterated with piperine. Liver tests should be followed. Additionally, turmeric may affect platelet aggregation so should be avoided in patients on anticoagulants.

B. Should I be drinking coffee?

Coffee consumption has been the subject of much debate. There have been studies suggesting a detrimental effect on cardiovascular health; however, simultaneously there is data suggesting an inverse relation between the two. A possible explanation may be that many of these studies did not consider smoking, which is a huge confounding factor associated with coffee intake.

The mechanism by which caffeine is postulated to affect the immune system is by inhibiting the cAMP phosphodiesterase, thus increasing intracellular cAMP and activating protein kinase A, which in turn affects many immunomodulatory pathways. There have been studies reporting an increase in the incidence of seropositive RA in patients who consume coffee in excess of four cups per day. However, these studies did not report this increase in tea drinkers bringing into question if the association is related to caffeine intake at all. There has been data about an increased incidence of osteoporosis with coffee intake of more than two cups per day. You could keep in mind the rule of "everything is fine in moderation" and recommend your nonpregnant patients to try and limit consumption to two cups per day.

C. Should I be eating more dark chocolate?

Chocolate is derived from the fermented, dried, and roasted leaves of the cacao tree, *Theobroma cacao*. In Central America, it has been traditionally considered to have therapeutic benefits. Cocoa, rich in polyphenols and low-molecular-weight flavanols, has direct and indirect antioxidant properties. The active extracts of cocoa play a role in downregulating IL-1 and IL-2 while upregulating IL-4, thus playing a regulatory role in innate and acquired immune systems. Dark chocolate as a small part of their diet should be fine (and they will love you for this advice)!

18. What CAM therapies have shown benefit in gout?

- **Cherry juice:** has phenolic compounds (anthocyanins) that are anti-inflammatory and inhibit cyclooxygenase and nitric oxide production. In addition, it increases uric acid excretion by inhibiting proximal tubular reabsorption of uric acid.
- **Vitamin C:** at a dose of 500 mg/day, it lowers uric acid by being a competitive inhibitor of uric acid reabsorption at the proximal tubule of the kidney.

19. What CAM therapies have been shown to be beneficial for fibromyalgia?

No oral or topical CAM therapy has been proven to be beneficial. Randomized trials have shown tai chi, hydrotherapy, and thermal therapies to be beneficial. Overall, an exercise program is the most therapeutic.

20. What CAM therapies have been shown to be beneficial for Raynaud's?

None. Notably, biofeedback has been shown not to be beneficial.

21. What is dimethyl sulfoxide (DMSO), methylsulfonylmethane (MSM), and SAM-e?

- **DMSO:** it is a byproduct of wood pulp processing. There is a medical grade that is safe and an industrial grade that is used in paint thinner and antifreeze. DMSO can be used as a solvent to transport molecules across cell membranes like the skin. DMSO taken internally or topically causes the person's breath to smell like garlic or oysters. DMSO is a prescription drug given by catheter to treat interstitial cystitis. Therefore, it cannot be sold over the counter. Patients getting it from vendors are taking industrial-grade DMSO, which is unsafe. There are reports supporting DMSO's ability to relieve pain and reduce inflammation.
- **MSM:** 15% of DMSO is broken down to MSM. MSM does not cause oyster-garlic smell. MSM is an organic sulfur compound that may contribute sulfur to the formation of connective tissue. Additionally, animal studies suggest that it may be anti-inflammatory, but there are no controlled scientific data to support its use. MSM has become popular after the actor James Coburn said that it works for his RA. Usual dose is 1000 to 3000 mg twice a day.
- **SAM-e:** this is already formed in the body from methionine and ATP. SAM-e is a methyl-accepting intermediate in homocysteine formation, which with the help of vitamin B_{12} will relinquish a methyl group to surrounding tissues (see Fig. 55.1, Chapter 55: Inborn Errors of Metabolism Affecting Connective Tissue). SAM-e is then broken down to sulfate groups, which may help cartilage formation. SAM-e is equivalent to NSAIDs in therapy of OA in controlled trials. Dose is 400 mg thrice a day and costs $40/month. It is also used to treat depression.

22. Are there any herbs believed to be unsafe?

- **Carcinogens**—borage, calamus, coltsfoot, comfrey, life root, sassafras.
- **Hepatotoxicity**—chaparral, germander, life root, skullcap, Jin Bu Huan, comfrey, kava kava, turmeric with piperine.
- **Other**—licorice (electrolyte imbalance), Ma Huang (hypertension, strokes, seizures), borage seed oil (seizures), red yeast rice/oyster or shiitake mushrooms (myositis), Spirulina as part of other supplements (myositis, skin rash) .

PEARL: Stop all herbs for at least 24 hours prior to surgery, since many have an anticoagulant effect.

23. What other CAMs have people tried?

- **Movement therapy**—Tai Chi has been shown to decrease falls in the elderly.
- **Magnets**—Static magnets cause a localized magnetic field. Theorized to interact with the body's nerve conduction and reduce pain perception. Magnet strength ranges between 300 and 4000 gauss (refrigerator magnet is 60 gauss). Little data to support use of this expensive therapy. May help localized joint pain.
- **Acupuncture**—Theory is that good health is maintained by circulation of vital energy (known as Qi) in the body. Illness is due to disruption of this flow. In order to correct this disruption, insertion of needles at defined points along meridians causes discomfort that is necessary to elicit Qi. Actually, it has been shown that acupuncture causes endorphin and serotonin release, which can help pain.

  Recently, there have been nine high-quality RCTs concerning acupuncture for patients with rheumatic diseases. Six RCTs reported no statistically significant difference between experimental and control groups, whereas the remaining three RCTs showed that acupuncture had beneficial effects for patients with rheumatic diseases, especially knee OA. For RA, the evidence seems to be clearly negative with all three available RCTs demonstrating no beneficial effects.

  There are also different modalities of acupuncture treatment, including traditional acupuncture without electricity, laser acupuncture, dry needling, gold bead implantation, electroacupuncture, and moxibustion. Moxibustion is a noninvasive procedure that involves burning moxa, the herb Artemisia vulgaris, at acupuncture points. Among patients with knee OA, moxibustion treatment may improve function and pain score. Similarly, laser acupuncture was reported to be beneficial for patients with knee OA. Dry needling, which involves placing needles at trigger points, was found to lower pain among patients with myofascial pain syndrome.

- **Shark cartilage**—reported to have anti-inflammatory properties and to inhibit angiogenesis. No data to support its use. Because it may inhibit angiogenesis, it should not be used in pregnancy, children, or patients undergoing surgery or with coronary artery disease.

24. Are manipulation techniques useful for the treatment of rheumatic diseases?

Many patients with soft-tissue rheumatism respond positively to physical therapy and manipulation from chiropractors and osteopaths. Manipulation has been shown to decrease joint pain, although the mechanism of action is not well understood. If these modalities are used appropriately, it often leads to a decrease in the need for systemic anti-inflammatories. They also give patients a sense of participation in their treatment program.

25. How does one report a potentially unsafe CAM remedy?

The Office of Consumer Affairs publishes the *Consumer's Action Handbook* that explains how to file a complaint. The publication is free through the website https://usa.gov/handbook.

26. In summary, how should CAM remedies be approached?

CAM remedies are widely used by patients with rheumatic diseases. Some are safe and harmless, and others can be deadly. Some remedies have therapeutic potential and may unlock the door to the next treatment for rheumatic disease; these deserve the attention of the medical community. I would encourage all healthcare providers to discuss their use with patients. There are several internet resources to get additional information. Two of these are the National Center for Complementary and Integrative Health at https://nccih.nih.gov and a website to look up a new supplement at https://ods.od.nih.gov.

BIBLIOGRAPHY

American College of Rheumatology Position Statement: Complementary and Integrative Medicine for Rheumatic Diseases. 2024. https://rheumatology.org. Accessed 4 March 2025.

Asher GN, Spelman K. Clinical utility of curcumin extract. *Altern Ther*. 2013;19:14–16.

Barnes PM, Bloom B, Nahin RL. Complementary and alternative medicine use among adults and children: United States, 2007. *Natl Health Stat Rep*. 2008;12:1–23.

Bhaskar A, Bell A, Boivin M, et al. Consensus recommendations on dosing and administration of medical cannabis to treat chronic pain: results of a modified Delphi process. *J Cannabis Res*. 2021;3:22.

Dahan S, Segal Y, Shoenfeld Y. Dietary factors in rheumatic autoimmune diseases: a recipe for therapy? *Nat Rev Rheumatol*. 2017;13:348–358.

De Silva V, El-Metwally A, Ernst E, et al. Evidence for the efficacy of complementary and alternative medicines in the management of fibromyalgia: a systemic review. *Rheumatol.* 2010;49:1063–1068.

England BR, Smith BJ, Baker NA, et al. 2022 ACR guideline for exercise, rehabilitation, diet, and additional integrative interventions in rheumatoid arthritis. *Arthritis Rheumatol.* 2023;75:1299–1311.

Ernst E. Herbal medicine in the treatment of rheumatic diseases. *Rheum Dis Clin North Am.* 2011;37:95–102.

Ernst E. Complementary treatments in rheumatic diseases. *Rheum Dis Clin North Am.* 2008;34:455–467.

Fitzcharles M-A, Clauw DJ, Ste-Marie PA, Shir Y. The dilemma of medical marijuana use by rheumatology patients. *Arthritis Care Res.* 2014;66:797–801.

Fouladbakhsh J. Complementary and alternative modalities to relieve osteoarthritis symptoms. *AJN.* 2012;112:S44–S51.

Goldbach-Mansky R, Wilson M, Fleischmann R, et al. Comparison of Tripterygium wilfordii hook F versus sulfasalazine in the treatment of rheumatoid arthritis. *Ann Int Med.* 2009;151:229–240.

Gorelick DA. Cannabis-related disorders and toxic effects. *NEJM.* 2023;389:2267–2275.

Jubair WK, Hendrickson JD, Severs EL, et al. Modulation of inflammatory arthritis by gut microbiota through mucosal inflammation and autoantibody generation. *Arthritis Rheumatol.* 2018;70:1220–1233.

Juraschek SP, Miller ER, Gelber AC. Effect of oral vitamin C supplementation on serum uric acid: a meta-analysis of randomized controlled trials. *Arthritis Care Res.* 2011;63:1295–1306.

Macfarlane GJ, El-Metwally A, De Silva V, et al. Evidence for the efficacy of complementary and alternative medicine in the management of rheumatoid arthritis: a systematic review. *Rheumatology.* 2011;50:1672–1683.

Malenfant D, Catton M, Pope JE. The efficacy of complementary and alternative medicine in the treatment of Raynaud's phenomenon: a literature review and meta-analysis. *Rheumatology.* 2009;48:791–795.

Michalsen A. The role of complementary and alternative medicine (CAM) in rheumatology—it's time for integrative medicine. *J Rheumatol.* 2013;40:547–549.

Nelson KM, Dahlin JL, Bisson J, et al. The essential medicinal chemistry of curcumin. *J Med Chem.* 2017;60:1620–1637.

Nugent SM, Morasco BJ, O'Neil ME, et al. The effects of cannabis among adults with chronic pain and an overview of general harms: a systemic review. *Ann Int Med.* 2017;167:319–331.

Panush RS. American College of Rheumatology position statement. *Rheum Dis Clin N Am.* 2000;26:189–192.

Phang JK, Kwan YH, Goh H, Ching VI. Complementary and alternative medicine for rheumatic diseases: a systematic review of randomized controlled trials. *Complement Ther Med.* 2018;37:143–157.

Quandt SA, Chen H, Grzywacz JG, et al. Use of complementary and alternative medicine by persons with arthritis: results of the National Health Interview Survey. *Arthritis Care Res.* 2005;53:748–755.

Rubenstein SM, van Middelkoop M, Kuijpers T, et al. A systematic review on the effectiveness of complementary and alternative medicine for chronic nonspecific low-back pain. *Eur Spine J.* 2010;19:1213–1228.

Schönenberger KA, Schüpfer AC, Gloy VL, et al. Effect of anti-inflammatory diets on pain in rheumatoid arthritis: a systematic review and meta-analysis. *Nutrients.* 2021;13:4221.

Strand N, D'Souza RS, Karri J, et al. Medical cannabis: a review from the American Society of Pain and Neuroscience. *J Pain Res.* 2023;16:4217–4228.

Tekin L, Akarsu S, Durmuş O, Çakar E, Dinçer Ü, Kıralp MZ. The effect of dry needling in the treatment of myofascial pain syndrome: a randomized double-blinded placebo-controlled trial. *Clin Rheumatol.* 2013;32:309–315.

Vadell AKE, Bärebring L, Hulander E, Gjertsson I, Lindqvist HM, Winkvist A. Anti-inflammatory Diet in Rheumatoid Arthritis (ADIRA): a randomized, controlled crossover trial indicating effects on disease activity. *Am J Clin Nutr.* 2020;111:1203–1213.

Wipfler K, Simon TA, Katz P, Wolfe F, Michaud K. Increase in cannabis use among adults with rheumatic diseases: results from a 2014 to 2019 United States observational study. *Arthritis Care Res.* 2022;74:2091–2099.

Zeng L, Yang T, Yang K, et al. Curcumin and Curcuma longa extract in the treatment of 10 types of autoimmune diseases: a systemic review and meta-analysis of 31 RCTs. *Front Immunol.* 2022;13:896476.

FURTHER READING

https://nccih.nih.gov.
https://ods.od.nih.gov.
https://usa.gov/handbook.

CHAPTER 92

History, the Arts, and Rheumatic Diseases

Sterling G. West, MD

The more you know about the past, the better prepared you are for the future.

—Theodore Roosevelt (1858–1919)

1. What is the derivation of the word *rheuma*?

Rheuma is derived from the Greek term indicating "a substance which flows," a humor that originates in the brain and causes various ailments. Guillaume Baillou claimed that "what arthritis is in a joint is what rheumatism is in the whole body," raising the idea that arthritis is but one manifestation of systemic processes. In 1940, Bernard Comroe coined the term *rheumatologist*, and in 1949, Joseph Hollander used the term *rheumatology* in his textbook *Arthritis and Allied Conditions*.

2. Who described and coined the term *rheumatoid arthritis* (RA)?

Augustin-Jacob Landre-Beauvais is credited with the first clinical description in 1800. He called it a variant of gout—"goutte asthenique primitif." Benjamin Brodie described the slow progression from synovitis to bursal and tendon sheath involvement. Sir Alfred Garrod introduced the term "rheumatic gout" and separated it from classic gout using the "thread test" for urate in synovial fluid from 1858 to 1859. Archibald Garrod, the fourth son of Sir Alfred, coined the term "rheumatoid arthritis" in 1890.

3. Which famous French painters were afflicted with RA?

Pierre Auguste Renoir (1841–1919), the popular French impressionist, developed a severe form of RA beginning around 1890. Despite his increasing disabilities, he continued to paint, supported his family, and devised his own exercises and adaptive equipment. By 1912, he was bedridden and unable to transfer. Just before his death, he developed vasculitis in his fingertips.

Raoul Dufy (1877–1953), the talented Fauvist who explored "the miracle of imagination in color" in paintings, watercolors, ceramics, tapestries, and stage and mural designs, exhibited his first attack of RA at the age of 60 years. Within 13 years, when he became dependent on his crutches and wheelchair, he was invited to Boston to participate in one of the first drug studies that utilized different steroid preparations for the treatment of RA. He underwent a remarkable recovery, returned to his painting with vigor, but also suffered the consequences of the steroids, including a buttock abscess and a gastrointestinal bleed before his death.

4. What other famous people had RA?

Performers who developed RA include Edith Piaf, the French chanteuse, motion picture actresses Rosalind Russell, Lucille Ball, and Kathleen Turner, motion picture actors James Coburn and Jamie Farr, lead *Eagles* singer Glenn Frey, and TV show host Matt Iseman (*American Ninja Warrior*). Other notables with RA include the cardiac surgeon Sir Christiaan Barnard, Los Angeles Dodgers' pitcher Sandy Koufax, and US Presidents Thomas Jefferson, James Madison, and Theodore Roosevelt.

5. Who is credited with the early naming and descriptions of systemic lupus erythematosus?

1230—Rogerius Frugardi, a surgeon at the medical school in Salerno, used the term *lupus* (latin for "wolf") to describe ulcerative skin lesions that were reminiscent of what would be caused by a wolf's bite. Most of these referred to lesions on extremities (not the face) and were probably due to tuberculosis, syphilis, or cancer.

1500–1800—Paracelsus and others used the term *lupus* to describe ulcerative skin lesions from any cause. Attempts made at identifying subtypes.

1808—Robert Willan, considered the founder of British dermatology, describes *lupus vulgaris* due to tuberculosis causing lesions with ulcerations on the face.

1833— Laurant Biett with student Pierre Cazenave described and published description of discoid lupus on the face and called it "erythema centrifugum."

1845—Ferdinand von Hebra described the butterfly rash on the nose and cheeks. Separates skin lupus from lesions caused by tuberculosis and syphilis.

1852—Pierre Cazenave coined the term *lupus erythemateux.* Published it in the first dermatology textbook (1856), *Atlas of Skin Diseases.*

1872—Moritz Kaposi, who was a student and son-in-law of von Hebra, separated discoid lupus from systemic "disseminated" lupus.

1895–1903—Sir William Osler describes the systemic features under the name *"erythema exudativum multiforme with visceral injuries."* Describes renal and central nervous system involvement.

1904–1940— Other lupus manifestations described: pulmonary (1908), Libman-Sacks endocarditis (1923), leukopenia and photosensitivity (1939).

1948—Malcolm Hargraves described the lupus erythematosus cell in bone marrow aspirates.

1949— J.R. Haserick reported that the "LE cell factor" are immunoglobulins in lupus patients' sera reacting with bone marrow cells.

1954—Peter Miescher described the absorption of the "LE cell factor" by cell nuclei.

1957—Multiple investigators including Henry Kunkel described antibodies against dsDNA in lupus sera.

1958—George Friou described the method of identifying antinuclear antibodies by labeling with fluorescent antihuman globulin.

1950s-1960s—CL Conley (1952) identified circulating lupus anticoagulant; JE Moore (1952) identified false positive VDRL; EJ Bowie (1963) describes paradox of lupus anticoagulant associated with thrombosis.

1959–1975—Henry Kunkel and his investigators at the Rockefeller identified antibodies reacting with "extractable nuclear antigens" including Sm, Ro, and La. Morris Reichlin identified anti-RNP (1971).

6. Name some famous people who had systemic lupus erythematosus.

- Southern authoress Flannery O'Connor.
- Former Philippine President Ferdinand Marcos.
- TV journalist Charles Kuralt; TV show host Nick Cannon.
- Lucy Vodden—subject of Beatles' song *Lucy in the Sky with Diamonds.*
- Singers: Toni Braxton, Selena Gomez, Seal (discoid LE).
- Baseball player Tim Raines.
- Women's Olympic soccer player Shannon Box.

7. Who is credited with the early descriptions of systemic sclerosis?

i. 400 BCE—Hippocrates described "persons in whom the skin is stretched, parched, and hard, the disease terminates without sweats."

ii. 1842—English physician W.D. Chowne described a child with clinical features.

iii. 1846—English physician James Startin described an adult with clinical features.

iv. 1860—French clinician Elie Gintrac coined the term *sclerodermie.*

v. 1862—Maurice Raynaud described the vasospastic phenomenon of painful, cold-induced acrocyanosis.

vi. 1964—Richard Winterbauer, while a medical student, described the CRST syndrome of calcinosis, Raynaud phenomenon, sclerodactyly, and telangiectasia. The E for esophageal dysmotility was added subsequently (CR**E**ST).

8. What famous Swiss painter and printmaker had systemic sclerosis?

Paul Klee (1879–1940), the complex and incredibly talented Swiss artist who completed more than 9000 works in diverse media, was stricken with systemic sclerosis at age 56 years. His last paintings include "Ein Gestalter" (the Creator) as he recovered his desire and energy to paint;

"Stern Visage," which described the skin changes; "Death and Fire," as he painted his requiem; and "Durchhalten" (Endure), a line drawing that described the dysphagia prompting his final admission to the sanitorium.

9. Who is credited with the early descriptions of spondyloarthropathies?

In 1691, the Irish physician Bernard Connor described a skeleton with ankylosing spondylitis. In 1818, the English physician Benjamin Brodie provided the first clinical description of a patient with ankylosing spondylitis and iritis. In the late 1890s, the Russian physician Vladimir von Bechterew, the German–Russian physician Adolf Strumpell, and the French physician Pierre Marie described the clinical features of ankylosing spondylitis before the development of severe deformities. In the early 1900s, the German physician Hans Reiter and the French physicians Noel Fiessinger and Emile Leroy described the clinical characteristics of reactive arthritis. The association with the class I gene, *HLA-B27*, is credited to the Americans Lee Schlosstein, Rodney Bluestone, and Paul Terasaki, and the English persons Derrick Brewerton, David James, Maeve Caffrey, and Anne Nicholls.

10. Name some famous personages who had ankylosing spondylitis.

- Egyptian pharaoh Amenhotep II (1439–1413 BCE) (controversial, may be DISH).
- Olympic gold medalist swimmer Bruce Furniss.
- Cricket captain Mike Atherton.
- Television emcee Ed Sullivan.
- Renowned cellist Gregor Piatigorsky.
- American political journalist Norman Cousins.
- Motion picture actor Boris Karloff (All of the stiff walking in his Frankenstein role may not have been acting!).
- *Motley Crue's* guitarist Mick Mars.
- *Imagine Dragon's* lead singer Dan Reynolds.

11. Do any notable people have psoriasis or psoriatic arthritis?

Psoriasis is a common disease with a strong hereditary predisposition. King Herod built his fortresses close to the Dead Sea so he could be close to the healing waters for his psoriasis and arthritis. Benjamin Franklin suffered with severe psoriasis. Fleet Admiral William "Bull" Halsey, Jr., could not command the Third Fleet during the WWII Battle of Midway due to a severe attack of psoriasis. Phil Mickelson, winner of the 2010 Masters and 2013 British Open, has psoriatic arthritis and has been a spokesperson for the success of etanercept therapy. Performers Art Garfunkel (musician), Kathryn Hepburn (actress), LeAnn Rimes (singer), and Jerry Mathers *(Leave it to Beaver)* all had psoriasis and served as spokespersons for the disease. Kim Kardashian (reality TV star), Dara Torres (swimmer, Olympic medalist), and John Updike (novelist) also had psoriasis. Famous villains with psoriasis include Russian dictator Joseph Stalin and drug lord Pablo Escobar.

12. What spondyloarthropathy did Christopher Columbus possibly have?

Reactive arthritis. According to written accounts in 1494, Christopher Columbus developed lower extremity arthritis following a diarrheal illness (? Shigella). He had a relapse in 1498 of lower extremity arthritis associated with severe conjunctivitis, at which time he wrote, "I have never had an affliction of my eyes with hemorrhage and pain as in this time."

13. What persons are credited with the early descriptions of gout?

5th century BCE—although gout was reported in medieval medicine as *gutta*, Latin for "a drop" of a poisonous noxa, Hippocrates first described the clinical features of gouty arthritis ("the unwalkable disease") following dietary excesses in sexually active men and postmenopausal women.

Late 1600s—Thomas Sydenham described the clinical features, and Anton van Leeuwenhoek described the microscopic appearance of uric acid recovered from a tophus.

1703—Treaty of Metheun. England signed an accord with Portugal to export wool in exchange for importing Portuguese wines. These wines were fortified with brandy and stored in lead casks for shipping. Lead levels were increased 3 to 19 times, leading to saturnine gout in England.

1797—WH Woolaston, an English chemist, demonstrated that urate is the chemical compound that makes up a tophus. He took samples for analysis from tophi on his own ear.

1814—John Want reported the effectiveness of colchicine in the treatment of 40 patients with gout. Colchicine had been used by others since the 6th century CE but felt to be too toxic by many because it was a strong purgative/laxative.

1857—A.B. Garrod developed an assay ("thread test") that detected uric acid in synovial fluid in patients with acute gouty arthritis. He also demonstrated uric acid on the cartilage of those with gout and formulated the current hypotheses that lead to gouty arthritis.

1961—Joseph Hollander and Daniel McCarty demonstrated monosodium urate in the synovial fluid cells of those with gout using compensated polarized light.

1964—Michael Lesch, as a medical student, wrote the clinical description of a patient with neurobehavioral changes for his mentor, William Nyhan, who described the complete deficiency of hypoxanthine-guanine phosphoribosyl transferase, the enzyme that catalyzes the salvage reactions of purines (Lesch–Nyhan syndrome).

1950s–present—development of medications for therapy: probenecid (1951), allopurinol (1963), febuxostat (2008), pegloticase (2010), and lesinurad (2015).

14. Which famous Flemish painter had gout?

Peter Paul Rubens (1577–1640), the portrayer of Baroque, developed attacks of fevers and arthritis that put him to bed at the age of 49 years. Within 10 years, his attacks were continuous, and he had difficulty painting and ambulating. He died of "ague and the goutte" at the age of 63 years. Some interpret the stylistic paintings of the hands as deformities that resembled RA.

15. Which American Presidents and English Kings suffered from gout? Any other notable diplomats who had gout?

English Kings (gout was the "Disease of Kings"): Henry VIII (1491–1547), George III (1738–1820).

American Presidents: James Buchanan (1791–1868), Martin van Buren (1782–1862).

There were probably multiple diplomats who suffered from attacks of gout. Some of these gout attacks may have affected history:

- William Pitt the Elder (1708–1778). British statesman who was against taxation of the American colonists. Gout attacks prevented him from arguing in Parliament against the Stamp Act (1765) and duty on colonial tea (Boston Tea Party, 1773), which helped precipitate the American Revolutionary War (1775–1783).
- Benjamin Franklin (1706–1790). He missed many meetings due to gout attacks when the Declaration of Independence was being written (1776).

16. What was Beethoven's disease?

Ludwig von Beethoven (1770–1827) noted hearing loss at the age of 26 years, was "stone deaf" at 49 years, and died at 57 years. His deafness is popularly attributed to otosclerosis or eighth nerve compression from Paget disease. More in-depth studies included records of attacks of rheumatism. A postmortem by Wagner and Rokitansky described "dense half-inch-thick cranial vault, shrunken auditory nerves, wasted limbs, with cutaneous petechiae, cirrhosis with ascites, a large spleen, and chalky deposits in the kidneys." These findings led to the differential diagnosis of meningovascular syphilis, sarcoidosis, and Whipple disease.

17. What were the rheumatic diseases in the Civil War era?

Medical records of the American Civil War recorded 160,000 cases of "acute rheumatism," mainly acute rheumatic fever, perhaps infectious arthritis or gout. More than 260,000 cases of "chronic rheumatism" were recorded, probably chronic rheumatic fever and reactive arthritis, of which 12,000 were discharged. The validity of these clinical diagnoses on the war front may temper some of these data, and more recent data of war-related rheumatic syndromes give a better perspective.

In 1863, General Robert E. Lee described paroxysms of chest pains radiating to the left shoulder and back, which was diagnosed as rheumatic pericarditis. He was given quinine. By 1870, because the pains occurred at rest, these attacks were probably advancing coronary atherosclerosis.

18. Which famous persons had their lives affected by rheumatic fever?
- Bobby Darin (singer).
- Andy Warhol (artist).
- Donald Sutherland (actor).
- Lou Costello (comedian).
- Robert Burns (Scottish poet).
- Amadeus Mozart (composer).
- Carson McCullers (writer).

19. Did Abraham Lincoln have a genetic disease?
The debate on whether the American President Abraham Lincoln had **Marfan syndrome,** the autosomal dominant disorder of connective tissue, reached national proportions when an advisory committee in the 1990s ruled against proposed molecular genetic testing of his tissue, which is preserved at the National Museum of Health and Medicine at the Armed Forces Institute of Pathology. Most geneticists do not feel he had the disease because of his excellent eyesight and normal vasculature throughout his 56 years of life.

20. What was Henri de Toulouse Lautrec's disease?
Henri de Toulouse Lautrec (1864–1901) developed growing pains at the age of 8 years, was hospitalized for rehabilitation at 10, and fractured his femurs following minimal trauma at 14 and 15 years. The clinical geneticists Maroteaux and Lamy noted the parental consanguinity and short stature and proposed the diagnosis of pyknodysostosis, an autosomal recessive disease character-ized by mutations of the *cathepsin K* gene on chromosome 1. This retrospective diagnosis has been disputed and other bone diseases proposed.

21. What musicians may have been "helped" by their proposed connective tissue disease?
Nicolo Paganini (1782–1840) of Genoa, Italy, was a violin virtuoso who had a flair for the dra-matic and ostentatious. Although he had extraordinary musical talent, he also had extraordinary manual dexterity and hypermobility believed to be due to Ehlers–Danlos syndrome or Marfan syndrome. This enabled him to play notes that most ordinary mortals could not.

Sergei Rachmaninov (1873–1943) was known to have hands so large that they "covered the keyboard like octopus tentacles." He was believed to have had Marfan syndrome.

22. What other celebrities have true connective tissue diseases?
- Marfan syndrome: actor Vincent Schiavelli who starred in *One Flew over the Cuckoo's Nest*, among others. The Olympic Silver Medalist in women's basketball, Flo Hymen, died of an aortic dissection and serves as a reminder that this disease can be lethal. Notably, the Olympic Gold Medalist in swimming, Michael Phelps, does **not** have Marfan syndrome.
- Osteogenesis imperfecta: actors Michael J. Anderson *(Carnivale)* and Atticus Shaffer *(The Middle).*

23. What is the purpose of recognizing "famous autoimmune and rheumatic diseas" personalities?
Many patients who suffer from an autoimmune disease take comfort in knowing that they are not alone and that other people, both average and famous, are afflicted with their disease. It is particularly helpful when a famous person who has an autoimmune or rheumatic musculoskeletal disease or a loved one with the disease becomes a spokesperson to raise awareness as well as funds for research and treatment. Some notable spokespersons for the disease they have:
- Sjögren's syndrome: tennis great Venus Williams, TV's *Dancing with the Stars* judge Carrie Ann Inaba.
- Systemic sclerosis: Fox News sports reporter Matt Napolitano.
- Sarcoidosis: basketball great Bill Russell, comedian Bernie Mac, and football star Reggie White, before their deaths from the disease.
- Fibromyalgia: actors Morgan Freeman and Michael James Hastings; singers Lady Gaga and Sinead O'Connor.
- Lyme disease/post-Lyme syndrome: actor Alec Baldwin, model Bella Hadid.
- Stiff-person syndrome: Celine Dion

BIBLIOGRAPHY

Appelboom T, de Boelpaepe C, Ehrlich G, Famaey JP. Rubens and the question of antiquity of rheumatoid arthritis. *JAMA*. 1981;245:483–486.

Ball GV. The world and Flannery O'Connor. In: Appelboom T, ed. *Art, History and Antiquity of Rheumatic Diseases*. Brussels: Elsevier Librico.

Benedek T. History of the rheumatic diseases. In: Schumacher HR, ed. *Primer on the Rheumatic Diseases*. 10th ed. Atlanta, GA: Arthritis Foundation.

Bollet AJ. Rheumatic diseases among Civil War troops. *Arthritis Rheum*. 1991;34:1197–1203.

Brewerton D, Caffrey M, Nicholls A. Ankylosing spondylitis and HLA-27. *Lancet*. 1973;i:904–907.

Buchanan WW, Kean WF, Rainsford KD, et al. Reactive arthritis: the convoluted history of Reiter's disease. *Inflammopharmacology*. 2023. doi:10.1007/s10787-023-01336-4.

Deshpande S. History of rheumatology. *Med J DY Patil Univ*. 2014;7:119–123.

Francke U, Furthmayr H. Marfan's syndrome and other disorders of fibrillin. *N Engl J Med*. 1995;330:1384–1385.

Frey J. What dwarfed Toulouse-Lautrec? *Nature Genet*. 1995;10:128–130.

Gelb BD, Shi GP, Chapman HA, Dresnick RJ. Pycnodysostosis, a lysosomal disease caused by cathepsin K deficiency. *Science*. 1996;273:1236–1238.

Homburger F, Bonner CD. The treatment of Raoul Dufy's arthritis. *N Engl J Med*. 1979;301:669–673.

Louie JS. Renoir—his art and his arthritis. In: Appelboom T, ed. *Art, History and Antiquity of Rheumatic Diseases*. Brussels: Elsevier Librico.

Mainwaring RD. The cardiac illness of General Robert E. Lee. *Surg Gynecol Obstet*. 1992;174:237–244.

Maroteaux P, Lamy M. The malady of Toulouse-Lautrec. *JAMA*. 1965;191:715–717.

Marx R. *The Health of the Presidents*. New York: G.P. Putnam's Sons.

Palferman TG. Beethoven: medicine, music, and myths. *Int J Dermatol*. 1994;33:664–671.

Parish LC. An historical approach to the nomenclature of rheumatoid arthritis. *Arthritis Rheum*. 1963;6:138–158.

Schlosstein L, Terasaki P, Bluestone R. High association of an HLA antigen, w27, with ankylosing spondylitis. *N Engl J Med*. 1973;288:704–706.

Sharma OP. Beethoven's illness: Whipple's disease rather than sarcoidosis? *Int J Dermatol*. 1994;87:283–286.

Shearer PD. The deafness of Beethoven: an audiologic and medical overview. *Am J Otol*. 1990;11:370–374.

Smith CD, Cyr M. History of lupus erythematosus from Hippocrates to Osler. *Rheum Dis Clin North Am*. 1988;14:1–14.

Smith RD, Worthington JW. Paganini. the riddle and connective tissue. *JAMA*. 1967;199:820–824.

Young DAB. Rachmaninov and Marfan's syndrome. *Br Med J*. 1986;293:1624–1626.

INDEX

Note: Page numbers followed by "*f*" indicate figures, "*t*" indicate tables, and "*b*" indicate boxes.